Histology

Histology
third edition

Roy O. Greep

*John Rock Professor of
Population Studies
Harvard School of Public Health
and
Director of the Laboratory
of Human Reproduction
and Reproductive Biology
Harvard Medical School*

Leon Weiss

*Professor of Anatomy
The Johns Hopkins University
School of Medicine*

McGRAW-HILL BOOK COMPANY
A Blakiston Publication

*New York   St. Louis   San Francisco   Düsseldorf   Johannesburg
Kuala Lumpur   London   Mexico   Montreal   New Delhi   Panama
Rio de Janeiro   Singapore   Sydney   Toronto*

HISTOLOGY

4 5 6 7 8 9 0   VHVH   7 9 8 7 6 5

Library of Congress Cataloging in Publication Data

Greep, Roy Orval, 1905–   ed.
    Histology.

    Includes bibliographies.
    1. Histology. I. Weiss, Leon, joint ed.
QM551.G73 1973   599'.08'2   72-3483
ISBN 0-07-024371-9

This book was set in Galaxy by York Graphic Services,
Inc. The editors were Diane Drobnis and Norma Frankel;
the designer was Ben Kann; and the production super-
visor was John A. Sabella.
The printer and binder was Von Hoffmann Press, Inc.

Contents

List of Contributors

Russell J. Barrnett, M.D.
Department of Anatomy
Yale University
School of Medicine
New Haven, Connecticut 06510

Leonard F. Bélanger, M.D.
Histology and Embryology
Faculty of Medicine
University of Ottawa
Ottawa 2, Canada

Richard J. Blandau, Ph.D., M.D.
Department of Biological Structure
University of Washington
School of Medicine
Seattle, Washington 98105

Edward H. Bloch, M.D., Ph.D.
Department of Anatomy
Case Western Reserve University
School of Medicine
Cleveland, Ohio 44106

Ruth Ellen Bulger, Ph.D.
Department of Pathology
University of Maryland
School of Medicine
Baltimore, Maryland 21201

David G. Cogan, M.D.
Howe Laboratory of Ophthalmology
Harvard University
School of Medicine
Boston, Massachusetts 02114

Åke Flock, M.D., Ph.D.
King Gustaf V Research Institute
Stockholm 60, Sweden

Robert M. Frank, D.D.S., M.D.
École Nationale de Chirurgie Dentaire
University of Strasbourg
Strasbourg, France

William U. Gardner, Ph.D.
Department of Anatomy
Yale University
School of Medicine
New Haven, Connecticut 06510

Geraldine F. Gauthier, Ph.D.
Laboratory of Electron Microscopy
Wellesley College
Wellesley, Massachusetts 02181

Roy O. Greep, Ph.D.
Laboratory of Human Reproduction
   and Reproductive Biology
Harvard University
School of Medicine
Boston, Massachusetts 02115

Nicholas S. Halmi, M.D.
Department of Anatomy
The University of Iowa
College of Medicine
Iowa City, Iowa 52240

Elizabeth D. Hay, M.D.
Department of Anatomy
Harvard University
School of Medicine
Boston, Massachusetts 02115

Susumu Ito, M.D.
Department of Anatomy
Harvard University
School of Medicine
Boston, Massachusetts 02115

Albert L. Jones, M.D.
Division of Electron Microscopy
Veterans Administration Hospital
San Francisco, California 94121

Toichiro Kuwabara, M.D.
Howe Laboratory of Ophthalmology
Harvard University
School of Medicine
Boston, Massachusetts 02114

Aaron J. Ladman, Ph.D.
Department of Anatomy
The University of New Mexico
School of Medicine
Albuquerque, New Mexico 87106

John A. Long, Ph.D.
Department of Anatomy
University of California
School of Medicine
San Francisco, California 94122

A. Gedeon, Matoltsy, M.D.
Department of Dermatology
Boston University
School of Medicine
Boston, Massachusetts 02118

Robert S. McCuskey, Ph.D.
Department of Anatomy
University of Cincinnati
School of Medicine
Cincinnati, Ohio 45219

Elinor Spring Mills, Ph.D.
Division of Electron Microscopy
Veterans Administration Hospital
San Francisco, California 94121

Helen A. Padykula, Ph.D.
Laboratory of Electron Microscopy
Wellesley College
Wellesley, Massachusetts 02181

Jean-Paul Revel, Ph.D.
Division of Biology
California Institute of Technology
Pasadena, California 91109

Willard D. Roth, Ph.D.
Department of Biological Sciences
Union College
Schenectady, New York 12308

Marcus Singer, Ph.D.
Department of Anatomy
Case Western Reserve University
School of Medicine
Cleveland, Ohio 44106

Reidar F. Sognnaes, D.M.D., Ph.D.
School of Dentistry
The Center for the Health Sciences
University of California
Los Angeles, California 90024

Sergei P. Sorokin, M.D.
Department of Physiology
Harvard University
School of Public Health
Boston, Massachusetts 02115

John S. Strauss, M.D.
Department of Dermatology
Boston University
School of Medicine
Boston, Massachusetts 02118

Leon Weiss, M.D.
Department of Anatomy
The Johns Hopkins University
School of Medicine
Baltimore, Maryland 21205

Preface to the third edition

This textbook, the third edition of Greep's HISTO-LOGY, has as its plan the presentation of the microscopic and submicroscopic structure of the mammalian body, with some emphasis on human tissues. This presentation depends primarily upon results obtained with bright field microscopy and transmission electron microscopy, but it calls upon an extraordinary number of morphologic and chemical techniques in order to present a complete picture of our subject. These techniques include autoradiography, histochemistry, tissue culture, freeze fracture etch, scanning electron microscopy, and techniques in such related fields as endocrinology and immunology. We write at that fortunate time histologists have long anticipated, when it is clear not only to morphologists but to our colleagues in other fields that without the knowledge provided by our discipline—knowledge which we attempt to transmit in this book—the functions of the body from the level of tissue to molecular organization cannot be understood.

We and the other contributors come to this text as a group of 29 experienced teachers and investigators, prepared to offer an authoritative treatment of each of our subjects. We treat our subjects in depth but not, we hope, with undue detail. While we continue to direct this text to students in the medical sciences, we have broadened our treatment and wish to serve graduate students in the biological sciences and advanced undergraduate students. Indeed, we have sought to provide enough background so that students with only introductory courses in biology and chemistry can use this book profitably. In general, the order of treatment is light microscopy, electron microscopy, histochemistry, and histophysiology, although we have departed from this order where the nature of the subject has warranted it. As editors we are aware that the price a reader may have to pay for the authority provided by a multiple-author text is an unevenness in treatment. But by plan, editorial control, and, most important, by selection of the contributors, we hope we have achieved not only an authoritative book but also a coherent and pleasing one.

Doctors Barrnett, Cogan, Gardner, Halmi, Hay, Ito, Kuwabara, Padykula, Roth, Singer, Sognnaes, and Sorokin remain with us from the second edition. We welcome Drs. Bélanger, Blandau, Bloch, Bulger, Flock, Frank, Gauthier, Jones, Ladman, Long, Matoltsy, McCuskey, Mills, Revel, and Strauss as new colleagues. This revision has been thoroughly revised in both illustration and text. To an even greater degree than in earlier editions we have been dependent upon outside colleagues for illustrations. It is a considerable pleasure as well as a responsibility to acknowledge this necessary help.

We are indebted to Dr. Burton Guttman of the Evergreen State College, Olympia, Washington, who read the entire manuscript and made invaluable suggestions in regard to style, redundancy, and cross referencing, as well as matters of scientific accuracy; to Edda Rasekhy, who has worked with us on every phase of the book's preparation; to Norma Frankel, who, as the editor dealing with the manuscript at McGraw-Hill, has put the book together: and to Diane Drobnis, who has been with this book from a critical reading of the second edition to the sponsoring editorship of this one.

Roy O. Greep
Leon Weiss

Preface to the second edition

This second edition of *Histology*, like the first, is designed to cover in some depth, but not in detail, the available knowledge in this area of medical science. It is a modern text which has taken cognizance of the contributions of other disciplines to morphology, and is offered in the confident belief that a reasonably thorough knowledge of tissue *structure* is fundamental, important, and in fact indispensable to an understanding of *function* and therefore of human biology in health and disease.

In essence this is a much revised, rewritten, and updated version of the first edition of *Histology*. The extent to which individual chapters were revised depended in large measure on the amount of new information available since publication of the first edition eleven years ago. Most chapters were extensively revised, some are wholly new, and a few required only minor changes. The major additions in most instances have arisen from the necessity of including fine structure (electron microscopy). Colored illustrations have been employed where color is critical and has some special meaning.

The usual order of presentation of subject matter within chapters has been basic histology (light microscopy), fine structure, histophysiology, and histogenesis. Some flexibility has been allowed, however, as not every subject lends itself well to this pattern of treatment.

I am personally most grateful to the contributors for their genial collaboration and for their critical reading of the manuscripts for one or more chapters relating to their particular fields of interest. A special note of gratitude goes to Dr. Nicholas S. Halmi, who read the manuscripts for nearly every chapter and made many valuable suggestions as to style and content. To all those who have kindly furnished illustrations for this work, I wish to extend, personally and on behalf of the contributors, sincere appreciation of their help. Each such contribution is acknowledged in the text. I also wish to thank the many publishers who have given us permission to duplicate illustrations from the literature.

I wish to thank Dr. Don W. Fawcett, Chairman of the Department of Anatomy, Harvard Medical

School, for being helpful in many ways. For assisting me in revising the chapter on the parathyroid gland I am indebted to Dr. Sanford I. Roth of the Department of Pathology, Harvard Medical School. Also, I join Dr. George Odland in thanking Dr. George Szabó of the Department of Dermatology, Harvard Medical School, for providing text material on melanocytes and melanin pigmentation; and Dr. Helen Wendler Deane in expressing appreciation to Dr. Jacques Padawer and to colleagues in the Department of Biochemistry at the Albert Einstein College of Medicine, especially Dr. Betty L. Rubin, for assistance with the chapter on histochemistry and cytochemistry. To Mrs. Vivian Kiel, my secretary, who read the entire manuscript in typescript and proof and contributed immeasurably to its final form, it is a pleasure to acknowledge my gratitude; whatever merit the book may have, it is certainly a better one for her constant interest and painstaking efforts. The cooperation given all contributors by the publisher has been a source of genuine satisfaction.

Roy O. Greep

chapter 1   The cell   LEON WEISS

The cell is a physical entity that constitutes the unit of living structure. The tissues that form the body consist entirely of cells and of extracellular material elaborated by cells. The cell, moreover, can carry out an independent existence whereas none of its constituents can do so. Indeed, an entire phylum, the Protozoa, is unicellular, and isolated metazoan cells may be maintained in tissue culture. Furthermore, growth, reproduction, continued responsiveness to stimuli, and other attributes of life are characteristics of cells and not of their parts.

Most mammalian cells are microscopic, although in some instances they reach macroscopic visibility. The limits of cell size are exemplified by bacteria or bacteria-like organisms, which may be less than 1 μm in largest dimension, and by avian egg cells, measured in centimeters (Fig. 1-1).

A cell is an intricate, complex, aqueous gel that consists chemically of protein, carbohydrate, fat, and nucleic acids as well as inorganic materials.

Protein is the major structural element of the cell. By itself or in combination with fat, as lipoprotein, or with carbohydrate, as glycoprotein or mucoprotein, it constitutes the substantive structural element both of the cell and of extracellular substances. Enzymes, large molecules which catalyze all essential metabolic reactions, are proteins. Products and secretions of cells may be proteins.

Carbohydrate is the major source of energy in mammalian cells. It is present as *glucose*, a monomeric utilizable form, and as *glycogen*, a polymeric storage form. Carbohydrates, built into complexes with protein, are the key to linking cells or com-

Figure 1-1 Equivalent measurements.

10 angstroms (Å) =	1 millimicrometer (mμm) or 1 nanometer (nm)
10,000 angstroms =	1 micrometer (μm)
1,000 microns =	1 millimeter (mm)
10 millimeters =	1 centimeter (cm)
100 centimeters =	1 meter (m)

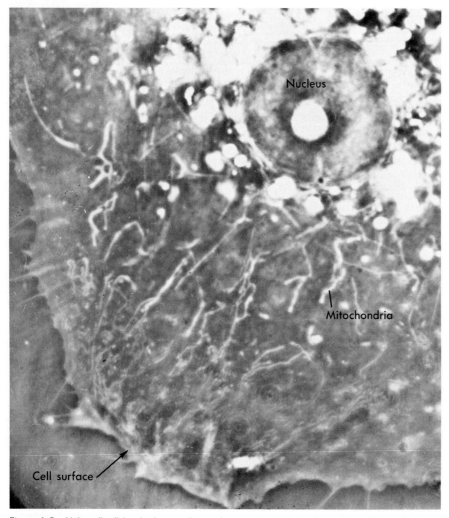

Figure 1-2   Hela cells, living in tissue culture; phase-contrast photomicrograph.   Hela cells were derived by Dr. George Gey from a carcinoma of the uterine cervix explanted in tissue culture and are maintained as a cell strain in tissue culture and used in a variety of experimental procedures. The cell border is ruffled and in places retracted, resulting in spine-like processes. The nucleus is spherical, surrounded by refractile clear bodies. Mitochondria are evident as irregular linear structures.   × 1,200. (From the work of Dr. G. Gey.)

pounds together and have significant structural properties. They may serve as distinctive surface receptors necessary for such phenomena as cell to cell recognition and cell homing.

Fat, too, may be a source of energy to the cell and may exist as a storage form. Two major constituents of fat are glycerol and fatty acid. Fatty acids vary in length of carbon chain and in degree of hydrogen saturation. They constitute the principal storage form of fat and are an efficient depot of energy. Fatty substances confer distinctive properties on many cellular structures. In the cell membrane they permit relatively easy passage of fat-soluble substances.

Inorganic materials may be present in cells in a variety of combinations. They may be associated with enzymes and with other proteins or fats, or they may be free of combination with organic chemicals. They influence the adhesiveness and other physical properties of cells and extracellular materials. Thus calcium contributes to the rigidity of bone, to the adhesiveness of the constituents of the subcellular particles, the ribosomes, and to the capacity of cells to aggregate.

It is one of the achievements of microscopic anatomy that selective chemical reactions revealing the presence and location of different chemical moieties may be carried out in microscopic preparations of tissue. Chapter 2 is devoted to *histochemistry*, the term given to this division of histology.

There are two major classes of cells: prokaryotes and eukaryotes. Prokaryotes, exemplified by bacteria, contain aggregated nuclear material which lies free in the cell protoplasm. In eukaryotes, represented by fungi and higher forms, a true nucleus is present, bounded by a membrane and thereby separated from the cytoplasm. The nucleus is typically a prominent central spherical or ovoid structure. It contains the chromosomes, which harbor the genetic material, and typically one or more nucleoli, which are concerned with the synthesis of protein. The cytoplasm surrounds the nucleus and typically contains many distinctive, highly ordered organelles, which are the structural

parts of the cytoplasm. These include *mitochondria, lysosomes, Golgi apparatus, endoplasmic reticulum, centrioles, microtubules, microfilaments, ribosomes, secretory granules,* and other structures which will be considered presently. The cytoplasm is limited by a membrane termed the *cell membrane, plasma membrane,* or *plasmalemma* (Figs. 1-2 to 1-4). Certain substances, often containing a carbohydrate, may lie on the outside surface of the plasmalemma. In addition to these relatively large, organized vesicular, membranous, tubular, and fibrillar structures, both nucleus and cytoplasm contain an apparently amorphous ground or matrix, the *karyolymph* and *hyaloplasm,* respectively.

Metazoa consist of cells organized into tissues and organs, and the specializations developed in these cells are remarkable (Figs. 1-5 and 1-6). In man cells vary in shape and size from spherical blood cells 6 μm in diameter to branched nerve cells whose processes may reach a meter or more in length. Cells may display pronounced internal variation as well. Striated muscle cells are packed with cross-banded contractile filaments, adipose cells are distended with fat, and secretory cells are filled with granules or other cell products. Osteoclasts may contain 25 or more nuclei, interstitial cells of the testis are packed with endoplasmic reticulum, parietal cells of the stomach have rich infoldings of plasma membrane, renal tubular cells

Figure 1-3   Human bone marrow cells. This field shows immature white blood cells (myelocytes) which contain large indented nuclei and cytoplasmic granules. Erythrocytes are also present (see Chap. 12). Nucleated cells are numbered. Erythrocytes, lacking a nucleus, are not. ×1,300. (From the work of G. A. Ackerman)

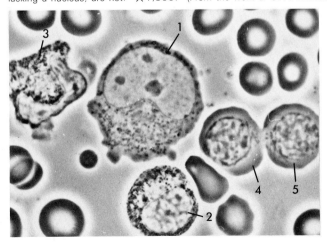

Figure 1-4   Diagram of a cell, showing structures revealed by electron microscopy.   The cell is enclosed by a membrane, the plasmalemma.   The cell surface in this model is quite irregular.   It is thrown up into microvilli (Mvl) and displays deep infoldings which "pocket" mitochondria (Mit).   It is active in pinocytosis (Pin) and phagocytosis (Pha).   The nucleus lies near the center of the cell and is indented by the cytocentrum which contains centrioles (Cen) and Golgi apparatus (Gol).   A spherical nucleolus is present.   Chromatin is aggregated into heterochromatic masses (Chr).   The nuclear membrane is a double membrane bearing nuclear pores (n.p.).   The outer nuclear membrane is continuous with the endoplasmic reticulum in the cytoplasm.   The endoplasmic reticulum may be entirely membranous or smooth (SER), or it may bear ribosomes on its outside surface (GER).   Ribosomes are also present as clusters, polyribosomes (PRib), free in the cytoplasm unassociated with endoplasmic reticulum.   The Golgi apparatus consists of stacks of membranes with the concave or distal face directed away from the nucleus and the convex or proximal face toward the nucleus.   The edges of the sacs are expanded, and vesicles bud from the Golgi, increase in size, and lie free in the cytoplasm (LGr).   These may be secretory granules or lysosomes.   Pinocytotic (or phagocytotic) vesicles may fuse with these Golgi-produced vesicles.   The Golgi is continuous with endoplasmic reticulum, and the endoplasmic reticulum may be continuous with the plasma membrane.   Small packets of Golgi membranes and vesicles lie in the cytoplasm elsewhere than the centrosome.   This diagram is representative of a free or unattached cell such as a macrophage.   When cells lie next to one another in forming tissues, their contour is modified by contiguous cells and they may bear modifications of their cell surface, as discussed in Chap. 3.

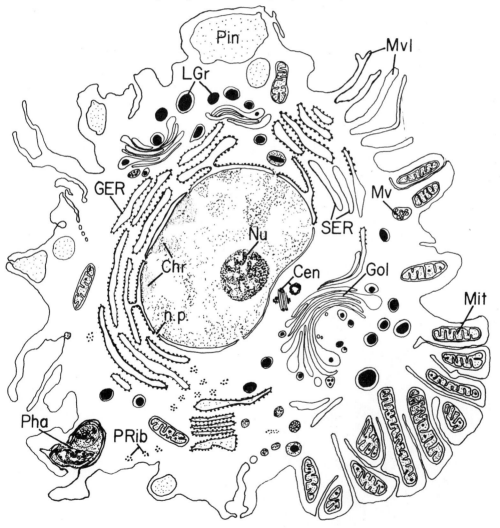

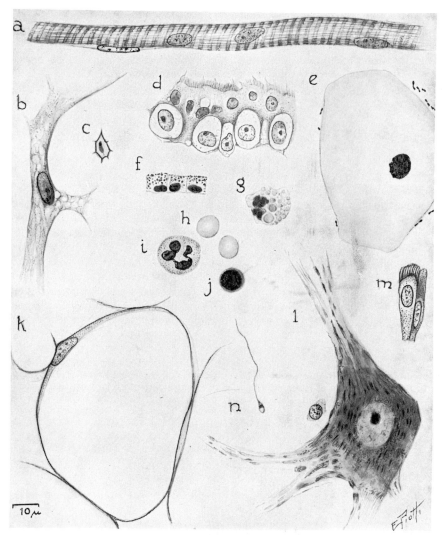

Figure 1-5 Variety of cells from the human body. a, Portion of a striated muscle fiber. b, Fibroblast from the umbilical cord. c, Osteocyte within a bone lacuna. d, Portion of the placental chorion, showing syncytial trophoblast and underlying cytotrophoblast cells. e, Squamous epithelial cell and bacteria from a vaginal smear. f, Three pigmented epithelial cells from the first layer of the retina. g, Macrophage in bone marrow, which has ingested masses of blood pigments. h, Two red blood cells; i, poly-morphonuclear neutrophil; and j, small lymphocyte, all from a blood smear. k, Fat cell from loose connective tissue. l, Large motor neuron and adjacent small glial cell (process not revealed) from a hypoglossal nucleus in the medulla. m, Adjacent ciliated and secretory epithelial cells from the oviduct. n, Mature spermatozoon from semen. Cells a and d are multinucleate; g is binucleate; e has a pycnotic nucleus; c, f, j, and n have dense nuclei; the nucleus of l is extremely vesicular; i has a lobulated nucleus; the nuclei of a, g, and k are displaced by the cell contents. Some of the cells are rounded or polygonal, but a is extremely elongate, b and c have short processes, and the neuron in l has long processes (cut off here). The syncytium in d has a brush border; one cell in m has cilia; n has a flagellum. Cells a and l display cytoplasmic fibrils; f, pigment granules; g, phagocytized masses; l, specific granules; k, a space left by dissolved fat; j and the neuron in l, conspicuous amounts of cytoplasmic basophilia. [The diameter of the red blood cells (approximately 7.5 μm) provides a useful measure of the other cells.] All × 700. (Prepared by H. W. Deane and E. Piotti.)

and brown fat may contain extraordinarily large numbers of mitochondria, and immature blood cells may be unusually rich in ribosomes. Indeed, such variations in cell structure and function constitute a major theme of this book. Despite pronounced and significant variations in cell structure, cells have considerable similarity of structure and of function. This chapter will explore some of these general features of cells. However, we first consider some of the techniques used by morphologists.

Microscopy

To be suitable for most kinds of microscopic study, a tissue must be sufficiently thin to transmit light and its parts must have sufficient contrast or color difference for one part to be distinguishable from another. But beyond the simple identification of cell structures, there is considerable physical, chemical, and ultrastructural information to be obtained from cells. In quest of this information, refined methods of tissue preparation have been worked out, and phase, fluorescent, dark-field, interference, polarizing, and electron microscopes have been developed.

TYPES OF MICROSCOPY

In most microscopy of biologic material, a thin piece of tissue modifies light passing through it. This modified light contains information inherent in the specimen, and the function of the lens systems in any microscope is to amplify that information to a form discernible by eye.

The human eye is sensitive to the contrast of light and dark and to differences in color. A light train may be represented as electromagnetic sine waves, color being a function of wavelength and intensity a function of amplitude. In order to render

Figure 1-6 Various cytoplasmic organelles and cell inclusions. Because of their specific physical and chemical properties, these objects are not generally demonstrated by routine methods and are rarely revealed together. A. Cytocentrum in a cell of grasshopper testis, showing paired centrioles. B. Golgi material in a pancreas cell of guinea pig, as demonstrated with osmic acid fixation. (Redrawn from E. V. Cowdry (ed.), "Special Cytology," 2d ed., Paul B. Hoeber, Inc., New York, 1932.) C. Mitochondria in a hepatocyte of a dog, stained with hematoxylin. (Weatherford.) D. Crystal within the nucleus of a hepatocyte of a dog. (Weatherford.) E. Spaces in a young fat cell left by dissolved fat. F. Secretory granules in a human pancreas cell. Below and lateral to the nucleus lies ergastoplasm.

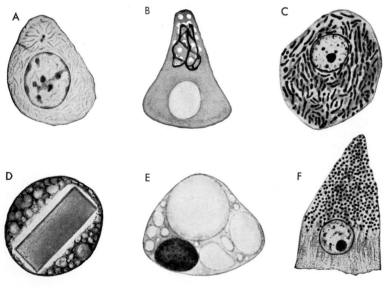

visible the disturbance in the light train induced by a biologic preparation, the light must be modified in color or intensity. Thus some wave frequencies must be absorbed more than others so that the preparation will be seen to contain materials of different colors, or there must be a change in the amplitude of a wave so that the preparation will be seen to consist of darker and lighter parts. Because unstained tissue generally does not absorb light differentially and does not modify its amplitude to a useful degree, numerous staining techniques have been developed.

Bright-field microscopy The *bright-field microscope* is a complex optical instrument consisting of three lens systems, a stage on which to place the preparation, and controls to permit focus, control of lens aperture, and centering of lenses and of light (Fig. 1-7). The light, coming in parallel rays, is focused upon the preparation by the condenser lens. It passes through the specimen, where it is modified, and this modified beam enters the objective lens system. An image is formed in the focal plane of the objective. In that image lies whatever resolution the instrument is capable of providing. The bright-field microscope is theoretically capable of resolving points approximately 0.2 μm apart. The ocular or eyepiece then magnifies the image formed by the objective, presenting it to the eye as a visible magnified image.

The primary purpose in staining histologic preparations is to induce differential absorption of light so that various structures may be seen. Staining has expanded from this elementary function until it has become possible to stain many chemical compounds selectively and specifically (see Chap. 2).

Phase microscopy Although unstained material does not absorb light, it does affect light by *retarding* some wave trains more than others. Thus the light may enter a specimen in phase, that is, with peaks and troughs of the component sine waves in register. But the components of the specimen, having different optical densities, retard the sine waves differentially, putting them out of phase with one another. These phase differences are not perceivable by the eye. The function of the *phase* microscope is to convert phase differences into

amplitude differences by matching the retarded waves with out-of-phase waves so as to cancel or diminish the amplitude of the retarded waves. The phase microscope thus permits one to observe considerable detail in unstained material and hence is suited to the study of living cells (Figs. 1-2 and 1-3).

Dark-field microscopy The *dark-field microscope* is also able to provide contrast in unstained material. Its effectiveness depends upon excluding the central light train that comes into the objective from the condenser in the conventional bright-field microscope. Instead, the specimen is illuminated by light coming in from the side. Should there be objects of greater optical density than their surroundings in the field, such as bacteria moving in a fluid medium, they will deflect light into the microscopic objective and appear as light objects against a dark background. The effect is similar to motes visualized on a sunbeam in a darkened room (Tyndall effect) (Fig. 10-4). Little or no internal structure of the lighted particles is revealed. This technique, eminently suited to such examinations as the detection of bacteria in fluid, has been superseded by phase-contrast microscopy in many situations.

Interference microscopy The *interference microscope* provides not only contrast in unstained preparations but additional information on the physical properties and the submicroscopic organization of tissue. Like the phase microscope, the interference microscope depends upon phase differences induced in transmitted light by differences in optical densities in the parts of the biologic preparation. But this is a quantitative instrument in which the light trains subject to phase retardation are compared with a reference beam. Since the optical density and phase retardation are in proportion to specimen mass, the mass of different components of the cell may be calculated.

Fluorescence microscopy The *fluorescence microscope* depends upon exciting the emission of visible light in a specimen irradiated with ultraviolet light. Certain biologic substances, such as vitamin A, are autofluorescent; that is, they can absorb light of one frequency and emit light of another. In practice, light within one frequency range, usually in the

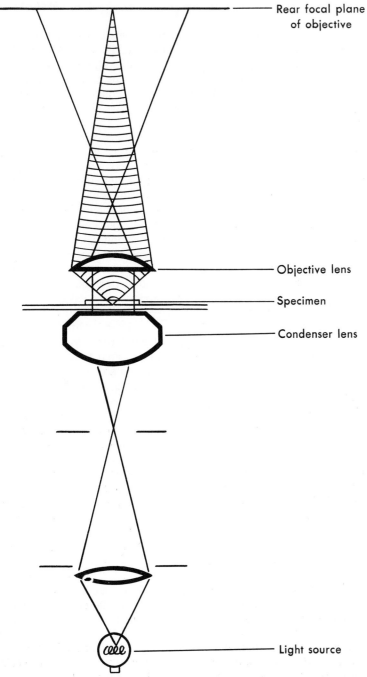

— Rear focal plane
of objective

— Objective lens

— Specimen

— Condenser lens

— Light source

Figure 1-7   Diagram of the paths of light beams in the light microscope.   Light focused on the specimen by the condenser is diffracted by the specimen and is traced by the cross-hatching.   In the image plane this diffracted light is imposed on direct light, and the two provide the distribution of light intensity recognized as the microscopic image.   In this diagram the light pathway is traced from the light source to the rear focal plane of the objective.   In the practice of microscopy, the image in the rear focal plane of the objective is then magnified and viewed through another lens, the ocular.   (Prepared by P. Bartels.)

ultraviolet spectrum, is focused upon the specimen, care being taken to protect the observer's eyes from this damaging radiation. This light is absorbed by certain structures within the specimen which then emit light within the visible range, the wavelength of the emitted light being dependent upon the chemical nature of the emitting substance. Although the autofluorescence of materials like vitamin A permits the use of this microscope with unstained material, the value of the technique is enormously enhanced by staining the tissue with fluorescent reagents. (See Fig. 1-8 and Chaps. 2 and 13.)

Ultraviolet microscopy The *ultraviolet microscope*, like the fluorescence microscope, is built around the use of ultraviolet light instead of visible light. Its optical system is usually made of quartz which efficiently transmits ultraviolet light. The image-bearing ultraviolet light coming from the ocular of the ultraviolet microscope is recorded on a photographic film, since ultraviolet is both invisible and damaging to the eye. The value of the ultraviolet microscope lies in the fact that certain highly significant cellular structures, notably those containing nucleic acids, absorb ultraviolet light of specific wavelength and can therefore be demonstrated. Because the wavelength of ultraviolet is shorter than that of visible light, this microscope offers somewhat higher resolution than the bright-field microscope.

Polarizing microscopy The *polarizing microscope* permits one to determine whether biologic materials have different refractive indices along different optical axes. Such materials are *birefringent* or *anisotropic*. They have the capability of converting a beam of linear polarized light to elliptical polarized light, one axis of which can be transmitted by an analyzer and visualized. In the polarizing microscope, light is polarized below the stage of the microscope by a Nicol quartz prism or other suitable polarizer. This polarized light is passed through the specimen. An analyzer is placed at the ocular; like the polarizer, it is made of material capable of transmitting only polarized light in one plane or axis. By rotating the analyzer, the polarization of the light transmitted by the specimen may be determined and any change from the character of

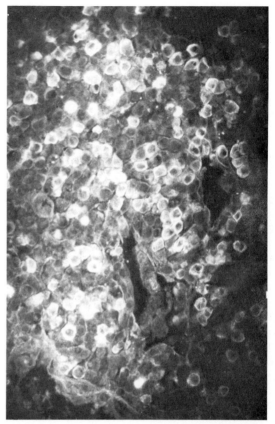

Figure 1-8 Fluorescence microscopy. A lymph node of a rabbit in the fourth day of a secondary antibody response to the antigen bovine serum albumin. The antibody, which has been tagged with a fluorescent tracer and is white in this photomicrograph, is present in the cytoplasm of plasma cells and lymphocytes. The nuclei are seldom stained and are present as negative (dark images). See Chaps. 2 and 14. ×500. (From the work of A. H. Coons.)

polarization of the source detected. Those substances incapable of affecting polarized light are termed *isotropic*. The capacity of biologic material to change linear to elliptical polarized light requires that submicroscopic particles which are asymmetric be present, and that these particles be oriented in an ordered nonrandom manner. *Thus, change of linear to elliptical polarized light by biologic material indicates that its submicroscopic structure consists of oriented asymmetric molecules.*

Filaments, fibers, and linear proteins are gran-

typically birefringent. Lipoprotein complexes, such as those composing membranes, may display complex polarizing properties. Typically the orientation of the lipid molecules, and hence their rotation of polarized light, is at right angles to that of the protein component. Polarization optics have been fruitfully applied to the study of muscle, connective tissue fibers, cell membranes, and the achromatic mitotic apparatus (Fig. 1-64).

Electron microscopy The *electron microscope,* in contrast to all light microscopes, uses a beam of electrons in place of a beam of visible light. Additional differences follow from the special properties of electrons. Electron beams are streams of negatively charged particles incapable of passing through or being refracted by glass. Hence the lenses of an electron microscope are electromagnetic coils which surround the beam at different levels, somewhat like a set of collars. The strength of these electromagnetic lenses may be changed by varying the current passing through their coils. By varying the strength of the projector lens (the counterpart of the ocular of the light microscope), the magnification of the image formed by the objective lens is changed.

Electrons are charged particles, and since collision with charged molecules of air will absorb electrons and distort the beam, the optical system of an electron microscope must be evacuated of air. The electron stream is produced by heating a tungsten filament. It is directed and impelled by a high voltage, usually ranging from 40,000 to 100,000 V. Since electron beams are invisible to the eye, the images they form are revealed by causing them to strike a fluorescent screen, and they are then recorded on a photographic plate. Indeed, the eye and the whole body of the operator must be protected from the electron beam, not only because of the damage it can do but because it produces x-rays, which are also damaging.

Stability of the specimen is always a major consideration, and efforts must be made to protect the structure of the specimen against sublimation, distortion, and other damage by the electron beam. Extreme thinness of the specimen is required so that the electrons, so easily absorbed, may pass through it and create an image on the fluorescent screen and photographic plate. Electron-microscopic sections are approximately $\frac{1}{40}$ μm (250 Å) thick. Obtaining sections of tissues this thin has required the development of new slicing machines, ultramicrotomes, and a new or highly modified technology of fixation and embedding of tissues.

The value of the electron microscope lies in its great resolving power. *Resolution* of a microscope, measured as the distance between the closest two points it can resolve as two separate points, depends upon the wavelength of the radiation. An electron train has wave characteristics in addition to the characteristics of charge and mass. Its wavelength is small enough so that resolution of about 2 Å is possible and of about 30 Å is routine. This means that a useful magnification of more than 500,000 is possible. The bright-field microscope is capable of resolution of approximately 0.2 μm and useful magnification of 2,000. It has not proved practicable, so far, to examine living tissue by electron microscopy because of the vacuum and the damaging effects of electrons. However, the development of modified specimen chambers may permit this. New cytochemical techniques that make it possible to obtain histochemical information at electron-microscopic resolutions have made electron microscopy increasingly productive. Moreover, quantitative analytic methods are also being introduced.

Variations on the transmission electron microscope characterized above have been made. High-voltage electron microscopes capable of exceptionally high resolution exist. Scanning electron microscopy, wherein a remarkably detailed three-dimensional view of the surface of a specimen is obtained, is increasingly useful (Fig. 1-9). New methods of preparing tissues, as discussed below, have considerably enhanced the versatility of electron microscopy.

BIOLOGIC MICROSCOPIC PREPARATIONS

Study of living cells Living cells may be maintained in *tissue culture* for long periods and examined by microscopy while in culture through the use of suitable culture vessels. Tissue culture permits control over the environment of cells and isolation of single cells or of clones, which are colonies derived from proliferation of a single cell.

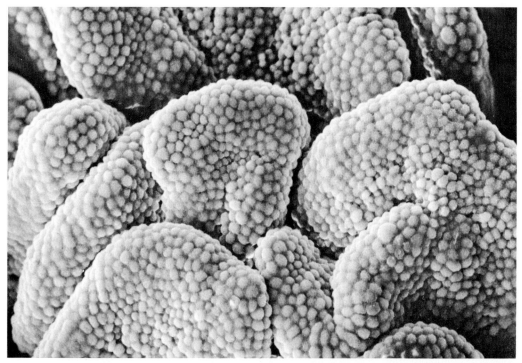

Figure 1-9   Scanning electron microscopy of the surface of the yolk sac. Note the three-dimensional character of the scanning electron micrograph. The surface is thrown up into folds, and each of the folds is beset with many cobblestone-like protuberances. The surface drips down around these protuberances. The appearance of this surface by light microscopy and transmission electron microscopy is presented in Chap. 25. (From B. King, Jr., and A. C. Enders, Amer. J. Anat., **127**:397, 1970.)

Maintenance of cells in tissue culture requires considerable attention, involving nutritive media, temperature control, and sterility. For short-term investigation, living cells such as leukocytes from a drop of blood may be placed on a clean slide, covered with a cover slip, sealed with petroleum jelly to prevent evaporation, placed on a warming stage, and studied under the microscope. This type of preparation is called *supravital* in distinction to more stable, longer-lasting preparations, such as whole animals or long-term tissue cultures, which are called *vital preparations*. Thus living cells may be observed with the conventional bright-field microscope or with the phase, interference, polarizing, or fluorescence microscopes. Living material may be studied unstained or it may be stained and remain alive, but such vital or supravital staining offers limited structural detail and damages the cells. Although it is of value in special situations (Chap. 10), it is not generally used.

The nucleus, cytoplasm, mitochondria, Golgi apparatus, and centriole may all be observed in the living state, as may such cell functions as motility of whole cells and the movement of structures within the cell. The behavior of the plasma membrane is rewardingly studied in living material. The membrane is in active movement and may be associated with such processes as pinocytosis and phagocytosis. The study of living material offers certain satisfactions. Any scientific study induces artefacts, or departures from the natural state of things. A question that a scientist must always consider is whether or not the artefacts he has induced in his material are consistent, repeatable, and significant. Intuitively, one thinks that what is seen in the living cell is less apt to be an uncontrolled or misleading artefact and nearer to the undisturbed life of the unscrutinized cell than what can be inferred from killed, sectioned, and stained tissue. For example, for years the existence of the

Golgi element was in doubt because it was not unequivocally identified in living cells.

In order to obtain greater resolution and more chemical and other information about the structure and function of cells, it is necessary to kill them by fixation, section them into thin slices, and stain them. The nature of these procedures will now be considered.

Fixation Fixation is a step wherein a certain structure or function of interest in a cell or tissue is preserved. Fixation is usually accomplished by immersing the tissue in a solution of chemicals. It is important to realize that, although there are fixatives which may be of general use, fixation may be quite selective. Thus, if an investigator wishes to study the structure of fat droplets, he may fix the tissues in formaldehyde or other materials which stabilize the fat and avoid the use of alcohol or other organic solvents which extract fats. Fixatives that fix or coagulate protein are widely used because they preserve the general structure of nucleus and cytoplasm. Greater resolution and less distortion of cellular structures are obtained with a fixative that produces a fine coagulum than with one that produces a coarse one. Thus glutaraldehyde and osmium tetroxide, which cause a very fine precipitation of protein, permit high resolution without appreciable distortion of structure. Indeed, so finely do they fix tissue that they are the most widely used fixatives for electron microscopy. Phosphotungstic acid is a coarse protein precipitant which causes the cell to be thrown into heavy strands. For general work, therefore, phosphotungstic acid is used little, but one consequence of its drastic action is that it may expose more reactive groups. Thus more sulfhydryl groups are free to react after the coarse fixation with phosphotungstic acid than with fixatives that induce a finer coagulation of protein, and so for the special purpose of detecting sulfhydryl groups in tissue section this otherwise unsatisfactory chemical may be the fixative of choice.

It is important to emphasize that fixation is a chemical process. Thus fixatives containing heavy metals, such as Zenker's fluid, which contains mercuric chloride, may react with the carboxyl groups of tissue proteins and influence their subsequent staining. Staining methods are now available for detecting enzyme activity. The fixative used for this purpose must be very gentle; most chemical fixatives tend to damage enzymes so much that they become inoperative and therefore undetectable. It is possible, by freezing fresh tissue under certain conditions, or by freezing and treating very briefly in dilute formaldehyde or other fixative, to preserve enzyme activity. In such methods of fixation many cellular structures are destroyed and distorted and the general fixation is poor.

Fixation is thus a procedure wherein a given cellular structure is preserved or stabilized, often at the expense of other structures, for subsequent viewing in microscopic preparations. Fixation may be achieved by immersing the tissue in a solution of chemicals, the form most commonly employed, or it may be physical, as heat denaturation, freezing, or air drying.

Embedding and sectioning After the tissue is fixed, it is necessary to section it into sufficiently thin slices so that the detail it contains can be inspected by microscopy. Only in exceptional cases, as in spreading out a drop of blood on a slide, can the required thinness of tissue be obtained without slicing. The slices must be thin enough to allow light or electrons, in the case of electron microscopy, to pass through them. Moreover, since the depth of focus of microscopic objectives is shallow, clarity of detail is favored by thin sections. For light microscopy, section thickness varies from less than 1 μm to about 100 μm. Most preparations are about 5 μm thick. Slices this thin are made with an instrument known as a *microtome,* which consists of a chuck that holds the tissue, a knife, and an advance mechanism. However, tissue after fixation often is pulpy or brittle and impossible to cut into thin slices. In order to cut tissue successfully for microscopy, it must be infiltrated with a material which is stiff and of a consistency that can be cut. Most of these infiltrating or embedding agents are fatty waxes, immiscible with the aqueous cytoplasm. Most fixing solutions, moreover, are aqueous. Therefore, to embed in the most commonly used embedding agents, which are paraffin or celloidin for light microscopy and the acrylic or epoxy resins for electron microscopy, the fixed tissues must be dehydrated. To this end the tissues are passed through a series of increasingly concentrated aqueous solutions of ethyl alcohol, acetone, or other dehydrating agent which is miscible with both water and fat. Thus the tissue may be passed through 50, 70, 80, 95 percent, and then into absolute ethanol. From here, either directly or through an intermediate organic solvent like toluene, the tissue is placed in the embedding agent in a liquid phase. The embedding agent replaces the solvent and thus thoroughly infiltrates the tissue.

Paraffin is made fluid by temperatures above the melting point, usually about 60°C, and the dehydrated tissue is allowed to steep in molten paraffin. The preparation is then cooled. Having infiltrated the interstices of the tissue, the paraffin becomes solid, forming a block that can be cut.

In plastic embedding for electron or light microscopy, the plastic is introduced in the fluid monomeric state. With sufficient steeping, it infiltrates the tissue. Then, by means of heat or ultraviolet light, the plastic is polymerized and becomes, like paraffin, a solid in which the tissue lies thoroughly infiltrated and embedded.

But a price must be paid to obtain such stable infiltrated blocks of tissue capable of being cut into microscopic sections. The alcohols employed to dehydrate tissues before infiltration extract fat, coagulate protein, and effect other chemical changes in a tissue. In order to infiltrate with paraffin, moreover, the tissue must be subjected to temperatures high enough to inactivate many enzymes. As plastic polymerizes, heat is given off and may damage the tissue undergoing embedding. Moreover, paraffin and other embedding agents may shrink and thereby distort the structure of tissues. For these reasons, alternatives to these convenient types of embedding are often employed. Water-soluble embedding agents are available which circumvent the need for dehydration so that fatty materials may be preserved.

Some enzymatic activities, however, are so fugitive that they do not withstand infiltration with an embedding agent. In such circumstances the tissue may be frozen, and the frozen block of tissue has sufficient rigidity, elasticity, and other physical properties to permit sectioning. Freezing may speed up the processing of tissues, saving the time required for embedding. When speed is essential, as in the operating room where a surgeon awaits the decision of the pathologist as to the benignancy or malignancy of excised tissue before going ahead with surgery, tissues are frozen and sections obtained in minutes.

More specialized methods of fixation and embedding have been developed.

Freeze-drying is a significant refinement over fixation by freezing or chemical means because it allows minimal distortion and displacement of tissues, minimal chemical extraction, and maximal preservation of enzyme activity for light microscopy. A small block of tissue is quick-frozen or quenched by immersion in isopentane in liquid nitrogen at a temperature of -150 to $-160°C$. It is then placed in a vacuum and dried by sublimation of H_2O, thereby avoiding liquid H_2O which causes displacement and extraction of cellular components. The dried tissue, while still in vacuo, may be infiltrated with molten paraffin.

Tissues that have been quenched may have their sublimated water replaced by a chemical fixative in vapor form; this type of fixation is designated *free substitution*. It offers the results of freeze-drying coupled with chemical fixation. A valuable new electron-microscopic technique is the *freeze-fracture-etch* method (Fig. 1-10). The living tissue is quenched in isopentane and liquid nitrogen and placed in a vacuum. There the tissue is fractured, and its broken surface is permitted to sublimate, causing a relief or etched surface where sublimated water leaves hollows. A thin film of platinum is evaporated over this surface, forming a tough, metallic, transparent replica. Out of the vacuum this replica is floated free and then studied in the transmission electron microscope. Details in the structure of membranes, heretofore unavailable, have been obtained with this technique. Resolution of approximately 30 Å (the grain of the platinum replica) can be obtained.

In scanning electron microscopy a three-dimensional image of the specimen is obtained by detecting secondary emissions induced by an electron beam striking the surface of a tissue. The tissue is fixed, dried, and then coated or shadowed with a metal layer; the surface is studied with considerable depth of field. (Fig. 1-9).

Mounting and staining   After the tissue is sectioned it is usually mounted on a glass slide and

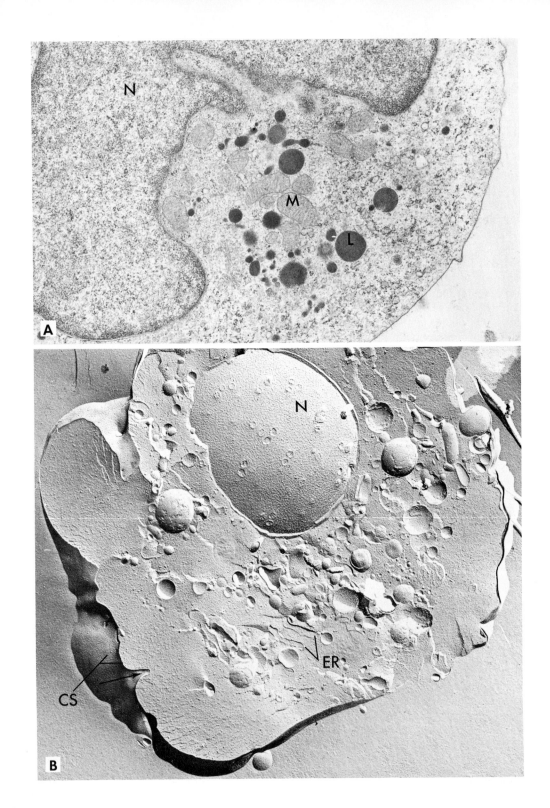

stained, although, as with living cells, it is possible by the use of the phase-contrast or the interference microscope to study unstained tissue. The primary purpose of staining is to induce some parts of the cell to appear darker or of different color than others so that they can be recognized. Staining, however, is a chemical procedure, and it has been refined to a degree that it provides considerable information on the chemical constitution of the parts of cells (consult Chap. 2). Staining procedures have been developed for the electron microscope and are being added to at a rapid rate.

DISRUPTIVE AND MICROCHEMICAL TECHNIQUES

The morphologic procedures outlined above have been amplified by techniques wherein the cell is disrupted and its constituent parts isolated and analyzed, and by microchemical methods wherein sections are analyzed by chemical procedures adapted to minute quantities. In the analysis of constituent parts of a cell, the main elements of the procedure are as follows. Fresh tissue is sliced into small pieces or run through a meat grinder, placed in a mortar, and ground in fine sand with a pestle or in a mill in which a glass piston rides in a test tube, or the tissue may be homogenized in a blender. The grinding reduces the tissue to a pulpy, apparently homogeneous liquid which actually contains disrupted cells and their constituent parts, extracellular material, and other debris. This homogenate is centrifuged, and, depending upon the force of the centrifugal field, different components are isolated. The nucleus is a relatively large, heavy structure and is concentrated in fields of low gravity. Mitochondria, ribosomes, lysosomes, and other cellular elements may also be separated. An isolated component may be studied by electron microscopy to confirm its nature, determine the damage, if any, done in its disruption and concentration, and determine the cleanness of separation. The pellet may also be studied chemically or by other means. Rich correlative chemical and morphologic data have been obtained by these procedures.

Microchemical methods have evolved from an extraordinary refinement of chemical methods. Thus it has been possible to take a section of a tissue and study it under the microscope and then take the section next to it and analyze it for inorganic salts, oxidative enzymes, or other components. It is possible, moreover, to dissect sections and carry out chemical analyses on small groups of similar cells or even upon single cells.

The structure of the cell

THE NUCLEUS

The nucleus is the fundamental part of a cell that encodes the information from which the structure and function of the organism derive. The information is encoded in the genetic material, deoxyribonucleic acid (DNA), complexed to simple basic proteins, histones, to form deoxyribonucleoprotein (DNP). With some exceptions, notably mitochondria, DNA lies exclusively in the nucleus. DNA is capable of replicating itself, thereby providing precise copies of the genetic code that are passed on to daughter cells by cellular division and also augment the synthetic processes of a cell in the nondividing or interphase state (see discussion of ploidy below).

The nucleus further plays a central role in synthesizing proteins and polypeptides from the genetic information it carries. All the nucleated cells of the body contain the same genes, yet cells differ in their structure, function, and products. The nucleus differentially controls the use of this information from cell to cell by repressing or derepressing the

Figure 1-10   Guinea pig macrophage. A. A cell which has been fixed and sectioned and photographed in the electron microscope after staining with heavy metals. Nucleus (N), mitochondria (M), lysosomes (L), and the plasma membrane are visible by this standard technique. ×13,500. B. A freeze-fractured-etched macrophage, showing the nucleus (N), bearing nuclear pores, numerous globular profiles, two cisternae of the ER (ER), and an invagination (arrow) at the cell surface (CS). ×19,000. (From W. Th. Daems and P. Bredero, in R. van Furth (ed.), "Mononuclear Phagocytes," p. 29, F. A. Davis Company, Philadelphia, 1970.)

action of various genes. The nucleus, moreover, actually initiates the translation of its encoded information into the synthesis of proteins by means of ribonucleic acids (RNAs), a group of nucleic acids different in base composition and other critical respects from DNA. Some RNAs are complexed to proteins to form ribonucleoprotein (RNP). The RNAs are produced in or under the control of the nucleus and are released to the cytoplasm where they actually engage in protein synthesis. The "machine" which assembles proteins from amino acids is a complex of RNAs and protein, the *ribosome*, whose constituents are produced largely in a nuclear subdivision termed the *nucleolus*. The nucleus, in summary, encodes genetic information, determines in any cell type which information is to be used in differentiation and maturity, and initiates and effects the utilization of this information in cellular synthesis. Moreover, it possesses mechanisms for replicating its DNA and passing it on to its progeny or utilizing it for augmented cellular activities (see *ploidy* below).

A nucleus is present in virtually all differentiated metazoan cells, being absent only from mammalian erythrocytes and a few other end-stage cell types. Certain cell types have many nuclei or are polyploid (see below), thereby multiplying the number of genes and other elements in the protein-synthesizing apparatus of a cell, and permitting it to produce a greater volume of product. Hepatocytes, particularly with age, may develop two or more nuclei, and renal tubular cells may be binucleate. Giant cells with 100 or more nuclei may exist as osteoclasts or foreign-body giant cells. A mechanism wherein nuclear function is increased without increasing nuclear number is *polyploidy,* an increase in the number of chromosomal pairs within a single nucleus. Most somatic cells are diploid (2n), having one pair of each chromosome characterizing its species, but cells may develop two pairs (4n) or more. Hepatocytes tend to increase in ploidy with age, in old rats often being 8n and 16n. Megakaryocytes, giant cells of the bone marrow containing a giant polymorphous nucleus, regularly become 32n or 64n. A more restricted mechanism for increasing nuclear components is that of increasing the number of nucleoli in certain oocytes, with a concomitant increase in ribosomal RNA production. The foregoing adaptations increase nuclear

activities without increasing the number of cells.

The nucleus may occur in a dividing (mitotic or meiotic) state, during which it reproduces itself, or in a nondividing or interphase state. The interphase nucleus is that most frequently encountered, since nuclear division takes only 1 hr or more whereas, even in actively dividing cells, 8 hrs or more elapse between divisions.

The interphase nucleus is, in most cell types, a round or ovoid structure several micrometers in diameter (Figs. 1-11 to 1-16 and 1-18 to 1-22). It is deformable and hence may be pressed into a reniform or horseshoe shape. In contracted smooth muscle, the nucleus may be twisted like a corkscrew (Fig. 1-12). In the leukocytes of blood and connective tissues, the nucleus is lobulated and hence termed *polymorphous* (see Chaps. 10 and 11).

The interphase nucleus typically contains several distinctive structures. These include *chromatin, nuclear sap* or *karyolymph,* and one or more *nucleoli.* The protoplasm of the nucleus is termed *nucleoplasm* or *karyoplasm.*

Chromatin, by light microscopy, consists of irregular clumps or masses which, although not highly constant, tend to be characteristic in texture,

Figure 1-11   Nucleus, isolated from an oocyte of *Xenopus laevis.* The nucleus was dissected from the oocyte, flooded with cresyl violet stain, and photographed. The deeply stained spots are those of the hundreds of nucleoli which are in the plane of focus. (From D. D. Brown and I. B. Dawid, Science, **160:**272, 1968.)

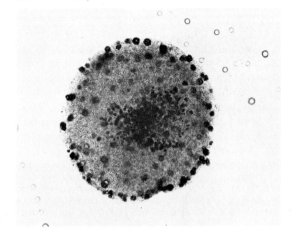

quantity, and size in any given cell type. These clumps, sometimes termed *karyosomes,* have an affinity for basic dye because chromatin is a DNA-protein complex, DNP. DNA confers other distinctive staining reactions upon chromatin. In preparations stained with methyl green–pyronin, chromatin binds methyl green. In Romanovsky preparations which are stained with methylene blue and azures, chromatin masses are stained violet (Chap. 10). A highly significant staining reaction is the selective staining of DNA in the Feulgen reaction (Chap. 2). These distinctive staining reactions are abolished by pretreatment of the specimen with the enzyme *deoxyribonuclease.*

Chromatin is the representation in the interphase nucleus of the DNP of the chromosomes. The chromosomes in the interphase nucleus are very slender, long, thread-like structures lying in a rather tangled mass. It is impossible to delineate individual chromosomes from this tangle. Indeed it was at one time thought that this mass was a continuous single thread instead of individual interlaced chromosomes, and the name *spireme* was applied to it.

In the early phases of mitosis, however, the chromosomes become highly coiled, so that in light-microscopic preparations they become shorter, broader, densely stained, and clearly visible (see later discussions of mitosis). Masses of chromatin visualized in the interphase nucleus by light microscopy represent the persistence of coiling along a segment of a chromosome. The dense chromatin is termed *heterochromatin* in contrast to the uncoiled or extended *euchromatin.* Thus, whereas DNA is present along the length of chromosomes, it is not visible by light microscopy in the extended chromosomes of interphase (euchromatin), being too finely dispersed. It is visible only where the coiling of a chromosome brings it to an aggregate size, above the limit of resolution of the light microscope, 0.2 μm (heterochromatin).

Figure 1-12 Contracted muscle cell. The nucleus has been twisted into a corkscrew spiral. On relaxation, the nucleus will untwist and be cigar-shaped.

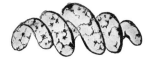

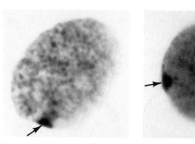

Figure 1-13 Sex chromatin of a human female. The chromatin lies against the nuclear membrane (arrows). This formation of sex chromatin appears to be due to the persistent coiling in interphase in one of the X chromosomes. Human buccal mucosa. ×4,000. (From the work of B. R. Migeon.)

Heterochromatin masses, moreover, may be an index to a cell's activity. Cells with large blocks of heterochromatin tend to be relatively inactive in at least an early stage of protein synthesis, production of mRNA (see p. 33). In the extended chromosome there is optimum exposure of its functional surface for transcription of mRNA. In certain cell types a characteristic mass of chromatin represents one of the female sex chromosomes which remains clumped through interphase. It may lie against the nuclear membrane or in other positions and is termed the *sex chromatin* or, after the discoverer, the *Barr body* (Fig. 1-13). It permits the determination of the genetic sex of an individual, a procedure of value in certain endocrinopathies or congenital disturbances in which the genetic sex may not be apparent. The Y (male) chromosome may be demonstrated in interphase nuclei by a special fluorescence staining method.

In addition to chromatin, nuclei may contain discrete RNA-rich bodies, nucleoli (see below). The clear space in the nucleoplasm between chromatin and nucleoli is the nuclear sap or karyolymph. The nucleus is bounded by a well-defined *nuclear membrane* (see below).

The elements of the interphase nucleus, namely chromatin, nucleoli, karyolymph, and nuclear membranes, are readily identified by electron microscopy (Figs. 1-14 to 1-26). But the correlation of electron-microscopic observations of interphase nuclei with what is inferred of the structure of chromosomes and other nuclear structures from genetic and other data is, at this time, rudimentary. It is known, for example, that an uncoiled chromosome

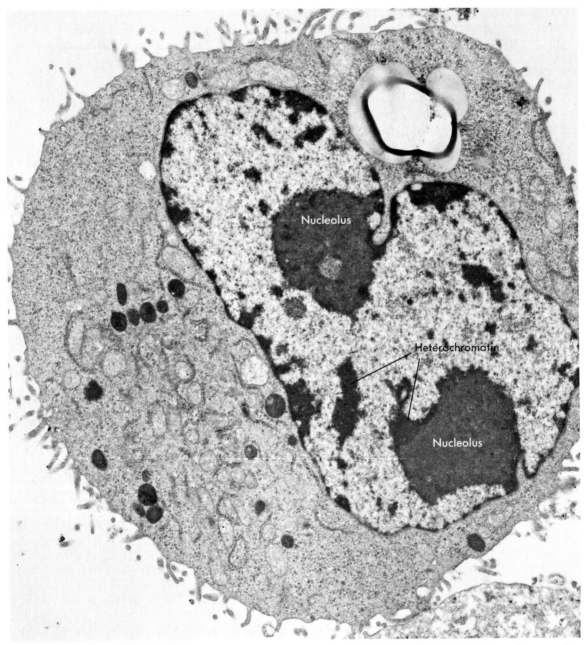

Figure 1-14   Tumor cell (Ehrlich's ascites tumor).   The nucleus is somewhat irregular in shape and deeply indented at one point. Heterochromatin, densely stained, is present against the inner surface of the nuclear membrane and upon the nucleolus.   Two nucleoli are present.   They are darkly stained, but not as dense as the chromatin.   The cell has been fixed in glutaraldehyde and osmium tetroxide and stained with both lead and uranyl acetate.   ×13,000.   (From the work of A. Monneron.)

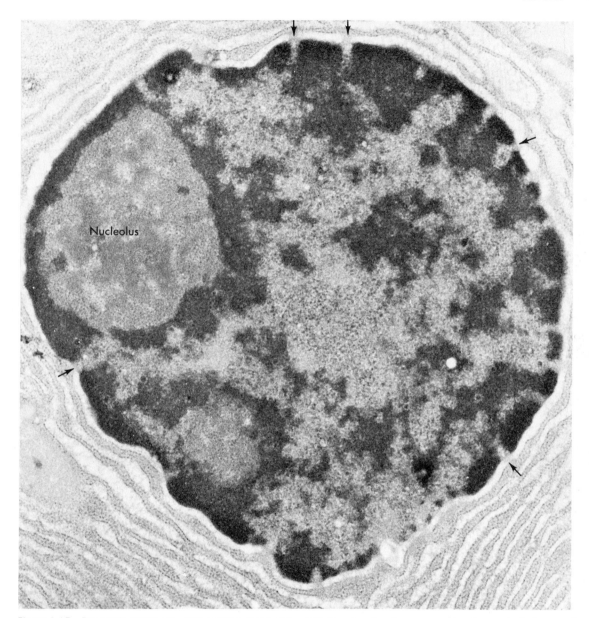

Figure 1-15 Pancreatic acinar cell. The nucleus of this cell, which secretes digestive enzymes, has been selectively treated to enhance the staining of DNA and to reduce the staining of the nucleoli and other RNA-containing structures. Chromatin is densely stained. Much of it is marginated on the inner surface of the nuclear membrane. Nuclear pores are prominent (arrow), their location marked by the lightly stained aisles between heterochromatin masses. The section was treated with picric acid, uranyl acetate, and lead. ×30,000. (From the work of A. Monneron.)

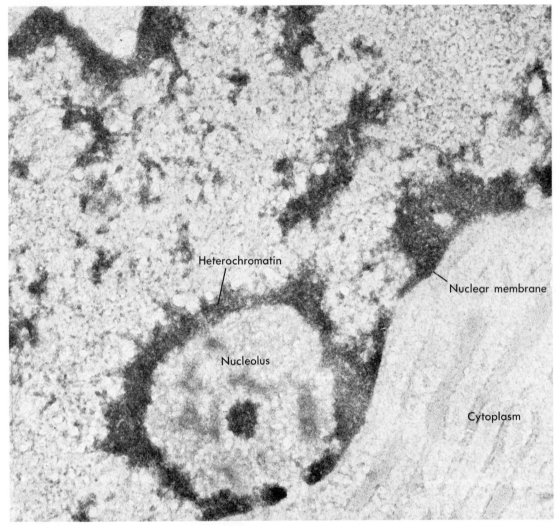

Figure 1-16   Pancreatic acinar cell.   The chromatin stands out sharply in this nucleus, having been stained with uranyl acetate and lead.   The nucleolus and other RNA-containing structures are poorly stained because the section was treated with ribonuclease which digested away the RNA.   The tissue was embedded in water-soluble methacrylate, an embedding medium which permits penetration of the ribonuclease.   ×30,000.   (From the work of A. Monneron.)

may be of the order of 10,000 times the largest dimension of the nucleus.   But it is difficult to gain any appreciation in sections of nuclei of the nature of the immense amount of folding and coiling which the chromosomes must undergo. Such inferences as electron microscopy affords come from preparations in which chromosomes are floated out of disrupted nuclei, dried down on supporting membranes, and examined whole.   Here high degrees of coiling and folding are evident.   Pure DNA may be prepared and examined as whole, unsectioned filaments by electron microscopy.   The filaments in such preparations are approximately 20 Å in diameter.   DNA can be identified in sectioned interphase nuclei on the basis of selective staining.   It is present in filaments of varying diameter, the slimmest being about 100 Å in diameter.   The greater thickness of DNA in sections must be due to such factors as coiling, folding, or intertwining of DNA filaments or complexing of DNA with histones or other substances.

NUCLEOLUS

A nucleolus is a discrete intranuclear structure consisting largely of protein and RNA whose function is the synthesis of the major components of ribosomes.   The nucleolus is well developed in cells active in protein synthesis.   Such cells typically contain several nucleoli.   In cells inactive in protein synthesis, as spermatocytes and muscle cells, a nucleolus may not be evident.   Nucleoli appear at certain specific sites in certain chromosomes, the nucleolar organizing sites.   These sites are secondary constrictions in the chromosomes.   They represent the location on the chromosomes of the gene sequences (cistrons) which encode the genetic information for the synthesis of ribosomal RNA. Nucleoli remain attached to the chromosomes at nucleolar organizing sites.   See Figs. 1-17 to 1-20.

Light microscopy   Nucleoli by light microscopy are often dense, clearly outlined structures up to 1 μm or more in size.   They have a characteristic structure dependent upon cell type and activity.   Often they are spherical, but they may be oval or even bow-tie-shaped.   They are usually compact and sharply outlined, but they may be porous with fuzzy borders.   Nucleoli may lie at random in the nucleus or against the inside of the nuclear membrane, an efficient location for the discharge of substances into the cytoplasm.

Nucleoli are demonstrated cytochemically by methods for RNA.   Thus the nucleolus absorbs at about 2600 Å, in the ultraviolet.   It is stained with pyronin in the methyl green–pyronin mixture and is blue in Romanovsky blood stains.   RNA contains the characteristic nucleotide base uracil, in contrast to DNA, and so if radioactive uracil is given an animal, autoradiography of its cells shows positive nucleoli, because of the high concentration of RNA in nucleoli and the selective uptake of uracil.   Selective demonstration of nucleoli by staining or other means is not possible after pretreatment of the section with ribonuclease.   Occasionally a nucleolus may be closely associated with, or ringed

by, DNA.   This represents the nucleolar-associated chromatin at the nucleolar organizer site and is stained by the Feulgen reaction.   A thread-like structure, the *nucleolonema*, may be demonstrated in the nucleolus by silver or other selective stain. Although its composition is not yet known, and its significance in doubt, it may be predominantly RNA.

Electron microscopy   By electron microscopy, nucleoli contain two forms of RNA.   One is granular, approximately 150 Å in diameter, similar, but not identical, to ribosomes.   This form is typically the dominant nucleolar structure.   The second form of RNA is fibrillar, 50 to 80 Å in thickness; the fibrils are probably precursor to the granules.   Poorly defined granular material, probably protein, occurs throughout nucleoli.   Rarefied vacuolar zones, not membrane-bounded, occur.   Nucleoli are not confined by a membrane.

Ribosomes have several subunits (see below). In mammalian cells ribosomes have a sedimentation constant of 80S.   They are divisible into two fractions: the heavy, sedimenting at 60S, and the light, at 40S.   The RNA component of the light fraction has a sedimentation constant of 18S. Several RNA components of the heavy fraction exist, with sedimentation constants of 28S, 5S,

Wild type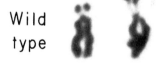

Hetero-zygote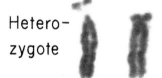

Figure 1-17   Chromosomes containing nucleolar organizing sites from the clawed toad *Xenopus laevis*.   They are taken from the metaphase karyotype (see text).   Each of the chromosomes in the wild type contains very slender zones, the nucleolar organizing sites.   In the heterozygote, on the other hand, only one pair of chromosomes contains this site.   The result in heterozygotes, as discussed in the text, is nucleolar-deficient mutants. (From the work of D. D. Brown.)

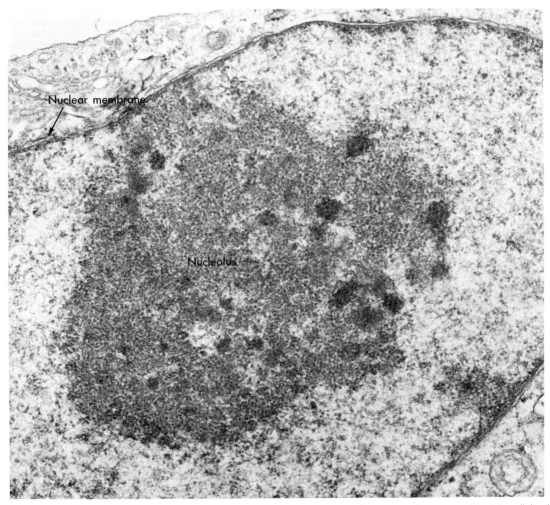

Figure 1-18   Rhesus kidney cell (strain MA 104) in culture.   The nucleolus, stained with uranyl acetate and lead, is well developed. ×40,000.   (From the work of A. Monneron.)

and 7S. It appears, on the basis of isolation of nucleoli and sedimentation analysis, that they produce at least the 18S and 28S components of RNA of ribosomes and release them to the cytoplasm. It is likely that the release to the cytoplasm is facilitated by the nucleolus moving against the nuclear membrane and discharging through nuclear pores. Once in the cytoplasm, the nucleolar-produced ribosomal components may mature further, perhaps by adding certain proteins, and combine to form ribosomes.

Support for the role of nucleoli in ribosomal synthesis comes from the work of Brown and his associates (1965) on amphibian mutants lacking nucleoli (Figs. 1-11 and 1-17). The embryo of the clawed toad, *Xenopus laevis*, synthesizes few ribosomes before the tail bud stage, the ribosomes from the oocyte serving until that time. A lethal anucleolate mutant of *Xenopus* may be bred from a spontaneously occurring heterozygote mutant with but one nucleolus per cell, instead of the normal two. Development of the anucleolate embryos is retarded after hatching. The embryos are microcephalic and edematous and die before feeding.

The mutation which prevents the formation of a normal nucleolus also prevents the synthesis of 28S and 18S ribosomal RNA, as well as high-molecular-weight ribosomal RNA precursor molecules.

The correlation between ribosome production and nucleoli is evident in multinucleate amphibian oocytes where the DNA specifying the sequences for 28S and 18S ribosomal RNAs is selectively replicated. As many as 1,000 nucleoli may occur per oocyte (Fig. 1-17)! Each of these nucleoli is analogous to the nucleoli of somatic cells and is an autonomous site for the synthesis of ribosomal RNA.

Figure 1-19   Hepatocyte. In this preparation RNP is preferentially stained and chromatin is bleached. The nucleolus stands out sharply. Stained granules, presumably containing RNA, lie outside the nucleolus in association with the chromatin. There are large (400 to 500 Å) perichromatin granules and small (200 Å) interchromatin granules. × 27,000. (From the work of A. Monneron; see also W. Bernhard, J. Ultrastruct. Res., **27:**250, 1969.)

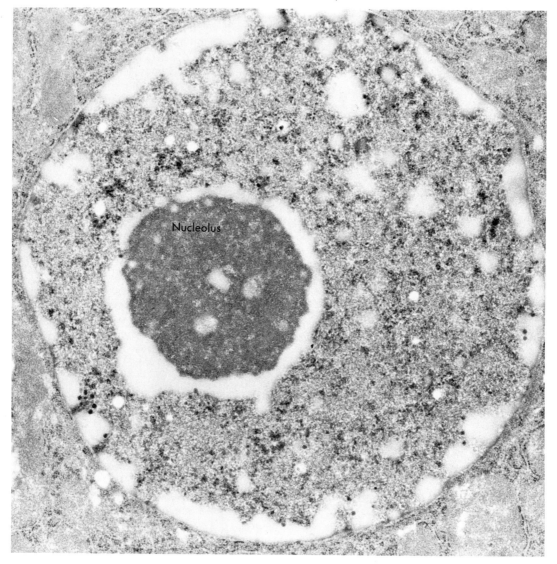

Nucleolus

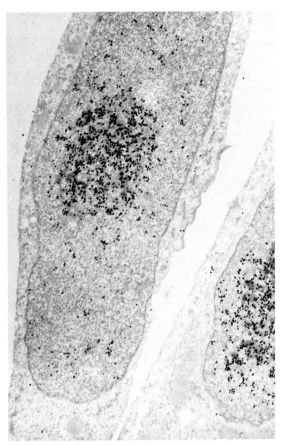

Figure 1-20   Monkey kidney cells (strain BSC). These cells, in tissue culture, were exposed to [³H] uridine (a precursor of RNA) for 30 min and then fixed and processed for EM autoradiography. The distribution of silver grains is only over the nucleus and mainly over the nucleolus. ×25,000. (From A. Monneron, J. Burglen, and W. Bernhard, J. Ultrastruct. Res., **32**:370, 1970.)

Nucleoli are not the only sites of RNP in the nucleus. Particles of different sizes and filaments of RNP lie against and between chromatin. It is likely that some of this widely dispersed nuclear RNA is mRNA (see below) produced on extended segments of DNA (euchromatin).

Functions   The nucleolus, a site of considerable molecular traffic, is a center for the synthesis of ribosomes. The size and number of nucleoli depend upon the level of ribosomal RNA synthesis. In actively synthesizing secretory cells (pancreatic acinar cells) the nucleoli are large and multiple whereas in cells showing a low level of protein synthesis (muscle cells, certain small lymphocytes) nucleoli may be small or absent.

NUCLEAR ENVELOPE

The nuclear membrane or envelope stands for a major evolutionary change, the development of eukaryotic organisms. In prokaryotic organisms such as bacteria, nuclear material, although zonal, lies unseparated from the remainder of the protoplasm. In the higher fungi and on, the eukaryotes, the nucleus becomes a discrete unit bounded by a complex discriminatory envelope.

The envelope consists of two concentric unit membranes. Each is approximately 70 Å in thickness, the inner one somewhat thinner. The space or cisterna between inner and outer nuclear membranes varies in size and content. It is commonly about 150 Å wide and lucent. The outer nuclear membrane is continuous with the ER, both rough and smooth. The continuity of the outer nuclear membrane with the ER establishes the cytoplasmic character of these membranes. This character is underscored in the re-formation of nuclear membranes in the telophase. The nuclear membranes are clearly formed by segments of ER which line up around the reconstituted nuclear mass. In cells synthesizing protein the nuclear envelope may, like the rough ER, contain the protein product. Thus, in antibody-producing cells the nuclear envelope may be distended with antibody and, indeed, is among the first places antibody accumulates. The chromosomes during the first meiotic prophase may be attached to the nuclear surface of the inner membrane and nucleoli may lie there (see above). Although the nuclear envelope cannot be resolved by light microscopy, its location is often revealed as a definite line representing the sum of the nuclear membranes, nuclear cisterna, and adherent material.

Regularly spaced on the nuclear envelope, accounting for nearly 10 percent of its surface, are *nuclear pore complexes*. (Fig. 1-21). At these locations the inner and outer nuclear membranes fuse to form a complex about 600 Å in diameter. The pore appears blocked by a thin diaphragm consisting of a matrix in which fine filaments and small granules are embedded. The disposition of the

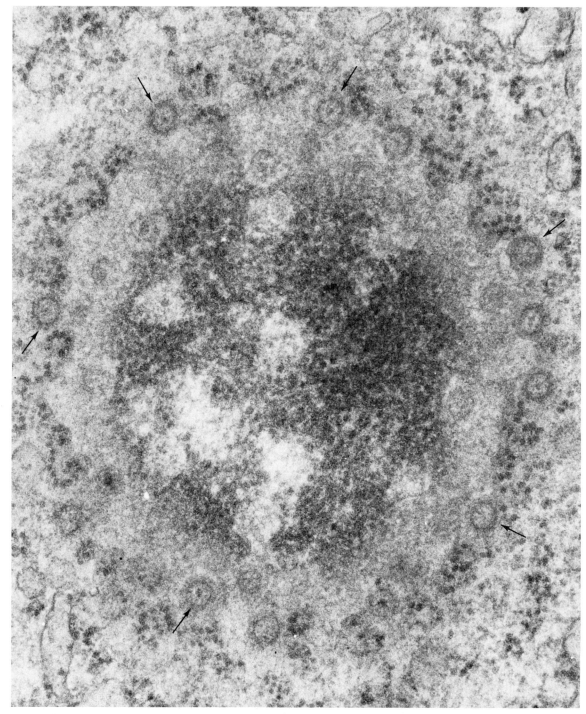

Figure 1-21   Rat hepatocyte.   This is a tangential section of the nucleus, revealing nuclear pores all around (arrow), some with a dark central granule.   Note that polyribosomes are in close association with the pores.   This preparation is stained with uranyl acetate and lead.   ×140,000.   (From the work of A. Monneron.)

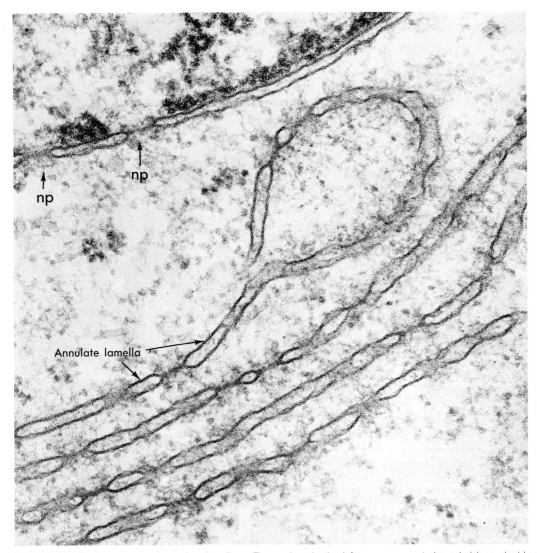

Figure 1-22 Nuclear pores and annulate lamellae. The nucleus in the left upper corner is bounded by a double membrane, each component consisting of a unit membrane (see text). Within the nucleus, densely stained chromatin is arranged against the nuclear membrane, in which two nuclear pores (np) are present. Within the cytoplasm, occupying much of the field, are stacks of annulate lamellae. These appear identical in structure with the nuclear membrane and, like the nuclear membrane, have frequently spaced pore complexes. ×65,000. (From G. Maul, J. Cell Biol., **46:**604, 1970.)

ules and filaments is subject to variation. The granules commonly aggregate to form a central granule. The filaments may be arranged radially. In human melanoma cells, ring structures, approximately 40 and 125 Å in diameter, are usually in the center of the pore.

The rim of the pore is typically modified or asso-

ciated with a complex thickening often octagonal on surface view, the *annulus*. The annulus may be quite large, with an outside diameter of more than 1000 Å. The inside diameter may be about 600 Å, but it may be smaller, thus reducing the diameter of the pore.

The pores are passageways between nucleus and

cytoplasm. Thus RNP granules occur in the pores and are probably en route to the cytoplasm. The considerable variation in the morphology and arrangement of the material covering pores probably represents different functional states in their control of nuclear-cytoplasmic exchange. See also Fig. 1-37

ANNULATE LAMELLAE
In many cell types stacks of membranes which exactly resemble portions of nuclear membranes, pore complexes and all, may be found in the cytoplasm (Figs. 1-22 and 1-23). In certain germ cells they may be present in nucleoplasm. These membranes are termed *annulate lamellae* and are especially common in germ cells. They may be present in varying concentrations and in different parts of the cytoplasm and may be continuous with the endoplasmic reticulum (see below). Their significance is not known. It has been suggested that they may exercise a type of nuclear control in parts of the cytoplasm distant from the nucleus.

THE CYTOPLASM
The cytoplasm surrounds the nucleus and is bounded by the plasma membrane or plasmalemma. The cytoplasm is capable of energy formation and release, of protein synthesis, growth, motility, phagocytosis, and diverse other functions. It is dependent upon the nucleus for direction, renewal, and regeneration. Thus isolated units of cytoplasm, exemplified by blood platelets and mature erythrocytes, are capable of protein synthesis and of such specific functions as respiration and the retraction of blood clots, but they cannot adapt to their environment. The volume of cytoplasm in proportion to the nucleus, the *nuclear-cytoplasmic ratio,* varies considerably from cell type to cell type. In some cells, as the spermatozoa, the cytoplasm is scant and, structurally, highly specialized, whereas in others, such as the lymphocytes, it is scant and apparently unspecialized. In most cells the cytoplasm is relatively abundant, exceeding the nuclear volume by a factor of 3 to 5 or more. The cytoplasm possesses several distinctive organelles with specialized functions of protein synthesis, energy production, etc. They lie in the ground substance or hyaloplasm. The volume of cytoplasm and its functions are determined by the number and nature of its organelles.

Several zones may be recognized in cytoplasm. The cytoplasm in the center of the cell, next to the nucleus, may be gelated. It contains the centrioles and centrosphere but is usually clear of other organelles, and it is surrounded by the Golgi element. Often it pushes the nucleus aside, deforming it into a U-shaped or reniform structure. This zone is designated the *cell center* or *cytocentrum.* Peripheral to this is a rather solvated part of the cell in which many vacuoles and granules, mitochondria, and elements of the endoplasmic reticulum are present. Active cytoplasmic streaming occurs here, carrying the cytoplasmic organelles in rapid movement. This zone is designated *endoplasm.* The peripheral cytoplasm in many cell types, particularly in free or motile cells, is gelated and free of organelles. This zone is the *ectoplasm.* The cytoplasm is capable of rapid sol-gel transformations. Areas of gelation of the ectoplasm may break down, particularly in motile cells or cells extending pseudopodial processes, and the solvated endoplasm bearing organelles then flows in.

Figure 1-23 Annulate lamellae. In this face-on section, surface views of the pore complexes (pc) are presented. The pores appear limited by a unit membrane and have a complex, regular internal structure. ×65,000. (From G. Maul, J. Cell Biol., **46:**604, 1970.)

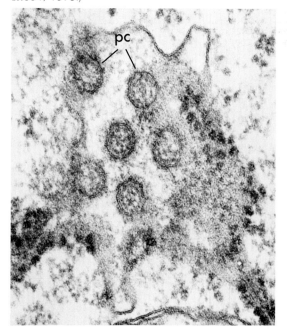

THE PLASMA MEMBRANE AND
OTHER CYTOPLASMIC MEMBRANES

The plasma membrane or plasmalemma is a selectively permeable membrane which limits the cell. It is often about 70 Å in thickness but may be as thick as 100 Å. Too thin to be resolved by light microscopy, its location may nonetheless sometimes be determined under the light microscope where it is tightly folded on itself to form a cuticular or brush border or where mucoprotein or other substance coats its surface. Often a carbohydrate-rich coat lies on the outside surface of the plasma membrane and has been recognized as a *glycocalyx* (Chap. 3).

Plasma membranes have been isolated by differential centrifugation of a number of cell types. The

Figure 1-24   Erythrocyte, peripheral cytoplasm. Note the trilaminar character of the plasmalemma, there being two dark laminae separated by a light one. This membrane is a unit membrane. ×280,000. (From the work of J. D. Robertson.)

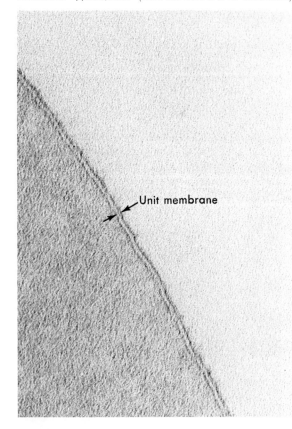

Unit membrane

membrane fraction of hemolyzed erythrocytes is relatively simple to obtain. By chemical analysis of such fractions, membranes have been found to be complex structures. Protein accounts for approximately 60 percent of their composition, fat about 35 percent, and carbohydrate 5 percent.

Protein is present in linear and globular forms. Enzymes are present in the plasma membrane. They include Mg^{2+}-, Na^+-, and Ca^{2+}-dependent adenosine triphosphatase (ATPase) and other enzymes which permit a discriminatory passage of materials across the plasma membrane. Adenosine triphosphate (ATP) and other compounds constituting energy sources are also present in the membrane. The combination of selective permeation and energy consumption in crossing a membrane against a concentration gradient (''uphill'') is designated as *active transport,* in contrast to *passive transport,* a nondiscriminatory, ''downhill'' transfer due to diffusion. The fat in the membrane is mostly phospholipid. The activity of many membrane-bound enzymes depends upon fat, as does the ready passage of certain molecules, notably the fat-soluble ones. Carbohydrate-containing compounds occur preferentially on the outer surface; they include the sialic acids which probably play a role in cell homing and cell recognition in cell-to-cell interaction. The carbohydrates are good antigens and the basis of immunologically sorting cells, as in the blood (erythrocyte) cell types. It is the elaboration of carbohydrate-containing materials that results in the glycocalyx. The materials in certain cell types, such as intestinal epithelium, may form a conspicuous felted layer, *fuzz* or the *fuzzy layer.* These layers may be sufficiently developed to render the location of the plasma membrane visible by light microscopy. They may, by electron microscopy, be selectively stained by *ruthenium red* (Fig. 1-25).

By electron microscopy of conventionally fixed (that is, glutaraldehyde, osmium tetroxide, or potassium permanganate) and sectioned material the plasma membrane may be recognized as a three-layered structure, the *unit membrane* (Figs. 1-24 and 1-25). The outer layers are electron-dense, and each measures approximately 20 Å in thickness. The central lucent layer is about 30 Å thick. Occasionally it is possible to resolve certain structures within the unit membranes. Thus in

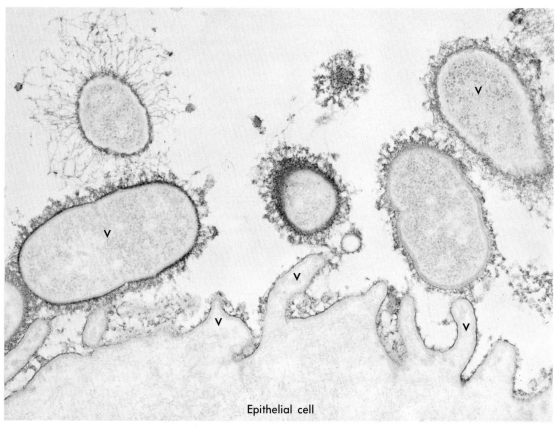

Epithelial cell

Figure 1-25   Cell surface, human buccal epithelium; electron micrograph.   The free surface of an epithelial cell having large and small villi (v) is shown.   A surface coat has been stained selectively with the dye ruthenium red.   The coat, where it lies upon the plasmalemma, is relatively dense.   On its free surface, on the other hand, the surface coat has a flocculent or filamentous character.   ×40,000.   (From John Luft, Anat. Rec., **171**:347, 1971.)

some locations discrete or globular structures may make up the inner membrane, or strands of dense material may cross the lucent central layer.

The unit membrane may be seen not only as the plasma membrane.   Many intracellular structures are fabricated of unit membranes; thus Golgi membranes, endoplasmic reticulum, and nuclear and mitochondrial membranes are unit membranes, but important variations in membrane structure exist. The thickness of the unit membrane varies characteristically.   In the Golgi the unit membrane may be but 50 to 60 Å in thickness on the forming face whereas in the plasmalemma it may be 100 Å thick.   The inner mitochondrial membrane may reveal a globular pattern, particularly well shown after negative staining.   However, it is well known that membranes in different places differ in chemical composition and function, and it is remarkable that they look so much alike in conventionally fixed and sectioned electron micrographs.

Membrane heterogeneity has been well demonstrated in the valuable technique of freeze-fracture (Fig. 1-26).   The fracture line in this technique tends to follow membranes, and, preferentially, to run within a membrane, exposing its core.   By freeze-fracture-etch techniques discrete granular structures are found that differ from membrane to membrane and may assume rather regular patterns.   For example, there is a characteristically regular pattern of granules within red cell membranes.   The outer

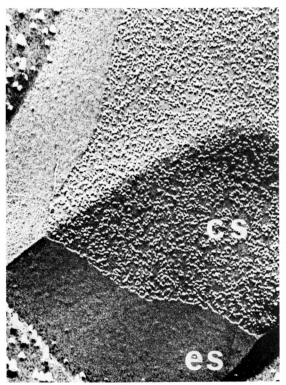

Figure 1-26   Human red cell; platinum replicas of freeze-etched preparation.   Normal ghost membranes freeze-cleaved and deep-etched.   The face of the membrane exposed by the cleavage process (cs) is covered by globular particles which are distributed uniformly over the surface membrane of the cell. The true external surface of the cell (es) is exposed by deep etching.   The carbohydrate portions of the glycoproteins are present on this surface, but they cannot be recognized. × 50,000.   (From V. T. Marchesi, T. W. Tillack, R. J. Jackson, J. P. Segrest, and R. E. Scott, Proc. Nat. Acad. Sci., **69:**1445, 1972.)

mitochondrial membrane has a regular pattern, moreover, whereas the inner one does not.   These granules or particles are of the size of enzymes in many cases and probably represent enzymes or enzyme complexes.   Work in freeze-fracture-etch has scarcely begun, but its value appears great. It is providing information about membrane heterogeneity at relatively high resolution (about 30 Å is the resolution possible in replicas) in unfixed material.   The heterogeneity, moreover, fits well with chemical data.   See also Fig. 1-54.

Many models have been proposed for the ar-

rangement of the constituents of membranes. These take into consideration such evidence as the presence of carbohydrate groups on the outer surface, the lipid solubility of many materials which cross the membranes readily, the globular nature of many of the membrane-bound proteins and their ability to move in the membrane to some degree, and the linear or structural nature of other proteins.   These models remain tentative.

ENDOPLASMIC RETICULUM

The endoplasmic reticulum (ER) is a cytoplasmic system of tubules, vesicles, and sacs or cisternae fashioned of unit membranes.   The ER is subject to characteristic variations in complexity and extent, depending upon cell type and cell function.   It is continuous with the outer membrane of the nuclear envelope (Fig. 1-27) and with the Golgi membranes and may be continuous with the plasmalemma (Figs. 1-39 and 1-40).

The ER has been defined by electron microscopy, although it has been observed by light microscopy in some cells, notably as the *sarcoplasmic reticulum,* the specialized ER of striated muscle.   The ER was first described in electron micrographs of fibroblasts in tissue culture examined as whole mounts without sectioning.   Ordinarily whole cells are too thick for electron-microscopic study, but cells in culture may put out cytoplasmic processes thin enough to pass an electron beam.   In such preparations a cytoplasmic network, the endoplasmic reticulum, may be seen (Fig. 1-28).

The ER is subject to specialization.   Perhaps the most important is the differentiation of *rough* or *granular* ER (Fig. 1-29), with ribosomes on its outside surface, and *smooth* ER, whose surface is free of ribosomes.   Ribosomes synthesize protein (see below) and need not be associated with ER.   The association of ER and ribosomes occurs in cells which either secrete the protein they synthesize or isolate it within membrane-bounded sacs.   Thus in *polychromatophilic erythroblasts* which synthesize the pigmented respiratory protein *hemoglobin* that remains free in the cytoplasm, ribosomes are plentiful but little ER is present.   In plasma cells, on the other hand, which synthesize and secrete large volumes of antibody protein, rough ER is abundant.   Probably peptides or larger molecules are synthesized in the ribosomes and sent across the

ER membrane into the lumen of the ER (see below). The ER thereby isolates synthesized material from the rest of the cytoplasm, permits further assembly of peptides into larger molecules, facilitates complexing with other compounds, and chan-

Figure 1-27 Connective tissue cell from human embryo spleen. Here the continuity of the outer nuclear membrane and the smooth ER is evident. Thus the perinuclear space and the lumen of the ER are continuous. ×12,000.

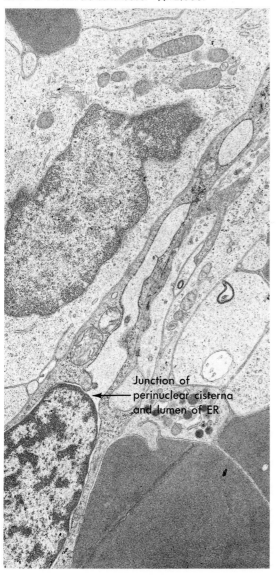

Junction of perinuclear cisterna and lumen of ER

nels it into the Golgi where further synthesis, aggregation, complexing, and packaging occur. Although rough ER is well developed in secretory cells, it is also abundant in certain phases in the life cycle of cells which synthesize a protein product and hold it membrane-bounded within their cytoplasm, as in blood leukocytes and in macrophages which contain enzyme-rich membrane-bounded granules. The formation of these granules parallels the formation of a secretory vacuole, except that the granules tend to be retained rather than released (secreted).

In nerve cells rough ER exists as large, flattened sacs lying upon one another in lamellated fashion to form masses, *Nissl bodies*, identifiable by light microscopy. Hepatic parenchymal cells contain smaller blocks of rough ER. In plasma cells the rough ER is rather uniformly distributed through the cytoplasm, except for the region of the cytocentrum. It may be tubular, vesicular, or flattened, depending upon the phase of antibody secretion. Rough ER occupies the base of the pancreatic acinar cell, its development varying with the secretory cycle. This rough ER, recognizable in light microscopy as basophilic material (because of the affinity of ribosomes for cationic dye), was termed *ergastoplasm* (see Ribosomes, below).

Smooth ER occurs in a number of cell types and may have diverse functions. It may well have a role in the production of steroid hormones since it is abundant in such cells as the Leydig cells of the testis which produce the steroid testosterone. It may be active in the detoxification of certain drugs, becoming very prominent in the inactivation of phenobarbital by the liver, for example. In striated muscle, smooth ER is distinctively organized as the sarcoplasmic reticulum whose functions include the delivery of high concentrations of Ca^{2+} and other ions to critical places in the sarcomere for muscular contraction and relaxation. Smooth ER in megakaryocytes delimits platelet zones in the cytoplasm and, by fusing, frees platelets from the megakaryocyte. Glycogen synthesis is associated with smooth ER and the Golgi apparatus. The reformation of the nuclear membrane in telophase is accomplished by smooth ER.

The smooth ER may be continuous with rough ER. Possibly the rough ER synthesizes the smooth. It is likely that ER is a dynamic system whose tubules

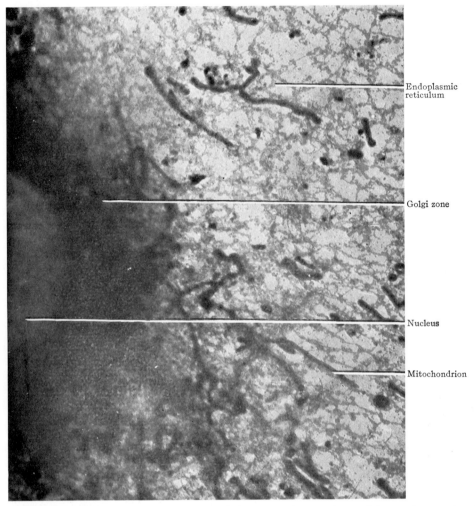

Endoplasmic reticulum

Golgi zone

Nucleus

Mitochondrion

Figure 1-28 Fibroblast; tissue culture. The preparation in this electron micrograph has not been sectioned. It is a whole mount of the cell, and only the peripheral region is sufficiently thin to permit passage of the electron beam. (From the work of K. R. Porter.)

may extend or retract and which may dilate into cisternae or separate into vesicles or vacuoles that lose continuity with the main body. Indeed, the membranes of the ER appear to possess a self-healing capacity when disrupted. When ultra-centrifugation fractions rich in ER are recovered from disrupted cells, the ER is found as small sphe-roid vesicles (*microsomes*) (Fig. 1-30). Evidently the tubular system is fragmented, but the mem-branes reunite or "heal" to form small vesicles.

After fixation with osmium tetroxide, the tubular T system of sarcoplasmic reticulum is revealed as a system of vesicles—another example of the readi-ness with which the tubules of ER may be broken up and re-formed as small vesicles. See Chap. 7.

RIBOSOMES

Light microscopy A single ribosome is below the limit of resolution of the light microscope, but in aggregate, ribosomes can be seen. Owing, in all likelihood, to their PO_4^{3-} groups, they have a pronounced affinity for cationic or basic dyes such as methylene blue$^+$. As a result, cells rich in ribosomes are basophilic; this basophilia may be abolished by pretreatment of the tissue with ribonuclease. The intensity and disposition of the basophilia are highly characteristic of cell type. The material by light microscopy has been designated *chromidial substance* or *ergastoplasm*. Consult the description of the *pancreatic acinar cells, lymphocytes,* and *erythroblasts* for a description of the patterns of chromidial substance.

Electron microscopy   Ribosomes are flattened, spheroidal, complex cytoplasmic particles measuring approximately 150×250 Å which synthesize protein (Figs. 1-31 to 1-35). They consist of RNA and protein. Their RNA is classed as *ribosomal RNA*, which accounts for 85 percent of the RNA of the cell. In addition to this form of RNA, there is *messenger RNA* (mRNA) and *transfer RNA* (tRNA). The instruction for protein synthesis is encoded in DNA. This information is transcribed to messenger RNA which is about 300 to 600 nm long, depending upon the protein. Messenger RNA is produced in the nucleus, on a template of un-

Figure 1-29   Hepatocyte of a rat. In this portion of the cytoplasm most of the cisternae of the rough ER were cut transversely (top), and others tangentially. In the latter (arrow) the membrane of the ER and the attached polysomes are seen *en face*. A section of a mitochondrion (mit) is present.   ✕64,000. (From the work of G. E. Palade.)

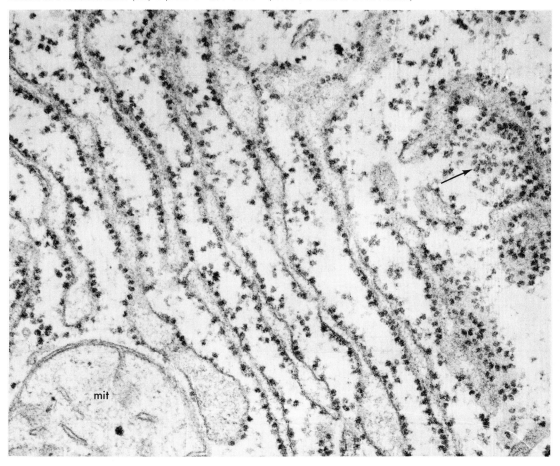

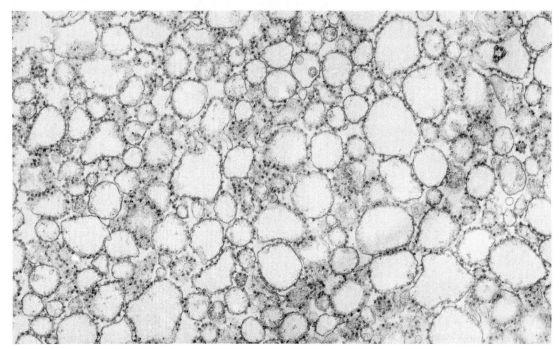

Figure 1-30   Microsomes of rat liver.   The liver was disrupted and various fractions recovered by ultracentrifugation.   This is the microsome fraction.   It consists almost entirely of rough ER which had been disrupted and ''healed'' as vesicles.   Ribosomes remain attached to the outer surface.   ×40,000.   (From the work of D. Sabatini and M. Adelman.)

Figure 1-31   Ribosomes, hepatocyte, of a guinea pig.   Ribosomes at high magnification show a larger and smaller component.   When associated with the ER, the larger component lies upon the membrane.   In this field a single cisterna (c) of the ER is present.   The arrows indicate the position and orientation of the partitions separating the large from the small subunits of the ribosomes.   Note that these partitions lie generally parallel to the surface of the membranes (m).   This specimen was fixed in osmium tetroxide, embedded, sectioned, and stained with uranyl acetate.   ×270,000.   (From the work of D. Sabatini, Y. Toshiro, and G. E. Palade.)

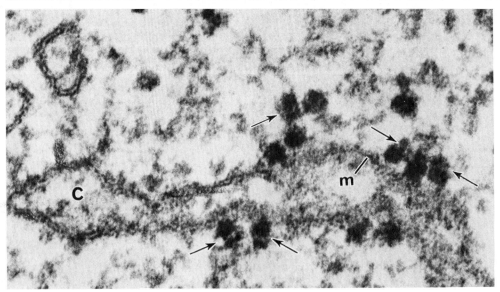

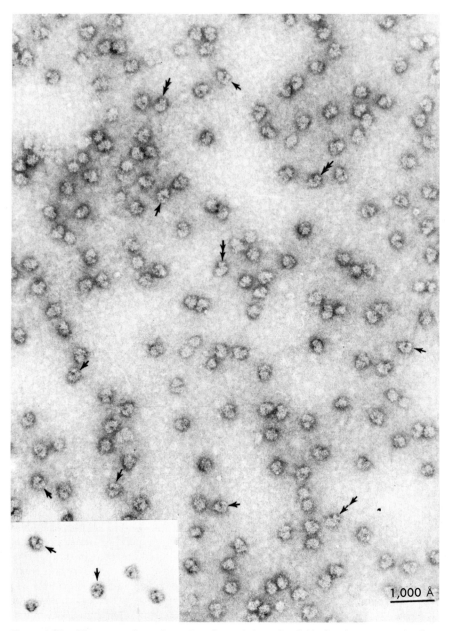

Figure 1-32   Ribosomes of a guinea pig.   General view of a field of native monomeric ribosomes.   Several image types are predominant.   Frontal images (arrows) have an elongated small subunit profile and a dense spot toward the side of the separation between subunits.   All frontal images in the field have this spot to the left of the observer if the particle image is oriented with the elongated small subunit horizontally and toward the top.   In lateral images (double arrows) the small subunit produces a small rounded or rectangular profile toward one side of the large subunit profile.   The insert shows images of monomeric ribosomes, reconstituted in vitro from the isolated large and small subunits.   This preparation was made from ribosomes isolated by differential centrifugation of disrupted cells.   The ribosomes were then floated on a membrane-covered electron-microscopic grid, dried, and negatively stained with phosphotungstic acid.   ×125,000.   (From the work of D. Sabatini, Y. Nonomura, and G. Blobel.)

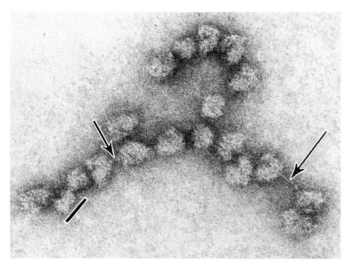

Figure 1-33   Ribosomes of a guinea pig. Here a strand of messenger RNA (arrows) links ribosomes into a polyribosomal unit. The mRNA runs between the small and large subunits. ×240,000. (From the work of D. Sabatini, Y. Nonomura, and G. Blobel.)

Figure 1-34   Polyribosomes from reticulocytes. These polyribosomes have been isolated by differential centrifugation of disrupted reticulocytes, spread on a grid, shadowed by evaporating heavy metal over them from one direction, and photographed in the electron microscope without sectioning. Note that the polyribosomes consist of clusters of about five ribosomes. The polyribosomes in intact reticulocytes form similar clusters (see Chap. 10). ×100,000. (From the work of A. Rich, J. R. Warner, and H. M. Goodman.)

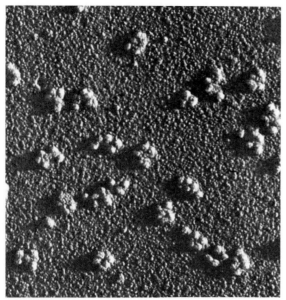

coiled DNA. It moves to the cytoplasm where it associates itself with ribosomes that lie along the mRNA like beads on a necklace. Ribosomes occurring singly in the cytoplasm are not active; only when they are linked by mRNA to form *polyribosomes* do they play a part in protein synthesis. The ribosomes are the small machines which receive the amino acid constituents of protein, assemble them into peptide chains, and release these chains into the cytoplasm or into the lumen of the ER where they continue to aggregate to form protein. The amino acids are brought to the ribosomes by tRNA, a low-molecular-weight compound (see below) that may be produced in the nucleolar region of the nucleus, as is ribosomal RNA, and passes out of the nucleus into the cytoplasm. There is a different tRNA for each of the amino acids. In protein synthesis, a ribosome moves along mRNA and reads the genetic message which has been transcribed from DNA. As the ribosome translates the message it condenses on its surface the proper activated amino acyl-tRNA and synthesizes the peptide linkage of this amino acid to the earlier ones.

The peptide chain grows larger as the ribosome moves along the mRNA and, as the ribosome slides off the mRNA, it releases the peptide chain. As one ribosome slides off one end of the mRNA another slides onto the other end and several ribosomes "read" or translate the mRNA at any time. The ribosomes lie on the mRNA approximately 340 Å apart (Fig. 1-33). For a polypeptide chain of hemoglobin 150 amino acids long, 1 to 1½ min is required for the ribosome to run the length of mRNA.

The ribosome is divisible into two major components: a larger one that, in eukaryotic cells, has a sedimentation constant of 160S and a molecular weight 1.25×10^6, and a smaller unit, 40S and MW of 6×10^5, that lies like a flattened cap on the larger one. mRNA threads its way between smaller and larger units.

Polyribosomes may lie free in the cytoplasm, releasing their peptide chains into the cytoplasm for further combination and complexing. This is the means by which hemoglobin is synthesized. Where the ribosomes attach to the outer surface of ER it is the larger unit which maintains attachment. The mRNA and the ER membranes are parallel. Further, there may be a canal which runs through the larger ribosomal component at right angles to the mRNA and the ER. This canal has been postulated to run through the membranous wall of the ER, with the result that the amino acids, in peptide linkage, are "spun out" by the ribosomes directly into the lumen of the ER (Fig. 1-35).

The smaller and larger components may be well visualized by negative staining. It is evident that each of these components is divisible into a number of smaller segments. The major components of the ribosomes are dependent, for their union, on the concentration of Mg^{2+}. Below a critical concentration the components are dissociated. They reassociate on restitution of a sufficient concentration of Mg^{2+}. It is possible to make hybrids of ribosomes by such alterations of Mg^{2+}. Even where there are interspecies hybrids, ribosomes may synthesize peptides from a messenger RNA of one of the constituents of the hybrid, indicating that ribosomes are "machines" amenable to a wide range of instruction.

Ribosomes probably have but a short life-span. With cessation of protein synthesis they are quickly metabolized and disappear.

GOLGI APPARATUS

The Golgi apparatus is a system of membranes and vesicles, usually located in the region of the cytocentrum, whose functions include the packaging of cellular products and the modification of these products, especially by the addition of carbohydrates. The Golgi may be continuous with the ER.

Light microscopy The Golgi has a characteristic appearance by light microscopy. It is often juxtanuclear and, in the intestinal epithelium, for example, lies toward the apical surface. Its size fluctuates with cell type and cell activity. It is well developed in secretory cells, especially in the

Figure 1-35   Model of the relationship between ribosomes and ER membrane. Attachment by the large subunits and orientation of the partition separating the two ribosomal subunits are strongly suggested by the evidence presented. The central channel in the large subunit and the discontinuity in the subjacent ER membrane are tentative features of the model, included only to indicate a possible pathway for the release of the newly synthesized protein in the cisternal space. (From the work of D. Sabatini and G. Blobel.)

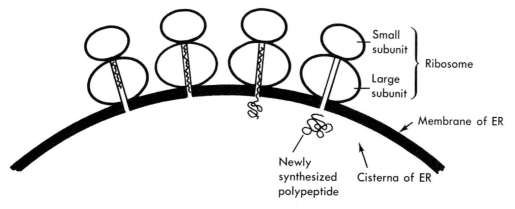

mucus-producing intestinal epithelial cells which elaborate a product rich in carbohydrate. It is subject to waxing and waning during the secretory cycle. The Golgi has the capacity to reduce metal salts, such as salts of osmium and of silver (Figs. 1-6 and 1-36). It may be a small compact structure or a widely dispersed internal reticular apparatus as initially defined by C. Golgi in nerve cells.

Electron microscopy   By electron microscopy the Golgi is fabricated of unit membranes about 60 Å thick, thinner than the plasmalemma and even the ER (Figs. 1-37 to 1-40). The proximal membranes (those facing the nucleus) are thinner than the distal (those facing out toward the bulk of the cytoplasm), which are more like those of plasmalemma and ER. The Golgi apparatus contains large flat sacs or cisternae lamellated on one another. They are relatively compressed at their centers and somewhat dilated peripherally. The sacs tend to be bowed, presenting a convex proximal face and concave distal face. The cisternae communicate with one another at places along their contiguous surfaces. These cisternae thus form bowl-shaped structures. At the edge of the lamellated sacs, near their expanded peripheries, vesicles 400 to 800 Å in diameter are typically present. Some contain dense lipoidal material. Similar vesicles may also be abundant at the distal face. These vesicles may be seen attached to the superficialmost sac by hollow stalks, suggesting they are being produced and released from the face of that sac. The vesicles vary in size and probably fuse to form larger vesicles. These vesicles, like the lateral ones, may contain a dense material. The proximal face is relatively free of vesicles and has been termed the *forming face,* but in certain cell types, notably leukocytes, this face is active in a distinct type of membrane-bounded granule formation. The distal face, which is typically engaged in granule and vacuole formation, has been termed the *maturation face.* The Golgi is continuous with the ER and even the outer nuclear membrane. The connection may be best seen at the lateral edges and the forming face.

A highly characteristic disposition of the Golgi is to lie in the cytocentrum rather toward its periphery, its concave face partially enclosing the centrioles. A cell may contain several packets of Golgi membranes and vesicles of the type described above, and some may well be found outside the clear cytocentrum in the contiguous endoplasm.

Many functions have been laid to the Golgi. Its conspicuous development in secretory cells and its change in size and form with different phases of the secretory cycle clearly accord it secretory functions. Modern studies using electron microscopy and autoradiography indicate that proteins synthesized in the ER move into the Golgi where they are "packaged," that is, they are bounded in a membrane and discharged as a vesicle which may remain in the cytoplasm, as, for example, the granules of a leukocyte, or may be secreted from the cell, such as the secretory granule of the pancreatic acinar cell. This packaging isolates, segregates, or concentrates certain materials from the remainder of the cell. There is evidence from tracer, isolation, and autoradiographic studies that the Golgi synthesizes carbohydrates and complexes them to the proteins coming in from the ER. For example, the antibody molecules have carbohydrate moieties attached; these are affixed and presumably synthe-

Figure 1-36   Golgi material in cells of guinea pig uterus. The Golgi material was blackened with silver by the method of Da Fano. Large quantities of it lie above the nuclei of the glandular cells (GC); smaller amounts lie next to the nuclei of the stromal cells (SC). ×500.

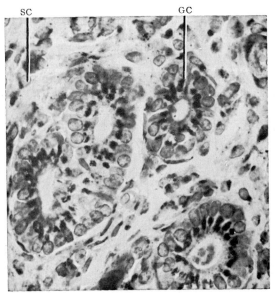

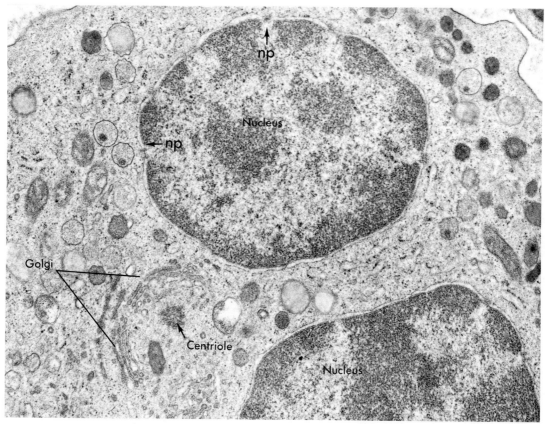

Figure 1-37 Human myelocyte. In this developing blood cell (see Chap.11) the nucleus is lobed. Nuclear pores (np) are present. The cytoplasm contains granules, vesicles, rough and smooth ER, mitochondria, and free ribosomes. A Golgi apparatus is present, partially surrounding a centriole. ×26,000. (From the work of G. A. Ackerman.)

sized in the Golgi. The Golgi is particularly well developed and active in the secretion of such carbohydrate-protein complexes as mucus. The Golgi may be active in lipoprotein synthesis (Figs. 1-39 and 1-40). The Golgi is unusually prominent in certain cells, such as the sperm where the prominent *acrosome* is a much-modified Golgi. In hormone-producing cells the hormone, or its precursor, is isolated by Golgi, and pigment is managed similarly. In macrophages the *primary lysosomes* are first produced by the Golgi. Pinocytotic vesicles containing environmental material fuse with these lysosomes to produce the *secondary lysosome,* a demonstration of the interaction of Golgi vesicles with plasmalemma-derived vesicles. In the production of leukocytic granules, evidence of large-

scale fusion of Golgi vesicles and the activity of both convex and concave faces has been obtained. Thus variations in the fundamental theme of Golgi packaging are encountered.

The Golgi has been isolated by differential centrifugation and characterized cytochemically. It consists of approximately equal parts of lipid and protein and tends to be unusually rich in nucleoside diphosphatases. Histochemical demonstration of these phosphatases may serve as a marker for Golgi membranes.

MITOCHONDRIA

Mitochondria are membranous cytoplasmic organelles capable of releasing chemical energy present in compounds obtained from food and of fixing that

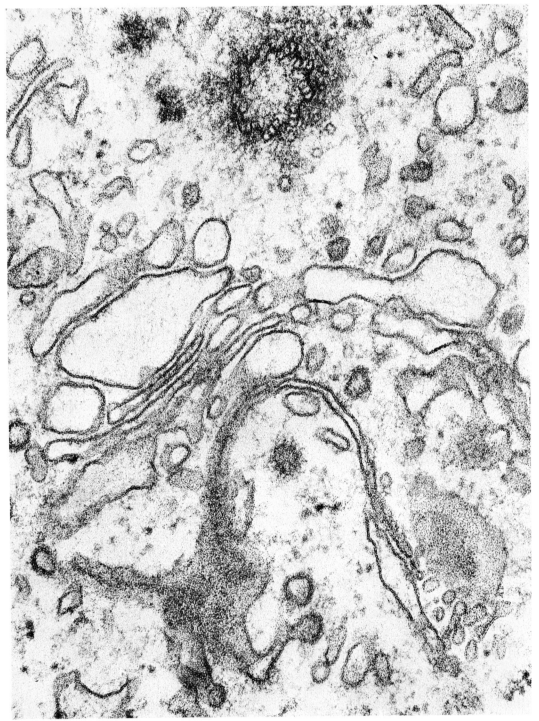

Figure 1-38 Golgi complex. It is evident, in this field, that the Golgi membranes and vesicles are made of the trilaminar unit membrane. A centriole is also present. (From the work of E. D. Hay and J. P. Revel.)

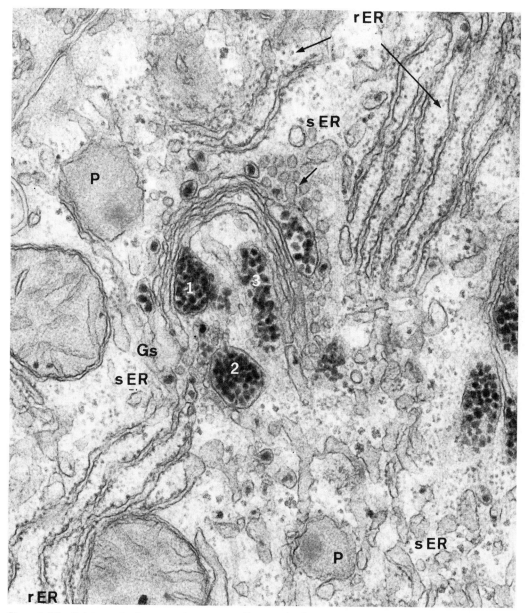

Figure 1-39   Golgi complex from a rat hepatocyte.   The complex lies near the center of this field.   The forming face of the Golgi, where the development of secretory product is initiated, is at the convex side of the apparatus, with extensions from the smooth ER network (sER) piling up from below and above, along the curved structure.   This smooth ER is probably produced by the rough ER (rER) which surrounds the Golgi and is continuous with the smooth ER.   A cluster of small vesicles, on top of the Golgi structure and next to a concentrating or secretory vesicle, is interpreted as representing cross sections of tubular, smooth ER extensions, with one of them (arrow) connecting with the concentrating vesicle.   At the concave or maturing face of the Golgi three concentrating or secretory vesicles (1 to 3) are present.   Each contains many small granules.   At (P), there are two peroxisomes (see text).   Compare this process of lipoprotein granule formation with that of the formation of granules within leukocytes, described in Chap. 11.   ×56,500.   (From A. Claude, J. Cell Biol., **47**:745, 1970.)

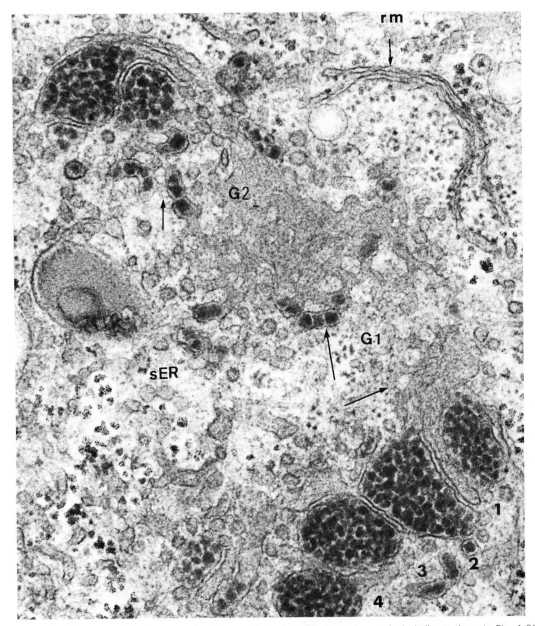

Figure 1-40 Golgi complex from a rat hepatocyte. Smooth-surfaced membranes (rm) similar to those in Fig. 1-39 are cut in cross section. As they are traced to the right they are continuous with rough ER. At G_2 Golgi membranes at the forming surface are cut in a plane parallel to their surface. These membranes are fenestrated and, in all probability, are formed by coalescence of smooth ER (sER) tubules (arrows) carrying rows of dense lipoprotein granules. Four large concentrating or secretory veiscles are present (numbered 1 to 4). These would develop from the maturing face of the Golgi, corresponding to the concave portion in Fig. 1-39. $\times 67,800$. (From A. Claude, J. Cell Biol., **47**:745, 1970.)

energy in a form readily utilizable by the cell. They are present, in suitably prepared light-microscopic sections, as punctate or linear structures just within the resolving power of the microscope (Figs. 1-6 and 1-41). By electron microscopy they are tubular structures bounded by one membrane and containing an internal folded membrane (Figs. 1-42 to 1-45).

A cell obtains energy from substrates derived from food. Thus amino acids derived from protein, fatty acids from fat, and glucose from carbohydrate may be sources of energy, but the major source is glucose. Glucose is broken down in the cell by *glycolytic* enzymes to form pyruvic acid, which is then oxidized to *acetyl coenzyme A*. This compound then proceeds to a cycle of further oxidations, the *Krebs tricarboxylic acid cycle,* which has as its end products carbon dioxide and water. Approximately 686,000 calories of energy per mole lie in the chemical bonds of glucose. Its oxidation to pyruvate yields approximately 40,000 calories per mole, but its complete oxidation to carbon dioxide and water through the Krebs cycle yields approximately another 650,000 calories per mole. The energy-capturing mechanism of cells is at best only about 50 percent efficient, however, losing half the energy as heat, so that the total caloric content of glucose is never available. Only about 350,000

Figure 1-41   Light micrograph of a portion of the stomach lining. The preparation has been stained for NAD+-dependent isocitric dehydrogenase activity (consult Chap. 2). This constitutes a selective stain for mitochondria. Nuclei are present in negative image. Two cell types are present. One, the parietal cell, is rich in granular mitochondria and carries out active transport. The second, the chief cell, has relatively few filamentous mitochondria and is concerned with the synthesis of protein. These cell types are discussed in Chap. 18.   ×1,500.   (From the work of D. G. Walker.)

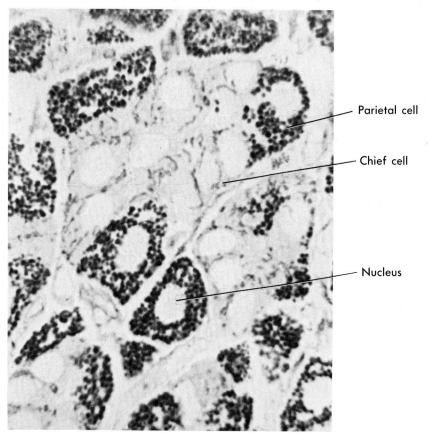

Parietal cell

Chief cell

Nucleus

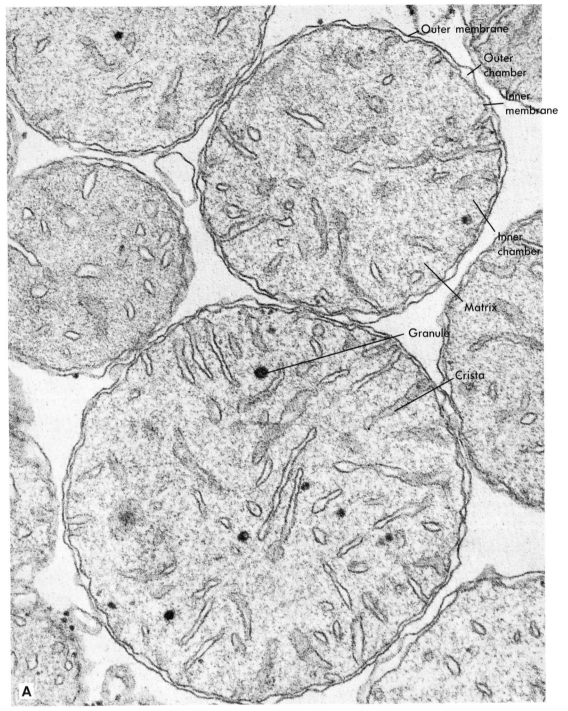

Outer membrane

Outer chamber

Inner membrane

Inner chamber

Matrix

Granule

Crista

A

Figure 1-42 Mitochondria of a rat hepatocyte. Mitochondria undergo reversible ultrastructural transformations between a condensed and an orthodox conformation in relationship to the level of oxidative phosphorylation (see text). These changes may be observed in isolated mitochondria and in tissue section. Mitochondria are isolated from disrupted hepatocytes and sectioned.

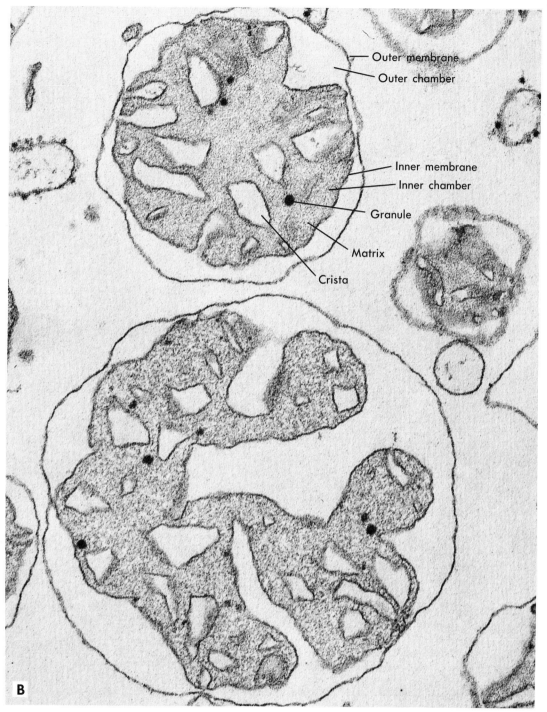

Outer membrane
Outer chamber

Inner membrane
Inner chamber

Granule

Matrix

Crista

B

A. The conventional conformation, the outer membrane, outer chamber, inner membrane with cristae, and inner chamber containing matrix and granules may be seen.   B. The condensed state; the outer chamber is considerably enlarged and the inner membrane and matrix thereby condensed.   Each ×110,000.   (From C. R. Hackenbrock, J. Cell Biol., **37**:345, 1968.)

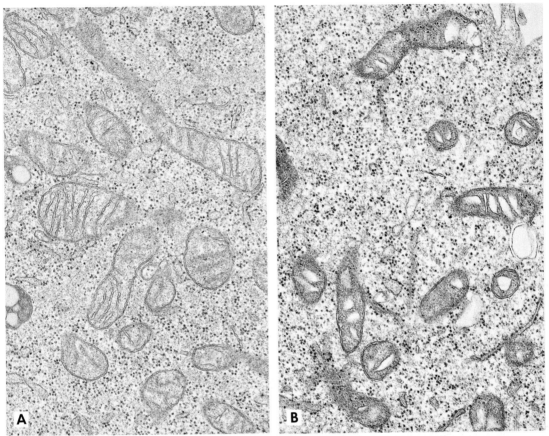

Figure 1-43   Mitochondria of an ascites tumor cell.   A. Mitochondria are present in the orthodox conformation.   A mitochondrion is enclosed in an outer membrane.   The inner membrane is folded into cristae which extend into the matrix of the inner chamber. ×26,800.   B. The condensed form, wherein the outer chamber is expanded, is evident.   The cytoplasm also contains polyribosomes and rough ER.   ×26,800.   (From C. R. Hackenbrock, T. G. Rehn, E. C. Weinbach, and J. J. Lemasters, J. Cell Biol., **51:**123, 1971.)

calories per mole are useful to the cell.   The glycolytic breakdown of glucose to lactic acid is anaerobic—that is, it does not utilize oxygen—in contrast to the mechanism of the Krebs cycle which does require oxygen, and is, therefore, respiratory in nature.   The oxidation through the Krebs cycle is clearly of great importance, as indicated by its caloric yield; indeed, it is necessary to life.   Blocking this system, as can be done with fluoroacetate, causes death.   *The Krebs cycle enzymes are present in mitochondria.*

The oxidation of pyruvate to carbon dioxide and water by itself, however, would yield only heat.

Another enzyme system is coupled into the Krebs cycle.   This is an *electron transfer system* of cytochromes which accepts the energy liberated in each of the steps of the Krebs cycle and incorporates it into so-called *high-energy phosphate compounds,* notably *adenosine triphosphate,* or ATP.   This is accomplished by the conversion of adenosine diphosphate (ADP) to ATP.   The additional phosphate bond so formed represents approximately 7,300 calories of stored energy.   *The cytochrome electron transfer system capable of fixing the energy obtained from the oxidations of the Krebs cycle into ATP lies in mitochondria.*   The ATP appears to diffuse from mitochondria into surrounding cytoplasm. Its energy is released by ATPases which lie at different locations in a cell. One depot rich in ATPase is the cell membrane. Here the energy obtained from the conversion of ATP to ADP is used in the active transport of compounds across the cell membrane.

Mitochondria may be observed in living cells by phase-contrast microscopy. They are quite pliant and appear to be carried passively in cytoplasmic streams, twisted, bent, and changing shape. On occasion they appear contractile or motile. They are subject to swelling in certain physiologic states.

Mitochondria may be vitally stained with Janus green B, pinacyanole, or other vital dyes which exist in a colored oxidized form and colorless reduced form. Because of their oxidative enzymes, mitochondria are capable of maintaining the dye in its oxidized form (a green or blue in the case of Janus green B) whereas the remainder of the cytoplasm is, in most instances, unable to do so.

In fixed and stained light-microscopic preparations, mitochondria are usually demonstrated by virtue of the phospholipid contained in their membranous walls. For this reason, solvents which extract phospholipid must be avoided in making these preparations or the subsequent staining will be markedly reduced or absent. The reason for using iron hematoxylin, an excellent stain for mito-

Figure 1-44 Mitochondria of a rat hepatocyte. Freeze-fracture-etch of isolated mitochondria. The fracture line exposed the inner surface of the outer membrane and the inner surface of the inner membrane. Note the rather regularly arranged system of granules on the inner surface of the outer membrane. The granules are the size of certain enzymes and may represent membrane associated enzymes. ×110,000. (From the work of C. R. Hackenbrock.)

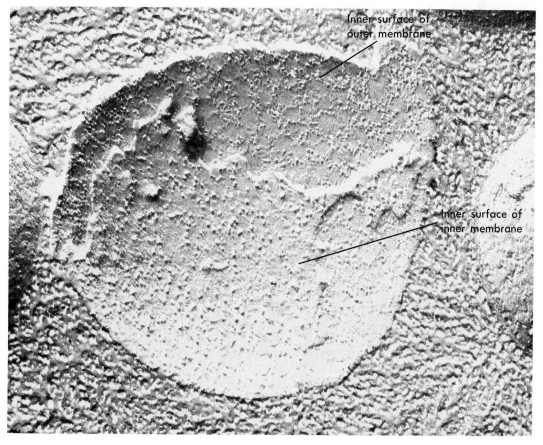

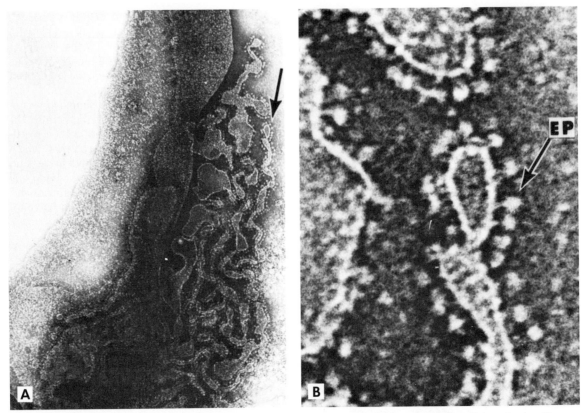

Figure 1-45   Mitochondrion from beef heart; negatively stained electron micrograph.   A. The cristae of the mitochondrion are outlined at a magnification of 62,000.   Note that small bodies (arrow) appear on the outer cristal membrane facing the interior of the mitochondrion.   B. Under 420,000 magnification these small bodies, the elementary particles (EP), are seen attached to the cristal membrane by a slender stalk.   (From H. Fernández-Morán, T. Oda, P. V. Blair, and D. E. Green, J. Cell Biol., 22:63, 1964.)

chondria utilized in the Regaud, Baker, and other methods, is the staining of phospholipid.   Sudan black B or other dyes which dissolve in lipid stain mitochondria faintly.

Mitochondria may also be demonstrated with light microscopy by histochemical staining of the activity of their enzymes (Fig. 1-41).   Thus stains for succinic dehydrogenase, malic dehydrogenase, isocitrate dehydrogenase, fumaric dehydrogenase, and other oxidative enzymes are effective.   The cells must be carefully fixed to limit diffusion of enzymes and to achieve good morphology; even slightly prolonged fixation destroys enzyme activity and renders the methods valueless.   These methods also provide valuable physiologic information.   For example, mitochondria may appear identical by methods dependent upon phospholipid staining, by supravital staining, or by phase microscopy.   Yet in such mitochondria Krebs cycle enzymes may have different activities, and by staining for a variety of these enzymes, different functional classes of mitochondria may be recognized on the basis of different intensities of staining.

By electron microscopy, mitochondria may be recognized as distinctive tubular structures made of inner and outer unit membranes (Figs. 1-41 to 1-45).   The outer limiting membrane is unfolded. The inner membrane is typically corrugated or folded to form cristae which extend into the center of the mitochondria.   In most mammalian cells the cristae are plates or shelves which extend partway across the internal cavity of the mitochondrion.

Some variation in cristal pattern is evident. In cardiac muscle there may be many cristae which reach across the mitochondrion, whereas in macrophages there are usually few cristae, and these are short. In kidney tubular cells the cristal pattern is quite regular, and the cristae reach almost all the way across the interior of the mitochondrion. In cells secreting steroid hormones, the cristae may be tubular rather than shelflike.

The unit membrane is modified in the cristae of mitochondria. The membrane surface which is exposed to the inner chamber of the mitochondrion possesses knob-like repeating units attached to a basal membrane by slender stalks (Fig. 1-45). These units, designated *elementary particles,* are revealed at high magnification with negative staining after osmotic shock. Their significance has not been established, although they may contain the enzymes associated with the electron transfer system. It is possible, moreover, that these particles, under normal conditions, are embedded in the membrane rather than projecting from it.

The inner chamber (the space enclosed by the inner membrane) of the mitochondrion contains finely granular material called *matrix*. It may contain dense granules.

Mitochondria are, however, subject to conformational change (Figs. 1-42 and 1-43). The *orthodox form* just described is typical of mitochondria in tissue section when the level of ADP is low and the mitochondria inactive in oxidative phosphorylation. If oxidative phosphorylation is induced in isolated mitochondria by the addition of ADP to a mitochondrial pellet, or if suitable measures are taken to preserve mitochondria in the process of oxidative phosphorylation in tissue sections, a condensed conformation is revealed. Here the crests of the inner membrane are not present. Instead, the outer chamber (the space between the inner and outer membranes) is increased to approximately 50 percent of the volume of the organelle.

Methods for demonstrating oxidative enzymes by electron microscopy have been developed. With them, cytochrome oxidase activity and the activity of related enzymes have been demonstrated within mitochondria.

Mitochondria may be isolated with relative ease from cells by a technique which requires disruption of cells and then centrifugation of the fragments.

In density gradient centrifugation, the mitochondria form a tan-colored stratum lying between the nuclei below and the lysosomes and ribosomes above.

Mitochondria isolated under these circumstances exhibit the various reactions delineated above. In addition, they may be studied by standard chemical and microchemical methods. They may be dissociated by application of deoxycholate and other surface-active agents, and by this method it has been ascertained that the electron transfer system of cytochromes appears firmly bound to membranes whereas the enzymes of the Krebs tricarboxylic acid cycle are not.

Freeze-fracture-etch methods have been used to reveal granules on mitochondrial membranes (Fig. 1-44). Both orthodox and condensed forms may be seen. Granules are seen within both inner and outer membranes. Those on the inner membrane are numerous and may constitute the enzymes of the electron transfer chain.

In ameboid free cells, mitochondria have no special distribution aside from being excluded, as a rule, from the cell center and the gelated cytoplasm of the ectoplasmic zones. In cells which maintain a marked polarity, as the renal tubular cells which present an apical surface to the lumen of a tubule and a basal surface to blood vessels, the mitochondria may have a characteristic location. In these cells the mitochondria are concentrated in the basal portion of the cell, lying at right angles to the basal surface between folds of the invaginated cell membrane.

The number of mitochondria is subject to variation. Hepatic cells may contain around 1,000 to 1,500 mitochondria. At the other extreme, mature erythrocytes, totally dependent for energy upon glycolysis, contain none.

Mitochondria may bear characteristic relationships to other organelles and cell structures. This relationship is often of great functional significance, as the mitochondrion is the primary source of energy in a cell. Thus in cells synthesizing protein, mitochondria may occur close to ribosomes (see below). In cells engaged in large-scale active transport of materials across a cell membrane, as in the parietal cell of the stomach (which pumps protons across a membrane in the production of hydrochloric acid) or the salt gland parenchymal cell of marine birds (which pumps sodium ions) the plasma membrane dips into the cell in many folds. Closely enveloped in this plasma membrane are mitochondria. In striated muscle cells, which contain myofilaments associated with contraction, the mitochondria are present in characteristic relation to the contractile elements. In the development of fat cells, the minute fat droplets which form and then coalesce are intimately associated with mitochondria.

As has been discussed, mitochondria possess a primary respiratory function. They may display other activities as well, notably the concentration of cations. The dense granules of the mitochondrial matrix in the inner chamber may represent concentrations of Ca^{2+}.

Mitochondria may constitute an extraordinary symbiotic event. Mitochondria, on first discovery by Altmann, were believed to be intracellular parasites termed *bioblasts,* a conception considered unacceptable then. However, mitochondria have now been found to contain DNA and RNA, of types typical of prokaryotes. Moreover, although the method of mitochondrial biogenesis has not been definitively resolved, there is evidence that existing mitochondria may produce new mitochondria. It thus must be considered possible that, in the evolution of eukaryotes, ancestral prokaryote structures established a felicitous symbiotic relationship which has become established and, indeed, permitted the considerable eukaryotic evolution which has occurred. A similar but far less fully documented case can be made for centrioles.

LYSOSOMES, PEROXISOMES, AND MULTIVESICULAR BODIES

Lysosomes are a class of cytoplasmic particle 50 to 80 Å in diameter, bounded by a unit membrane and containing hydrolytic enzymes active at acid pH. Lysosomes may be isolated by differential centrifugation of disrupted cells. They lie in the fraction centripetal to mitochondria. In electron micrographs they are oval or round membrane-bounded bodies containing variably dense granular material (Figs. 1-46 and 1-47). They may be identified cytochemically by reactions for acid phosphatase, a commonly used marker, or by reactions for other enzymes they contain. In such cytochemical preparations they may be visualized as punctate structures by light microscopy. Only under the electron microscope can their detailed structure be resolved.

The lysosomes of liver cells have been isolated and extensively studied. They contain a dozen or more hydrolytic enzymes. It is evident that even within a given tissue, as the liver, subclasses of lysosomes may be isolated, each somewhat different in enzymatic constitution. An hepatocyte may contain about 200 lysosomes.

Lysosomes occur in a number of states, accounting for heterogeneity of appearance. The *primary lysosome* or *storage body* is produced at the Golgi apparatus. Its genesis involves production of its enzymes in the rough ER, their movement into and packaging by the Golgi, and their release as enzyme-rich membrane-bounded particles. Lysosomes, with their complement of hydrolytic enzymes, are digestive organelles, and their heterogeneity must be understood in relationship to the incorporation of outside substances into the cell. A cell may engulf particulate matter (*phagocytosis*) or imbibe fluid (*pinocytosis*). Pinocytosis may be of a macrotype visible by light microscopy or of a microtype seen only in the electron microscope. In any case, the invaginated plasmalemma forms a membrane-bounded cytoplasmic vacuole, termed a *phagosome* or *pinosome.* On moving into the cytoplasm, phagosomes or pinosomes may meet primary lysosomes and fuse by coalescence of their membranes to form a *secondary lysosome, heterolysosome, heterophagosome,* or *definitive lysosome.* These structures may be stable structures, as in macrophages, which are notably effective later in fusing with new phagosomes and digesting their

Table 1-1   Enzymes present in rat liver lysosomes[*]

Acid ribonuclease
Acid deoxyribonuclease
Acid phosphatase
Phosphoprotein phosphatase
Cathepsin
Collagenase
α-Glucosidase
β-N-Acetylglucosaminidase
β-Glucuronidase
β-Galactosidase
α-Mannosidase
Aryl-sulfatase

[*] From C. de Duve, "The Lysosome Concept," Ciba Foundation Symposium, Little, Brown and Company, Boston, 1963.

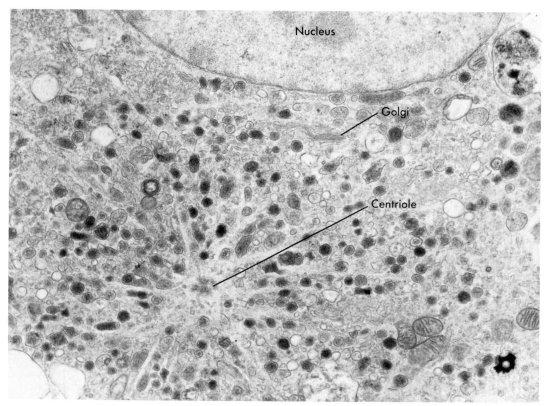

Figure 1-46 Lysosomes of the epithelioid cell of chicken. In this cell, derived from a macrophage, the cytoplasm is filled with lysosomes. They crowd out the centrosome. From the centriole, rays of gelated cytoplasm free of organelles radiate. At one place a small pocket of Golgi membranes is present. (From J. Sutton and L. Weiss, J. Cell Biol., **28**:303, 1966.)

contents. Indeed, following fusion of the primary lysosome to form a heterolysosome, new substances and heightened hydrolytic enzyme activity may become apparent. At the end of their development, secondary lysosomes become *residual bodies*. These are membrane-bounded structures containing pigment, myelin bodies, lipid, and variegated materials: the residues of incompletely digested materials. These bodies may be expelled from the cell, as in macrophages and many invertebrate cells. On the other hand, they may accumulate as indices of "wear and tear" or ageing.

Another group of secondary lysosomes is *autophagocytic vacuoles* or *cytolysosomes*. These are membrane-bounded structures containing some of the cells' own mitochondria, ribosomes, etc. They may originate from segments of smooth ER which curve about some cytoplasm and fuse to enclose it in a vacuole. These vacuoles may then fuse with primary lysosomes just as phagosomes do. Another mechanism may be the incorporation of some cytoplasm directly into a lysosome. The formation of autophagosomes may well be a mechanism of "internal policing" of a cell, removing damaged or senescent cell substance.

Although such end-stage structures as residual bodies may result from secondary lysosomes, many of the substances brought into lysosomes may be digested and their products released to the cytoplasm, and the lysosome, with the selective addition of certain materials and with augmented enzyme activity, may constitute a relatively long-lived, active cellular component.

Lysosomes constitute a product similar in many ways to secretory granules. However, lysosomes are typically not released but remain within the

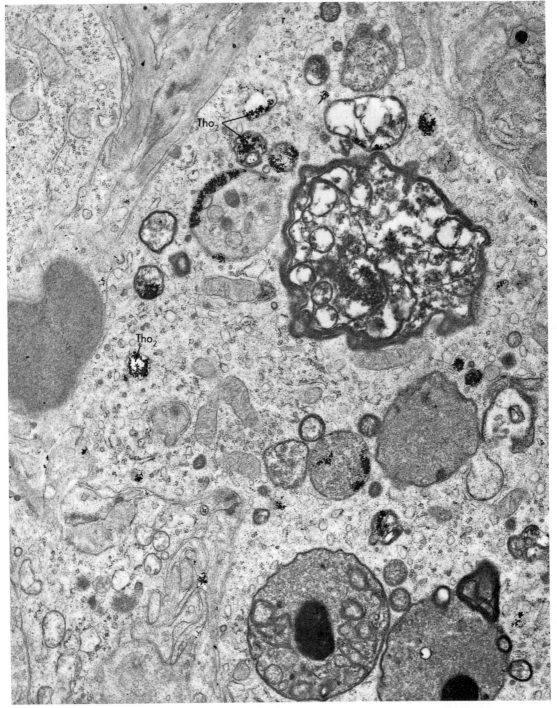

Figure 1-47 Lysosomes of a macrophage from a rabbit. This animal was given thorium dioxide (ThO$_2$) and electron-dense salt of the heavy metal shortly before this cell was fixed. Heterolysosomes, considerably different in appearance, are present. Many contain some ThO$_2$. ×40,000. (From L. Weiss, Bull. Hopkins Hosp., **115**:99, 1964.)

cytoplasm. It is likely, however, that macrophages in such loci as the red pulp of the spleen do selectively release lysosomes.

The membrane limiting the lysosome must protect the cell against the lytic effect of lysosomal enzymes, and so the lysosome represents an adaptation whereby a cell may concentrate powerful digestive enzymes without undergoing autodigestion (except in the controlled way associated with the development of autophagosomes). Cell death and postmortem autolysis may result largely from lysosomal disruption. That point at which the membrane of a lysosome is maintained or disrupted is clearly a critical matter. A number of diseases have been identified in which the lysosomal membrane in leukocytes is untowardly resistant to breakdown, such as the Chediak-Higashi disease and chronic granulomatous disease of childhood in which the control of bacteria is impaired and affected individuals die of infection.

Peroxisomes or *microbodies* are membrane-bounded particles somewhat larger than lysosomes, distinctive in containing peroxidase and catalase, D-amino acid oxidase, and urate oxidase. They can both synthesize and degrade peroxide. They have a variegated granular internum which may be crystalline. They are present in liver, kidney, macrophages, and a number of other cell types. The granules in polymorphonuclear heterophils may represent a type of peroxisome. See also Fig. 24-20.

Multivesicular bodies are found in liver and relatively few other cell types. They are somewhat larger than lysosomes and consist of a number of small clear vesicles lying within a larger vesicle. Their relationship to lysosomes and peroxisomes is not known.

MICROTUBULES

Microtubules are major structures in prokaryotic and eukaryotic cells. They play a part, as a cytoskeleton, in creating cell shape and may be required for movement, particularly for the movement of structures within the cell.

Microtubules appear as hollow, nonbranching cylinders 210 to 240 Å in diameter and many micrometers long (Figs. 1-48 and 1-49; see also succeeding figures on centrioles and mitosis). Their dense wall appears to be fabricated of globular subunits 40 Å in diameter, arranged in a helix with 13 subunits per turn. The center zone is lucent in most microtubules, giving the structures the appearance of hollow cylinders. Microtubules often appear in groups of 30 or 40 or more and may be connected by slender bridges.

Microtubules are the basis of such complex and well-defined structures as centrioles and cilia. In addition, there are bands of microtubules in the axons of nerve cells (neurotubules), beneath the plasma membrane of many cylindrical or asymmetric cells, within the endoplasm of such cells as macrophages, and constituting the achromatic mitotic apparatus. The foregoing groups of microtubules are less stable than those in cilia and centrioles. They disappear on fixation in the cold and after fixation with many fixatives such as osmium tetroxide. Microtubules are relatively easily dispersed by the action of colchicine and by hydrostatic pressure. Only relatively recently, with the introduction of glutaraldehyde and fixation at room temperature, has the wide distribution of microtubules been appreciated.

Microtubules may be isolated and disaggregated and reassembled. Their subunits may assume other forms than the standard 240-Å-diameter microtubule; they may form a tubule of about 350 Å in diameter and possibly filaments of two classes: one 100 Å in diameter and the other approximately 50 Å in diameter. Microtubules may originate from nucleating or initiating sites in the cell. The centriole is a nucleating site for microtubular structures such as the cilia and achromatic apparatus.

The composition and function of microtubules have been revealed by the use of selective agents. Thus the dispersal of microtubules follows treatment of a cell by colchicine or vinblastine. As the drug effect wears off, the microtubules re-form. With the disappearance of microtubules, asymmetric cells, unless held in a certain form by external pressures, become radially symmetric. With reappearance of microtubules, asymmetry is restored. Much of cellular differentiation depends upon the assumption of asymmetric shapes, and this can be severely interfered with by agents which disrupt microtubules. Thus the proper development of axons appears to depend upon the alignment of great numbers of microtubules in the axonal process; if the microtubules are disaggregated, the axon fails to form.

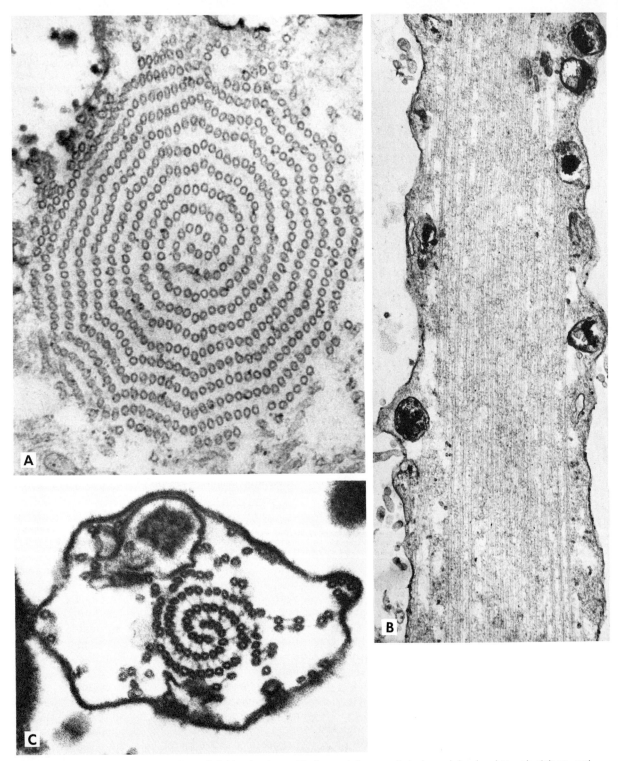

Figure 1-48 Microtubules in axoplasm of *Echinoshaerium*. Much correlative morphologic work in chemistry, physiology, and morphology has been done on invertebrates. A. Transverse section of an axoneme at the base of an axopodium. There are 12 sections of microtubules in cross section. ×70,000. B. Longitudinal section of an axoneme. Peripheral to the parallel array of microtubules constituting the axoneme are dense granules which undergo saltations. ×40,000. C. Transverse section of an axoneme heavily stained with MnO_4 to emphasize the bridges which connect the microtubules. ×110,000. (From L. G. Tilney and K. R. Porter, Protoplasma, **60**:317, 1965.)

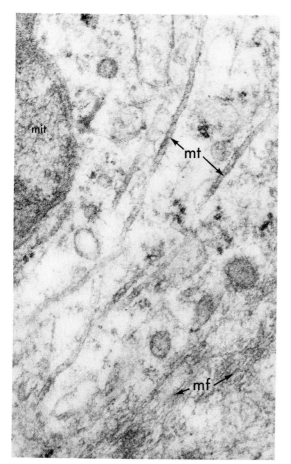

Figure 1-49   Microtubules of a human splenic reticular cell.
This field is from the peripheral cytoplasm and contains sections
of microtubules (mt), microfilaments (mf), and a mitochondrion
(mit). ×90,000. (From L. T. Chen and L. Weiss, Amer. J.
Anat., **134**:425, 1972.)

Microtubules appear to be important in intracellular transport. A fluid interface betweeen the
microtubular surface and the surrounding cytoplasm
may facilitate the directed and rapid movement of
large molecules. The movement of organelles,
such as mitochondria, often in a saltatory or jump-
like fashion, appears directed along microtubules.

CENTRIOLES

Centrioles are minute cylinders, 0.25 to 2 μm in
length and 0.1 to 0.2 μm in diameter, whose walls
are composed primarily of microtubules. Centrioles

lie in the cytocentrum or centrosome, and may be
surrounded by microtubules which can radiate out
into the cytoplasm. Diploid metazoan cells contain
two centrioles. Multinucleate cells may contain
many centrioles: In osteoclasts and foreign-body
giant cells, which may have 50 or more nuclei, the
central regions of the cells are comprised of fused
cytocentra strewn with centrioles. Higher plants
are exceptional in lacking centrioles.

Centrioles are active in mitosis, in the genesis
of cilia, and in the production of new centrioles.
Such activities may depend upon a role in the production and orientation of microtubules. Unlike
other cytoplasmic structures, centrioles are duplicated synchronously and precisely with division of
the nucleus.

Light microscopy   By light microscopy, centrioles
are resolved as minute rods. They are well stained
with a number of dyes, of which iron hematoxylin
is the most commonly used (Fig. 1-6).

Electron microscopy   The centriolar wall is made
up of nine vanes or blades, each consisting of three
fused microtubules (Figs. 1-50 to 1-52). The nine
blades are set next to one another, their long axes
parallel; the edge of one is slightly shingled beneath
the edge of its neighbor, curving about to form the
cylinder which is the outer wall of the centriole.
In cross section, this array of the vanes resembles
a pinwheel.

The fused microtubules, making up each of the
blades, extend the length of the centriole and lie
almost in a plane, with the result that the long
blades they form are slightly curved from side to
side. In addition, each of the blades, as one follows along its length, is subject to a slight twist
about its long axis. Each of the microtubules is
approximately 250 Å in diameter. Its wall is 45
Å in thickness. The lumen of the tubule, about 160
Å in diameter, is clear.

The principal structure within the lumen of the
centriole is a 75-Å filament wound into a helix
curving against the inside surface of the wall, apparently held in place by small spurs. The lumen
of the centriole may also contain a large clear vesicle. An end of the centriolar cylinder may show
spokes, radiating from a hub out to the wall.

Satellites, amorphous masses about 750 Å in

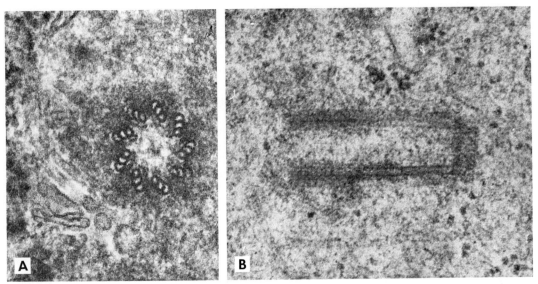

Figure 1-50   Centrioles of a Chinese hamster fibroblast.   A. The centriole is cut in cross section (from an interphase cell). B. The centriole is cut in longitudinal section (from a metaphase cell).   ×100,000.   (From the work of B. R. Brinkley.)

diameter, may be observed close to the surface of centrioles, near the end, and may be material from which new centrioles are assembled.

Duplication   A new centriole is assembled at an end of each extant centriole a few hours before DNA replication.   It is oriented at right angles to the parent centriole and requires several hours to complete.

In its development a centriole is preceded by a procentriole, a cylinder 150 nm in diameter with nine single microtubules in its wall.   These singlets probably develop into the triplets of the centriole. The procentrioles are themselves preceded by small, dense procentriolar precursor bodies which are apparently transformed into procentrioles by the stimulation of ''procentriole organizers,'' dense amorphous surrounding masses.

Functions   Centrioles are associated with cell division.   They separate, move to opposite poles, and become foci for the arrangement of the mitotic apparatus.   Centrioles move beneath the cell surface and, as basal bodies, initiate the formation of cilia.   Flagella are similarly related to centrioles. Basal bodies are structurally different from centri-

oles, primarily in possessing a basal plate which closes the end directed toward the cell membrane. The other end, directed toward the nucleus, is open and may contain spokes.   In spermatocytes, a centriole may be involved in both the mitotic apparatus and the flagellum.   Microtubular formations other than the mitotic apparatus, cilia, and flagella may send bundles of microtubules into the cytocentrum in characteristic alignment with centrioles.

The role of the centriole in microtubular formation is not known but it is likely that centrioles induce and direct the formation of microtubules.

MICROFILAMENTS

Several populations of microfilaments exist within cells.   Some may be the dispersed forms of microtubules; others, specialized forms of RNP or other proteins.   Some may have skeletal functions (see Chap. 3).

A most important class of microfilaments is encountered in large amounts in many cells (Figs. 1-53 and 1-54).   They are about 50 Å in diameter and are fabricated of the contractile protein actin.   They lie beneath the plasma membrane and account for such important phenomena as ruffling of the cell membrane, pinocytosis and phagocytosis, and for ameboid motion. They are attached to the inside surface of the tips of microvilli of epithelial cells and permit the microvilli to move about. These filaments are disaggregated and rendered functionless by the antibiotic *cytochalasin B*. The use of cytochalasin B in living cells has provided insight into the many functions of this class of microfilaments.

The life cycle of cells

Two major types of cell may be recognized: *somatic cells,* which are the diverse cells making up the somatic structure of the body, fated to die with or before the individual they constitute; and *gonadal cells,* which are the gametes capable of uniting sexually with those of another individual to form a new individual.

A somatic cell begins its life-span as one of the daughter cells of a mitotic division. Directly after this division the cell may undergo a period of in-

Figure 1-51   Centriole of a Chinese hamster fibroblast. The centriole is cut in cross section. Paracentriolar material (pc) is evident around the lower half of the centriole. Microtubules (mt) are also present, particularly in the upper half of the field.   ×92,000. (From B. R. Brinkley and E. Stubblefield, in D. M. Prescott, L. Goldstein, and E. McConkey (eds.), "Advances in Cell Biology," vol. 1, Appleton Century Crofts, New York, 1970.)

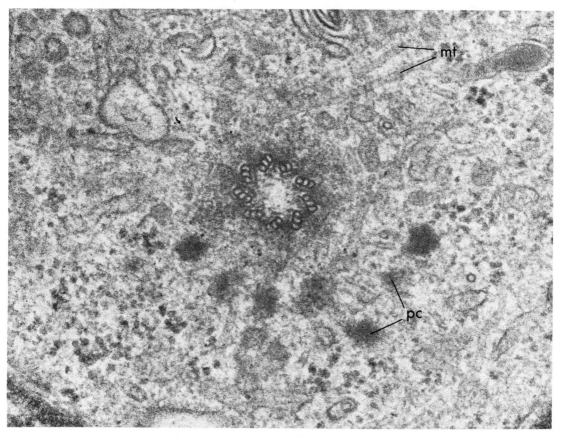

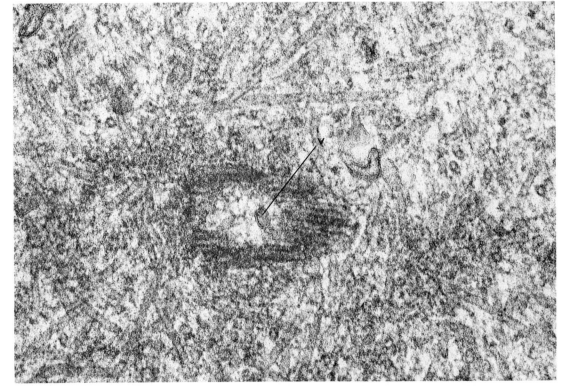

Figure 1-52 Centriole of a melanoma cell. The centriole is cut in oblique section. It contains a small vesicle (v). The field surrounding the vesicle abounds in microtubules. ✕120,000. (From the work of G. G. Maul.)

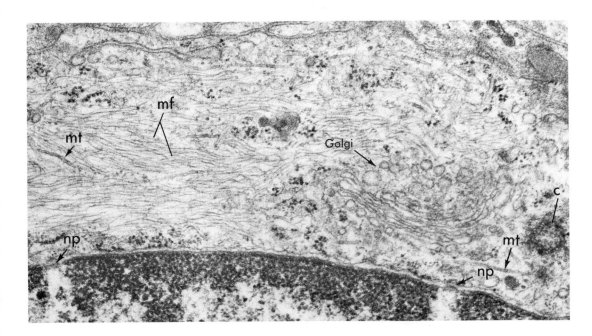

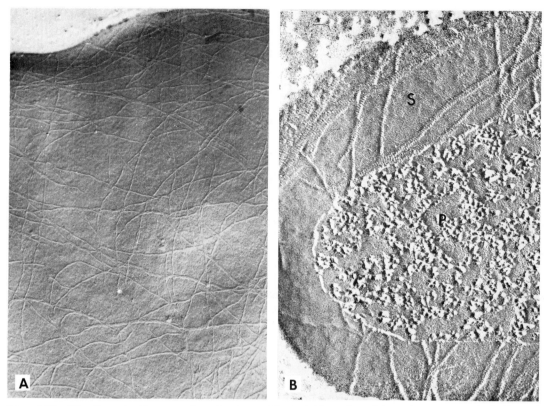

Figure 1-54   Microfilaments of human erythrocytes, freeze-etched.   A. The surface of the erythrocyte was etched without cleavage. Actin microfilaments are exposed just beneath the outer surface of the erythrocyte's plasma membrane.   ×40,000.   (From the work of V. T. Marchesi.)   B. This cell was freeze-cleaved and deep-etched.   The cleaved central area (P) is deep in the membrane and contains particles 85 Å in diameter.   The outer zone (S) is the uncleaved smooth portion of the cell as in A.   It is crisscrossed by strands of actin.   Those strands run only on the superficial part of the membrane in a narrow plane since they are sharply cut off at the junction of smooth and particulate faces.   The fibrous actin shows a periodicity of approximately 50 Å. Actin is a contractile protein.   The erythrocyte membrane is actively pinocytotic, and this activity probably depends upon these filaments.   ×75,000.   (From T. W. Tillack and V. T. Marchesi, J. Cell Biol., 45:649, 1970.)

tense protein synthesis, as a result of which emerge those granules, filaments, or other specific structures which mark the cell as mature and specialized.   As the cell matures and morphologic signs of specialization occur, the cell is differentiating from a primitive, perhaps multipotential cell, into a highly specialized unit of limited cellular potency. But although a cell may appear undifferentiated, its direction of maturation may be fixed and limited genetically, only time being required to disclose the nature of the differentiation by the appearance of morphologic specializations.   In short, a cell which appears morphologically undifferentiated may, in fact, be highly differentiated.

The frequency of mitotic division varies with the cell type and tissue.   Tissues may be classified as

Figure 1-53   Microfilaments of human spleen, endothelium or lining cells of arterial capillary.   The cytoplasm is filled with microfilaments (mf) 50 Å in width.   Although the identity of these filaments has not been established in these vessels, it is likely they are made of actin and are contractile.   They would thereby control blood flow through the control of the caliber of the vessel by contractility of the endothelium.   Some microtubules (mt), nuclear pores (np), a Golgi complex, and centriole (c) are also present. ×60,000.   (From L. T. Chen and L. Weiss, Amer. J. Anat., 134:425, 1972.)

showing no mitotic division, resulting in no renewal (nervous tissue); little division, resulting in slow renewal (liver, skin, thyroid); and active division, resulting in fast renewal (gastrointestinal tract, hematopoietic tissue). Some slowly renewed tissues may be termed ''conditional renewal'' systems because their renewal rate can be considerably increased under certain circumstances. After partial hepatectomy, for example, the remaining hepatocytes divide very actively, providing fast renewal. Even some cells showing no mitotic division may, with appropriate stimulation, proliferate and differentiate. Certain small lymphocytes (T cells) may circulate and recirculate for many years in man without dividing, but when stimulated by the appropriate antigen they may divide rapidly, producing clones of immunologically competent cells. In neurons, mitosis occurs only in embryonic and neonatal years until the full number of neurons is reached. Thereafter, no replacement occurs; a cell lost diminishes the total number and its absence may cause functional impairment. The cells in tissues undergoing slow renewal tend to be long-lived. The relatively low levels of mitotic division provide new cells to replace those dying off or to permit the growth and increased functional capacity of the tissue. The increase in genetic material in certain tissues by increased nuclear number and polyploidy has been discussed above. Rapidly renewing tissues are characterized by short-lived cells replaced by active cell division, so that a rather stable number of cells results. In the replacement of intestinal epithelial cells, new cells formed in the depths of the intestinal glands appear to move up the wall of the gland with unremitting pressure, toppling the apparently still viable topmost cells into the detritus of the gut lumen. As a result, the entire intestinal epithelium is renewed in a span of days. The kinetics of hematopoietic tissues, particularly of the granular leukocytes, also exemplifies this pattern.

It is possible to define a *generation time* for a population of similar cells, relating the interphase state, the period of DNA replication, and the process of mitotic division. A series of four periods follows mitosis: G_1, S, G_2, and M. G_1 is an interval or gap which follows cell division; S is the period of DNA replication; G_2 is the gap between replication of DNA and the start of mitosis; and M is mitosis.

The duration of G_1 varies greatly with cell type and mitotic turnover. In rapidly dividing cells it may be a matter of several hours. In nonrenewing tissues it may last the life of the organism. Such prolonged G_1 periods may be designated G_0. S is demonstrated by autoradiography. Indeed, it is the ability to delineate the S period by this means that makes possible the determination of the whole of the generation time. In a rapidly renewing tissue S is approximately 7 hr. It is a matter of great interest that the DNA in a given chromosome does not all replicate at the same time. Instead, different segments of the chromosome replicate at different times in the S, and in a characteristic sequence. G_2 is very short in rapidly renewing tissues, in time about an hour. In cells destined to be polyploid, G_2 may last indefinitely. The whole of the cycle in such rapidly dividing rodent tissues as germinal centers or thymus may be about 12 hr. In the gastrointestinal tract in man G_2 is 1 to 7 hr, the S phase 10 to 20 hr, G_1 10 to 20 hr, and the whole of the cycle 1 to 2 days. In rodents this cycle may take but a third of this time.

The sequences in the generation cycle may be illustrated as follows*:

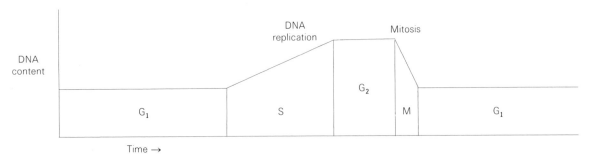

Time →

*After L. F. Lamerton, in R. J. M. Fry, M. L. Griem, and W. H. Kirsten (eds.): ''Normal and Malignant Cell Growth,'' Springer-Verlag, New York, 1969.

After functioning as a mature cell for varying lengths of time, a cell dies, its death often presaged by a period of senescence. Perhaps the best-studied case history of this sort is that of the erythrocyte, whose life-span in the circulation of man is approximately 120 days. Near the end of its life-span, the activity of glucose 6-phosphatase and certain other enzymes declines, and the cell becomes mechanically more fragile. There are no morphologic concomitants of these senile changes.

In other cell types, however, morphologic changes may signify senescence and coming cell death. These include, in muscle cells, attenuation, decrease in specific functional elements such as contractile filaments, and accumulation of pigment. Other changes include diminution in mitochondria, accumulation of fat, and vacuolization of cytoplasm and nucleus. Dead cells may disappear by lysis, by phagocytosis, or by displacement from the tissue, as exemplified by desquamated skin cells, respiratory cells, and intestinal cells.

CELL DIVISION

The division of one cell into two virtually identical cells is the basis of the continuity of life and underlies the complexity of metazoan organisms. The life-span of an individual protozoon is limited, but by cell division the line of Protozoa goes on. In Metazoa, division provides the cells constituting these organisms, provides replacement of lost cells, underlies the phenomena of cellular differentiation and specialization, and permits the continuity of the species despite the death of individuals. Several types of cell division exist. We shall consider *mitosis, amitosis,* and *meiosis.* Cell division may be separated into two events: *karyokinesis,* or nuclear division, and *cytokinesis,* or cytoplasmic division. As indicated above, karyokinesis may occur without cytokinesis, resulting in binucleate or multinucleate cells.

Mitosis   DNA is capable of precise replication, ensuring constancy of genetic information from generation to generation and, thereby, maintenance of the characteristics of the species. (Occasionally, however, the replication of DNA is inexact and a change or *mutation* in a cell line results.) Mitosis is a complex, highly ordered process wherein the original and replicated molecules of

DNA are separated from one another and distributed to two nuclei. Cytokinesis typically follows karyokinesis and two cells result. The DNA with associated protein is organized as chromosomes, whose number is highly characteristic for a species. These chromosomes are typically matched in pairs or homologues.

The human nucleus contains 46 chromosomes, paired as 23 homologues. The partners in 22 of these pairs, the *autosomes,* are morphologically alike. The remaining two chromosomes in the female are also matched and alike; they are the X chromosomes. In the male, however, these two chromosomes are morphologically different from each other; they are the X and Y or sex chromosomes. Chromosomes in the interphase nucleus are so long and thin that it is not possible to recognize 46 of them.

The first phase of mitosis is *prophase* (Figs. 1-55, 1-56, 1-59, and 1-60). Here the extended chromosomes characteristic of the interphase become progressively thicker and more and more tightly coiled. The coils may undergo secondary coiling. As perceived by light microscopy, the individual chromosomes emerge from the nuclear substance as strands which appear progressively shorter, thicker, and more intensely stained. Moreover, as prophase goes on, one can see that each of the chromosomes is split longitudinally into precisely equal halves, or *chromatids.* This longitudinal splitting of the chromosome actually occurs in the S and G_2 phases just preceding mitosis, but it becomes apparent only in late prophase. Through most of prophase the individually emerging chromosomes remain confined within the nuclear envelope and are too bunched together to be clearly characterized as to size and shape. Near the end of prophase, when the chromosomes are maximally contracted, the nuclear membrane disappears and so do the nucleoli.

In prophase the centriole divides, if it had not divided preceding mitosis, and the two centrioles diverge from one another and move to opposite poles of the cell. From the polar centrioles, radiating toward the center of the cell, into and around the mass of chromosomes, is a system of poorly stained fibers, the *spindle.* Some of these, the discontinuous fibers, attach to chromosomes. Others, the continuous fibers, pass around the

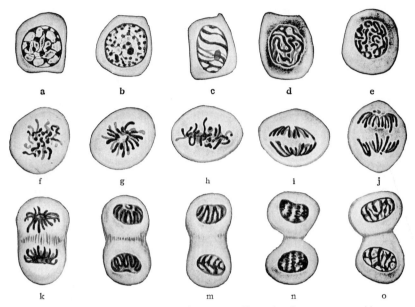

a   b   c   d   e

f   g   h   i   j

k   m   n   o

Figure 1-55   Mitosis. Epidermal cells of a mouse. These drawings are arranged in sequence from early prophase into telophase. A to F. Prophase. G and H. Metaphase. I and J. Anaphase. K to O. Telophase. Bouin fixation: iron hematoxylin. (From the work of Ortiz-Picón.)

chromosomes, going from one centriole to the other. In addition, a set of fibers radiates about each centriole, forming an *aster*. The fibers of the spindle and of the asters are actually microtubules, as may be observed in electron micrographs. They are designated the *achromatic apparatus,* because of their lack of affinity for dyes, and are thus distinguished from the deeply stained ensemble of chromosomes, termed the *chromatic apparatus* (Figs. 1-55 to 1-64).

In the next phase of mitosis, *metaphase,* the chromosomes arrange themselves in an equatorial plane, forming an *equatorial plate* (Figs. 1-55, 1-56, 1-61 to 1-64). Viewed from the side, this plate appears like a somewhat irregular, dense line transecting the cell. Viewed from one of the poles, the chromosomes form a circlet. It is in polar view that the morphology of the chromosomes may best be studied in histologic preparations. Metaphase

chromosomes are linear, densely stained structures. Each chromosome is constricted at one place along its length. An unstained zone, the *centromere* or *kinetochore,* lies at this place. The two chromatids of the chromosomes are free of one another except at the centromere, and the spindle fibers also attach there. Chromosomes may be divided into three groups, depending upon the location of the centromere. If the centromere divides the chromosomes into segments of equal length, the chromosome is *metacentric*. Those chromosomes separated into larger and smaller limbs by the centromere are *submedian*. Those in which the centromere is almost at the end of the chromosomes, so that there is virtually only one limb, are *telocentric*.

The chromatic material of the chromosome may have another *secondary constriction* in one of the limbs. This constriction may have some length,

Figure 1-56   Mitosis. Human leukocytes. Only the chromosomes are stained. Each chromosome is seen to consist of two chromatids joined at the kinetochore. Note the secondary constrictions in several of the chromosomes and the presence of satellites (arrows). Note, too, the coiling evident in several of the chromatids. In anaphase, two chromosomes lie near the equatorial plane, lagging behind the others in joining the two diverging masses of chromosomes. This happens frequently. Note the sharp separation furrow in telophase. Aceto-orcein stain. ×4,000. (From the work of B. R. Migeon.)

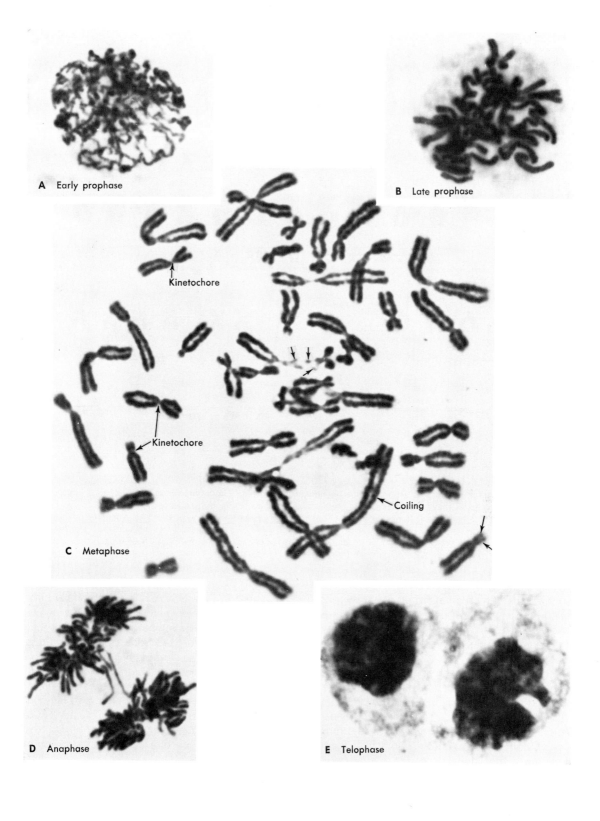

A Early prophase

B Late prophase

Kinetochore

Kinetochore

Coiling

C Metaphase

D Anaphase

E Telophase

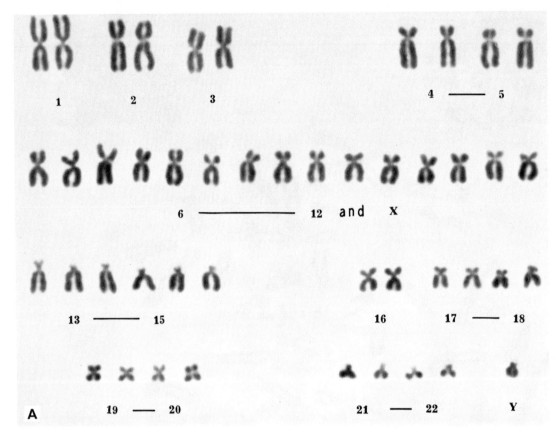

Figure 1-57   A. Human karyotype.   Metaphase chromosomes have been arranged into morphologically similar groups of paired chromosomes and numbered.   Pairs 1, 2, 3, and 16 can be identified as different from other chromosomes.   It is impossible to separate 4 from 5, but 4 and 5 may be separated from the remainder. Similarly it is impossible to separate 6, 7, 8, 9, 10, 11, 12, and the X chromosome as different from one another, but this large group may be recognized as different from the other chromosomes.   Chromosomes 13, 14, and 15; 17 and 18; 19 and 20 form similar groups.   This individual is male, having an X and Y chromosome.   B. The metaphase from which the karyotype was prepared.   An interphase nucleus is present for comparison of size.   Aceto-orcein stain.   ×2,400.   (From the work of B. R. Migeon.)

and so it isolates the chromatic material at the end of the chromosome into a *satellite*.   Typically, nucleoli develop in certain zones of constriction in satellited chromosomes on reconstitution of daughter nuclei.

The chromosomes of each species may be classified on the basis of the location of the centromere, the size and shape of the limbs, and the presence of secondary constrictions and satellites.   These characteristics make up the *karyotype*, or the morphology of the metaphase chromosomes singly and in aggregate.   The karyotype of the human male

is presented in Fig. 1-57A.   The metaphase plate from which the karyotype was prepared is shown in Fig. 1-57B.   The karyotype is prepared by cutting out the chromosome pairs from a photograph of a squash preparation of a metaphase cell selectively stained with a dye such as aceto-orcein.   The cut-out chromosomes are then arranged in clusters of similar chromosomes.   It is not possible to differentiate chromosomes occurring within a cluster by the standard aceto-orcein procedure.   Thus, in the human male karyotype one cannot separate chromosomes 6, 7, 8, 9, 10, 11, 12, and the X chro-

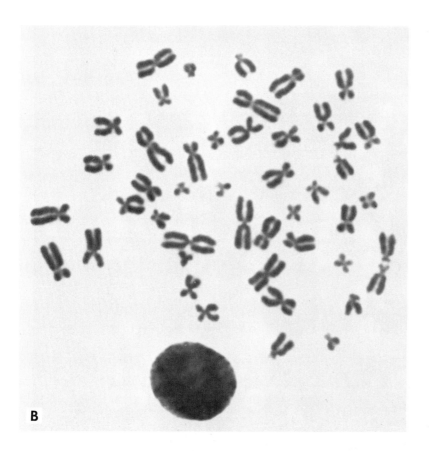

B

mosome from one another. Recently, however, it has been found that certain fluorochromes produce a banded staining pattern in each of the chromosomes (Fig. 1-58). By this means it has proved possible to identify chromosomes not differentiable otherwise. Correlations of genetic diseases such as Down's syndrome (mongolism) and leukemia with abnormal karyotypes are being made in increasing number. The fluorochrome method is providing impetus for such correlation with individual chromosomes. Very recently, it has been possible to visualize this banding by the use of giemsa stain at a pH of about 6.8.

At the beginning of metaphase, the chromatids of a chromosome are connected only at the centromere. At the end of metaphase the centromeres divide and each of the chromatids, now a daughter chromosome and attached to the spindle by its own centromere, moves outward from the metaphase plate toward one pole of the cell. Thus, in human somatic cells, one set of 46 chromosomes moves to one centriole and the other set to the other. This divergent movement constitutes the *anaphase* of mitosis (Figs. 1-55, 1-56, and 1-59C). The spindle fibers attached to the centromeres are responsible, to a considerable degree, for the characteristic orderly diverging movement of the chromosomes in anaphase. The drug colchicine interferes with the spindle by breaking up microtubules, leaving dividing cells suspended in metaphase and unable to complete the cell division.

Anaphase is concluded when the two chromosomal masses have moved to opposite poles of the cell. There now begins the final stage of nuclear division, *telophase* (Figs. 1-55, 1-56, and 1-59), during which two daughter nuclei are formed. Nuclear membranes form about each of the chromosomal masses, nucleoli appear at the satellite-

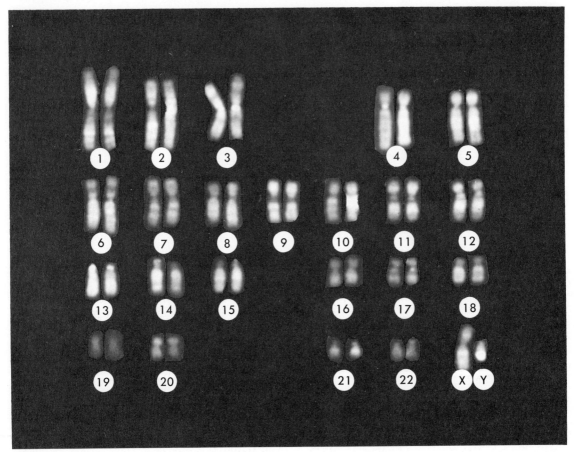

Figure 1-58   Karyotype of normal male (XY) cultured human leukocyte, showing quinacrine fluorescence patterns.   Note the bandings present in each of the chromosomes.   Although the significance of this banding is not understood, it has proved useful in differentiating chromosomes which are morphologically alike.   Compare with the conventional karyotype in Fig. 1-57A and B. ×2,500.   (From the work of W. R. Breg.)   Very recently it has proved possible to obtain a similar banding pattern by staining a chromosomal preparation with a giemsa stain at a pH of about 6.8.   The latter is a relatively easy procedure and may become more widely used than fluorescence staining.

Figure 1-59   Electron micrograph of mitosis in a human Hela cell in tissue culture.   These cells, originally derived from a carcinoma of the uterine cervix, form a strain of cells maintained in tissue culture.   (A through D from E. Robbins and N. K. Gonatas, J. Cell Biol., **21:**429, 1964.)   A. In early prophase, the chromatin becomes clumped because of the condensation of chromosomes (Cr).   The nuclear membrane is still intact, and the centriole (C) and multivesicular bodies (MB) are prominent.   Approximately ×3,850.

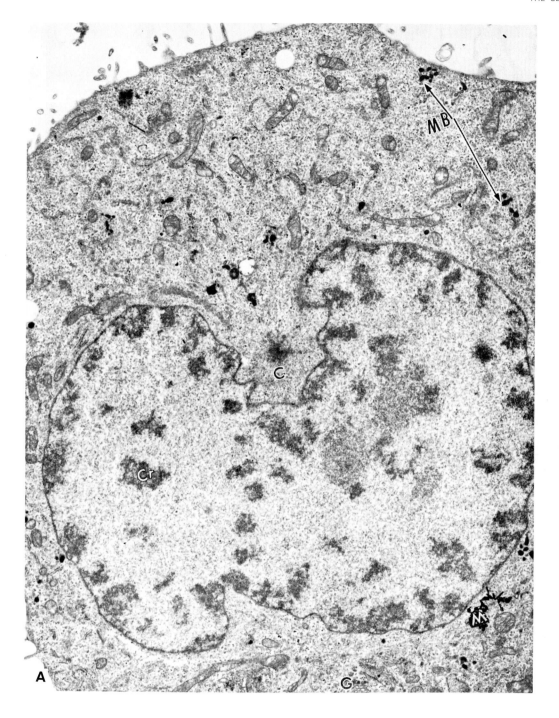

A

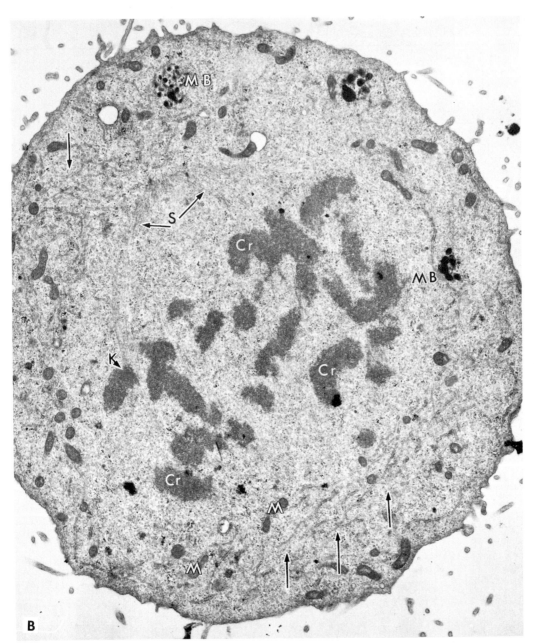

Figure 1-59 (continued)   B. In later prophase the chromosomes are close to the equatorial plate and metaphase.   The spindle fibers (S) are seen radiating from the centriole and attached to a chromosome at the kinetochore (K).   Approximately ×5,640.

C. In late anaphase, the two chromosomal masses have moved apart.   They are already surrounded by a double nuclear membrane. At the lower pole, a portion of a centriole and spindle fibers may be seen.   Note how the spindle fibers are present, together with some mitochondria, in the constriction between what will be the two daughter cells.   Note, too, the blebs of cytoplasm (BL) about the periphery of these cells, indicating the frothing that occurs in this phase.   Approximately ×5,225.

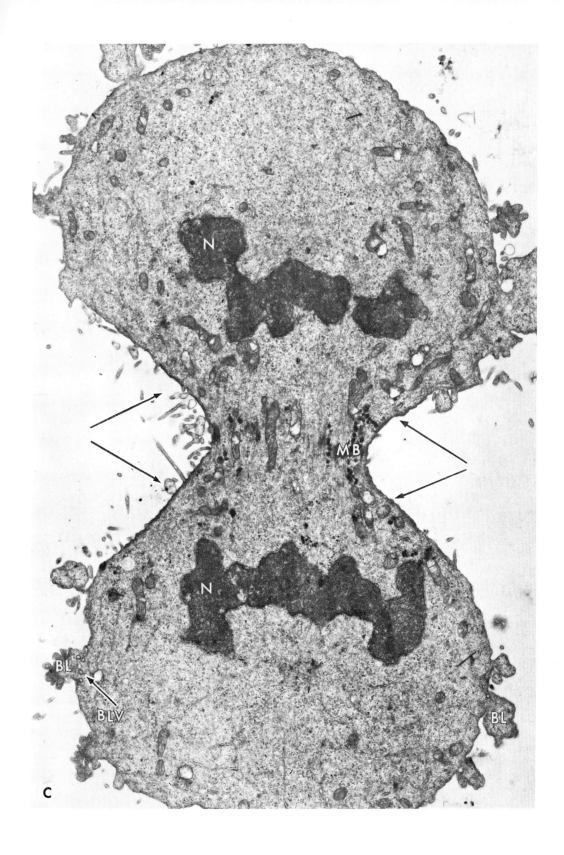

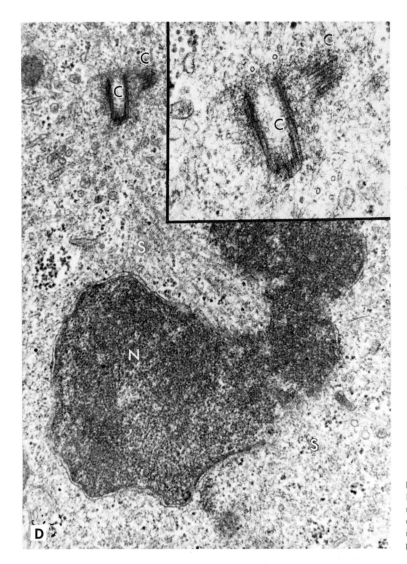

Figure 1-59 (continued) D. Telophase. Note the presence of a double nuclear membrane about a daughter nucleus. The centriole (at higher magnification in the insert) has already been duplicated. Approximately ×13,750 (insert ×30,800).

bearing chromosomes, and segments of the chromosomes uncoil to become euchromatin.

Although primary attention must be accorded the nucleus in mitosis, characteristic changes occur in the cytoplasm. The division of the centrioles and the formation of the achromatic apparatus in prophase have already been discussed. In anaphase, frothing or bubbling of the cytoplasm occurs as the putative daughter nuclei separate. This is an index of the considerable change in solvation and gelation that attends mitosis. With the separation of the nuclear masses in anaphase, a partition of cytoplasmic constituents occurs. Mitochondria, lysosomes, ribosomes, and cytoplasmic membranes become distributed in approximately equal amounts about the two newly formed nuclei. As the nuclear membrane is reconstituted, the cytoplasm becomes deeply constricted between the two masses of chromosomes; as the nuclei form, the cytoplasm divides, forming two equal daughter cells. For a

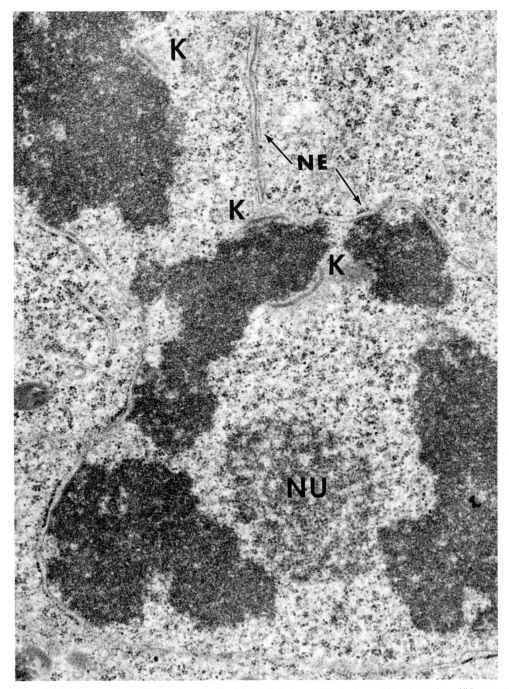

Figure 1-60 Late prophase, Chinese hamster fibroblast. Fully formed kinetochores (K) and a nucleus (NU) are present. The nuclear envelope (NE) is almost completely intact. (From B. R. Brinkley and E. Stubblefield, in D. M. Prescott, L. Goldstein, and E. McConkey (eds.), "Advances in Cell Biology," vol. 1, Appleton Century Crofts, New York, 1970.)

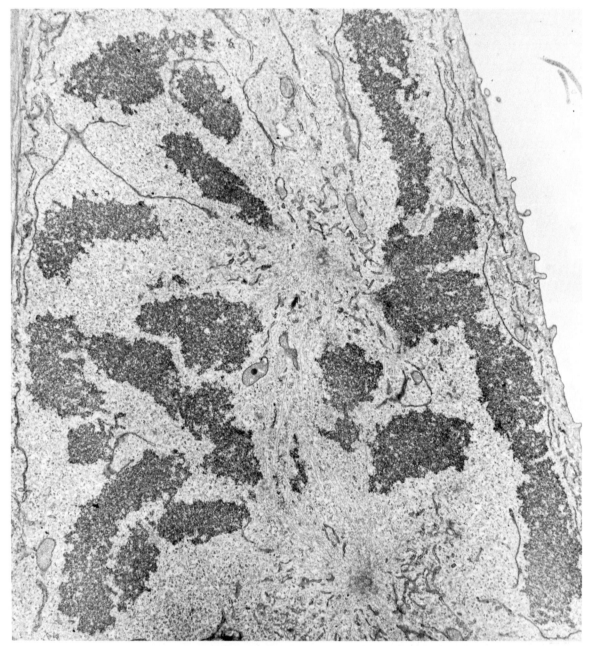

Figure 1-61 Prometaphase, rat kangaroo fibroblast. Here each of the chromosomes is tightly coiled and, although not evident, split into two chromatids. The chromosomes are moving to take positions on the metaphase plate. A centriole and microtubules are present in the cytoplasm. ×14,000. (From the work of B. R. Brinkley.)

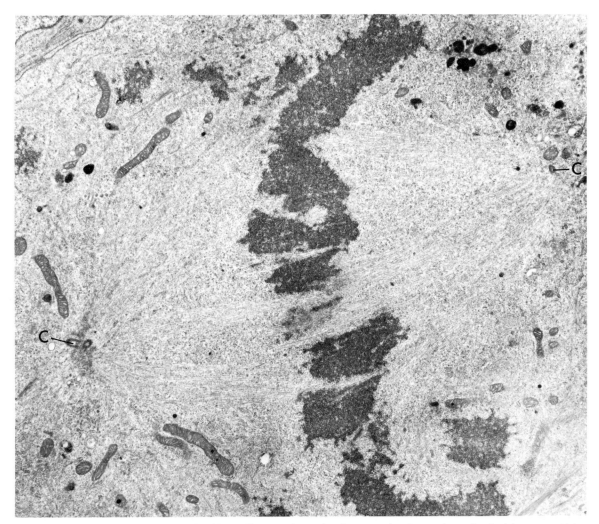

Figure 1-62 Metaphase, rat kangaroo fibroblast. The metaphase plate is present in edge-on view. On the left, two centrioles (C) may be observed; on the right, one centriole. The microtubules of the spindle radiate from the centrioles. Both chromosomal (attached to kinetochore) and continuous (pole to pole) microtubules are present. × 10,350. (From B. R. Brinkley and J. Cartwright Jr., J. Cell Biol., **50:**416, 1971.)

short time, the spindle may persist as a transient bridge between daughter cells. In the latter part of telophase, a cytocentrum and Golgi elements are formed.

The electron microscope has elucidated several aspects of mitosis despite its disappointingly scanty information on chromosomal structure. The tubular nature of the spindle fibers and structural details of the centromere and attachment of the spindle

are among these findings. An observation of particular interest relates to the formation of the nuclear membranes in telophase. Here the masses of chromosomes, before they are aggregated into a single mass, are surrounded by membranes similar to the nuclear membranes, derived from the ER. Later, when the chromosomes unite into a single zone to become the nucleus, the membranes formed about each of the dispersed chromosomal

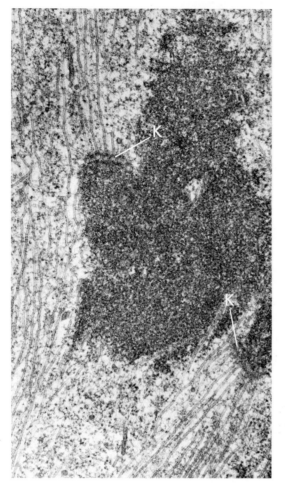

Figure 1-63 Metaphase, rat kangaroo fibroblast. Chromosomal microtubules are inserted into kinetochores (K). Note the double nature of the kinetochore. Continuous microtubules pass between the chromosomes running from pole to pole without insertion into kinetochores. ×30,800. (From B. R. Brinkley and J. W. Cartwright, J. Cell Biol., **50**:416, 1971.)

groups coalesce to form a definitive nuclear membrane.

Amitosis Occasionally forms of somatic nuclear division besides mitosis occur; these are grouped under the term *amitosis* (Fig. 1-65). Amitosis may occur in terminal or highly transient cell types such as certain cells of the placenta or of the blood. It may also occur in some multinucleated cells, as the giant cells of the connective tissue. In amitosis

the nuclear membrane appears to constrict deeply and a single nucleus becomes pinched into two. Although equal-sized daughter nuclei may sometimes result, it is clearly impossible that a precise separation of chromosomal material can thus be achieved.

Polyteny and Poliploidy DNA replication may occur without nuclear division. It is characteristic of certain cell types, as the salivary gland cells of diptera, that DNA replication occurs without subsequent chromosomal division, resulting in *polytene* chromosomes. These are chromosomes which replicate themselves many times over. But the replicates remain together rather than move apart into separate chromosomes and thereby form giant chromosomes. Polytenic chromosomes readily show a type of banding which requires fluorochromes or special giemsa staining (pp. 65–66) to demonstrate in other chromosomes. DNA replication may occur with subsequent chromosomal duplication but without karyokinesis, resulting in polyploid nuclei (p. 16). Polyploid nuclei thus contain more than a diploid number of chromosomes, and may become larger than diploid nuclei as in some hepatocytes and megakaryocytes.

Meiosis Meiosis is a type of nuclear division, restricted to gametes, that is, spermatocytes and oocytes, wherein the number of chromosomes characteristic of somatic cells, the *diploid* number (2n), is halved to the *haploid* number (1n). For this reason meiosis is termed reduction division. The haploid nuclei of the gametes unite and the diploid number of chromosomes is restored in the process of fertilization. The fertilized ovum, and all its descendants except the gametes, divide by mitotic division, and the diploid number is thereby maintained in somatic cells. But meiosis has the second major function of providing genetic variation by the exchange of segments of homologous chromosomes and the random selection of one of the two homologues during the reduction division.

Meiosis involves two successive nuclear divisions with only one division of chromosomes (Figs. 1-66 and 1-67). The first meiotic division is characterized by a prolonged prophase. In this prophase the homologous chromosomes come to lie together, closely and exactly paired in a point-for-

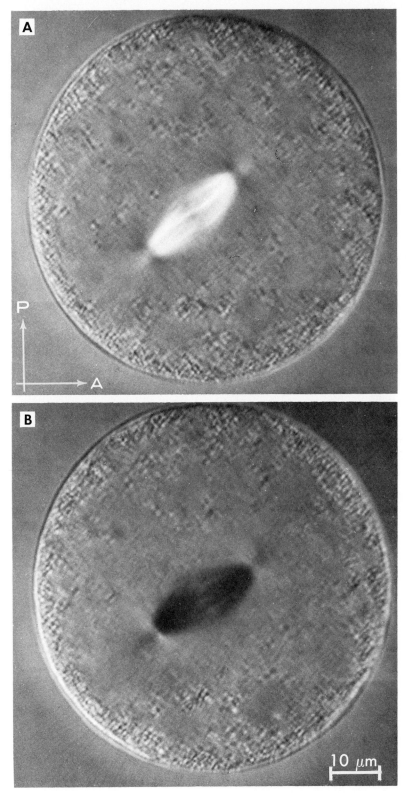

Figure 1-64   Metaphase spindle.   Oocyte of *Pectinaria goulde*.   The birefringence of the spindle is evident in these fields photographed by polarization microscopy.   P represents the axis of polarized light and A corresponds to the direction of the analyzer. A. The optical axes of the polarizing plates (analyzer and polarizer) are crossed.   B. Optical axes are parallel.   See text under Polarizing microscopy.   (From H. Sato and S. Inové, J. Gen. Physiol., **50:**259, 1967.)

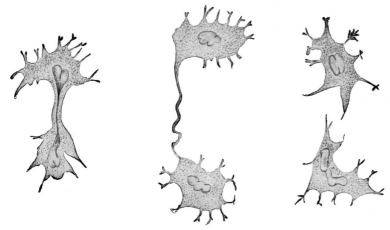

Figure 1-65   Amitosis in a histiocyte of a frog. The drawing is prepared from a cell in tissue culture. (From the work of Arnold.)

point correspondence along their entire length (*synapsis*). During the process the chromosomes shorten by coiling, but not as much as in the prophase of mitosis. Moreover, each of the chromosomes is observed to be longitudinally split into two chromatids. The homologous paired chromosomes, termed a *bivalent,* therefore consist of four chromatids. A spindle forms and the bivalents arrange themselves on a metaphase plate. The divergent movement of anaphase begins as the homologues, consisting of two chromatids each, move apart to opposite poles and are then separated into daughter cells at telophase. Thenceforth, after the first meiotic division, each of the daughter cells contains one of the homologous chromosomes. It is of great significance that in the first meiotic division the kinetochore does not divide, as it does in mitosis, and so the chromatids remain together. A second meiotic division ensues in which the chromosomes become arranged in a

Figure 1-66   The stages of meiosis I and II shown schematically. A pair of homologous chromosomes, one dark and the other light, is followed through meiosis I. Then chromatids of a daughter cell are traced through meiosis II. The events are as follows:
   Prophase I. Leptotene: The chromosomes become apparent as thin linear structures. Zygotene: Homologous chromosomes line up and pair with one another point to point (synapsis). Pachytene: With pairing completed, the chromosomes become shorter and thicker, and each longitudinally splits into chromatids, the centromere remaining single. The four chromatids of the two chromosomes constitute a bivalent. Chromatids from each of the homologous chromosomes may cross over one another, forming a chiasma. Diplotene: The chromosomes further shorten and broaden; they also coil. Homologous chromosomes begin to move apart but are held together at the chiasma. Diakinesis: The chromosomes become broader, thicker, more tightly coiled; they move further apart.
   Metaphase I. The chromosomes are on the equatorial plate.
   Anaphase I. The chromosomes diverge, exchanging chromosomal segments at the site of the chiasma.
   Telophase I. Each chromatid pair, joined by a single centromere, lies in a daughter cell. The chromatids uncoil and lengthen to some extent.
   Chromatids in the left-hand daughter cell pass through the following stages in meiosis II:
   Prophase II. This stage is transient and possibly absent, since the chromatids may move directly to metaphase II.
   Metaphase II. Chromatids become shorter, broader, and coiled. The centromere divides.
   Anaphase II. Chromatids separate and move to opposite poles.
   Telophase II. Each of the chromatids is now a daughter cell.
   Thus in the course of these two divisions the four chromatids forming the bivalent of prophase I are separated, first into two daughter cells of telophase I, each containing two chromatids ($4n \rightarrow 2n$), and then into two daughter cells again in telophase II, each containing one chromatid ($2n \rightarrow 1n$). A total of four daughter cells is produced, each having the haploid ($1n$) number of chromosomes. In a male individual four sperms are produced; in a female, one ovum and three polar bodies. On fertilization the diploid ($2n$) number is restored.

MEIOSIS I

MEIOSIS II

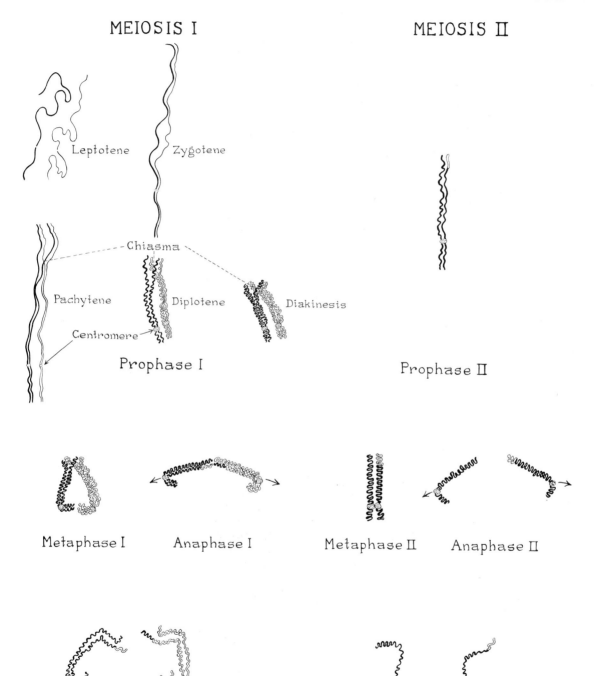

Leptotene

Zygotene

Chiasma

Pachytene   Diplotene   Diakinesis

Centromere

Prophase I

Prophase II

Metaphase I   Anaphase I   Metaphase II   Anaphase II

Telophase I   Telophase II

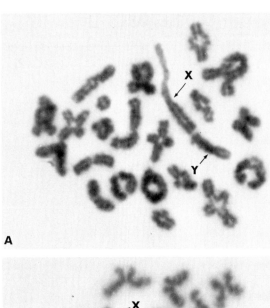

A

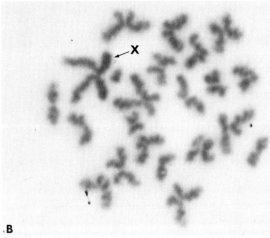

.B

Figure 1-67 Meiosis in the golden hamster, *Mesocricetus auratus*. A. Primary spermatocyte showing the 22 bivalents at the first meiotic metaphase. The X and Y chromosomes are associated terminally, the X being distinguished by its length. The autosomal bivalents demonstrate chiasmata in various stages. Note the coiling of the chromatids. B. Secondary spermatocyte at the second meiotic metaphase, containing the haploid number of 22 chromosomes. This cell has received the X chromosome. At this stage, the chromosomes show "relic" spirals, which are probably remnants of coiling from the first meiotic division. Aceto-orcein stain. ×2,200. (From the work of M. Ferguson-Smith.)

metaphase plate and the kinetochores divide. The chromatids which make up each of the chromosomes are now free of one another and diverge from the metaphase plate in an anaphase movement.

Later in telophase they form daughter nuclei and then daughter cells. The two meiotic divisions have thus sorted the four homologous chromatids present in prophase of the first meiotic division into four separate gametes, each of which has the haploid number of chromosomes. In a male, four functional spermatozoa will result from the two meiotic divisions. Curiously, the completion of cytokinesis in the spermatozoa may be delayed so that four otherwise mature spermatozoa may remain linked in Siamese-quadruplet style. In a female four ova are produced as well, but the cytoplasmic division leaves virtually all the cytoplasm with one nucleus. The remaining nuclei, surrounded by minimal cytoplasm, cannot survive and are termed *polar bodies*. This unequal cytoplasmic division provides one nucleus with sufficient cytoplasm to support fertilization and embryogenesis. Each of the gamete nuclei contains 23 chromosomes. In female gametes one of these is an X chromosome, whereas in male gametes one is either an X or a Y. During fetal life in a human female, oocytes migrate into the ovary, proliferate a short time, and then enter prophase of the first meiotic division, and remain in that state until shortly before ovulation. Since a woman may ovulate until about 45 years of age, oocytes may remain in meiosis for more than 45 years. It may well be that the first meiotic prophase constitutes a particularly stable state for DNA.

The second major function of meiosis is to provide genetic variation. It will be recalled that in diploid cells one chromosome in a homologous pair is contributed by the spermatozoon and the other by the oocyte. When the homologous chromosomes are arranged upon the first meiotic metaphase plate, it is a matter of chance whether the homologue contributed by the sperm or the homologue contributed by the ovum faces a given pole. As a result, in each cell produced in the first meiotic division, the number of chromosomes derived from the sperm and the number derived from the egg are a matter of chance. This random separation is one mechanism of genetic mixture. A second mechanism is the exchange, by homologous chromosomes, of corresponding segments. This exchange occurs when the homologues are in synapsis during the early phases of meiotic prophase I. The extent of the exchange becomes apparent as the homologues pull away from their synaptic union. It is then seen that they frequently remain attached in one or more places. This persistent link between diverging chromosomes is termed a *chiasma*. The exchange of segments is termed *crossing over*.

The stages in meiosis are as follows:

1. The first prophase, prophase I, is long and may be divided into five stages. In *leptotene* the chromosomes are long and thin. In *zygotene* the homologous chromosomes move toward one another and pair, lying in close touch with one another in a point-for-point correspondence along their length (synapsis). In *pachytene* the chromosomes coil considerably, appearing shorter and thicker. At about this time it becomes apparent that each of the chromosomes of the bivalent contains four chromatids. The centromere does not split. In *diplotene* the chromosomes begin to separate from one another, but the separation is incomplete, with chiasmata forming. The separation continues into the *diakinesis*, a stage which shows the chiasmata and the thickened, coiled, partially separated chromosomes to good advantage. The nuclear membrane disappears.

2. In metaphase I the bivalent chromosomes are arranged upon an equatorial plate. There are two centromeres, one for each of the chromosomes, and these are attached to spindle fibers.

3. In anaphase I the chromosomes, each of which consists of two chromatids, move to opposite poles.

4. Telophase I follows, but the chromosomes may remain in a shortened form.

In the first meiotic division, therefore, the diploid number of chromosomes has been reduced to the haploid number; an exchange of genetic information may have occurred between the chromosomes; the distribution of chromosomes of a given bivalent to each pole has been a matter of chance, further increasing genetic variation; and each of the chromosomes is longitudinally split to form two chromatids.

5. Interphase, or *interkinesis,* is brief.

6. In prophase II a spindle forms, the nuclear membrane breaks down, and the chromosomes move equatorially.

7. In metaphase II the chromatids are arranged upon an equatorial plate and their centromeres divide and become attached to spindle fibers.

8. In anaphase II the chromatids, now daughter chromosomes, move to opposite poles.

9. Telophase II finds the appearance of a nuclear membrane, uncoiling of the chromosomes, and the development of daughter cells.

References

GENERAL

BAKER, J. R.: "Principles of Biological Microtechnique: A Study of Fixation and Dyeing," John Wiley & Sons, Inc., New York, 1958.

BRACHET, J., and A. E. MIRSKY (eds.): "The Cell." I. Biochemistry, Physiology, Morphology; II. Cells and Their Component Parts; III. Mitosis and Meiosis; IV. Specialized Cells, pt. 1; V. Specialized Cells, pt. 2, Academic Press, Inc., New York, 1961.

BROWN, W. V., and E. M. BERTKE: "Textbook of Cytology," The C. V. Mosby Company, Saint Louis, 1969.

COWDRY, E. V. (ed.): "Special Cytology," 2d ed., vols. 1–3, Paul B. Hoeber, Inc., New York, 1932.

DE ROBERTIS, E. D. P., W. W. NOWINSKI, and F. A. SAEZ: "Cell Biology," 5th ed., W. B. Saunders Company, Philadelphia, 1970.

DOWBEN, R. M.: "Cell Biology," Harper & Row, Publishers, Incorporated, New York, 1971.

GOMORI, G.: "Microscopic Histochemistry," The University of Chicago Press, Chicago, 1952.

LOEWY, A. G., and P. SIEKEVITZ: "Cell Structure and Function," Holt, Rinehart and Winston, Inc., New York, 1963.

PORTER, K. R., and M. A. BONNEVILLE: "An Introduction to the Fine Structure of Cells and Tissues," 2d ed., Lea & Febiger, Philadelphia, 1964.

SPECIFIC ASPECTS OF CYTOLOGY

ACKERMAN, G. A.: Histochemistry of the Centrioles and Centrosomes of the Leukemic Cells from Human Myeloblastic Leukemia, *J. Biophys. Biochem. Cytol.*, **11**:717 (1961).

ADELMAN, M. R., G. G. BRISY, M. L. SHELANSKI, R. C. WEISENBERG, and E. W. TAYLOR: Cytoplasmic Filaments and Tubules, *Fed. Proc.*, **27**:1186 (1968).

BAKER, J. R.: The Cell-theory: A Restatement, History, and Critique, *Quart. J. Micr. Sci.*, **89**:103 (1948); **90**:87 (1949); **93**:157 (1952).

BARR, M. L.: Sex Chromatin and Phenotype in Man, *Science*, **130**:679 (1959).

BENEDETTI, E. L.: Cell Membrane Organization, *First Int. Sympos. Cell Biol. Cytopharmacol.*, Venice, July, 1969.

BENSLEY, R. R., and I. GERSH: Studies on Cell Structure by the Freezing-Drying Method. I. Introduction; II. The Nature of the Mitochondria in the Hepatic Cell of Amblystoma; III. The Distribution in Cells of the Basophil Substances, in Particular the Nissl Substance of the Nerve Cell, *Anat. Rec.*, **57**:205, 217, 369 (1933).

BENSLEY, R. R., and N. L. HOERR: Studies on Cell Structure by the Freezing-Drying Method. VI. The Preparation and Properties of Mitochondria, *Anat. Rec.*, **60**:449 (1935).

BRANDT, P. W., and G. D. PAPPAS: An Electron Microscopic Study of Pinocytosis in Ameba. I. The Surface Attachment Phase, *J. Biophys. Biochem. Cytol.*, **8**:675 (1960).

BRINKLEY, B. R.: The Fine Structure of the Nucleolus in Mitotic Divisions of Chinese Hamster Cells in vitro, *J. Cell Biol.*, **27**:411 (1965).

BRINKLEY, B. R., and E. STUBBLEFIELD: Ultrastructure and Interaction of the Kinetochore and Centriole in Mitosis and Meiosis, in D. M. Prescott, L. Goldstein, and E. McConkey (eds.), "Advances in Cell Biology," vol. 1, Appleton Century Crofts, New York, 1970.

BROWN, D. D., and J. B. GURDON: Absence of Ribosomal RNA Synthesis in the Anucleate Mutant of *Xenopus laevis,* in E. Bell (ed.), "Molecular and Cellular Aspects of Development," Harper & Row, Publishers, Incorporated, New York, 1965.

BUSCH, H., and K. SMETANA: "The Nucleolus," Academic Press, Inc., New York, 1970.

DALTON, A. J., and M. D. FELIX: A Comparative Study of the Golgi Complex, *J. Biophys. Biochem. Cytol.*, **2**:79 (1956).

DE DUVE, C.: Lysosomes and Phagosomes, *Protoplasma,* **63**:95 (1967).

DE DUVE, C.: Lysosomes, a New Group of Cytoplasmic Particles, in T. Hayashi (ed.), "Subcellular Particles," The Ronald Press Company, New York, 1958.

DE DUVE, C.: The Enzymic Heterogeneity of Cell Fractions Isolated by Differential Centrifuging, *Sympos. Soc. Exp. Biol.*, **10**:50 (1957).

ESSNER, E., A. B. NOVIKOFF, and B. MASEK: Adenosine Triphosphatase and 5-Nucleotidease Activities in the Plasma Membrane of Liver Cells as Revealed by Electron Microscopy, *J. Biophys. Biochem. Cytol.*, **4**:711 (1958).

FAWCETT, D. W.: Cilia and Flagella, in J. Brachet and A. E. Mirsky (eds.), "The Cell," vol. 2, Academic Press, Inc., New York, 1961.

FELDHERR, C. M.: The Nuclear Annuli as Pathways for Nucleocytoplasmic Exchanges, *J. Cell Biol.*, **14**:65 (1962).

FERNANDEZ-MORAN, H., T. ODA, P. V. BLAIR, and D. E. GREEN: A Macromolecular Repeating Unit of Mitochondrial Structure and Function Correlated Electron Microscopic and Biochemical Studies of Isolated Mitochondria and Submitochondrial Particles of Beef Heart Muscle, *J. Cell Biol.*, **22**:71 (1964).

FREEMAN, J. A., and B. O. SPURLOCK: A New Epoxy Embedment for Electron Microscopy, *J. Cell Biol.*, **13**:437 (1962).

GOSS, R. T.: Turnover in Cells and Tissues, in D. M. Prescott, L. Goldstein, and E. McConkey (eds.), "Advances in Cell Biology," vol. 1, Appleton Century Crofts, New York, 1970.

GRISHAM, J. W.: Cellular Proliferation in the Liver, in R. J. M. Fry, M. L. Griem, and W. H. Kirsten (eds.), "Normal and Malignant Cell Growth," Springer-Verlag New York Inc., New York, 1969.

HARRIS, E. J.: Transport through Biological Membranes, *Amer. Rev. Physiol.*, **19**:13 (1957).

HOLTER, H.: Pinocytosis, *Int. Rev. Cytol.*, **8**:481 (1960).

HUGHES, A.: "The Mitotic Cycle," Academic Press, Inc., New York, 1952.

INOUÉ, S.: On the Physical Properties of the Mitotic Spindle, *Ann. NY Acad. Sci.*, **90**:529 (1960).

ITO, S.: The Endoplasmic Reticulum of Gastric Parietal Cells, *J. Biophys. Biochem. Cytol.*, **11**:333 (1961).

KARNOVSKY, M. J.: Simple Methods for "Staining with Lead" at High pH in Electron Microscopy, *J. Biophys. Biochem. Cytol.*, **11**:729 (1961).

LAJTHA, L.: Proliferative Capacity of Hemopoietic Stem Cells, in R. J. M. Fry, M. L. Griem, and W. H. Kirsten (eds.), "Normal and Malignant Cell Growth," Springer-Verlag New York Inc., New York, 1969.

LAMERTON, L.: General Introduction, in R. J. M. Fry, M. L. Griem, and W. H. Kirsten (eds.), "Normal and Malignant Cell Growth," Springer-Verlag New York Inc., New York, 1969.

LEBLOND, C. P., and Y. CLERMONT: The Cell Web, a Fibrillar Structure Found in a Variety of Cells in Animal Tissues, *Anat. Rec.*, **136**:230 (1960).

LEBLOND, C. P., and B. E. WALKER: Renewal of Cell Populations, *Physiol. Rev.*, **36**:255 (1956).

LESHER, S., and J. BAUMAN: Cell Proliferation in the Intestinal Epithelium," in R. J. M. Fry, M. L. Griem, and W. H. Kirsten (eds.), "Normal and Malignant Cell Growth," Springer-Verlag New York Inc., New York, 1969.

LIMA-DE-FARIA, A. (ed.): "Handbook of Molecular Cytology," North-Holland Publishing Company, Amsterdam, 1969.

MAUL, G. G.: On the Relationship between the Golgi Apparatus and Annucleate Lamellae, *J. Ultrastruct. Res.*, **30**:368 (1970).

MAZIA, D.: Mitosis and the Physiology of Cell Division, in J. Brachet and A. E. Mirsky (eds.), "The Cell," vol. 3, Academic Press, Inc., New York, 1961.

MC QUILLAN, K.: Ribosomes and Synthesis of Proteins, *Progr. Biophys. Biochem.*, **12**:69 (1962).

MIRSKY, A. E., and S. OSAWA: The Interphase Nucleus, in A. E. Mirsky and J. Brachet (eds.), "The Cell," vol. 2, Academic Press, Inc., New York, 1961.

MITCHELL, J. S. (ed.): "The Cell Nucleus," Academic Press, Inc., New York, 1960.

NEUTRA, M., and C. P. LEBLOND: The Golgi Apparatus, *Sci. Amer.*, **220**:100 (1969).

NOVIKOFF, A. B.: Mitochondria (Chondriosomes), in J. Brachet and A. E. Mirsky (eds.), "The Cell," vol. 2, Academic Press, Inc., New York, 1961.

NOVIKOFF, A. B.: Lysosomes and Related Particles, in J. Brachet and A. E. Mirsky (eds.), ''The Cell,'' vol. 2, Academic Press, Inc., New York, 1961.

PALADE, G. E.: Functional Interrelations of Cytoplasmic Organelles: Current Concepts and Outlook, *First Int. Sympos. Cell Biol. Cytopharmacol.,* Venice, July, 1969.

PALADE, G. E.: A Small Particulate Component of the Cytoplasm, *J. Biophys. Biochem. Cytol.,* **1:**59 (1955).

PALADE, G. E.: A Study of Fixation for Electron Microscopy, *J. Exp. Med.,* **95:**285 (1952).

PALADE, G. E., P. SIEKEVITZ, and L. G. CARO: Structure, Chemistry and Function of the Pancreatic Exocrine Cell,'' in A. V. S. de Reuck and M. P. Cameron (eds.), ''The Exocrine Pancreas,'' Ciba Foundation Symposium, Little, Brown and Company, Boston, 1962.

PELC, S. R.: Labelling of DNA and Cell Division in So-called Non-dividing Tissues, *J. Cell Biol.,* **22:**21 (1964).

PORTER, K. R., and G. E. PALADE: Studies on the Endoplasmic Reticulum. V. Its Form and Differentiation in Striated Muscle Cells, *J. Biophys. Biochem. Cytol.,* **3:**269 (1957).

PORTER, K. R., and E. YAMADA: Studies on the Endoplasmic Reticulum. V. Its Form and Differentiation in Pigment Epithelial Cells of the Frog Retina, *J. Biophys. Biochem. Cytol.,* **8:**181 (1960).

PRESCOTT, D. M.: Structure and Replication of Eukaryotic Chromosomes, in D. M. Prescott, L. Goldstein, and E. McConkey (eds.), ''Advances in Cell Biology,'' vol. 1, Appleton Century Crofts, New York, 1970.

RHOADES, M. M.: Meiosis, in J. Brachet and A. E. Mirsky (eds.), ''The Cell,'' vol. 3, Academic Press, Inc., New York, 1961.

RICH, A., J. R. WARNER, and H. M. GOODMAN: The Structure and Function of Polyribosomes, *Cold Spring Harbor Sympos. Quant. Biol.,* **28:**269 (1963).

ROBBINS, E., and N. K. GONATAS: The Ultrastructures of a Mammalian Cell during the Mitotic Cycle, *J. Cell Biol.,* **21:**429 (1964).

ROBERTSON, J. D.: The Unit Membrane, in J. D. Boyd, F. R. Johnson, and J. D. Lever (eds.), ''Electron Microscopy in Anatomy,'' The Williams & Wilkins Company, Baltimore, 1961.

SIEGEL, B. M. (ed.): ''Modern Developments in Electron Microscopy: The Physics of the Electron Microscope; Techniques; Applications,'' Academic Press, Inc., New York, 1964.

SJÖSTRAND, F. S.: The Structure of Cellular Membranes, *Protoplasma,* **63:**248 (1967).

STERN, H.: Function and Reproduction of Chromosomes, *Physiol. Rev.,* **42:**271 (1962).

STRAUS, W.: Occurrence of Phagosomes and Phagolysosomes in Different Segments of the Nephron in Relation to the Reabsorption, Transport, Digestion, and Extrusion of Intravenously Injected Horseradish Peroxidase, *J. Cell Biol.,* **21:**295 (1964).

TAYLOR, J. H.: The Duplication of Chromosomes, in P. von Sette (ed.), ''Probleme der biologischen Reduplikation,'' Springer-Verlag OHG, Berlin, 1966.

TAYLOR, J. H.: The Time and Mode of Duplication of Chromosomes, *Amer. Naturalist,* **91:**209 (1957).

VALENCIA, J. I., and R. F. GRELL (eds.): Genes and Chromosomes, Structure and Function, *Nat. Cancer Inst. Monogr.* 18, 1965.

WATSON, M. L.: Staining of Tissue Sections for Electron Microscopy with Heavy Metals, *J. Biophys. Biochem. Cytol.,* **4:**475 (1958).

WEISS, J. M.: The Ergastoplasm; Its Fine Structure and Relation to Protein

Synthesis as Studied with the Electron Microscope in the Pancreas of the Swiss Albino Mouse, *J. Exp. Med.,* **98:**607 (1953).

WHITE, M. J. D.: "The Chromosomes," 5th ed., Methuen & Co., Ltd., London, 1961.

WILBRANDT, W., and T. ROSENBERG: The Concept of Carrier Transport and Its Corollaries in Pharmacology, *Pharmacol Rev.,* **13:**109 (1961).

WOLSTENHOLME, G. E. W., and M. O'CONNOR, (eds.): "Principles of Biomolecular Organization," Ciba Foundation Symposium, J. & A. Churchill, London, 1966.

chapter 2   Histo-chemistry and cyto-chemistry

HELEN A. PADYKULA

Histochemistry-cytochemistry is a biological approach which permits a precise interpretation of the chemistry of cells and tissues in relation to structural organization. A student of histology quickly becomes aware of the intrinsic heterogeneity in the structure of multicellular organisms. Biochemical analysis alone is inadequate because homogenization of an organ obscures the structural heterogeneity, which extends to the molecular level. In histochemistry-cytochemistry, by using tissue sections, morphologic relationships are maintained. In its current stage of development, it is primarily a qualitative science, although significant advances in quantitation in situ have been made. The principal question asked by the cytochemist is the following: Where, within the organized framework of the cell, is a particular chemical component located? To identify and localize the component, a specific procedure derived from well-established reactions in inorganic or organic chemistry is used to yield a reaction product visible with microscopes. The result offers qualitative and spatial precision; for example, it has been established that glucose-6-phosphatase is localized in the rough and smooth endoplasmic reticulum as well as in the nuclear envelope of the hepatocyte and that galactose is incorporated into mucoprotein in the Golgi complex of the intestinal goblet cell. Such information is essential to an understanding of cell physiology.

Another major approach to the chemical characterization of cells and tissues is the isolation of cellular and tissue components by ultracentrifugation. Current procedures of ultracentrifugation and electron microscopy are so refined that ultrastructural entities (for example, the outer mitochondrial membrane or the Golgi complex) can be isolated, recognized, and characterized quantitatively. A limitation of this powerful methodology is that cell and tissue organization is dismantled with consequent loss of the interrelationship of component parts. Thus, the two major approaches to chemical characterization of cells are complementary in terms of the kinds of information yielded.

The potential for study of biological organization

unleashed by the electron microscope's resolving power of 2 Å offers an exciting challenge to cytochemistry. Already many significant chemical localizations have been made at the ultrastructural level. The new impetus provided by electron microscopy is extending most of histochemistry (intratissue localizations) to cytochemistry (intracellular localizations).

Many significant biological concepts have emerged from the application of histochemistry and cytochemistry, only a few examples of which are cited here. Concepts of the mechanism of cellular defense have been shaped in part from information gained through the cytochemical study of phagocytosis (via identification of lysosomal derivatives by localization of acid phosphatase) and by identification of antibody-producing cells by fluorescent and other labels. Interpretations related to cell differentiation, migration, and replacement have been heavily dependent on information gained through radioautography, which permits visualization of the location of an incorporated radioactive label. The characterization of chemical differences along the nephron is accomplished mainly through histochemistry, since the complex histologic organization of the kidney makes biochemical analysis exceedingly difficult. Modern exploration of the heterogeneity of vertebrate skeletal muscle fibers received its direction from histochemical observations; zonation of the hepatic lobule is largely a histochemical concept. In all problems involving multicellular systems, some information can be derived through histochemistry. It is necessary, however, for an observer to have an adequate background in microscopic anatomy as well as in chemistry.

General principles of histochemistry

1. The essential first step is the preservation and immobilization of the chemical substance by appropriate fixation and processing. Cellular structure and selected chemical features must survive the procedures required to prepare a suitable tissue section for transmission microscopy. Special fixation is usually required to ensure retention of the chemical entity with its characteristic reactivity. In fixation for morphologic purposes, only the macromolecular protein framework (for example, nucleoproteins, lipoproteins, glycoproteins) is retained, since the proteins are denatured and new crosslinkages are established which render them insoluble. Thus, the cytochemistry of macromolecules is more readily approached than that of small molecules, such as simple sugars, amino acids, and electrolytes, which are usually washed out of tissue sections. To preserve triglycerides and other lipids, organic solvents such as acetone, chloroform, and xylol must be avoided. The fact that glycogen is soluble in water but insoluble in concentrated ethanol should be considered in selecting an appropriate fixative. Most enzymes are inactivated to some degree by fixation, and some enzymes, in addition, are soluble. Thus, fixation preceding a cytochemical demonstration of enzymatic activity usually represents a compromise between the quality of morphologic preservation and the degree of activity.

2. A specific chemical-identifying reaction is needed which will yield an insoluble product that is composed of particles small enough to be localized among the tissue and cell components and large enough to be resolved by light and electron microscopes. In addition, the reaction product should be visible by virtue of its color (ordinary light microscope), fluorescence (ultraviolet microscope), or high electron opacity (electron microscope).

3. The specificity of the histochemical test must be defined by the appropriate use of control preparations. The importance of this principle cannot be overemphasized, since the tissue section is a heterogeneous system with highly varied chemical reactivity. Common control preparations are ones in which a significant reagent has been omitted from the reaction or ones in which the reactive substance has been removed or masked.

4. The accuracy of the localization of the reaction product must be evaluated to eliminate the possibility that one of the reagents may have been bound nonspecifically to a tissue component or that the reaction product may migrate or be soluble in adjacent cell inclusions, such as lipid droplets.

5. The sensitivity of the histochemical test must be considered when evaluating results. There must of course, be enough material to be detected. One can never safely say that a substance is completely absent; negative results might mean that the material is not present or that an interfering substance is present, that the substance has been chemically altered, that the substance has been lost from the tissue during preparation, or that there is too little for detection.

To introduce the rationale of the histochemical-cytochemical approach, these principles are illustrated in a few commonly employed procedures. For more information about these and other procedures, the books by Barka and Anderson, Pearse, Gomori, and Burstone should be consulted.

Acidophilia and basophilia

Staining with a basic (cationic) dye and an anionic (acid) dye is the principal way of creating the color contrasts necessary for morphologic study (see Chap. 1). The designations *acidophilia* and *basophilia* are primary distinctions drawn to characterize cellular and tissue components. Here we shall consider how these cationic and anionic dyes may be used as histochemical reagents to characterize the cell. Figure 2-1 illustrates the chemical structure of a representative anionic (so-called *acidic*)[1] dye, orange G, and a representative cationic (*basic*)[1] dye, methylene blue. Many substances in the protein scaffolding of the tissue section—simple proteins, nucleoproteins, glycoproteins, and lipoproteins, as well as many lipids, glycolipids, and mucopolysaccharides—have ionizable radicals that allow formation of electrostatic (salt) linkages with these dyes.

This staining capacity is most easily appreciated in relation to the chemical structure of proteins. A protein is a polymer of a variety of amino acids; it is amphoteric because of the side groups of these acids, since some residues contain additional anionic functions (for example, phenolic hydroxyl or carboxyl groups) and others have additional cationic

functions (for example, amino, imidazole, or guanidine) (Fig. 2-2). The basis of the amphoteric property is illustrated in Fig. 2-3, which indicates that the charge of an amino acid depends on the pH of the medium. Thus, the protein as a whole may act either as an anion or cation, depending on the algebraic sum of its positive and negative charges at the pH of its environment. The pH at which the protein approaches electrical neutrality is known as the *isoelectric point.*

The fixed proteins of a tissue section retain their amphoteric properties but they are modified by denaturation. Actually fixation causes increased affinity for stains, since secondary groups are ruptured and become available for combination with the dye molecules. Certain fixatives (for example, those containing osmium or mercury) combine with

Figure 2-1   Formulas of a typical anionic ("acid") dye, orange G, and a typical cationic ("basic") dye, methylene blue.

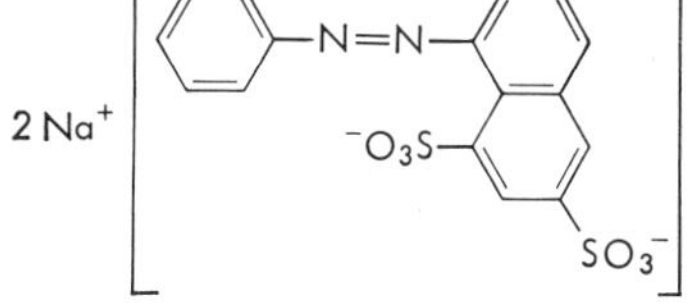

Disodium orange G

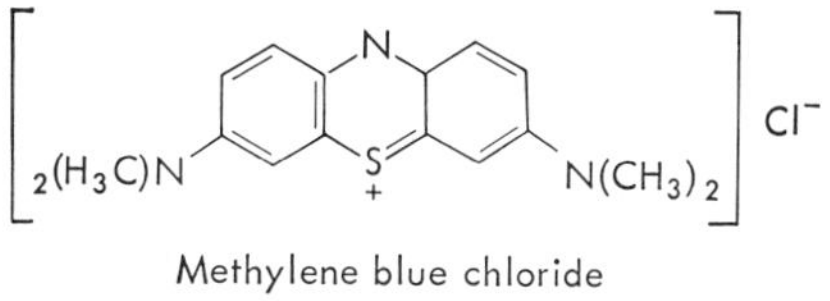

Methylene blue chloride

[1]The designations *acidic* and *basic* dyes are inherited ones which, unfortunately, do not conform to current chemical definitions for an acid and a base (that is, an acid is a substance capable of donating protons and a base is capable of accepting protons.) Thus, *through histochemical usage,* an acidic dye is one capable of forming a salt linkage with a positively charged tissue group; therefore, the dye molecule is negatively charged (anionic). A basic dye is positively charged (cationic) and hence forms a salt with a negatively charged tissue group. This usage is analogous to the naming of the nucleic acids and their constituents.

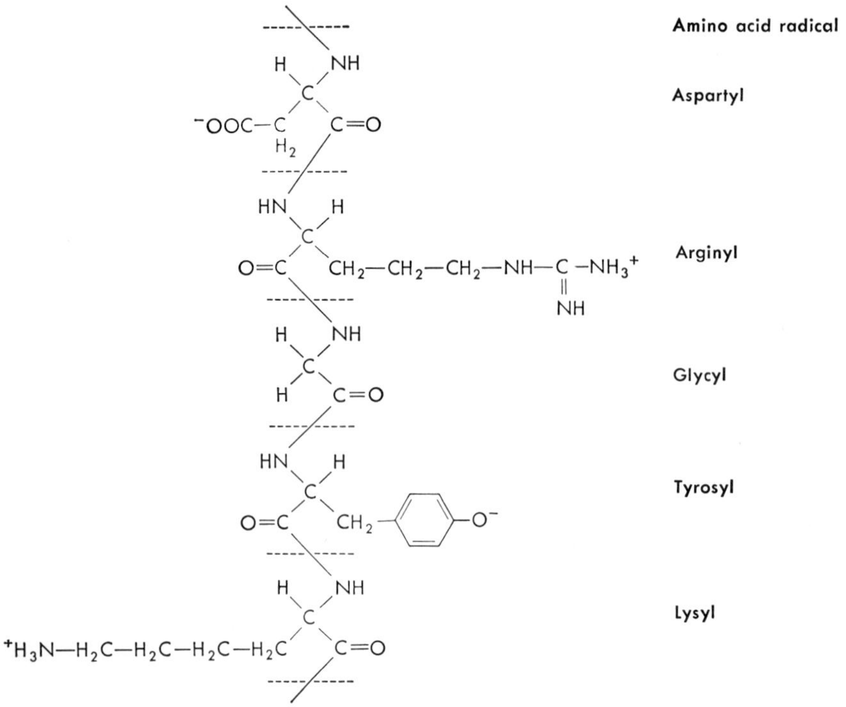

Figure 2-2 Structural formula of a portion of a hypothetical protein chain, showing the presence of ionizable radicals.

various reactive groups in the tissue and can influence subsequent stainability considerably.

Evidence that the binding of acid (anionic) and basic (cationic) dyes by proteins is principally an electrostatic phenomenon can be obtained by experiments involving the dye-binding of a single pure protein, fibrin, at various pH levels (Fig. 2-4). The intensity of staining at each pH—that is, the amount of light absorbed—can be measured with a photometer, and when plotted against pH, curves representing the acidophilia and basophilia of the protein can be drawn. Study of Fig. 2-4 shows that the least binding of cationic and anionic dyes occurs near pH 6.0, which is near the isoelectric point of fibrin. Below its isoelectric pH, the fibrin is acidophilic (that is, it binds the anionic orange G) by virtue of its overall positive charge, as $-NH_2$ ionizes to NH_3^+. Above the isoelectric point, the fibrin is basophilic (that is, it binds the cationic methylene blue) because of its overall negative charge as $-COOH$ ionizes to $-COO^-$.

A tissue section, however, contains a myriad of proteins that differ in their amino acid composition and thereby have different isoelectric points, so at a pH that creates good color contrast for morphologic study, certain tissue components will show a relative acidophilia (for example, mitochondria, collagen, hemoglobin of red blood cells) while others

Figure 2-3 The amino acid zwitterion: the net charge is zero at the isoelectric point. Above the isoelectric point the substance is anionic and below it is cationic.

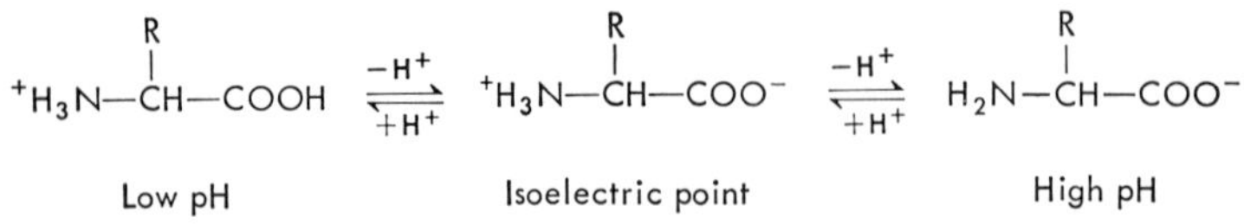

Low pH Isoelectric point High pH

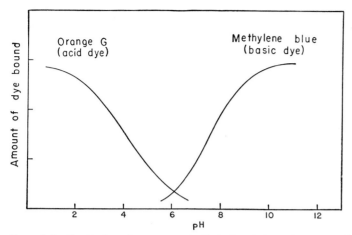

Figure 2-4   Dye binding of a pure protein, fibrin, in solutions of constant salt and dye concentration.   The amount of dye bound is calculated from the light absorption of the stained protein.   For further explanation, see the text.   (Courtesy of M. Singer.)

display a relative basophilia (for example, chromatin, nucleoli, and ergastoplasm). However, the dye-binding of proteins is not related only to their amino acid content but is also profoundly affected by the presence of associated groups, such as the phosphoric acid of the nucleoproteins (Fig. 2-5). Much of the cellular basophilia commonly observed in the chromatin, nucleoli, and endoplasmic reticulum (Fig. 2-6) is based on the dissociation of the phosphate groups of DNA and RNA to form negative radicals, even at relatively low pH (Fig. 2-7). Other highly basophilic structures (granules of mast cells and blood basophils, cartilage matrix, mucus of goblet cells) contain sulfated mucopolysaccharides; the high electronegativity of the sulfate group causes a basophilia that persists even at pH 2 (Fig. 2-7).

To identify basophilia originating from nucleoproteins, other information is required which can be derived from control preparations.   For example, if the cytoplasm exhibits marked basophilia, a control section may be exposed to the action of the enzyme ribonuclease before staining.   RNase will hydrolyze and thus remove RNA present in the control, so areas in the section whose dye affinity is due to RNA will not be basophilic after such treatment.   Similarly, DNase can be used to remove DNA from control preparations.   Also, useful information concerning the relative basophilia of various radicals on protein molecules can be uncovered

rather simply by staining at different pH levels, as shown in Fig. 2-7.   The basophilia caused by the carboxyl groups of muscle proteins will be extinguished at a higher pH than that originating from the phosphate groups of ribonucleoprotein.   Baso-

Figure 2-5   Structure of a portion of DNA, the component responsible for the basophilia of chromatin, is its content of phosphate radicals.   The arrow indicates the point between the purine and deoxyribose residues where acid hydrolysis occurs, an essential step in the Feulgen nuclear reaction.

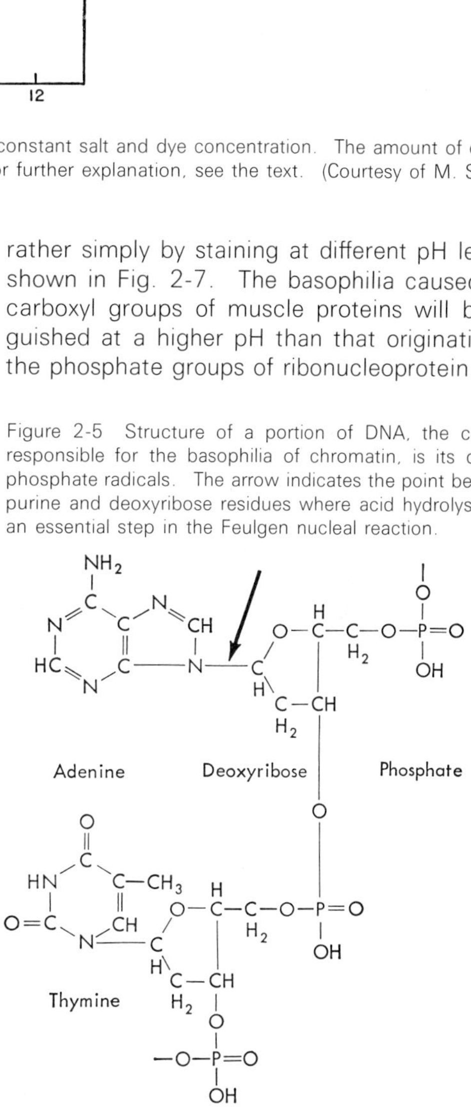

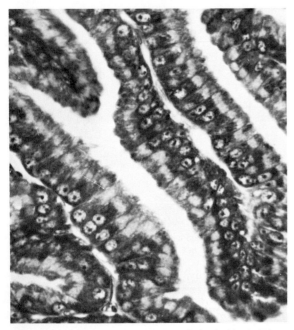

Figure 2-6   Epithelium, prostrate, rat.   Stained with methylene blue and eosin.   Dark areas represent basophilia, whereas pale areas mark acidophilia.   In the nuclei, the basophilia of the nucleoli and associated strands is evident.   Most of the cytoplasm is strongly basophilic, except for a supranuclear acidophilic region, which is occupied by the Golgi complex.

philia persisting at pH 2 is usually indicative of the presence of the sulfate group, as in the heparin (Fig. 2-8) of mast cells or chondroitin sulfate of cartilage matrix.   There are, of course, still other procedures for distinguishing among basophilic substances.

Intense acidophilia over a wide pH range may reflect the presence of certain proteins.   For example, red blood cells are strongly acidophilic because they are rich in hemoglobin, which contains an abundance of the amino acid lysine.   The eosinophilic leukocytes obtain their name from the presence of strongly acidophilic (eosinophilic) cytoplasmic granules that contain arginine.   It should be added, however, that there are also substances, such as elastic fibers, which are relatively chromophobic and which therefore show little reactivity toward these aqueous dyes.

Since the dyes hematoxylin and eosin are commonly used in routine study, it should be noted that the color-bearing moiety of the hematoxylin is actually an anionic substance called hematein that is bound (or chelated) to tissue components by a multivalent metallic cation, such as aluminum or iron, which is known as a mordant.   The hemateinmordant *complex* (referred to as a *lake*) carries a positive charge.   Although it behaves generally as a cationic dye, certain hematoxylin mixtures will

Figure 2-7   Staining characteristics, or ''signatures,'' of several basophilic constituents of tissues.   Methylene blue staining was employed under constant conditions of salt and dye concentration.   (Courtesy of M. Singer.)

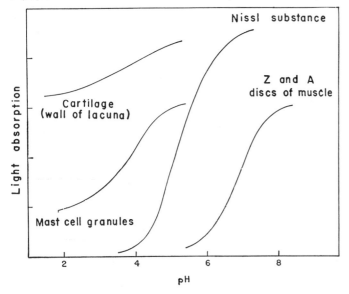

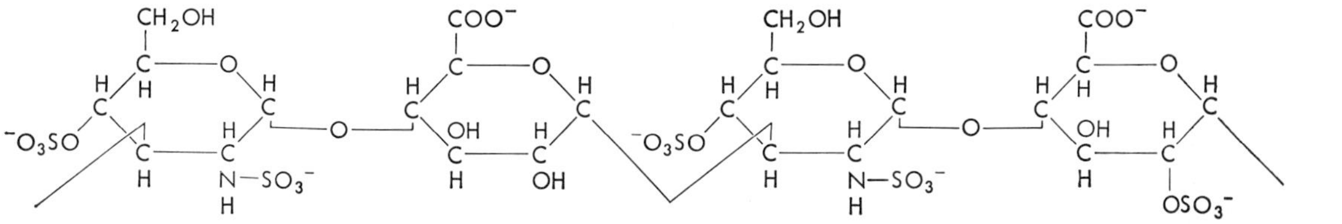

Figure 2-8 Tetrasaccharide unit of one type of heparin, showing the presence of sulfated radicals, which account for the marked basophilia and the metachromatic staining, and also of an unsubstituted uronic acid residue, which apparently accounts for the moderate PAS-reactivity of this substance.

stain mitochondria and other structures which are not basophilic under the conditions previously described. For critical distinction between acidophilic and basophilic structures, the use of methylene blue and eosin at controlled pH levels yields more histochemical information than a hematoxylin and eosin preparation.

Some special staining mixtures (Mallory's trichrome, Heidenhain's azan, Masson's trichrome) employ combinations of acid dyes, and the mechanism of their differential staining of tissue structures is still largely unanalyzed. In each mixture, however, one dye (light green, aniline blue) shows a particular affinity for collagen after the preparation has been pretreated with a tanning agent such as phosphotungstic or phosphomolybdic acid. This produces selective staining although not specific staining.

Metachromasia

In a tissue section, *metachromasia* signals the change in the absorption spectrum of certain basic dyes when they are bound to polyanionic polymers, such as heparin (Fig. 2-8), other acid mucopolysaccharides, and nucleoproteins. Thiazine dyes (such as toluidine blue, thionine, and to a lesser extent, methylene blue) are *orthochromatic* blue when seen in a dilute solution where they exist in a monomeric state; however, when they are concentrated in a solution, they aggregate as dimers and polymers which absorb at a lower wavelength and thus appear *metachromatic* red. Thus, different colors may be obtained from a single thiazine dye, depending on the state of aggregation of the molecules, and this state may be altered by the tissue components themselves.

For a histochemical demonstration of metachromasia, a tissue section is exposed to a dilute solution of toluidine blue. This cationic dye will bind electrostatically with anionic sites. Wherever the anionic sites are close enough, as in polyanionic polymers, the dye molecules will be aggregated by certain constituents of the tissue (Fig. 2-9). Their interaction on the surface of the polyanion will result in a shift in absorption that creates the metachromatic effect. It is postulated that the distance between dye molecules should be about 5 to 7 Å for such interaction and that the presence of water is essential. Metachromasia is illustrated in Fig. 25-30; here the nuclei stain an orthochromatic blue, but the ground substance of the connective tissue is metachromatic red. Under certain conditions, nucleoproteins will also stain metachromatically but less obviously than the acid mucopolysaccharides. For the expression of metachromasia, the chemical nature of the binding site does not seem so important as the distribution and frequency of the negative charges (Fig. 2-9). For a stimulating analysis of metachromasia, see Bergeron and Singer (1958).

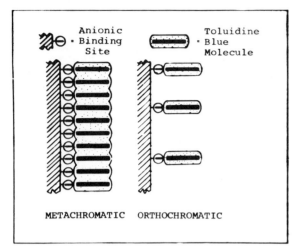

Figure 2-9 Hypothesis concerning the basis of metachromasia in tissue sections. The polyanionic polymer on the left possesses a series of closely, uniformly spaced negative sites which react electrostatically with cationic molecules of toluidine blue. This alignment allows interaction of dye molecules that results in a metachromatic shift (red). On the right, the anionic sites are more widely and irregularly spaced; this results in an orthochromatic effect (blue). (Modified from Bradley and Wolf. Proc. Nat. Acad. Sci., **45**:944, 1959.)

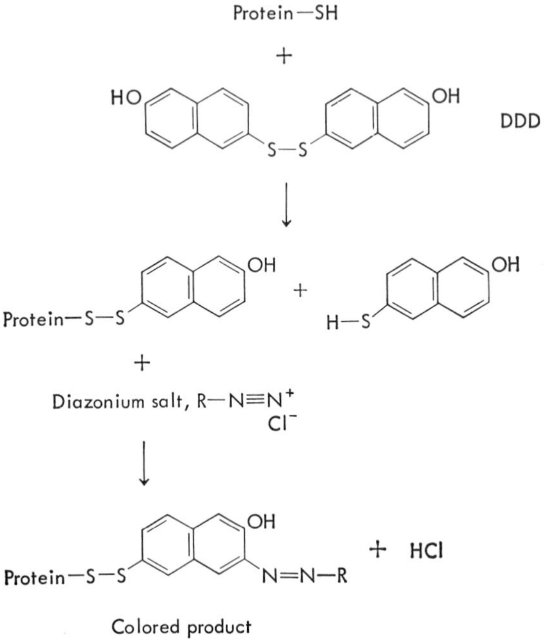

Figure 2-10 The azo dye principle in a procedure demonstrating protein-based sulfhydryl groups. The reaction is between the reagent DDD and an —SH-containing compound. It gives a naphtholic product able to react with a diazotized compound to yield a colored azo dye. (Barrnett and Seligman)

Special end-group reactions

To characterize proteins beyond the properties of acidophilia or basophilia, it often becomes necessary to use tests for certain radicals such as the sulfhydryl (cysteine), guanidyl (arginine), and phenyl (tyrosine) groups. Certain proteins contain a sufficient number of one of these amino acids to be detectable cytochemically. A single example of this type of reaction, one for protein-bound sulfhydryl (—SH) groups, is included here; many other examples may be found in the texts of Barka and Anderson and of Pearse.

The amino acids possessing —SH groups are cysteine and, after reduction of S—S bonds, cystine. Many important proteins contain a large number of —SH or S—S groups—for example, the keratin of epidermis, myosin of muscle, growth hormone, and insulin. A highly specific cytochemical reaction for these groups is based on the fact that, at alkaline pH, only the —SH groups of proteins are oxidized by disulfides. A cytochemical sequence for localizing —SH groups is illustrated in Fig. 2-10. The DDD (dihydroxy dinaphthyl disulfide) reagent of Barrnett and Seligman can "oxidize" (that is, form a disulfide with) —SH groups and thereby attach naphtholic radicals to the sites of protein-bound sulfhydryl. Color is then produced by coupling with a diazonium salt. The final reaction product, an azo dye, is insoluble in water and in organic solvents.

Control preparations for this reaction include the use of reagents capable of blocking —SH groups. Moreover, it must be shown that the diazonium salt does not produce color with tissue components other than the bound naphtholic reagent.

The application of this procedure to the study of hair growth in particular has yielded information about the site of formation of disulfide bonds during keratin synthesis.

Reactions of the Schiff reagent with aldehyde groups

THE PERIODIC ACID–SCHIFF (PAS) REACTION

The histochemistry of carbohydrates centers around the periodic acid–Schiff reaction, a procedure used routinely in most histology and pathology laboratories. It permits the localization of carbohydrate-rich macromolecules such as glycogen, mucoproteins, and glycoproteins. Glycogen is the principal storage form of carbohydrate in animals, and its identification and localization is often important.

The specificity of the PAS reaction is derived from the sequential use of two selective reagents, periodic acid (HIO_4) and the Schiff reagent. Periodic acid oxidizes the free hydroxyl groups on two adjacent carbon atoms, such as the 1,2-glycol linkage in hexoses or the adjacent hydroxyl and amino groups in hexosamine (Fig. 2-11). The hydroxyl groups are converted to aldehydes, the carbon bond is cleaved, and under the conditions of the PAS procedure, the oxidation does not proceed further. The resulting aldehydes react readily with the Schiff reagent to produce a stable colored complex. The usual Schiff reagent is leukofuchsin, or fuchsin-sulfurous acid, a chromogenic bisulfite compound which, when it forms an additional product with aldehydes, produces a stable red product (Fig. 2-12).

Numerous substances, especially in the epithelia and connective tissues, are reactive in the PAS method. Common reactive tissue components are glycogen, some epithelial mucins, the Golgi apparatus, cell coats (see Fig. 2-13, color insert, and Fig. 7-47), basement membranes, and mucosubstances occurring in the ground substances of the various connective tissues. To establish that the PAS-reactive material is glycogen, a control preparation is used which has been predigested with α amylase, an enzyme which hydrolyzes glycogen specifically (Fig. 2-14). The sorting out of the PAS-reactive substances not digested by amylase is a more difficult task, since many of the carbohydrate-rich substances that have been localized histochemically have not yet been characterized biochemically (see Spicer et al., 1967).

Another characterization of a carbohydrate-rich substance that can be easily made is the determination of its degree of basophilia (Fig. 2-7), which indicates the presence of associated sulfate or sialic acid groups. However, it must be appreciated that some carbohydrate units built into cellular and extracellular materials fail to stain by the PAS procedure, including several of the hyaluronic acids and most chondroitin sulfates.

An important application of the PAS reaction will be encountered in Chap. 27; the identification of the cells producing the glycoprotein hormones FSH, LH, and TSH is facilitated by this histochemical reaction. At the ultrastructural level, carbohydrate macromolecules may be detected by oxidation with periodic acid followed by silver methenamine as a substitute for the Schiff reagent, which yields a final reaction product of sufficient electron opacity.

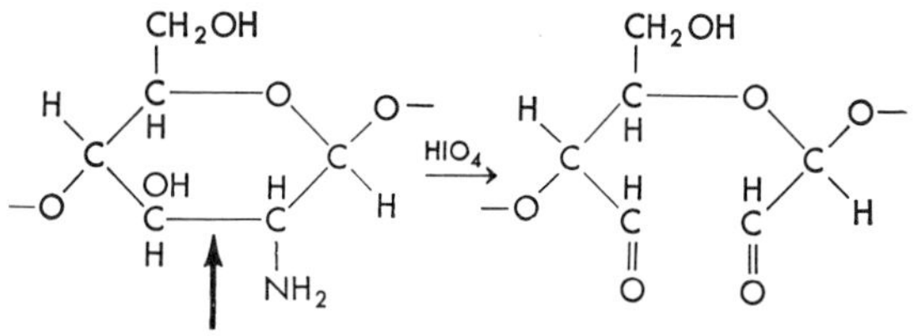

THE FEULGEN REACTION FOR DNA

A highly specific reaction for the cytochemical localization of DNA was devised by Feulgen and Rossenbeck in 1924. This widely used technique permits the localization of high-polymer DNA, and this can be followed by quantitative estimation using microspectrophotometry. The specificity is derived from the presence in DNA of a unique sugar, deoxyribose.

Figure 2-11 Oxidation of hexosamine residue of a polysaccharide or glycoprotein by periodic acid to form dialdehydes. The point of attack is shown by the arrow.

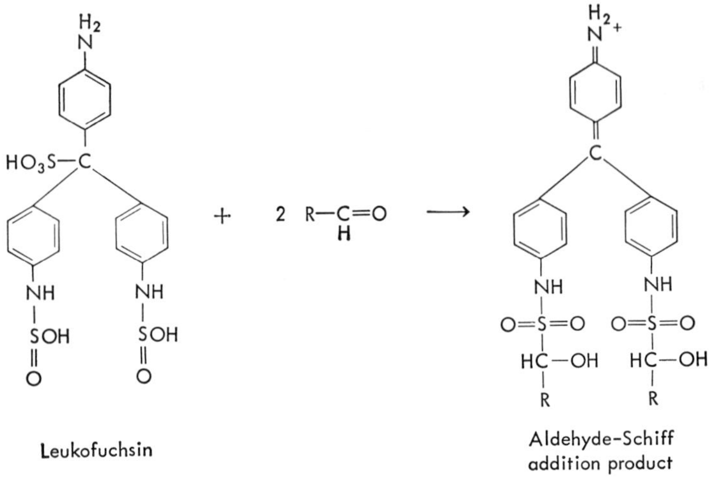

Leukofuchsin

Aldehyde-Schiff
addition product

Figure 2-12   Reaction of colorless leukofuchsin with a dialdehyde to form a magenta-colored complex (see Fig. 2-13, color insert).

The procedure involves the hydrolytic removal of the purine groups by *mild* acid hydrolysis (Fig. 2-5). The furanose ring of deoxyribose thus opens and forms an aldehyde group which can react with Schiff reagent. A magenta-colored product marks the locus of DNA. One control for this test involves predigestion of the section with deoxyribonuclease; this control preparation is then stained in parallel

Figure 2-14A   Glycogen synthesis in liver slices. Radioautographs of sections stained with PAS and hematoxylin. These three sections were taken from a single liver slice (obtained from a rat fasted for 24 hr) that had been incubated in a medium containing [³H] glucose for 15 min. In the control, silver grains overlay PAS-positive material, especially at the periphery of the hepatocytes. That this reactive material is glycogen is demonstrated by its complete removal by α amylase. The amylase of saliva removes the glycogen only partially. ×680. (From Coimbra and Leblond, J. Cell Biol., **30:**151, 1966.)

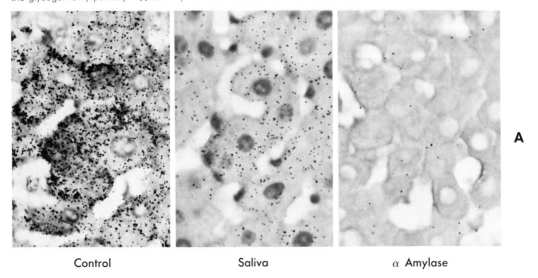

Control   Saliva   α Amylase

A

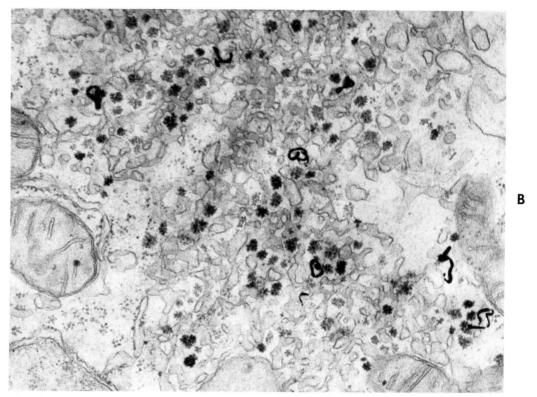

B

Figure 2-14B   Electron-microscopic radioautograph of a portion of the cytoplasm of a hepatocyte (from liver of a fasted rat 1 hr after administration of glucose-^{3}H).   Most of the field is occupied by a glycogen area composed of profiles of smooth endoplasmic reticulum and dense alpha particles of glycogen in the cytoplasmic matrix.   Note that the curled silver grains occur primarily in the glycogen area and not over mitochondria.   ×63,000.   (From Coimbra and Leblond, J. Cell Biol., **30:**151, 1966.)

with a standard preparation.   A comparison of the two preparations allows identification of the DNA.

In most normal cells, the material reactive in the Feulgen test is limited to nuclear chromatin.   Although mitochondria contain DNA, the amount is too low for the sensitivity of this procedure.   Usually the same material is basophilic, but in some instances the high isoelectric point of the protein (a protoamine) associated with the DNA competes with the cationic dye and prevents any expression of basophilia.

Sudanophilia of lipids

The most common cellular lipids are triglycerides and phospholipids.   Triglycerides are metabolic reserves that occur in droplet form in cells, and their fluctuations within a tissue can be followed cytochemically.   Phospholipids are structural components of membranes and are more difficult to localize visually.   Lipids are usually preserved by formalin fixation, and frozen sections are then prepared to avoid the extraction of lipids that occurs in the routine paraffin technique.

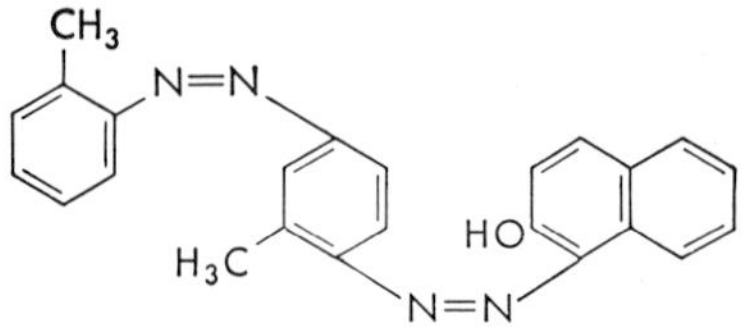

Figure 2-15   Sudan IV; representative oil-soluble dye.

A widely used procedure for localizing lipids is based on the properties of the Sudan dyes. These lipid "stains" are weakly ionizable and hence can be dissolved only in nonaqueous media (Fig. 2-15). The carrier for the Sudan dye is an organic solvent in which lipids are relatively insoluble, such as 70% ethanol or propylene glycol. The dye should also be only moderately soluble in this carrier but more soluble in lipids, so "staining" occurs with substances in which the dye is partitioned, as in a separatory funnel. The stained sections are then mounted in glycerol or some other water-soluble medium to avoid extraction of either the dye or the lipid. Sudanophilia therefore depends on solubility rather than salt formation or the reactivity of certain end groups. The Sudan dyes will dissolve in droplets containing triglycerides and color them intensely (see Chap. 5, Fig. 5-3).

Sudan black is widely used because of its color and its ability to demonstrate lipoprotein structures such as mitochondria and myelin. Structures containing polymerized lipids, such as lipofuscin granules, can also be stained with Sudan dyes, but crystallized lipids cannot be colored. One type of control preparation consists of extraction prior to staining with an organic solvent such as acetone or chloroform plus methanol. Such extraction would remove triglycerides and cholesterol but not the phospholipids. Another important control is based on the extraction of the Sudan dye from the stained tissue section by excess solvent; this helps identify any chemical binding that might occur.

Special techniques are available for localizing cholesterol and other lipids. For a critical discussion of the cytochemistry of lipids, see the review by Deane (1958).

Specific proteins: enzymes, antigens, and antibodies

The inherent specificity of an enzyme for its substrate, or of an antibody for its antigen, constitutes the basis for precise cytochemical localizations, some of which can now be performed at the ultrastructural level. A colored reaction product is needed for a light microscopic localization, whereas visualization with the electron microscope requires an electron-opaque product, such as one containing a heavy metal. Furthermore, the great resolving power of the electron microscope demands that reaction products be composed of exceedingly fine particles, ideally as close as possible to the limit of resolution.

ENZYMATIC ACTIVITY

In cytochemical localizations, *the enzyme itself is not directly visualized, but rather, as a result of its catalytic activity, a visible reaction product is formed that marks its site.* A typical cytochemical reaction for hydrolases and oxidoreductases can be formulated, in simple fashion, as follows: *AB* is the *substrate*, which undergoes an enzyme-catalyzed reaction to *A* + *B*. In the presence of *R*, a reagent capable of precipitating one of the products of the enzymatic reaction (in this case *A*), an insoluble complex *AR* is formed:

$$AB \xrightarrow[R]{\text{enzyme}} AR\downarrow + B$$

The initial insoluble complex *AR* may itself be colored or electron-opaque and hence readily visualized; more frequently, it is insoluble but not colored and must usually be converted secondarily to a colored precipitate for visualization with the light microscope. During incubation, conditions favorable for enzymatic activity—proper pH, ionic composition, and temperature—are maintained as closely as is compatible with the requirements for visualizing the product.

The choice of fixative is critical, since most fixatives inhibit enzymatic activity to some degree. Enzymes vary in their sensitivity to fixation as well as in their solubility; these properties present problems to the cytochemist. To avoid denaturation and other inhibition, frozen sections of fresh tissue are prepared, usually in a cryostat (a refrigerated chamber held usually at -15 to $-20°C$ and containing a microtome). The frozen sections are incubated in an appropriate medium for demonstrating enzymatic activity. Usually the activity of fixed and unfixed sections is compared. Fixation is generally necessary, particularly at the ultrastructural level, to preserve the macromolecular structure during the subsequent cytochemical processing. Aldehydic fixatives such as formalin or glutaraldehyde are most frequently used, the latter being especially effective for dual preservation of cellular structure and protein reactivity.

As representatives of this principle of histochemistry, two examples will be cited: the Gomori procedure for phosphatases and a method for a pyridine nucleotide–dependent dehydrogenase.

PHOSPHATASES

A valuable cytochemical approach was introduced by Gomori in 1939 for localizing phosphatase activity, and it possesses a versatility that is still being explored. Phosphatases hydrolyze the ester linkages of natural organic phosphates such as ATP, glucose-6-phosphate, or glycerophosphate, and liberate phosphate ions as one of the reaction products (Fig. 2-16). The released phosphate ions are then trapped, ideally at the site of the enzyme, by either lead or calcium ions, to form a relatively insoluble primary reaction product, lead or calcium phosphate, which lacks color. Therefore, for light microscopy, lead phosphate is customarily converted to lead sulfide, which is black (Fig. 2-17, see color insert). However, the interference or the phase-contrast microscope can be used to detect the primary product; also for electron microscopy, the second step is unnecessary since lead phosphate itself is electron-opaque (Fig. 2-18A and B). Calcium phosphate is converted in a two-step reaction to cobalt sulfide, a brown-black precipitate for light-microscopic study. The Gomori principle is thus termed metal-salt visualization.

This rationale permits localization of phosphatases over a wide range of pH. Below pH 8, lead is the trapping ion. Though lead is useful for both light and electron microscopy, it tends to combine with hydroxyl ions about pH 8 and precipitates from the medium, so calcium is used as the capture agent above pH 8. To localize acid phosphatase, which has a pH optimum near 5, the incubating medium would contain the substrate (for example, glycerophosphate), buffer (for example, tris maleate), and lead ion as the capture reagent (Fig. 2-16). The morphologic identification of lysosomal derivatives rests heavily on this ultrastructural cytochemical demonstration of the presence of acid phosphatase. In contrast, the muscle protein myosin has ATPase activity with an alkaline pH optimum; thus, frozen sections are incubated with ATP, barbital buffer (pH 9), and calcium ion as the capture agent. Phosphatases with a pH optimum near 7, such as glucose-6-phosphatase or mitochondrial ATPase, can be demonstrated by suitable adjustment of buffer and substrate. In addition, known activators can be incorporated to enhance catalysis and specificity.

Because it yields an electron-opaque, lead-containing reaction product, the Gomori procedure has had widespread use in ultrastructural localizations. The great resolving power of the electron microscope carries a more stringent requirement for morphologic preservation than that needed for cytochemistry at the light-microscopic level. It became apparent in early attempts at ultrastructural cyto-

Figure 2-16 The Gomori acid–phosphatase reaction, pH 5.0, performed in two steps, the first yielding lead phosphate, the second, lead sulfide, both of which are insoluble.

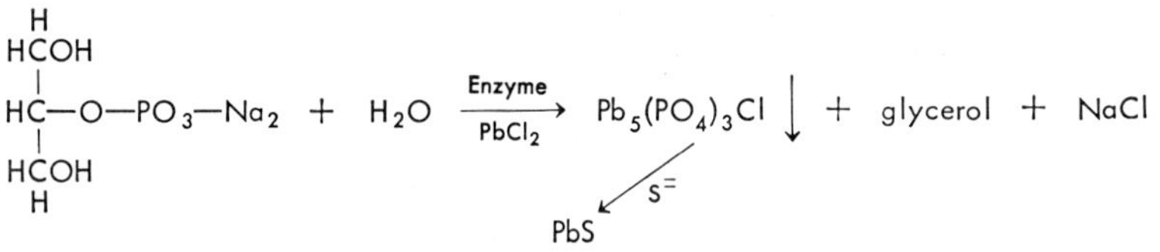

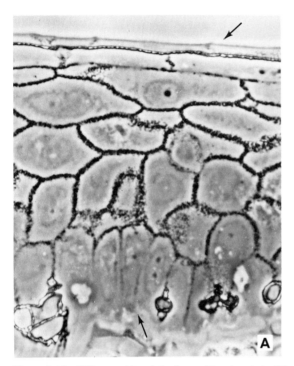

Figure 2-18   ATPase activity of the frog epidermis.   A. In this photomicrograph, the shapes of the cells comprising the stratified squamous epithelium are evident because the lead sulfide reaction product, which reflects ATPase activity, is located at most of the cell boundaries.   It is absent, however, from the free and basal surfaces of the epithelium (see arrows).   Dendritic portions of pigment cells are also reactive in the deeper layers of the epidermis.   Glutaraldehyde-fixed tissue, incubation in a Gomori-type medium for ATPase activity at pH 7.2, post fixation in OsO_4, araldite section 1 μm treated with $(NH_4)S$ to produce PbS $\times$900.   (From Farquhar & Palade, J. Chem. Biol., **30**:359, 1966).

chemistry that osmium tetroxide, although an excellent preserver of ultrastructure and a creator of contrasting densities, is a potent inhibitor of enzymes.   To circumvent this problem, two different kinds of fixation are employed.   Initial fixation by glutaraldehyde preserves ultrastructure while retaining the reactive groups of many enzymes, antibodies, and other proteins (Sabatini et al., 1963).   Then a cytochemical demonstration, such as that of the Gomori procedure, may be performed, preferably on tissue slices.   Such aldehyde-fixed tissues tend, however, to be too low in contrast for morphologic examination, and a second fixation (or

postfixation) with osmium tetroxide is performed to create the usual density contrasts associated with the ultrastructural image (Fig. 2-18B).

Various controls are required to ensure that the reaction product is a result of enzymatic activity and that its location accurately reflects the site of the enzyme.   The most common control preparation is one in which the substrate has been omitted; a positive reaction here would signify the presence in vivo of metallic precipitates such as calcium or iron salts or nonspecific binding of the capture reagent.   Diffusion of a reaction product to another locus is also a possibility that must be considered.   In addition, special problems sometimes arise; for example, lead ion at certain concentrations can hydrolyze ATP and thus contribute a nonenzymatic component to the reaction product (Rosenthal et al., 1969).   Generally the specificity of enzymatic localization and identification is greatest for enzymes that are tightly bound to cellular organelles and that also have a high substrate specificity or are selectively inhibited or activated by certain compounds.

It should be pointed out that hydrolases can also be demonstrated through the so-called *azo-dye procedures* which depend on a different principle.   For example, acid phosphatase can be demonstrated by using an artificial substrate, such as naphthyl phosphate.   The primary reaction products are naphthol and phosphate, but in this system, the naphthol instead of the phosphate is visualized by precipitation with a chromogenic diazonium compound.   An azo dye is thereby formed as the final reaction product.   This principle is illustrated in Fig. 2-10 for demonstration of the —SH groups of proteins.   Numerous histochemical methods can be derived from the azo dye principle since a great variety of naphthol-containing substrates or compounds can be synthesized.   For additional information consult the texts by Burstone (1962), Pearse (1968), and Barka and Anderson (1963), and the publications of Seligman, Nachlas, et al.

REPRESENTATIVE OXIDOREDUCTASE REACTION
This class of enzymes catalyzes the transfer of hydrogen and electrons.   Many biologic oxidations take place with loss of hydrogen and electrons and without the addition of oxygen; the enzymes cata-

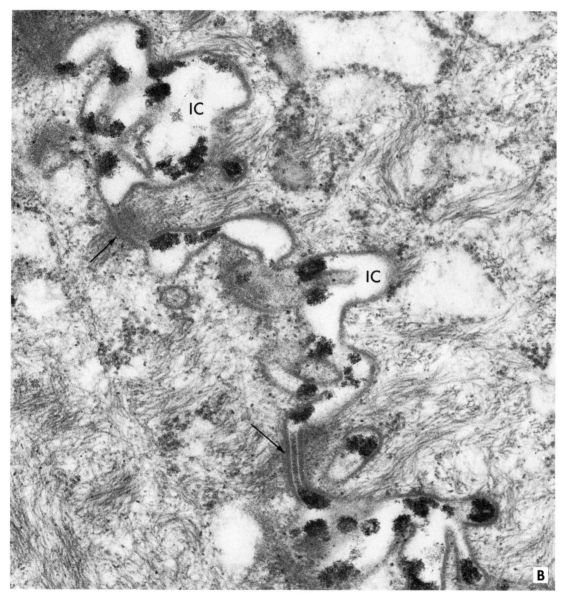

B. Electron micrograph of the junction of two cells of the stratum corneum. Lead phosphate deposits occur as aggregates of small particles (approximately 50 Å) which are located irregularly along the apposed cellular surfaces as well as in the intercellular spaces (IC). No reaction product occurs at the site of the desmosome (arrows). Fixation in glutaraldehyde, incubation in a Gomori-type medium for ATPase activity at pH 7.2, postfixation in OsO_4, and embedding in araldite. ×72,000. (From Farquhar & Palade, J. Cell Biol., **30**:359, 1966.)

lyzing such oxidations are called *dehydrogenases*. The majority of the available histochemical methods employ a reagent known as a *tetrazolium salt*. Such compounds are nearly colorless, water-soluble substances that become insoluble and colored formazans upon reduction (Figs. 2-19 and 2-21).

Chemically, the reduction of tetrazoles requires quite vigorous reducing agents acting at high pH and temperature, but in the presence of specific enzymes and substrates, the reaction will proceed at biologic temperature and pH. Normally, when substrates are oxidized, hydrogen ions and electrons are transferred through a pyridine nucleotide coenzyme (NAD or NADP) to cytochrome *c* and thence through the electron-transport chain to oxygen. The tetrazolium can substitute for the cytochrome *c*. The enzyme capable of transferring hydrogen ions to the tetrazolium from the reduced pyridine nucleotide is called a diaphorase, or more specifically in the histochemical reaction, a tetrazolium reductase.

A representative reaction, using lactate as the initial hydrogen donor, a pyridine nucleotide coenzyme (NAD) as the initial hydrogen acceptor, and a tetrazolium salt as the final acceptor, involves a minimum of two linked enzymes, lactate-NAD oxidoreductase (lactate dehydrogenase) and $NADH_2$–tetrazolium reductase (diaphorase) (Fig. 2-20). Thus, histochemically, one is demonstrating the activity of the second, not the primary, enzyme, although the primary one is necessary for obtaining reduced coenzyme.

Figure 2-19 Reduction of a tetrazolium salt to its formazan, which is insoluble in aqueous solution and is colored. R is a substituted phenolic radical.

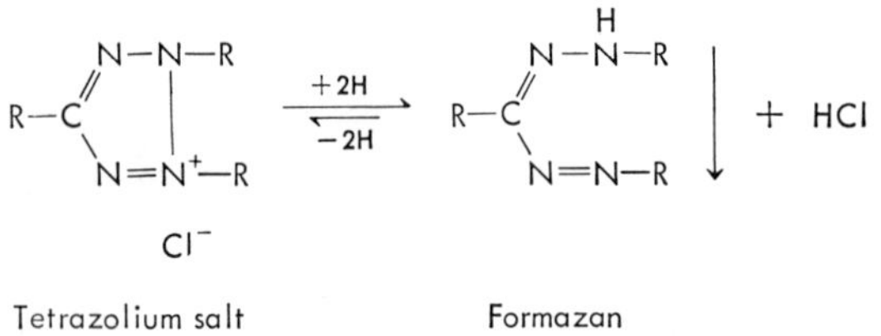

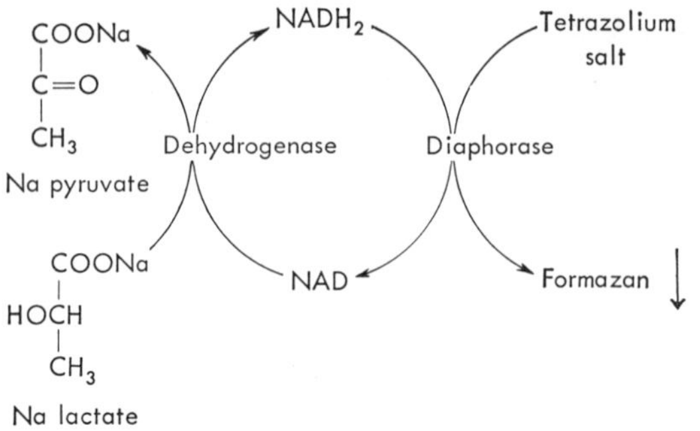

Figure 2-20   Production of a formazan deposit as the end result of the oxidation of sodium L-lactate, with nicotinamide-adenine dinucleotide (NAD) serving as the coenzyme.

The reaction in which $NADH_2$ itself is supplied as substrate may be used to demonstrate the locations of the $NADH_2$–cytochrome *c* reductases. The insoluble dehydrogenases, those capable of reliable visualization, reside in mitochondria and, in some cell types, also in the endoplasmic reticulum.

Control procedures to confirm the enzymatic nature of the reaction and to establish that the provided substrate is the source of the hydrogen ions include (1) inactivation by pretreatment with heat or an —SH reagent such as *p*-chloromercuribenzoate (since like most dehydrogenases, lactate dehydrogenase is —SH dependent) and (2) omission of the primary substrate or of the coenzyme from the incubation medium. Control preparations to confirm the location of the enzyme are more complex, especially in this example, where one is, at best, localizing the second of two enzymes.

A major problem in the use of tetrazoles in histochemistry has been the frequency of false localization of the formazans owing to their solubility in lipids. This difficulty has now been largely overcome by the substitution of additional water-soluble radicals on tetrazolium salts, rendering their formazans virtually insoluble in lipids. Illustrations in this book have used nitro-blue tetrazolium (nitro-BT) and tetranitro-blue tetrazolium, both of which yield

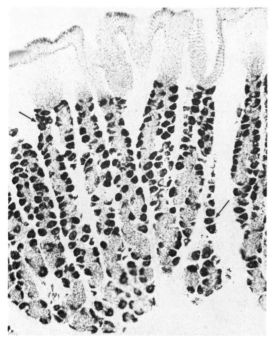

Figure 2-21   Succinic dehydrogenase activity, gastric glands of the cat. This cryostat section was incubated with succinate and neotetrazolium at pH 7.5 for 10 min. The diformazan deposits reveal various levels of succinic dehydrogenase activity in the cells of the gastric epithelium. The most reactive cells are the parietal cells (arrows), which have numerous mitochondria. The mucous cells of the gastric surface and pits are considerably less reactive.   × 150.

highly insoluble formazans. With the tetrazoles that yield highly insoluble formazans composed of fine particles, attempts have been made to localize enzymatic activity with the electron microscope.

The diaphorase reaction is of key importance for many biologic processes, since oxidative metabolism of nutrients provides energy. Many of the oxidative enzymes are located within mitochondria, presumably in a spatial organization that permits ordered activity.

Other methods utilizing tetrazoles as hydrogen-ion acceptors from oxidative enzymes are those for the succinate oxidase system (Fig. 2-21) and mono-amine oxidase. These reactions do not require pyridine nucleotides as coenzymes. In addition, at high pH, tetrazoles can accept hydrogen ions from —SH and ketol groups.

IMMUNOCYTOCHEMISTRY: ANTIGENS AND ANTIBODIES

Our understanding of the immune response in lymphatic organs and elsewhere in the body has been significantly advanced by the techniques of immunocytochemistry. The high specificity that resides in the mutual recognition of an antigen and its antibody makes these cytochemical identifications potentially the most precise. This powerful approach was introduced in 1941 by Albert H. Coons who, in essence, adapted immunologic procedures for use with tissue sections. *The technique is based on the use of a specific antibody that carries a label capable of being visualized.* In his highly original investigations, Coons conjugated a fluorescent dye in vitro with an antibody and thus labeled it without destroying its ability to form a complex with its antigen. The corresponding antigen could then be identified in tissue sections by ''staining'' with the fluorescein-labeled antibody and then studying the preparation with an ultraviolet microscope to localize the characteristic fluorescence of the dye-immune complex. Fewer molecules of a fluorescent dye are required for detection than of a visible dye, giving this method great sensitivity. A modification of this procedure allows recognition of the cells that produce antibody to a given antigen. Antibody is usually localized by an indirect approach which involves exposing the antibody-containing tissue section first to the corresponding antigen and then allowing the attached antigen to be ''stained'' with a fluorescein-labeled antibody. The specificity of the reaction is only as good as the purity of the antigen used for immunizing the animal that supplies the antibody. In addition, several types of control preparations are required to establish valid identifications.

The importance of immunocytochemistry extends beyond study of the immune response because it is theoretically possible to localize any *endogenous* protein that can be isolated and highly purified so that specific antibody can be prepared to it. Significant applications of immunocytochemistry to the identification and localization of endogenous proteins have already been made in relation to the origin and location of myosin in developing muscle (Holtzer, 1970); see Chap. 7, Figs. 7-15 and 7-16, and the cellular origin of the various protein hormones of the anterior pituitary (Nakane, 1967; see Chap. 27).

Ultrastructural localizations have also been effected by using antigens that can be seen with the electron microscope. The protein ferritin is identifiable ultrastructurally and has been used as an antigenic stimulus to identify antibody-producing cells (de Petris et al., 1963). The ferritin molecule (MW 650,000) contains ferric hydroxide micelles arranged in a tetrahedral lattice, so it is opaque to electrons and has a characteristic ultrastructure. When ferritin is introduced as an antigenic stimulus into the footpad of a rabbit, antibody to ferritin is produced by plasma cells in the popliteal lymph node; then exposure of tissue sections of lymph node to ferritin reveals the presence of antiferritin antibody in the cisternae of the rough endoplasmic reticulum, including the nuclear envelope, of the plasma cell. Ferritin has also been used as an ultrastructural tag for antibodies, in a manner comparable to the use of fluorescent dyes as labels in light microscopy.

Immunocytochemistry has recently received considerable impetus from the use of horseradish peroxidase (MW 44,000) as an antigenic stimulus and also as a label for antibody. The use of an enzymatic label on an antibody increases the sensitivity of the identification since relatively few enzyme molecules can generate considerable reaction product. A valuable cytochemical procedure[2] introduced by Graham and Karnovsky for identifying peroxidase activity, uses diaminobenzidine as an oxidizable substrate. An electron-opaque reaction product is yielded which allows ultrastructural localization (Fig. 2-22). Antibodies labeled with horseradish peroxidase and other enzymes have been used as sensitive identifiers of cellular antigens (Nakane, 1970), and it is evident that the use of enzyme-labeled antibodies will have wide application to biologic problems.

Radioautography

Radioautography is a cytochemical procedure for localizing sites of radioactivity within biologic specimens, usually by using tissue sections. An animal is injected with a biologically important molecule that is labeled with a radioactive isotope, usually tritium (^3H), an isotope of hydrogen that emits particles of low energy and thus short range. For example, thymidine-^3H is injected to label DNA for a study of cellular origin and turnover; to investigate protein synthesis, a tritiated amino acid is used; or for a study of glycogen synthesis, [^3H]-glucose serves as the precursor for this carbohydrate macromolecule (Fig. 2-14A and B). After appropriate time intervals, the animal is sacrificed and tissue sections are prepared for light and electron microscopy. Such radioactive precursors are rapidly incorporated into macromolecules which can be readily preserved in tissue sections. Then in a darkroom, a very thin layer of photographic emulsion (suspension of silver halide crystals in gelatin) is placed on top of the tissue section (Fig. 2-23). During the subsequent period of exposure, β particles are emitted from the sites of radioactivity, and some of them pass through the photographic emulsion and hit some of the silver halide crystals to produce a latent image (that is, small sites within a crystal where ionic silver is converted to metallic silver). After an appropriate interval of exposure, chemical development is used to convert

---

[2] It is important to mention that horseradish peroxidase has been effectively applied to cytochemical investigations of protein transport, since it can be readily visualized both in the light and electron microscopes (that is, Straus, 1964; Karnovsky, 1967).

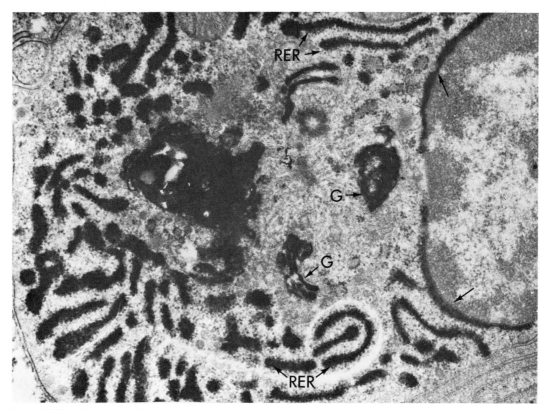

Figure 2-22   Ultrastructural localization of the antibody produced in response to the injection of horseradish peroxidase as an antigen. Local lymph nodes were fixed in paraformaldehyde, then exposed to a solution of horseradish peroxidase which binds specifically to its antibody: the procedure of Graham and Karnovsky was then used to visualize the enzymic activity of the anti-body-attached horseradish peroxidase; the reaction product was rendered electron-opaque by OsO_4.

In this immature plasma cell, antibody is located within the cisternae of the rough endoplasmic reticulum (RER) (including the perinuclear cisterna, see arrow), and also within the cisternae of the Golgi complex (G). ×23,000. (Leduc and Avrameas, Triangle, the Sandoz Journal of Medical Science, **9:**220, 1970.)

the entire silver halide crystal that has been hit by β particles into metallic silver (a true image). Finally, the unexposed crystals are dissolved out as silver thiosulfate complexes by the photographic fixer.

The reaction product is a pattern of metallic silver grains (Fig. 2-14A and B) which localizes the position of the isotope. A resolution of 0.1 μm can be achieved under good conditions, and this is certainly adequate for light microscopy. In the ultrastructural image, however, precise localization may require statistical analysis, since 0.1 μm can include a variety of structures. Resolution is influ-enced by geometric factors such as section and emulsion thickness, and also by the size of the silver halide crystal and the resulting developed grain.

Dynamic aspects of cellular and tissue morphology can be followed through radioautography, and many important concepts have been derived from such studies, only a few of which are noted here. Concepts of epithelial replacement, as in the gastro-intestinal tract, have been evolved from labeling dividing cell populations and following their subse-quent migration and differentiation. The first clue that galactosyl transferase might be an enzyme of the Golgi complex was obtained from the radio-

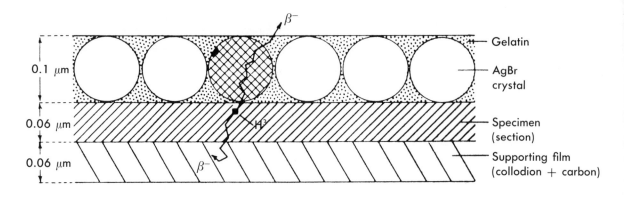

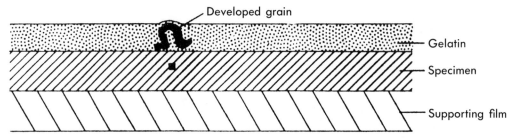

Figure 2-23   Diagram of a radioautographic preparation for electron microscopy.   Top.   A β particle emanating from a tritium source within a tissue section hits a silver halide crystal in the overlying gelatin photographic emulsion.   This exposure creates a latent image in that crystal.   Bottom.   After photographic processing, the exposed crystal has been converted to a true image of metallic silver (developed grain) whereas the unexposed crystals have been dissolved out by the hypo solution. (Caro).

autographic observation that galactose-^{3}H is incorporated in the Golgi region of intestinal goblet cells (Neutra and Leblond).   The site of macromolecular synthesis and the subsequent path of migration can be traced by ultrastructural radioautography, for example, the synthesis, storage, and secretion of digestive enzymes by the pancreatic acinar cell (Caro and Palade).

References

BARKA, T., and P. J. ANDERSON: "Histochemistry—Theory, Practice, and Bibliography," Hoeber-Harper, New York, 1963.

BARRNETT, R. J., and A. M. SELIGMAN: Histochemical Demonstration of Sulfhydryl and Disulfide Groups of Protein, *J. Nat. Cancer Inst.*, 14:769 (1954).

BERGERON, J. A., and M. SINGER: Metachromasy: An Experimental and Theoretical Reevaluation, *J. Biophys. Biochem. Cytol.*, 4:433 (1958).

BRADLEY, D. F., and M. K. WOLF: Aggregation of Dyes Bound to Polyanions, *Proc. Nat. Acad. Sci. USA*, **45:**944 (1959).

BURSTONE, M. S.: "Enzyme Histochemistry and its Application in the Study of Neoplasms," Academic, New York, 1962.

CARO, L. G.: High Resolution Autoradiography, in vol. 1 Chap. 16, David M. Prescott (ed.), "Methods in Cell Physiology," Academic, New York, 1964.

CARO, L. G., and G. E. PALADE: Protein Synthesis, Storage, and Discharge in the Pancreatic Exocrine Cell. A Radioautographic Study, *J. Cell Biol.*, **20:**473 (1964).

CONN, H. J.: "Biological Stains," 7th ed., Biotechnical Publications, Geneva, N.Y., 1965.

COONS, A. H.: Some Reactions of Lymphoid Tissues to Stimulation by Antigens, *Harvey Lectures*, Series L111, p. 113, 1959.

DEANE, H. W.: Intracellular Lipides: Their Detection and Significance, in S. L. Palay (ed.) "Frontiers in Cytology," Yale, New Haven, 1958.

DE PETRIS, S., G. KARLSBAD, and B. PERNIS: Localization of Antibodies in Plasma Cells by Electron Microscopy, *J. Exp. Med.*, **117:**849 (1963).

GOMORI, G.: "Microscopic Histochemistry," University of Chicago Press, Chicago, 1952.

GRAHAM, R. C., and M. J. KARNOVSKY: The Early Stages of Absorption of Injected Horseradish Peroxidase in the Proximal Tubules of Mouse Kidney: Ultrastructural Cytochemistry by a New Technique, *J. Histochem. Cytochem.*, **14:**291 (1966).

HOLTZER, H.: Proliferative and Quantal Cell Cycles in the Differentiation of Muscle, Cartilage, and Red Blood Cells, in H. A. Padykula (ed.), "Control Mechanisms in the Expression of Cellular Phenotypes," vol. 9, Sympos. Int. Soc. Cell Biol., Academic, New York, 1970.

KARNOVSKY, M. J.: The Ultrastructural Basis of Capillary Permeability Studied with Peroxidase as a Tracer, *J. Cell Biol.*, **35:**213 (1967).

KASTEN, F. H.: The Chemistry of the Schiff's Reagent, *Int. Rev. Cytol.*, **10:**1 (1960).

LEDUC, E. H., S. AVRAMEAS, and M. BOUTEILLE: Localization of Antibody in Plasma Cells by Electron Microscopy, *J. Exp. Med.*, **127:**109 (1968).

NACHLAS, M. M., A. C. YOUNG, and A. M. SELIGMAN: Problems of Enzymatic Localization by Chemical Reactions Applied to Tissue Sections, *J. Histochem. Cytochem.*, **5:**565 (1957).

NAKANE, P. K., and G. B. PIERCE, JR.: Enzyme-labeled Antibodies for the Light and Electron Microscopic Localization of Tissue Antigens, *J. Cell Biol.*, **33:**307 (1967).

NAKANE, P. K.: Classifications of Anterior Pituitary Cell Types with Immunoenzyme Histochemistry, *J. Histochem. Cytochem.*, **18:**9 (1970).

NEUTRA, M., and C. P. LEBLOND: Synthesis of the Carbohydrate of Mucus in the Golgi Complex, as Shown by Electron Microscopic Radioautography of Goblet Cells from Rats Injected with Glucose-H^3, *J. Cell Biol.*, **30:**119 (1966).

PEARSE, A. G. E.: "Histochemistry—Theoretical and Applied," vol. 1., 3d ed., Little, Brown, Boston, 1968.

ROSENTHAL, A. S., H. L. MOSES, C. E. GANOTE, and L. TICE: The Participation of Nucleotide in the Formation of Phosphatase Reaction Product: A Chemical and Electron Microscope Autoradiographic Study, *J. Histochem. Cytochem.*, **17:**839 (1969).

SABATINI, D. D., K. BENSCH, and R. J. BARRNETT: Cytochemistry and Electron Microscopy. The Preservation of Cellular Ultrastructure and Enzymatic Activity by Aldehyde Fixation, *J. Cell Biol.*, **17:**19 (1963).

SALPETER, M. M., L. BACHMANN, and E. E. SALPETER: Resolution in Electron Microscope Radioautography, *J. Cell Biol.*, **41:**1 (1969).

SINGER, M.: Factors Which Control the Staining of Tissue Sections with Acid and Basic Dyes, *Int. Rev. Cytol.*, **1:**211 (1951).

SPICER, S. S., T. J. LEPPI, and P. J. STOWARD: Suggestions for a Histochemical

Terminology of Carbohydrate-rich Tissue Components, *J. Histochem. Cytochem.*, **13:**599 (1965).

SPICER, S. S., R. G. HORN, and T. J. LEPPI: Histochemistry of Connective Tissue Mucopolysaccharides, Chap. 17 in "The Connective Tissue" Internat. Acad. Pathol. No. 7, Williams & Wilkins, Baltimore, 1967.

STRAUS, W.: Occurrence of Phagosomes and Phagolysosomes in Different Segments of the Nephron in Relation to the Reabsorption, Transport, Digestion and Extrusion of Intravenously Injected Horseradish Peroxidase, *J. Cell Biol.*, **21:**295 (1964).

SWIFT, H.: Cytochemical Techniques for Nucleic Acids, in E. Chargaff and J. N. Davidson (eds.), "The Nucleic Acids," vol. 2, Academic, New York, 1955.

chapter 3   Epithelium   ELIZABETH D. HAY

A *tissue* is defined by the histologist as a group of similar cells that work together to perform a role in the structuring and functioning of the body. For example, the tissue called muscle provides locomotion; nervous tissue integrates body activities; and connective tissue furnishes support and a source of mobile cells. *Epithelium* is the tissue that covers the free surfaces of the body, from the exposed external surface to the smallest free facets within the internal organs. The term, which was introduced in the eighteenth century by the Dutch anatomist Ruysch, probably refers to the fact that the tissue grows (G. *theleo*) upon (G. *epi*) another tissue. The cells are contiguous and rest upon a supporting extracellular layer, the *basement membrane*. There is very little intercellular material in the tissue. The free surface of the outer cells may exhibit small immobile cytoplasmic projections, called *microvilli,* and other structural specializations such as *cilia.* The total free surface of the tissue itself is frequently increased by means of folds,

tubules, and, in the intestine, by large multicellular projections called *villi.* The various epithelia of the adult originate from all three of the primary embryonic germ layers (ectoderm, mesoderm, endoderm).

The functions of the epithelia are related to the fact that the tissue usually lines free surfaces. *Protection* of underlying tissues is the main role of the epithelium covering the external surfaces and body orifices. *Surface transport* of mucus and other substances is performed by the ciliated epithelium which is found in the respiratory and genital ducts. The epithelium of the intestine, kidney, and certain other organs is concerned primarily with *absorption* and *secretion* of products into and from a lumen. The exocrine glands are devoted exclusively to the job of providing secretory materials that will reach a free surface. Most of the endocrine glands derive from epithelium, and in some cases the fundamental relation of the tissue to a free surface is retained (follicles of thyroid gland).

By virtue of their exposed position on free surfaces, epithelial cells are also natural candidates for a role in *sensory reception,* as in the case of the taste buds and olfactory mucosa.   Highly modified epithelia nourish and sustain the *reproductive cells* of the ovary and testis, but these very specialized epithelia will not be taken up in any detail in this chapter.

Classification of epithelia

An epithelium that consists of one cell layer is said to be *simple*.   A simple epithelium is usually found where transfer of materials must take place across the tissue, by secretion, absorption, or diffusion. On the other hand, the protective epithelia on exposed surfaces of the body are usually *stratified;* that is, they consist of two or more layers of cells. Simple epithelium is sometimes erroneously identified as stratified in oblique sections which pass through two or more adjacent cells.   It is a good idea to survey large areas of an epithelium before deciding that it is really stratified.

The simple and stratified epithelia are classified as *squamous, cuboidal,* or *columnar* according to the shape of the cells on the free surface of the tissue.   The cell form is actually more irregular than these terms imply, for the lateral cell surface usually has a dozen or more facets, and cell processes from adjacent cells often interdigitate to form numerous intercellular clefts.   In the stratified epithelium of the urinary tract, the shape of the cells varies continually as mechanical tension changes.   Nevertheless, the general differences in stratification and cell form make it convenient to subdivide the epithelia proper—that is, the sheets of contiguous cells lining free surfaces—into the following eight categories:

Simple epithelium

> Simple squamous epithelium
> Simple cuboidal epithelium
> Simple columnar epithelium
> Pseudostratified columnar epithelium

Stratified epithelium

> Stratified squamous epithelium
> Stratified cuboidal epithelium
> Stratified columnar epithelium
> Transitional epithelium

General structure and distribution of epithelia

SIMPLE SQUAMOUS EPITHELIUM

The cell in a simple squamous epithelium (Fig. 3-1) is shaped like a flat plate or "scale" (L. *squama*). Interdigitations of adjacent cell surfaces (Fig. 3-2) and specialized attachment plates along the cell facets keep the tissue intact as a sheet.   The *mesothelium* lining the body cavities and the *endothelium* of the blood and lymphatic vessels are simple squamous sheets of attenuated cells whose nuclei bulge into the lumen.   Good examples of simple squamous epithelium are also found in the air sacs of the lung, in the glomerulus and thin segment of the loop of Henle in the kidney, in the rete testis, and in certain small ducts of glands.

SIMPLE CUBOIDAL EPITHELIUM

A single-layered epithelium is said to be cuboidal if the height of each component cell is approximately equivalent to its width.   The increased height permits a more extensive development and more polarized arrangement of the cytoplasmic organelles.   Thus, it is not surprising to find that cuboidal cells often take a more active role in secretion and absorption than do the attenuated cells of the squamous epithelia.   The best examples of simple cuboidal epithelium in the adult occur in the kidney, ciliary body, and choroid plexus.   Many of the organs of the embryo are lined with a cuboidal type of epithelium (Figs. 3-1 and 3-3).

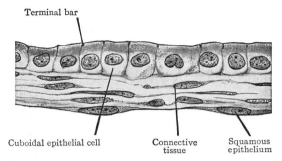

Terminal bar

Cuboidal epithelial cell   Connective   Squamous
                                     tissue   epithelium

Figure 3-1 Section showing simple squamous epithelium (below) and simple cuboidal epithelium (above) from adherent allantois and amnion of a pig embryo measuring 60 mm. At the surface of the allantois, terminal bars are evident. Zenker fixation; H&E.

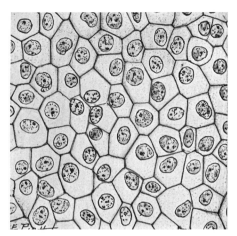

Figure 3-3   Surface view of allantois of a pig embryo. The cell outlines are more regular than those of the mesothelial cells in Fig. 3-2. The cell has on the average six lateral facets, and at each corner three cells meet.

SIMPLE COLUMNAR EPITHELIUM

The cells comprising a simple columnar epithelium are usually tall and prismatic in shape. The height exceeds the width of the cell. The absorptive epithelia of the intestine and the ciliated epithelia lining the uterine tubes and small bronchi of the lung are typical examples of simple columnar epithelium (Fig. 3-4). There are, of course, cells whose shape is intermediate between those of the typical columnar and typical cuboidal cells. The secretory cells of the exocrine glands are mostly low columnar or pyramidal in shape. In the thyroid gland and seminal vesicles, the epithelial cells vary in height from low cuboidal to columnar, depending on the degree

of hormonal stimulation. In general, the taller the gland cell, the more polarized the arrangement of its organelles and the greater its secretory activity are.

PSEUDOSTRATIFIED COLUMNAR EPITHELIUM

When a simple columnar epithelium lines a large tube, an additional layer of less differentiated cells

Figure 3-2   Surface view of mesothelial cells of cat mesentery. The cell outlines are demonstrated by silver nitrate impregnation. The serrated facets of the cells interdigitate extensively.

Figure 3-4   Section of simple columnar epithelium from intestinal mucosa of Necturus. The epithelial cells are of two types: (a) cells that absorb foodstuffs, (b) goblet-shaped cells that secrete mucus.

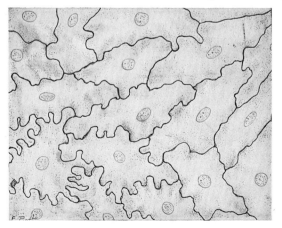

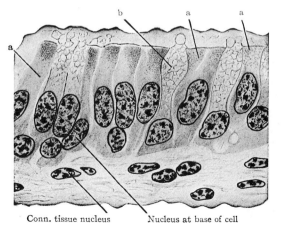

Conn. tissue nucleus   Nucleus at base of cell

is often added to the basal region (Fig. 3-5). The tissue usually does not become truly stratified. A careful dissection would reveal that the differentiated surface cells have retained their attachment to the basement membrane, even though their nuclei lie at different levels in the tissue. Such an epithelium is regarded as pseudostratified and is much more common than the truly multilayered columnar type. Pseudostratified columnar epithelium with cilia lines the large ducts of the respiratory tract, including the trachea, large bronchi, and much of the pharynx. Pseudostratified columnar epithelium also occurs in the vas deferens and epididymis, the male urethra, and large ducts of glands.

STRATIFIED SQUAMOUS EPITHELIUM

True stratification of an epithelium provides a complete basal layer of proliferating cells. The cells that will replace the superficial layer differentiate in the intermediate regions of the epithelium. The disadvantage is that the outer cells are displaced away from the vascular system in the underlying connective tissue. A ciliated or secretory cell on an epithelial surface might not function well if it were so far removed from its source of nutrition.

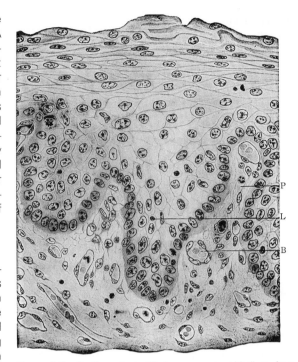

Figure 3-6   Section of stratified squamous epithelium from human esophagus. The cells are flattened at the surface, large and polygonal in the intermediate regions, and small and cuboidal at the base of the epithelium. The connective tissue under the epithelium forms projections (such as P) which are called papillae (L., nipple). Blood vessels are prominent in the connective tissue (such as B), but they do not extend into the epithelium. Cell L is a small lymphocyte that is migrating through the epithelium.

Figure 3-5   Pseudostratified columnar epithelium from the human trachea. All the cells rest upon the basement membrane, but not all reach the surface. The lateral cell membranes are difficult to distinguish. Three goblet cells are present, and three lymphocytes are seen migrating between the ciliated epithelial cells.

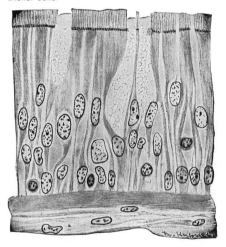

It is not surprising, then, to find that most of the truly multilayered epithelia in the adult are stratified squamous epithelia (Fig. 3-6) whose growing basal cells are cuboidal or even columnar in form, but whose *outer cells* are flattened and relatively inert metabolically.

In regions exposed to air, the outer cells lose their nuclei and transform into keratinized plates (skin). In regions covered with fluid (cornea, esophagus, mouth, vagina), the superficial cells generally do not lose their nuclei. Such epithelium is spoken of as *nonkeratinized* to distinguish it from the *keratinized* epithelium of the skin. The difference, however, is merely one of degree, since keratin occurs in both types of stratified squamous epithelia.

STRATIFIED CUBOIDAL AND STRATIFIED COLUMNAR EPITHELIUM

The two-layered epithelium of the sweat gland ducts and the epithelium in intermediate zones of the anal canal, conjunctiva, and female urethra are sometimes classified as stratified cuboidal, because the superficial cells are shaped more like cubes than squames.

Stratified columnar epithelium occurs in the intermediate zones between pseudostratified columnar epithelium and stratified squamous epithelium in the larynx, pharynx, and ducts of large glands (mammary, parotid). It is distinguished with difficulty from the more common pseudostratified columnar epithelium; if the plane of sectioning is perpendicular to the long axis of the cells, the regular appearance of the outer row of cells can be used as an identifying characteristic of the stratified epithelium. Both stratified cuboidal and stratified columnar epithelia occur more extensively in the embryo (Fig. 3-7) than in the adult.

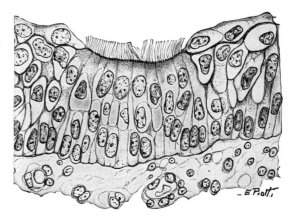

Figure 3-7 A section of stratified epithelium from the esophagus of a 4-month-old human fetus. In the central portion the superficial cells are ciliated and columnar, whereas laterally the epithelium is stratified cuboidal.

TRANSITIONAL EPITHELIUM

The arrangement of the cells in transitional epithelium is a truly remarkable adaptation for the special tensions that may develop in the bladder, ureters, and upper part of the urethra. When the bladder is relaxed, the multilayered epithelium resembles a nonkeratinized stratified squamous or cuboidal type. The large surface cells are round and bulge into the lumen; the basal cells are smaller and they interdigitate with the overlying cells. It was once believed that the cells slide past each other to become a flattened, seemingly simple layer when the wall is stretched. It now seems more likely that the cells do not move over one another during distension of the organ but only become more flattened, with less interdigitation of cell processes.

The interdigitations of cell processes and folding of the luminal surface that occur in transitional epithelium are best appreciated in electron micrographs (Fig. 3-8). The cells rest on a connective tissue substratum which is not organized into rigid layers, for it also must be adapted to stretching. A rather unusual feature of the cytoplasm of bladder epithelium is the presence of numerous membrane-bounded oblong vacuoles (inset, Fig. 3-8). These may serve as reservoirs of membranous material for expansion of the cell surface, or perhaps they play a role in water exchange across the epithelium.

Cytological features of epithelia

The most fundamental property of epithelial cells is their tendency to cover surfaces and maintain closely knit sheets. Structural specializations of the cytoplasm and the *lateral and basal surfaces* of the cells help to maintain cell contiguity and to give strength to the epithelial sheets. Such specializations are particularly well developed in epithelia that have a protective role, as in the skin and oral mucosa. The keratin of the epidermis protects the body surface from desiccation and abrasion. The dense tonofibrils and terminal webs of the superficial cells in the stratified squamous and transitional epithelia also protect against abrasion. Simple epithelia subject to wear and tear likewise have a tough superficial *cytoskeleton*, as in the gastrointestinal tract. Secretory and absorptive cells and ciliated cells usually have a highly specialized *free surface* and are more strikingly *polarized*. The lat-

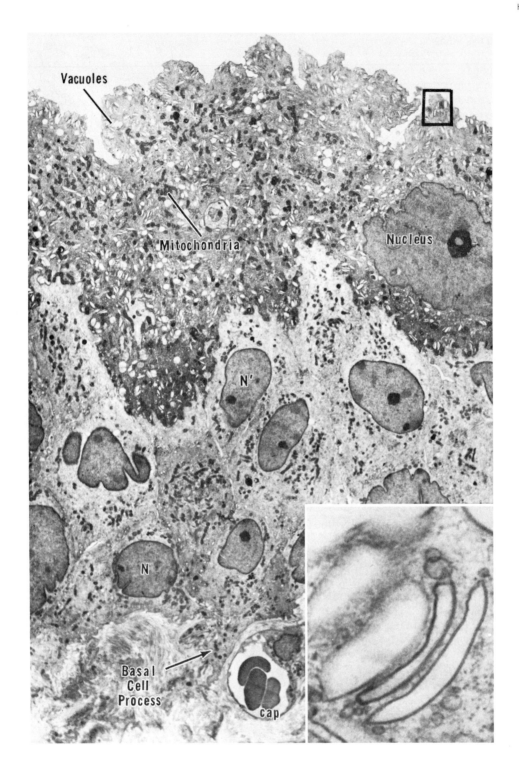

Vacuoles

Mitochondria

Nucleus

N'

N

Basal
Cell
Process

cap

eral surface may also be greatly modified by extensive interdigitations. In the discussion below, the various cytological features of the epithelial cells and their immediate environment will be considered in the following order:

1. Specializations of the lateral surface
2. The cytoskeleton
3. Specializations of the basal surface
4. Specializations of the free surface
5. Polarity of the cells

SPECIALIZATIONS OF THE LATERAL SURFACE

Intercellular junctions Epithelial cells are linked on their lateral surfaces by several kinds of intercellular junctions. Two of these contribute greatly to the strength of the adhesion between the cells and are called adhering junctions: (1) the *macula adhaerens* or *desmosome,* which is plate-shaped and is widely distributed along the intercellular facets; and (2) the *zonula adhaerens,* which is belt-shaped and occurs around the juxtaluminal border of certain epithelia where it is the principal component of the *terminal bar.* A third type of junction, the *zonula occludens,* seals the intercellular space from contact with the lumen, and a fourth, the *gap junction* or *nexus,* seems to play a role in intercellular communication.

Maculae adhaerentes (desmosomes) are particularly well developed in the epidermis, where they occur on intercellular bridges between the cells (D, Fig. 3-9). There was considerable debate among light microscopists as to whether or not the cytoplasm of adjacent cells was continuous through the bridges containing the desmosomes. Microdissection studies by Chambers and Rényi showed the desmosome to be a point of very strong attachment at the very least. Electron-microscopic studies have now demonstrated that the intercellular bridge

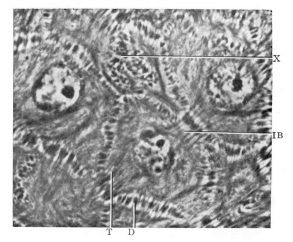

Figure 3-9   Light micrograph showing desmosomes (D) and tonofibrils (T) in stratified squamous epithelium. Tonofibrils course through the cells and into the intercellular "bridges" (IB). The midpoint of each bridge is marked by a dense body known as a desmosome. At X, the desmosomes are cut in cross section. Buccal epithelium. Zenker Formalin fixation, photographed unstained under a phase-contrast microscope. ×1,500. (Courtesy of P. H. Ralph.)

is not a region of actual cytoplasmic continuity between cells (Fig. 3-10). The intercellular space, however, is narrow (about 200 Å) between the two halves of the desmosomes and is filled by extracellular material of low density, often bisected by an electron-opaque central or intermediate line (arrow, Figs. 3-11 and 3-12). Both the extracellular intermediate line and the amorphous material are believed to contain sialic acid, acid mucopolysaccharide, and protein which together presumably act as a glue. The most characteristic intracellular morphologic feature of the desmosome is the dense *attachment plaque* in the cytoplasm next to each apposed plasma membrane (DP, Figs. 3-11 and 3-12). Tonofilaments (see Cytoskeleton) are inserted into the attachment plaque. Within

Figure 3-8   Low-magnification electron micrograph of transitional epithelium from empty bladder of a mouse. The superficial cells in transitional epithelium are large and vary from cuboidal to squamous in shape, depending on the degree to which the bladder is distended. The surface cells of the mouse bladder (above) have large nuclei and are probably polyploid. Superficial cells are characterized by the presence of numerous mitochondria and oblong vacuoles. Several of these vacuoles are shown at high magnification in the inset. The square on the larger picture indicates approximately the area that appears in the inset. The nuclei of the cells in the intermediate layer (N') and basal layer (N) are diploid and are smaller than nuclei in the superficial layer. A basal cell process extends into the connective tissue near a capillary (cap). Osmium fixation; lead tartrate stain. ×1,600; inset, ×50,000. (Courtesy of J. Rhodin.)

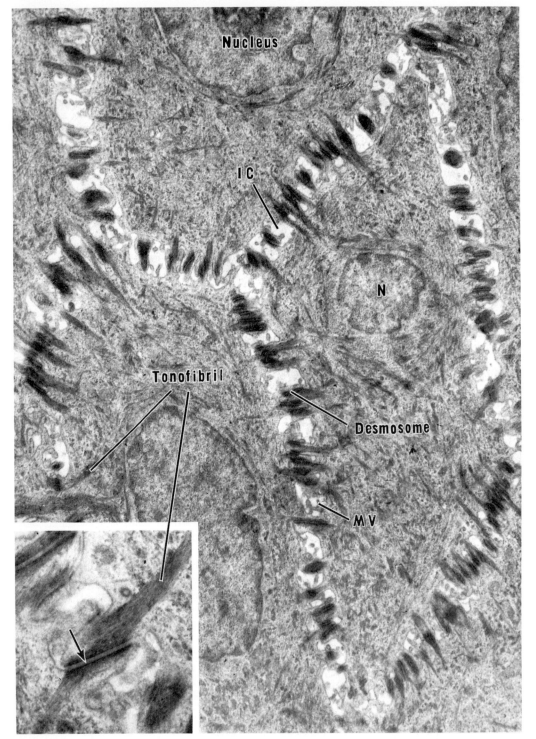

Figure 3-10   Electron micrograph of tonofibrils and desmosomes in stratified squamous epithelium of human oral mucosa.   The desmosome is resolved as consisting of two dense attachment plates into which the tonofibrils of adjacent cells insert.   The tonofibrils do not pass from cell to cell; the intercellular space, however, is very narrow between the two "halves" of the desmosome. One of the opposed plasmalemmas is labeled here (arrow, inset).   The lateral surface of the epithelial cells have a few microvilli (MV) which project into the interfacial canals (IC).   Osmium fixation.   ×10,000; inset, ×30,000.   (Courtesy of M. A. Listgarten.)

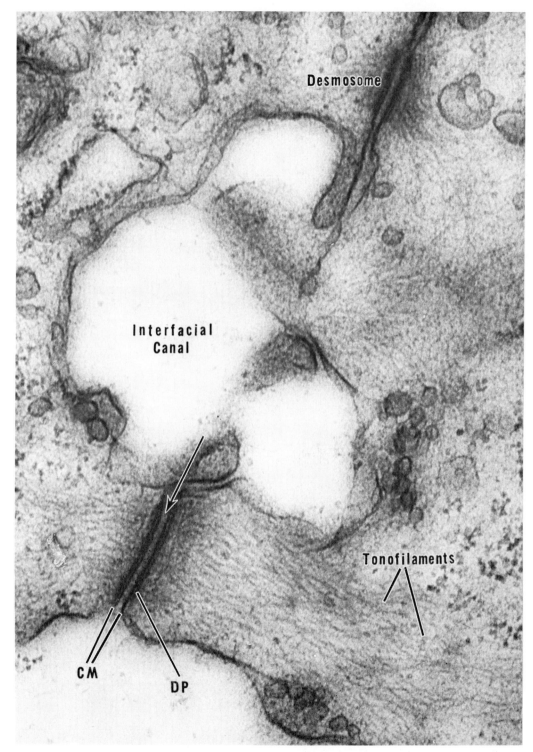

Figure 3-11 Electron micrograph at higher magnification showing two desmosomes and a large interfacial canal in salamander epidermis. A plaque of dense intracellular material (DP) is seen subjacent to the cell membrane (CM) on each side of the desmosome. The rather vague electron-opaque "line" (arrow) in the intercellular space may represent condensed ground substance. The component filaments of the tonofibril (tonofilaments) are resolved clearly at this magnification. They appear to be firmly anchored in the cytoplasm adjacent to the dense plaques of the desmosomes. Osmium fixation; lead hydroxide stain. ×75,000.

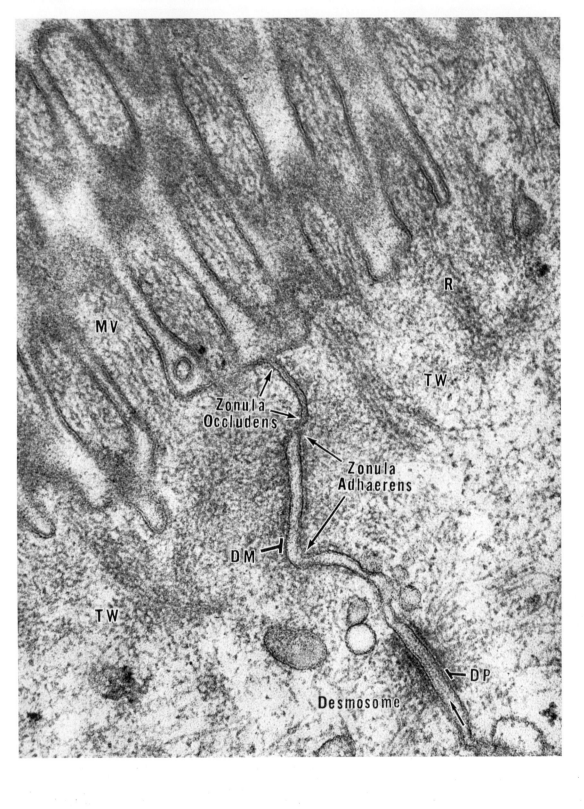

the plaque, each filament makes a hairpin loop and then passes back into the cytoplasm. Desmosomes can be broken by the enzymes trypsin, collagenase, and hyaluronidase; they are also sensitive to ethylenediaminetetraacetic acid (EDTA) and low levels of calcium. The intracellular attachment plaques can be digested by pepsin and chymotrypsin and thus are probably rich in protein. The bipartite structure of desmosomes is demonstrated by their mode of development. In the embryonic corneal epithelium, hemidesmosomes have been described as forming first between the cells; the halves are subsequently joined to make whole desmosomes.

The *zonula adhaerens* surrounding the lateral surface of epithelial cells near the junction of their luminal borders is similar in some respects to the desmosome (Fig. 3-12). The apposed cell membranes are separated by a very regular extracellular space, 200 Å wide, in the contact zone. The dense extracellular intermediate line of the macula adhaerens is not found in the zonula adhaerens. A well-developed attachment plaque does not occur, but a moderately dense material associated with filaments of the *terminal web* is usually present in the cytoplasm next to the plasmalemma of the adjacent cells (DM, Fig. 3-12). This cytoplasmic component of the zonula adhaerens probably contributes to the darkly staining, or chromophilic, component of the terminal bar that can be visualized with the light microscope around the luminal borders of epithelial cells (Fig. 3-1).

The outermost component of the terminal bar can only be appreciated with the electron microscope and is called the *zonula occludens*. At low magnification, the zonula occludens may appear to be an area where the outer leaflets of the plasma membranes of the apposed cells are broadly fused (Fig. 3-12). Higher-magnification micrographs of

thin sections show that membranes are in contact only at points within the zonula occludens (arrows, inset, Fig. 3-13). These close contacts have been called tight junctions because outer leaflets of the two apposed membranes appear as a single line and the total distance between inner leaflets is less than the sum of the width of two membranes, suggesting that the membranes really do fuse at these points. Freeze-cleave preparations reveal the three-dimensional disposition of the seemingly punctate contacts. Each contact point in fact represents a tiny ridge that, together with other ridges, forms an anastomosing network (Figs. 3-13 and 3-14). The zonula occludens network extends completely around the apical border of the cell to seal the underlying intercellular clefts from contact with the outside environment. Electron-dense tracers placed in the tissue space do not reach the free surface of the tissue (Fig. 3-15C). Interestingly, such a tracer may pass into the zonula occludens between incomplete ridges, but it is invariably stopped by the final ridge in the assembly before it reaches the cell surface. Alternatively, one can place an electron-dense tracer in the lumen and show that the material cannot penetrate directly into the extracellular space within the epithelium.

The term *junctional complex* is used to refer to the assortment of cell junctions along the lateral interfaces next to the lumen of an epithelium. In simple columnar epithelia subjected to wear and tear, such as the intestinal epithelium, the junctional complex is especially well developed and includes, in addition to the belt-like zonula adhaerens and the zonula occludens, a band of desmosomes (Figs. 3-12 and 3-17). In other epithelia, the zonula occludens may be the only component of the junctional complex present at the luminal border (Figs. 3-13 and 3-14). In some

---

Figure 3-12   Electron micrograph of the junctional complex between two epithelial cells of the rat intestine. The tight junction (zonula occludens) and the intermediate junction (zonula adhaerens) form an attachment belt which extends around the luminal surfaces of the cells. A row of desmosomes disposed under the zonula adhaerens may be present as a third component of the junctional complex. The terminal bar visualized by the light microscope corresponds to the zonula occludens and zonula adhaerens together. A dense material (DM) is usually associated with the cell membranes in attachment belts. It is similar to but not so well developed as the dense plaque (DP) of the desmosome. Intercellular material (arrow) also is more prominent in the desmosome. The terminal web (TW) is a filamentous meshwork in the apical cytoplasm of columnar and cuboidal cells. Anchoring filaments (R) extend into the web from the cores of the microvilli (MV) of intestinal cells. Osmium fixation; stained with lead hydroxide.   ×100,000.   (Courtesy of M. G. Farquhar and G. E. Palade.)

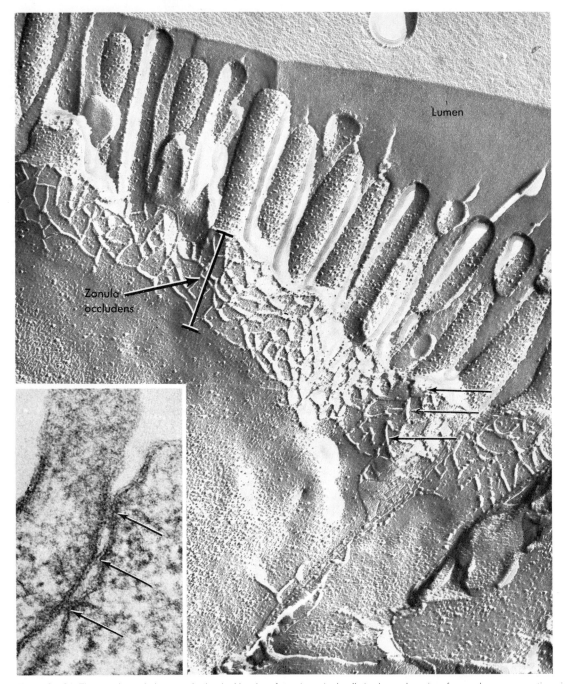

Figure 3-13 The zonula occludens on the luminal border of two intestinal cells is shown here in a freeze-cleave preparation viewed in the electron microscope. Numerous microvilli broken in different planes can be seen across the top of the cells. It is believed that the cell membrane cleaves through the middle, thus exposing the two inside surfaces of the plasmalemma. The surface viewed in this electron micrograph is studded with many small particles and therefore is probably the outside surface (face A) of the inner lamella (LM 1) of the plasma membrane (Fig. 3-14). The ridges (arrows, main picture) correspond to what in thin section appear to be points of tight contact (arrows, inset). An electron-dense marker, such as lanthanum entering from below, can penetrate partly into the zonula occludens by passing between incomplete ridges, but it is eventually stopped before it reaches the lumen (Fig. 3-15C). Were the other cleaved surface of the plasmalemma visible (face B), it would be seen generally to be smooth except for a few particles and, in the area of the zonula occludens, rows of indentations (Fig. 3-14). ×75,000 (Courtesy of J. P. Revel); inset ×200,000 (Courtesy of R. L. Trelstad, E. D. Hay, and J. P. Revel.)

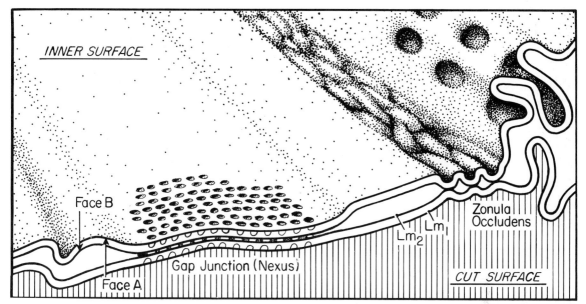

INNER SURFACE

Face B

Gap Junction (Nexus)

Face A

Lm₂ Lm₁ Lm

Zonula
Occludens

CUT SURFACE

Figure 3-14   This diagram depicts the junctional specializations adjacent to the bile canaliculus (BC) of a liver cell.   The bile canaliculus is an example of an intercellular canaliculus (Fig. 3-27); it represents an extension of the free surface between two cells for the purpose of collecting secretory products.   As for any free surface, a zonula occludens seals the adjacent lateral cleft. In routine sections, the zonula occludens is seen as a series of tiny membrane contacts immediately adjacent to the free surface. In three dimensions (inner surface, above), it is represented by a web-like array of ridges.   The gap junction, or nexus, is seen in routine sections as an area of close membrane apposition where the outer leaflets of the apposed cell membranes are separated by a very regular 20 Å gap.   The so-called gap is filled by a polygonal array of subunits located in the narrow extracellular space. Freeze-cleave techniques reveal additional subunits within each apposed plasma membrane adjacent to the subunits in the extracellular gap (see Fig. 3-15).   The artist has taken some freedom in depicting the inner surface of the cell above.   Freeze-cleave preparations view the outer side (face A) of the inner leaflet (LM 1) or inner face (face B) of the outer leaflet (LM 2) of the plasmalemma, and so the real inner cell surface is probably never visualized.   (Diagram based on an unpublished illustration by D. A. Goodenough.)

epithelia, even the zonula occludens seems to be poorly developed or absent; the rather permeable endothelium lining capillaries is an example of this kind.   Sometimes the terms *terminal bar* and *junctional complex* are used synonymously, but this is not quite correct because the terminal bar is the belt-like zone around the lateral surface of epithelial cells which can be visualized in the light microscope after appropriate staining.   It probably corresponds principally to the zonula adhaerens and zonula occludens (Fig. 3-17), whereas the junctional complex is any combination of one or more juxtaluminal contacts.   Since the zonula occludens and zonula adhaerens are specializations of the juxtaluminal surface of epithelia, they obviously do not occur as such in tissues lacking a lumen.   However, the intercalated disc of cardiac muscle is so similar to

an epithelial-adhering junction that it has been called a *fascia adhaerentes*.   Moreover, punctate tight junctions have been described in sections of connective tissue cells and incompletely developed desmosomes occur in fibroblasts, cardiac muscle, and possibly other cell types.

Still another kind of junction has now been demonstrated in epithelium and in all other tissues that exhibit electrotonic coupling between component cells.   Termed a *gap junction,* or *nexus*, this contact specialization is a rather large plate-like junction which occurs on the deep lateral surfaces of epithelial cells.   It has been widely misnamed a tight junction because the minute gap (20 Å wide) between apposed cell membranes is obscured by the lead stains routinely used in electron microscopy, thus giving the false impression that the outer regions of the membranes are fused in the area. However, the distance between the inner leaflets of the apposed membranes is greater than the width of two fused membranes. In thin sections stained with uranyl acetate and viewed at high magnification, the so-called *gap* can be seen (arrows, Fig. 3-15A). The fact that the outer leaflets of the plasma membranes are not fused in this widely distributed junction has now been conclusively demonstrated with electron-dense tracers. Tracers such as lanthanum or peroxidase can and do penetrate into the gap (Fig. 3-15B). The presence of such a tracer, interestingly, reveals the existence of an unexpected subunit within the gap, which accounts for its highly uniform width. In preparations treated with lanthanum, the minute subunit is revealed in areas where the plane of section passes tangential to the plasma membrane (Fig. 3-15B). The term *gap junction* initially used to describe these contacts, then, is incorrect in the sense that the term implies that a blank space separates the membranes. Each of the extracellular subunits is arranged hexagonally around the others and each contains a central density (arrow, Fig. 3-15B). The distance from the center of one subunit to the next is 90 Å. Lipids occur in these junctions and acetone dissolves the hexagonal extracellular component, thereby obliterating the 20 Å gap. Goodenough and Revel (1970) have suggested that protein and carbohydrate as well as lipid are the structural components of the polygonal lattice. With the freeze-cleave technique, moreover, it can be shown that still another polygonal lattice exists in the gap junction, within the plasma membrane of each apposing cell (Fig. 3-16). These subunits appear as small particles, and again, the distance between the centers of the subunits is 90 Å. Thus, it is likely that the particles within the plasma membrane are situated in some definite relationship to the acetone-extractable subunits within the extracellular gap.

The gap junction, or nexus, has received particular attention recently because of the possibility that it is the principal or even the only junction which mediates electrical (electrotonic) coupling between cells. Furshpan and Potter (1968) and Loewenstein (1967) have shown that most normal epithelial cells are electrically coupled by placing a stimulating electrode in one cell and a recording electrode in an adjacent cell. Current passed through the first electrode meets less resistance going from cell to cell than it would if it had gone via the surrounding extracellular space. Electrical coupling between cells does not imply that currents normally are passing from one cell to the other, but rather shows that regions exist for preferential exchange of small ions between cells. Moreover, there is now evidence that molecules of large dimensions (up to 10,000 MW) can pass preferentially from one cell to the other, presumably through gap junctions. It has been speculated that the small hole in the middle of the subunit (arrow, Fig. 3-15B) is the pore through which molecules flow. The gap junction seems to mediate impulse transmission in electrical synapses within the nervous system and may have a similar function in smooth and cardiac muscle. The myocardium beats and electrotonic coupling between heart cells persists as long as gap junctions are intact, even though desmosomes and intercalated discs are disrupted by calcium removal. When cells tear away from each other, the gap junctions do not split in half but go with one cell or the other, and coupling is lost. Loewenstein (1967) has stressed the correla-

Figure 3-15   Fine structure of the gap junction as seen in thin sections. A. Two trilaminar unit membranes are closely apposed along most of their length in this view. A gap 20 Å wide can be made out between the outer leaflets of the two apposed membranes (arrows). B. A section at the same magnification showing tissue which had been soaked in lanthanum while fixing. The electron-dense marker has filled the extracellular space and penetrated the gap junction. The junction is cut tangential to the cell membrane along part of its length, and this plane of section reveals the hexagonally arrayed subunits that occupy the gap. The electron-dense dye has penetrated around the subunits, making them easy to see. The significance of the dot in the center of each 90 Å subunit (arrow) is unknown; it could mark the location of a tiny canal linking the cells. C. A lower-magnification view of a section of a piece of liver that had been soaked in lanthanum while fixing. The bile canaliculus at the top of the figure is an extension of free surface between two cells. The electron-dense marker, which entered from below, has passed around the gap junction cut tangentially near the bottom of the figure. It penetrated the zonula occludens, presumably through incomplete ridges in the zonula meshwork, but it was finally stopped by the outermost tight contact (arrow). A and B, ×300,000; (Courtesy of A. J. Hudspeth and J. P. Revel.) C, ×170,000; (Courtesy of D. A. Goodenough and J. P. Revel.)

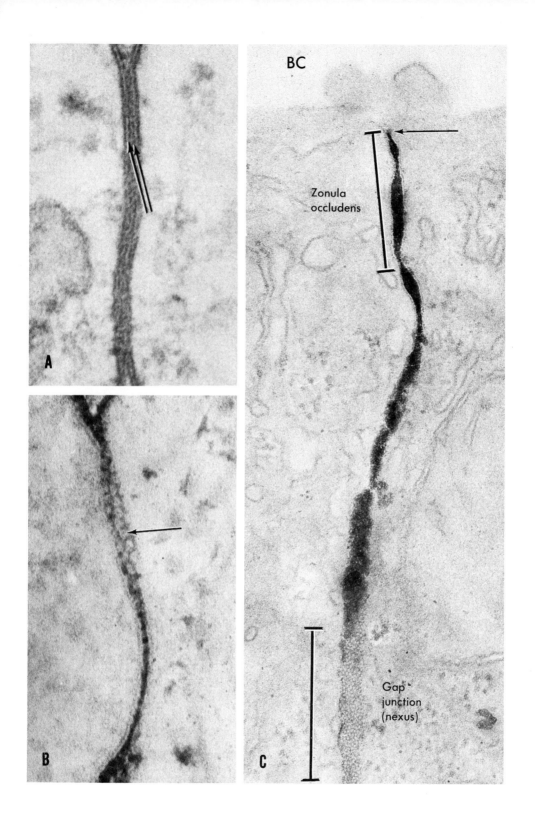

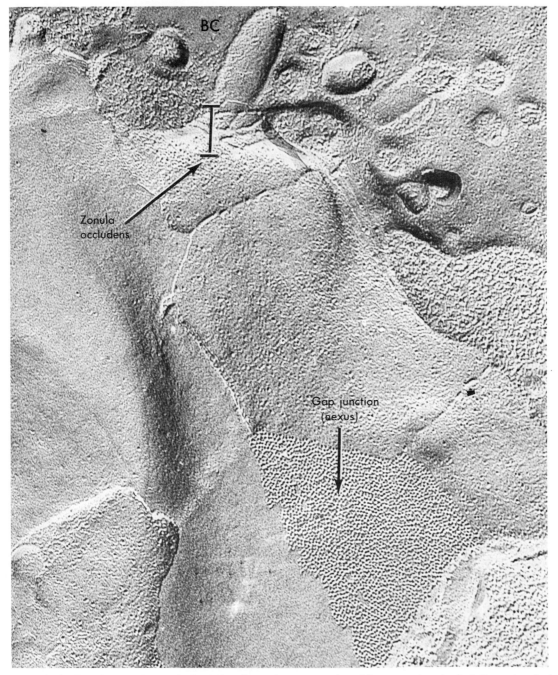

Figure 3-16   This electron micrograph shows, in a freeze-cleave preparation of liver, a portion of cell similar to that depicted in Fig. 3-15C. The bile canaliculus (BC) at the top of the picture is flanked by microvilli cleaved longitudinally and obliquely. The small part of the zonula occludens included in the plane of cleavage can be seen to have a typical web-like structure. Several microns below the luminal surface, a gap junction (nexus) can be seen. The surface of the membrane visualized above is the outer side (face A) of the inner leaflet (LM 1); it contains numerous closely packed particles that are more evident when the micrograph is viewed in the proper orientation, which is upside down from the way it is mounted here (carbon was sprayed onto the cleaved surface from above). The particles in the membranes of the nexus are spaced approximately 90 Å apart, as are the subunits visible in the extracellular space, or so-called gap (Fig. 3-15B and C). It is likely that each particle within the plasmalemma is situated next to one of the subunits within the extracellular space.   ×90,000; (Courtesy of J. P. Revel.)

tion between loss of intercellular communication of this kind and neoplasia, and he has also presented evidence that electrical coupling accompanies contact inhibition of movement when migrating cells meet during wound repair.

The lateral extracellular compartment   The lateral extracellular compartment in many epithelia is narrow (200 to 300 Å), even in regions lacking junctions, suggesting there are invisible bonds holding the cells together along their entire opposed surfaces. Such bonds may be contributed by the mucopolysaccharides demonstrated by Leblond to coat all the surfaces of the cells, and they may even be the same bonds that bring disaggregated epithelial cells together so specifically. In some epithelia, the lateral extracellular compartment may be quite large in its dimension. In stratified squamous epithelia, for example, the intercellular spaces are so dilated they are referred to as *interfacial canals* (Figs. 3-10 and 3-11). It is likely that nutrients are circulated to the middle of the thickened epithelium through these canals between the cell facets. It is a characteristic of true epithelia that neither blood nor lymphatic vessels are present between the cells. White blood cells and macrophages can be found migrating through the intercellular spaces of epithelia on exposed surfaces of the body, particularly in the oral mucosa. Processes of unmyelinated sensory nerves extend into the interfacial canals of the epithelium of the cornea and the lip.

Interdigitation of lateral cell processes occurs to some extent in all epithelia and probably contributes to contiguity. In stratified squamous epithelia subjected to abrasion, the desmosomes are dispersed along interlocking lateral cell processes (Fig. 3-10), an arrangement which may help to spare the plasmalemma from shearing forces. In the kidney, particularly in the distal renal tubule, the epithelial cells interdigitate so extensively with one another that it is difficult to tell where one cell ends and the next begins. The interdigitations of renal tubule cells enormously increase the lateral surface membrane, which presumably plays a role in water and salt transfer across the cells. Salt-secreting cells in birds have the same highly elaborate interdigitating cell processes, and so do the cells of the secretory ducts of salivary glands and sweat glands

and the lining epithelium of the ciliary body, gall bladder, and choroid plexus. Diamond (1964) has postulated a standing osmotic gradient between such epithelial cells caused by active pumping of sodium by the cells from the lumen into the intercellular space. He suggests that osmotic pressure causes water to flow passively across the cells into the same space. Transport of water out of the epithelium into underlying capillaries is thought to result from hydrostatic pressure caused by swelling of the water-filled extracellular compartment. Kaye et al. (1966) have shown by electron microscopy that the extracellular clefts become enormously dilated during water transport by the gall bladder epithelium.

Intercellular canaliculi often connect the lateral facets of secretory epithelial cells to the free surface (Figs. 3-17 and 3-27). They are bounded by a zonula occludens which seals the rest of the lateral extracellular compartment from contact with their contents. Within such a canaliculus (BC, Fig. 3-14), microvilli project as on a typical free surface. Thus, the intercellular canaliculus is really an extension of the free surface into the tissue.

CYTOSKELETON

It is tempting to think that mechanical tension developing at the desmosome or terminal bar is not borne by the cell membrane alone but is transmitted to the tough fibrous elements of the cytoplasm. Cytoplasmic filaments approximately 50 Å in diameter form thick bundles called *tonofibrils* in stratified squamous epithelia (Fig. 3-10). The filaments are developed to some extent in most epithelial cells, and they usually insert into the dense placodes of the desmosomes (Fig. 3-11). The *terminal web* in the apical cytoplasm of the intestinal absorptive cell is composed of a meshwork of small filaments, which seem to be attached to the zonula adhaerens (TW, Fig. 3-12). The individual cytoplasmic filaments have been called *tonofilaments*, and they comprise what might be termed the cytoskeleton of the epidermal cell (see Chap. 1). They are responsible for the birefringence of epidermal cells and are probably composed of the fibrous protein keratin in its less highly cross-linked form. This fibrous protein is rich in sulfhydryl, whereas the true keratin of the outer cornified layers of the epidermis contains disulfide bonds (see Chap. 16).   On the other hand, the small filaments in the intestinal microvilli may be composed of actin.   The tonofilaments of the epidermis, the small filaments of the terminal web, and other cytoplasmic filaments 50 Å or less in diameter may be considered together as *microfila-*ments, but they probably comprise a heterogeneous class with respect to protein composition and possible function.   In addition to microfilaments, *microtubules* help maintain the shape of some epithelial cells and thus can be classified as part of the cytoskeleton (Chap. 1).

Figure 3-17   Diagram illustrating the principal surface specializations that would be found on a simple columnar epithelial cell. The junctional complex at the luminal surface consists of a zonula occludens and zonula adhaerens (together they form a terminal bar) and a row of desmosomes.   Under the row of desmosomes, gap junctions occur.   Other desmosomes and gap junctions are located deeper in the tissue.   The intercellular canaliculi are bound off from the rest of the lateral cell compartment by zonulae occludentes.   Canaliculi are, in fact, extensions of the free surface and communicate with it.   Microvilli therein and on the free surface are covered with a glycoprotein "fuzzy" coat.   The basal surface of the cell rests on another glycoprotein layer called the basement or basal lamina, which is the main component of the basement membrane.

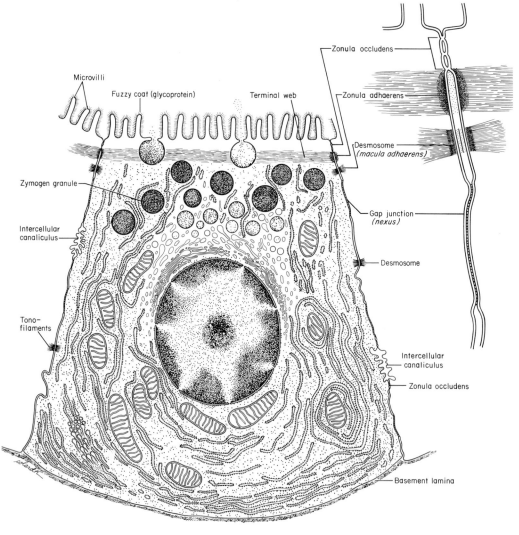

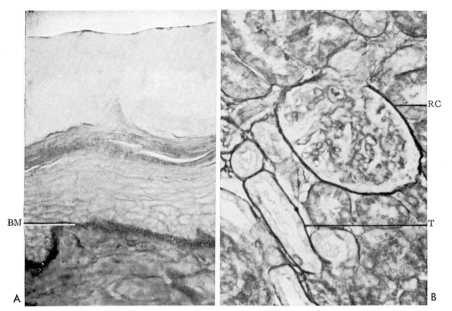

Figure 3-18   Basement membranes taken from different sites in adult monkey tissue and viewed with the light microscope.   × 300. A. Palmar skin, showing thick basement membrane (BM) underlying epidermis: stained by the PAS procedure for carbohydrate-containing complexes.   B. Kidney, showing relatively thin membranes around renal corpuscles (RC) and various tubules (T): stained by Pap's ammoniacal–silver nitrate method, illustrating the argyrophilia of reticular fibers in basement membranes.   (Courtesy of H. W. Deane.)

SPECIALIZATIONS OF THE BASAL SURFACE

The *basement membrane* is an extracellular condensation of mucopolysaccharide and proteins that occurs under the basal surface of all epithelia (Fig. 3-18).   It reaches its greatest width under epithelia that are subject to abrasion, such as the epidermis.   In addition to providing support, the basement membrane undoubtedly serves as a semipermeable filter under the epithelium.   Its most consistent component is a dense filamentous sheet 500 to 1,000 Å thick, called the *basement lamina* (*basal lamina*).   This layer seems attached to the plasmalemma of the basal epithelial cell and to the underlying reticular tissue (Fig. 3-19).   The underlying tissue, or *reticular lamina,* of the basement membrane is composed of condensed ground substance and small irregular bundles of collagen fibrils termed *reticular fibers* (Fig. 3-19).   In the trachea, elastic fibers are also present in the reticular lamina of the basement membrane.   In certain epithelia, the basement membrane is so poorly developed

that it seems to consist only of basement lamina (Fig. 3-20).

Some electron microscopists refer to the basement lamina alone as the basement membrane, even when describing tissue such as the epidermis.   This practice leads to confusion, because it ignores the reticular lamina, which is usually the component visualized with the light microscope (Fig. 3-18).

Neutral mucopolysaccharide and collagen are present in the reticular lamina of the basement membrane and in the basement lamina.   It is, of course, difficult to study the chemistry of the narrow basement lamina.   In the renal glomerulus, the basement lamina is fairly broad, and light microscopy reveals that it does stain with the periodic acid–Schiff (PAS) technique for mucopolysaccharide (Fig. 3-20).   Chemical studies of the isolated glomerular basement lamina show that the main structural protein is an amorphous form of collagen.

There is considerable evidence that the epithelium makes its own basement membrane.   Broad-

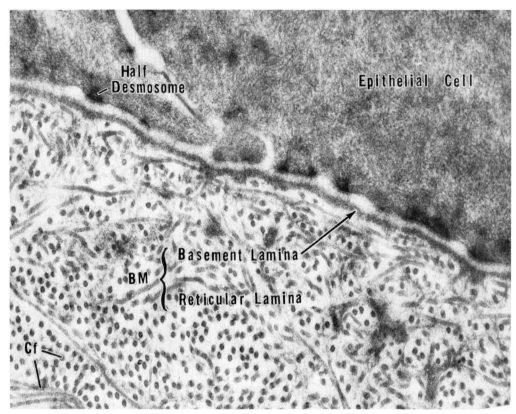

Figure 3-19   Electron micrograph of the basal surface of corneal epithelium of the albino rabbit.   Basal attachment plates called half desmosomes help to anchor the epithelial cells to the basement lamina.   The basement lamina is a glycoprotein layer about 0.1 μm thick, composed of fine filaments, and is seen to be intimately related to the epithelium and to the underlying collagen fibrils.   The collagen fibrils (Cf) are embedded in ground substance and are arranged in a condensed network, the reticular lamina. The reticular lamina and the basement lamina together correspond to the basement membrane (BM) usually visualized in the light microscope.   It is known that the corneal epithelium makes the basement membrane shown here.   Stained with phosphotungstic acid in block after osmium fixation.   × 15,000.   (Courtesy of M. Jakus, relabeled according to the nomenclature suggested by Fawcett.)

ening of the renal glomerular basement lamina in nephrosis is accompanied by hypertrophy of the epithelial cells, which acquire the secretory organelles that would be needed to produce large amounts of collagen and mucopolysaccharide. Although it is likely that underlying fibroblasts, when present, contribute to the formation of the reticular lamina, Dodson and Hay (1971) have shown that isolated corneal epithelium in vitro can produce the collagenous reticular component, as well as the basal lamina of the basement membrane, in the complete absence of fibroblasts.

Basal cell processes that extend into the under-lying connective tissue increase the attachment surface of the basal epithelial cells, particularly in stratified squamous and transitional epithelia (Fig. 3-8).   Adhesion plates that occur on the basal plasmalemma in certain stratified epithelia are called *hemidesmosomes* because there is no matching counterpart in the underlying connective tissue (Fig. 3-19).

SPECIALIZATIONS OF THE FREE SURFACE
Microvilli are narrow (0.1 μm) cylindrical cytoplasmic processes that project from the free surface of the cell.   They compose the *brush border* of the

absorptive cells of the proximal renal tubule, the choroid plexus, and the placental epithelium. The so-called *striated border* of the intestinal epithelium (Fig. 3-21A) has essentially the same structure as a brush border. The free surface of one absorptive cell may contain as many as 2,000 of the minute cytoplasmic projections which give the border a refractile, brush-like or striated appearance as viewed in the light microscope. The plasmalemma of the microvillus is an extension of the cell membrane. The moderately dense cytoplasm within the microvillus may contain microfilaments which connect with the underlying terminal web (Fig. 3-12).

The increased free surface provided by microvilli undoubtedly contributes to the absorptive function of cells. The brush border of the intestine contains enzymes which hydrolyze sugar phosphate esters and disaccharides to monosaccharides. Active transport mechanisms exist in or near the microvilli (see Chap. 18). In the kidney, the microvilli are quite long and may fill the entire lumen of the proximal tubule. The urine must filter through the cytoplasmic processes of these epithelial cells. Large molecules such as hemoglobin, which sometimes traverse the glomerulus to reach the lumen of the proximal tubule, are taken up through membrane-bounded invaginations at the base of the microvilli. The same kind of process occurs between the microvilli of intestinal cells during lipid absorption (see Chaps. 1 and 18).

Figure 3-20   High-power electron micrographs of the junction between renal epithelium and capillary endothelium in rat glomerulus. Foot processes of the renal epithelium (Epi) rest on the basement membrane (arrow). The basement membrane in this case represents the combined basement laminas of the capillary endothelium (End) and the renal epithelium. There is no reticular lamina throughout most of the glomerulus, for the narrow adepithelial layer is the effective filter between the blood and nephron cavities. The inset shows basement membrane under higher magnification. Osmium fixation; stained with lead citrate and uranyl acetate. ×75,000; inset, ×150,000. (Courtesy of E. Reynolds.)

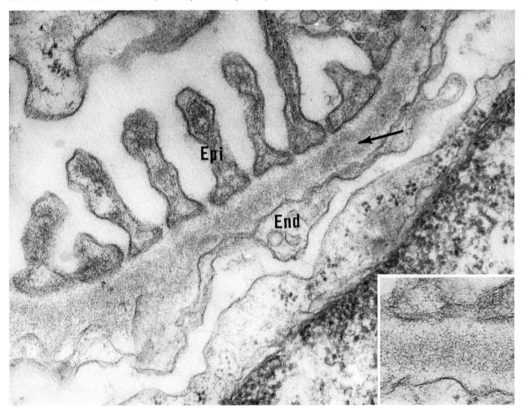

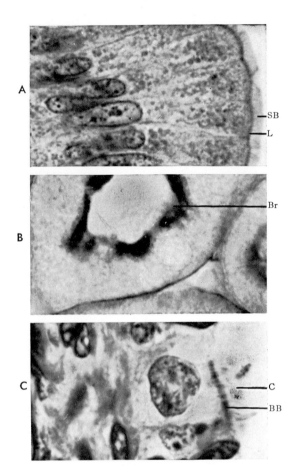

Figure 3-21   Specializations of free surface of epithelial cells as viewed with light microscope. A. Striated border (SB) of cells covering duodenal villus of monkey. The dense line (L) corresponds to the outer portion of the terminal web. H&E. B. Brush border (Br) of cells lining proximal convoluted tubule of mouse. The border is stained by the PAS method for demonstrating glycoprotein. C. Cilia (C) emerging from a cell lining human oviduct. The basal bodies (BB) can be seen. Iron alum hemtoxylin. All ×1,600. (Courtesy of H. W. Deane.)

Stereocilia are very long microvilli which are quite numerous on the surface of the epithelial cells lining the epididymis and vas deferens (Fig. 3-22). This epithelium regulates the specialized environment in which the spermatozoa mature, and perhaps the stereocilia play a role in secretion as well as absorption of the surrounding medium. The secretory cells of exocrine glands possess a few microvilli on their free surface.

Glycoprotein surface coats cover the luminal surface of the microvilli in the proximal renal tubule (Fig. 3-21B) and can be demonstrated in the intestine (inset, Fig. 3-23). When present, they give the brush and striated borders a positive PAS reaction and probably contribute to the gel-like rigidity of the regular array of microvilli on such surfaces. The surface glycoprotein coat has been called *fuzz* by Ito (1965) and *fluffy coat* by Farquhar and Palade (1963) because it is filamentous in its fine structure (Fig. 3-23).

Cilia are motile cell processes with a complex inner structure adapted for contractility (Fig. 3-21C). They are not to be confused with microvilli. Viewed in cross section in the electron microscope, each cilium is seen to contain two central fibrils and nine peripheral fibrils enclosed in the plasmalemma (Fig. 3-24). Each peripheral fibril is actually composed of two smaller fibrils. The fibrils run from the tip of the cilium to the basal body, where the central fibrils terminate (Fig. 3-25). The nine outer fibrils originate next to nine longitudinal fibrils in the peripheral wall of the basal body. Fibrous rootlets, which may be striated, extend from the basal body into the apical cytoplasm (Fig. 3-25). The basal body is a modified centriole and often an additional centriole is oriented more or less perpendicular to it (Fig. 3-25). During development of the multiciliated cell, the centrioles, which give rise to the cilia, are duplicated a hundred or more times. In other cell types, a single centriole lying close to the plasmalemma may give rise to an isolated cilium of no apparent function. In developing cells, newly forming fibrils within the cilium can be disrupted by colchicine and thus resemble ordinary microtubules (Chap. 1). In fully formed cilia, the fibrils are considered to be modified microtubules because they are insensitive to colchicine treatment.

The cilium is within the resolution of the light microscope in diameter (0.2 μm) and is 5 to 10 μm in length, much longer than the usual microvillus (1 to 2 μm). Thus, the living cilia of the cells of the respiratory and genital epithelia can be resolved fairly readily with the light microscope and ciliary action observed directly. During the forward of *effective stroke*, the cilium is rigid and curved slightly forward. The return or *recovery stroke* is slower, and to effect it the cilium curves backward

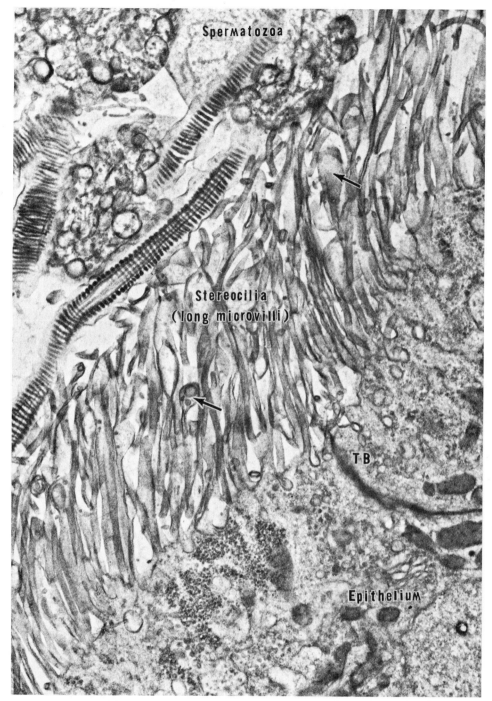

Figure 3-22 Electron micrograph of the free border of the epithelium of the epididymis of bat. Stereocilia are unusually long microvilli that extend from the free surface of the epithelium into the lumen. The microvilli are often dilated (arrows) and may contain secretory products. A terminal bar between two epithelial cells is obliquely sectioned at TB. Osmium fixation; no counterstain. ×12,000. (Courtesy of A. Mitchell.)

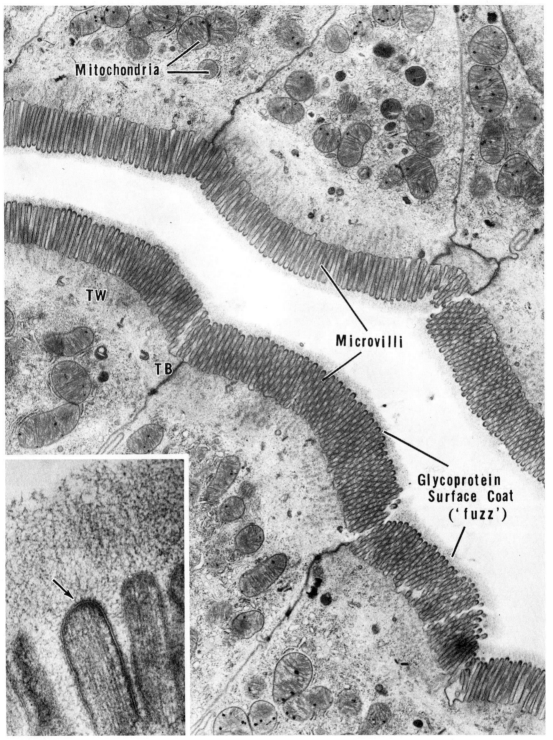

Figure 3-23 Electron micrographs of intestinal epithelium, showing the filamentous glycoprotein surface coat which covers the surface of the microvilli. Glycoprotein surface coats are particularly well developed in the bat intestine (large micrograph), cat intestine (inset), and human intestine (not illustrated). They account for the positive staining of the striated border with Schiff's reagent after periodic acid oxidation (Fig. 2-21B). The filaments of "fuzz" (arrow, inset) are closely related to the cell membrane. In the large micrograph the terminal bar (TB) and terminal web (TW) in the apical cytoplasm are shown to good advantage. Osmium fixation; stained with uranyl acetate and lead citrate. ×8,000; inset, ×100,000. (Courtesy of S. Ito.)

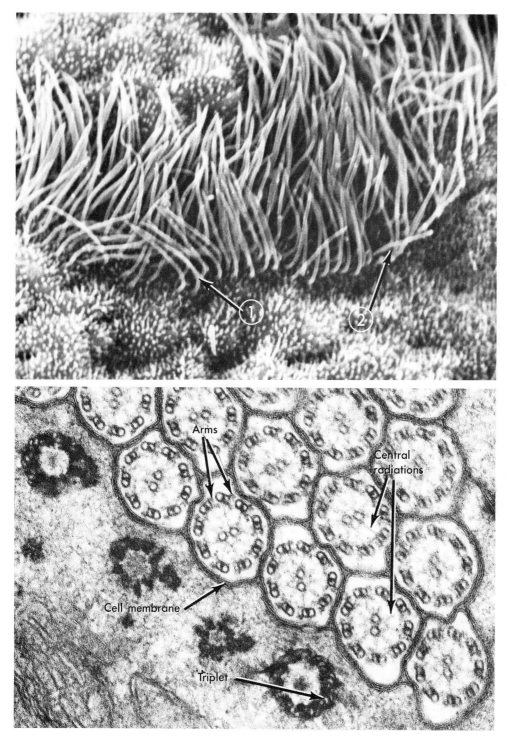

Figure 3-24   A (top). Low-power scanning electron micrograph reveals the three-dimensional configuration of a group of cilia on the outer surface of a planarian.   Some cilia seem to have been caught by the fixative while in their forward stroke, as at 1, others while in their back stroke, as at 2.   The smaller protrusions are microvilli.   B (bottom). Higher-magnification transmission electron micrograph reveals a group of closely apposed cilia in cross section.   Each cilium has two central fibrils or microtubules from which fine condensations (central radiations) pass toward the peripheral fibrils.   Each of the nine peripheral fibrils is a pair of microtubules.   The arms on the fibrils contain ATPase and are thought to cause sliding of the fibrils during ciliary contraction. Several centrioles in an adjacent cell appear on the left.   Unlike the cilium, the centriole has no central fibrils.   Each of its nine peripheral fibrils is a triplet of microtubules.   A, ×4,000; B, ×90,000.   (Courtesy of S. J. Coward and R. O. Vitale-Calpe.)

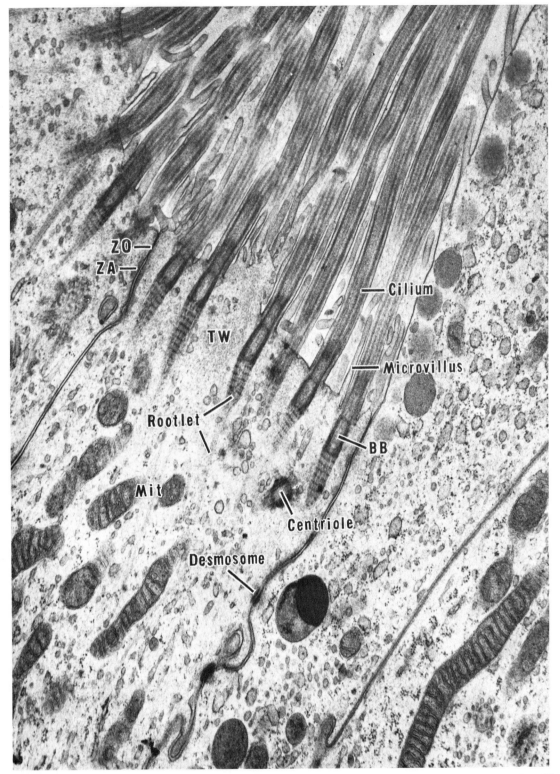

Figure 3-25 Electron micrograph of a longitudinal section through the apex of a ciliated cell in human fallopian tube. Cilia and microvilli are shown to good advantage. The centriole adjacent to the basal body (BB) of one cilium appears but is obliquely sectioned. Note the moderately well-developed terminal web (TW). Also shown are the zonula occludens (ZO) and zonula adhaerens (ZA) of a terminal bar, Mit, mitochondrion. Osmium fixation; stained with lead hydroxide. ×25,000. (Courtesy of N. Bjorkman and B. Fredricsson.)

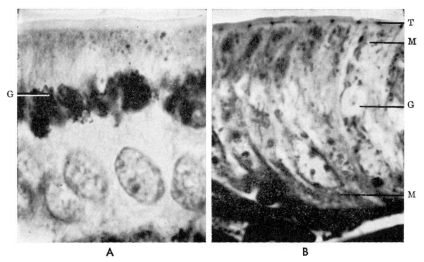

Figure 3-26. Intestinal cells viewed in the light microscope. A. The supranuclear Golgi net, (G) small intestine of guinea pig. Da Fano's silver nitrate method. B. Mitochondria in rat intestine. M, mitochondria; G. negative image of Golgi apparatus; T, terminal bar. Compare with electron micrograph shown in Fig. 3-20. Iron alum—hematoxylin stain. Both ×1,600. (Courtesy of H. W. Deane.)

and then progressively stiffens from base to tip. It has been suggested that the impulse causing the movement first spreads from the basal body to the forward-placed peripheral fibrils. These fibrils may then slide along the central fibrils via the so-called arms of the fibrils, much as actin filaments slide past myosin filaments in muscle. Gibbons has called the protein composing the arms of the fibrils *dynein*. Dynein has a molecular weight (600,000) similar to myosin (500,000), but it polymerizes into dimers that are ultrastructurally amorphous instead of tubular. It nevertheless resembles myosin in that it has ATPase activity. The protein (*tubulin*) of the outer fibrils resembles actin in that it binds nucleotides and plays a role in a motile system involving interaction with ATPase. The morphologic assembly of tubulin (into microtubules rather than filaments), the molecular weight (60,000 as against 46,000 for actin), and the composite peptide units are not the same as in actin. In spite of these differences in the composition of the underlying proteins, a similar sliding mechanism of contraction may exist in cilia and muscle. Glycerin-extracted cilia will beat if supplied with ATP, and ciliary fibrils remain the same length during the ciliary beat, as if the outer fibrils were sliding along the central core.

The cilia of the columnar epithelia of the respiratory tract, oviduct, and uterus do not beat synchronously; rather, they exhibit a *metachronal rhythm*, which results in forward-spreading ciliary waves that effectively move mucus or other materials over the free surface of the organ. Acetylcholine and acetylcholinesterase occur in ciliated cells, and it has been speculated that the coordinated metachronal rhythm is caused by a propagated impulse passing from cilium to cilium and cell to cell.

POLARITY OF THE EPITHELIAL CELLS
An epithelial cell whose apex differs from its base is said to be *polarized*. The most striking examples of polarity occur in the columnar epithelia. In the absorptive epithelial cells of the intestine (Fig. 3-26A), digested lipid enters the apical cytoplasm, where it is processed by the Golgi complex and then transported to the intercellular space. Mitochondria tend to be preferentially located in the apical cytoplasm of intestinal epithelial cells (Fig. 3-26B) and ciliated columnar cells (Fig. 3-25). Mitochondria also show striking polarity in the simple cuboidal and columnar epithelium associated with water and electrolyte transport. In the secretory ducts of the salivary gland (Fig. 18-24) and con-

voluted tubules of the kidney (Figs. 24-13 and 24-18), they are concentrated in the basal cytoplasm. Their striking orientation parallel to the long axis of the cell gives the basal cytoplasm its characteristic striated appearance as viewed in the light microscope. The highly interdigitated lateral cell membranes of these cells are intimately related to the mitochondria.

In exocrine gland cells, the well-developed endoplasmic reticulum is located primarily in the basal cytoplasm. The Golgi apparatus, or "packaging" center, occurs in the apical juxtanuclear cytoplasm (Fig. 3-17). Mitochondria tend to be disposed to the base of the cell, particularly when secretory product has accumulated in the apical cytoplasm (Fig. 3-30).

Regeneration of epithelia

Epithelia on exposed surfaces of the body and the epithelia of the intestinal tract, holocrine glands, and female genital tract exhibit a remarkable degree of physiologic regeneration. In most of the stratified squamous epithelia, the relatively undifferentiated cuboidal cells of the basal layer proliferate to supply new cells which move to the outer surface. The cells differentiate along the way, a process called *cytomorphosis.* The continuing growth of hairs and nails involves a similar proliferation of basal epithelial cells which subsequently are converted to hard keratin plaques. In *holocrine glands,* such as the sebaceous gland, the cells are secreted as part of the product and so must be renewed constantly. In the alimentary tract, relatively undifferentiated cells in the intestinal crypts and necks of the gastric glands serve as a reservoir of new cells to replace surface epithelia. The epithelium of small intestinal villi is entirely replaced every 2 to 4 days.

In addition to its capacity for physiologic regeneration, epithelium in general shows considerable ability to proliferate after a traumatic wound. If a lesion occurs in the epidermis, for example, the basal cells adjacent to the wound migrate over the underlying connective tissue as a single sheet of contiguous cells which gradually increases in thickness as more cells move in. Interestingly enough, the migrating cells do not usually divide. The synthesis of new DNA and mitosis occur in the epithelium at the margin of the wound. It seems likely that in exocrine glands, regeneration is accomplished by proliferation of the relatively undifferentiated cells of the ducts. In the bladder, the less differentiated basal cells seem to have the greatest proliferative capacity. Nevertheless, the relation between degree of differentiation and ability to divide is not an absolute one. Some highly differentiated epithelial cells do retain the capacity to proliferate after injury, as, for example, in the liver.

Classification of glands

The glands of the body fall into two major groups: the exocrine glands, which secrete products that reach a free surface, and the endocrine glands, which produce hormones that enter the bloodstream.

The *endocrine glands* usually arise as invaginations of the surface epithelium but later lose their connection with the surface and thus are ductless. In some cases, typical epithelial characteristics are retained by the secretory cells (thyroid gland). In most cases, the "epithelial" nature of the tissue

is difficult to recognize. The cells may be arranged in anastomosing sheets or as irregular cords. Such cells are often said to be *epithelioid,* because they resemble epithelium in that they are contiguous; however, other epithelial characteristics, such as a free surface, are not present. Certain endocrine cells are more like fibroblasts (the interstitial tissue of testis, the theca interna of ovarian follicles). The cytology of endocrine cells will be considered in subsequent chapters.

Exocrine glands are usually classified according

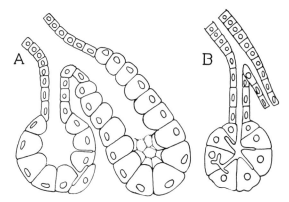

Figure 3-27   Diagrams of glands.   A. Duct ending in alveolus and tubule with wide lumina, as in a mixed serous and mucous gland.   B. Duct ending in alveolus with narrow lumen, as in a purely serous gland.   Intercellular canaliculi are shown.

to the branching of the ducts and shape of the secretory units.   In some cases, the gland cells are dispersed throughout a lining epithelium as single units, called *unicellular* glands.   More commonly, the secretory cells are arranged in *tubules* or sac-like endpieces called *alveoli* (*acini*), which connect to a duct (Fig. 3-27). If the duct goes directly to the surface without branching, the gland is considered to be a *simple tubular* or *simple alveolar* gland (Fig. 3-28).   If the duct branches, connecting more than one secretory unit to the surface, the gland is a *compound tubular* or *compound alveolar* gland.   Both tubular and alveolar secretory units are present in a *compound tubuloalveolar* gland.

An exocrine gland is said to be *holocrine* if whole cells are secreted (sebaceous gland); *apocrine* if protrusions of apical cytoplasm are lost; and *merocrine* if no actual cytoplasm is lost.   Most secretory cells are merocrine.   The "part" (G. *meros*) that is secreted is a protein synthesized in the endoplasmic reticulum and combined with oligosaccharide or polysaccharide as it passes through the Golgi zone (see Chap. 1).

The secretory cells of merocrine glands are usually classified as serous or mucous.   *Serous cells* are common in glands of the alimentary tract. *Mucous cells* occur as unicellular glands throughout the gastrointestinal and respiratory tracts and are a prominent component of many of the salivary glands.   In some of the salivary glands serous and

mucous cells occupy the same endpieces.   The serous cells are pushed away from the lumen to form a crescent, or *demilune,* at the periphery of the alveolus or tubule (Fig. 3-29).

Serous cells produce a secretion which is watery but high in enzyme content.   The protein precursor accumulates in the apical cytoplasm in the form of small zymogen or "preenzyme" granules.   Nuclei are round and located near the base of the cell (Fig. 3-29).   The abundant endoplasmic reticulum gives the basal cytoplasm a strong affinity for basic dyes. Cell borders are indistinct as viewed with the light microscope, and the lumen of a typical serous acinus or alveolus is usually quite narrow (Fig. 3-29).   The serous secretion is rich in protein and contains some mucopolysaccharide.

Mucous cells produce a protein secretion richer in sugar and more viscous than the serous secretion.   It forms large masses in the apical cytoplasm of the mucous cell and compresses the flattened nucleus to the basal surface (Fig. 3-30).   Secretion extruded from the cells often dilates the lumen of the secretory alveolus.   In the unicellular mucous gland, the *goblet cell* (Fig. 3-31, see color insert), the accumulated mucus in the apical cytoplasm gives the appearance of the "globe" of a goblet; the narrow, compressed basal cytoplasm is the "stem."   Mucus usually stains poorly in routine histologic preparations and so the cells often appear empty with well-defined borders (Fig. 3-29).   Endoplasmic reticulum is present in the basal cytoplasm when the cells are making the protein component of mucus.   Examples of cells that make products intermediate between typical mucous and serous secretions can be found (Brunner's glands of the

Figure 3-28   Diagrams of simple and compound forms of tubular and alveolar glands, including a compound tubuloalveolar gland.

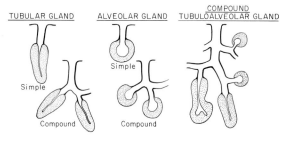

TUBULAR GLAND   ALVEOLAR GLAND   COMPOUND TUBULOALVEOLAR GLAND

Plasma cells

Lumen,
serous
alveolus

Lumen,
mucous
tubule

Serous
demilune

Serous
cell

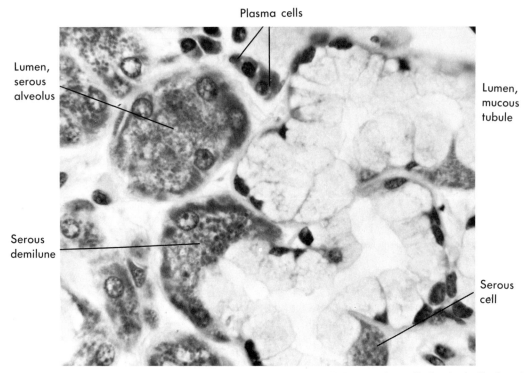

Figure 3-29   Light micrograph showing typical serous and mucous alveoli in human submandibular gland.   The irregular, branching mucous endpieces are often so elongate that they are called tubules instead of alveoli, and the gland is said to be tubuloalveolar. Serous cells may form caps (demilunes) on the ends of mucous tubules.   Isolated serous cells also occur in mucous tubules in a mixed salivary gland such as the submandibular.   The plasma cells located in the connective tissue adjacent to the glandular alveoli (upper part of picture) are commonly seen in organs associated with the gastrointestinal tract.   Bouin's fixation; H&E. ×850.

Figure 3-30   Mucous cells from the sublingual gland of a dog in various phases of secretion.   The mitochondria appear as blackened filaments; the mucous droplets have been dissolved out and are represented by empty vacuoles.   Potassium dichromate and formaldehyde fixation; mitochondria stained by acid fuchsin. (Hoven.)

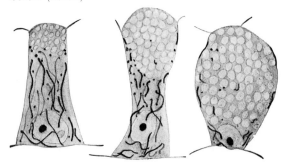

duodenum, mucous neck cells of the stomach).

It will become apparent in subsequent chapters that secretion of protein and mucoid products is not an exclusive property of the typical exocrine gland cells discussed above.   *Connective tissue cells* secrete mucopolysaccharide and protein to form the extracellular matrix that surrounds these cells, and certain *neurons* produce neurosecretory materials which are rich in polypeptides and polysaccharides.   The connective tissue cells that form the bone matrix, the osteoblasts, are often arranged in sheets and are said to be epithelioid, so closely do they resemble true epithelial cells.   It might be pointed out, too, that even *muscle* can take on so-called epithelial characteristics where contiguity is essential to function; true desmosomes and modified adhering zonules called *intercalated disks* occur in cardiac muscle.   The distinction between the epithelia and other tissues of the body is, in last measure, an arbitrary one, a matter of the degree to which the cells express the criteria that we assign to a particular tissue category.   Our classification of the tissues, then, should never become so rigid that it leaves us unprepared to recognize similarities among cells of apparently diverse origin and function.

References

SPECIALIZATIONS OF THE LATERAL SURFACE

CHAMBERS, R., and G. S. RÉNYI: The Structure of the Cells in Tissues as Revealed by Microdissection. I. The Physical Relationships of the Cells in Epithelia, *Am. J. Anat.*, **35:**385 (1925).

DIAMOND, J. M.: The Mechanism of Isotonic Water Transport, *J. Gen. Physiol.*, **48:**15 (1964).

DOUGLAS, W. H. J., R. C. RIPLEY, and R. A. ELLIS: Enzymatic Digestion of Desmosomes and Hemidesmosome Plaques Performed on Ultrathin Sections, *J. Cell Biol.*, **44:**211 (1970).

FARQUHAR, M. G., and G. E. PALADE: Junctional Complexes in Various Epithelia, *J. Cell Biol.*, **17:**375 (1963).

FURSHPAN, E. J., and D. D. POTTER: Low Resistance Junctions between Cells in Embryos and Tissue Culture, in "Current Topics in Developmental Biology," vol. 3, Academic Press, New York, 1968.

GOODENOUGH, D. A., and J. P. REVEL: A Fine Structural Analysis of Intercellular Junctions in the Mouse Liver, *J. Cell Biol.*, **45:**272 (1970).

HAY, E. D., and J. P. REVEL: "Fine Structure of the Developing Avian Cornea," vol. 1, "Monographs in Developmental Biology," A. Wolsky and P. S. Chen (eds.), S. Karger, Basel, 1969.

KAYE, G. I., H. O. WHEELER, R. T. WHITLOCK, and N. LANE: Fluid Transport in the Rabbit Gall Bladder. A Combined Physiological and Electron Microscopic Study, *J. Cell Biol.*, **30:**237 (1966).

LOEWENSTEIN, W. R.: On the Genesis of Cellular Communication, *Dev. Biol.*, **15:**503 (1967).

MCNUTT, N. S., and R. S. WEINSTEIN: The Ultrastructure of the Nexus. A Correlated Thin-section and Freeze-cleave Study, *J. Cell Biol.*, **47:**666 (1970).

MUIR, A. R.: The Effect of Divalent Cations on the Ultrastructure of the Perfused Rat Heart, *J. Anat.*, **101:**239 (1967).

RASH, J. E., J. W. SHAY, and J. J. BIESELE: Urea Extractions of Z-bands, Intercalated Discs, and Desmosomes, *J. Ultrastruct. Res.*, **24:**181 (1968).

SPECIALIZATIONS OF THE BASAL SURFACE

DODSON, J. W., and E. D. HAY: Secretion of Collagenous Stroma by Isolated Epithelium Grown in Vitro, *Exp. Cell Res.*, **65:**215 (1971).

KEFALIDES, N. A.: Comparative Biochemistry of Mammalian Basement Membranes, in E. A. Balazs (ed.), "Chemistry and Molecular Biology of the Intercellular Matrix," p. 535, Academic Press, New York, 1970.

SPECIALIZATIONS OF THE FREE SURFACE

CRANE, P. K.: Structure and Functional Organization of an Epithelial Cell Brush Border, in K. B. Warren (ed.), "Intracellular Transport," p. 71, Academic Press, New York, 1966.

GIBBONS, J. R.: The Structure and Composition of Cilia, in K. B. Warren (ed.), "Formation and Fate of Cell Organelles," p. 99, Academic Press, New York, 1967.

ITO, S.: The Enteric Surface Coating of Cat Intestinal Microvilli, *J. Cell Biol.*, **27:**475 (1965).

SATIR, P.: Studies on Cilia. II. Examination of the Distal Region of the Ciliary Shaft and the Role of the Filaments in Motility, *J. Cell Biol.*, **26:**805 (1965).

SLEIGH, M. A.: Metachronism and Frequency of Beat in the Peristomial Cilia of *Stentor, J. Exp. Biol.*, **33:**15 (1956).

STEPHENS, R. C.: On the Apparent Homology of Actin and Tubulin, *Science,* **168:**845 (1970).

GENERAL

BENNETT, G., and C. P. LEBLOND: Formation of Cell Coat Materials for the Whole Surface of Columnar Cells in the Rat Small Intestine, as Visualized by Radioautography with L-Fucose-^{3}H, *J. Cell Biol.*, **46:**409 (1970).

MESSIER, B., and C. P. LEBLOND: Cell Proliferation and Migration as Revealed by Radioautography after Injection of Thymidine-H^3 into Male Rats and Mice, *Am. J. Anat.*, **106:**247 (1960).

chapter 4   Connective tissue

JEAN-PAUL REVEL

The connective tissues, which we consider here from a general viewpoint, are composed of cells (free or fixed) separated by large amounts of extracellular materials such as collagen, elastic and reticular fibers, and a ground substance. The connective tissues provide a three-dimensional framework which supports the epithelia and other tissues, and play a major role in transport, storage, protection, and repair. In a way, they are the *milieu intérieur* of the body. They form a continuum, interposed between the blood vasculature and the epithelia which face the outside world, such as the skin, the lining of the intestine, and that of the urinary bladder. All exchanges between "inside and outside" must therefore take place across connective tissues, which are reduced to minimum thickness in areas where the exchanges are particularly critical, such as in the lungs or the kidneys.

Tissues such as fat, cartilage or bone, or even blood, can be considered as connective tissues but are so specialized that they are best discussed separately. Even within the connective tissue proper, however, there are great variations in the relative amounts of the various component elements. These variations are closely related to the function of the particular tissue under consideration. Thus, in loose areolar tissue, the connective tissue type discussed in greatest detail here, all the elements are well represented, whereas in dense collagenous connective tissue (as in a tendon, for example) collagen fibers predominate, and in mucous connective tissue (as in the umbilical cord), the ground substance is quantitatively the most important structure.

The extracellular elements of connective tissue

The extracellular matrix of the connective tissues consists of collagen and reticular fibers, elastic fibers, and an amorphous ground substance, each of which will be discussed in turn. These elements play a major role in fulfilling the supporting function of the connective tissues, but as we will see they also contribute significantly to the other functions.

COLLAGEN FIBERS

Microscopic appearance The most abundant and characteristic connective tissue fibers are the collagen fibers. They are very flexible but resist stretching and have a tensile strength comparable with that of steel. Collagen can be studied in the natural state in teased fragments of fresh subcutaneous connective tissue, or in a piece of mesentery spread on a slide. Examined under the light microscope in such preparations, the collagen fibers appear as wavy, interlacing strands of various thicknesses (Fig. 4-1). The large fibers are really bundles of the more slender ones which come together or separate, giving the appearance of branching. Collagen is colorless in its fresh state, and it is hard to distinguish in histologic prepara-

tions unless stained. With hematoxylin and eosin, it appears pink (as do most other proteins). It is brilliantly colored by aniline blue dye in Mallory's stain for connective tissue and by light green in Masson's. It can be stained red by the combination of picric acid and acid fuchsin employed in the Van Gieson procedure. None of these stains is specific in the sense that it will stain only collagen, but each is selective enough to be very useful in analyzing the distribution of collagen in particular tissues.

When examined in the polarizing microscope, collagen fibers are birefringent, suggesting a regular underlying arrangement of asymmetric substructures. With the electron microscope one finds that the fiber bundles and the apparently individual fibers detected with the light microscope can be resolved into even smaller fibrils (Fig. 4-2). A typical fibril is some 40 to 50 mμm wide and of indeterminate length. Depending on where in the body the connective tissue is taken from, the fibrils vary somewhat in thickness. Some of the most delicate fibrils (in the cornea) measure only 30 mμm or less, but they may range up to 100 mμm and more in a big tendon. A very constant feature of collagen fibrils everywhere is a pattern of cross striations which repeats every 64 mμm (Fig. 4-3).

Molecular anatomy of the collagen fibril Treatment with dilute acid causes the collagen fibers to swell and eventually to dissolve. In young animals or in actively growing tissues, collagen can also be solubilized by using salt solutions at physiologic pH (neutral salt solutions). Collagen solutions consist of tropocollagen, a rod-like molecule 290 mμm long and 1.5 mμm wide. Each tropocollagen has a molecular weight of 300,000 and consists of three polypeptides (α chains) helically coiled about each other (Fig. 4-4). The amino acid composition of these chains is remarkable; 30 percent of the residues are glycine and 30 percent, either proline or hydroxyproline. There is no cysteine. Besides hydroxyproline, collagen also contains another rare amino acid, hydroxylysine, to which a few carbohydrate residues (typically 1 to 5 per 1,000 amino acid residues) are bound. The three spiraling polypeptides of tropocollagen are so arranged that the

Figure 4-1 Collagenous fibers appear as wavy interlacing strands in this spread-out piece of rat mesentery. The preparation was stained, but is reproduced as a negative to further enhance the contrast. ×450.

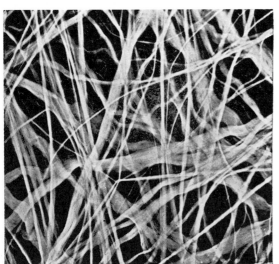

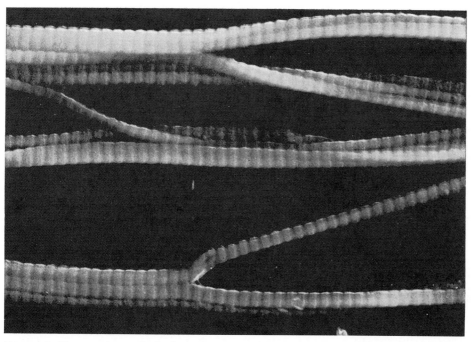

Figure 4-2 Electron micrograph of collagen fibrils from rat tail tendon. The individual fibrils, each of which carries a characteristic cross-banding, associate with each other to form thicker strands.   ×45,000. (Courtesy of Gibbins.)

glycine residues, with no side chains, lie inside the triple helix, whereas the bulky rings of proline and hydroxyproline and the side chains of other amino acids are directed toward the outside.

The tropocollagen isolated from normal collagen consists of two α_1 chains and one α_2 chain, which has a different amino acid composition. In gelatin, which like tropocollagen has a MW of 300,000 and is obtained by boiling collagen-containing tissues, all three chains are present but are not coiled about each other. When dealing with such denatured but still cross-linked collagen, one speaks of a γ component. Partial disruption of three-chained molecules such as tropocollagen or gelatin yields β components (MW 200,000) consisting either of two identical α chains ($\beta_{1,1}$) or of an α_1 and an α_2 ($\beta_{1,2}$). The chains which make up tropocollagen are held together by intramolecular bonds. Besides hydrogen bonds there are also covalent cross-links whose formation involves the aldol condensation of aldehyde derivatives of lysine side chains. By appropriate manipulation native tropocollagen can be caused to reaggregate into fibrils. Normal collagen

Figure 4-3 Collagen fibrils seen at high magnification in longitudinal section The typical periodicity is well displayed. Within each period there is a complex set of subbands which results from the precise staggering of tropocollagen within the fibrils. ×250,000. (Courtesy of Joan Rosenblith.)

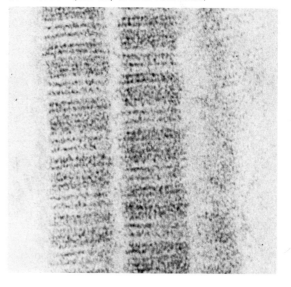

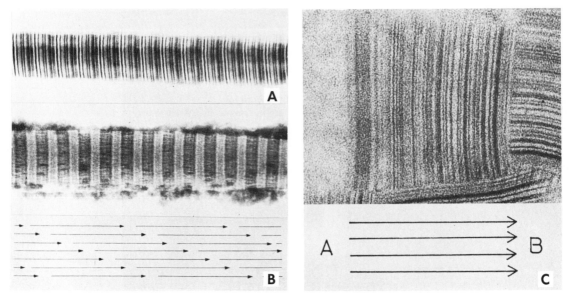

Figure 4-4   A. Normal collagen fibrils stained positively with phosphotungstic acid and uranyl acetate to demonstrate the periodicity and asymmetric cross-banding which results from the precise staggering of tropocollagen in the fibrils.   (Courtesy of Kühn.)
B. Normal collagen fibril seen in negative staining.   Regions of the fibril where molecules are tightly packed because of head to tail overlap are relatively impermeable to the stain and appear light.   Looser regions contain much stain and appear dark.   Note that one can distinguish thin longitudinally oriented structures in the dark areas.   Those correspond to the tropocollagen units in the fibril.   Each tropocollagen extends for 4.4 periods as shown in the diagram.   (Courtesy of Kühn.)   C. SLS tactoids essentially yield a "map" of the location of staining groups along the molecule and have been very useful in the analysis of the molecular structure of tropocollagen.   (Courtesy of Kühn.)

fibrils with 64 mμm banding are formed, as a result of the side-by-side aggregation of staggered tropocollagen all oriented in the same direction and with an overlap of about 10 percent of their length (Fig. 4-4).   By varying conditions so that end-to-end aggregation of tropocollagen is inhibited, small segments rather than fibrils are formed.   This is called SLS (segment long spacing) and is a tactoid 290 mμm long, that is, of the same length as tropocollagen itself.   The SLS form of collagen has been particularly useful in analyzing the structure of tropocollagen, since the chains are parallel to each other and in register.   Thus the asymmetric cross striations visible on SLS tactoids in the electron microscope can be successfully identified as representing the location of amino acid residues stained by the contrasting agent used.   Other conditions of reaggregation can lead to the formation of a variety of different structures.

In vivo origin of collagen fibers   In most cases (but not all, see Chap. 3) collagen precursors are synthesized by fibroblasts.   The polypeptide chains are assembled on ribosomes attached to the endoplasmic reticulum and seem to follow the same route as that established for other "export" proteins, although there are indications that some of the collagen may not necessarily pass through the Golgi area.   Since there are no transfer RNAs for the hydroxyamino acids, the hydroxyproline and hydroxylysine residues so characteristic of collagen arise from the hydroxylation of proline and lysine, after they have been incorporated into chains.   Collagen has to be hydroxylated before it can be secreted.   The hydroxylation reaction is complex and requires oxygen, iron, and ascorbic acid.   Collagen metabolism is severely impaired in scurvy, which is caused by an ascorbic acid deficiency.   Most workers believe, although there is as yet little

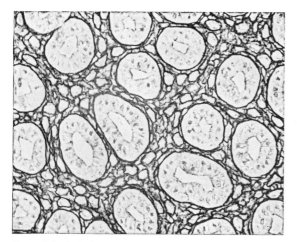

Figure 4-6   Reticulum and basement membranes in the medulla of the kidney.   Photomicrograph of a section of a dog's kidney stained by Pap's silver method.   ×400.

direct proof, that it is tropocollagen that is secreted by the cells.[1]   This soluble collagen then aggregates to form fibrils in vivo, as it does in vitro.   With time, intermolecular links form between tropocollagen molecules.   Although neutral salt solutions suffice to dissolve newly laid-down collagen fibrils, it becomes increasingly difficult to solubilize fibrous collagen which is allowed to stand ("age").   If it is indeed tropocollagen that is secreted, the formation of fibrils is controlled by the environment surrounding the cells, not by some intracellular mechanism.   Once deposited as fibrils, collagen normally turns over very little in most adult tissues; an important exception is the periodontal ligament which holds the teeth in their sockets.

RETICULAR FIBERS

Reticular fibers are a family of very fine collagenous fibers which have all the properties of collagen but can also be stained with the periodic acid–Schiff (PAS) reaction for polysaccharides and by silver stains (hence the name *argyrophilic fibers*).   Long thought to be radically different from collagen, reticular fibers are now recognized as a variant of this

[1] Recent evidence indicates that it is a procollagen that is secreted, of higher molecular weight than the α chains to which it will give rise perhaps after proteolytic cleavage (G. Bellamy, and P. Bornstein: *Proc. Nat. Acad. Sci. USA*, **68:**1138, 1971).

protein which is substituted by more numerous carbohydrate residues.   Reticular fibers, as seen in the light microscope, are very thin and form delicate meshworks intimately associated with cells (Fig. 4-5, see color insert).   They enclose fat cells, are found under the endothelium of capillaries, and surround smooth muscle cells.   They constitute the fibrous framework of lymphoid and blood-forming tissues and are an important part of the stroma of pancreas, liver, and other parenchymatous organs.   In the electron microscope one finds a few very fine fibrils where reticular fibers are expected.   It is believed that much of the reticulin does not form fibrils but exists as an amorphous matrix which can be stained with silver salts and recognized as "fibers" only with the light microscope.

Reticular fibers are closely associated with the basement lamina of various epithelia (Fig. 4-6).   The basement lamina itself also consists of a collagenous protein, but one that is even more heavily substituted by carbohydrate residues than reticular fibers.   This protein does not form fibrils and is thought to be secreted by the epithelial cells that rest on it rather than by connective tissue cells.   They are described in detail in Chap. 3.

Figure 4-7   Network of elastic fibers in rat mesentery.   The preparation was stained with resorcin fuchsin, and the photomicrograph printed as a negative.   ×450.

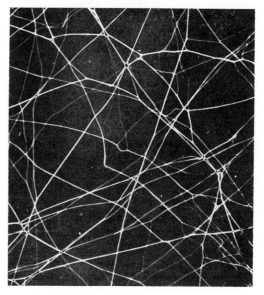

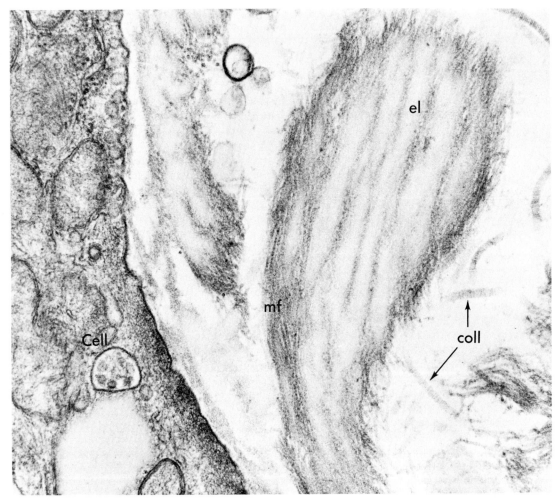

Figure 4-8 Electron micrograph of an elastic fiber in a developing human aorta. The elastic fibers seen in the extracellular space consist of an amorphous, lightly stained component (el) surrounded by numerous microfibrils (mf). Scattered collagen fibrils can be seen in the background (coll). (Part of a cell is seen on the left of the illustration.) ×50,000. (Courtesy of R. Ross.)

ELASTIC FIBERS

In fresh preparations of loose connective tissue, elastic fibers are very thin, highly refractile strands which branch and anastomose freely to form a taut network (Fig. 4-7). When broken, as is often the case in teased preparations of connective tissue, the elastic fibers appear kinked and curled as the tension on them is released. They have a yellow color visible where they are particularly thick or abundant, as in the intervertebral ligaments of man or the neck ligaments which help to support the heads of grazing animals. In the walls of arteries, the elastic component occurs as fenestrated sheets, rather than as fibers.

Elastic fibers are optically homogeneous and are best demonstrated in fixed preparations by staining with the resorcin-fuchsin or aldehyde-fuchsin procedures. In the electron microscope elastic fibers are seen to consist of two morphologically distinct components. One, usually described as amorphous, is the elastic protein elastin. The other consists of "microfibrils," very thin fibrils which surround strands of elastin and are interspersed between them (Fig. 4-8). Little is yet known of the microfibrils, but they appear to consist of a glycoprotein, which differs from collagen in important respects: it is sensitive to trypsin and chymotrypsin, rich in polar amino acids and cysteine, and lacks either hydroxyproline or hydroxylysine. The amorphous elastin is particularly rich in nonpolar amino acid residues. Elastin consists of peptide chains, connected by cross-links such as desmosine or other similar molecules. The desmosine cross-links apparently arise from the condensation of four lysine residues to form a complex ring structure. Copper is somehow involved in cross-link formations, and the degenerative changes observed in the elastic tissues of the aorta in lathyrism may be the result of interference with desmosine formation by an agent (β-aminopropiononitrile) contained in sweet peas.

It has recently been shown that smooth muscle cells in tissue culture can synthesize both of the electron-microscopically recognizable components of elastic fibers. It is likely that where smooth muscle cells are absent, fibroblasts are involved in the synthesis.

GROUND SUBSTANCE

Filling the spaces between the extracellular elements we have just discussed and the cells that we will discuss later in this chapter, one finds an optically homogeneous material that contains much water, salts, and other low-molecular-weight materials, as well as very low concentrations of proteins. The principal components, however, are "acid mucopolysaccharides," now more properly called *glycosaminoglycans*. The high concentration of these molecules is responsible for the viscosity of the ground substance, and it accounts for the fact that bacteria introduced into the connective tissue cannot move freely through the seemingly wide-open spaces separating the formed elements. In the fresh state the ground substance is optically homogeneous and transparent. It is not seen in routine preparations of areolar connective tissue, and it can only be preserved by using specialized techniques such as freeze-drying. The ground substance of cartilage, however, is easily preserved and has therefore been intensely studied. Many of the glycosaminoglycans in the ground substance are rich in negatively charged groups, such as carboxyls and sulfate residues. The dye Alcian Blue is often used to stain ground substance components because it seems to bind preferentially to extracellular molecules. Another favorite staining procedure employs the "basic dye" toluidine blue, which is blue when randomly bound to negatively charged compounds. With many glycosaminoglycans, however, the bound dye molecules are evenly and closely distributed because of the regular and close spacing of negative groups so they can interact with each other, with a resultant color shift to longer wavelengths (from blue to red or pink). Often in a given region there will be some dye with the blue (or orthochromatic), as well as with the pink (or metachromatic) color, so that intermediate shades of purple can also be observed.

Hyaluronate   One major glycosaminoglycan of connective tissue is hyaluronic acid, a linear polymer of a disaccharidic unit formed of glucuronic acid linked to N-acetylglucosamine. At one end of the chain there is a small peptide sequence. The molecular weight of hyaluronic acid is on the order of 10^6. Each *molecule* is therefore approximately 2.5 μm long (Fig. 4-9). In tissue, of course, such a huge molecule as hyaluronate does not exist in an extended form but as a random coil about 0.4 μm in diameter. It is clear that even at low concentrations there will be some overlap between the "domains" of neighboring molecules, and as a result of such entanglement the viscosity of a hyaluronate solution is high. Besides being found in connective tissue in general, hyaluronate is the major component of synovial fluid.

Chondroitin sulfates   Another major class of glycosaminoglycans are the chondroitin sulfates. The form found in loose areolar connective tissue, formerly called chondroitin sulfate A, is now referred to as *chondroitin-4-sulfate*. The basic structure here is also a repeating disaccharide unit containing galactosamine and glucuronic acid. The amino

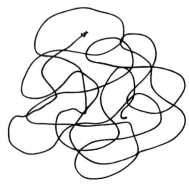

Figure 4-9   An idealized hyaluronic acid molecule.   The thickened end represents the protein moiety and the thin strand, the carbohydrate chain.

chondromucoprotein as the protein backbone is split, and the relatively small carbohydrate sequences disperse.   The "wilting" of a rabbit's ears after injection of papain is the result of in vivo degradation of the protein core of chondroitin-6-sulfate of ear cartilage ground substance.

Biology of ground substances   The high molecular weight and sheer bulk of the glycosaminoglycans in ground substance are responsible for many of its important properties.   Three tropocollagens would weigh the same as one molecule of hyaluronic acid, but the latter occupies a volume of $330{,}000 \times 10^{-19}$ ml, as against only 4.3×10^{-19} ml for the tropocollagen.   The glycosaminoglycans are therefore very efficient space fillers.   They do this, however, without interfering with the passage of small molecules, which see only a very wide meshwork. Molecules of the size of serum albumin, whose dimensions are 4×15 mμm, can diffuse rather freely through solutions of hyaluronate.   Larger structures are increasingly restricted and the movement of particles 30 to 300 mμm in diameter is distinctly limited, while bacteria ($1 \times 0.5 \ \mu$m) are essentially immobilized by the ground substance.   Some bacteria overcome this barrier by producing enzymes (hyaluronidase) which depolymerize glycosaminoglycans and thus reduce the viscosity of the ground substance.

sugar is esterified by sulfate in position 4.   The chondroitin sulfates have molecular weights even larger than that of hyaluronic acid on the order of 5×10^{6}.   The native molecules are really "protein polysaccharides."   They have a protein backbone to which some 100 polysaccharide chains, each of a molecular weight of 5×10^{4}, are attached like the bristles to the stem of a bottle brush.   A specific carbohydrate sequence containing xylose forms the link between protein and carbohydrate side chains.   Exposure to proteolytic enzymes causes a precipitous drop in the viscosity of the

Connective Tissue Cells

Many different cells are found in the connective tissue.   Some of these belong to the connective tissue proper, but others represent blood or other cell types also found as normal constituents of the connective tissue.   A detailed discussion of all cell types would be cumbersome here, and we will emphasize only those types that are typical of the connective tissue, referring the reader to appropriate chapters for more information about the others.   The normal cellular complement of the connective tissue includes fibroblasts, adipose cells, mast cells, some "fixed" macrophages, and free cells such as monocytes, or "free" macrophages, eosinophils, lymphocytes, and plasma cells.

FIBROBLASTS
The fibroblast is one of the most common cell types found in the connective tissue.   Its appearance may change drastically depending on its state of activity.   It is usually a fusiform or spindle-shaped cell whose nucleus shows a finely granular chromatin with one or two nucleoli.   In normal, mature connective tissue the cytoplasm is often so attenuated that it may be difficult to distinguish it in sections. As seen in the electron microscope, the thin cytoplasmic extensions contain some mitochondria, some endoplasmic reticulum cisterns, and some elements of the Golgi apparatus.   This appearance is characteristic of a resting, or quiescent, cell, sometimes described as a *fibrocyte* (Fig. 4-10) to

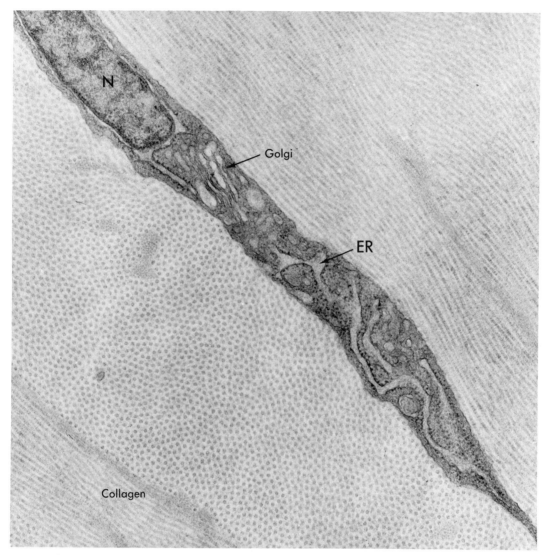

Figure 4-10 A "resting" fibroblast in the cornea of a chick. The cell is squeezed between thick arrays of precisely oriented collagen fibrils. In this particular cell, many of the organelles of an active cell can well be recognized, albeit in small amounts. In completely inactive fibroblast, the organelle complement may be even more scanty. Compare with Figs. 1-26 and 1-27. ×34,000. (Courtesy of Hay and Revel.)

distinguish it from the fibroblast of growing connective tissue, where the cells have all the appearances of being synthetically active, with much cytoplasm filled with organelles.

The behavior of active fibroblasts can be studied to good advantage in growing animals or in tissue culture. Fibroblasts migrate out from a tissue explant placed in a culture dish, clearly revealing their shape (Fig. 4-11). Although they are considered as fixed cells, in the sense of not leaving the connective tissue, fibroblasts are capable of gliding movements, undulating their fan-like ruffled membrane. Observed in a transparent chamber mounted in a rabbit's ear, fibroblasts have been

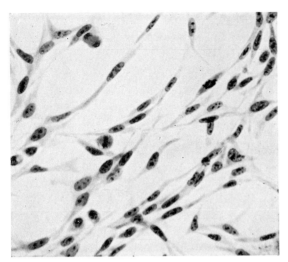

Figure 4-11 Fibroblasts in a 4-day-old culture of mouse embryo skin. Several cells are in different phases of mitotic division. Harris Hematoxylin; ×300.

seen to migrate at speeds of 8 μm per hr. In tissue culture migration rates of as much as 33 μm per hr have been recorded. Fibroblasts in culture can divide rapidly. They also divide actively in the tissue of growing animals or after appropriate stimulation (such as wound repair). Fibroblasts are only poorly phagocytic; they will only ingest foreign material (trypan blue) if very large doses are injected into animals.

In healing wounds, resting fibroblasts take on the appearance of actively secreting fibroblasts. As seen in the light microscope, their cytoplasm grows dramatically and becomes intensely basophilic because of the presence of many ribosome-studded endoplasmic reticulum cisterns. That fibroblasts have as one important role the synthesis and deposition of collagen is beyond question. They produce characteristic collagen fibrils in vitro and in their active form have the cytoplasmic machinery necessary for the synthesis of proteins (rough endoplasmic reticulum) and for its transport to the extracellular environment (Golgi apparatus) (Fig. 4-12). Microsomal fractions (which represent isolated endoplasmic reticulum) incorporate amino acids into newly synthesized (neutral salt soluble) collagen. Autoradiographic studies with labeled precursors also support this secretory role of fibro-

blasts. Fibroblasts also secrete the polysaccharide components of the ground substance, such as hyaluronic acid, although the synthesis of glycosaminoglycans has been studied in more detail in cells of the synovial membranes of joints (hyaluronate) and of cartilage (chondroitin sulfate). The protein moiety of the glycosaminoglycans is probably synthesized in the endoplasmic reticulum; although some of the sugar residues may also be incorporated at the level of this organelle, it is likely that the bulk of the carbohydrate component of the glycosaminoglycans is actually synthesized and sulfated in the Golgi apparatus. Besides these roles, there is reason to believe that fibroblasts may also be involved in the synthesis of elastic fibers when smooth muscle cells are absent.

In some areas of the body, particularly the lymphoid organs, one finds reticular cells, closely associated with the branching and anastomosing network of argyrophilic reticular fibers. The cells are stellate in shape and form a cellular network lining the lymph sinuses and enclosing large numbers of cells of the lymphoid or myeloid series. Reticular cells have large pale nuclei and abundant, moderately basophilic cytoplasm. Long thought to be stem cells, they are now believed to be similar to fibroblasts, playing roles in the formation of reticular fibers and being able to phagocytize under restricted conditions. They are described more fully in Chap. 14.

FAT CELLS
These cells are discussed in greater detail in Chap. 5. In connective tissue they are encountered either singly or in small clumps, particularly near small blood vessels. In fresh tissue they resemble oil droplets. Closer inspection reveals that they are large spherical cells in which the cytoplasm is reduced to an exceedingly thin film enclosing a single large vacuole of stored lipid. The nucleus, which is greatly flattened, occupies a thickened area in the peripheral film of cytoplasm. In either fresh or Formalin-fixed tissue, the lipids of fat cells can be stained with the fat-soluble Sudan dyes, but in most histologic preparations the lipid is extracted, leaving behind only the delicate cytoplasmic envelopes and an empty vacuole. Fat cells are nonmotile and nonphagocytic. They appear incapable of mitotic division. New fat cells appar-

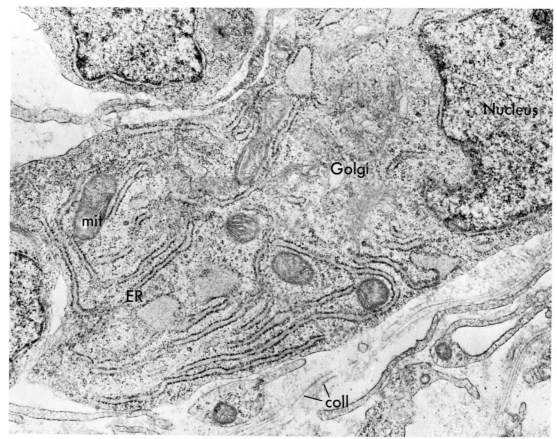

Figure 4-12 An active fibroblast in a very young chick cornea. This cell displays the organelles expected in a state of active formation and secretion of extracellular materials. It has a nucleus with a dispersed chromatin, many cisterns of the endoplasmic reticulum (ER) studded with ribosomes and a well-developed Golgi apparatus. It is actively involved in collagen secretion and probably is the synthesis of other extracellular matrix components as well. ×40,000. (Courtesy Hay and Revel.)

ently arise only by further differentiation of more primitive cellular elements in the connective tissue. The number of fat cells present in areolar tissue depends upon the state of nutrition. They are abundant in the well-nourished and virtually absent in emaciated individuals. Some fat cells (synovial fat pads) which have supportive roles rather than triglyceride storage roles do not disappear even in starved animals.

MAST CELLS

These cells were discovered by Ehrlich, the "father of pathology," who thought they were especially abundant in well-fed animals (German, *mast*, well-fed). They are large, often oval or elongated cells which tend to congregate along small blood vessels (Fig. 4-13A). After appropriate fixation and staining with a basic dye the mast cells display intensely staining granules which may be so numerous as to obscure the smallish, dense, and round nucleus. These granules are metachromatic when stained with dyes such as thionin or toluidine blue, indicating the presence of numerous and closely packed negatively charged sites (Fig. 4-13B). The cells are motile and may sometimes leave a trail of granules as they move.

The mast cell granules have been shown to contain heparin, a heavily sulfated glycosaminoglycan

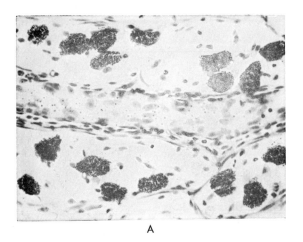

A

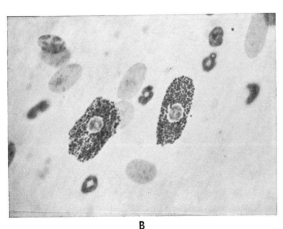

B

carry a net positive charge and are bound to the negatively charged heparin of mast cell granules from which they can be released by physiologic salt solutions. Histamine released into the tissues causes a vasodilation and induces leaks in the blood vasculature, particularly in the venules. Release of biologically active amines from mast cells near the capillaries takes place under various conditions of trauma, mechanical or other, as well as in immunologic reactions, and is a prime factor in tissue reaction to injury.

MACROPHAGES AND MONOCYTES

The macrophages play a major protective role in the body. They occur as fixed in the connective tissues or as wandering cells. Their precursors are the monocytes, which pass into the connective tissue from the blood. The macrophages are very difficult to differentiate from fibroblasts in ordinary preparations, but their nuclei are somewhat smaller, with a more condensed chromatin. Such cells may move about in the connective tissue (and also in culture dishes) with blunt pseudopodia extending in various directions (Fig. 4-14). Their random movements can become directed toward the locus of an attractant. This attraction phenomenon is described by the term *chemotaxis,* but we understand very little of its mechanism. Macrophages have a great capacity for ingesting particulate matter, and one may take advantage of this property to distinguish them from fibroblasts. If an

Figure 4-13 Mast cells in the rat mesentery. A. The cells are clustered along a small blood vessel. They stain intensely with toluidine blue because of the characteristic metachromatic granules. ×300. B. The basophilic granules and small round nucleus are seen better at this higher magnification. The pale oval nuclei in the background are probably those of fibroblast whose cytoplasm has not stained. The doughnut-shaped nuclei near the mast cells are those of rat eosinophils. May-Grünwald-Giemsa stain. ×650.

Figure 4-14 Macrophages migrating through a plasma clot. Tissue culture of mouse lung. May-Grünwald-Giemsa stain; ×550.

(which derives its name from the fact that it was first found in the liver of dogs, whose connective tissue is very rich in mast cells). Although heparin is an anticoagulant, it is not believed to play an important role as such in the body. When mast cells are osmotically shocked or induced to degranulate by the action of pharmacologic agents, histamine is released. This vasoactive amine and other similar compounds such as 5-hydroxytryptamine

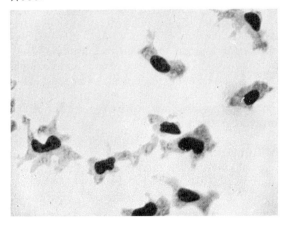

animal is injected with vital dye such as trypan blue, the dye is phagocytized by macrophages and concentrated in large granules within their cytoplasm, whereas fibroblasts and other cell types take up very little dye (Fig. 4-15, see color insert). Because of their motility and phagocytic activity, macrophages are important agents in the body's defense. Acting as scavengers, they engulf extravasated blood, dead cells, bacteria, and inert foreign bodies. Organic material which they ingest is destroyed by the action of intracellular proteolytic enzymes, but foreign matter which resists digestion may remain in their cytoplasm for a long period. The carbon particles of inhaled soot, for example, are taken up by macrophages which accumulate in great numbers in connective tissue septa of the lungs of city dwellers. Tattoos consist of dyes introduced into the connective tissues and ingested by macrophages and also by fibroblasts. Around objects too large to be ingested, numerous macrophages may gather and coalesce to form multinucleated cellular masses known as *foreign body giant cells*. These become very large and may contain as many as 80 or 90 nuclei. Monocytes of the blood and macrophages of tissue appear to be different functional phases of the same cell type. Transitional forms can be recognized upon careful examination of connective tissue, and transformation of monocytes into macrophages and even multinucleate giant cells can be observed in tissue cultures of leukocytes. The monocytes have but scanty lysosomal enzymes. These enzymes characterize macrophages and clearly distinguish them from the polymorphonuclear leukocytes of blood which are early invaders of the connective tissues at sites of infection. The polymorphs already have stores of digestive enzymes as granules in their cytoplasm and form the first line of defense. The macrophage's important role in the protection of the body by ingestion of foreign materials takes place later in the defensive process, for they evidently process certain foreign material in order to induce large-scale antibody synthesis by immunologically competent cells.

LYMPHOCYTES

The smallest of the free cells of connective tissue are lymphocytes, the majority being 7 to 8 μm in diameter. The nucleus, round and rich in heterochromatin, occupies much of the cell. The narrow rim of cytoplasm is basophilic, containing many free ribosomes, but with a sparsely developed endoplasmic reticulum and few mitochondria. Observed in tissue culture, lymphocytes move about quite rapidly with the aid of very fine pseudopodia.

Lymphocytes are not found in large numbers in connective tissue generally but are numerous in the submucosa of the alimentary and respiratory tracts. They are greatly increased in chronic inflammation and in the vicinity of injected foreign protein. They are concerned with antibody formation and are also active in cell-mediated immunity. Lymphocytes emigrate from the capillaries into the submucosa of the stomach, jejunum, ileum, and colon, and leave the body by passing through the epithelium into the lumen of the gastrointestinal tract. They are described in detail and illustrated in Chaps. 10 and 14.

PLASMA CELLS

These round or oval cells (10 to 20 μm in diameter) characteristically have abundant cytoplasm. The nucleus, which is usually eccentric in position, contains coarse, angular clumps of deeply stained chromatin that are in contact with the nuclear membrane and may be arranged in a pattern suggesting spokes of a wheel. Most of the cytoplasm of plasma cells is deeply basophilic. There is typically a rather lightly stained area adjacent to the nucleus, representing the Golgi area and centrioles. Living plasma cells exhibit sluggish ameboid movements. In the electron microscope, the plasma cell typically shows many of the characteristics of cells known to be active in the synthesis of protein for secretion, including a rough endoplasmic reticulum whose cisternae are filled with a fine granular material.

Plasma cells are relatively uncommon in normal connective tissues but become plentiful in chronic inflammation. They secrete antibody. They are often found in close association with lymphocytes, and it is believed that some lymphocytes may become plasma cells. Further discussion of the role of plasma cells and their interrelation with lymphocytes is found in Chap. 14.

EOSINOPHILS

The human tissue eosinophil closely resembles the eosinophilic leukocyte of the blood (see Chap. 10). The nucleus is usually kidney-shaped but may have two lobes connected by a narrow isthmus. The eosinophils in rats have a ring-shaped nucleus (Fig. 4-15, see color insert). The cytoplasm of the eosinophil contains highly refractile granules which are preserved by all the common fixatives and stain vividly with acid dyes (eosin). As observed in electron micrographs, they show a characteristic dense band. These granules are now known to be lysosomes that contain hydrolytic enzymes, and there is evidence that eosinophils may preferentially ingest antigen-antibody complexes (Chap. 10).

Eosinophils probably migrate into the connective

tissues from the blood. There are marked species differences in their number. In the rat it has been estimated that the subcutaneous tissues contain 25 times as many eosinophils as the circulating blood. They are not nearly so numerous in human subcutaneous tissue but are plentiful in the connective tissue stroma of the lactating breast and beneath the epithelium of the respiratory and gastrointestinal tracts. They accumulate in the blood and tissues in certain parasitic diseases and allergic disorders, indicating that they are related in some way to the phenomenon of hypersensitivity.

Types of connective tissue

The character of connective tissue varies greatly in different parts of the body depending upon the relative proportions and arrangement of its cellular, fibrous, and amorphous components. The different kinds of connective tissue are given names which describe their organization and/or indicate which of the components are predominant.

Loose, or areolar, connective tissue is found most abundantly in subcutaneous and intermuscular tissue. It occurs also in the tunica propria and submucosa of the respiratory and gastrointestinal tracts and beneath the serosal linings of the pleural and peritoneal cavities and constitutes the stroma of many organs. It is moderately cellular, is soft and pliable in texture, and contains numerous blood vessels and nerves which supply it or course through it to their ultimate distribution in epithelial, muscular, or skeletal tissues.

Networks of lymphatics are generally present in connective tissue, but they are especially extensive in the subserous and submucous areolar tissues. In the latter, wandering cells are unusually plentiful, and focal accumulations of lymphoid tissue are common.

In *adipose connective tissue*, fat cells are the most abundant cellular element. A fair number of mast cells and eosinophils are scattered along the blood vessels, but other free cells are uncommon. Each adipose cell is enmeshed in a web of fine reticular fibers. There are relatively few coarser

collagenous and elastic fibers. Adipose tissue may develop almost anywhere that areolar tissue abounds, but in man the commonest sites of fat accumulation are the subcutaneous and retroperitoneal connective tissues, the mesenteries, and the omentum. Adipose tissue arises from areolar tissue and serves a supporting function in some regions of the body (for example, in joints). Its principal function, however, is the storage and metabolism of lipid nutrient material.

In *dense collagenous connective tissue,* the collagenous fibers greatly predominate over all other components and are gathered into coarse bundles. These may be interwoven without recognizable pattern in their orientation, as in the dermis of the skin, in the periosteum of bone, and in the fibrous capsules of various organs. On the other hand, in structures subject to tension, the collagenous fibers show a very orderly parallel arrangement. Thus, in ligaments which connect bones and in aponeuroses which afford attachment for muscles, parallel bundles of collagenous fibers form broad, tough sheets. In tendons the bundles are compactly bound together into strong fascicles with very little intervening ground substance and relatively few cells. The cells are undoubtedly a form of fibroblast, but they are so different in shape that they are usually given the name *tendon cells.*

Dense elastic connective tissue is seen in its most typical form in the massive ligamentum nuchae of grazing animals.   It consists of coarse (10 to 15 μm) parallel fibers of elastic tissue in tight bundles which are bound together by areolar tissue. Typical fibroblasts are associated with the areolar tissue.   The individual elastic fibers are enclosed by a delicate argyrophilic reticulum.   The ligamentum nuchae has an important function in sustaining the weight of the head in quadrupeds, but it is rudimentary in man and its elastic component is not so well developed.   Dense elastic connective tissue also occurs in the ligamenta flava of the vertebral column and in various parts of the larynx.   In the superficial fascia covering the lower part of the abdominal wall, connective tissue constitutes a separate layer, Scarpa's fascia, which aids in supporting the viscera.   The corresponding layer in the large quadrupeds, the tunica abdominalis, is an extensive yellow sheet of typical dense elastic tissue several millimeters in thickness.

Mucous connective tissue occurs principally in the umbilical cord.   It is noteworthy for its abundant content of the slippery ground substance known as Wharton's jelly.   The abundance of metachromatic ground substance in the umbilical cord had made this a favorite object in which to study the staining reactions and chemical properties of this connective tissue component.   Collagen fibers are plentiful but reticular, and elastic fibers are rare or absent except in the umbilical vessels. The cells of mucous connective tissue are larger and more stellate in shape than the cells of adult areolar tissue.

Reticular tissue is not simply a variant of areolar tissue in which reticular fibers predominate.   It is a special form of connective tissue in which the cells (reticular cells) have distinctive properties which set them apart from common fibroblasts. It constitutes the supporting framework of the bone marrow, thymus, spleen, lymph nodes, tonsils, adenoids, and other lymphoid organs and is composed of branching and anatomosing reticular fibers closely associated with reticular cells (see Chaps. 14 and 15).

Functions of connective tissue

The principal functions of connective tissue are support, transport, storage, protection, and repair. Although we have already discussed various functional aspects of different connective tissue elements, we will here examine roles of the connective tissue as a whole.

The function of *supporting* and binding together the structures of the body involves principally the fibrous components of connective tissue. Reticular fibers, the most delicate of these, chiefly support coherent groups of cells.   They surround capillaries and sinusoids and, with the basement lamina discussed earlier, form the basement membranes of various epithelia.   The basement membranes enclose groups of parenchymatous cells which constitute the functional units of organs.   Collagen fibers bind these units together and form the septa and the capsules of the organs.   Collagen fibers are major components of the tendons and provide for the attachment of muscles to the skeletal framework of the body.   Elastic fibers allow the tissues to spring back after they have been deformed by a mechanical force.

The organization of the various components of connective tissue differs greatly from one region to another, depending upon the local structural requirements.   Where mobility of parts is important, slender collagenous fibers run in all directions, interwoven in a loose connective tissue that is rich in ground substance and interstitial fluid.   Thus the skin is attached by the subcutaneous areolar tissue but is permitted to move freely over the underlying structures, and the intermuscular areolar tissue allows one muscle to glide over another during contraction.   On the other hand, where tensile strength is of primary importance, there are usually few cells and little ground substance.   Instead, coarse collagenous fibers predominate and are compacted into dense sheets or cords with their fiber bundles oriented so as to resist most effectively the local mechanical stresses.   The fascias, aponeuroses, and ligaments so formed provide great strength while preventing or limiting motion of the parts.

Networks of elastic fibers are plentiful in the walls of hollow viscera prone to periodic distension, as in the lung, which is subject to rhythmic expansion. The recoil of the pulmonary elastic tissue is largely responsible for emptying the lungs in the passive expiratory phase of respiration. In the subcutaneous connective tissue, elastic fibers ensure the return of the skin to its normal position after it is displaced or stretched. With advancing age elastic tissue gradually loses its resiliency, leading to progressive loss of tone and wrinkling of the skin in senility. The elastic rebound of blood vessel walls is essential for the maintenance of normal circulation. The calcification and fragmentation of arterial elastic tissue, which occur with aging, are therefore important factors in the pathogenesis of arteriosclerosis and hypertension.

Connective tissue is involved in the *transport* of metabolites to the extent that substances diffusing from the bloodstream must pass through the ground substance of the perivascular tissues. It has been suggested that the ground substance, rather than constituting a barrier, may actually facilitate transport of metabolites. It is possible that soluble materials may diffuse in the fluid interface between connective tissue fibers and the matrix, as well as through the ground substance. In any case, it is reasonable to suppose that the state of hydration of the ground substance, as well as other factors, influences the exchange of materials between the blood and tissues.

The role of connective tissue in *storage* is not limited to adipose tissue (see Chap. 5). The connective tissue ground substance may, under certain conditions, also store water and electrolytes in excess of its normal content. We have also seen that mast cells play a role in the storage of vasoactive amines such as histamine.

Cellular, fibrous, and amorphous components of connective tissue all participate in the important functions of *protection* and *repair*. Although substances in solution readily permeate the ground substance, the latter constitutes a mechanical barrier against the spread of pathogenic microorganisms, and thus affords a degree of protection against infection. It is interesting that the invasiveness of bacteria can be correlated with the production of hyaluronidase, which is an enzyme that splits both hyaluronic acid and some of the chondroitin sulfate residues of the protein polysaccharides.

The connective tissues respond to injury by the complex protective reaction known as inflammation. The mast cells release histamine, thus increasing vascular permeability and producing a local edema. Leukocytes emigrate from the bloodstream to attack the bacteria. Eventually macrophages ingest dead cells, bacteria, and organic debris. Repair of the tissue involves fibroblasts, which multiply and begin to synthesize extracellular components. Collagenous fibers develop, filling the defect with dense fibrous scar tissue. In certain chronic infections when the best efforts of leukocytes, blood-borne antibodies, and tissue phagocytes are insufficient to eradicate the invading bacteria, excessive production of fibrous tissue around the lesion protects the rest of the body by walling off and thus isolating the infectious tissues. Just how bacterial damage to tissues or mechanical injury initiates a prompt proliferative response in fibroblasts and what factors bring about a cessation of cellular proliferation when healing is complete are intriguing problems which still await solution. Inflammation is further discussed in relationship to blood vessels (see Chap. 10).

Connective tissues have recently been the subject of intensive study in relation to a group of human diseases characterized by pathologic changes in the collagen and ground substance. These diseases include rheumatic fever, rheumatoid arthritis, lupus erythematosus, and polyarteritis. Interest in the relation of the endocrine glands to the connective tissue has been particularly stimulated by the discovery that adrenocorticotropic hormone of the pituitary gland and cortisone, a hormone of the adrenal cortex, both have a beneficial effect on the distressing symptoms of these diseases, symptoms which appear to be due in part to an exaggeration of the protective and reparative functions of connective tissue. Although the mechanism of their action is still poorly understood, there is experimental evidence that administration of an excess of either of these hormones suppresses the inflammatory reaction and delays fibroplasia. Alterations in the extracellular components of connective tissue are also found in hypothyroidism and hypogonadism, and it is now apparent that the endocrine system normally influences in varying degree the growth and maintenance of all the mesenchymal tissues.

References

COLLAGEN, RETICULAR, AND ELASTIC FIBERS

GROSS, J.: Organization and Disorganization of Collagen, *Biophys. J.*, **4** (Suppl.):63 (1964).

HERINGA, G. C., and A. WEIDINGER: Reticulin and Collagen, *Acta Neerl. Morph.*, **4**:291 (1941–1942).

HODGE, A. J.: Chemistry of Collagen, in Ramachandran, G. N. (ed.), "Treatise on Collagen I," Chap. 4. Academic Press, New York, 1967.

HODGE, A. J., and F. O. SCHMITT: The Tropocollagen Macromolecule and Its Properties of Ordered Interaction, in M. V. Edds, Jr. (ed.), "Macromolecular Complexes," Ronald Press, New York, 1961.

KRETSINGER, R. H., G. MANNER, B. S. GOULD, and A. RICH: Synthesis of Collagen on Polyribosomes, *Nature,* **202**:438 (1964).

KUHN, K.: The Structure of Collagen, in P. N. Campbell and G. D. Greville (eds.), "Essays in Biochemistry," vol. 5, p. 59, Academic Press, New York, 1969.

PETRUSKA, J. A., and A. L. HODGE: A Subunit Model for the Tropocollagen Macromolecule, *Proc. Nat. Acad. Sci. USA*, **51**:871 (1964).

PORTER, K. R.: Repair Processes in Connective Tissues, in C. Ragan (ed.) "Connective Tissues, Trans. *2nd Conf.*" Josiah Macy, Jr. Foundation, 1952.

PORTER, K. R., and G. D. PAPPAS: Collagen Formation by Fibroblasts of the Chick Embryo Dermis, *J. Biophys. Biochem. Cytol.*, **5**:153 (1959).

REVEL, J. P., and E. D. HAY: An Autoradiographic and Electron Microscopic Study of Collagen Synthesis in Differentiating Cartilage, *Z. Zellforsch.*, **61**:110 (1963).

ROSS, R., and E. P. BENDITT: Wound Healing and Collagen Formation. III. A Quantitative Radioautographic Study of the Utilization of Proline-H[3] in Wounds from Normal and Scorbutic Guinea Pigs, *J. Cell Biol.*, **15**:99 (1962).

ROSS, R., and P. BORNSTEIN: Studies on the Components of the Elastic Fiber, in E. A. Balasz (ed.), "Chemistry and Molecular Biology of the Intercellular Matrix," p. 641 Academic Press, New York, 1970.

ROSS, R., and P. BORNSTEIN: The Elastic Fiber. Separation and Partial Characterization of Its Macromolecular Components, *J. Cell Biol.*, **40**:366 (1969).

SCHMITT, F. O., C. E. HALL, and M. A. JAKUS: Electron Microscope Investigations of the Structure of Collagen, *J. Cell. Comp. Physiol.*, **20**:11 (1942).

SPIRO, R. G.: The carbohydrate of collagens, in E. A. Balasz (ed.), "Chemistry and Molecular Biology of the Intercellular Matrix," p. 195, Academic Press, New York, 1970.

STEARNS, M. L.: Studies on the Development of Connective Tissue in Transparent Chambers in the Rabbit's Ear, *Amer. J. Anat.*, **66**:133 (1948).

GROUND SUBSTANCE

BENSLEY, S. H.: On the Presence, Properties, and Distribution of the Intercellular Ground Substance of Loose Connective Tissue, *Anat. Rec.*, **60**:93 (1934).

DEMPSEY, E. W., H. BUNTING, M. SINGER, and G. B. WISLOCKI: The Dye-binding Capacity and Other Chemo-histological Properties of Mammalian Mucopolysaccharides, *Anat. Rec.*, **98**:417 (1947).

DURAN-REYNALS, F.: Studies on Certain Spreading Factor Existing in Bacteria and Its Significance for Bacterial Invasiveness, *J. Exp. Med.*, **58**:161 (1933).

GERSH, I., and H. R. CATCHPOLE: The Organization of Ground Substance and Basement Membrane and Its Significance in Tissue Injury, Disease, and Growth, *Amer. J. Anat.*, **85**:451 (1949).

GODMAN, G. C., and K. R. PORTER: Chondrogenesis Studied with the Electron Microscope, *J. Biophys. Biochem. Cytol.*, **8:**719 (1960).

HAMERMAN, D.: Synovial Joints: Aspects of Structure and Function, in E. A. Balasz (ed.), "Chemistry and Molecular Biology of the Intercellular Matrix," p. 1259, Academic Press, New York, 1970.

LAURENT, T. C.: Structure of Hyaluronic Acid, in E. A. Balasz (ed.), "Chemistry and Molecular Biology of the Intercellular Matrix," p. 703, Academic Press, New York, 1970.

MC MASTER, P. D., and R. J. PARSONS: Physiological Conditions Existing in Connective Tissue. I. The Method of Interstitial Spread of Vital Dyes, *J. Exp. Med.*, **69:**247 (1939).

MC MASTER, P. D., and R. J. PARSONS: Physiological Conditions Existing in Connective Tissue. II. The State of the Fluid in the Intradermal Tissue, *J. Exp. Med.*, **69:**265 (1939).

REVEL, J. P.: Role of the Golgi Apparatus of Cartilage Cells in the Elaboration of Matrix Glycosaminoglycans, in E. A. Balasz (ed.), "Chemistry and Molecular Biology of the Intercellular Matrix," p. 1485, Academic Press, New York, 1970.

SCHUBERT, M.: Intercellular Macromolecules Containing Polysaccharides, *Biophys. J. (Suppl.)*, **4:**119 (1964).

FIBROBLASTS AND MACROPHAGES

CARREL, A., and A. H. EBELING: The Fundamental Properties of the Fibroblast and the Macrophage. I. The Fibroblast, *J. Exp. Med.*, **44:**261 (1926).

CLINE, M.: Monocytes and Macrophages, in T. J. Greenwalt and G. A. Jamieson, (eds.), "Formation and Destruction of Blood Cells," Lippincott, Philadelphia, 1970.

COHN, R. A., M. E. FEDORKO, and J. G. HIRSCH: The *in Vitro* Differentiation of Mononuclear Phagocytes. IV. The Ultrastructure of Macrophage Differentiation and V. The Formation of Lysosomes, *J. Exp. Med.*, **123:**767 and 757 (1966).

EVANS, H. M., and K. J. SCOTT: On the Differential Reaction to Vital Dyes Exhibited by the Two Great Groups of Connective Tissue Cells, *Carnegie Inst. Contrib. Embryol.*, **47:**1 (1921).

HARRIS, H.: Chemotaxis and Phagocytosis, in MacFarland and Robb-Smith (eds.), *"Functions of the Blood,"* p. 413, Academic Press, New York, 1961.

LEWIS, M. R.: The Formation of Macrophages, Epithelioid Cells and Giant Cells from Leucocytes in Incubated Blood, *Amer. J. Pathol.*, **1:**91 (1925).

LEWIS, W. H.: Macrophages and Other Cells of the Deep Fascia of the Thigh of the Rat, *Carnegie Inst. Contrib. Embryol.*, **116:**193 (1929).

MOVAT, H. Z., and N. V. P. FERNANDO: The Fine Structure of Connective Tissue. I. The Fibroblast, *Exp. Molec. Path.*, **1:**509 (1962).

WEISS, L., and D. W. FAWCETT: Cytochemical Observations on Chicken Monocytes, Macrophages and Giant-cells in Tissue Culture, *J. Histochem. Cytochem.*, **1:**47 (1953).

MAST CELLS

BENDITT, E. P., and D. LAGUNOFF: The Mast Cell: Its Structure and Function, *Progr. Allerg.* **8:**195 (1964).

BLOOM, G. D.: Electron Microscopy of Neoplastic Mast Cells: A Study of the Mouse Mastocytoma Mast Cell, *Ann. N.Y. Acad. Sci.*, **103:**53 (1963).

EHRLICH, P.: Beitrage zur Kenntnis der Anilinfarbungen und Ihrer Verwandung in der Mikroskopischen Technik, *Arch. Mikr. Anat.,* **13:**263 (1877).

FAWCETT, D. W.: An Experimental Study of Mast Cell Degranulation and Regeneration, *Anat. Rec.* **121:**29 (1955).

FAWCETT, D. W.: Cytological and Pharmacological Observations on the Release of Histamine by Mast Cells, *J. Exp. Med.* **100:**217 (1954).

HOLMGREN, H., and O. WILANDER: Beitrag zur Kenntnis der Chemie und Funktion der Mastzellen, *Z. Mikr. Anat. Forsch.* **42:**242 (1937).

RILEY, J. F.: "The Mast Cells," Livingstone, Edinburgh, 1959.

UVNAS, B.: Release Processes in Mast Cells and Their Activation by Injury, *Ann. N.Y. Acad. Sci.* **116:**880 (1964).

OTHER CELLS

ARCHER, G. T., and J. G. HIRSCH: Motion Picture Studies on Degranulation of Horse Eosinophils during Phagocytosis, *J. Exp. Med.,* **118:**287 (1963).

EVERETT, N. B., and R. W. TYLER: Quantitative Aspects of Lymphocyte Formation and Destruction, in T. J. Greenwalt and G. A. Jamieson (eds.), "Formation and Destruction of Blood Cells," p. 264, Lippincott, Philadelphia, 1970.

LITT, M.: Eosinophils and Antigen-antibody Reactions, *Ann. N.Y. Acad. Sci.,* **116:**964 (1964).

NAPOLITANO, L.: Observations on the Fine Structure of Adipose Cells, *Ann. N.Y. Acad. Sci.,* **131:**34 (1965).

chapter 5   Fat

RUSSELL J.
BARRNETT

Adipose tissue, or fat, is the storage of reserve lipid nutrients which occurs in aveolar connective tissue. In mature, domesticated animals of average nutrition, it accounts for approximately 15 percent of the gross weight. It should be recognized, however, that the amount of ordinary fat varies greatly with the nutritional state. In most mature animals, two types of adipose tissue can be recognized. The most widespread type is *yellow* or *white fat* or, more specifically, *unilocular adipose tissue,* the cells of which usually contain a single large vacuole of stored lipid. The second variety, more restricted in distribution and amount, is called *multilocular adipose tissue,* or *brown fat;* the lipid is present in multiple small droplets within its cells.

Distribution of adipose tissue

In man, unilocular adipose tissue is the common form, and in well-nourished individuals it forms a more or less continuous subcutaneous layer, the *panniculus adiposus,* which in part is responsible for sex difference in body contours. Unilocular adipose tissue is particularly well developed in the axillary and episcapular regions, over the lower abdomen and lower back, and on the buttocks and thighs. Fat of this sort is also abundant in the omentum and mesenteries and in the retroperitoneal regions. In primates, it has a yellow color owing to the presence of carotenoids and other lipochrome pigments. In some rodents, on the other hand, it is nearly white. In adult human beings multilocular adipose tissue is relatively uncommon; however, fatty tissue closely resembling

159

the brown fat of rodents occurs in human fetuses and in newborns in the interscapular region, axillae, posterior triangle of the neck, and along the major blood vessels. In mature rodents, brown fat is confined to certain localities, the bulk of it being located in the interscapular region on either side of the midline. Small, discrete lobules of brown fat also occur in the mediastinum adjacent to the thymus and along the major vessels of the thorax and abdomen. Some animals show peculiar species distribution of adipose tissue, such as that in the hump of the camel or in the tail of Merino sheep. In fish, the liver serves as the main depot for fat storage, in contrast to the minor role it plays in most terrestrial forms.

Origin of fat cells

One of the most fundamental problems, the cell of origin of adipose tissue, has not yet been conclusively solved. Part of this difficulty is due to the fact that in man and in some experimental animals brown and white fat cannot be clearly distinguished morphologically during embryonal lipogenesis. The transformation of mesenchymal cells into adipose tissue of both varieties is initiated by the gradual deposition of fat globules; that is, embryonal adipose tissue is multilocular. Despite this fact, it is likely that adipose tissue in all mammals arises by two different developmental processes and these differences correspond to the two types of fat. The adipose anlagen, therefore, can be distinguished mainly by anatomic position. This opinion has been arrived at as a result of transplantation and tissue culture experiments as well as by morphologic observation.

Concerning the origin of white adipose tissue, there are still differing opinions that parallel those expressed by Toldt and by Fleming in the last century. Toldt first stated that fatty tissue of mammals was a specific organ, entirely distinct from connective tissue in which it most frequently occurs. Fleming, in the other hand, contended that adipose tissue was merely ordinary connective tissue in which fat has been deposited. This old argument appears only slightly modified in the twentieth-century literature. The present consensus is that white or yellow fat cells are of a definite type, formed by the differentiation of primitive mesenchymal cells. According to most investigators, fat cells were not fibroblasts, nor were they derived from fibroblasts, and in emaciation they do not revert to fibroblasts. Others indicate that fat cells are derived from cells that are "fibroblast-like" in appearance. It is noteworthy that fat is not laid down equally in all the connective tissues but shows a predilection for certain regions. In addition, there are parts of the body (eyelid, external ear, penis, dorsum of the hand, etc.) which contain connective tissue but which never develop a significant number of adipose cells, regardless of the degree of obesity of the animal. This selective deposition of fat has been interpreted as evidence favoring the origin of adipose tissue from specific cells with a definite distribution, rather than from fibroblasts which are abundant in connective tissue everywhere.

In miduterine life, white adipose tissue begins to develop in certain areas of vascular parenchyma called *fat islands* (Fig. 5-1). Small lipid droplets appear in the cytoplasm of stellate or fusiform mesenchymal cells. As the lipid droplets accumulate in the cytoplasm, the cell becomes round. The droplets of lipid enlarge and coalesce to form a single large lipid accumulation that displaces the nucleus to the periphery of the cell. Small lipid droplets continue to arise in the cytoplasm near the nucleus and join the large lipid accumulation, until in the mature cell it is many times the diameter of the original cell. Fully formed fat cells are unable to divide; this may be looked upon as evidence of their high degree of specialization. New adipose tissue develops in postnatal life, as it does in the fetus, from spindle-shaped, undifferentiated mesenchymal cells in loose connective tissue, especially near small vessels. This process can be seen macroscopically by examination of the mesentery of small rodents of different ages. In young animals, single fat cells lie along the small mesenteric

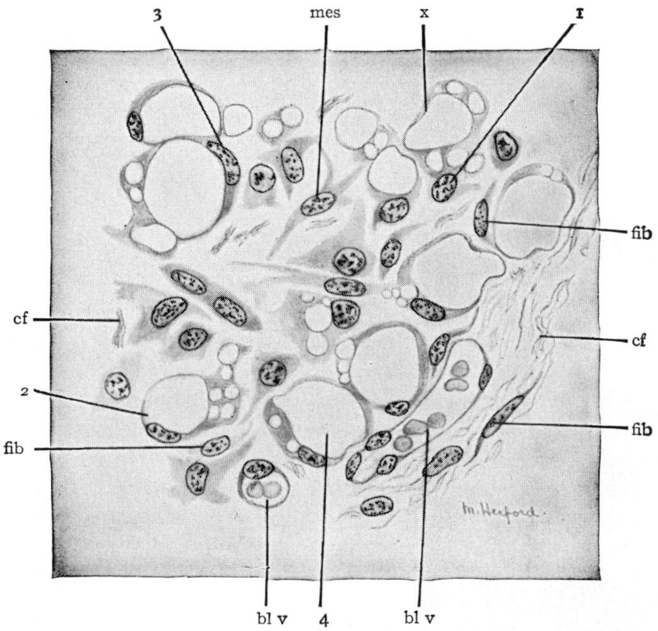

3   mes   x   1

fib

cf

cf

2

fib

fib

bl v   4   bl v

M. Hexford.

Figure 5-1   Fat island from subcutaneous tissue of a human embryo of 4 months; mes, mesenchymal cell; fib, young fibrocyte; 1, 2, 3, 4 are stages in the development of fat cells; x, young fat cell cut without showing nucleus; cf, collagenous fibers; bl v, blood vessel.

vessels; as the animal grows older, more fat cells appear until they finally form a sheath which completely surrounds the vessels (Fig. 5-2).

Some workers have stressed that this relationship of primitive fat cells to small blood vessels suggests that the undifferentiated mesenchymal cells from which adipose cells develop may be related to elements of the reticuloendothelial system. Evidence in favor of this point of view also stems from the observations that under certain pathologic conditions some undifferentiated cells in adipose tissue seem able to reestablish the function of blood cell formation, that inactive hematopoietic tissue in the bone marrow is fatty, and that in the embryo fat lobules contain hematopoietic foci. In addition, both brown and white fat cells will take up and store vital dyes, which is a well-known property of the cells of the reticuloendothelial system.

Brown adipose cells appear to have a different developmental process. These cells are also derived from undifferentiated, spindle-shaped mesenchymal cells, but these assume a characteristic epithelioid appearance and become arranged in

Figure 5-2   Adipose cells of rat mesentery. Mesentery was fixed in alcohol and stained by the May-Grünwald-Giemsa method. The lipid has been extracted from the central vacuole, and only the thin rim of cytoplasm is visible. ×150.

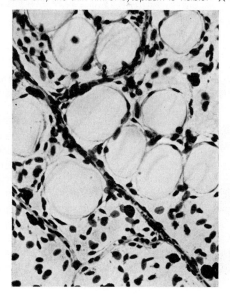

gland-like lobules before they begin to accumulate lipid. This process occurs only in embryos and results in the formation of multilocular fat, which occurs, as previously stated, in distinctly confined regions. Apparently no brown fat is formed in adult animals, and there is no transformation of one type to the other. However, in some pathologic conditions yellow adipose cells may attain a multilocular appearance. In fact, some fatty tumors of man and other mammals, called *lipomas*, may bear a striking resemblance to the brown fat of rodents.

Morphology of fat cells

UNILOCULAR ADIPOSE TISSUE

Unilocular fat cells are very large (more than 100 μm in diameter) because of the quantity of lipid which accumulates in them. In fresh preparations, isolated fat cells, as in the mesentery, are spherical (Figs. 5-2 and 5-3). When crowded together they deform one another and become oval or polyhedral (Fig. 5-4). In ordinary histologic paraffin sections, from which the soluble fats have been lost during the process of dehydration of the tissue prior to embedding and sectioning, the cells are frequently collapsed or there is distortion of their contours (Fig. 5-5). There is some degree of variation in the size of individual fat cells, not only from one region of the body to another but even in the same area. The size of the fat cell may be a reflection of its metabolic activity, and the variation in size may be

an indication that fatty tissues do not necessarily function as one unit. This idea is supported by the work of Gage and Fish, who fed animals fat-soluble dye and found that the dye was not deposited in different depots with equal intensity. In addition, fat cells at different sites become depleted of lipid at different rates on starvation, and they accumulate lipid at different rates on refeeding.

According to the classic descriptions of white adipose tissue, the cytoplasm surrounding the central lipid accumulation is little more than a thin film. The nucleus is flattened and displaced to the periphery of the cell, where it occupies a thickened area of cytoplasm (Figs. 5-2 and 5-5). The nucleus, which does not contain a nucleolus, is oval and frequently indented, and the chromatin is dispersed and dustlike. Because of the unusually large size of these cells, a histologic section of usual thickness includes only a thin segment of those fat

Figure 5-3 Isolated fat cells in rat mesentery. After Formalin fixation, the lipid of these cells was stained with Sudan black B. Compare the size of fat cells with red blood cells in small vessels. A number of eosinophils are also stained, because of lipid coating of their granules. ×150.

Figure 5-4 Adipose tissue stained with Sudan black B. When adipose cells are crowded they are mutually compressed into polygonal forms. Peripheral cytoplasm of cells unstained. ×275.

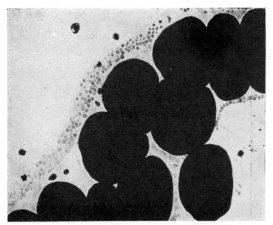

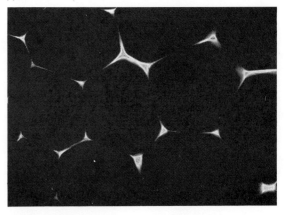

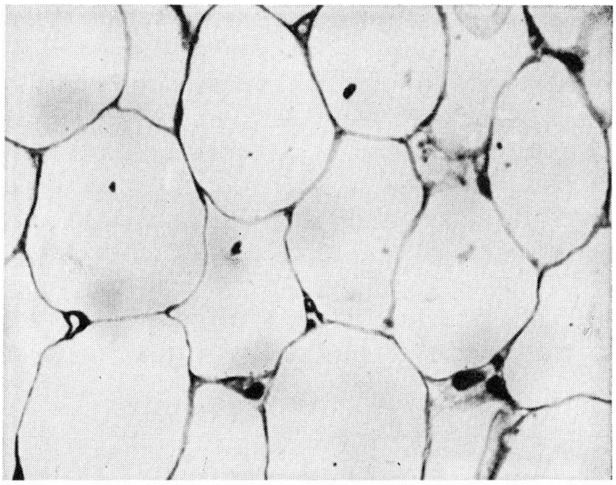

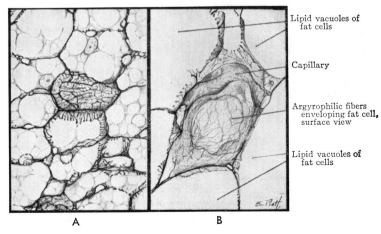

Figure 5-5   Subcutaneous adipose tissue of a rat. The cytoplasm of the cell is reduced to a narrow rim around a single vacuole. ×350.

especially concentrated in the cytoplasm adjacent to the nucleus, but they also occur in the other portions of the cytoplasm. A small, flattened Golgi apparatus is found near the nucleus. Occasionally small lipid droplets may be seen in the thickened portion of the cytoplasm, which also may contain glycogen (Fig. 5-7). The lipid in the large central vacuole consists mainly of a mixture of triglycerides. This lipid is retained in frozen sections and other special preparations and can be stained with Sudan dyes and other histochemical methods that will demonstrate lipid (Figs. 5-3 and 5-4).

Unilocular adipose tissue is divided into ill-defined lobules by thin connective tissue septa. Except for these interlobular septa, the stroma consists mainly of delicate reticular fibers which also form close networks that surround the capillaries (Fig. 5-6). White fat has been generally regarded as a poorly vascularized tissue (Fig. 5-8). Nevertheless, each fat cell, despite its large size, is in contact with at least one capillary. It should be borne in mind that the metabolic activity of a fat cell is confined to its narrow rim of cytoplasm, and this constitutes only a very small fraction of the total volume of the cell. If the ratio of capillary surface to volume of active, nonlipid protoplasm is calculated, it is found that the capillary bed, in proportion to the amount of cytoplasm, is actually as rich in adipose tissue as it is in skeletal muscle. Thus,

cells which are transected, and the plane of the section may by chance include the nucleus of only a few (Fig. 5-5). Around each individual fat cell, forming a coat around the plasma membrane, is a delicate, felt-like network of reticular fibers which are stained by either the PAS method or a silver method (Fig. 5-6). With special cytologic or histochemical methods, rod-shaped and filamentous mitochondria can be demonstrated. These are

Figure 5-6   Argyrophilic reticulum of fat cells (Pap's silver method).   A. Brown adipose tissue of rat.   B. White adipose tissue of rat.   Portions of six cells are shown. The one in the center is seen in surface view and shows the delicate network of reticular fibers which cover the cell surface.   Camera lucida, 4 × ocular 1.3 oil.

Lipid vacuoles of fat cells

Capillary

Argyrophilic fibers enveloping fat cell, surface view

Lipid vacuoles of fat cells

A   B

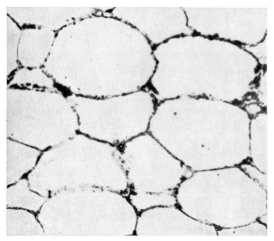

Figure 5-7   Glycogen in white fat cells of a rat fed after a period of fasting.   Note darkly stained granular deposits of glycogen in the thin layer of cytoplasm.   PAS method.   ×300.

cells (for example, those in the mesentery), the central lipid vacuole becomes smaller.   If fasting continues, all the lipid may be mobilized and the fat cells become stellate or fusiform and look superficially like fibroblasts.   Upon refeeding, lipid reappears in these cells, after a transient appearance of glycogen.   It should be noted that not all adipose tissue gives up its lipid easily as a result of starvation.   In general, fat cells in which lipid is most easily deposited are the ones which give up lipid most readily.   The fat pads in the orbit, in the major joints, and in the sole of the foot, however, are very slowly depleted of lipids.   These fat pads are also histologically different in that they have heavy connective tissue capsules and septa and are presumed to have a structural function rather than a metabolic one.

MULTILOCULAR ADIPOSE TISSUE

Brown fat, differing from ordinary white or yellow fat, has a distinct lobulated appearance.   In histologic sections, the lobules of brown fat are composed of fairly large polygonal cells, which are surrounded by a network of fine to moderately coarse argyrophilic fibers (Fig. 5-6) as well as a few col-

in spite of its appearance of relatively poor vascularity, adipose tissue has sufficient blood supply to support a very active metabolism.

As lipid is depleted by starvation from depot fat

Figure 5-8   Unstained, thick celloidin section of brown and white adipose tissue in a rat in which india ink was injected into the circulatory system.   Compare the richness of the vascular bed of the brown fat (above) with that of the white fat (below).   ×50.

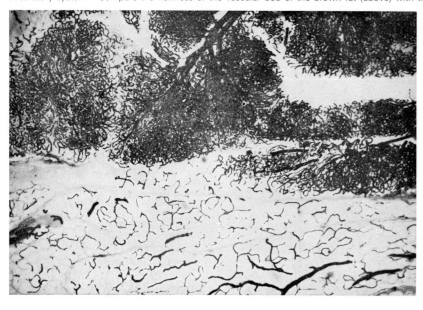

lagenous fibers. The cytoplasm in brown fat cells is much more abundant than that in white fat cells and appears more granular in ordinary histologic sections (Fig. 5-9). It contains multiple small lipid droplets and numerous large spherical mitochondria, but the Golgi apparatus is small and inconspicuous. The nucleus of these cells occupies a slightly eccentric position and contains one or more nucleoli. The chromatin is somewhat coarser than that in the nuclei of white adipose cells.

Brown fat appears much more vascular than white fat (Fig. 5-8). Because of its vascularity, its lobular, gland-like appearance, and brown color, it was originally thought that brown fat, extensively developed in species which hibernate, was an endocrine gland, functionally related to winter dormancy. For this reason, it was sometimes called the *hibernating gland*. However, fatty tissue having the same gross structure and microscopic appearance is found in nonhibernating mammals, including primates. The evidence to date does not seem to warrant the designation of this controversial tissue either as a gland of internal secretion or as an organ of hibernation. Instead, it probably should be looked upon as a special form of adipose tissue which does not play a significant role in general lipid metabolism. Nutritional states have less effect on brown fat than on ordinary fat. On prolonged starvation, the lipid droplets in brown fat slowly disappear and the tissue becomes a highly vascular organ which bears little resemblance to adipose tissue.

It was previously assumed that the function of adipose tissue was unrelated to the nervous system,

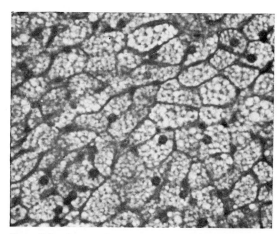

Figure 5-9   Brown adipose tissue from an interscapular fat pad of a rat. Cells are polygonal in shape and have a relatively abundant cytoplasm and multiple small lipid vacuoles.   ×350.

despite the fact that clinical observations suggested that localized fat deposition and depletion may, in part, be governed by nervous factors. As a result of laboratory experiments, particularly comparing a denervated brown fat pad with the contralateral innervated one (and these results presumably apply to white fat also), it was shown that the denervated adipose cells accumulated lipid and glycogen more rapidly than innervated controls. Furthermore, denervated fat cells lose their lipid more slowly on starvation than do innervated adipose cells. Fibers innervating adipose tissue are probably autonomic in origin and play an important role in lipid mobilization.

Cytology and histochemistry of adipose cells

Since the cytoplasm of white and yellow adipose cells exists as such a thin rim, ordinary light-microscopic observations are not suitable for histophysiologic experiments, and in most instances electron-microscopic or histochemical observations are necessary for additional important data. Several details pertinent to the submicroscopic structure of adipose cells will be covered in this section because they suggest a relationship of fine-structural elements to cellular function.

In electron micrographs, the plasma membrane

is surrounded by a clear layer about 150 Å wide separating it from the basement membrane or lamella, which is composed of amorphous dense material. Delicate connective tissue fibers insert in the outer surface of the lamella (but do not penetrate). The lamella is a special morphologic and functional differentiation at the border of adipose cells and is important in uptake of marker particles which attach to the basement membrane prior to incorporation into the cell.

The mitochondria of adipose cells are rather

distinctive and have a dense matrix in which are embedded cristae that extend the full width of the organelle (Fig. 5-10). This is especially prominent in the mitochondria of brown fat where the cristae are quite close together, suggesting a close packing of respiratory enzymes.

Mitochondria of brown fat are very special since they are incapable of oxidation phosphorylation. Since this process is usually coupled to oxidative metabolism, these mitochondria appear to be incapable of capturing the energy released during oxidation. They are, therefore, strictly heat pro-

Figure 5-10   Electron micrograph of a white adipose cell of a rat showing nucleus (lower left) and central fat vacuole (lower right). Morphologic features are typical of a fat cell not synthesizing or mobilizing lipid. Cytoplasm is granular, containing pleomorphic mitochondria. At the surface (top) basement membrane overlies the plasma membrane. ×48,000. (From R. J. Barrnett, in L. W. Kinsell (ed.), "Adipose Tissue as an Organ," Charles C Thomas, Publisher, Springfield, Ill., 1962.)

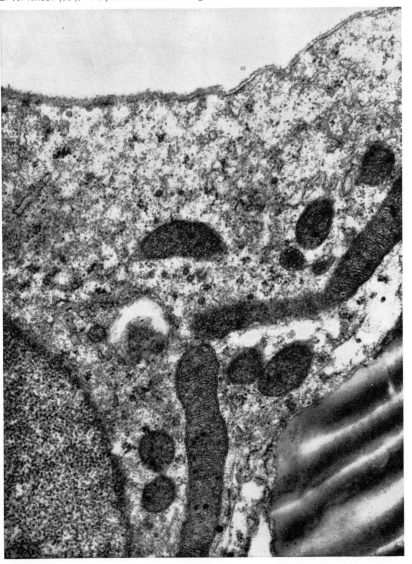

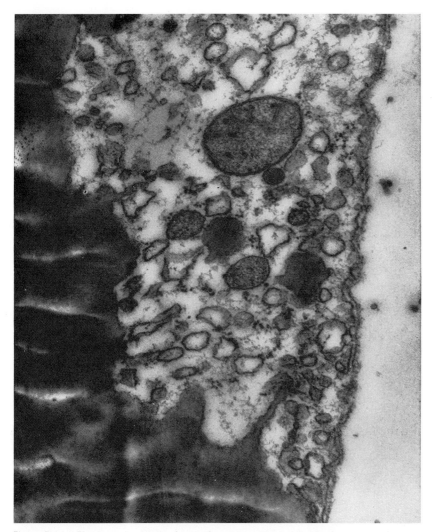

Figure 5-11   Electron micrograph of part of a white adipose cell stimulated to synthesize lipid.   Cytoplasm is less granular than in the resting state (Fig. 5-10) and contains numerous profiles of smooth ER and lipid droplets.   Central lipid vacuole at bottom and left.   ×56,000.

ducers.   In fact, recent findings suggest that the major function of brown fat is the rapid production of heat under a variety of physiologic circumstances, including arousal from hibernation.

Another prominent feature of white adipose cells is the smooth endoplasmic reticulum (ER) which forms tortuous channels and fills the deep portion of the cytoplasm close to the central lipid vacuoles (Fig. 5-12).   These structures are noted especially in the thick portion of the cytoplasm near the nu-

cleus.   Rough ER and free ribosomes are only occasionally present.   In unilocular adipose tissue that is rapidly synthesizing lipid from glucose, an event that occurs in the presence of trace amounts of insulin, numerous smooth-surfaced profiles of discontinuous ER abound in the cytoplasm (Fig. 5-11), close to small, irregular, presumably newly synthesized lipid droplets which rapidly fuse with the central lipid vacuole.

In multilocular adipose cells, small lipid droplets

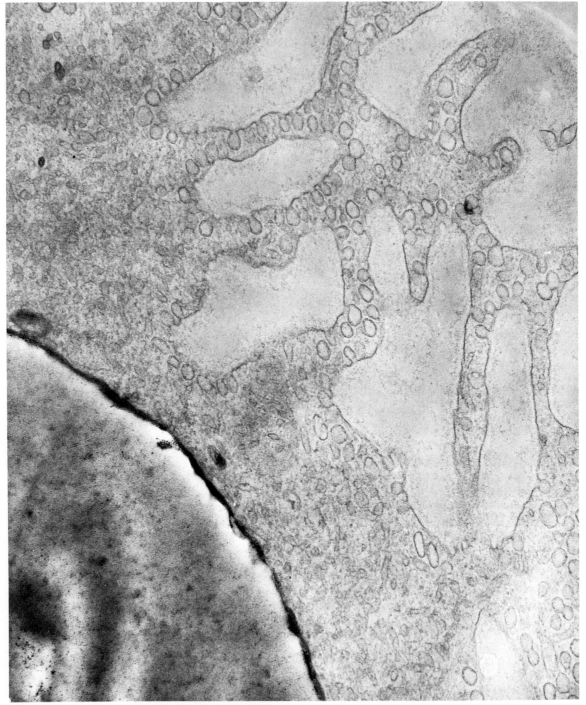

Figure 5-12 Electron micrograph of the surface of an adipose cell of a fasted animal. Central lipid vacuole (lower right) is not depleted of triglyceride. Cytoplasm is thrown into finger-like projections, and numerous pinocytic invaginations stud the surface. Note, especially, the profiles of smooth ER in the cytoplasm. ×60,000.

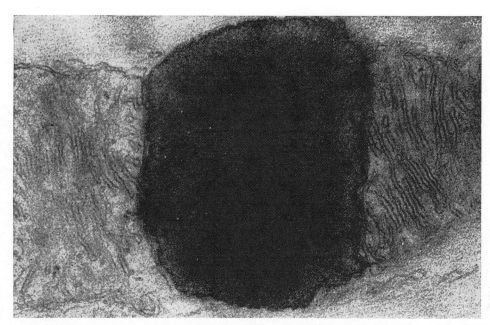

Figure 5-13   Micrograph indicating the relationship of lipid droplet to muscle mitochondria.   In some regions the mitochondria abut directly on the lipid droplet, and the outer mitochondrial membrane cannot be visualized.   This morphologic situation is indicative of lipid utilization by mitochondria.   ×72,000.

in the cytoplasm are the rule, and some of these droplets ordinarily bear a close relationship to mitochondria, being partially or completely surrounded by these organelles.   This occurrence of lipid droplets in relation to mitochondria is not seen in unilocular adipose cells, but it is common in a variety of other tissues of starved animals, especially in striated muscle (Fig. 5-13). The latter morphologic relationship is considered indicative of the utilization of lipid, since the mitochondria contain enzymes for fatty acid oxidation.

Histochemically, both brown and yellow adipose tissue have similar qualitative characteristics but show distinctive quantitative differences.   Glycogen may be demonstrated in the cytoplasm of both, especially upon refeeding after starvation; this is a more prominent occurrence in brown fat (Fig. 5-14).   The amount of glycogen detectable histochemically appears to have an endocrine dependence.   Neutral fat droplets (or the central fat vacuole in yellow fat) stain with Sudan or other oil-soluble dyes (Figs. 5-3 and 5-4).   The lipid in the droplets of brown fat is more saturated than that of yellow fat, but in both fats the storage form

of the lipid is triglyceride.   Brown fat contains more phospholipid, presumably because of a greater content of mitochondria.   Glycolipids have also been detected and are in greater abundance in yellow fat.

Figure 5-14   Glycogen in brown fat cells of a rat fed after a period of fasting.   Note the large glycogen content in comparison with white fat (Fig. 5-7).   PAS method.   ×350.

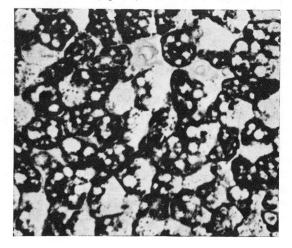

A number of enzymes have been studied in adipose tissue. One or more carboxylic acid esterases (or lipases) occur in the cytoplasm of white fat cells. This enzyme presumably functions in the splitting of triglycerides (the storage form of fat) to yield free fatty acids which are released from the fat cells. One or more phosphatases are associated with the surface and cytoplasm of some adipose cells and with capillary endothelia in fat pads. Oxidative enzymes, such as succinic dehydrogenase, can be demonstrated in the mitochondria. Brown adipose tissue is exceedingly rich in this enzyme (as well as cytochrome oxidase) and is surpassed in such content only by cardiac muscle. This observation correlates well with the number of mitochondria, the arrangement of their cristae, and the metabolic studies which indicate that brown fat has a greater oxygen consumption and a more rapid phosphorus turnover than white fat.

Cytophysiology of fat cells

For many years it was thought that ordinary fat had little metabolic activity of its own. Modern biochemical studies show that adipose tissue can no longer be regarded as an inert site of fat storage or as a tissue without specific or interesting metabolic activities. The use of isotopes to follow the synthesis, transport, and utilization of fat shows that the lipids of the fat depots are not static reserves but are constantly being drawn up and renewed. It is now generally accepted that adipose tissue is actively and continually involved in metabolism, even though it may be difficult to consider the thin rim of cytoplasm around a yellow fat cell as the site of complex metabolic reactions.

In the past 10 years, there has been a great increase in the studies of the physiology and biochemistry of white or yellow adipose tissue which can be correlated with its fine structure. The first major function of adipose tissue is to store triglyceride. This is derived from two sources. The first is uptake from the circulation. Circulating triglyceride also has two sources: dietary triglyceride, which is carried as chylomicrons, and endogenous triglyceride, which is synthesized by the liver and carried in the blood in the form of low-density lipoproteins. The second source of triglyceride is its synthesis in the fat cell itself, usually from glucose. The second major function is the mobilization of stored triglyceride. This occurs after hydrolysis to give free fatty acids which leave the cell and are carried in the blood bound to albumen. The hydrolysis of stored triglyceride is subject to close hormonal control so that the free fatty acids released into the blood closely parallel the caloric requirements of the body. With regard to lipid storage, 95 percent of the total weight of an adipose cell is triglyceride. Morphologically, this can be accounted for solely by the central lipid vacuole.

Considering the uptake of triglyceride from the blood, little work has been done on the low-density β-lipoprotein form of lipid carriage. Chylomicrons, on the other hand, move from the intestinal absorptive cells into the lymph and thence into the blood circulation. The most plausible explanation of the transport across the capillary into fat cells is that the chylomicron triglyceride is broken down, probably to free fatty acid and glycerol, at the surface of the capillary, and the products of this hydrolysis pass through the endothelial cells. This is supported by evidence that intravenously injected chylomicrons, labeled with both ^{14}C in the glycerol part and ^{3}H in the fatty acid part of the triglyceride, result in incorporation of ^{3}H-labeled fatty acid into the adipose cells and a loss of the ^{14}C glycerol. This suggests that hydrolysis of the glyceride occurs outside the fat cell and that the water-soluble glycerol is lost to circulating fluid. Interestingly, all tissues which take up the chylomicron triglyceride have an enzyme, lipoprotein lipase, which uses chylomicrons as its natural substrate and hydrolyzes the triglyceride to yield free fatty acid and glycerol. This enzyme is loosely associated with structure and is easily dissociated; that is intravenous injection of heparin or dextran causes lipoprotein lipase to be released into the blood plasma. This occurs very rapidly and, since dextran cannot leave the vascular compartment, this suggests that the enzyme is located on the surface of the endothelial cells of blood vessels. The level of lipoprotein lipase in adipose and in muscle tissues varies with the nutritional state. In the fed state, when most dietary triglyceride is stored, the adipose tissue level of the enzyme rises and that of the muscle falls. In the fasting state, when muscle uses dietary fat as a source of calories, lipoprotein lipase regulates the level of tissue utilization of dietary triglyceride as the requirements of the tissue are altered. This may be an important factor in the control of triglyceride deposition in adipose tissue.

As indicated, the second source of stored triglyceride is synthesis from endogenous sources, mainly glucose from the blood. Glucose enters the cell and is activated to glucose-6-phosphate. Thereafter, there are two major sources for the breakdown of glucose; one is the glycolytic pathway that yields acetyl-CoA, which could be fed into the Kreb cycle or, alternatively, used for the biosynthesis of fatty acids. Additionally, the pentose phosphate shunt may be used, one of the products of which is dihydroxyacetone phosphate which is converted enzymatically to α-glycerophosphate. Thus, the metabolism of glucose yields both fatty acid CoA derivatives and α-glycerophosphate which are the substrates for the synthesis of triglyceride. The limiting step in this whole process is the entrance of glucose into the adipose cells, which are ordinarily impermeable to the molecular process. However, the entrance is facilitated by insulin, which increases the utilization of glucose by the fat cell as triglyceride is synthesized. While these events are being monitored biochemically, corresponding morphologic observation indicates that fat pads incubated in the presence of insulin and glucose contain an increased number of pinocytic vesicles in the plasma membrane of the fat cell at a time when there is a great increase in glucose utilization. These results could be interpreted that glucose is taken into the cell by pinocytosis; however, there are definite structural requirements for the uptake of glucose with regard to the glucose molecule configuration, and it is probable that the glucose molecule enters the cell by a molecular mechanism. It is possible that insulin causes an increase in cell surface in order to facilitate this movement.

The third role of adipose tissue is to mobilize stored triglyceride. This occurs after the hydrolysis of the triglyceride by a lipase which responds to hormones such as norepinephrine, released from autonomic nerve endings. Products of hydrolysis are free fatty acids; these are released from the cell into the tissue spaces where they become complex with plasma albumen which is necessary for the release of fatty acids and is probably the carrier of free fatty acid between the adipose tissue and the tissue using these substrates. The hormones initiate the mobilization of lipids by activating the enzyme adenyl cyclase probably present in the fat cell plasma membrane. This produces cyclic AMP from ATP, and the cyclic AMP moves into the cell activating the "hormone-sensitive lipase" and causing it to produce free fatty acid. Adenyl cyclase occurs in all tissues acted on by these hormones, and the action of cyclic AMP is a mediator believed to provide the general mechanism for hormone action. The other product of hydrolysis of triglyceride is glycerol, which is not reused for resynthesis of triglyceride. Therefore, the rate of hydrolysis of triglyceride regulates the rate of utilization of α-glycerophosphate which, in turn, is produced from glucose. Hydrolysis of stored triglyceride is, therefore, a potential method of regulation of triglyceride deposition; if this exceeds the rate of availability of α-glycerophosphate, mobilization rather than synthesis will occur.

If an animal is starved for a period of time, there is a reduction in the size of the central lipid vacuole in adipose cells. After 5 days of starvation, most of the triglyceride is depleted. The fat cell now assumes a stellate shape with numerous pseudopodia and an increase in pinocytic vesicles on the surface which are probably a compensatory response of surface activation of a tissue seeking substrate (Fig. 5-15). It should be noted, however, that under normal physiologic circumstances, when the animal is in a steady state, the turnover of triglyceride still occurs, and there is a steady flux of fatty acid from the fat cells. As the physiologic requirements for the free fatty acids alter, so do the hormone concentrations in the plasma; these, in turn, alter the action of the hormone-sensitive lipase via adenyl cyclase. Fatty acids apparently leave the cell via a smooth ER which exists as tortuous channels in the cytoplasm and is increased during lipid mobilization (Fig. 5-12). So far as the localization of the lipase is concerned, the fat cell apparently has two: one at the surface of the fat cell and the other at the surface of the central lipid vacuole in association with the smooth ER.

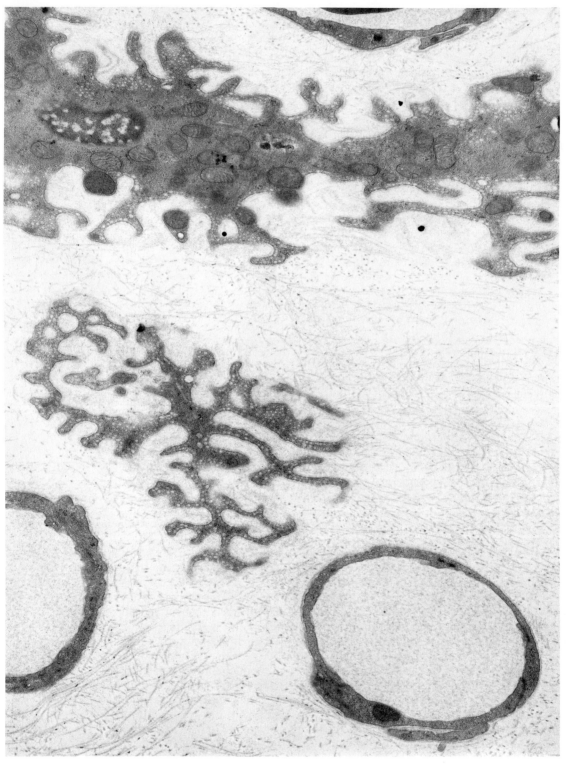

Figure 5-15   Electron micrograph of stellate adipose cells of a fasted animal.   Note numerous pinocytic invaginations and vesicles at the surface of fat cells.   In connective tissue spaces three capillaries (top and bottom) are close to adipose cells.   ×6,000.

References

BARRNETT, R. J.: The Morphology of Adipose Tissue with Particular Reference to Its Histochemistry and Ultrastructure, in L. W. Kinsell (ed.), "Adipose Tissue as an Organ," Charles C Thomas, Publisher, Springfield, Ill., 1962.

BARRNETT, R. J., and E. G. BALL: Metabolic and Ultrastructural Changes Induced in Adipose Tissue by Insulin, *J. Biophys. Biochem. Cytol.*, **8**:83 (1960).

CLARK, E. R., and E. L. CLARK: Microscopic Studies of the New Formation of Fat in Living Adult Rabbits, *Amer. J. Anat.*, **67**:255 (1940).

CUSHMAN, S. W.: Structure Function Relationships in the Adipose Cell, *J. Cell Biol.*, **46**:326 (1970).

FAWCETT, D. W.: A Comparison of the Histological Organization and Cytochemical Reactions of Brown and White Adipose Tissue, *J. Morph.*, **70**:363 (1952).

GERSH, I., and M. A. STILL: Blood Vessels in Fat Tissue. Relation to Problem of Gas Exchange, *J. Exp. Med.*, **81**:219 (1945).

HAUSBERGER, F. X.: Quantitative Studies on the Development of Autotransplants of Adipose Tissue in Rats, *Anat. Rec.*, **122**:507 (1955).

HAUSBERGER, F. X.: Ueber die Innervation der Fettorgane. *Z. Mikr. Anat. Forsch.*, **36**:231 (1934).

JEANRENAUD, B.: Dynamic Aspects of Adipose Tissue, *Metabolism*, **10**:535 (1960).

JOHANSSON, B.: Brown Fat: a Review, *Metabolism*, **8**:211 (1959).

MENG, H. C.: "Lipid Transport," Charles C Thomas, Publisher, Springfield, Ill., 1964.

MENSCHIK, Z.: Histochemical Comparison of Brown and White Adipose Tissue of Guinea Pigs, *Anat. Rec.*, **116**:439 (1953).

NAPOLITANO, L.: The Differentiation of White Adipose Cells. An Electron Microscope Study, *J. Cell Biol.*, **18**:663 (1963).

NAPOLITANO, L., and D. W. FAWCETT: The Fine Structure of Brown Adipose Tissue in the Newborn Mouse and Rat, *J. Biophys. Biochem. Cytol.*, **4**:685 (1958).

RENOLD, A. E., and C. F. CAHILL: "Adipose Tissue," American Physiological Society, Washington, 1965.

RODAHL, K., and B. ISSWEUTZ: "Fat As a Tissue," McGraw-Hill Book Company, New York, 1964.

SIDMAN, R. L.: Histogenesis of Brown Adipose Tissue *in vivo* and in Organ Culture, *Anat. Rec.*, **124**:581 (1956).

WASSERMAN, F.: Die Fettorgane des Menschen; Entwicklung; Bau und systematische Stellung des sogenannten Fettgewebes, *Z. Zellforsch.*, **3**:235 (1926).

WASSERMAN, F., and T. F. MACDONALD: Electron Microscopic Study of Adipose Tissue (Fat Organs) with Special Reference to the Transport of Lipids between Blood and Fat Cells, *Z. Zellforsch.*, **59**:326 (1963).

WELLS, H. G.: Adipose Tissue, a Neglected Subject, *J. Amer. Med. Ass.*, **114**:2177 (1940).

WILLIAMSON, J. R.: Adipose Tissue. Morphological Changes Associated with Lipid Mobilization, *J. Cell Biol.*, **20**:57 (1964).

chapter 6

The skeletal tissues

LEONARD F.
BÉLANGER

Skeleton is a Greek word which refers to the dry object of sometimes equally dry anatomical lessons. To the gross anatomist, it is a bilaterally symmetrical series of jointed structures arranged along and around the vertebral axis. To the classical histologist, it consists of only a few types of microscopic entities—dense fibrous tissue, chordoid, cartilage, bone—which form complex functional units between themselves. To the physiologist and to the biochemist, these tissues, especially bone, represent an important reservoir of essential electrolytes which control many of the vital functions. To the pathologist and to the sociologist, the skeleton has revealed a great deal about the nutrition, customs, diseases, and even the religion of contemporary and historical man. To the anthropologist, the skeleton has been the most important—sometimes the only—record of the progressive evolution of ancient man and of the gradual growth of his brain. A few scholars of the vertebrate skeleton (Romer, 1946 and 1963; Urist, 1964; Tarlo and Tarlo, 1965; Urist and van de Putte, 1967; McLean and Urist, 1968) have in recent time brought to life the fascinating story of the origin of bone, its progressive adaptation, and its regulating mechanisms. Through them we have learned that the cartilaginous fish were not, as we believed, the earliest of vertebrates. One million years before them were the Ostracoderms, fishes with a dermal skeleton, a protective armor against dominant invertebrate predators (Romer, 1963). The loss of armor for better mobility and the subsequent development of the endoskeleton in softwater teleosts, the synthesis of vitamin D, and the development of the branchial hormone-producing derivatives (thyroid, parathyroid, and ultimobranchial gland) are only a few aspects of this marvelous story.

Minor varieties

CHORDOID TISSUE

Chordoid tissue is an ancestral remnant in vertebrates. In man, it is represented by only the embryonic notochord. This tissue consists of large, contiguous cells filled with fluid and forming in their ensemble a compartmented "water bag" that provides some structural support. There is practically no intercellular substance between the chordal cells.

DENSE FIBROUS TISSUE

This variety of connective tissue is generally not described in this chapter. However, the fact that it can become mineralized "by the addition of a new matrix to the collagen bundles" (Weidenreich, 1930; Johnson, 1960), as is the case for the turkey leg tendon, makes it a primitive form of skeletal tissue. The new matrix consists of polysaccharides and lipids in part (Johnson, 1960). A "chemical metaplasia" also occurs in the collagen bundles. The fibers become enlarged, they lose their waviness, their staining properties are modified; eventually they become mineralized. In the turkey tendon,

these changes lead to the adjacent formation of true cartilage or true bone. Thus, we learn that the occurrence of these two main forms of skeletal tissues was probably the result of persistent local conditions such as the quantity and quality of mucopolysaccharides in the matrix, the amount of oxygenation and hydration, and possibly also some local mechanical irritant (Hall, 1970).

FIBROCARTILAGE

Special mechanical conditions seem to be provided by the large, mobile articulations. In some of the dense fibrous tendons and ligaments which surround them, a regularly occurring change leads to the formation of single rows of large, rounded cells surrounded by matrix rich in mucopolysaccharides (Fig. 6-1). These conditions are characteristic of cartilage, and the tissue in its ensemble is known as *fibrocartilage*.

CHONDROID

A primitive tissue commonly found in cyclostomes and other early vertebrates has been described as

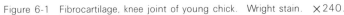

Figure 6-1   Fibrocartilage, knee joint of young chick.   Wright stain.   ×240.

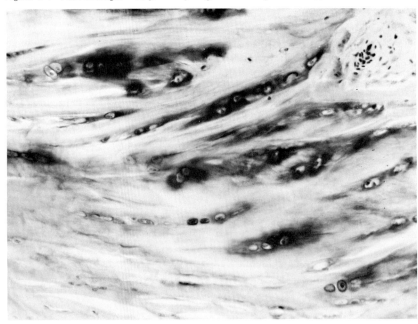

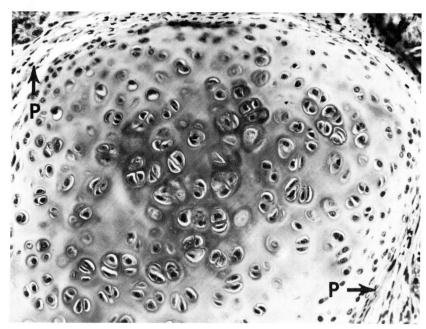

Figure 6-2   Hyaline cartilage, a part of the nasal choanae of a young cat; P, perichondrium; hematoxylin-phloxine-orange stain. ×240.

pseudocartilage, or *chondroid.* It consists of closely adjacent vesicular cells surrounded by a thin capsule rich in collagen fibers but poor in mucopolysaccharides.

Cartilage

DEVELOPMENT

Cartilage in the human embryo appears during the fifth week of life. Different inducers, such as the notocord and cells migrating from the neural crest, have been proposed by the early embryologists. More recently, Anderson (1967) has shown that injections of cultured amnion cells can provoke the formation of heterotopic cartilage and bone. The mother tissue is, of course, the versatile and multi-talented mesenchyme.

The first histologic evidence of the new tissue consists of variously shaped agglomerations of closely apposed, rounded cells. These units or *centers of chondrification* at first resemble the chondroid of more primitive species. They will grow from then on by division of already differentiated cartilage cells (*interstitial growth*) or by addition of more mesenchymal elements at the periph-ery of the unit (*appositional growth*). After a time, an envelope, the *perichondrium* (Fig. 6-2, P), consisting of densely arranged flattened cells and fibers, will form around the unit, separating it from the mesenchyme. This envelope is not only protective but is also a growth regulator. Appositional development will occur from then on through cellular differentiation at the inner surface of the perichondrium.

The main property of cartilage resides in the ability of its cells to secrete a *complex protein-polysaccharide mixture* which gels as it accumulates in the intercellular matrix (Figs. 6-2 and 6-3), producing the solid yet resilient consistency characteristic of this tissue.

A variety of technical procedures and especially electron microscopy have revealed that *fibrillo-genesis* goes on inside the cartilage masses as well

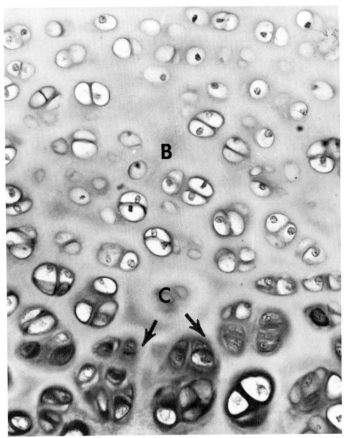

Figure 6-3 A portion of hyaline cartilage of a young cat; B, chondroblasts; C, chondrocytes. Hematoxylin-phloxine-orange stain. ×370.

as outside. In most cartilage units, the fibers are of the white, collagenic variety. These are optically homogeneous with the environmental amorphous matrix and consequently invisible by light microscopy (Figs. 6-2 and 6-3). This type of cartilage is known as *hyaline.*

A few cartilage pieces, however, such as those of the external ear, the auditory canal, the epiglottis (Fig. 6-4) and certain small laryngeal units, contain yellow *elastic* fibers. These are optically different from the fundamental substance and thus easily recognized in routinely stained preparations (Fig. 6-4).

ADULT CARTILAGE

Cells In the *appositional growth* process, the new cartilage cells originate from the inner portion of the perichondrium. They are, at first, flattened elements (Fig. 6-2) which are progressively dispersed by their secretory activity that results in the production of the new hyaline matrix (Figs. 6-2 and 6-3). In routinely stained preparations where a combination of acid dyes such as eosin, phloxine B, and orange G is used in combination with the basic dye haematoxylin, the matrix which is proximal to the perichondrium is stained with the acid dyes and is described as *acidophilic.* The immature small cells in this peripheral area are sometimes referred to as *chondroblasts* (Figs. 6-2 and 6-3, B).

Farther inward, the cells are progressively larger and the matrix around them preferentially takes up the basic dye (Figs. 6-2 and 6-3, C). This difference in staining behavior has long been thought to be related to the progressive acquisition of secretory

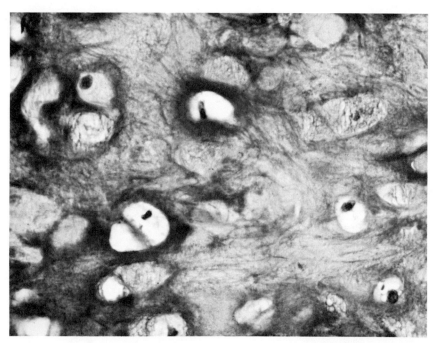

Figure 6-4   A portion of the epiglottis cartilage of an adult man.   The elastic fibers are quite prominent.   H & E.   ×370.

ability by the cartilage cell through the completion of its differentiation (chondrocytes).

At the light microscope level, the cytoplasma of the *chondrocytes* exhibits progressive staining affinity for the acid dyes along with maturation.   The adult cells often show accumulation of metaplastic masses of carbohydrates and lipids.   Technical dehydration is mainly responsible for the shrunken, sometimes crenated appearance of these cells.

Viewed through the electron microscope (Fig. 6-5), the chondrocytes exhibit a membrane system "characteristic of cells responsible for discharge of protein secretion" (Davies et al., 1962); the rough endoplasmic reticulum and portions of the Golgi complex are prominent.   Granular material (Godman and Porter, 1960; Anderson, 1967) (Fig. 6-5) and fine nonperiodic filaments (Revel and Hay, 1963) have been identified within the enlarged vesicles of the Golgi complex (Anderson, 1967) (Fig. 6-5).   The mitochondria are surprisingly abundant and apparently capable of "well-marked glycolysis" (Bywaters, 1937).   The accumulation of intracytoplasmic glycogen is apparently related to senescence (Silberberg et al., 1964).

Ground substance   Following the introduction of the integrated process of radioautography (Bélanger and Leblond, 1946), which allows the simultaneous visualization of tissue tracers and their photographic record (Fig. 6-6), dynamic histology has rapidly advanced.   One of the early achievements was the demonstration of the role of the chondrocytes in mucopolysaccharide and protein secretion.

Radioactive sodium sulfate injected into young rats was thus found incorporated into a stable compound present in considerably greater proportion within the larger cells (Fig. 6-7) a short time after the treatment and subsequently into the surrounding matrix (Bélanger, 1954).   The existence of a hyaluronidase-resistant sulfated fraction and its localization at the site of insertion of tendons and ligaments (Fig. 6-8) also was revealed by combining $^{35}SO_4$ radioautography with enzyme incubation (Bélanger, 1954).

Isogenic groups, capsule, lacuna   *Interstitial growth* occurs through division of adult chondrocytes.   The result is manifested histologically by the presence of closely apposed large cells in groups of two or

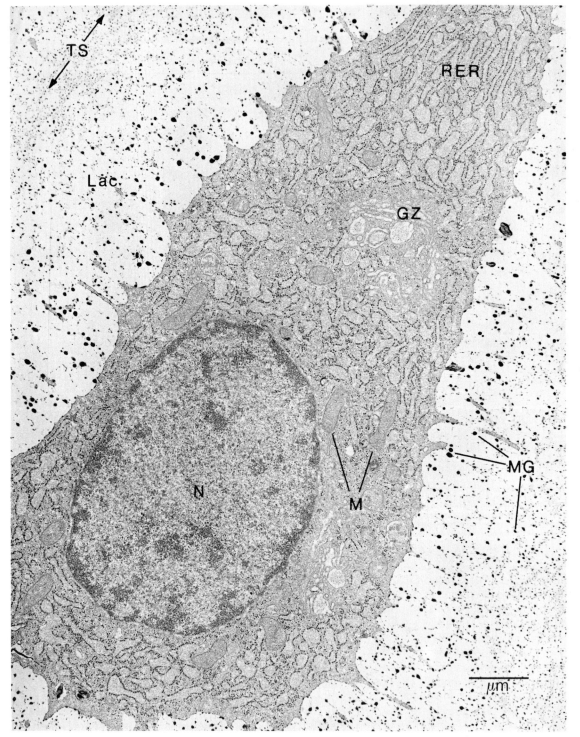

Figure 6-5 Electron micrograph of an early hypertrophic chondrocyte of rabbit epiphysis, showing a lacuna (Lac), matrix granules (MG), and a portion of transverse matrix septum (TS). (Courtesy of Dr. H. Clarke Anderson.)

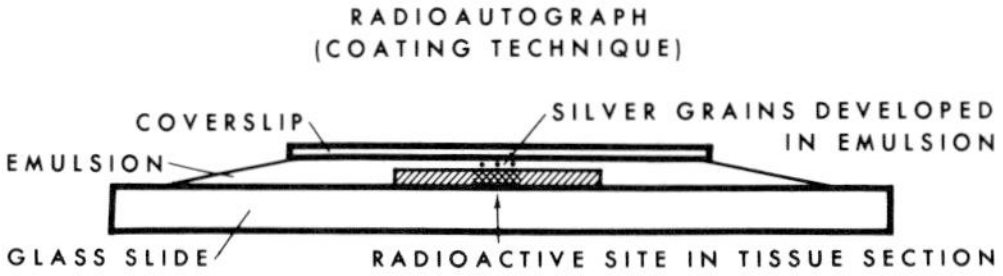

RADIOAUTOGRAPH
(COATING TECHNIQUE)

COVERSLIP   SILVER GRAINS DEVELOPED
EMULSION   IN EMULSION

GLASS SLIDE   RADIOACTIVE SITE IN TISSUE SECTION

Figure 6-6 Diagram representing the components of an integrated radioautograph.

more located deep inside the cartilage piece (Figs. 6-2 and 6-3). These groups are called *isogenic* or are said to form *nests* because they are often surrounded by a common dense basophilic layer termed *capsule* by the early histologists. This term was motivated by the fact that the layer was considered as an outer wall of the chondrocyte. Inside the capsule, the often shrunken cartilage cell occupies a space called the *lacuna.*

The *capsule* is a pericellular zone of concentrated chondromucoprotein. The presence of sulfated mucopolysaccharides in that area has been revealed histochemically by Revel (1964) with his thorium reaction (Fig. 6-9).

The basophilia of the adult cartilage matrix is not always maintained. With age and with a critical increase in size of the cartilage mass, centrally located areas of some cartilage pieces lose their basophilia. This is due to a decrease in the secretion of sulfated mucoprotein and also to the accumulation in the matrix of an *albuminoid* chemically related to keratin, a strongly acidophilic substance.

Collagen Histologic procedures for staining cartilage have placed a great deal of emphasis on the mucopolysaccharides and the protein components of ground substance. However, the masked collagen forms an important component of this tissue: up to 40 percent of the dry weight is collagen. Recent electron microscope radioautographic studies of a collagen precursor, [3H]proline (Revel and Hay, 1963), have revealed the presence of this substance inside the endoplasmic reticulum of the chondrocytes and its rapid passage into the surrounding matrix. Apparently there are fibrils of different sizes in cartilage and also fibrils with a

Figure 6-7 Radioautograph of $^{35}SO_4$ incorporation and synthesis into sulfated mucopolysaccharide by the cartilage cells. The label is located mostly in the large chondrocytes 2 hr after administration. ×50.

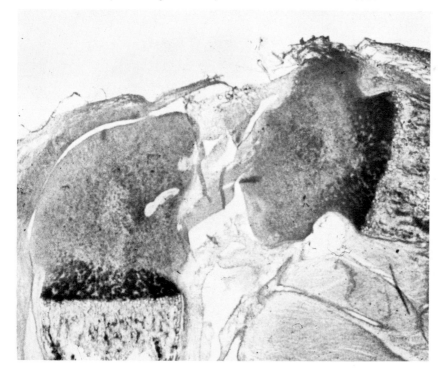

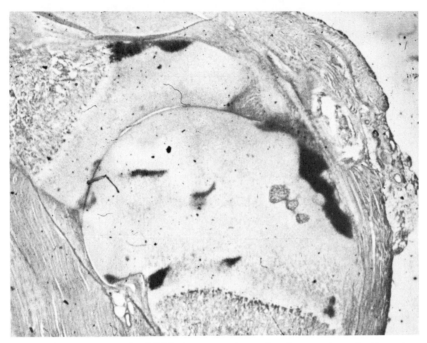

Figure 6-8 Radioautograph of $^{35}SO_4$ incorporated as sulfated mucopolysaccharide and secreted into the matrix. The section has been treated with hyaluronidase which has removed the label except in sites of insertion of tendons and ligaments where presumably a hyaluronidase-resistant mucopolysaccharide is present. ×50.

Figure 6-9 Electron micrograph of a portion of mouse cartilage. The section has been stained with colloidal thorium to show the presence of acid mucopolysaccharides. A perilacunar concentration is apparent. ×10,000. (Courtesy of Dr. J. P. Revel and Journal de Microscopie.)

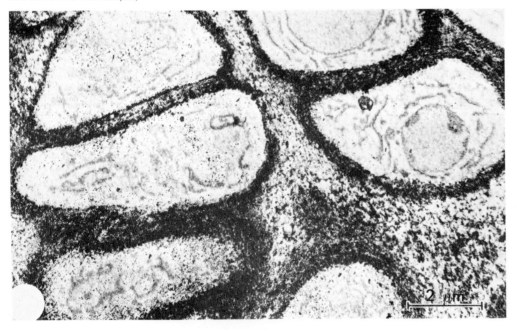

varying periodicity (Anderson, 1967; Fahmy et al., 1969) which may possess different physiologic properties.

Collagen fibers are said to be randomly distributed in the matrix. There are, however, local concentrations in the immediate vicinity of the lacuna (capsule). The same is true of elastic fibers (Fig. 6-4). In some cartilage pieces, an apparently organized network of fibers seem to radiate from a nutritional zone containing blood vessels to surrounding lacunae (*interlacunar network*, Fig. 6-10; Bélanger, 1959; Bélanger and Migicovsky, 1961).

Blood vessels   Cartilage is essentially an avascular tissue. In contrast to most other tissues (another remarkable exception is the cornea), it has *no capillary network of its own*. It must draw its nutrition from fluids which are capable of diffusing through its matrix. The fluid content of this matrix is on the order of 75 percent of the fresh weight, a finding surprising to the morphologist.

It has been said that interstitial growth is stimulated by the need for the hinterland chondrocytes to increase their surface in order to maintain their oxygen supply from a progressively poorer environment as these cells become located farther away from the blood vessels. When interstitial growth is no longer possible, often the cells cannot maintain their normal metabolic activities. They degenerate and die.

GROWTH AND MAINTENANCE FACTORS
Nutritional   Severe deficiency in the nutritional supply of protein precursors, minerals, and vitamins such as A, C, and D, leads to abnormal growth and maturation of cartilage.

Vitamin A   Very little information is as yet available on the skeletal effects of vitamin A deficiency in man. Nevertheless, in birds, where Wolbach and Hegsted (1952) have studied this problem particularly well, the maturation of the epiphyseal cartilage was irregular and less extensive than normal. Mitotic activity was arrested, but continuous secretion associated with lack of maturation led to the formation of a broad zone of immature tissue.

Vitamin C   This vitamin is apparently needed for the production of collagen, if not for its maintenance (Ham and Elliot, 1938). According to Bourne (1956), it also has a role in the production of

Figure 6-10   A portion of the articular cartilage of the tibia of a young chick, stained by the PAS reagent. The fibers of the interlacunar network are apparent.   ×550.

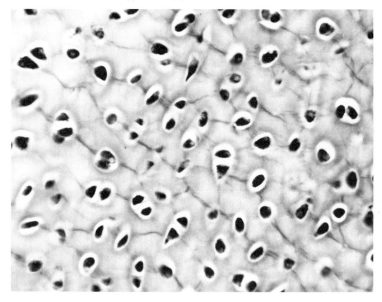

ground substance through its stimulation of the oxidative enzymes which preside over the oxidation of organic sulfur to sulfate as part of the process of chondroitin sulfate synthesis.

Vitamin D   Rickets (''die Englische Krankeit,'' Glisson, 1650), was a prominent disease of the Northern countries in days gone by.   The use of cod-liver oil as a cure in man dates back to the end of the eighteenth century (Harris, 1956).   However, the synthesis of vitamin D and its abundance in the liver of the teleost fish recall dramas of survival which occurred millions of years ago as the bony fishes migrated into mineral-poor ponds and streams (McLean and Urist, 1968).

The search for the intimate effects of vitamin D has ''frustrated the efforts of so many for so long'' (DeLuca, 1967) until this substance was recently recognized as involved in inducing the synthesis of enzymes ''responsible for the formation of a calcium transport protein'' (DeLuca, 1970).   The main problem is one of a deficient supply of calcium and potassium to mineralizing tissues (*Nutrition*

Reviews, 1968).   The morphologic manifestations of rickets include a *subsequent* retardation of maturation but not of growth of the cartilage pieces. This leads to cartilage hypertrophy and eventual degeneration.

Hormones   Several hormones have an important role in the growth and maintenance of cartilage.

Somatotropin   The growth hormone of the *adenohypophysis,* this hormone is essential for the proper growth of cartilage and for the maintenance of the secretory activity of the chondrocytes.   In a young rat surgically deprived of its hypophysis, the thickness of the epiphyseal plate of the long bones is most affected (Fig. 6-12).   As compared with that of a normal littermate (Fig. 6-11), the cartilaginous plate is thinner, the cells are flattened and less numerous (Fig. 6-12), their mitotic activity decreases (Bois et al., 1963), and the matrix looses its metachromasia (Fig. 6-12), an indication that its sulfated mucopolysaccharide content has considerably decreased.   Treatment of an hypophysec-

Figure 6-11   A portion of the epiphyseal plate of the tibia of a young rat.   A. zone of resting or reserve cartilage; B. zone of young proliferating cartilage; C. zone of maturing cartilage; D. zone of calcifying cartilage.   Toluidine blue stain.   ×120.

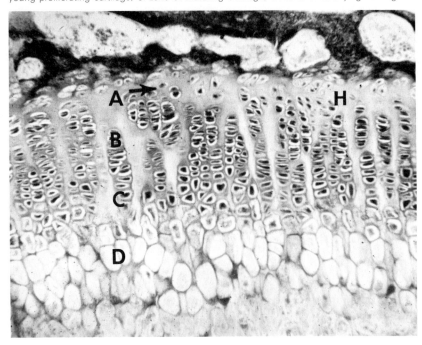

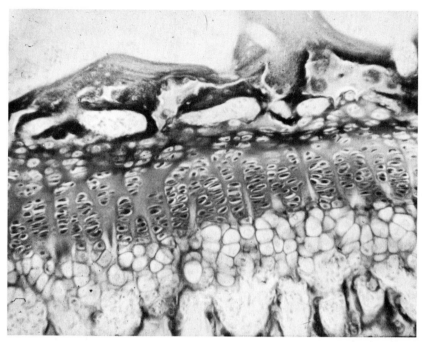

Figure 6-12   An area comparable to that of Fig. 6-11, but from an hypophysectomized littermate.   The plate is thinner; the cartilage cells have practically stopped secreting.   ×120.

tomized animal with growth hormone fully restores the normal size, histologic appearance (Fig. 6-12), and mitotic (Bois et al., 1963) and secretory activity (Fig. 6-13) after 3 days.

Thyroid   The thyroid gland apparently is synergistic with the hypophysis in promoting normal skeletal growth (Turner, 1966).   Removal of either the hypophysis or the thyroid in a young animal produces *dwarfism*.   An exaggerated amount of growth hormone during the period of growth promotes *gigantism*.   In the absence of the hypophysis, the thyroid hormone thyroxine promotes erosion of the cartilage and its replacement by bone.

Male sex hormone   Testosterone, the male sex hormone, is an anabolic factor and promotes protein synthesis.   Thus, in principle, it favors cartilage growth.   However, since it has been found to promote maturation at the same time (Silberberg and Silberberg, 1956; Joss et al., 1963), the net result is harmonious maintenance.

Estrogens   "Present knowledge concerning the relationship of oestrogens to postfetal osteogenesis is obscure" (McLean and Urist, 1968).   Fahmy et al. (1969) have recently observed that fibrillogenesis in cartilage is stimulated by this type of hormone.

Cortisone   The anti-inflammatory hormone of the adrenal cortex, cortisone apparently retards the maturation of cartilage and its replacement by bone at the epiphyseal plate.   It interferes somehow with the metabolism of the sulfated mucopolysaccharides (Kowalewski, 1958; Bélanger and Migicovsky, 1960).

DEGENERATION AND CALCIFICATION

When the chondrocytes can no longer maintain their production of sulfated mucoprotein, the water content of the matrix decreases and albuminoid appears as mentioned above.   The matrix sometimes takes on a fibrous appearance ("asbestfaserung," amiantine degeneration) and precipitation of mineral salts occurs.   These events add insult to

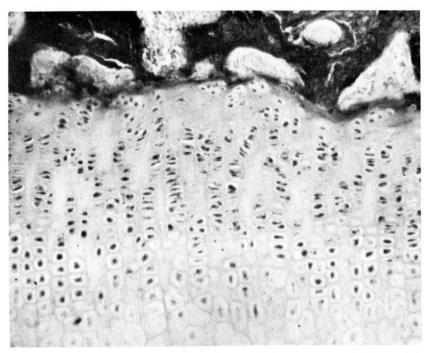

Figure 6-13 The epiphyseal plate of an hypophysectomized young rat treated with growth hormone. Growth and secretion have been resumed.   ×120.

injury; separated further from their vital supplies, the chondrocytes rapidly lose their glycogen reserves and soon degenerate and perish. These various episodes of cartilage degeneration are far less frequent in elastic cartilage than in the hyaline variety.

The factors responsible for mineral precipitation have been under intense scrutiny by researchers from various disciplines. In recent time, a greater collaboration between morphologists, physiologists, and biochemists has led to considerable learning. According to Hirschman and Dziewiatkowski (1966), ''during or just preceding calcification, protein-polysaccharide or its protein component is lost or drastically altered.'' The relationship of collagen to mineralization has been revealed through the beautiful electron micrographs of Robinson and Watson (1952), Jackson (1957), Glimcher et al. (1957), and Nylen et al. (1960): the crystals of hydroxyapatite in the form of little needles line themselves up along the collagen

fibers, starting at the periodically repeated ''nodes'' of the fibers.

The exact role of the mucopolysaccharides has been much less evident until very recently. Anderson (1967) and Bonucci (1967) described ''roundish bodies forming near both maturing and hypertrophic cells'' containing glycoprotein and ''changing as crystallites are laid in them'' (Bonucci, 1967). Matukas and Krikos (1968) have also suggested that protein-polysaccharide changes take place at the level of these matrix bodies. Anderson (1969) and Ali et al. (1970) have been able to demonstrate that these bodies could be resolved as vesicles (Figs. 6-5 and 6-14) and state that these are probably extruded by the chondrocytes and, furthermore, that these particles which contain enzymes, lipids, and a membrane ''could locally concentrate calcium and/or phosphate ions to the point of crystallization.'' Thus these extracellular membranes would be primarily responsible for the initiation of mineralization in the carti-

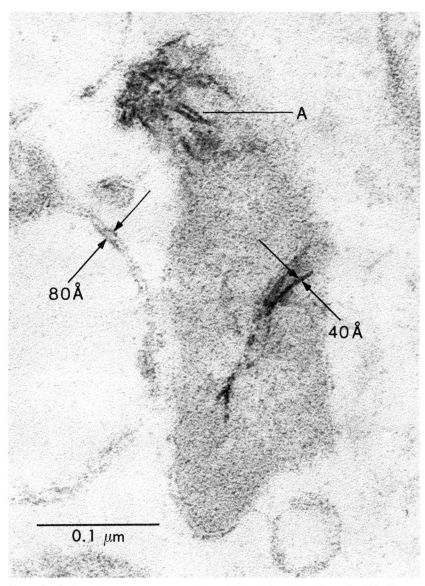

Figure 6-14   Vesicles within the matrix of calcifying epiphyseal cartilage of rabbit. These vesicles appear to be the initial site of deposition of calcium phosphate in the form of hydroxyapatite and/or fluorapatite (A).   The apatite needles measure approximately 40 Å in width and the unit membrane which invests the vesicles measures approximately 80 Å in overall thickness. The photograph shows an early stage of calcification with typical deposition of needles within the substance of a vesicle and also adjacent to the vesicular membrane. Glutarldehyde fixation with postosmication and lead citrate and uranyl acetate staining. ×333,000.   (Courtesy of Dr. H. Clark Anderson).

lage matrix, a last protective effort of the dying chondrocyte.

REPAIR, TRANSPLANTATION, ANTIGENICITY, SELF-INDUCTION

The chondrogenic activity of the perichondrium is limited to the period of youth and active growth. When injury occurs in an adult cartilage piece, cells from the perichondrium proliferate but generally produce dense fibrous tissue which may then change slowly and only in part into cartilage.

Cartilage is considered a good candidate for *transplantation* in autografts and even in allografts.

The chondrocytes, because of their low metabolic activity in a normally avascular environment, are well adapted to surgical transfer. On the other hand, the host is protected against their antigens, which cannot diffuse easily through the matrix. It seems from recent observations that cartilage antigenicity is very low at any rate (Peacock et al., 1960). On the other hand, a cartilage allograft in the connective tissue of a young growing animal, even if it dies after a time, often induces a chondrogenic or osteogenic persistent reaction from the host (McLean and Urist, 1968).

Bone

ORIGIN

The sharks, which have an endoskeleton entirely composed of cartilage, have calcium deposits in the interior of their vertebrae which apparently are highly reactive and constitute a mineral bank of a sort (McLean and Urist, 1968). In the majority of modern fishes, in amphibians, and in terrestrial

Figure 6-15   Head of a human embryo of $3\frac{1}{2}$ months gestation. Stained with alizarin and cleared to reveal the trabeculae radiating from the centers of intramembranous ossification in the frontal and parietal bones.   ×1.5

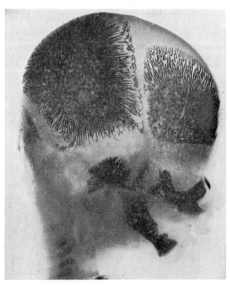

vertebrates, however, the organism depends for support and for storage of minerals on the ancestral armor tissue known as bone. Although in a few species such as the turtle the *exoskeleton* or dermal type of bone persists, in most the dermal skeletal pieces have disappeared; they have been replaced by a well-developed internal bony framework, the *endoskeleton*. The endoskeleton is of mesodermic origin. It sometimes arises directly from the primitive cells of mesenchyme as in the case of a small number of flat bones located close to the surface known as *membrane* bones. More often, bone is preceded in the embryo by a cartilage template which it replaces totally or partially; all the long bones arising through this *replacement process* are thus described as *endochondral*.

These traditional appellations have caused a great deal of confusion. It is now suggested that they be replaced by the following: (1) The bones of direct connective tissue origin could be called mesenchymal bones. (2) Those that arise by partial replacement of a prior cartilage anlage would then be known as osteochondral complexes.

BASIC STRUCTURAL COMPONENTS

Mesenchymal bones   *Mesenchymal bones* arise at *ossification centers* (Fig. 6-15). These are areas in which the loosely arranged mesenchymal cells of the embryo are seen to increase in number through a local acceleration of the mitotic rate.

The new cells soon show a modified microscopic appearance: they become enlarged and their cytoplasm shows an affinity for the basic dyes. Soon they will line up in single or double rows (Fig. 6-16), and as a result of a newly acquired secretory activity, a layer of modified intercellular substance will appear (Fig. 6-16).

Bone matrix New matrix called *bone matrix* contains densely arranged collagen fibers soon obliterated from the microscopic picture as they become embedded in amorphous ground substance rich in mucopolysaccharides. Almost immediately also, mineral salts consisting mainly of a crystalline form of *calcium phosphate* known as *hydroxyapatite* precipitate into the newly formed bone matrix.

The early bone histologists (Pommer, 1885) used to describe a zone of nonmineralized matrix, which they called osteoid, at the border of the bone matrix. McLean and Bloom (1940), using the silver nitrate method of von Kossa to demonstrate microscopically the bone minerals, concluded that "the matrix may be regarded as calcifiable as soon as the tissue is recognizable as bone" (McLean and Bloom, 1940). Current observations with the electron microscope have shown, on the other hand, that "there is a thin layer of 1 μ or less of uncalcified preosseous tissue, during the formation of bone even in animals with an optimum intake of minerals" (McLean and Urist, 1968).

Recent electron-microscope and crystallographic studies indicate that mineralization is not an immediate process, but that it depends on the presence of extracellular vesicular extrusions rich in polysaccharides and capable of providing cationic binding sites for calcium (Bernard and Pease, 1968). These buds "are also aggregating agents for collagenous fibrils" (Matthews et al., 1970). They are apparently preformed inside the osteoblasts (Pautard, 1966). These descriptions seem to match those previously reported in this chapter for mineralizing cartilage.

Figure 6-16 Intramembranous bone formation in the maxilla of a cat fetus. Osteoblasts are aligned along a trabeculum of new bone. ×1200. (Nonidez and Windle.)

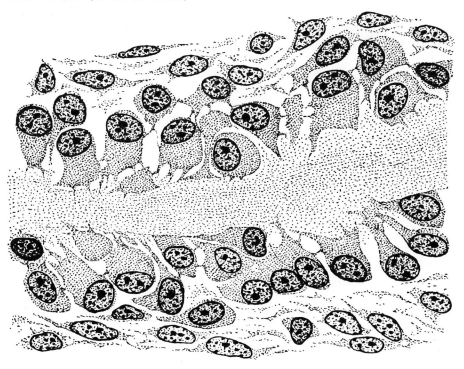

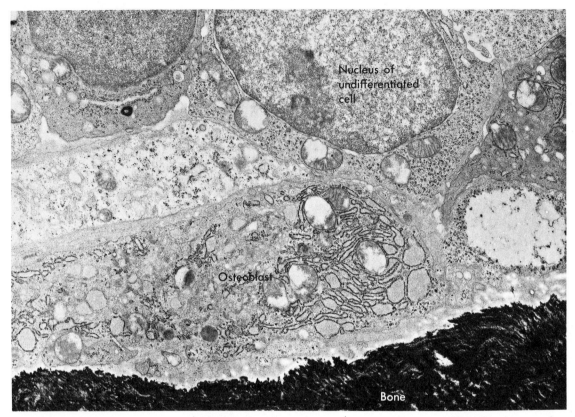

Figure 6-17   Electron micrograph showing an osteoblast (B) immediately adjacent to the bone surface.   Development of rough ER and Golgi is great compared with that in undifferentiated cells above.   Almost no unmineralized bone is visible.   ×6,000. (Courtesy of Dr. Stephen B. Doty.)

Osteoblasts   The cells with the new osteogenic potential are called *osteoblasts*.   These highly basophilic elements closely apposed in an epithelial-like fashion (Fig. 6-16) show in the electron microscope a typical secretory development of the rough endoplasmic reticulum (Fig. 6-17) and the Golgi (Fig. 6-17).   Sometimes large confluent vesicles are present at the apical pole of the cell (Fig. 6-17), which faces the new mineralized matrix.

Osteocytes   As subsequent rows of osteoblasts differentiate behind the original one, the new osteoblasts will start secreting and the cells of the first row will now be imprisoned in bone matrix which will segregate them generally as single cells in lacunae (Fig. 6-18), as was the case for cartilage.

However, here there are two major differences: (1) The imprisoned cells, now called osteocytes, will rarely divide, so that growth of bone will be strictly by the appositional process.   (2) The osteocytes will not be isolated in their lacunae.   Through a large number of *processes* they will remain in close membrane contact with adjacent osteocytes and with the surface osteoblasts.   The processes under normal conditions maintain their integrity inside channels known as *canaliculi* (Fig. 6-19).

In electron micrographs young osteocytes resemble osteoblasts.   However, a gradual decrease in the amount of endoplasmic reticulum and a diminution in the size of the Golgi complex occurs (Jande and Bélanger, 1971.   Fig. 6-20).   Fine filamentous processes appear under the plasma membrane.   These extend into the processes,

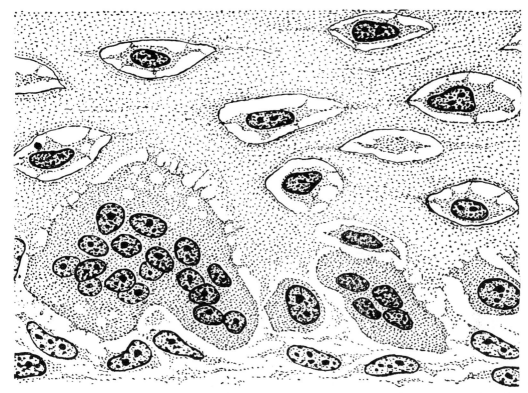

Figure 6-18   Osteoclasts.   The large one is in a Howship's lacuna, on a trabeculum of fetal jawbone.   Osteoblasts, osteocytes, osteoclasts, fetal jaw bone.   ×1,200.   (Nonidez and Windle.)

Figure 6-19   Portion of a rat tibia stained with picrothionine to show the canaliculi.   ×550.

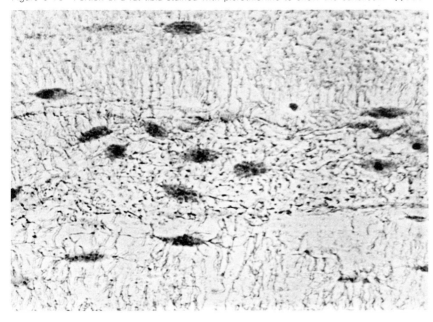

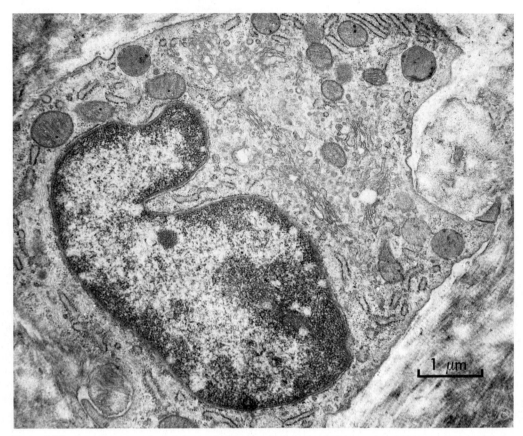

Figure 6-20 A young osteocyte showing endoplasmic reticulum, the Golgi complex, and lysosomes.

where they become the main constituents (Fig. 6-20). A few membrane-bound dark bodies also appear in the young osteocytes. These are probably lysosomes; they will be discussed later. The pericellular space separating the plasma membrane of the osteocyte from the border of the lacuna is quite small at first (Fig. 6-20).

Trabeculae As more rows of primitive cells differentiate into osteoblasts and new bone is laid down, the new tissue will not grow into a uniform mass like cartilage, but spider-like threads will radiate away from the centers of ossification (Fig. 6-15). These bone threads are called trabeculae. They are the units of mesenchymal or membranous bone.

Blood vessels A very interesting observation was

made by Harris and Ham (1956) in their study of fracture repair and the conditions which made bone transplants viable. It had been known for some time that bone grafting, even in autotransplants, was a far more hazardous affair than cartilage transplantation. One important factor was the more critical requirement for blood circulation. As new layers of bone are being added to preexisting surfaces, "this must be accomplished . . . so that no bone cell is removed more than a fraction of a millimeter from a capillary" (Harris and Ham, 1956). In his textbook (1969), Ham emphasizes this point: "In the experience of the author, trabeculae of more than one fifth of a millimeter in thickness generally have blood vessels disposed in canals near their middles to provide the more deeply disposed bone cells with nourishment. Accordingly the thickness of solid trabeculae is limited."

Osteoclasts When the growing trabeculae reach a critical thickness, when there is a need for the bone unit to adopt a special form in order to conform to regional requirements, or if something happens to the nutritional supply or to the regulating agents so that abnormal bone formation occurs, a new type of cell will enter the scene. This new cell will always appear at the periphery of the trabecula. Generally it will be located next to the bone surface itself. It is sometimes found half buried in indentations known as Howship's lacunae (Figs. 6-18 and 6-21). It is easily distinguished from adjacent osteoblasts or preosteoblasts: it is several times larger than these and contains several nuclei (Figs. 6-18 and 6-21). The cytoplasm of these multinucleated cells stains with either the basic or the acid dyes, sometimes with both. On the surface which touches the bone, *a ruffled border* is seen; underneath it, the cytoplasm is frothy as if intense gas bubbling were occurring. The bone surface of the Howship's lacuna is also modified. It often shows patches of lower density in microradiographs. It is not surprising that Kölliker (1873) from the very beginning considered these cells as bone-destroying rather than bone-building elements and called them "Ostoklast," which later became *osteoclast,* the bone-eating cell.

In recent times, electron microscopists have confirmed the classic status of these bone eaters. The ruffled border was shown to be constituted by microvilli (Fig. 6-22A and B). Between these, mineral particles and microfibrils of collagen have been detected (Hancox and Boothroyd, 1963). Within the cells, membrane-bound dense bodies rich in lytic enzymes have been identified as lysosomes (Fig. 6-22A).

Radioautography of a DNA precursor, [^{3}H] thymidine, has revealed that a flow of new nuclei enters constantly into these cells as older nuclei degenerate (Bélanger and Migicovsky, 1963; Bélanger and Drouin, 1968). The new nuclei are apparently contributed by adjacent primitive cells which fuse with the osteoclasts. Once inside the osteoclast, the nuclei seldom divide but have a limited life-span of only a few days (Bélanger and Drouin, 1968) while the large multinucleated cells, capable of renewing their nuclei, seem to enjoy a very long life.

Cancellous bone, marrow spaces Mesenchymal bone or trabecular bone is the original form of bone in the embryo. When considered as a tissue, it constitutes what is referred to in anatomy textbooks as *cancellous bone* or *spongy bone.* This type of

Figure 6-21 A portion of a trabecula from the jawbone of a horse which has been fed an exaggerated amount of phosphate for 30 weeks. The newly formed bone is fibrillar and poorly mineralized. The trabeculae are surrounded by a large number of osteoclasts. Wright stain. ×360.

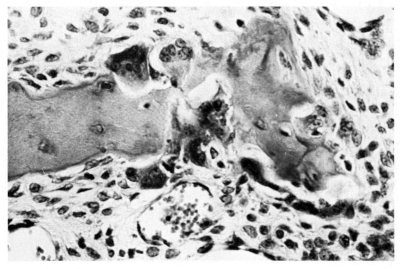

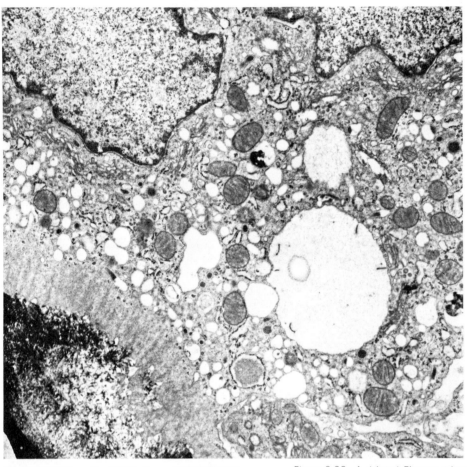

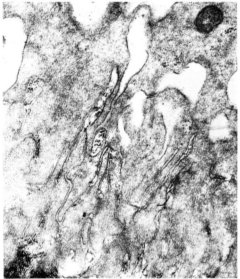

Figure 6-22 A. (above) Electron micrograph of a portion of an osteoclast showing the brush border (B) and a variety of intracellular constituents such as vacuoles (V), lysomes (L), mitochondria (M), the Golgi (G), and portions of the nucleus (N). ×6,000. B. (left) A portion of the brush border of the above at ×25,500. Individual infoldings (B) in immediate proximity to the bone are visible. Behind these are found many large vacuoles. (Courtesy of Dr. Stephen B. Doty.)

bone tissue represents the ensemble of mesenchymal bone even in adult life. In the more numerous osteochondral complexes which are the long bones, the trabecular, cancellous type of bone will represent a general embryonic condition. As the more adult type, known as *compact bone,* develops (Fig. 6-23), the cancellous trabeculae will persist within the deeper regions of the extremities (Fig. 6-23). In fresh preparations, these trabeculae are easily recognized by the honeycomb, spongy appearance of the bone and by the intense red color of the tissue in between. In the early days of cancellous bone, it seems that this new tissue has an inducing influence on the immediately adjacent mesenchyme: In the highly protected little locular spaces between the branching trabeculae, the hematopoietic marrow will differentiate. The spaces then become known as *primary marrow spaces.* Cancellous bone will retain its precious hematopoietic red marrow throughout life.

Periosteum As each unit of mesenchymal bone becomes constituted and takes shape, as with the previously described pieces of cartilage, it becomes surrounded by a distinct membrane, the *periosteum.* Histologically it is possible to distinguish two regions in the periosteum, especially during the period of growth of the bone: an *outer* portion, made of tough, fibrous tissue, and an *inner* region, called the *cambium,* more loosely arranged and better vascularized, from which the bone-forming osteoblasts will differentiate.

The osteochondral complexes All the bones of the body are of mesenchymal origin. Nevertheless, most bones will develop around and eventually within a cartilage primordium. In some rare instances, as in the case of Meckel's cartilage of the lower jaw, the new tissue will completely replace the preexisting cartilage piece. In the majority of cases, the osseous tissue will replace the cartilage

Figure 6-23 Section of the upper end of the human femur and x-ray picture (right) showing weak area of neck. (Courtesy of Dr. William J. Tobin.)

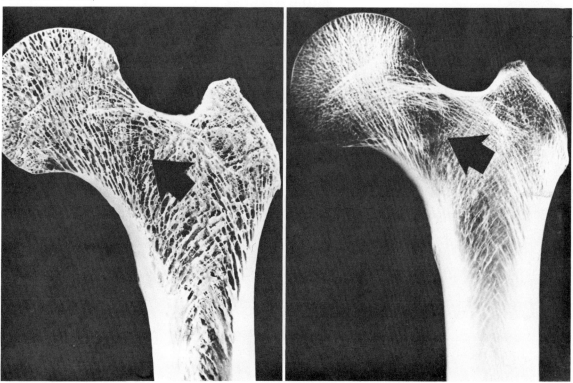

only in part—thus the term *osteochondral complex,* which is now proposed for this variety, classically known as *endochondral bone.*

Ossification of the cartilage primordium begins very early. For instance, the human femur begins to ossify when the embryo is only 7 weeks old and 17 mm long. The general shape of the early embryonic femur closely resembles that of the adult. Its main features are the two extremities, the proximal and distal *epiphyses,* and the elongated, roughly cylindrical midpiece, the *diaphysis.*

The diaphyseal phase: PERICHONDRAL OSSIFICATION

The cartilage primordium belongs to the hyaline variety. Although wider, the epiphyseal portions do not grow at the same rate as the diaphyseal portion. In the latter, the newly formed cells align themselves in rows between which only a small amount of matrix forms (Fig. 6-24A). The first mature chondrocytes occupy the middiaphysis. They will rapidly degenerate (Fig. 6-22B), and the adjacent matrix will become mineralized. At this moment, the surrounding perichondrium *changes its potential:* from chondrogenic it becomes osteogenic.

Figure 6-24 Diagrams of the ossification of a long bone. A. Early cartilaginous stage. B. Stage of eruption of the periosteal bone collar by an osteogenic bud of vessels. C. Older stage with a primary marrow cavity and early centers of calcification in the epiphyseal cartilages. D. The condition shortly after birth with epiphyseal centers of ossification. Calcified cartilage in all diagrams is black; *b,* periosteal bone collar; *m,* marrow cavity; *p,* periosteal bone; *v,* blood vessels entering the centers of ossification. (Nonidez and Windle.)

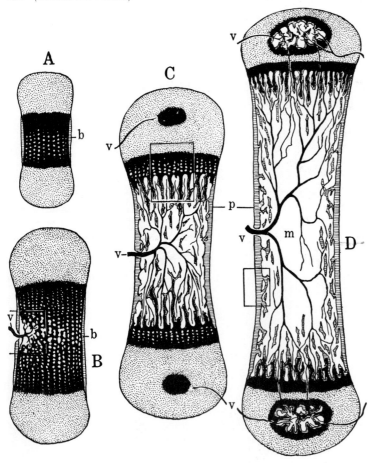

The initial bone deposition will be in the form of a *middiaphyseal ring* surrounding the area of cartilage degeneration and calcification. Some years ago, Lacroix (1949) postulated an induction effect from the modified cartilage in the form of a secretory product (''osteogenin'') capable of influencing the perichondrial cells (or for that matter, connective tissue cells anywhere in the body) so they would be programmed toward manufacturing bone. Further work has failed to reveal a specific inducer; it seems that a variety of chemical substances can trigger the phenomenon of bone growth.

SUBEPIPHYSEAL BONE GROWTH   As the initial peripheral bone ring enlarges by further perichondrial-periosteal conversion toward the epiphyses (Fig. 6-24C), the cartilage inside seems to accelerate its degeneration (Fig. 6-24C). Blood vessels (Fig. 6-24C and D) will invade the spaces created by the cartilage breakdown and will colonize the inner portion of the degenerating primordium, stretching their network until they reach the subepiphyseal area where accompanying cells will turn into osteoblasts and lay down bone onto calcified remnants of cartilage matrix. The result will be a subepiphyseal bone colony in which the units will be linear, fragile, pencil-like outgrowths known as *spicules,* consisting of a small layer of bone investing an acellular, calcified cartilage core (Fig. 6-24C and D). While this subepiphyseal colony is being established, the peripheral periosteal growth continues (Fig. 6-24C and D). Since growth has originated at the middiaphysis, it is not surprising to find that the bone is thickest in that area, tapering down to the epiphyseal limits where a circular depressed area (notch of Ranvier) marks the zone of transition.

In normal vertebrate bones, the length of the subepiphyseal spicules and the thickness of the periosteal bone are constantly kept in check by osteoclasts which appear in the *central cavity.* This cavity, like the primary marrow spaces, will soon become filled with hematopoietic and adipose-rich *marrow* (Fig. 6-24D, m).

EPIPHYSEAL BONE CENTERS; ARTICULAR CARTILAGE; EPIPHYSEAL PLATE   The next major step in the establishment of a long bone is the development within the epiphyses of one or more ossification centers. This phenomenon is marked by the development of blood vessels which will occasionally penetrate the epiphyseal cartilage radiating toward its center (Fig.

6-24C and D, v. Apparently, these hasten the degeneration and calcification of cartilage which precedes bone formation (Fig. 6-24C and D).

The epiphyseal bone centers will undergo limited growth only. Throughout life, in most instances, a cartilage vault will persist over this bone-marrow center and will take part in the mobile relationship with adjacent bone units; this permanent feature of the bone head is the *articular cartilage.*

Underneath the epiphyseal bone center, cartilage will also remain, separating the epiphyseal bone colony. This cartilaginous disc is the *epiphyseal plate* (Fig. 6-24D; also Figs. 6-12–6-14). The epiphyseal plate will persist until the adult length for each individual bone has been reached. In the human species, the life-span of the epiphyseal plate is, on the average, 3 years shorter for the female than for the male. In the male, most of the plates have disappeared by the twentieth year.

THE METAPHYSIS: ENDOSTEAL BONE GROWTH   In the bony fishes and the amphibians, only periosteal bone develops. When a long bone of these early vertebrates is boiled and all organic matter is destroyed, a hollow, diaphyseal cylinder is the only thing that remains. In reptiles, birds, and mammals, the diaphyseal cylindrical shaft is united to the much wider epiphysis by a tapered conical portion (Fig. 6-25) known as the *metaphysis.* This strong and graceful additional supporting structure, akin to the capitals of columns in architecture, was developed at a time when the body lost the buoyancy of its original aquatic environment as the reptiles became the conquerors of the earth.

The metaphysis appears late in the embryo as it does in the history of bone. It grows through the establishment of an osteoblastic colony, probably originating from the subepiphyseal center. However, as this *endosteal* colony has to cope with the problem of maintaining a relationship between a slowly expanding diaphysis and a rapidly enlarging epiphysis, metaphyseal growth must occur according to a *gradient* progressively accelerated toward the epiphysis. That this is actually the case was demonstrated in recent time by radioautography (Leblond et al., 1950) (Fig. 6-25).

THE EPIPHYSEAL PLATE   The role of the epiphyseal plate in controlling growth in length was recognized early in the eighteenth century by Hales (1727) and by Duhamel (1743a) through simple experiments

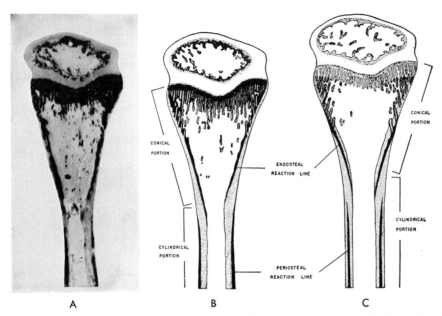

A   B   C

Figure 6-25   A. Radioautograph of the head of the tibia of a young growing rat killed a few hours after injection of ³²P.   The blackened areas of the photographic emulsion reveal the location of the radioactive phosphorus in the underlying section of the bone. The phosporus is incorporated at the sites of active bone deposition.   (Radioautograph by C. P. Leblond, G. W. Wilkinson, L. F. Bélanger, and J. Robichon reproduced from a review by J. Gross et al., Amer. J. Roentgen., 65:443, 1951.)   B. Diagram interpreting the radioautograph.   Black areas indicating the sites of incorporation of ³²P are found overlying the zone of provisional calcification in the epiphyseal cartilage, the trabeculae of the metaphysis, the endosteal surface of the conical portion, and the periosteal surface of the cylindrical portion of the shaft.   C. Diagram showing distribution of the radioisotope in the tibia of an animal killed several days after injection of ³²P.   As a result of growth subsequent to the injection, the reactive material is now found in trabeculae well below the epiphyseal cartilage and in the interior of the compacta in the shaft.   (B and C, after C. P. Leblond, G. W. Wilkinson, L. F. Bélanger, and J. Robichon, Amer. J. Anat. 86:289, 1950.)

in which *metal implants* above and below the plate of young animals became progressively separated, while two implants, both located below the plate, retained a constant relationship.   Duhamel (1743b) apparently also recognized the mechanism of peripheral accretion as responsible for the increase in diaphyseal thickness.   This observation was the result of intermittent feeding of madder, a plant which contains a red coloring agent that attaches itself to newly formed bone.   Thus, red rings alternating with white and originating at the periosteal surface marked the period of madder-labeling in the growing bones.   *Intravital color labeling* is still widely used in contemporary bone investigation.   In the nineteenth century, interstitial metal implants were employed by John Hunter to demonstrate that interstitial growth does not exist in bone.

A variety of growth mechanisms have been ob-

served in recent time by the use of *x-ray* (Fig. 6-23), a method which still yields considerable information in the case of individual children as to their skeletal response to nutritional, hormonal, genetic, climatic, and even economic factors (Harris, 1933; Lacroix, 1949).

Endosteal accretion in the metaphysis and the existence of the growth gradient at that level have been revealed by *radioautography* of labeled bone precursors (Leblond et al., 1950) (Fig. 6-25).

Recently, alizarin, the bone-coloring substance extracted from the madder plant, has been found to fluoresce brightly in ultraviolet light.   Other substances, such as antibiotic cyclines, porphyrin, and carotenoids, have the same property and have been utilized for bone labeling.   Krook et al. (1970), using a triple *fluorochrome label* in dogs, have recently mapped the transit of the variously colored fluorescent lines in long bones of dogs over a period of 41 weeks. Such studies have led the authors to conclude ''that these tissues are in a state of constant flow.''

In the functional epiphyseal plate responsible for the growth in length of the osteochondral complex, four zones are described, extending from the epiphyseal side toward the subepiphyseal ossifying portion:

ZONE OF RESTING OR RESERVE CARTILAGE These cells (Fig. 6-11A) consist of only a few rows of small cells, mostly immature and evenly distributed in the intercellular matrix.

THE ZONE OF YOUNG PROLIFERATING CARTILAGE The cells in this zone are bunched in linear piles like coins (Fig. 6-11B). In spite of the known function of this zone, mitotic figures are rare in routinely prepared specimens. However, when a DNA tracer such as [3H]thymidine has been administered, radioactive, newly synthesized DNA, mostly located in the first few rows of cells in this zone, is revealed by radioautography (Fig. 6-26).

THE ZONE OF MATURING CARTILAGE This area is thinner than the former one; the cells are larger (Fig. 6-11C), and they secrete and accumulate carbohydrates and lipids; they show a strong alkaline phosphatase activity (Fig. 6-27).

THE ZONE OF CALCIFYING CARTILAGE This zone contains mainly degenerating and dead chondrocytes (Fig. 6-11D). The lacunae are considerably enlarged and the thin intercellular bands of matrix are calcified as demonstrated by the von Kossa procedure, whereby calcium phosphate is transformed into a silver phosphate from which a black silver precipitate is obtained by treatment with a reducing agent (Fig. 6-28).

SIGNIFICANCE AND FATE OF THE EPIPHYSEAL PLATE Comparisons between bone radiographs taken at two successive periods of growth indicate clearly that with time the epiphyseal plate is displaced in relation to the diaphysis (Fig. 6-29). The distance between the two positions indicates the growth in length. It is also evident that in the meantime the metaphysis has undergone a complex remodeling (Fig. 6-29) as the result of the teamwork of the bone-forming and bone-destroying cells.

The significance of the spicules hanging like stalactites from the epiphyseal plate is at first mysterious. However, comparative histology has re-

Figure 6-26 Radioautograph of [3H]thymidine incorporation into some of the cells of the proliferating zone of the epiphyseal plate of the tibia of a young rat. ×370.

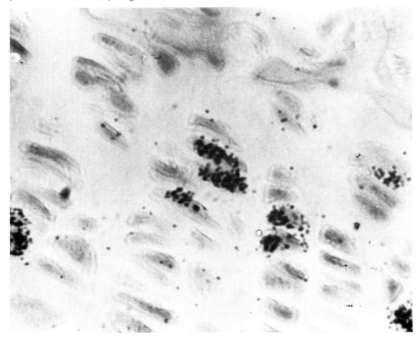

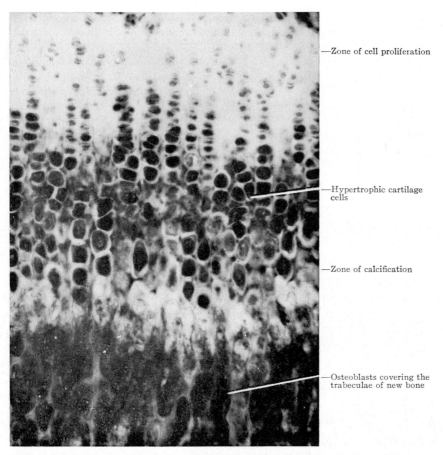

—Zone of cell proliferation

—Hypertrophic cartilage cells

—Zone of calcification

—Osteoblasts covering the trabeculae of new bone

Figure 6-27 Epiphyseal cartilage of a rat's tibia stained for alkaline phosphatase. Only traces of activity are found in the zone of proliferation, but a strong reaction occurs in the zone of calcification and in the osteoblasts covering the trabeculae of the metaphysis. Gomori method glycerophosphate substrate. ×200. (Courtesy of R. O. Greep.)

vealed that in female birds these spicules grow to fill the entire marrow cavity (medullary bone) at the time when the large mineralized eggs are produced.

BLOOD VESSELS AND NERVES

The main artery, the *medullary or nutrient artery,* reaches the marrow cavity from the periosteum. It is accompanied by one or two veins. The branches of these vessels distribute themselves proximally and distally to reach all the nutritive spaces in the bone.

Little is known about lymphatics, but they have been seen accompanying the larger blood vessels (Goss, 1959). Recently, channels that were in striking contrast to the blood capillaries have been observed by Cooper (Fig. 6-30; Cooper, 1972) in about 3 percent of the osteonic canals of immature dogs. These are presumably the first intraosseous lymphatic capillaries reported. There was already indirect evidence of the existence of a lymphatic circulation in bone. "India ink injected into the peritoneal cavity can be traced across small cortical channels to the endosteal surface of bone. Three or four percent of bone sarcomas metastasize to regional lymph nodes" (Cooper).

Nerves are abundant in the periosteum. Unmyelinated branches located in the depth of the small nutritive spaces have been observed recently through the electron microscope (Cooper et al., 1966).

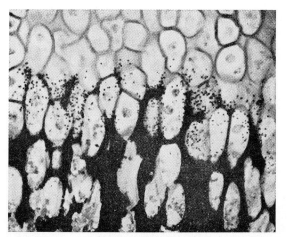

Figure 6-28 Section through the zone of calcification in the epiphyseal cartilage at the proximal end of the tibia of a normal rat, age 28 days. The granular deposits of bone salts are stained black. Undecalcified section; silver nitrate-hematoxylin-eosin. ×295. (Courtesy of F. McLean and W. Bloom, Anat. Rec. **78**:357, 1940.)

COMPACT BONE: GROWTH AND REMODELING

As the organisms have grown bigger and heavier, new stresses and strains occurred in the bones, necessitating increased support. This need has apparently been met by the transformation of trabecular, spongy bone into compact bone (Amprino, 1965). As this operation begins in the young bone, a large number of osteoblasts appear in the nutritive spaces. These cells deposit at the border of the space concentric rings of new bone (lamellae) separated by narrow bands of less mineralized interlamellar substance. This operation continues until the nutritive space reaches a critical diameter of approximately 20 μm and then the growth ceases. The unit of the new compact bone is called an *osteon* (Figs. 6-31 and 6-32). The small, remaining nutritive space is now an *osteonic canal* (Figs. 6-31 and 6-32).

The original osteons are known as *primary osteons*. Since their nutritional support is apparently critical, some of this bone becomes necrotic. Nature responds by initiating *remodeling*.

According to Currey (1968), remodeling begins in areas of the osteons in which a considerable number of osteocytes are "in a bad way." Remodeling tunnels are filled with osteoclasts followed by blood vessels and connective tissue cells. These soon differentiate into osteoblasts that lay down new concentric lamellae, which comprise a group of *secondary osteons*. The remnants of the primary osteons are now represented by the filling substance between the secondary osteons and are described as *interstitial lamellae* (Fig. 6-31). Several successive orders of smaller and smaller osteons are thus formed until the bone acquires adequate strength. Then the growth of compact bone, dealing only with normal turnover, becomes very slow. Frost (1963) states that whereas remodeling is of the order of 200 percent per year in young children, this rate falls to 1 percent in the adult.

RESORPTION CAVITIES: OSTEOPOROSIS

In older people, a variety of conditions such as negative salt balance, sex hormone deficiency, hypercorticoadrenalism, thyrotoxicosis, or simply

Figure 6-29 Superimposed tracings of two radiographs of the tibial head taken 1 year apart. The epiphysis has become displaced upward by growth. The underlying metaphysis has undergone remodeling as indicated by the stippled areas. (Courtesy of Dr. Pierre Lacroix and Masson & Cie.)

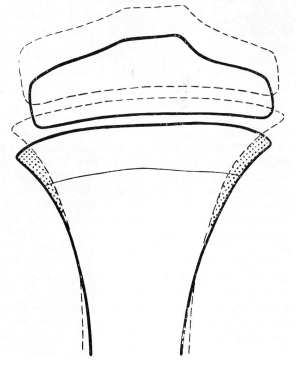

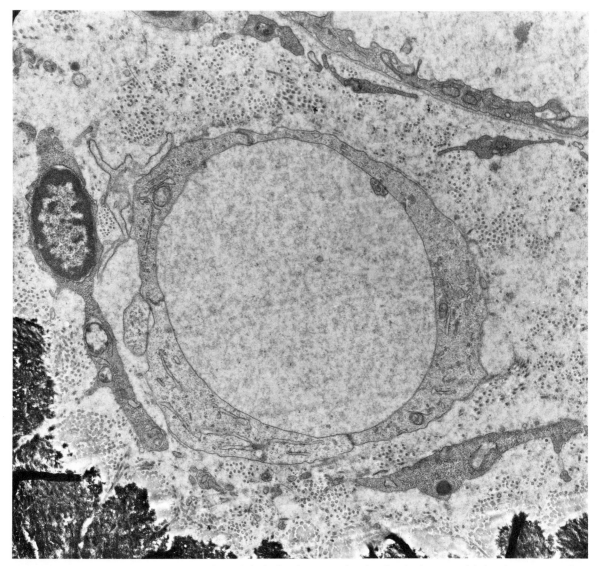

Figure 6-30   An osteonic canal from the midfemoral shaft of an immature dog showing, in the upper right-hand corner, a portion of a capillary wall with typical endothelial cells and surrounding basement membrane.   The large channel in the center, presumably a lymphatic vessel, does not have a basement membrane and the fluid in its lumen consists only of precipitated protein.   ×10,000. (Courtesy of Dr. Reginald R. Cooper.)

prolonged immobilization will cause an increased amount of bone resorption.   In compact bone, this phenomenon is marked by the appearance of local resorption cavities (Fig. 6-33) and an overall re-modeling resulting in a thinner diaphyseal cortex and a progressively enlarged marrow cavity (Duncan and Jaworski, 1970).   This phenomenon is clini-cally described as *osteoporosis*.

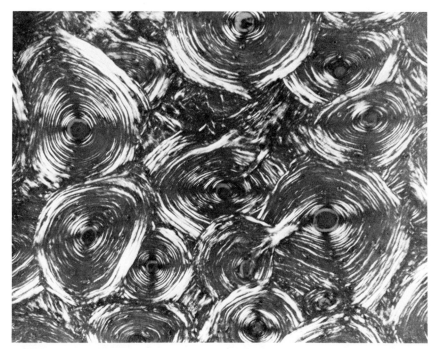

Figure 6-31 A portion of a nondemineralized cross section of the humeral diaphysis of a horse, photographed in polarized light. ×130. (Courtesy of Dr. Lennart Krook.)

Figure 6-32 Ground cross section of typical osteon of human femur. ×225.

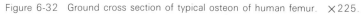

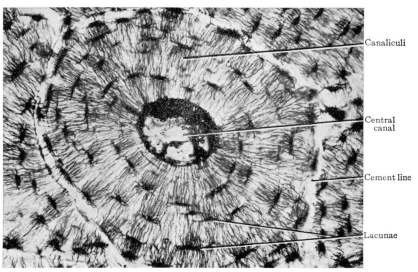

Canaliculi

Central
canal

Cement line

Lacunae

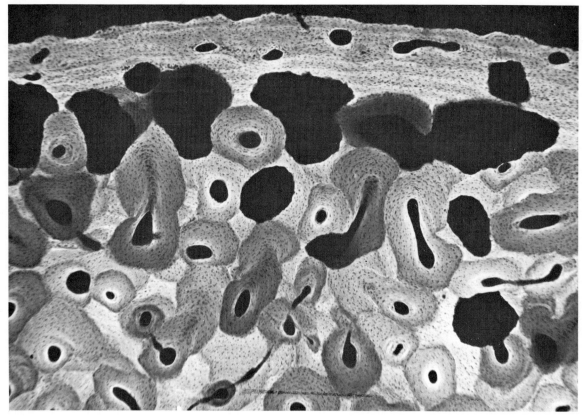

Figure 6-33   Microradiograph of a 200-μm-thick cross section of bone from a normal 19-year-old male. Secondary Haversian bone is actively replacing non-Haversian bone which is seen on the periosteal (upper) surface.   New, low-density bone in Haversian systems appears gray, whereas high-density bone appears white and is seen largely in interstitial areas.   ×57. (Courtesy of Dr. Jenifer Jowsey.)

PHYSIOLOGICAL CONTROL OF CALCIUM HOMEOSTASIS; OSTEOCYTIC OSTEOLYSIS

The constant supply of calcium to the blood and its regulation are so important that nature has devised the enormous reservoir of bone along with specific endocrine glands to preside over its output.

Recent observations demonstrate that the maintenance of a constant plasma concentration (homeostasis) is the result of the antagonistic action on bone of the parathyroid hormone and a thyroid product known as calcitonin, causing a controlled release of salt followed by growth replacement ("bone flow," Krook et al., 1970). This physiologic turnover seems to occur mainly in trabecular cancellous bone where the replacement rate is high (Bélanger and Migicovsky, 1963). In this tissue, the larger osteocytes, located in the midtrabecular region, are apparently instrumental in this bone breakdown, described as *osteocytic osteolysis* (Bélanger, 1969) (Fig. 6-34). These cells acquire lysosomes as they mature. Under parathyroid stimulation, the lysosomes (Fig. 6-35) release their lytic enzymes to the surrounding bone substance. The breakdown of collagen is accompanied by the release of the minerals and their transit toward the bloodstream. The intimate effects of calcitonin on bone cells are not yet fully understood. Bélanger and Rasmussen (1968) have recently established, however, that when this substance is introduced into the organism at the same time as parathyroid hormone, it inhibits the osteolytic activity of the osteocytes.

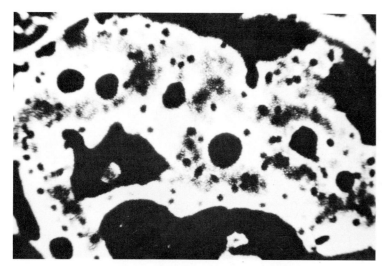

Figure 6-34 A portion of a cross section of the metaphysis of the tibia of a young rat. Several areas of osteocytic osteolysis show enlarged confluent lacunae surrounded by low-density matrix. Alpharadiograph. ×120.

Figure 6-35 An osteocyte in the resorptive phase. Here endoplasmic reticulum is represented by only a few cisternae; the Golgi complex is well developed. Several lysosomes and autophagic vacuoles are seen. Outside the cell, some flocculent material (*), a breakdown product of the pericellular bone matrix, is seen.

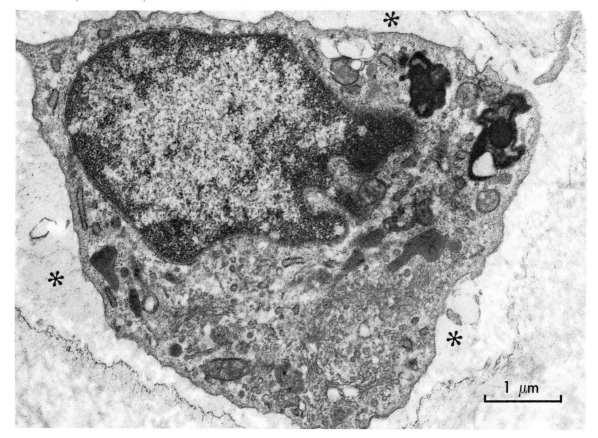

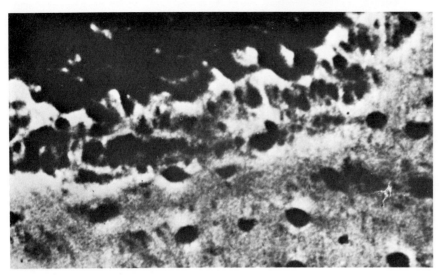

Figure 6-36   Alpharadiograph of a demineralized section showing a portion of the border of a resorption cavity in the tibia of a horse which had been fed a diet rich in phosphate for 30 weeks. Several enlarged and confluent lacunae are indicative of an increase in osteocytic osteolysis preceding osteoclasia. ×370. (Courtesy of Dr. Lennart Krook.)

High-power microscopy of microradiographs has revealed that the border of the resorption cavities (Fig. 6-33) often shows a characteristic pattern of enlarged and confluent lacunae (Fig. 6-36), pointing to the sequence of events in bone breakdown.

ULTRASTRUCTURAL EVENTS OF BONE MINERALIZATION

According to Kashiwa (1968), the osteoblasts and osteocytes can concentrate calcium. Furthermore, Talmage (1969) has recently postulated that these cells act as pumps to promote the transit of ca-

tions. The mitochondria have been shown to contain concentrations of calcium (Baud, 1962; Matthews et al., 1970). Hydroxyapatite is apparently formed inside cytoplasmic calcification vesicles. These are extruded, and as they reach the collagen fibrils at the periphery of the lacunae, they transfer their crystals to the collagen, where they become parallelly oriented (Bernard, 1969). The presence of mucopolysaccharides in the perifibrillar particles has been demonstrated recently by ruthenium red staining (Fig. 6-37; Cooper and Laros, 1972).

Joints

The site of union between two or more bones is called a *joint* or *articulation*.

SYNARTHROSES

Some of these joints, which are quite rigid, are called *synarthroses*. The inventory of the whole skeleton has revealed that the synarthroses represent a variety of histologic components: (1) The sutures of the skull consist of dense fibrous tissue (Fig. 6-38) and are thus referred to as *syndes-*

moses. (2) Between some of the bones of the face, cartilage is the unifying tissue. These pieces of cartilage, unlike the epiphyseal plate, show two or more calcifying surfaces. This type of joint is a *synchondrosis*. (3) When a synchondrosis eventually becomes completely ossified, it is then a *synostosis*. (4) In a few areas, such as between the mandibles or the pubic bones, the articulation consists of two plates of cartilage united by dense connective tissue. This type of joint is a *symphy-*

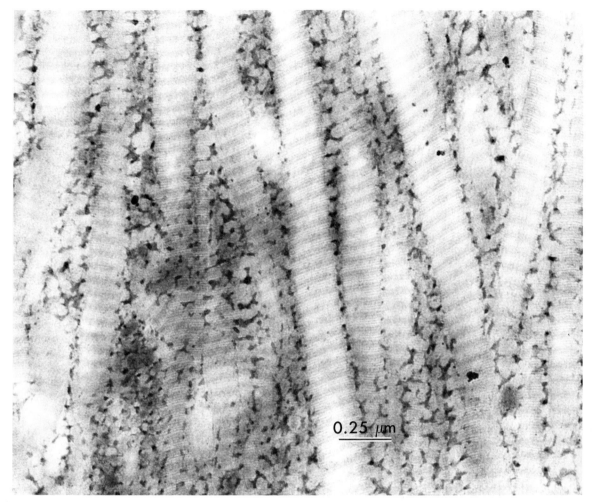

Figure 6-37 Perifibrillar particles stained by ruthenium red, indicative of mucopolysaccharides. (Courtesy of Dr. Reginald R. Cooper and Dr. Gerald Laros.)

sis. In certain species of mammals, there is considerable disparity between the size of the pelvic birth canal and the full-term fetus (Crelin, 1969). In the free-tailed bat, the pelvic joint "stretches to more than 15 times its original length" (Crelin, 1969).

The *intervertebral disc* is a specialized type of symphysis. Between the cartilage plates covering adjacent vertebrae, the dense fibrous tissue encloses a space filled with semifluid material rich in hyaluronic acid. This is the *nucleus pulposus,* which provides increased resiliency for the spine and thus cushions the upper nerve centers against trauma. Ruptures of the intervertebral disc followed by herniation of the nucleus pulposus are common in this era of mechanized crafts of all sorts.

MOBILE JOINTS

Joints that allow great mobility of the bones are called *diarthroses.* They consist of a joint cavity, mobile surfaces and envelopes, the inner synovial membrane, and the outer protective components.

In the embryo, the *joint cavity* appears in an original *interzone* densely packed with mesenchymal

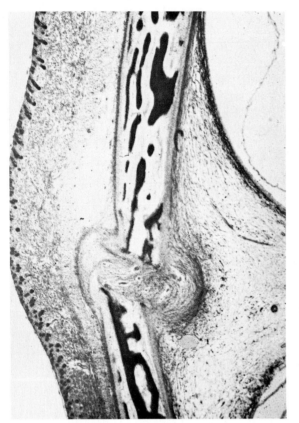

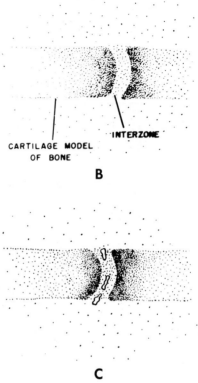

Figure 6-38 Section through the roof of a fetal calf skull showing the formation of a fibrous joint (syndesmosis). ×30.

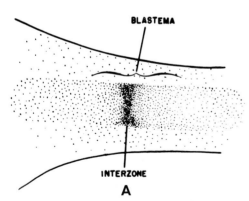

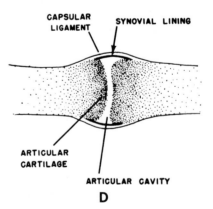

Figure 6-39 Diagram showing the main steps in the development of a diarthrosis. A. Early limb formation showing the blastema,
already segmented. B. The cartilage model of bone is well outlined and there is loosening of the cellular material in the interzone.
C. Early cleft formation. Coalescence of the miniclefts has begun. D. Mature joint. The opposed articular surfaces are covered
by articular cartilage, while synovial lining is present around the periphery of the joint. (Courtesy of Dr. D. B. Drachman.)

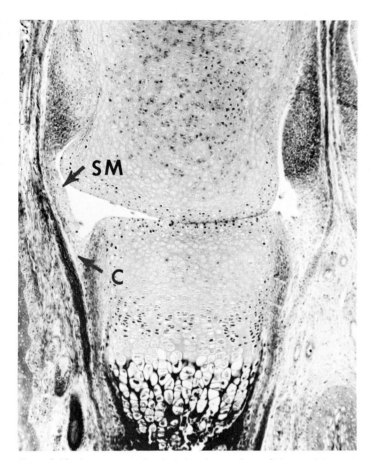

Figure 6-40   Intermetacarpal articulation, human fetus; SM, synovial membrane; C, capsule.   Mallory stain.   ×62.

cells (Fig. 6-39A).   Early cleft formation is characterized by loosening of the cellular material in the interzone (Fig. 6-39B).   This is followed by the appearance and coalescence of several *miniature spaces* (miniclefts, Fig. 6-39C).   The end result is a single joint space (cavitation phase; Figs. 6-39D and 6-40).   According to Drachman and Sokoloff (1966), the final modeling phase is dependent on skeletal muscle contractions occurring during the intrauterine life.   A marked decrease in muscle activity would lead to fusion of the mobile joint (ankylosis) or deformity.

The *articular surfaces* of a diarthrosis consist of hyaline cartilage (Fig. 6-40) that normally persists throughout life.   According to Mankin (1967), "there is ample evidence" that this articular carti-

lage "differs considerably in basic structure, chemical composition and metabolism" from cartilage located elsewhere.

The articular surfaces decrease rapidly in thickness in young organisms, as shown by comparative studies of rabbits 2, 6, and 18 months old (Mankin, 1967).   In the adult, four zones can be recognized in routine histologic preparations (Fig. 6-41): (1) at the surface, a narrow layer of flattened cells, called the gliding layer or *tangential zone*; (2) underneath, a *transitional zone* consists of ovoid or rounded cells randomly distributed; (3) beneath this, cells arranged in short columns, the *radial zone*; followed by (4) the cone of calcified cartilage.

The articular cartilage matrix is 70 to 85 percent water.   Collagen makes up 50 percent of the dry

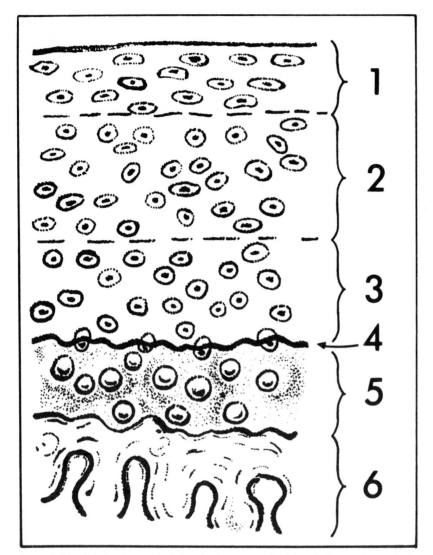

Figure 6-41 Artist's diagram depicting the four zones of adult articular cartilage. At the surface is a narrow layer of flattened cells called the gliding layer or tangential zone (1). Beneath this is the transitional zone (2) in which the ovoid to rounded cells are randomly distributed. Short irregular columns are noted deep to this in the radial zone (3), which is separated from the zone of calcified cartilage (5) by the "tidemark" (4), a thin wavy basophilic line. The bony end plate below is mature cortical bone with well-defined Haversian systems (6). (H&E). (Courtesy of Dr. H. J. Mankin.)

mass; the rest is a protein-mucopolysaccharide complex. The metabolism in articular cartilage is normally very low and the turnover of its components consequently slow.

The articular surfaces are naked (Fig. 6-43, AS). No limiting membrane of any kind has been seen even with the electron microscope (Cameron and Robinson, 1958).

The *synovial membrane*, the inner layer of the protective membranes, lines the joint everywhere except over the articular surfaces (Figs. 6-39D and 6-40, SM). It is somewhat like the cambium:

made of loose connective tissue (Fig. 6-40, SM) in which adipose cells are present in some areas. Elsewhere, such as at the site of attachment of the synovial membrane to the periphery of the articular cartilage, dense fibrous tissue is present (Fig. 6-40).

The surface cells of the synovial membrane are arranged in an epithelial-like fashion; when stretched, they appear squamous, but otherwise they look cuboidal. The surface cells sometimes undergo temporary outfolding. Some outward folds, however, are stable components called *villi* that are generally rich in capillary blood vessels. Infoldings of the surface form pediculated sacs called *bursae* which can become obstructed and distended with synovial fluid, causing discomfort.

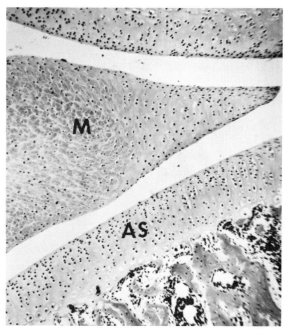

Figure 6-43 A portion of the knee joint of an adult rat. Notice the naked articular surfaces (AS) and the medial meniscus (M) made of fibrous tissue and cartilage. Hematoxylin-phloxine-orange stain. ×40.

Figure 6-42 Ligament insertion into cartilage of articular surface. Notice deep penetration of dense fibrous tissue. Alpha-radiograph. ×300.

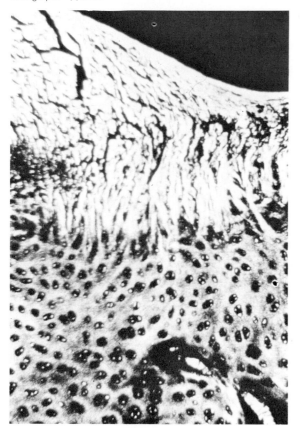

The joint cavity is filled with *synovial fluid,* generally considered to be an exudate of the blood to which mucopolysaccharides, particularly hyaluronic acid, are added, probably through the secretory activity of the cartilage cells of the articular surfaces. The term *synovial* (G., *syn ovum*) refers to this viscous fluid, which reminded the ancients of egg white.

The outer covering of the diarthrosal joint is known as the *capsule* (Fig. 6-40C). It is continuous with the outer periosteum and similarly composed of dense fibrous tissue. Cord-like thickenings of the capsule are called *ligaments.* They are sometimes made of fibrocartilage. Alpharadiography (Bélanger and Bélanger, 1959) has particularly well revealed their deep insertion in the articular cartilage (Fig. 6-42).

The *menisci* are also derivatives of the capsule found in some articulations, such as the knee joint. They are crescent-shaped discs of fibrocartilage attached marginally to the capsule and ending in a free edge inside the joint cavity (Fig. 6-43).

References

ALI, S., S. W. SADJERA, and H. C. ANDERSON: Isolation and Characterization of Calcifying Matrix Vesicles from Epiphyseal Cartilage, *Proc. Nat. Acad. Sci. USA,* **67:**1513 (1970).

AMPRINO, R.: Bone Structures and Functions, in W. Bargmann (ed.), "Werkstatt der Anatomen," Georg Thieme Verlag, Stuttgart, 1965.

ANDERSON, H. C.: Electron Microscopic Studies of Induced Cartilage Development and Calcification, *J. Cell Biol.,* **35:**81 (1967).

ANDERSON, H. C.: Vesicles Associated with Calcification in the Matrix of Epiphyseal Cartilage, *J. Cell Biol.,* **41:**59 (1969).

BAUD, C. A.: Morphology and Inframicroscopic Structure of Osteocytes, *Acta Anat. (Basel),* **51:**209 (1962).

BÉLANGER, L. F.: Autoradiographic Visualization of the Entry and Transit of S^{35} in Cartilage, Bone and Dentine of Young Rats and the Effect of Hyaluronidase in Vitro, *Canad. J. Biochem. Physiol.,* **32:**161 (1954).

BÉLANGER, L. F.: Observations on the Manifestations of Osteolathyrism in the Chick, *J. Bone Joint Surg.,* **41B:**581 (1959).

BÉLANGER, L. F.: Osteocytic Osteolysis, *Calcif. Tissue Res.,* **4:**1 (1969).

BÉLANGER, L. F., and C. BÉLANGER: Alpharadiography: A Simple Method for Determination of Mass Concentration in Cells and Tissues, *J. Biophys. Biochem. Cytol.,* **6:**197 (1959).

BÉLANGER, L. F., and P. DROUIN: A Radioautographic Survey of the Formation and Fate of Connective Tissue Giant Cells in Selye's Granuloma Pouch, in G. Jasmin (ed.), "Endocrine Aspects of Disease Processes," p. 325, Warren H. Green Inc., St. Louis, 1968.

BÉLANGER, L. F., and C. P. LEBLOND: A Method for Locating Radioactive Elements in Tissues by Covering Histological Sections with a Photographic Emulsion, *Endocrinology,* **39:**8 (1946).

BÉLANGER, L. F., and B. B. MIGICOVSKY: Comparative Effects of Vitamin D, Calcium, Cortisone, Hydrocortisone and Norethandrolone on the Epiphyseal Cartilage and Bone of Rachitic Chicks, *Develop. Biol.,* **2:**329 (1960).

BÉLANGER, L. F., and B. B. MIGICOVSKY: Comparison between Different Mucopolysaccharide Stains as Applied to Chick Epiphyseal Cartilage, *J. Histochem. Cytochem.,* **9:**73 (1961).

BÉLANGER, L. F., and B. B. MIGICOVSKY: Histochemical Evidence of Proteolysis in Bone: The Influence of Parathormone, *J. Histochem. Cytochem.,* **11:**734 (1963).

BÉLANGER, L. F., and H. RASMUSSEN: Inhibition of Osteocytic Osteolysis by Thyrocalcitonin and Some Anti-growth Factors, in R. V. Talmage and L. F. Bélanger (eds.), "Parathyroid Hormone and Thyrocalcitonin (Calcitonin)," p. 156, Excerpta Medica Foundation, Amsterdam, 1968.

BERNARD, G. W.: The Ultrastructural Interface of Bone Crystals and Organic Matrix in Woven and Lamellar Endochondral Bone, *J. Dent. Res.,* **48:**781 (1969).

BERNARD, G. W., and D. C. PEASE: An Electron Microscopic Study of Initial Intra-membranous Osteogenesis, *Amer. J. Anat.,* **125:**271 (1969).

BOIS, P., and L. F. BÉLANGER, and J. LE BUIS: Effect of Growth Hormone and Amino-acetonitrile on the Mitotic Rate of Epiphyseal Cartilage in Hypophysectomized Rats, *Endocrinology,* **73:**507 (1963).

BONUCCI, E.: Fine Structure of Early Cartilage Calcification, *J. Ultrastruct. Res.,* **20:**33 (1967).

BOURNE, G. H.: Vitamin C and Bone, in G. H. Bourne (ed.), "The Biochemistry and Physiology of Bone," p. 539, Academic Press, New York, 1956.

BYWATERS, E. G. L.: The Metabolism of Joint Tissues, *J. Path. Bact.*, **44**:247 (1937).

CAMERON, D. A., and R. A. ROBINSON: Electron Microscopy of Epiphyseal and Articular Cartilage Matrix in the Femur of the Newborn Infant, *J. Bone Joint Surg.* [*Amer.*], **40A**:163 (1958).

CLARK, I., and L. F. BÉLANGER: The Effects of Alterations in Dietary Magnesium on Calcium, Phosphate and Skeletal Metabolism, *Calcif. Tissue Res.*, **1**:204 (1967).

COOPER, R. R.: Personal communication, 1972.

COOPER, R. R., and G. LAROS: Personal communication, 1972.

COOPER, R. R., J. W. MILGRAM, and R. A. ROBINSON: Morphology of the Osteon. An Electron Microscopic Study., *J. Bone Joint Surg.* [*Amer.*], **48A**:1239 (1966).

CRELIN, E. S.: The Development of the Bony Pelvis and Its Changes during Pregnancy and Parturition, *Trans. N.Y. Acad. Sci.*, **31**(8): Series II, p. 1049 (1969).

CURREY, J. D.: Biology of Hard Tissue, in Ann M. Budy (ed.), NASA SP-161. National Aeronautics and Space Administration, Washington, 1968.

DAVIES, D. V., C. H. BARNETT, W. COCHRANE, and A. J. PALFREY: Electron Microscopy of Articular Cartilage in the Young Adult Rabbit, *Ann. Rheum. Dis.*, **21**:11 (1962).

DELUCA, H. F. Mechanism of Action and Metabolic Fate of Vitamin D, *Vitamins Hormones* (NY), **25**:315 (1967).

DELUCA, H.: The Metabolism and Mechanism of Action of 25 Hydroxycholecalciferol. Franklin C. McLean Commemorative Workshop Conference on Cell Mechanism for Calcium Transfer and Homeostasis, Portsmouth, N.H., September 1970.

DRACHMAN, D. B.: Normal Development and Congenital Malformation of Joints, *Bull. Rheum. Dis.*, **19**:536 (1969).

DRACHMAN, D. B., and L. SOKOLOFF: The Role of Movement in Embryonic Joint Development, *Develop. Biol.*, **14**:401 (1966).

DUHAMEL, H. L.: Cinquième Mémoire sur les Os, dans Lequel on Se Propose d'Éclaircir Comment Se Fait le Crûe des Os Suivant Leur Longeur. *Mém. Acad. Roy. Sci.*, **56**:111 (1743a).

DUHAMEL, H. L.: Quatrième Mèmoire sur les Os. Dans Lequel on Se Propose de Rapporter de Nouvelles Preuves Qui Établissent que les Os Croissent en Grosseur par l'Addition de Couches Osseuses Qui Tirent Leur Origine du Périoste, *Mém. Acad. Roy. Sci.*, **56**:87 (1743b).

DUNCAN, H., and Z. F. JAWORSKI: "Osteoporosis. Tice's Practice of Medicine," vol. 5, Chap. 52. Harper & Row, New York, 1970.

FAHMY, A., W. HILLMAN, P. TALLEY, and V. LONG: Fibrillogenesis in the Epiphyseal Cartilage of Adult Rats, *J. Bone Joint Surg.*, **51A**:802 (1969).

FROST, H. M.: A Unique Histological Feature of Vitamin D Resistant Rickets Observed in Four Cases, *Acta Orthop. Scand.*, **33**:220 (1963).

GLIMCHER, M. J., A. J. HODGE and F. O. SCHMITT: Macromolecular Aggregation States in Relation to Mineralization: The Collagen-hydroxyapatite System as Studied in Vitro, *Proc. Nat. Acad. Sci. USA*, **43**:860 (1957).

GLISSON, F.: "De Rachitide," London, 1650.

GODMAN, G. C., and K. R. PORTER: Chondrogenesis, Studied with the Electron Microscope, *J. Biophys. Biochem. Cytol.*, **8**:719 (1960).

GOSS, C. M.: "Gray's Anatomy," 27th ed., Lea & Febiger, Philadelphia, 1959.

HALES, S.: "Statistical Essays," W. Innys, London, 1727.

HALL, B. K.: Differentiation of Cartilage and Bone from Common Germinal Cells:

I. The Role of Acid Mucopolysaccharides and Collagen, *J. Exp. Zool.,* **173:**383 (1970).

HAM, A. W.: "Histology," 6th ed., Lippincott, Philadelphia, 1969.

HAM, A. W., and H. C. ELLIOTT: The Bone and Cartilage Lesions of Protracted Moderate Scurvy, *Amer. J. Pathol.,* **14:**323 (1938).

HANCOX, N., and B. BOOTHROYD: Structure-function Relationships in the Osteoclast, in R. F. Sognnaes (ed.), "Mechanisms of Hard Tissue Destruction," p. 497. A.A.A.S., Washington, 1963.

HARRIS, H. A.: "Bone Growth in Health and Disease," Oxford University Press, London, 1933.

HARRIS, L. J.: Vitamin D and Bone, in G. H. Bourne (ed.), "The Biochemistry and Physiology of Bone," p. 581, Academic Press, New York, 1956.

HARRIS, W. R., and A. W. HAM: The Mechanism of Nutrition in Bone and How It Affects Its Structure, Repair and Fate on Transplantation, in G. E. W. Wolstenholme and C. M. O'Connor (eds.), "Bone Structure and Metabolism," p. 135, Ciba Foundation Symposium, J. & A. Churchill Ltd., London, 1956.

HIRSCHMAN, A., and D. D. DZIEWIATKOWSKI: Protein-polysaccharide Loss during Endochondral Ossification: Immuno-chemical Evidence, *Science,* **154:**393 (1966).

JACKSON, S. F.: The Fine Structure of Developing Bone in the Embryonic Fowl, *Proc. Roy. Soc. Lond. (Biol.),* **B146:**270 (1957).

JANDE, S. S., and L. F. BÉLANGER. Electron Microscopy of Osteocytes and the Pericellular Matrix in Rat Trabecular, *Bone. Calcif. Tissue Res.* (in press).

JOHNSON, L. C.: Mineralization of Turkey Leg Tendon. I. Histology and Histochemistry of Mineralization, in R. F. Sognnaes (ed.), "Calcification in Biological Systems," p. 117, A.A.A.S., Washington, 1960.

JOSS, E. E., K. A. ZUPPINGER, and E. H. SOBEL: Effect of Testosterone Propionate and Methyl Testosterone on Growth and Skeletal Maturation in Rats, *Endocrinology,* **72:**123 (1963).

KASHIWA, H. K.: The Glyoxal BIS (2-hydroxyanil) Method for Differential Staining of Intracellular Calcium in Bone, in R. V. Talmage and L. F. Bélanger (eds.), "Parathyroid Hormone and Thyrocalcitonin (Calcitonin)," p. 198, Excerpta Medica Foundation, Amsterdam, 1968.

KÖLLIKER, A.: "Die Normale Resorption des Knochengewebes und Ihre Bedeutung fur die Entsechung der Typischen Knochenformen," Vogel, Leipzig, 1873.

KOWALEWSKI, K.: Uptake of Radiosulphur in Growing Bones of Cockerels Treated with Cortisone and 17-ethyl-19-nortestosterone, *Proc. Soc. Exp. Biol. Med.,* **97:**432 (1958).

KROOK, L., L. F. BÉLANGER, P.-A. HENRIKSON, L. LUTWAK, and B. E. SHEFFY: Bone Flow, *Rev. Canad. Biol.,* **29:**157 (1970).

LACROIX, P.: "L'Organisation des Os," Masson & Cie, Paris, 1949.

LEBLOND, C. P., G. W. WILKINSON, L. F. BÉLANGER, and J. ROBICHON: Radioautographic Visualization of Bone Formation in the Rat, *Amer. J. Anat.,* **86:**289 (1950).

MANKIN, H. J.: The Structure, Chemistry and Metabolism of Articular Cartilage, *Bull. Rheum. Dis.,* **17:**447 (1967).

MATTHEWS, J. L., J. H. MARTIN, K. KUETTNER, and C. ARSENIS: The Role of Mitochondria in Intracellular Calcium Regulation, Franklin C. McLean Commemorative Workshop Conference on Cell Mechanisms for Calcium Transfer and Homeostasis, Portsmouth, N.H., September 1970.

MATUKAS, V. J., and G. A. KRIKOS: Evidence for Changes in Protein-polysaccharide Associated with the Onset of Calcification in Cartilage, *J. Cell Biol.*, **39**:43 (1968).

MC LEAN, F. C., and W. BLOOM: Calcification and Ossification: Calcification in Normal Growing Bone, *Anat. Rec.*, **78**:333 (1940).

MC LEAN, F. C., and M. R. URIST: "Bone. Fundamentals of the Physiology of Skeletal Tissue," 3d ed., The University of Chicago Press, Chicago, 1968.

Nutrition Revue: An Hypothesis for the Action of Vitamin D on Bone, **26**:183 (1968).

NYLEN, M. U., D. B. SCOTT, and V. M. MOSLEY: Mineralization of Turkey Leg Tendon. II. Collagen-Mineral Relations Revealed by Electron and X-ray Microscopy, in R. F. Sognnaes (ed.), "Calcification in Biological Systems." p. 129, A.A.A.S., Washington, 1960.

PAUTARD, F. G. E.: A Biomolecular Survey of Calcification, in H. Fleisch, H. J. J. Blackwood, and M. Owen (eds.), "Calcified Tissues," p. 108, Springer-Verlag, New York, 1966.

PEACOCK, E. E. JR., P. M. WEEKS, and J. M. PETTY: Some Studies on the Antigenicity of Cartilage, *Ann. N.Y. Acad. Sci.*, **87**:175 (1960).

POMMER, G.: "Untersuchungen über Osteomalacie und Rachitis, nebst Beiträgen zur Kenntnis der Knochenresorption und Apposition in Verschiedenen Altersperioden und der Durchbohrenden Gefässe," F. C. W. Vogel, Leipzig, 1885.

REVEL, J.-P.: A Stain for the Ultrastructural Localization of Acid Mucopolysaccharides, *J. Microscopie* **3**:535 (1964).

REVEL, J.-P., and E. D. HAY: An Autoradiographic and Electron Microscopic Study of Collagen Synthesis in Differentiating Cartilage. *Z. Zellforsch.*, **61**: 110 (1963).

ROBINSON, R. A., and M. L. WATSON: Collagen-crystal Relationship in Bone as Seen in the Electron Microscope, *Anat. Rec.*, **114**:383 (1952).

ROMER, A. S.: The Early Evolution of Fishes, *Quart. Rev. Biol.*, **21**:33 (1946).

ROMER, A. S.: The "Ancient History" of Bone, *Ann. N.Y. Acad. Sci.*, **109**:168 (1963).

SILBERBERG, M., and R. SILBERBERG: Steroid Hormones and Bone, in G. H. Bourne (ed.), "The Biochemistry and Physiology of Bone," p. 623, Academic Press, New York, 1956.

SILBERBERG, R., M. SILBERBERG, and D. FEIR: Life Cycle of Articular Cartilage Cells: An Electron Microscope Study of the Hip Joint of the Mouse, *Amer. J. Anat.*, **114**:17 (1964).

TALMAGE, R. V.: Calcium Homeostasis—Calcium Transport—Parathyroid Action. The Effects of Parathyroid Hormone on the Movement of Calcium between Bone and Fluid, *Clin. Orthop.*, **67**:210 (1969).

TARLO, B. J., and L. B. H. TARLO: The Origin of Teeth, *Discovery*, **26**:1 (1965).

TURNER, C. D.: "General Endocrinology," 4th ed. Saunders, Philadelphia, 1966.

URIST, M. R.: The Origin of Bone, *Discovery*, **25**:13 (1964).

URIST, M. R., and K. A. VAN DE PUTTE: Comparative Biochemistry of the Blood of Fishes, in P. W. Gilbert, R. F. Mathewson, and D. P. Rall (eds.), "Sharks, Skates and Rays," p. 271, Johns Hopkins Press, Baltimore, 1967.

WEIDENREICH, F.: Das Knochengewebe, in W. von Möllendorff (ed.), "Die Gewebe, Handbuch der Mikorskopischen Anatomie des Menschen," p. 391, Julius Springer, Berlin, 1930.

WOLBACK, S. B., and D. M. HEGSTED: Vitamin A Deficiency in the Chick, *Arch. Pathol.*, **54**:13 (1952).

chapter 7 Muscular tissue

GERALDINE F.
GAUTHIER

The function of movement in multicellular organisms is usually assumed by specialized cells, called muscle fibers, which contract upon appropriate stimulation. This property is also manifested in other structures such as cilia and flagella. These various motile systems have in common the ability to transform chemical into mechanical energy through the enzymatic splitting of ATP, and each possesses a precisely arranged filamentous component. In muscle cells, filaments are oriented parallel to the direction of movement, and because of their precise arrangement, constitute the actual contractile machinery of the cell. In the vertebrate body, there are three types of muscle based on the appearance and location of their constituent cells: smooth, skeletal, and cardiac. All three types are composed of asymmetric cells, or fibers, with the long axis arranged in the direction of movement.

Smooth muscle, which is the simplest in appearance of the three types, consists of narrow and relatively short, tapering cells, each with a single centrally located nucleus. This type of muscle occurs in the walls of the viscera and hence is often

referred to as *visceral* or *involuntary* muscle. *Skeletal* muscle is associated, as the name implies, with the body skeleton. The cells are greatly elongated, and each contains numerous peripheral nuclei. Because of the conspicuous transverse striations of the individual cells, skeletal muscle is also referred to as *striated* muscle. It is controlled by the somatic nervous system and hence is often called *voluntary* muscle. *Cardiac* muscle is a highly specialized form of *involuntary striated* muscle found only in the heart and, in some species, in the walls of the pulmonary vein. It is similar to skeletal muscle in that the cells are transversely striated and multinuclear, but as in smooth muscle, the nuclei are centrally located.

In the descriptions which follow, emphasis will be placed on the appearance of muscle as it occurs in the mammal. Reference will be made to other vertebrate classes, however, particularly where information is otherwise limited. Discussion will be concerned with skeletal muscle in particular, since it has been the primary source of data concerning the relationships between structure and function.

217

Skeletal muscle

GENERAL FEATURES

Skeletal muscle (Fig. 7-1) consists of long bundles of more or less parallel cells called *muscle fibers.* Cross-sectional dimensions (Fig. 7-7) vary from about 10 to 100 μm. In longitudinal section, these cells are clearly marked by transverse striations (Figs. 7-2 and 7-3), and nuclei are located just beneath the cell membrane, or *sarcolemma.* The fibers contain smaller parallel units about 1 to 3 μm in diameter, the *myofibrils,* which are also transversely striated (Figs. 7-1 and 7-4) and are composed, in turn, of *myofilaments* that are visible only with the electron microscope (Fig. 7-5). The myofilaments are not transversely striated but are responsible for the striations because of their arrangement within the myofibril (Fig. 7-6).

Skeletal muscles are attached to bony structures by tendons, which are continuous with a connective tissue covering over the entire muscle, the *epimysium.* This outermost connective tissue extends into the muscle and surrounds bundles, or *fascicles,* of muscle fibers, forming the *perimysium,* which eventually divides into a delicate sheath of reticular fibers around each muscle fiber called the *endomysium.* Blood vessels and nerves follow these sheaths into the interior of the muscle, and a rich capillary network closely invests each muscle fiber.

Skeletal muscle fibers also contain a cytoplasm, or *sarcoplasm,* which occupies the limited space between the abundant myofibrils. Muscle fibers are conventionally depicted in longitudinal section, and emphasis is usually placed on the myofibrillar

Figure 7-1 Longitudinal organization of skeletal muscle. Dimensions are based on rabbit psoas muscle. (From H. E. Huxley, in J. Brachet and A. E. Mirsky (eds.), "The Cell," vol. 4, Academic Press, Inc., 1960.)

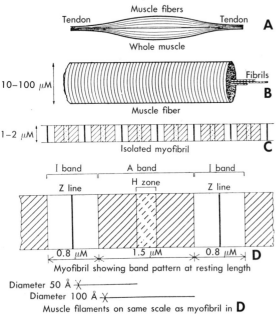

Figure 7-2 Longitudinal section of several skeletal muscle fibers (cat tongue). Each fiber is characterized by a transverse pattern of alternating dark A bands and light I bands, repeated along the length of the fiber. In certain areas, individual myofibrils can be recognized by their longitudinal orientation. Nuclei (N) are located at the periphery of the fibers. Angular structures (arrows) between fibers are distorted red blood cells present within capillaries, which closely invest individual muscle fibers. Iron-hematoxylin. ×560.

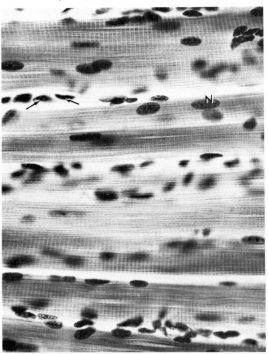

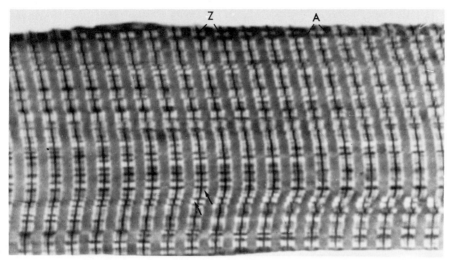

Figure 7-3   Longitudinal section of a single muscle fiber (guinea pig plantaris). The transverse banding pattern is clearly resolved, and part of a peripheral nucleus is visible at the upper left of the fiber. A bands are dark; I bands are light and are bisected by a very dark, narrow Z line. The precise alignment of paired mitochondria (arrows) in transverse rows over the I bands, on either side of each Z line, creates the impression of an additional interrupted dark band in this position. Toluidine blue.   × 1,900.

component. However, mitochondria are usually conspicuous components of the sarcoplasm (Figs. 7-7 and 7-8). Interfibrillar mitochondria are arranged in pairs at regular intervals in relation to the banding pattern of the myofibrils (Figs. 7-3 and 7-4). These paired mitochondria, which are characteristic of mammalian skeletal muscle fibers in general, encircle the myofibrils at the level of the I bands. Their arrangement is readily visible in transverse sections of the muscle fibers (Fig. 7-9), where they appear as filamentous profiles. In longitudinal sections of the fibers (Figs. 7-3 and 7-4), these mitochondria are usually sectioned transversely and thus appear as elliptical profiles on either side of the Z line. In a tangential section through a myofibril, mitochondrial profiles extend transversely across the I bands (Fig. 7-29). In certain types of fibers, mitochondria also form more continuous longitudinal rows and subsarcolemmal aggregations (Fig. 7-36), which are apparent in transverse as well as in longitudinal sections (Figs. 7-7 and 7-8).

The sarcoplasm also contains an elaborate membrane system, the *sarcoplasmic reticulum,* which surrounds individual myofibrils (Figs. 7-9 and 7-10). This system will be discussed in a later

section. In addition, a Golgi apparatus is present in the perinuclear sarcoplasm. Glycogen, in the form of β particles, is abundant between myofibrils, particularly in the region of the I bands, and it occurs within the myofibrils as well (Figs. 7-5, 7-9, and 7-10). Lipid droplets are frequently closely associated with large mitochondria (Fig. 7-36). Both lipid and glycogen provide metabolic fuel for the contractile machinery.

COMPOSITION OF THE MYOFIBRIL

The banding pattern of the skeletal muscle fiber reflects the ultrastructural organization of each myofibril, and knowledge of this pattern is fundamental to an understanding of the mechanism of contraction. *The two largest bands are named according to their appearance in polarized light* (Figs. 7-11 and 7-12). Certain bands exhibit positive birefringence, which reflects a parallel arrangement of asymmetric subunits. These birefringent or anisotropic bands are called *A bands* and are bright when viewed with the polarizing microscope (Fig. 7-12). They alternate with dark isotropic *I bands,* and the pattern is repeated along the length of the myofibril. Each A band has a less birefringent central zone called the *H band,* and each

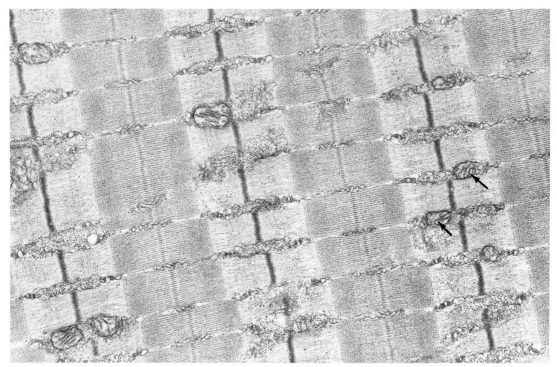

Figure 7-4   Electron micrograph of a portion of a fiber (rat semitendinosus).   Several myofibrils are present in this longitudinal section, and at least two sarcomeres are included in each myofibril.   The regular arrangement of transverse bands in each myofibril gives rise to the banding pattern of the whole fiber seen with the light microscope (Fig. 7-3).   Profiles of paired mitochondria (arrows) are present on either side of the electron-dense Z line (see also Fig. 7-5).   ×17,500.

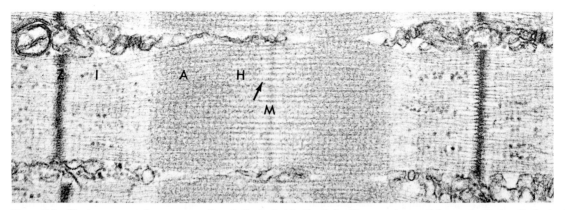

Figure 7-5   Single sarcomere from a preparation similar to that in Fig. 7-4.   The conspicuous Z line marks the longitudinal extent of this structural and functional unit.   The myofilaments, which comprise the myofibrils, are visible, but their arrangement is more readily apparent in Fig. 7-6.   All the major transverse bands can be seen in this micrograph, including the pseudo-H band (arrow), which is often confused with the H band.   Glycogen particles occur among the filaments of the I-band region.   ×48,000.

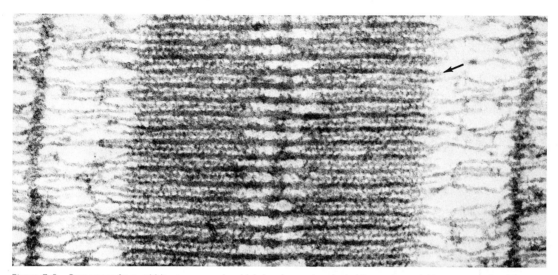

Figure 7-6 Sarcomere from rabbit psoas muscle which has been glycerinated to remove soluble components of the sarcoplasm. In this type of preparation, it is possible to discern the organization of myofilaments, which constitutes the ultrastructural basis of transverse banding in the myofibril. In the A band, there is a simple alternation of thick and thin filaments in this particular plane of section, and in the I band there are only thin filaments. The thick filaments extend to the limits of the A band, where their ends become tapered (arrow). The thin filaments extend from each Z line through both the I band and A band, but terminate at the H band. Bridge-like structures extend radially from the surfaces of the thick filaments. Six such structures are arranged in a helical pattern which is repeated every 400 Å along the thick filament (see Fig. 7-19). ×128,000. (From H. E. Huxley, 1957.)

I band is bisected by a distinct *Z line*. The *M line* marks the center of the H band, and in some instances (in insect muscle, for example), an N line is apparent on either side of the Z line. When viewed with phase-contrast optics (Fig. 7-11) or with ordinary light after staining with a cationic dye (Figs. 7-2 and 7-3), the banding pattern appears reversed. That is, the A band and Z line are basophilic or dark and the I and H bands are light. This is also the usual appearance of the various bands in electron micrographs (Figs. 7-4 and 7-5), but the appearance with polarized light is the basis for the more widely used nomenclature. The segment between two successive Z lines is called a *sarcomere* (Fig. 7-5) and is approximately 2 to 3 μm long, with the A band contributing about 1.5 μm and each full I band, about 0.8 μm. This structural and functional unit is repeated along the length of the myofibril.

Biochemical analysis has revealed that the myofibril consists of a number of proteins. Two of these, *myosin* and *actin,* account for most of the dry weight of the myofibril. Their interaction in the presence of ATP to form *actomyosin* is a fundamental feature of myofibrillar contraction. Three other proteins, *tropomyosin, troponin,* and *α-actinin* play a regulatory role in the contractile process. Troponin, in particular, can inhibit the formation of actomyosin when the calcium level is low. For a concise description of the functional role of these proteins, see Ebashi et al. (1969). It has been possible also to locate some of these proteins within the sarcomere. If, for example, the myosin is extracted from a preparation of myofibrils, the density of the A band is diminished (Figs. 7-13 and 7-14), which indicates that myosin is located in this region. The fluorescent antibody technique has also been a useful tool for the localization of muscle proteins. An antibody to myosin is prepared and combined with a fluorescent dye, and this complex is allowed to interact with a preparation of myofibrils. The complex becomes bound to the site where myosin is located, and the fluorescence serves as a visual marker. The site of fluorescence,

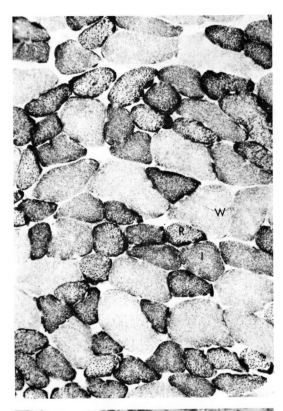

Figure 7-7   Transverse section of several muscle fibers (rat diaphragm), showing the localization of succinic dehydrogenase activity.   Reaction product reflects the location of mitochondria.   Small (red) fibers (R) are rich in mitochondria, especially along the periphery; large (white) fibers (W) have a low mitochondrial content; and intermediate fibers (I) have characteristics between the two.   ×200.

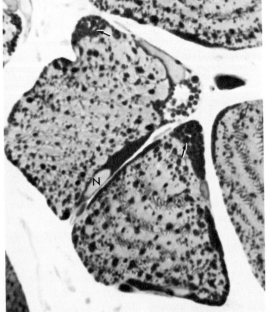

Figure 7-8   Transverse section of two red fibers (rat diaphragm), illustrating the distribution of mitochondria, which are stained darkly with toluidine blue.   The myofibrils appear relatively unstained.   Large circular profiles of mitochondria form conspicuous peripheral aggregations (arrows) at sites where enzymatic activity is demonstrated (Fig. 7-7) and are also abundant in the interior of the fibers.   Nuclei (N) appear in negative image. ×1,200.   (From G. F. Gauthier, 1970.)

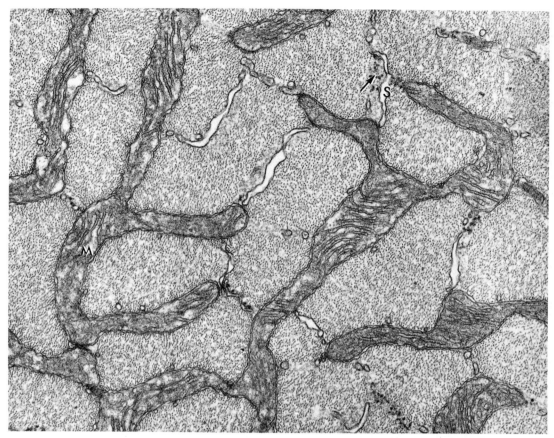

Figure 7-9   Electron micrograph of a transverse section (rat semitendinosus). The section passes through the I band and, therefore, through only the thin filaments which compose this part of the sarcomere. Bracelet-like mitochondria (M) encircle individual myofibrils; these mitochondria appear as paired elliptical profiles on either side of the Z line in longitudinal sections of a muscle fiber (Figs. 7-3 and 7-4). In addition, profiles of the sarcoplasmic membrane systems (S) surround individual myofibrils, and clusters of glycogen particles (arrow) occur close to them. ×42,000.

and therefore presumably of myosin, is the A band region of the myofibril (Figs. 7-15 and 7-16). By following similar procedures, actin can be demonstrated in the I band of the myofibril. Though localization of the other myofibrillar proteins is less certain, there is evidence that they are present in the I band or Z line (see below).

Ultrastructurally, the myofibril is composed of two major types of filaments, one type being thicker than the other (Figs. 7-6 and 7-10). When extracted myofibrils are examined with the electron microscope, loss of myosin is associated with loss

of the thick filaments, which indicates that the thick filaments are, in fact, myosin. The thin filaments, on the other hand, are composed of actin. In a classic ultrastructural study, H. E. Huxley (1957) demonstrated the exact arrangement of these filaments and established the ultrastructural basis of the banding pattern and of the contractile mechanism as well. In the A band, thick (100 Å) filaments alternate with thin (50 Å) filaments (Figs. 7-6 and 7-10). The thick filaments are 1.5 μm long and extend only to the limits of the A band, where their ends become tapered. The thin fila-

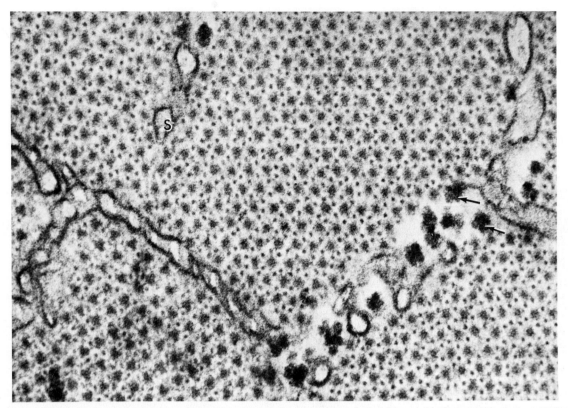

Figure 7-10 Transverse section through the A-band region (frog sartorius). Both thick and thin filaments are present, and each thick filament is surrounded by six thin filaments, giving rise to a precise hexagonal array. The presence of cross bridges imparts a rough surface to the thick filaments. Myofibrillar boundaries are marked by profiles of the sarcoplasmic reticulum (S) and by glycogen particles (arrows). ×150,000. (From H. E. Huxley, J. Molec. Biol., **37**:507, 1968.)

ments, however, extend from each Z line for a distance of 1 μm through the I band and into the A band. They are absent from the H band. The banding pattern is therefore the result of the presence or absence of overlap between the two sets of filaments (Figs. 7-6, 7-17, and 7-18). The A band, which is relatively dense when viewed with the light microscope, consists of both thick and thin filaments (Figs. 7-6 and 7-10). The less-dense I band consists only of thin filaments (Figs. 7-6 and 7-9), and the H band, only of thick filaments (Fig. 7-17a and c). The M line reflects the transverse extension of a series of projections from the centers of the thick filaments (Fig. 7-17a and e). The filaments are arranged, in transverse section, so that

they appear as more or less circular profiles in a remarkably precise hexagonal pattern. In the A band region, where the two sets of filaments overlap, each thick (myosin) filament is surrounded by six thin (actin) filaments (Figs. 7-10, 7-17b, and 7-18). In addition, a series of bridge-like structures extends radially from the thick filaments toward the thin filaments (Figs. 7-6, 7-10, 7-17b, and 7-18). There are six of these bridges arranged about each thick filament in a helical pattern which is repeated every 400 Å along the length of the thick filament (Fig. 7-19). The absence of bridges from the center of the H band produces an area of lower density often confused with the H band itself; this is called the L band, or *pseudo-H band* (Fig. 7-17a and d).

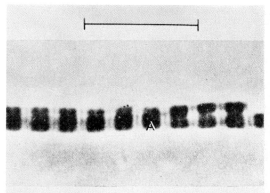

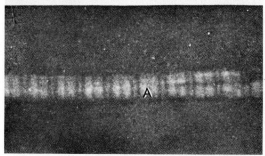

Figures 7-11 (upper) and 7-12 (lower)   A single isolated myofibril (glycerinated rabbit psoas), illustrating the banding pattern with phase-contrast optics and with polarized light. In the phase-contrast image (Fig. 7-11), the A band and Z line are dark and the I band is light. When viewed with polarized light (Fig. 7-12), the A band and Z line are bright and the I band is dark. (From J. Hanson and H. E. Huxley, Symp. Soc. Exp. Biol., **9:** 228, 1955.)

The bridges, which are part of the myosin molecule, possess the ATPase activity known to reside in this protein and presumably play a major role in the interaction of actin and myosin during contraction by forming a link between the two proteins.

Perhaps the least-understood structural component of the myofibril is the Z line. The thin filaments composing the I band are arranged so that in longitudinal sections of the myofibril, each thin filament on one side of the Z line faces the space between two thin filaments on the opposite side, and connecting elements appear to run obliquely across the Z line, creating a zigzag appearance (Fig. 7-20). In myofibrils sectioned transversely, filamentous components in the region of the Z line form a tetragonal pattern. On the basis of studies

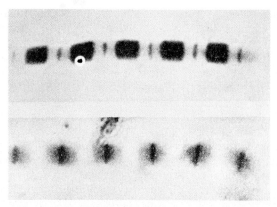

Figures 7-13 (upper) and 7-14 (lower)   Single myofibril (glycerinated rabbit psoas) photographed with phase-contrast optics showing the appearance before (Fig. 7-13) and after (Fig. 7-14) extraction of myosin. Following removal of myosin, the density of the A band is decreased, but that of the I band and the Z line remains. (From J. Hanson and H. E. Huxley, Symp. Soc. Exp. Biol., **9:**228, 1955.)

of amphibian muscle, it is believed that each terminating I-band filament forms the apex of a pyramid whose base is a square formed by four I-band filaments from the opposite side of the Z line. The sides of the pyramid are formed by the oblique structures composing the Z line itself. The arrangement in mammalian muscle is probably even more complex. The manner in which the I-band

Figures 7-15 (upper) and 7-16 (lower)   Myofibril (chicken breast muscle) treated with a fluorescent antibody to myosin and photographed using phase-contrast (Fig. 7-15) and fluorescence (Fig. 7-16) microscopy. The site of fluorescence (antimyosin) in Fig. 7-16 corresponds to the dark (A band) in Fig. 7-15. (From F. A. Pepe, J. Cell Biol., **28:**505, 1966.)

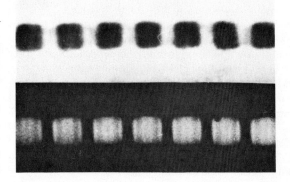

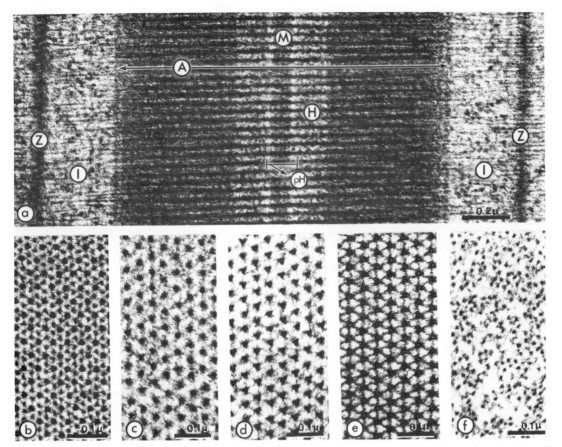

Figure 7-17 Single sarcomere (fish muscle) in longitudinal section (a), showing transverse banding pattern together with corresponding transverse sections through each of the bands. The A band (A) consists of both thick and thin filaments (b), the H band (H) and the bridge-free pseudo-H band (pH), only of thick filaments (c and d, respectively). The M band (M) also contains only thick filaments, but conspicuous transverse extensions are present as well (e). In the I band (I) only thin filaments are present (f). (From F. A. Pepe, 1971.)

filaments terminate at the Z line is not clear; it is possible, for example, that they actually continue into the Z line or that they form an entirely new structure. Evidence for the chemical nature of the Z line is conflicting also. Tropomyosin may be present along with other proteins, such as α-actinin. Both the chemical and structural composition of the Z line remains puzzling.

THE ULTRASTRUCTURAL BASIS OF CONTRACTION

Early observation with the light microscope showed that during contraction the length of the sarcomere was shortened. The I band in particular decreased in length, but there was no change in the length of the A band. The mechanism by which this occurs can be explained by the ultrastructure of the sarcomere. The extent by which the thick and thin filaments overlap can account for the change observed with the light microscope. X-ray diffraction data and direct observation with the electron microscope have established that, as the sarcomere shortens, the thin filaments of adjacent I bands are pulled toward the center of the A band, thereby obliterating the H band and decreasing the width of the I band (Fig. 7-21). The A band maintains

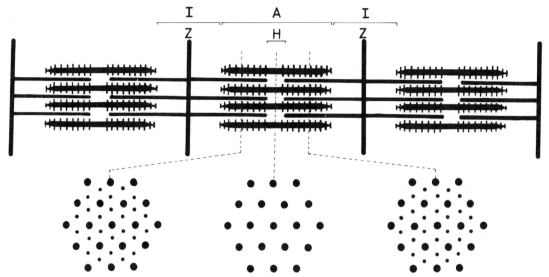

Figure 7-18 Diagrammatic interpretation of the organization of filaments giving rise to the transverse banding pattern. (From H. E. Huxley, 1969.)

Figure 7-19 Diagram illustrating the helical organization of cross bridges along the thick filament. The arrangement of six successive bridges corresponds to the 400-Å intervals observed in electron micrographs of sectioned muscle fibers. (From H. E. Huxley and W. Brown, J. Molec. Biol., **30**:383, 1967.)

Figure 7-20 Appearance of the Z line in a longitudinal section of a myofibril (rat semitendinosus). Each I-band filament on one side of the Z line faces the space between two filaments on the opposite side, and there appear to be filamentous structures connecting these filaments obliquely within the Z line itself. ×117,000.

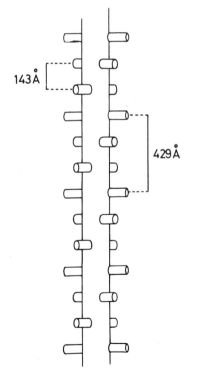

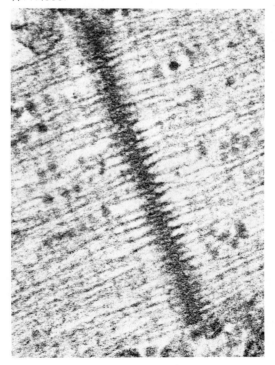

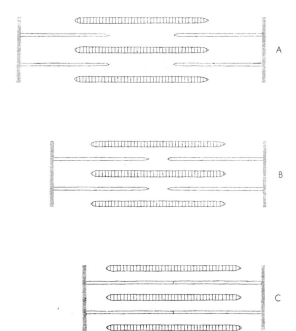

Figure 7-21   Diagram illustrating the manner in which the thin filaments of the I band may be pulled progressively toward the center of the A band during contraction, thereby decreasing the width of the I band (B and C) and eventually obliterating the H band (C). The sarcomere in B is at resting length, A is stretched, and C is contracted. (From H. E. Huxley, Sci. Am., **199**:No. 5, 1958.)

its original length, since the thick and thin filaments themselves do not shorten. The detailed events that take place as actin and myosin combine and chemical energy is converted to mechanical energy are not fully understood, but recent studies of the molecular basis of contraction are rapidly adding new information. The evidence suggests that the bridges actually move toward the actin filaments, engage them, and cause them to move along the myosin filament (see Huxley, 1969).

THE MOLECULAR CONFIGURATION OF THE MYOFILAMENTS

Myosin can be split into two major components, referred to as light meromyosin (LMM) and heavy meromyosin (HMM). The former is believed to form the linear "backbone" of the myosin molecule, whereas the latter projects outward from this "backbone" at regular intervals. Arrangement of LMM units parallel to one another but in a slightly staggered fashion (Fig. 7-23) would cause the HMM units to occur at intervals of about 400 Å, thereby accounting for the spacing of bridges observed with the electron microscope and the periodicity of skeletal muscle observed by x-ray diffraction (429 Å). Each visible bridge, therefore, reflects a single HMM unit. Electron micrographs of purified myosin confirm this arrangement. Such

Figure 7-22   Purified myosin, showing two examples of filaments aggregated at low ionic strength. Projections correspond to bridge-like structures seen in intact myofibrils (Fig. 7-6), and the bare central zone corresponds to the bridge-free pseudo-H band. ×145,000. (From H. E. Huxley, 1963.)

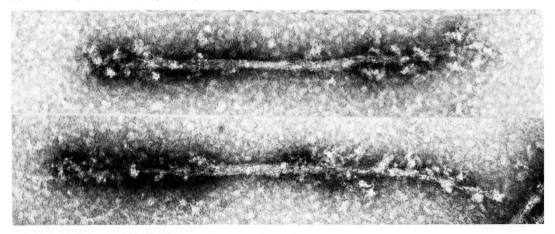

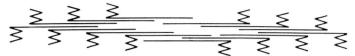

Figure 7-23 Diagrammatic interpretation of the arrangement of myosin molecules giving rise to the myosin filament, based on images such as those seen in Fig. 7-22. LMM units are parallel to the longitudinal axis of the filament, and HMM units extend at right angles from them. (From H. E. Huxley, 1963.)

preparations consist of tapered filaments, approximately 100 Å in diameter and 1.5 μm long, each resembling intact A-band filaments with their bridge-like projections (Figs. 7-22 and 7-23). Under certain experimental conditions, the molecules align with their HMM portions polarized toward either end of the filament, thereby leaving a bare zone that is most likely equivalent to the bridge-free zone in the intact sarcomere.

Preparations of pure actin consist of thinner filaments with dimensions comparable to intact I-band filaments. Each filament consists of a two-stranded helix with a turn about every 360 Å. The periodicity of actin is therefore close to but not equal to that of myosin. The individual strands (F-actin) composing the helix are actually a linear array of globular units called G-actin (Fig. 7-24). Although the periodicity of actin is 360 Å, that of the I band itself is actually greater, approximately 400 Å. This most likely reflects the presence of protein components other than actin. There is considerable evidence that some of the regulatory proteins are located in the I band, in close association with actin. It is believed that tropomyosin occupies the groove formed by the twisted double strands of actin and that troponin is confined to more circumscribed sites along the filament (Fig. 7-25).

When pure HMM is added to a preparation of F-actin, the HMM fragments attach precisely to the F-actin filaments (Fig. 7-26), and the complex has a 360-Å periodicity, which is characteristic of actin. This molecular interaction suggests that in whole muscle the HMM or bridge portion of the thick filament makes physical contact with the thin filament at the start of contraction. The polarity of the attachment, furthermore, is consistent with the ability of the two sets of filaments to slide past each other in a specific direction. The HMM portion of the myosin molecule actually consists of two

Figure 7-24   Purified F-actin showing the beaded appearance of several filaments and reflecting the helical arrangement of strands of G-actin monomers. ×525,000. (From J. Hanson and J. Lowy, 1963.)

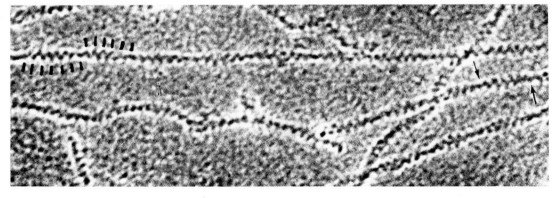

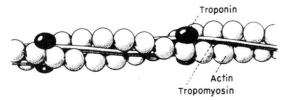

Figure 7-25   Diagrammatic interpretation of the organization of actin, troponin, and tropomyosin to form the I-band filament. Globular monomers of G-actin are arranged in rows forming a two-stranded helix which corresponds to the structures visible in Fig. 7-24.   (Courtesy of S. Ebashi.)

regions, one of which is attached in series to the LMM backbone of the myosin filament, with the other projecting outward at an angle to the major axis of the filament.   In this way, the HMM or bridge portion can swing out radially toward an adjacent thin filament while maintaining its base in the myosin filament (Fig. 7-27).

THE SARCOPLASMIC MEMBRANE SYSTEMS

Each myofibril is surrounded by an elaborate system of membranes aligned precisely with respect to the banding pattern of the myofibrils (Figs. 7-28 and 7-29).   It is apparent that a relationship exists between the sarcoplasmic membranes and the conduction of the impulse leading to contraction. The complex arrangement of tubules and cisternae which compose this system is best understood in the relatively simple form which exists in certain amphibian muscles (Fig. 7-28).   A parallel array of tubules is oriented along the long axis of the myofibril.   They extend along the full length of the A band and most of the I-band region of each

Figure 7-26   Isolated thin filaments treated with S_1 subunits of HMM.   The bridge-like units have become attached to the thin filaments at regular intervals, reflecting the periodicity of F-actin.   Note that the subunits project at an angle from the filaments and with a definite polarity, which is the same along the entire length of a given filament.   ×180,000.   (From P. B. Moore, H. E. Huxley, and D. J. DeRosier, 1970.)

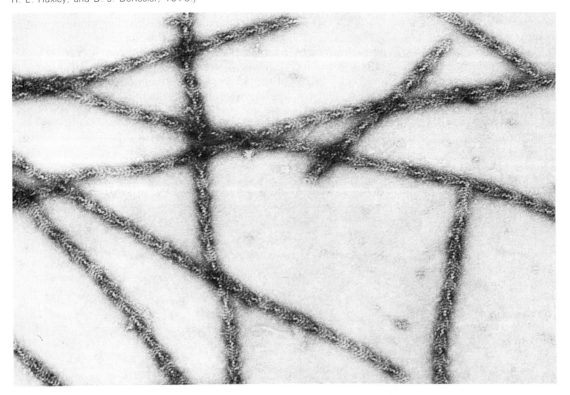

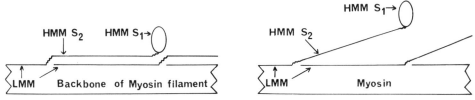

Figure 7-27   Diagram illustrating a possible mechanism whereby a HMM bridge can make contact with a nearby thin filament to bring about a sliding of the filaments with respect to each other.   The LMM unit remains as part of the thick filament itself, whereas the HMM portion swings out radially. The S_1 subunit of the latter is thus brought into contact with the thin filament. (From H. E. Huxley, 1969.)

Figure 7-28   Three-dimensional model of the sarcoplasmic membrane systems and their relationship to myofibrils in the frog sartorius muscle.   Note that triads (terminal cisternae of the sarcoplasmic reticulum plus the intervening T tubule) in this *amphibian* muscle, are aligned with the Z lines of the myofibrils.   Compare with Fig. 7-29.   (From L. D. Peachey, 1965.)

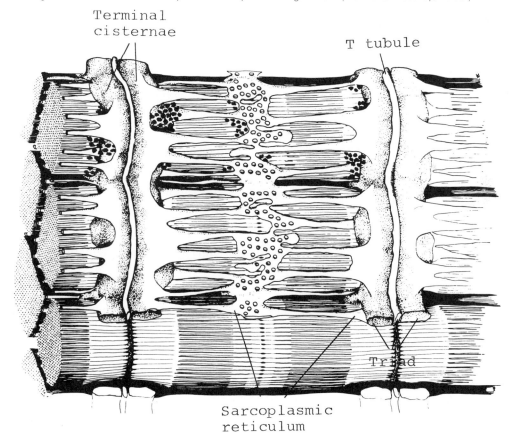

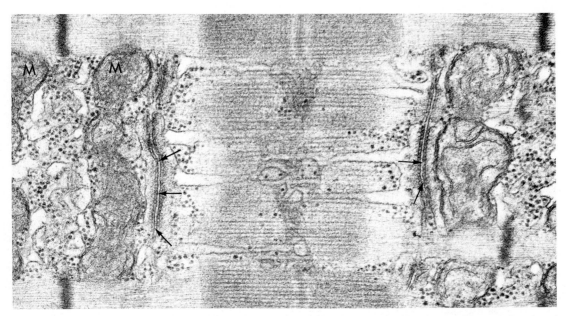

Figure 7-29   Electron micrograph showing tangential section of a single sarcomere (rat diaphragm). The sarcoplasmic reticulum extends over the A band and into the I band, and forms a tubular network in the region of the H band.   Longitudinal tubules give rise to terminal cisternae closely associated with the transversely oriented T tubule (arrows). The triads, in this *mammalian* muscle, are located near the junction of the A and I bands. That part of the sarcoplasmic reticulum which connects with that of the succeeding sarcomere is not fully included in this plane of section. Portions of it are visible between paired I-band mitochondria (M), which are closely aligned with the triads. See also Fig. 7-30. ×42,500. (Courtesy of H. A. Padykula.)

sarcomere and fuse in the region of the H band to form a fenestrated cisterna. As the tubules approach the Z lines at each end of the sarcomere, they join to form greatly expanded *terminal cisternae,* which run parallel to each Z line. Each terminal cisterna is faced by an equivalent structure on the opposite side of the Z line. This membrane complex is referred to collectively as the *sarcoplasmic reticulum.* It is associated with a transverse membrane system which originates at the cell surface. Between two terminal cisternae a tubular element runs transversely at the Z line. It extends through the sarcoplasm and is continuous, with comparable tubules at the same level of adjacent myofibrils. These transverse tubules compose the *T system,* which is separate from the sarcoplasmic reticulum. Two adjacent cisternae plus the intervening T tubule are referred to as a *triad.*

In mammalian skeletal muscle, the general arrangement of these two systems is similar except that triads are located, not at the Z line, but at the junction of the A and I bands. An additional network of tubules connects the terminal cisternae over the intervening I-band and Z-line regions (Fig. 7-29). In addition, the fused portion of the system over the H-band region may be either cisternal or tubular.

Although terminal cisternae and T tubules are separated from each other, they have a close apposition which is, at some points, reminiscent of the junctional complexes between certain epithelial cells. The membrane of each terminal cisterna is invaginated along the surface which faces the T tubule so that it appears "scalloped" in profile (Fig. 7-30). Between sites of invagination, the membrane of the terminal cisterna makes very close contact with that of the T tubule.

Various kinds of evidence indicate that the T system is continuous with the plasmalemma of the muscle cell, a structural relationship which facili-

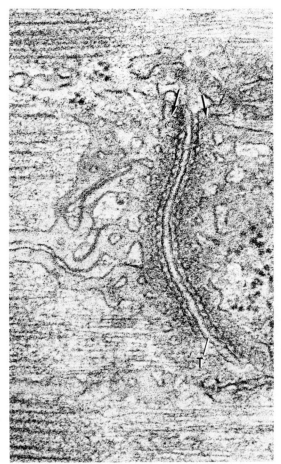

Figure 7-30 Single triad (rat semitendinosus). The membranes of both terminal cisternae (arrows) are "scalloped" along the surface that faces the T tubule (T). At the left, longitudinal tubules of the sarcoplasmic reticulum from the A-band region connect with one of the terminal cisternae. ×94,500.

wave of depolarization from the cell surface deep into the interior of the fiber to each myofibril. Comparative physiologic studies have shown, in fact, that those muscle fibers in which the triads are located at the Z line can be made to contract by means of a stimulating electrode placed at the Z line, whereas those fibers in which the triads are located at the A-I junction can be made to contract only if the same electrode is placed at the A-I junction. The manner in which a stimulus is transmitted from the T system along the length of the myofibril is less clear, but the close apposition of the T system to the terminal cisternae of the sarcoplasmic reticulum suggests that these are sites of low resistance across which an electrical impulse could pass to the sarcoplasmic reticulum.

THE NEUROMUSCULAR JUNCTION

The plasma membrane of the muscle cell or sarcolemma is structurally equivalent to the plasma

Figure 7-31 Single triad (fish muscle) illustrating the direct continuity between the membrane of the T system and the sarcolemma at the upper surface of the fiber (arrow). ×60,000. (From C. Franzini-Armstrong and K. R. Porter, 1964.)

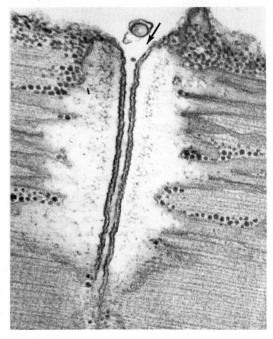

tates the inward conduction of the impulse that leads to contraction. Electron micrographs of certain fish muscles, for example, reveal a direct continuity between the T tubule and the sarcolemma (Fig. 7-31). In addition, when frog muscle fibers are immersed in a solution of ferritin, this electron-dense protein is subsequently observed within the T tubule (Fig. 7-32), which suggests a functional continuity as well. The form and distribution of the T system would thus permit rapid distribution of a

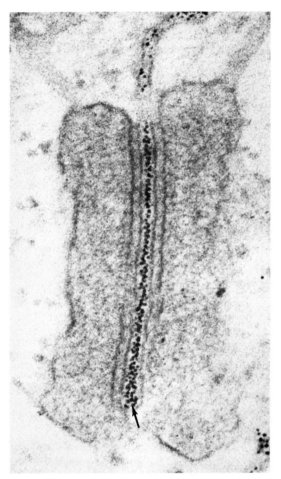

Figure 7-32   Triad from frog muscle fiber that had been immersed in a solution containing ferritin. Electron-dense particles of ferritin are present in the T system (arrow) but not in the sarcoplasmic reticulum, which suggests a functional continuity between the T system and the sarcolemma.   ×178,200. (From H. E. Huxley, 1964.)

(Figs. 7-33, 7-34, and 7-35). At all points, the plasmalemmae of the two cells remain separate, but the surface of the muscle fiber invaginates to form a shallow trough, the *primary synaptic cleft,* which receives the nerve terminal, or *axonal ending.* The sarcolemma invaginates further to form numerous deep *secondary synaptic clefts,* or *junctional folds,* which greatly increase the surface area of the muscle fiber (Fig. 7-34). The axon loses its myelin sheath as it approaches the neuromuscular junction, and its basal lamina, together with that of the Schwann cell (see Chap. 8), becomes fused with that of the muscle fiber. This cell coat extends into the primary synaptic cleft, as a single layer, separating nerve fiber from muscle fiber. It enters each junctional fold and forms a coating over its inner surface. That portion of the muscle fiber which contributes to the neuromuscular relationship is referred to as the *muscle sole plate,* or *motor end plate.* Nuclei and mitochondria are particularly abundant in this so-called *junctional sarcoplasm.* Cisternae of rough-surfaced endoplasmic reticulum and free ribosomes occur in this region also, suggesting that the synthesis of a receptor protein occurs there. The axonal ending is typically filled with vesicles, which may contain a neuromuscular transmitter or a trophic substance. Mitochondria are present, but filaments and microtubules, characteristic of the more proximal part of the axon, are absent.

Though myelin is absent from the axon at the neuromuscular junction, a Schwann cell remains closely associated with the axon and forms a covering over the junctional complex (Fig. 7-33). In this way, the axonal ending remains enclosed by the Schwann cell on one surface and by the muscle fiber on the other.

THE HETEROGENEITY OF SKELETAL MUSCLE FIBERS

In the mammal, measurements of physiologic properties such as speed of contraction have been limited, for the most part, to whole muscle, and interpretations of the data obtained have usually overlooked the fact that the component fibers are not alike. It has long been known that skeletal muscles differ in their color, with certain muscles being redder than others when viewed grossly. The

membrane of other cell types, and a typical basal lamina is applied to its outer surface. It is electrically polarized and, upon appropriate stimulation, usually by a nerve fiber, becomes depolarized, and contraction of the muscle fiber ensues. Branches of each motor nerve fiber terminate at specific sites along the muscle fiber; these are called *neuromuscular junctions.* The relationship between nerve fiber and muscle fiber is intimate and complex

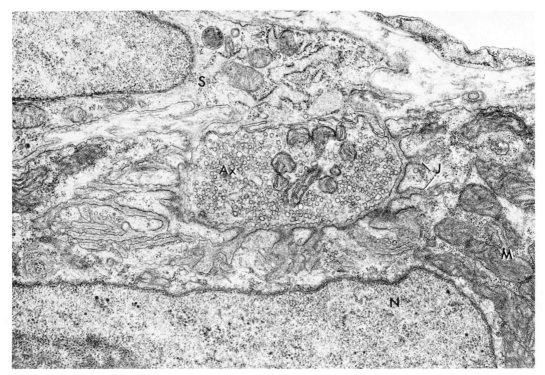

Figure 7-33   Neuromuscular junction of a red fiber (rat diaphragm).   The axonal ending (Ax) is located in a depression of the surface of the muscle fiber (primary synaptic cleft), and the surface is further invaginated to form junctional folds or secondary synaptic clefts (J).   Axonal vesicles and mitochondria are present in the axon.   Part of a Schwann cell (S) covers the upper surface of the axon, and a nucleus (N) and mitochondria (M) are present in the sarcoplasm below the axonal ending.   Structural organization is more readily apparent in the diagram in Fig. 7-35.   ×22,500.   (From G. F. Gauthier, 1970.)

fibers composing an individual muscle differ also, and the resulting heterogeneity is especially conspicuous following histochemical procedures for localizing enzymatic activity.   Fibers of the rat diaphragm, for example, differ in mitochondrial enzymatic activity, and this activity is, for the most part, inversely proportional to the cross-sectional dimensions of the fibers (Fig. 7-7).   In the mammal, small fibers, which are rich in mitochondria, are prevalent in red muscles and thus are referred to as *red fibers*.   Large fibers with a low mitochondrial content predominate in white muscles and thus are called *white fibers*.   Fibers with characteristics between the two, but which superficially resemble red fibers, are also prevalent in red muscles and are the so-called *intermediate fibers*.   It is possible to distinguish the three types of fibers by their ultra-

structural features also.   In the red fiber (Fig. 7-36), numerous large mitochondria with closely packed cristae form conspicuous aggregations beneath the sarcolemma and longitudinal rows between myofibrils.   The intermediate fiber is similar except that mitochondria tend to be smaller and their cristae less abundant than in the red fiber.   Also, the Z line is noticeably thinner in the intermediate than in the red fiber.   In the white fiber (Fig. 7-37), subsarcolemmal and interfibrillar mitochondria are sparse, and paired elliptical profiles at the I bands, which are present in all three fiber types, are the major form.   The Z line in the white fiber is about half as wide as that of the red fiber.   It is of interest that the red fiber, which is the smallest fiber, has the highest concentration of mitochondria, particularly at the cell surface.   These features

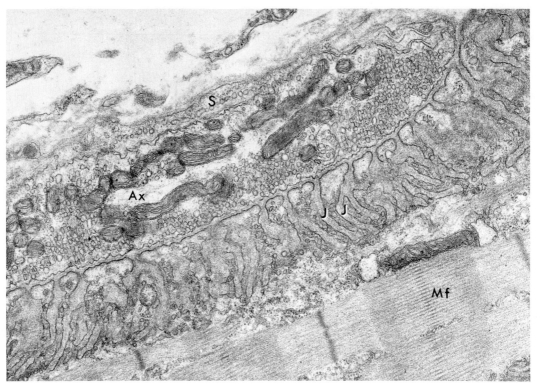

Figure 7-34   Neuromuscular junction of a white fiber (rat diaphragm).   Junctional folds are longer and more closely spaced than in the red fiber (Fig. 7-33), and axonal vesicles are more closely packed.   ×24,000.   (From H. A. Padykula and G. F. Gauthier, 1970.)

are consistent with a high rate of metabolic exchange.

Ultrastructural features of the neuromuscular junctions of red and white fibers indicate that differences exist also in the motoneurons serving these fibers.   In the white fiber (Fig. 7-34), the axonal ending is flat and elongated, and axonal vesicles are abundant.   Junctional folds are long and closely spaced.   In the red fiber (Fig. 7-33), the axonal ending is small and elliptical and contains fewer axonal vesicles.   The junctional folds are relatively short and sparse.   Experiments with cross innervation have shown that the microscopic distribution of fiber types as well as the physiologic and biochemical properties of the muscles are altered to a considerable extent when the nerve supplies are switched.   It has been demonstrated also that

stimulation of a particular motor neuron can bring about the cytochemical alteration of a single type of muscle fiber.   Current evidence suggests, therefore, that a motor unit is composed of a single type of muscle fiber.   These findings are consistent with the distinctive ultrastructural features of the muscle fibers and of their neuromuscular junctions.   Physiologic data indicate that red muscles contract more slowly than do white muscles.   Thus, it has been assumed that the red fiber is a slow fiber.   However, it is only through extrapolation that physiologic measurements have been associated with individual muscle fibers.   Most mammalian muscles consist of a mixture of fiber types, and the functional significance of the individual fibers is only beginning to be understood (see Gauthier, 1971).

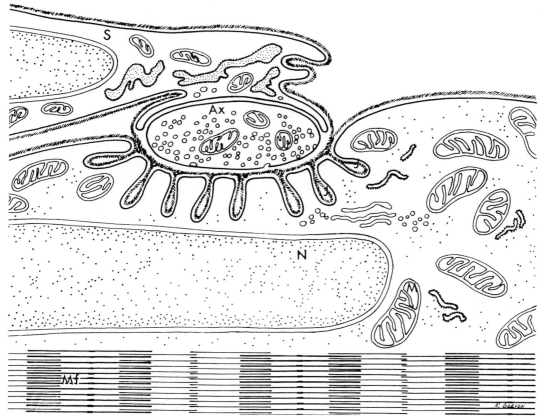

Figure 7-35 Generalized diagrammatic interpretation of the neuromuscular relationship. A Schwann cell (S) forms a covering over the axonal ending (Ax), and its basal lamina becomes fused with that of the muscle fiber, forming a coating which extends along the primary synaptic cleft and into each secondary synaptic cleft or junctional fold (J). Nuclei, mitochondria, free ribosomes, and rough endoplasmic reticulum occur characteristically in the junctional sarcoplasm.

Cardiac muscle

GENERAL FEATURES

The myocardium is composed of distinctive multinucleated striated fibers called *cardiac muscle fibers*. They are rich in mitochondria and are closely invested with an extensive capillary network. Although the nervous system is not required to initiate the heart beat, autonomic nerves are abundant. Nerve fibers appear to make contact with cardiac muscle fibers, but elaborate neuromuscular junctions such as those described for skeletal muscle fibers have not been observed.

Cardiac muscle is transversely striated, but unlike skeletal muscle, the fibers are branched and the nuclei are centrally located (Figs. 7-38 and 7-40). Bundles of myofilaments diverge as they approach the poles of the nucleus, leaving conical accumulations of sarcoplasm. Large mitochondria with closely packed cristae are abundant in the perinuclear sarcoplasm and form almost continuous longitudinal rows elsewhere in the fibers (Fig. 7-39). Paired I-band mitochondria, which are characteristic of skeletal muscle, are not present in cardiac muscle. The sarcoplasm is rich in glycogen and lipid (Fig. 7-39), which, as in skeletal

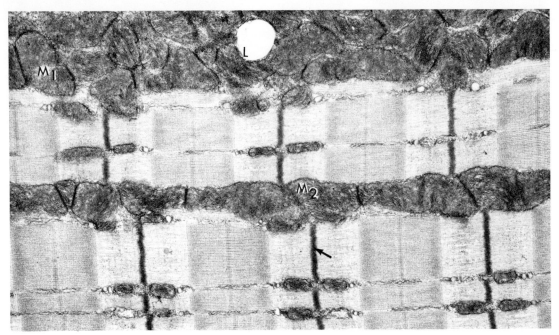

Figure 7-36   Longitudinal section of a typical red fiber (rat semitendinosus).   Large mitochondria (M_1) with closely packed cristae are aggregated just beneath the sarcolemma and in longitudinal interfibrillar rows (M_2).   The Z line (arrow) is relatively wide.   Compare with Fig. 7-37, which is at the same magnification. $\times 16,500$.   (From G. F. Gauthier, 1970.)

Figure 7-37   Typical white fiber (rat semitendinosus).   Subsarcolemmal and interfibrillar mitochondria are small and sparse.   Paired mitochondria (M_3) at the I bands, which are characteristic of mammalian skeletal muscle in general, are the predominate form in the white fiber.   The Z line (arrow) is about half as wide as in the red fiber (Fig. 7-36). $\times 16,500$.   (From G. F. Gauthier, Z. Zellforsch, **95:**462, 1969.)

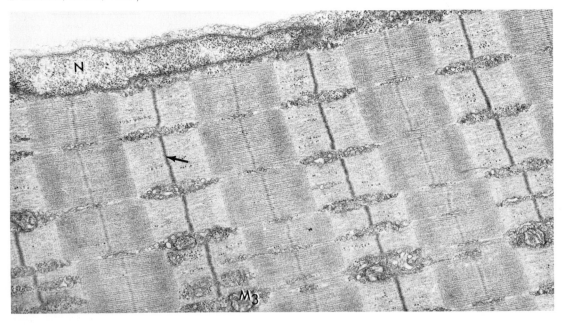

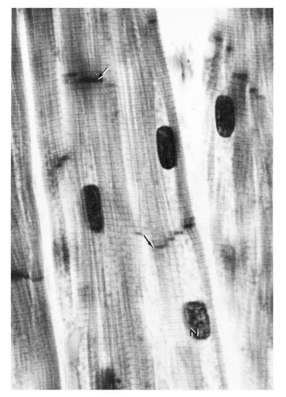

Figure 7-38 Longitudinal section of several cardiac muscle fibers. Nuclei (N) occupy a central position in these fibers, which are transversely striated. Bundles of filaments diverge as they approach the nucleus, leaving a conical region of sarcoplasm at each nuclear pole. Intercalated discs form conspicuous bands (arrows) which extend stepwise across the fibers, always at the level of a Z line. (H&E) ×1,200.

THE SARCOPLASMIC MEMBRANE SYSTEMS

Both the sarcoplasmic reticulum and the T system are present in mammalian cardiac muscle. The sarcoplasmic reticulum is less abundant and less elaborate than in skeletal muscle. An irregular network of tubules extends over the full length of the sarcomere, with no transverse specialization at the H band. Terminal specializations occur at the Z lines, that is, at a position comparable to that of the triads of amphibian skeletal muscle. However, the terminal cisternae are not so extensive or regularly arranged and thus make less frequent contact with the transverse tubules (Fig. 7-42). This leads to the appearance of so-called "dyads," or "couplings," where only one cisterna is apposed to a T tubule. The cisternae may also be apposed to the sarcolemma and, because of this relationship, are given the designation *subsarcolemmal cisternae*.

There are fewer T tubules in cardiac than in skeletal muscle, but they are larger in diameter (Fig. 7-42). The continuity of the T system with the sarcolemma is even more conspicuous than in skeletal muscle, and the basal lamina extends inward along with the membrane, forming a coating over the inner surface of the T tubule. The relationship between the cisternal membrane and that of the T tubule or the sarcolemma is similar to that observed in the triads of skeletal muscle, and this close relationship is believed to favor the transmission of an electrical stimulus carried by the T system.

INTERCELLULAR RELATIONSHIPS

Unlike skeletal muscle fibers, individual cardiac muscle fibers are associated in an end-to-end arrangement which produces the so-called *intercalated discs* at frequent intervals. The intercalated disc is a complex cell junction which consists of several transverse portions arranged stepwise at different levels across the fiber (Figs. 7-38 and 7-39). Two successive transverse portions are connected longitudinally by a continuation of the respective cell membranes, thereby creating a complete separation between cells. Therefore, contrary to early beliefs, the myocardium is not a synctium. The transverse cell surfaces are elaborately interdigitated and, in longitudinal sections

muscle, constitute metabolic fuels for contractile activity.

There are no apparent differences in the basic ultrastructural configuration of the contractile apparatus of skeletal and cardiac muscle fibers. The precise arrangement of thick and thin myofilaments produces a transverse banding pattern equivalent to that of skeletal muscle (Fig. 7-39). However, bundles of filaments are not aggregated transversely to form discrete myofibrillar units as in skeletal muscle fibers. The transverse continuity of myofibrillar material is interrupted only by the longitudinal rows of mitochondria and scattered profiles of the sarcoplasmic reticulum (Figs. 7-40 and 7-41).

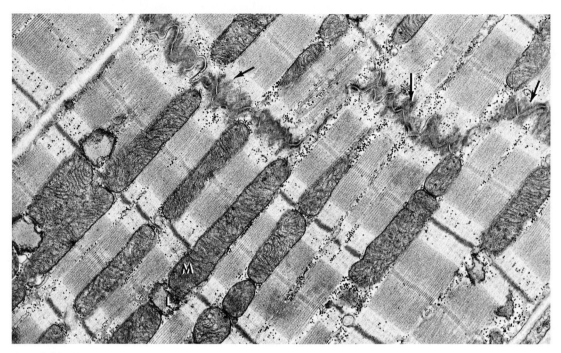

Figure 7-39   Electron micrograph of a longitudinal section from the ventricular papillary muscle of the cat.   The transverse banding pattern is similar to that of skeletal muscle.   Paired mitochondria are absent from the I bands, but large mitochondria (M) form almost continuous longitudinal rows, and lipid droplets (L) are closely associated with them.   A transverse cell junction is arranged in the typical stepwise pattern that constitutes the intercalated disc.   Parts of three transverse portions (arrows) of the intercalated disc are included in the section, together with the longitudinal portions that connect them.   ×15,000.   (From D. W. Fawcett and N. S. McNutt, 1969.)

Figure 7-40   Electron micrograph of portions of four fibers sectioned transversely (cat papillary muscle).   The central position of the nucleus (N) is apparent in one of the fibers.   Though discrete myofibrils are not apparent, the transverse continuity of myofibrillar material is partially interrupted by numerous large mitochondria (M).   ×6,700.   (From D. W. Fawcett and N. S. McNutt, 1969.)

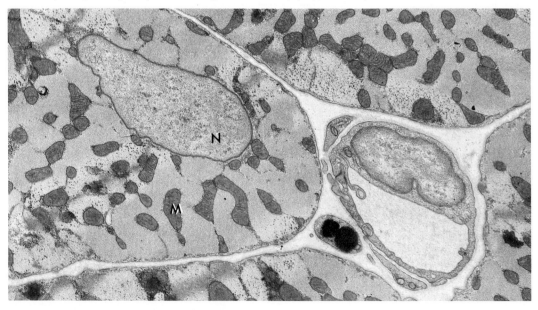

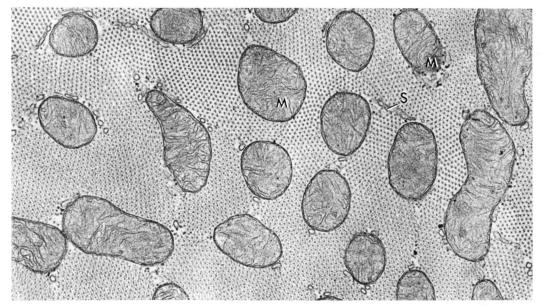

Figure 7-41   Transverse section similar to that in Fig. 7-40 showing the arrangement of myofilaments and sarcoplasmic organelles. The hexagonal array of thick and thin filaments is similar to that of skeletal muscle, but there is no organization into individual myofibrils.   Transverse sections of longitudinal rows of mitochondria (M) and profiles of sarcoplasmic membranes (S) form a discontinuous boundary between masses of myofilaments.   ×30,000.   (From D. W. Fawcett and N. S. McNutt, 1969.)

Figure 7-42   Three-dimensional model of the sarcoplasmic membrane systems of cardiac muscle.   The sarcoplasmic reticulum is less elaborate than in skeletal muscle.   T tubules, on the other hand, are even more prominent than in skeletal muscle, and their membranes are clearly continuous with the sarcolemma.   Note that they are located at the level of the Z line.   (From D. W. Fawcett and N. S. McNutt, 1969.)

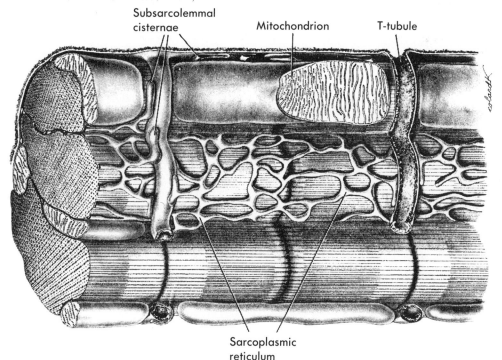

Subsarcolemmal cisternae   Mitochondrion   T-tubule

Sarcoplasmic reticulum

of the fibers, they have a characteristic undulating pattern (Figs. 7-39 and 7-43). The subsarcolemmal sarcoplasm contains dense masses of filamentous material into which the I-band filaments insert (Fig. 7-43). The appearance of the intercellular relationship at certain points is therefore similar to the desmosome or *macula adherens* observed in certain epithelia (see Chap. 3). In addition, the relationship may be more extensive than that of a typical desmosome, and is thus referred to as a *fascia adherens*.

At other sites, the intercellular space appears to be obliterated as in a typical tight junction or zonula occludens, but since this relationship is more circumscribed, it is referred to as a *macula occludens*. The longitudinal portion of the intercalated disc is continuous with the transverse portions. The longi-tudinal intercellular relationship is similar to the zonula occludens of epithelial cells, but is even more extensive, and thus comprises a *fascia occludens*. Both the macula occludens and fascia occludens comprise the so-called *nexus* of cardiac and smooth muscle. Recent technical advances in ultrastructural analysis have revealed that a narrow intercellular space (about 18 Å) exists at the nexus; therefore it is more correctly described as a *close junction*, or *gap junction*, rather than a tight junction. The gap junction is believed to be a site of low electrical resistance. Since electrical coupling between cells is a fundamental property of both cardiac and smooth muscle, the gap junction might constitute the structural basis for electrical transmission among cardiac- or smooth-muscle cells.

Figure 7-43   Part of a single transverse portion of an intercalated disc. The cell membranes at the extremities of the two fibers included in the micrograph are continuous at the left (arrow) with part of a longitudinal segment of the intercalated disc. The cell membranes pursue a wavy course but remain parallel to each other throughout the intercalated disc. I-band filaments above and below appear to insert into the dense sarcoplasmic material adjacent to the cell membranes. ×70,000. (From D. W. Fawcett and N. S. McNutt, 1969.)

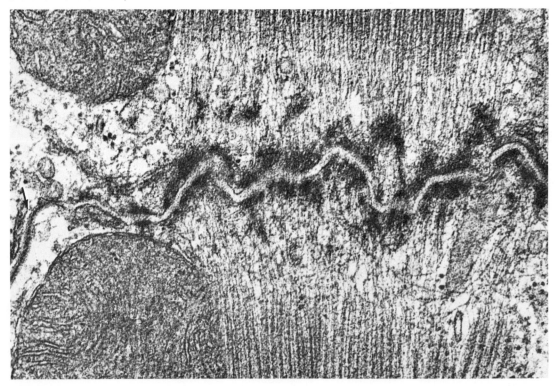

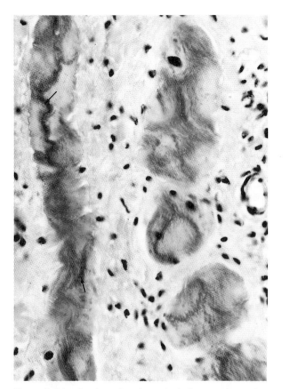

Figure 7-44   Section of ox heart including portions of several Purkinje fibers. The fiber at the left is sectioned longitudinally, and those at the right are sectioned transversely or somewhat obliquely. The fibers are large when compared with most ordinary cardiac muscle fibers (Fig. 7-38), and myofibrils (arrows) are relatively sparse. Most of the sarcoplasm is occupied by glycogen, which has been extracted from this preparation. (H&E)   ×480.

Most of the above description has been derived from the study of ventricular cardiac muscle, but atrial muscle shares many of the basic features. However, in the cat, at least, the atrial fibers tend to be smaller in diameter. The mitochondrial content tends to be even greater than in ventricular fibers, but T tubules are relatively sparse.

The origin and distribution of electrical activity leading to the characteristic rhythmical contraction of cardiac muscle reside in special forms of cardiac muscle fibers which compose the conducting system of the heart, namely the SA node, AV node, and AV bundle. These special fibers make contact ultimately with ordinary cardiac muscle fibers. Nodal fibers tend to be smaller, but those of the AV bundle tend to be larger, than ordinary cardiac

muscle fibers. The fibers of the AV bundle often acquire a distinctive appearance and may therefore be distinguished from ordinary cardiac muscle fibers. These special conducting fibers, or *Purkinje fibers*, are responsible for the final distribution of the electrical stimulus to the myocardium. Variable amounts of connective tissue separate these conducting fibers from one another, and this differs from species to species. Myofibrillar material tends to be less abundant than in ordinary cardiac muscle fibers, but this too varies with the species. In some species, notably among the ungulates, Purkinje fibers are extremely large, and massive amounts of glycogen are accumulated in the sarcoplasm. Only scattered strands of myofibrillar material are apparent in these fibers (Fig. 7-44).

Figure 7-45   Transverse section of frog intestine showing the typical appearance of the circular layer of smooth muscle adjacent to connective tissue (CT) of the submucosa. The fibers are arranged circumferentially with their narrow tapered ends adjacent to the wider central regions of nearby fibers. Nuclei are centrally located. Cell boundaries are somewhat difficult to distinguish. (H&E)   ×500.

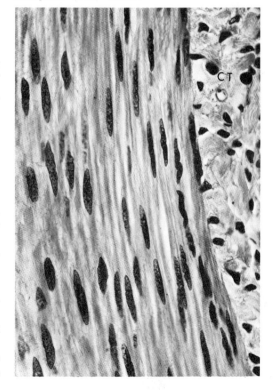

Smooth muscle

GENERAL FEATURES

Smooth muscle plays a critical role in the maintenance of the caliber of the lumens of the viscera and certain blood vessels. Through the appropriate degree of contraction or relaxation of the component fibers, physiologic processes such as digestion, respiration, and blood flow can be regulated. Accordingly, the fibers are arranged in characteristic directions, reflecting the functional activity of the organ (Fig. 7-45). Connective tissue, carrying blood vessels and autonomic nerve fibers, penetrates among individual fibers, but the amount of stroma varies among species and among the organ systems of a given species (for example, compare Figs. 7-45 and 7-46).

Smooth muscle fibers are narrow and tapering, and their length varies from about 20 μm in certain small blood vessels to 500 μm or more in the gestational uterus. The nucleus is centrally located, and there are no transverse striations (Figs. 7-46 and 7-47). A typical basal lamina is applied to the outer surface of the sarcolemma. In fact, when stained, the basal laminae facilitate the visualization of individual fibers (Fig. 7-47).

The arrangement of fibers is staggered so that the broad nuclear region of one fiber lies opposite the narrow tapered end of an adjacent fiber (Fig.

Figure 7-46 Longitudinal sections of several smooth-muscle fibers (lateral vaginal canal of the opossum). Because of the relative abundance of connective tissue in this bundle of smooth muscle, the cellular outlines are clearly distinguished. Nuclei occupy the broad central regions of these tapering fibers. (H&E) ×760.

Figure 7-47 Transverse section of smooth-muscle fibers (stomach of the grasshopper mouse), which has been stained by the periodic acid–Schiff reaction and with hematoxylin. The carbohydrate component of the conspicuous basal lamina is stained, and this facilitates visualization of individual fibers. Note that the plane of section passes through the broad nuclear regions of only certain fibers and through the narrow tapered ends of others. ×1,200.

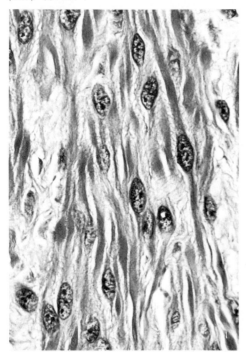

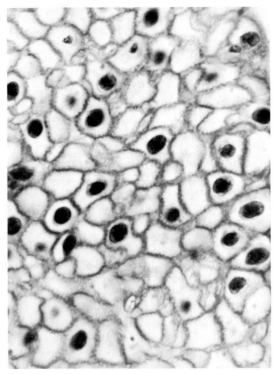

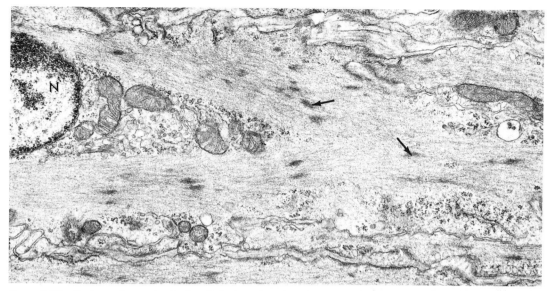

Figure 7-48   Electron micrograph of a longitudinal section of a smooth muscle fiber (ileum of a 13-day-old rat).   Part of the centrally located nucleus (N) is included at the left.   Mitochondria, a Golgi apparatus, and ribosomes are particularly abundant in the conical perinuclear region.   The remainder of the fiber is occupied by thin filaments and by dense bodies (arrows) into which the filaments appear to insert.   There are no transverse striations.   ✕17,220.

7-45).   A transverse section would therefore pass through the nuclear level of only certain fibers and through the tapered ends of those which intervene (Fig. 7-47).   At various points, adjacent fibers form an intimate association, called a nexus, or gap junction, where electrical coupling is believed to be facilitated as described earlier.

The cytoplasmic organelles, which include mitochondria, Golgi apparatus, scattered profiles of rough endoplasmic reticulum, and free ribosomes, are confined, for the most part, to a conical region at each pole of the nucleus (Fig. 7-48).   The remainder of the sarcoplasm is occupied by filaments which usually appear thin (Fig. 7-49).   Characteristic dense bodies, into which the thin filaments appear to insert, are distributed throughout the sarcoplasm (Figs. 7-48 and 7-49).

THE ULTRASTRUCTURAL BASIS OF CONTRACTION

Much less is known about the mechanism of contraction in smooth muscle than in striated muscle.

The absence of transverse banding has made application of the sliding filament model seem inappropriate.   Although both myosin and actin can be demonstrated in smooth muscle by chemical procedures, conventional ultrastructural preparations have ordinarily revealed a homogeneous population of filaments.   The dimensions of the filaments composing mammalian smooth muscle correspond closely to those of actin filaments.

Under precisely controlled conditions, myosin filaments can be prepared from homogenates of mammalian smooth muscle, and the ultrastructural appearance of these filaments closely resembles that of myosin filaments prepared from skeletal muscle.   Also, thick filaments have recently been observed in ultrathin sections of smooth muscle fibers that have been obtained in the contracted state (Fig. 7-50) or that have been fixed at a pH lower than that ordinarily used to preserve muscle fibers.   As in skeletal muscle, therefore, two types of filaments can be demonstrated.   It has been suggested (see Shoenberg, 1969) that, in smooth

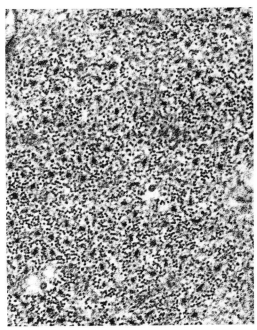

Figure 7-50   Transverse section of smooth muscle from the guinea pig intestine. This preparation was deliberately allowed to contract isometrically before fixation. Under these conditions, both thick and thin filaments are revealed, though the organization differs from that of striated muscle. ×91,840. (Modified from R. E. Kelly and R. V. Rice, 1969. Courtesy of R. E. Kelly.)

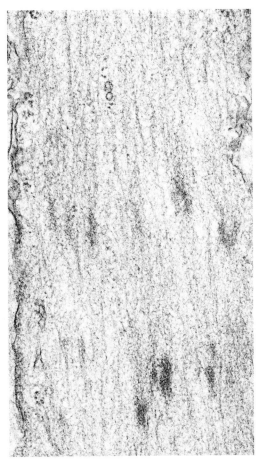

Figure 7-49   Longitudinal section similar to that in Fig. 7-48, illustrating the filamentous composition of the smooth-muscle fiber. There is an apparently homogeneous population of thin filaments with dimensions similar to those of actin filaments from striated muscle. Compare with Fig. 7-50. ×43,700.

muscle, myosin exists as very small aggregates in the relaxed state, and that, under conditions favorable for contraction, well-defined filaments are formed. It is thus possible that a sliding filament mechanism might be responsible for contraction in smooth muscle as well as in skeletal muscle.

References

DEVINE, C. E., and A. P. SOMLYO: Thick Filaments in Vascular Smooth Muscle, *J. Cell. Biol.,* **49:**636 (1971).

DEWEY, M. M., and L. BARR: A Study of the Structure and Distribution of the Nexus, *J. Cell Biol.,* **23:**553 (1964).

EBASHI, S., M. ENDO, and I. OHTSUKI: Control of Muscle Contraction, *Quart. Rev. Biophys.,* **2:**351 (1969).

FAWCETT, D. W., and N. S. MCNUTT: The Ultrastructure of the Cat Myocardium. I. Ventricular Papillary Muscle, *J. Cell Biol.,* **42:**1 (1969).

FRANZINI-ARMSTRONG, C.: Studies of the Triad. II. Penetration of Tracers into the Junctional Gap, *J. Cell Biol.,* **49:**196 (1971).

FRANZINI-ARMSTRONG, C.: Studies of the Triad. I. Structure of the Junction in Frog Twitch Fibers, *J. Cell Biol.*, **47**:488 (1970).

FRANZINI-ARMSTRONG, C., and K. R. PORTER: Sarcolemmal Invaginations Constituting the T System in Fish Muscle Fibers, *J. Cell Biol.*, **22**:675 (1964).

GARAMVÖLGYI, N., E. S. VIZI, and J. KNOLL: The Regular Occurrence of Thick Filaments in Stretched Mammalian Smooth Muscle, *J. Ultrastruct. Res.*, **34**:135 (1971).

GAUTHIER, G. F.: The Structural and Cytochemical Heterogeneity of Mammalian Skeletal Muscle Fibers, in R. J. Podolsky (ed.), "The Contractility of Muscle Cells and Related Processes," Prentice-Hall, Inc., Englewood Cliffs, N.J., 1972.

GAUTHIER, G. F.: The Ultrastructure of Three Fiber Types in Mammalian Skeletal Muscle, in E. J. Briskey, R. G. Cassens, and B. B. Marsh (eds.) "The Physiology and Biochemistry of Muscle as a Food," vol. II, The University of Wisconsin Press, Madison, 1970.

HANSON, J., and J. LOWY: The Structure of F-Actin and of Actin Filaments Isolated from Muscle, *J. Molec. Biol.*, **6**:46 (1963).

HUXLEY, H. E.: The Mechanism of Muscular Contraction, *Science,* **164**:1356 (1969).

HUXLEY, H. E.: Evidence for Continuity between the Central Elements of the Triads and Extra-cellular Space in Frog Sartorius Muscle, *Nature,* **202**:1067 (1964).

HUXLEY, H. E.: Electron Microscope Studies on the Structure of Natural and Synthetic Protein Filaments from Striated Muscle, *J. Molec. Biol.*, **7**:281 (1963).

HUXLEY, H. E.: The Double Array of Filaments in Cross-striated Muscle, *J. Biophys. Biochem. Cytol.*, **3**:631 (1957).

KELLY, D. E.: The Fine Structure of Skeletal Muscle Triad Junctions, *J. Ultrastruct. Res.* **29**:37 (1969).

KELLY, D. E.: Models of Muscle Z-band Fine Structure Based on a Looping Filament Configuration, *J. Cell Biol.*, **34**:827, 1967.

KELLY, R. E., and R. V. RICE: Ultrastructural Studies on the Contractile Mechanism of Smooth Muscle, *J. Cell Biol.*, **42**:683 (1969).

KELLY, R. E., and R V. RICE: Localization of Myosin Filaments in Smooth Muscle, *J. Cell Biol.*, **37**:105 (1968).

KNAPPEIS, G G., and F. CARLSEN: The Ultrastructure of the Z Disc in Skeletal Muscle, *J. Cell Biol.*, **13**:323 (1962).

MC NUTT, N. S., and D. W. FAWCETT: The Ultrastructure of the Cat Myocardium. II. Atrial Muscle, *J. Cell Biol.*, **42**:46 (1969).

MC NUTT, N. S., and R. S. WEINSTEIN: The Ultrastructure of the Nexus. A Correlated Thin-section and Freeze-cleave Study, *J. Cell Biol.*, **47**:666 (1970).

MOORE, P. B., H. E. HUXLEY, and D. J. DE ROSIER: Three-dimensional Reconstruction of F-actin, Thin Filaments and Decorated Thin Filaments, *J. Molec. Biol.*, **50**:279 (1970).

PADYKULA, H. A., and G. F. GAUTHIER: The Ultrastructure of the Neuromuscular Junctions of Mammalian Red, White, and Intermediate Skeletal Muscle Fibers, *J. Cell Biol.*, **46**:27 (1970).

PEACHEY, L. D.: The Sarcoplasmic Reticulum and Transverse Tubules of the Frog's Sartorius, *J. Cell Biol.*, **25** (3):209 (1965).

PEPE, F. A.: The Structural Components of the Striated Muscle Fibril, in S. N. Timasheff and G. D. Fasman (eds.), "Biological Macromolecules Series," vol. V, pt. A, Chap. 7, Marcel Dekker, New York, 1971.

PODOLSKY, R. J. (ed.): "The Contractility of Muscle Cells and Related Processes," Prentice-Hall, Inc., Englewood Cliffs, N.J., 1971.

PORTER, K. R., and G. E. PALADE: Studies on the Endoplasmic Reticulum.   III. Its Form and Distribution in Striated Muscle Cells, *J. Biophys. Biochem. Cytol.*, **3:**269 (1957).

RHODIN, J. A. G.: Fine Structure of Vascular Walls in Mammals, *Physiol. Rev.*, **42**(Suppl. 5):48 (1962).

ROBERTSON, J. D.: The Ultrastructure of a Reptilian Myoneural Junction, *J. Biophys. Biochem. Cytol.*, **2:**381 (1956).

SHOENBERG, C. F.: A Study of Myosin Filaments in Extracts and Homogenates of Vertebrate Smooth Muscle, *Angiologica* (*Basel*), **6:**233 (1969).

SHOENBERG, C. F.: An Electron Microscope Study of the Influence of Divalent Ions on Myosin Filament Formation in Chicken Gizzard Extracts and Homogenates, *Tissue Cell,* **1:**83 (1969).

SOMMER, J. R., and E. A. JOHNSON: Cardiac Muscle.   A Comparative Study of Purkinje Fibers and Ventricular Fibers, *J. Cell Biol.*, **36:**497 (1968).

chapter 8 Nervous tissue

MARCUS SINGER

The nervous system pervades most regions of the body (Fig. 8-1). If the nervous system, including all its microscopic subdivisions, could be viewed in a transparency, the pattern of nerves and their ultimate endings would reveal the outline of the body and its parts. Those surfaces most exposed to the environment would be shown best, especially the face, mouth, lips, tongue, and hands.

Another important feature of nervous anatomy is its continuity, resembling in this sense the vascular system, which is so arranged that blood flows from one region to another, continuously perfusing the whole body. The nerve cells and their processes are connected so intimately with one another that there is a continuous flow of information from one region of the body to another. If a nerve is traced centrally from a terminal twig, it will be seen to unite continuously to form larger and larger

nerves until the primary axis of the nervous system, the central nervous system, is reached (Fig. 8-1). Within the central nervous system one may trace any one of numerous internal pathways and then exit by one of many outlets, proceeding without break along a peripheral subdivision to one of its final terminations.

From widespread distribution and structural continuity emerge certain cardinal features of nervous function. The nervous system relates all parts of the body to one another and to events in the internal and external environment. In its response to the qualities of our environment it acts as an integrating unit which directs all our individual performances and attitudes against the background of widespread nervous activity.

In nervous tissue the cellular functions of irritability and conductivity attain their highest develop-

249

ment. *Irritability* is the ability of cells to react to various stimuli. Through *conductivity* the effects of stimulation are transmitted to distant parts of the cell or to adjacent cells. Nerve endings are stimulated by the external and internal environment; they transmit messages along the nerves to the central nervous system, where the information is sorted out and interrelated. On the basis of this sensory information and its central integration, messages are poured out through nerves to the muscles, causing movements of peripheral structures. Thus the basis of all our sensations and responses to sensations lies within the nervous system. Without the sensory functions of the nervous system the sensations of our environment and of our body itself could not be impressed upon us, and without the motor functions that move the body, we could not respond to these sensory experiences. The muscles may be thought of as the keyboard upon which the nervous system plays. Without the nervous system the instrument is silent.

Between the sensory and motor systems is the great central nervous system, composed of the brain and spinal cord, which interprets and elaborates the sensory stimuli and selects the appropriate motor expressions. Here there are various levels of integration, so that a stimulus may yield a simple muscle response or widespread body movements, or it may be stored away for a delayed response. The brain, particularly the cerebral cortex and thalamus, uses the information in higher functions of memory, symbolic thought, and language.

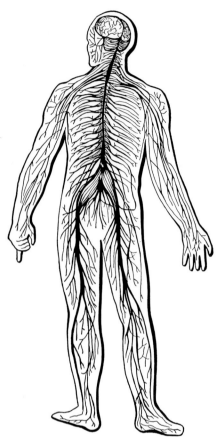

Figure 8-1   The central and peripheral nervous systems of the human being. (After Kimber, Gray, and Stackpole, "Textbook of Anatomy and Physiology," 12th ed., Macmillan, New York, 1938.)

Major divisions of the nervous system

For convenience in description, the nervous system may be divided into three major regions: the *central,* the *peripheral,* and the *autonomic.* The central nervous system, enclosed in the vertebral column and the cranium, consists of the spinal cord and the brain (Fig. 8-1). Since the detailed description of the conduction pathways and centers within each of these parts lies within the field of neuroanatomy, only certain aspects bearing upon the histology of central nervous structures will be touched upon in the ensuing pages.

The spinal and cranial nerves and their numerous branches constitute the peripheral nervous system

(Fig. 8-1). Except for the first cervical nerve, spinal nerves are connected to the central nervous system by two roots (Figs. 8-2 and 8-64): a posterior, or dorsal, root and an anterior, or ventral, one. In the exception only a ventral root is present. The roots themselves are often subdivided into rootlets. The dorsal and ventral roots join upon emerging from the spinal canal and form the trunk of the spinal nerve (Fig. 8-64). The dorsal root brings sensory impulses into the central nervous system, whereas the ventral root conducts motor impulses peripherally. The sensory root is characterized by a swelling (ganglion) containing nerve cell bodies.

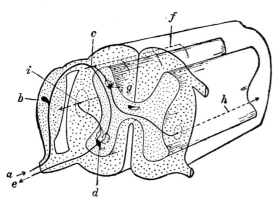

Figure 8-2 The spinal cord and roots of a spinal nerve. Visible are a sensory neuron, a and b; a motor neuron, e and d; and the connections with each other and with the brain, c, f, g, h, and i. The arrows denote the direction of impulse conduction.

The spinal nerve, being formed by the union of dorsal and ventral roots, therefore has mixed sensory and motor functions. The cranial nerves, unlike the spinal ones, arise by a single root or rootlets from one level of the brain axis (Fig. 8-66). The root may be mixed or may be devoted exclusively to motor or sensory function. Distally, the sensory part of both cranial and spinal nerves terminates either freely among peripheral tissues or upon receptors specialized to receive a particular stimulus, such as in the organ of Corti of the inner ear, which is specialized for receiving sound, and in the tactile corpuscles specialized for touch (see below).

The autonomic nervous system (Figs. 8-63, see color insert, and 8-64), also called the vegetative or interofective nervous system, is concerned mainly with visceral motility (smooth and cardiac musculature) and glandular secretions. The autonomic nervous system is commonly defined as a motor system, although sensory branches accompany the motor ones and sensations may initiate autonomic action. The autonomic nervous system consists of two subdivisions, the *sympathetic* and the *parasympathetic nervous systems*. The former is made up of two cords or "chains," of nervous tissue running the length of the spinal column on either side of the vertebral bodies. The cords are segmental in that they are periodically swollen with accumulations of nerve cell bodies called *sympathetic vertebral ganglia*. They are connected with each spinal nerve by a communicating branch, the *ramus communicans* (Fig. 8-63, see color insert). The rami communicantes bring information from the central nervous system via the ventral root to the sympathetic cords and conduct impulses from the sympathetics to the spinal nerve and thence to peripheral glands and to smooth muscle of hair follicles and blood vessels. In addition to the rami, numerous branches arise from the sympathetic trunks to supply the glands and the musculature of internal organs and blood vessels. In certain regions of the viscera they form complicated, interlacing networks (plexuses) of nerves which include scattered accumulations of parasympathetic nerve cell bodies. Still other branches that originate in the upper cervical region of the sympathetic chains follow the major blood vessels of the head to supply glands and smooth musculature of that region.

The parasympathetic system, unlike the sympathetic one, does not consist of cords; its general distribution is somewhat similar but is confined to visceral regions (Fig. 8-63, see color insert). It arises from four cranial nerves and, in general, two sacral spinal ones. The parasympathetic parts of these nerves separate from the rest of the nerve and are distributed to visceral structures; they tend to overlap the sympathetic system in distribution and contribute to the sympathetic plexuses. Further consideration will be given below to the structure and function of the autonomic nervous system and its parts.

Histology of the nervous system

The nervous system is a highly cellular structure whose parenchyma cells, the *nerve cells* or *neurons*, are the units of structure. All nervous functions have their basis in nerve cells and their interconnections. In addition to nerve cells, the nervous system also contains blood vessels and supporting and protecting tissue of various types. The supporting tissue differs for the central nervous system and for the peripheral and autonomic nervous systems. Among the differences is the presence of fibrous connective tissue in the last two and its absence within the central nervous system; moreover, the neuroglial tissue is unique to the central nervous system. Blood vessels are abundant within nervous tissue. They form a rich anastomosing network over the cord and brain and send numerous branches into the central nervous system. The latter are small-caliber and delicate structures with thinner walls than the vessels of other tissues, so they are more subject to hemorrhage. The arteries subdivide into a rich capillary network with many anastomoses that satisfies the heavy oxygen and nutritional demands of nervous tissue. The many small veins that leave the central nervous system form major channels which lie just outside.

THE NERVE CELL

The most striking feature of the neuron, which distinguishes it from all other cells, is the presence of greatly elongated cytoplasmic processes that, although microscopic in diameter, may extend in certain instances almost the length of the body. These long processes make up the essential structure of nerves and of tracts of the central nervous system. By means of these processes the neuron contacts other neurons, receptors, glands, or muscles and thus transmits or receives stimuli to or from them.

There are more than 10 billion neurons in the human nervous system, and by far the greatest number of these are located in the brain, particularly the cerebral cortex. Many types of neurons exist in the nervous system, but certain features are common to all of them. First, all neurons have a *cell body* (Fig. 8-3, see color insert). (The term *nerve cell* is frequently used synonymously with *cell body*.) The cell body is the swollen portion of the neuron and is irregularly round or oval. It contains abundant cytoplasm and a nucleus which is invariably large, round, or oval and usually centrally located. Second, all neurons have one or more cytoplasmic processes that arise from the cell body and are considerably smaller in diameter. Each process may terminate near the cell body or extend for a great distance (Figs. 8-3, see color insert, 8-4, 8-5, and 8-35). Because of the great length of some processes, it is rare that an entire neuron, even a small one, is included within a single histologic section, so the mature neuron with all its processes is seldom seen as a complete, isolated structure. Nevertheless, from what is known of the parts of a neuron, a diagram may be drawn of the

Figure 8-4 Two nerve cells from the central nervous system. A. Cell having a neuraxon ending at a considerable distance from the cell body. B. Neuraxon with many branches ending near the cell body. Golgi preparation. ×200.

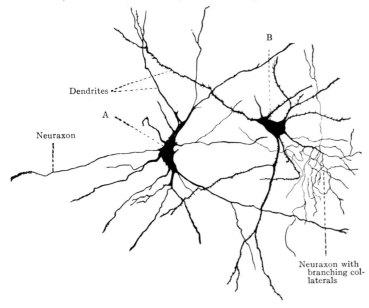

Dendrites

A

Neuraxon

B

Neuraxon with branching collaterals

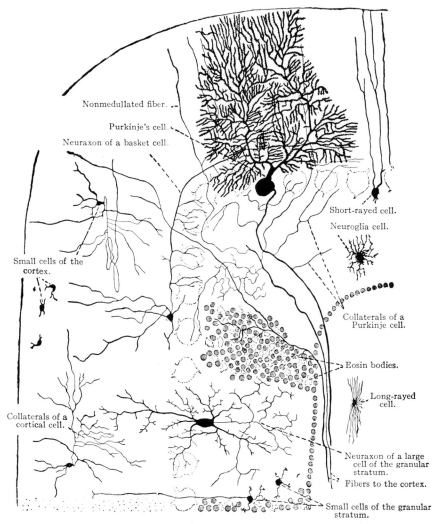

Figure 8-5 Section of the cortex of the cerebellum. Note the general differences in shape, size, and arrangement of neurons and their processes. Also note the complexity of the central nervous structure.

entire cell, such as the motor cell shown in Fig. 8-3, see color insert, which may serve as an idealized example of the structure of a neuron.

Axons and dendrites There are two major types of processes in neurons: the *axon,* or *axis cylinder* (also called *neuraxon*), and the *dendrite,* or *dendron* (Figs. 8-3, see color insert, 8-4, 8-5, and 8-35). Axons are present in all neurons. They are distinguished morphologically from dendrons by the fact

that they are generally longer, smoother processes and tend not to branch close to the cell body, although they may divide continuously and profusely more distally. To this definition of the axon is often added the physiologic one that axons conduct impulses away from the cell body. Although true for most neurons, this statement is not accurate for the peripheral process of the sensory neuron, which conducts impulses toward the cell body and is nonetheless called an axon. The term *axis cylinder* is more useful and accurate, although it is seldom employed since it does not imply a direction of conduction.

Most axonal processes gradually diminish in diameter along their length. In their distal course, they bifurcate occasionally or repeatedly so that each process may terminate in hundreds of twigs. Each branch is generally of smaller caliber than the mother process; yet the summed cross-sectional area of the branches exceeds that of the parent.

The second type of process is the *dendrite* (a term introduced by His in 1893) or *dendron* (which was probably derived from Kölliker's use in 1888 of the term *neurodendron* for the nerve cell to describe the branched processes found in many neurons after silver staining). These processes, unlike the axon, ordinarily do not run for long distances (Figs. 8-3, see color insert, 8-4, 8-5, and 8-35). They are less regular in contour than the axon and sometimes appear thorny (Fig. 8-35). They increase the surface of the cell body available for terminations of axis cylinders from other neurons, since the dendrons and the surface of the cell body from which they arise receive many axon endings (*axodendritic junctions*). There are instances in which a dendron may contact an adjacent dendron, and such contacts, believed to be functional, are now spoken of as *dendrodendritic junctions*. The dendrons have the granular structure of the cell body from which they extend, and were therefore originally named *protoplasmic processes*.

The terms dendron and axon are classic morphologic ones and are used in the original sense in modern light- and electron-microscopic studies. There is confusion when they are defined by the direction of conduction in a neuron. Dendrons do conduct toward the cell body. However, some neurons do not have dendrons; in some of these the cell body itself serves as the only receptive site. In other cases a long axis cylinder indistinguishable from an axon carries the impulse toward the cell body. For example, the long axis cylinder of sensory neurons, which extends from the cell body to the periphery and ends after branching among the peripheral receptors, is sometimes called a dendron because it conducts impulses toward the cell body from the receptors. Yet it is morphologically indistinguishable from the motor axon, which conducts centrifugally. Bodian suggests that the re-

ceptive site on a neuron, whether it be the peripheral ending of a sensory neuron or the synaptic surface of any other neuron, be called the *dendritic zone* and that the processes that conduct impulses away from the dendritic zone be termed *axons*. However, the term *dendron* is well established in the literature and will in all likelihood remain to mean the branching on cell bodies.

Although all neurons consist of a cell body and processes, these structures differ from one neuron to the next; and these structural differences, as well as functional ones, provide the basis for classifying neurons. In some neurons the cell body is very large. For instance, the motor cells (Fig. 8-3, see color insert) that supply striated muscle may be 125 μm or more in diameter, about the dimension of the human ovum. Other cell bodies, such as some in the olfactory bulb or the granule cells of the cerebellar cortex, are only a few micrometers in diameter. (Size differences are apparent in Figs. 8-5 and 8-10, see color insert.) The shape of cell bodies also varies widely. The body may be round, oval, or elliptical or a variant of these shapes; it may also be smooth or irregular because of many processes (compare Figs. 8-3, see color insert, 8-4, 8-5, 8-10, see color insert, and 8-35). Cell bodies also differ in the number of processes they produce. The body may be *unipolar* (*monopolar*) (Fig. 8-20) with a single process arising directly from it; *bipolar* (Figs. 8-69 and 8-70) with two processes; or *multipolar*, having many processes (Figs. 8-3, see color insert, 8-4, 8-5, 8-10, see color insert, and 8-35).

Axis cylinders (axons) may be relatively short and extend over only a microscopic distance, as many neurons of the central nervous system do (Fig. 8-4), or they may be very long. For example, there are motor axons that extend from the spinal cord to muscles of the foot (Fig. 8-3, see color insert) and sensory axons that lead from a peripheral receptor in the skin of the finger to the spinal cord and thence to the brain. The length of the long axons is all the more remarkable when one considers that their diameter is measured in micrometers and that despite their length they are part of a single cell.

Axons of different neurons vary greatly in diameter. The thicker ones conduct impulses rapidly and the fine fibers, very slowly. Diameter may also be related in a most general way to the distance the fiber travels, since fibers that have a longer course tend to be larger. Axons also vary according to the extent of their branchings, their position in the body, their relation to other neurons, and the functions they subserve, and they are classified accordingly.

Axis cylinders terminate on one of three structures. The most common ending is on the cell body and dendrons of other neurons. The region of termination of one neuron upon another is known as the *synapse* (Figs. 8-28 and 8-29). Since, as a rule, axons branch repeatedly, a single neuron may synapse with many other neurons. The recipient neuron, having an axon of its own, connects in turn with many other neurons, and rich and varied connections occur by way of cytoplasmic processes that form ever-expanding multiple chains of neurons within the nervous system. A second structure upon which processes of neurons, in this case sensory ones, terminate is the *receptor* (Figs. 8-41 to 8-44, 8-45, see color insert, and 8-46 to 8-49). Receptors are structures, often of nonnervous origin, which are specialized to receive energy in one form or another and to transmit the excitation to the associated sensory processes and thence to the central nervous system. Finally, there are the effector organs, such as muscle or glands (Figs. 8-32 and 8-37), upon which motor axons terminate, to call forth a response in the end organ. The structure and disposition of the processes of the neuron reflect well their function of conducting impulses from one part of the body to another. The neuronal processes have been likened to electric wires that carry messages over various distances and form relays (synapses) with other wire systems.

Investing neuronal membranes Neurons are protected throughout their entire course by investing structures of various types; these are not part of the neurons themselves. The cell body (Figs. 8-19 and 8-56) and dendrons are surrounded by supporting cells (neuroglia) and their processes; the axon is ordinarily enveloped by wrappings, although for a short distance near its origin from the cell body and at its termination it is naked. Axons in the peripheral nervous system are enwrapped by sequentially arranged Schwann cells. The sheath resembles a string of elongated beads strung on the axis cylinder. The region at which successive segments abut is called the *node of Ranvier*. Each Schwann cell wraps itself one or more times around the axon; repeated wrappings form a thick *myelin sheath* (Figs. 8-3, see color insert, and 8-21) on the outside of which is stretched the Schwann cell body. Before the advent of electron-microscopic studies the outermost layer alone of this sheath was considered part of the Schwann cell. It was called in the literature of that time the *neurilemma* or *sheath of Schwann* (as in Fig. 8-3, see color insert). The repeated wrappings, called the myelin sheath, were often considered a secretory product of the Schwann cell. Now that the neurilemma is known to be one with the myelin sheath, the term *myelin-Schwann sheath* may be most appropriate for the combined structure. In the central nervous system the *oligodendrocyte* bears the same relation to the central axons as the Schwann cell does to peripheral ones. It ensheaths the axon in a comparable manner and, together with its myelin, it may be called the *myelin-oligodendrocyte* sheath. The ultrastructure of these sheaths is described later. Outside of the myelin-Schwann sheath is a loose sheath of fibrous connective tissue, the *sheath of Henle* or *Key-Retzius* (Fig. 8-27).

THE LOCATION OF CELL BODIES

Cell bodies of neurons are found in localized concentrations both inside and outside the central nervous system. Within the central nervous system, cell bodies tend to form local aggregates or *nuclei* which are often quite discrete and identifiable (Fig. 8-9). Although there is a great variety of cell bodies within the central nervous system, those in each nucleus are generally quite similar and serve a similar function.

Collections of cell bodies outside the central nervous system are known as *ganglia*. A ganglion may be quite small, consisting of only two or a few cell bodies, as is commonplace in the autonomic system (Fig. 8-25D, see color insert), or it may be large and contain hundreds of cell bodies, as in the spinal and cranial nerves (Fig. 8-6). Both the peripheral and autonomic nervous systems contain ganglia. Peripheral ganglia are found as swellings on sensory cranial nerves (cranial nerve ganglia) and on the dorsal roots of spinal nerves (spinal nerve

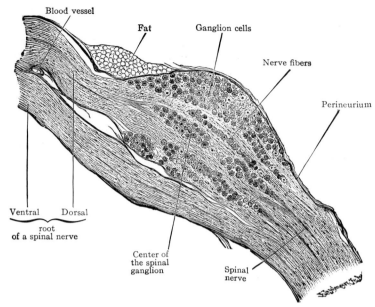

Figure 8-6   Longitudinal section through a spinal ganglion of a cat.

or posterior root ganglia) (Figs. 8-6 and 8-64 to 8-66). The autonomic system ganglia are found along the sympathetic cords and in the celiac and mesenteric plexuses (Fig. 8-63, see color insert). Less-discrete autonomic ganglia, consisting of scattered cells, are also found within the wall of the intestinal tract (Fig. 8-25D, see color insert), the heart, and other visceral organs. Although nuclei and ganglia are characterized by the accumulation of nerve cell bodies, they are traversed by many fibers (Fig. 8-6).

THE LOCATION OF NEURONAL PROCESSES

As noted previously, arborization of dendrons generally occurs within the immediate vicinity of the cell body (Figs. 8-4 and 8-5). Dendrons are found in the central and autonomic nervous system. Axons are distributed almost everywhere in the peripheral, autonomic, and central nervous systems.

NERVE FIBERS; NERVES; NERVE TRACTS

A *nerve fiber* may be defined as an axis cylinder plus its enveloping sheaths (Fig. 8-21). This definition also holds when the axon is naked, as it is during its development. The term *nerve fiber,* however, is often used loosely to mean any one of the neuronal processes without reference to the enveloping sheaths; for example, the axon may be called a nerve fiber.

A *nerve* is a collection of nerve fibers outside the central nervous system bound together by fibrous connective tissue and an outer epithelial sheath and containing blood vessels, generally of small caliber (Figs. 8-7 and 8-8). As previously noted, nerves are so widely distributed that they may be found in sections of most organs and tissues. The larger nerves, particularly the major trunks, consist of separate groups or cables of fibers embedded in connective tissue which binds them together (Fig. 8-7). Connective tissue uniting the several fascicles into one nerve is called the *epineurium.* In gross dissection it can be readily separated from overlying fascia. Its fibers are arranged semilongitudinally and are predominantly collagen with some scattered elastic fibers and fat cells; in it are contained blood vessels that supply the nerve. The sheaths immediately surrounding the individual cords of nervous tissue are called *perineurium* (Fig. 8-7). The perineurium is compact and forms a

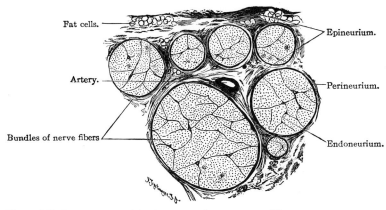

Fat cells.

Epineurium.

Artery.

Perineurium.

Bundles of nerve fibers

Endoneurium.

Figure 8-7   Cross section of the human median nerve.   ×20.

more or less dense and continuous membrane which is said by some investigators to contain spaces that eventually communicate with the subarachnoid spaces enclosed by the meninges of the central nervous system.   The collagen fibers within the nerve protect it from excessive stretch.   The subdivision of the nerve internally into cables of

Figure 8-8   Branching nerve stained with silver to show axis cylinders and Schwann nuclei. Bielschowsky method. (Courtesy of P. Stohr, Jr.)

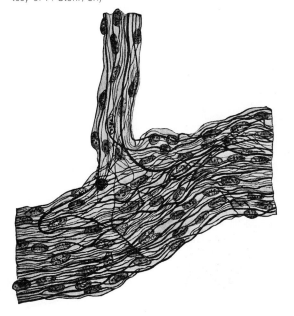

fibers surrounded by perineurium anticipates the lines of cleavage along which the nerve will branch as it proceeds distally (Fig. 8-7).   The perineurium is compact and consists of fibrous connective tissue covered by a continuous sheath of squamous epithelium, which Shantha and Bourne call the *perineural epithelium* (Bourne, 1968; 1969).   The epithelium is stratified in the larger nerves, and as many as 4 to 12 layers have been described. According to these authors, the perineural epithelium represents a continuation of the pia-arachnoid from the nerve roots distally to the very termination of the nerve fibers.   Indeed, they believe that the perineural epithelium contributes to the structure of the lamellae in receptor corpuscles, such as Pacinian corpuscles.   Moreover, they believe the system of epithelium enclosing the nerves and its branches to constitute a closed system channeling cerebrospinal fluid from the subarachnoid space to bathe the length of the nerve fibers to the end organs.

Surrounding the individual fibers within a large nerve is the *endoneurium*.   The term is often applied to the delicate reticular support lying outside of the myelin-Schwann sheath, and is synonymous with the sheath of Henle or Key-Retzius.   It consists of fine connective tissue fibers with their associated cells and represents the most intimate part of the general connective tissue framework of the nerve.   Microdissection studies of the sheath have shown that the fibers are elastic and can be readily manipulated and pulled without breakage

(Fig. 8-27). Examination by this means has revealed a reticular arrangement with major fiber orientation along the length of the axis cylinder. There is a sticky gelatinous matrix of ground substance between the reticular fibers, and the fibers are continuous with the fiber network of the perineurium. In the smallest nerves an endoneurium cannot be demonstrated.

As nerves proceed distally, they invariably divide into smaller and smaller ones containing fewer fibers and less connective tissue. In their course to the periphery, nerves may also unite to form a larger trunk. Although each nerve fiber may branch many times as it proceeds distally, division of a nerve generally means separation of groups of fibers, and there is no evidence of wholesale division of each fiber at the point of nerve branching (Fig. 8-8). The larger nerve trunks invariably contain both motor and sensory fibers. The motor fibers are destined for a number of muscles or muscle groups, and the sensory fibers for receptors of the skin, muscles, joints, and so forth. As the

nerve travels distally and subdivides, the diversity of motor and sensory fibers within each division is diminished. Each successive division becomes more restricted in its distribution and function until it consists only of motor or sensory fibers and, indeed, until only a certain muscle group, muscle, or mode of sensation is represented.

When examined fresh, in reflected light, nerves are seen to be of two sorts, formerly known as *white* and *gray* nerves. Similarly, sections of the brain and spinal cord are formed of white substance and gray substance. The obvious distinction in color is due to the abundance or relative absence of myelin, a fatty substance. Nerves that contain a large proportion of myelinated fibers appear white; those that have few are gray. All nerve fibers when first formed are *nonmyelinated* (*unmyelinated*), and most of the sympathetic nerves remain relatively so. Likewise, "central gray" refers to the nuclear centers of the brain and cord, since there is little myelin in these loci.

Except at their terminal ramifications, nerves are

Figure 8-9   Adjacent parasagittal sections of the human brainstem.   A. Section stained for cell bodies with cresyl violet (so-called Nissl stain).   B. Stained for fiber tracts with a modified Weigert myelin stain.   Nuclear centers appear dark with the basic stain and unstained with the myelin one; the reverse is true for the tracts.   ×0.75.

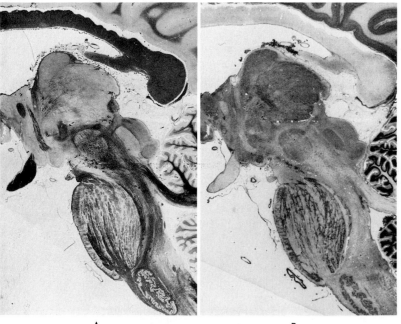

A   B

provided with intraneural blood vessels (*vasa nervo-rum*). Small nutrient arteries from nearby vessels pass into the epineurium and, after making anastomoses, form networks of arterioles within the perineurium from which are derived capillary plexuses with elongated meshes in the endoneurium. The capillary plexuses are drained by venules accompanying the arterioles and then in turn by small veins, which usually leave the nerve with the incoming arteries. Fine nerve fibers have also been described in the epineurium and perineurium, the *nervi nervorum*. Some of these are evidently sensory and terminate freely within the connective tissue, and others probably have a vasomotor function.

The fibers of most nerves take an irregularly wavy course so that frequently in transverse section groups of fibers may be cut lengthwise while adjacent ones are cut across. Because of the twisting course, the individual fibers are longer than the nerve as a whole (Figs. 8-8 and 8-25E, see color insert), which allows the nerve to stretch some before fiber injury occurs.

The term *tract* is reserved for the central nervous system and is defined as a collection of nerve fibers running together and often having a similar function (Fig. 8-9). A tract may be thought of as a nerve of the central nervous system. The fibers of a tract may have the same nucleus of origin and termination or they may arise from different nuclei and may sort out of the tract to form other tracts destined for various nuclei of termination. No common sheathing comparable to the epineurium of peripheral nerves binds the fibers of a tract together. An endoneurial sheath is also absent in the central nervous system, but processes and fibers of the neuroglia may be thought of as providing a comparable support.

The cytology and ultrastructure of nervous tissue

THE CELL BODY

As seen in the light microscope, the nucleus of the cell body is generally large and round or oval (Figs. 8-3, 8-10, 8-18, and 8-25D, all in color insert, and Figs. 8-13, 8-17, 8-19, and 8-28). It is centrally placed within abundant cytoplasm. Characteristically the nuclear sap is relatively free of stainable substance after common histologic techniques, except for a concentration of basophilic nucleoprotein which lines the inner margin of the well-defined nuclear membrane. Ordinarily, one or two large and heavily basophilic nucleoli are also evident.

The cytoplasm of the cell body (*neuroplasm*) contains a number of formed bodies, including the structures found in cells of other tissues, albeit in different arrangement and concentration. Notable among them are *Golgi formations, mitochondria, pigment, fat droplets, Nissl bodies,* and *neuro-fibrils.* The latter two most typify nerve cells.

Nissl substance   Named after the German histologist who described it in great detail, Nissl substance (Figs. 8-3 and 8-10, see color insert, and 8-53) is demonstrated with basic stains, such as methylene blue, cresyl violet, and toluidine blue, for which it shows great affinity. It also has a characteristic absorption peak in ultraviolet light in the region around 2600 Å, attesting to its nucleic acid content. It is striking in the large cell bodies of motor neurons that supply striated muscle, where the bodies are large, rhomboid, block-like masses separated by relatively unstained cytoplasm (Figs. 8-10, see color insert and 8-53). The striped pattern and arrangement the material sometimes assumes in motor cells has also given it the name of *tigroid* substance or bodies. The size, shape, disposition, and abundance of Nissl material differ among neurons and are identifying features for nuclear centers and ganglia. For example, the Nissl material in the cell bodies of sensory and autonomic ganglia, in contrast to that in somatic motor neurons, is usually diffusely distributed as fine granules; however, in the larger autonomic and sensory cell bodies the granules may be loosely aggregated to form bodies of medium size, not dense or sharply differentiated from the surrounding loose granules.

Nissl substance is found scattered throughout

the cell body and into the dendrites (Fig. 8-10, see color insert), but it does not occur—at least in obvious concentrations—in the axis cylinder. The neuroplasm subjacent to the *axon hillock*, the point at which the axon originates, is similarly devoid of Nissl substance, and this provides a way of distinguishing the axon, at its origin, from the cell body.

Since the affinity of Nissl substance for basic dyes resembles that of the nuclear chromatin, Nissl substance was once referred to as "cytoplasmic chromatin." In its staining properties, Nissl substance is also comparable to cytoplasmic inclusions of many other cells, such as the granules of the placental cytotrophoblast, liver cells, and serous cells of the pancreas. However, electron microscopy has now shown clearly that Nissl substance is a specialized form of rough endoplasmic reticulum and that its basophilia is due to its associated ribosomes. The membranes of this ER form vesicles, tubules, or interconnected, regular stacks of flat cisternae with luminae measuring 30 to 50 nm (Figs. 8-11 and 8-14); the usual configurations of free or attached polyribosomes are seen. The regularity of organization varies in different neurons.

Since rough ER is the site of protein synthesis, the abundance of Nissl substance presumably reflects a need to produce large amounts of protein. In neurons the volume of the cytoplasmic processes may exceed that of the parent body by hundreds of times. The processes are maintained by the cell body; parts that are separated from the cell body degenerate. Moreover, the processes may be considered ever-growing, since presumably their endings are reconstructed continuously and since they can under appropriate circumstances sprout to supply collateral fibers to adjacent regions. In recent years biochemical and autoradiographic studies have demonstrated a flow of labeled protein, synthesized in the cell body, into the axon and thence to its ending. The Nissl material presumably is the fountain of the synthesis. This would account for the striking changes undergone by Nissl material when axons are injured and during later repair and regeneration when a high level of protein synthesis would be expected (see Degeneration and Regeneration of Nerves). In addition to a function in maintaining and elaborating the processes, ribonucleic acid and protein metabolism are said to increase during conduction. Moreover, electric stimulation

has been reported to change the composition of the nucleic acids in brain cells. Some researchers have also implicated ribonucleoprotein in theories of memory and learning.

Neurofibrils and neurofilaments   *Neurofibrils* are fine filaments which are seen in abundance in fixed neuroplasm after it is treated with salts of silver or gold (Fig. 8-15). They run into the dendrites and axon and are sometimes seen also in synaptic endings. Neither the length of these threads nor their precise relations to one another has been definitely established. Although often difficult to demonstrate, they appear to be universal in neurons. Neurofibrils have been observed in the living cell body and axis cylinder of a few animals. They are found in all the ramifications of nerve processes and may be relatively coarse or exceedingly fine. Fine *neurofilaments* (60 to 100 Å in diameter) have been seen with the electron microscope (Figs. 8-11 and 8-12). They resemble the microfilaments found in many other cells. It is believed that the neurofilaments are the primary threads which tend to coagulate during fixation into larger units, the neurofibrils, which are then identifiable with the ordinary light microscope. Various functions have been ascribed to neurofilaments. Some believe that they are nutritive or supporting structures, or transient, reversibly polymerized neuroplasmic proteins. Recent suggestions are that they form the synaptic vesicles (see the discussion on the fine structure of the synapse under Terminations of Nerve Fiber) or that they are pathways for the transport of neurosecretions and other components of neuroplasm.

Golgi formations   Following staining with special procedures employing osmic acid or silver, an irregular interlacing network, the Golgi apparatus, is revealed within the neuroplasm around the nucleus of the cell body. Golgi formations are common to cells of all tissues and are richly represented in neurons. The Golgi apparatus of the nerve cell responds sensitively to damage of the neuron, perhaps even more so than does Nissl substance. It tends to disperse and during later regeneration or repair of the neuron, it is gradually reconstituted. The Golgi formation of the neuron and other cells has been identified with the electron microscope (Figs. 8-12 and 8-14). It is part of the smooth mem-

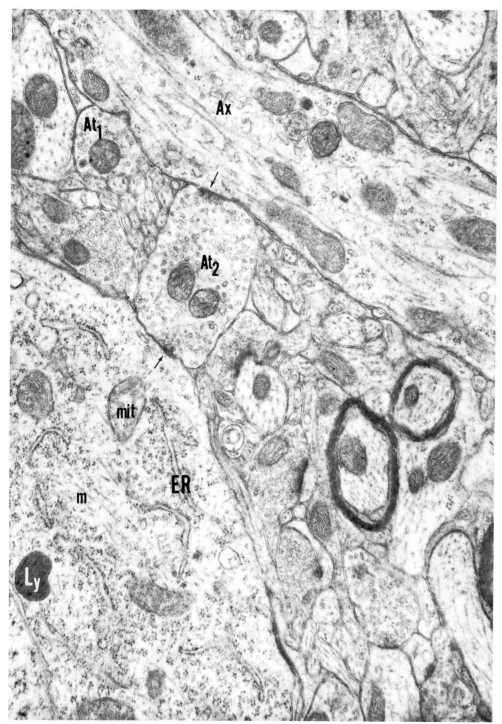

Figure 8-11 Axoaxonic and axosomatic synapses. Two axon terminals (At$_1$ and At$_2$) are shown in synaptic contact. The smaller (At$_1$) is synapsing with the axon (Ax) initial segment, and the larger (At$_2$) is synapsing at two different sites: with the Axon (Ax) initial segment and with the cell body of a pyramidal neuron, on the bottom left. Arrows indicate synaptic complexes on the larger axon terminal. The cell body of the neuron has several typical organelles: rough endoplasmic reticulum (ER), mitochondria (mit), microtubules (m), and an electron-dense body, probably a lysosome (Ly). ×14,500 (Courtesy of I. Kaiserman-Abramoff.)

branous endoplasmic reticulum of the cell. Golgi formations appear as closely packed parallel profiles of flattened sacs with small lumens (20 nm) and associated vesicles varying in diameter.

Mitochondria   The small granular, filamentous, or rod-like structures observed in all living cells may be demonstrated as well in neurons (Fig. 8-17). They are not confined to the cell body but exist within all the processes and are abundant at their terminations (Figs. 8-11, 8-12, 8-14, 8-29 to 8-31, and 8-33). In neurons they tend to be elongated. The electron microscope reveals a typical structure, with cristae arranged transversely or longitudinally. The mitochondrial matrix usually appears moderately dense in the electron microscope (Figs. 8-11, 8-12, 8-14, and 8-31).

Pigment   Melanin granules are normally observed in the cell bodies of certain neurons. They are abundant in some neurons; for example, those of the *substantia nigra,* a nucleus of the midbrain, which derives its name from the pigmentation. Pigment may accumulate in cell bodies in certain pathologic states.

Fat droplets   *Fat bodies* of various sizes, often containing a yellow pigment (Fig. 8-18, see color insert), may also be demonstrated in some nerve cell bodies, although not in the processes. Such accumulations increase in abundance and concentration with age and in certain pathologic conditions.

Other inclusions   Electron micrographs have revealed other inclusions. In some neurons there are membrane-bound inhomogeneous bodies containing dense granules. The inclusions resemble lysosomes (Fig. 8-14), described in neurons and other cells as sites of hydrolytic enzyme accumulations.

Membrane-bound packets of vesicles called *multivesicular bodies,* of unknown function, have also been reported in electron micrographs of nerve cells (Fig. 8-14).

THE NEURONAL PROCESSES
The axis cylinder tends to taper very gradually in its distal course. However, its diameter in any one region is not uniform. Instead, it may appear beaded or irregularly bulged, owing to intrinsic contractions or possibly to constrictions of the surrounding sheaths, as some believe. As the fiber approaches its termination, it divides with increasing frequency, and at the termination itself, it often ends in a spray of fibers. There generally is a small angle between the daughter fibers at the point of bifurcation. The size of the daughter fibers tends to be equal, but as already recounted, the sum of their cross-sectional areas invariably surpasses that of the parent axon. Here and there along the axon an occasional fiber of small diameter, termed a *collateral,* may leave approximately at right angles to the main axis. It generally arises at the node between successive myelin segments. Collaterals are found particularly in the central nervous system, and their function presumably is to send a sampling of neuronal activity to nuclei along the way.

The neuroplasm of the axon, most often called *axoplasm,* is continuous with that of the cell body, and there is now good evidence for a continuous discharge of neuronal cell products into the axon and a flow of axoplasm to the very terminations. Indeed, there is bidirectional streaming, with the centrifugal one apparently predominating, and there is evidence for subsidiary streams with different rates of flow. The fastest movements recorded in a component of axoplasmic flow are about 50 to 100 cm per day. The mechanism responsible for the movement is not known, but theories have implicated neurotubules and neurofilaments.

The plasma membrane of the axis cylinder (*axolemma*) is thin and smooth (Figs. 8-11, 8-23, 8-24, and 8-30), and the cytoplasm, as judged by microdissection, is viscous. The axolemma is separated from the surrounding sheath by a small fluid-filled space of about 20 nm. Embedded within the axoplasm are numerous vesicles and neurofibrils (80 to 100 Å in diameter) (Figs. 8-11 and 8-26) and occasional tubules (*neurotubules*) arranged parallel to the long axis of the cylinder. Thin, elongated mitochondria are scattered within the axoplasm (Fig. 8-11). Mitochondria also move, albeit slowly, to the terminations, where they may pile up. Nissl substance, Golgi, pigment, and fat are absent from the axon.

Dendrites are shorter, much more richly branched, and more irregular in contour than the

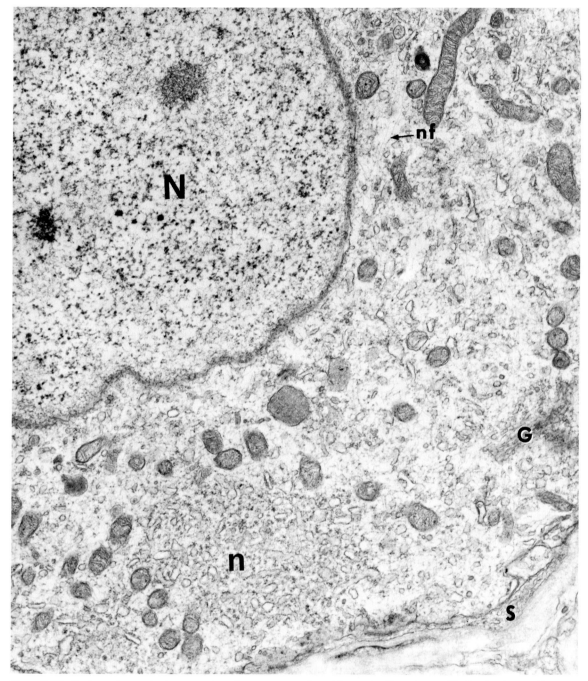

Figure 8-12   Electron micrograph of a neuron from the sensory ganglion of the newt.   N, nucleus; n, Nissl body; nf, neurofilaments; G, Golgi complex; S, satellite cytoplasm.   Approximately ×12,000.

axon. In addition, their surfaces may be thorny or spiny (Fig. 8-35) for the reception of synaptic terminations (Figs. 8-31 and 8-33). The contents of *dendroplasm,* unlike axoplasm, resemble that of the perikaryon. Neurotubules are abundant in electron micrographs of dendrons (Figs. 8-31 and 8-33). They are also larger and more distinct than in the axon—200 to 300 Å in diameter. The presence of large, distinct tubules provides a means of identifying dendrons from axons and glial processes in electron micrographs. Other distinguishing features are the presence of synaptic endings on the dendron and of dendroplasmic Nissl inclusions. These characteristics may be less striking at a great distance from the cell body. As pointed out previously, neurofilaments, mitochondria, and Nissl substance are present in dendrites.

THE INVESTING MEMBRANES OF THE CELL BODY AND DENDRONS

The cell bodies of spinal, cranial, and the large autonomic ganglia are enclosed within a capsule composed of *satellite cells,* which contain small, scattered, and flattened nuclei (Figs. 8-18, see color insert, and 8-19); some autonomic ganglia appear to be less completely encapsulated. The outer thickness of the capsule is a delicate layer of con-

Figure 8-13 Group of motor nerve cells in ventral horn of human spinal cord. The smaller nuclei are predominantly those of neuroglial cells. Methylene blue and eosin.

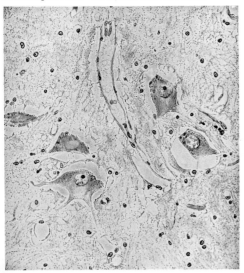

nective tissue comparable to the sheath of Henle. In addition, other connective tissue fibers enclosing a capillary network bind the capsules to one another and ensheath the entire ganglion (Fig. 8-6). Electron micrographs reveal an intimate contact between satellite and ganglion cells, with a separation of only 200 Å (Fig. 8-12); metabolic exchange between the cell body and vascular bed occurs through this space and possibly also via the cytoplasm of the satellite cell. As it leaves the cell body, the axis cylinder lies within the capsule, where it may wander in a tangle and give off curious end plates before escaping (Fig. 8-20). The sheath of satellite cells is continuous with the myelin-Schwann sheath at the region from which the axon exits. Futhermore, electron micrographs show that satellite and Schwann cells are very similar cytologically, and they have a common embryologic origin from the neural crest.

Cell bodies within the central nervous system are surrounded by oligodendroglia (Figs. 8-55 and 8-56), which develop from the neural tube, and by the processes of another neuroglial cell, the astrocyte (Figs. 8-42 and 8-55).

Dendrites are surrounded by a dense layer of supporting processes from neuroglial cells and a network of other dendrons and of axonal processes which ramify and end upon the dendrites (Figs. 8-42, 8-55, and 8-62). Other than these fibers, no special encapsulation like that of the axis cylinder is present.

THE INVESTING MEMBRANES OF AXONS

Most axons are enveloped by sheaths. In the central nervous system, the sheath is formed by *oligodendrocytes* (Fig. 8-57); in the peripheral and autonomic systems, the sheath is formed by *Schwann cells.* In both cases, the axon may be wrapped repeatedly to form the *myelin* of the sheath (Figs. 8-3, see color insert, 8-16, 8-21, and 8-23), on the outside of which the Schwann cell or oligodendrocyte body is stretched; these fibers are called *myelinated* (or *medullated*) fibers. The axon may also be wrapped only once or not at all (Fig. 8-24); these fibers are *nonmyelinated* (*nonmedullated*).

In the older literature of light microscopy, the outermost layer of the investing sheath in myelinated fibers was called the neurilemma (or sheath of Schwann for peripheral fibers); it was believed

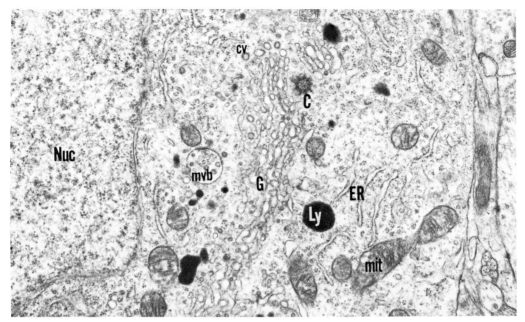

Figure 8-14   Cell body of a neuron.   Part of the perikaryon of a neuron in the rat visual cortex is shown here.   The nucleus (Nuc) is in the left of the field.   The perikaryal cytoplasm contains the following: A Golgi apparatus (G), a centriole (C), rough endoplasmic reticulum (ER), mitochondria (mit), coated vesicles (cv), lysosomes (Ly), and multivesicular body (mvb).   ×10,000.   (Courtesy of I. Kaiserman-Abramoff.)

Figure 8-15   Axis cylinders of a nerve after silver impregnation (Bodian method) to show neurofibrils.   Note the range in fiber diameter and the sheath nuclei.   Approximately ×1,000.

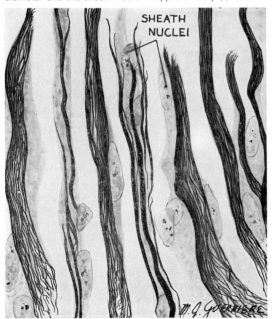

to be part of the Schwann cell, whereas the myelin was considered to be an extracellular secretion deposited between the neurilemma and the axon. Electron-microscope studies have now revealed that the myelin is only a specialized part of the investing cell, so the myelin sheath, neurilemma, and Schwann cell (or oligodendrocyte) are one. Consequently, the old terminology is no longer adequate, and there is confusion in the literature on the use of these terms; the following terminology is suggested to the student and will be used in the ensuing discussion:

myelin-Schwann sheath: the myelinated ensheathment around axons of the peripheral and autonomic nervous systems

myelin-oligodendrocyte sheath: the myelinated ensheathment around axons of the central nervous system

myelin-glial sheath: a general term for both of the above

myelin, or *myelin sheath:* the repeated wrappings around the axon, excluding the investing cell body

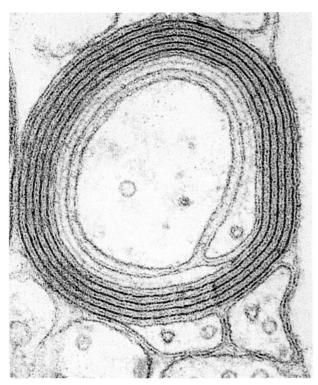

Figure 8-16 Myelinated axon from central white matter of the rat. Note the adaxonal cytoplasm, inner mesaxon, intermediate dense line of wrappings, and outer oligodendroglial processes. A single continuous spiral can be traced from the inner to the outermost layer.   ×166,000. (Courtesy of A. Hirano and H. M. Dembitzer, J. Cell Biol., **34:**555, 1967.)

The term *sheath of Schwann,* or *Schwann sheath,* may be used for the single wrapping of unmyelinated peripheral or autonomic fibers. The term *glial sheath* is sometimes used in modern literature in the most general way, to designate a sheath of any fiber, regardless of its structure. Of course, none of these definitions applies to the many axons without sheaths, as in the central nervous system, the epidermis, and the cornea.

Although the recommended terminology excludes the terms sheath of Schwann and neurilemma for the myelinated fiber, these terms persist in modern literature to mean the outermost wrapping of the myelin-glial sheath, including the Schwann cell body.

The *myelin-Schwann sheath* is a segmented tube enclosing the axon; it resembles a string of elongated beads, each derived from one Schwann cell whose spindle-shaped nucleus lies in the middle of each segment at the outer surface of the tube, with its long axis parallel to the fiber axis (see color Figs. 8-3 and 8-25B, E, and F; see Fig. 8-21A and C). The nucleus indents the myelin and is surrounded by cytoplasm. With common basic stains, the Schwann nuclei are readily visible; they resemble the nuclei of fibroblasts and smooth muscle, but the overall pattern they form is a distinguishing feature of nerve (Fig. 8-25E and F, see color insert). They appear at quite regular intervals. The segments of the myelin-Schwann sheath are about 0.8 to 1.0 mm long. In the light microscope the regions where successive segments abut appear as constrictions of the entire sheath and are known as the nodes of Ranvier (Figs. 8-3, see color insert, and 8-21). The axon is continuous at the node, but it may appear narrowed or enlarged. The internodal segments appear to be longest in fibers of large caliber; evidence suggests that the length

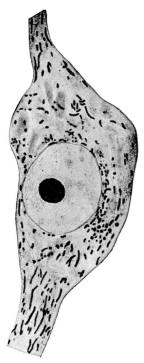

Figure 8-17 Mitochondria in a motor nerve cell of the spinal cord of the white mouse, after formaldehyde fixation and staining with acid fuchsin and methyl green. (Nicholson, from the Wistar Institute.)

is determined by the increase in length of the nerve after myelin is first laid down, so the myelin segments of facial nerve are shorter than those of limb nerves. The sheath and its nodes can be observed readily in fresh, teased nerve. The nodes are present in sheaths of axons in the central nervous system, although here the myelin-oligodendrocyte segments often do not abut one another and thus leave the axon bared for a short distance. Near its origin and termination the axis cylinder is also free of sheath. Branching of the axon occurs at the nodes of Ranvier. The thickness of the myelin sheath varies with the caliber of the axon (Fig. 8-50). Recently, the number of myelin layers has been correlated directly with the circumference of the axon; axons of fine caliber, such as those of the sympathetic postganglionic system, tend to be non-myelinated.

Myelin consists of about 40 percent protein and 60 percent lipids, including phospholipids, cerebrosides, sulfatides, and cholesterol. Studies employing x-ray diffraction and polarization optics indicate that the lipid and protein of myelin are arranged in alternate concentric layers, 170 to 180 Å apart. Myelin is one of the classic materials that formed the basis for the "unit membrane" model, for in myelin the lipids appear to be in bimolecular layers, oriented radially, and bound to adjacent layers of

Figure 8-19 Cell body and surrounding sheaths and connective tissue in semilunar ganglion of man.   ×600.   (von Mollendorff.)

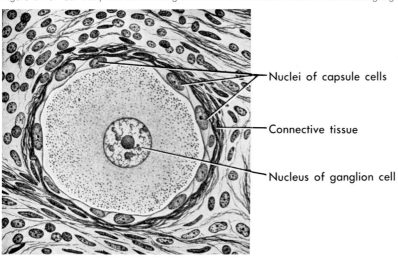

Nuclei of capsule cells

Connective tissue

Nucleus of ganglion cell

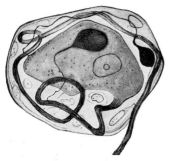

Figure 8-20   Sensory cell from the ganglion nodosum vagi with end-plate.   Observe the wanderings of the axon before it penetrates the capsule.   Collateral end-plates are occasionally seen. Silver preparation.   (Cajal.)

protein, possibly only one molecule thick and oriented somewhat circumferentially.

The appearance of the sheath in tissue sections prepared for light microscopy varies according to the method of fixation and staining (Fig. 8-50).

In fresh specimens or in those fixed and blackened with osmic acid, the *incisures* (*clefts*) *of Schmidt-Lanterman* (Fig. 8-21A) are readily identified. There may be as many as 20 incisures per myelin segment, partitioning the myelin sheath like a series of stemless funnels strung along the axis cylinder, not all pointed the same way.   With histologic treatments that employ a fat solvent such as alcohol, the fatty components of myelin are partly dissolved and the structural framework is considerably distorted (Fig. 8-25B and D, see color insert). There remains a *neurokeratin* network of protein fibrils with some bound lipid (Figs. 8-21C and D, 8-25A and B, see color insert) that is quite variable in pattern, depending on previous treatment; in cross sections of fibers, it may be arranged radially, like a cartwheel (Fig. 8-25A, see color insert), or concentrically.   In ordinary eosin and hematoxylin preparations, the neurokeratin net is hardly visible (Fig. 8-25E and F, see color insert).

Figure 8-21   Axons and their sheaths stained variously.   A. Osmotic acid preparation to reveal myelin: frog.   B. Silvered fiber of guinea pig (after Schaffer; below, after von Mollendorff).   C. Methylene blue: cat (after Nemiloff).   D. Neurokeratin network: cat.   (Cajal.)

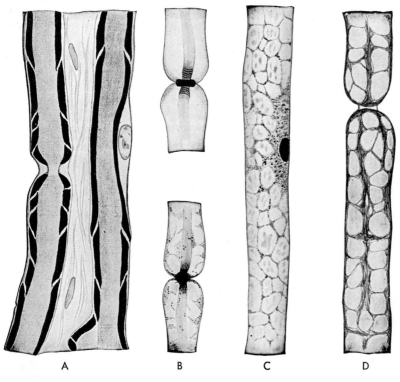

A   B   C   D

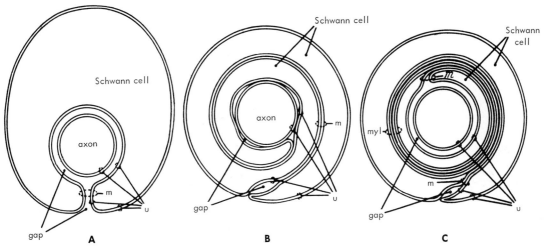

Figure 8-22   The formation of compact myelin in three stages (A to C). u, plasma membranes; m, mesaxon; myl, compact myelin.   (Courtesy of J. D. Robertson, Intern. Kongr. Elektronenmikroskopie, 4. Berlin, 1958, Proceedings, p. 163, 1960.)

When viewed with the electron microscope, after fixation with osmium tetroxide, the myelin is laminated with alternating concentric light and dark bands which repeat every 110 to 160 Å (Figs. 8-16 and 8-23).   With high resolution, a line of intermediate density is seen bisecting the less-dense band (Fig. 8-16).   In studies of developing myelin in fetal peripheral nerves, Geren (1954) first demonstrated that the myelin sheath is actually the plasma membrane of the surrounding Schwann cell wrapped around and around the axis cylinder in a spiral, like a bolt of cloth (Fig. 8-22B and C).   During development, the Schwann cell first enfolds the axis cylinder so the axon is surrounded, except on one side where a narrow space remains bounded by apposed Schwann cell membranes, known as the *mesaxon* (Figs. 8-16 and 8-22).   Although the details of the process are unknown, it is clear that the Schwann cell continues to wrap around the axon, leaving a spiral of mesaxon and some cytoplasm, with the Schwann cell nucleus and surrounding cytoplasm always on the surface of the sheath.   At first the wrappings are loose, but with maturation of the fiber they become tight.   The intervening cytoplasm is somehow extruded or dissipated and the cytoplasmic surface of the membranes contact each other to form the major dense line of the myelin profile (Fig. 8-22C).   The intervening less-dense line represents the original

apposed surfaces of the mesaxon.   The original first wrapping of the axon remains as a cytoplasmic layer (the *Mauthner's* or *adaxonal Schwann layer*).   The mesaxon persists internally in this adaxonal layer and externally in the outermost wrapping of the Schwann cell body.   The thickness of the myelin, of course, is simply a function of the number of spirals of Schwann cell membrane.

The morphology of the myelin-Schwann sheath and its parts may be envisioned best in a diagram of an imagined unrolled sheath drawn approximately to scale and showing the axon (Fig. 8-39).   In addition to the adaxonal Schwann layer, there are two regions in which the dense band does not form because Schwann cytoplasm is not extruded: the Schmidt-Lanterman clefts and the *paranodal spirals* at each end of the sheath (next to the nodes of Ranvier).   These two are therefore continuous spirals of modified Schwann cytoplasm that extend from the Schwann cell body to the adaxonal layer, and they are probably regions in which exchange can occur between the outside and the deeper regions of the myelin and indeed, even the axon itself.   There is now evidence that in living fibers the Schmidt-Lanterman clefts open and close with pulsations of the Schwann cell body, causing an active ebb and flow of cytoplasm to the adaxonal layer, which is sometimes highly swollen with cyto-

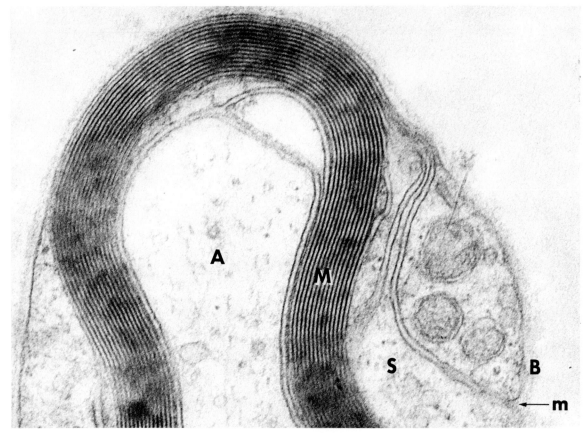

Figure 8-23   Myelinated nerve fiber from the acoustic ganglion of the rat.   A, axis cylinder; M, myelin; S, Schwann cell; B, basement membrane, m, external mesaxon.   Approximately ×64,000.   (Courtesy of J. Rosenbluth, J. Biophys. Biochem. Cytol., **12**:351, 1962.)

plasm.   Schmidt-Lanterman clefts are seldom seen in the central nervous system, although paranodal spirals and adaxonal cytoplasm are.   The imagined structure of the unrolled myelin-oligodendrocyte sheath is diagramed in Fig. 8-39B.

Where adjacent myelin-Schwann segments meet at the nodes of Ranvier (Fig. 8-26), the paranodal spirals appear as loops (Fig. 8-39A); the most peripheral loops of adjacent segments interdigitate and thus close the gap.   Surrounding the myelin-Schwann sheath is a thin, amorphous, submicroscopic membrane commonly called *basement membrane,* and outside this there is a loose sheath of fibrous connective tissue, the *sheath of Henle* or *Key-Retzius* (Fig. 8-27).   Fibers in the central nerv-ous system lack the basement membrane, and at the node, adjacent myelin segments do not interdigitate but leave a gap (Fig. 8-57) where the axon is exposed to the extracellular environment.

All peripheral and autonomic axons are ensheathed by Schwann cells.   However, non-myelinated axons are not enclosed beyond the initial enfolding stage or have only a minimum of subsequent wrappings, so the mesaxon is often quite obvious (Fig. 8-24).   Moreover, a single Schwann cell often enwraps a number of axons, and sometimes two or more axons share a single wrapping and mesaxon.   Loose or sparse wrappings around individual fibers are commonly seen in nerves of invertebrates, where successive layers

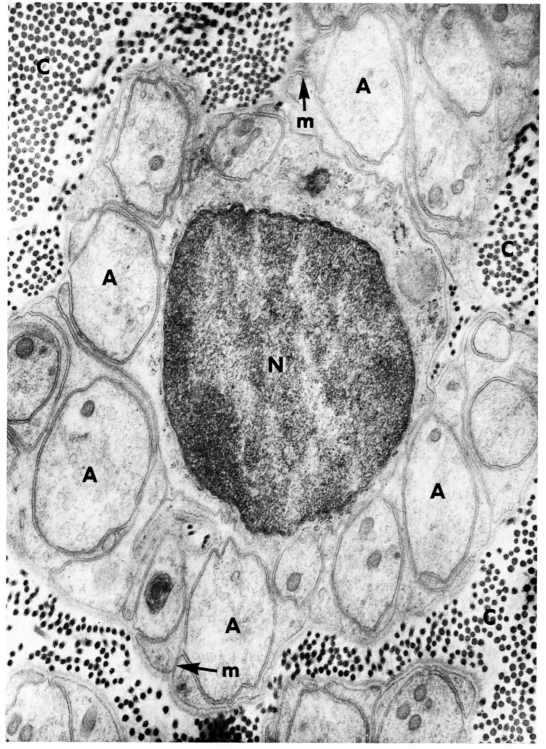

Figure 8-24   Nonmyelinated nerve fibers in cat splenic nerve.   Several fibers share the same Schwann cell.   A, axon; m, mesaxon; N, nucleus of Schwann cell; C, collagen.   Approximately ×25,600.   (Courtesy of L. G. Elfvin, J. Ultrastruct. Res., **7**:5, 1962.)

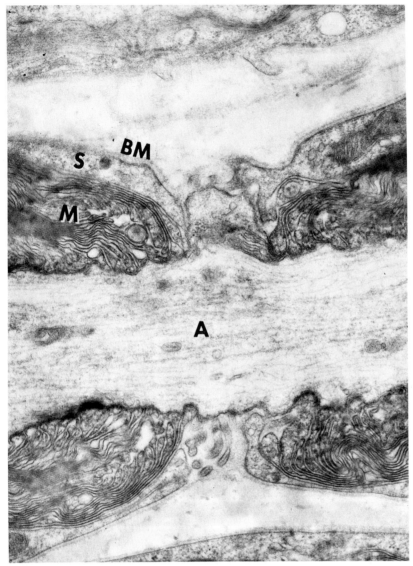

Figure 8-26 Node of Ranvier from acoustic ganglion in the rat. Lamellae of myelin terminate at the node, and the basement membrane is continuous across the node. A, axis cylinder; M, myelin; S, Schwann cell; BM, basement membrane. Approximately ×18,800. (Courtesy of J. Rosenbluth, J. Biophys. Biochem. Cytol., **12:**351,1962.)

Figure 8-27 A freshly isolated nerve fiber of the frog. The microneedle is lifting the Henle sheath, showing it to be composed of a homogeneous and viscous interfibrillar substance and to have a framework of more or less delicate fibrils. Approximately ×350. (After de Renyi, 1929.)

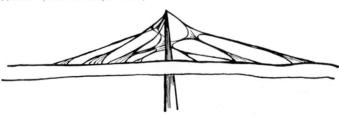

of Schwann membrane retain cytoplasm rather than compacting as in vertebrate myelin.

The Schwann cell and its wrappings extend partly along the roots of the cranial and spinal nerves proximal to the ganglia, except on the optic nerve, which is truly a brain tract and not a nerve. Still more proximally, the roots are devoid of schwannian elements, and the sheaths assume the characteristics of the glial sheaths of the central nervous system. Near the peripheral terminations of the fiber, the Schwann cell processes intimately contact the surface of the innervated structure.

The mechanism of myelin formation in the central nervous system is less generally agreed upon since the cell most commonly implicated, the oligodendrocyte, ensheaths a number of axons (Figs. 8-39B and 8-57). Some believe that central myelination occurs like peripheral myelination, through a wrapping of glial processes around the axons. An alternative theory proposes that central myelination occurs through a fusion of lipoprotein elements around the axon after it is embedded in the glial cytoplasm.

Various views are held concerning the function of myelin. Salient among these is the belief that myelin serves as an insulating material, preventing the spread of the impulse to adjacent axons. The speed of conduction has also been related to the extent of myelination. According to the theory of saltatory conduction, there is a discontinuous transmission of the nerve impulse from node to node in myelinated fibers; the longer the internodal segment, the more rapid the conduction. Finally, there is the recent evidence that myelin carries substances between the axon and the Schwann cell by way of the clefts and paranodal spirals and across the battery of myelin membranes. Moreover, there is now evidence for active metabolic turnover within the myelin layers, although myelin was previously thought to be inert.

The Schwann cells have a high metabolic rate and may provide energy for ionic movements, which are so necessary to maintain the resting potential of the fiber. They are of undoubted importance in regeneration of the fiber, since they serve as tubes that guide regenerating fibers to the periphery (see below) and undergo various structural changes in response to the regenerating fibers.

Terminations of nerve fibers

The axis cylinder and its branches terminate on other neurons, on muscle and glands, or on a variety of sensory receptors. The most abundant terminations are the first, the synapses where the process of one neuron contacts the process or cell body of another. These are largely responsible for the complexity of the central nervous system and for its function.

SYNAPSE

The synapse is the region in which conduction occurs from one neuron to another. The term is now frequently used also for terminations on muscle and other nonnervous tissue. Neuron to neuron connections are predominantly of axon to dendrite or to cell body. There are also, however, axoaxonal and dendrodendritic synapses. As the terminal fibers approach their endings on the cell body or dendrites of the next neuron, they lose their sheath. Occasionally they may wind about the

dendrites or the cell body before ending, and other fibers have been described which circle the axon hillock repeatedly to form a rich fibrous sleeve. At the very ending, the terminating fibers expand into enlargements, the *end-feet of Held*, also called *boutons terminaux, synaptic bulbs* (endings), and variants of these terms (Figs. 8-28, 8-29, 8-42, and 8-62). End-feet have also been described on the axon hillock and even farther along the axon (Figs. 8-11, 8-28, and 8-62). It has been suggested that such endings have an inhibitory function. Except for some size differences and ultrastructural details, end-feet are relatively similar in all vertebrate and invertebrate forms.

The end-feet show very rapid postmortem changes; they may retract from the surface of the second neuron and appear to be separated from it by a space. During fixation, the terminating fiber may also be torn near the end-foot. However, the relations of end-feet to cell bodies and dendrites

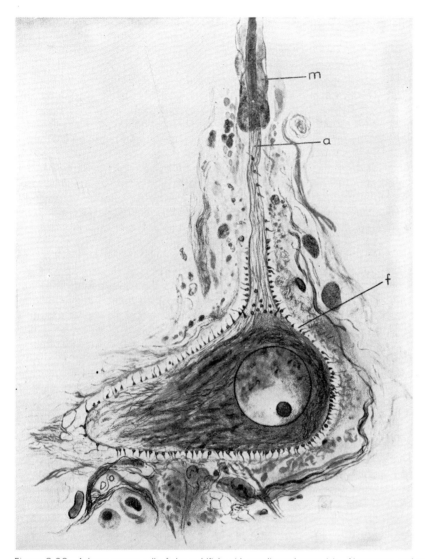

Figure 8-28   A large motor cell of the goldfish with myelinated axon (a).   Numerous and minute end-feet on the cell body and axon extend almost to the myelin sheath (m).   The pale zone (f) occupied by the end-bulbs is apparently not a shrinkage artifact, but a fiber-free zone characteristic of some of these cells.   Mallory-azan after Zenker-formol.   ×1,440.   (Courtesy of D. Bodian, J. Comp. Neurol., **73**:341, 1940.)

can be preserved by perfusion of fixatives through the arteries immediately upon death.

The end-feet are generally very small in contrast to the cell body and dendrites, and each neuron, in general, receives many end-feet.   The number of end-feet on the large motor cells of the spinal cord and the giant pyramidal cells of the cerebral cortex is estimated in the thousands (Fig. 8-62). The synapses on any one neuron ordinarily represent terminations from many neurons, although each contributing neuron may be represented by more than one of these endings.

The intimate relation between neural elements and the difficulty of defining the membrane boundaries of the synapse in light microscopy led to the early view that nervous tissue constitutes a true syncytium. This view is no longer tenable, since electron micrographs show the apposition of unbroken pre- and postsynaptic membranes separated, in most instances, by a space of 20 to 30 nm (Figs. 8-11, 8-31, and 8-33). The pre- and postsynaptic membranes, sometimes together called the *synaptolemma,* are increased in density so the synapse somewhat resembles a desmosome. The membranes adhere so strongly to each other that end-feet with postsynaptic membrane can be isolated as particles called *synaptosomes* by differential centrifugation of central nervous tissue homogenates. Accumulations of mitochondria and sometimes neurofibrils can also be seen in the presynaptic end-bulb (Figs. 8-11, 8-30, 8-33, and 8-42).

Each end-foot excites the second neuron or inhibits its excitation. It is now accepted that excitation or inhibition commonly occurs through the release of a chemical transmitter from the presynaptic membrane to change the properties of the postsynaptic membrane. An accumulation of *synaptic vesicles* 20 to 65 nm in diameter is usually found in the presynaptic end-bulb (Figs. 8-11, 8-31, and 8-33). The vesicles are believed by most investigators to contain the transmitter substance. The excitation induced by a single end-foot is not sufficient to raise the second neuron to the threshold necessary to induce an action potential;

instead, the simultaneous stimulation of many end-feet is required. Once excitation of the second neuron reaches the threshold level, a wave of induced excitation sweeps down it and all its divisions. Inhibitory endings make it more difficult to excite the second neuron; they block the excitation wave.

This description of the basic structure of the synapse applies to both the autonomic and central nervous systems. In the latter, the dendritic receptive sites may consist of local protuberances called *spines,* or *thorns* (Figs. 8-31 and 8-35). End-bulbs themselves may receive endings (axoaxonal synapses), and dendrites may form synaptic thickenings with other dendrites. Fused pre- and postsynaptic membranes are sometimes observed.

MOTOR AND SENSORY ENDINGS

Other than synaptic endings of one neuron upon another, there are two great groups of nerve terminations: the endings of motor fibers which originate in the central and autonomic nervous systems and the peripheral endings of sensory fibers.

Motor endings Motor nerve endings are the terminations of efferent axons on muscle fibers or on glands. Impregnation with gold or silver (Figs. 8-32 and 8-37) and supravital staining with methylene blue are most commonly used in light microscopy to demonstrate the endings.

As motor nerves approach and penetrate striated

Figure 8-29 Synaptic endings in acousticolateral centers of goldfish. On left, small end-bulbs from fine unmyelinated fibers on cell body. On right, large end-feet showing mitochondrial accumulations at terminal surfaces near cell bodies. Stained with the Bodian silver method and counterstained with Mallory-azan.

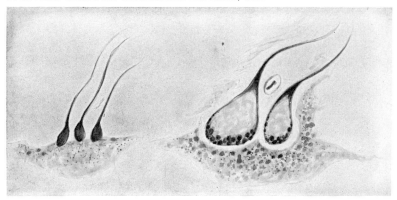

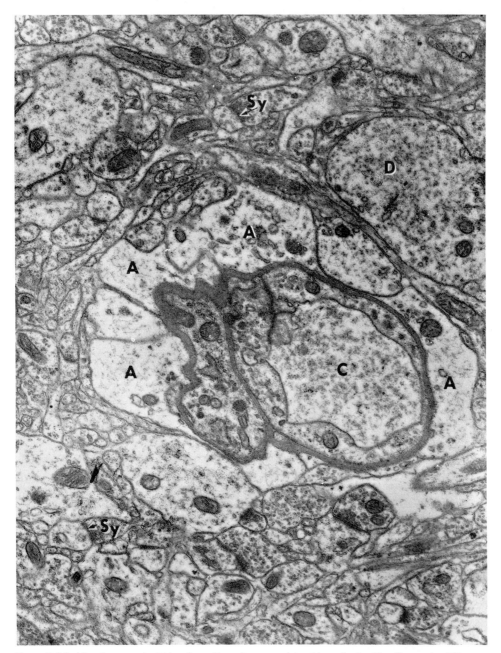

Figure 8-30 Visual cortex of rabbit. C, capillary; A, astrocytic end-feet; D, dendrite; Sy, axodendritic synapses. Approximately ×17,000. (Courtesy of H. Van der Loos.)

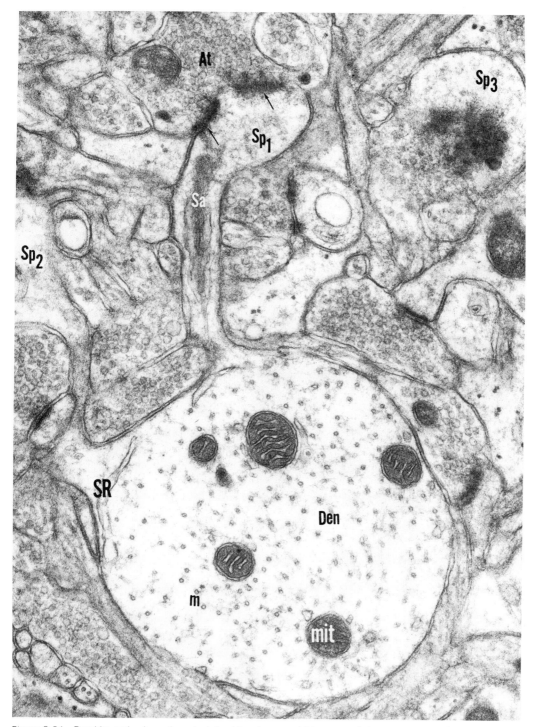

Figure 8-31 Dendrite and spine. An apical dendrite of a pyramidal neuron of the rat cerebral cortex occupies the larger portion of the field. The dendrite (Den) has cytoplasm with microtubules (m), smooth endoplasmic reticulum (SR), and mitochondria (mit). Two spines (Sp₁ and Sp₂) are arising from the upper and left portion of the apical dendrite and are forming synaptic junctions with axon terminals (At). Another spine (Sp₃) is shown on upper right of the field. A spine apparatus (Sa), which consists of a system of cisternae is contained inside the stalk of a spine (Sp₁). Two synaptic complexes (arrows) are also shown. ×49,500. (Courtesy of I. Kraiserman-Abramoff.)

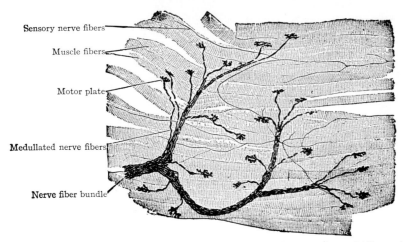

Sensory nerve fibers

Muscle fibers

Motor plate

Medullated nerve fibers

Nerve fiber bundle

Figure 8-32 Silvered preparation of motor nerve endings on intercostal muscle fibers of a rabbit. ×150.

Figure 8-33 Astrocytic sheaths. This field is part of the neuropil of the rat cerebral cortex. Dendrites (Den) filled with microtubules (m) are shown. On the upper right, a spine (sp) is in synaptic contact with an axon terminal (At). Filling the interstices of the various components of the neuropil are sheaths of astrocytic processes (As) containing particles of glycogen. ×38,000. (Courtesy of I. Kaiserman-Abramoff.)

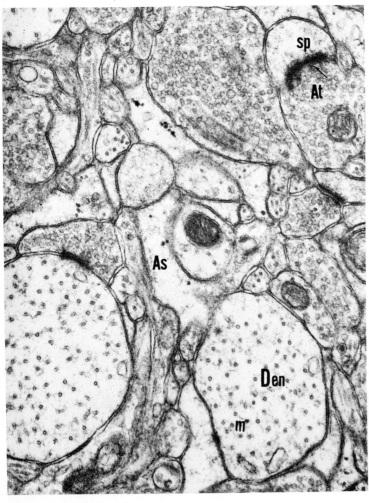

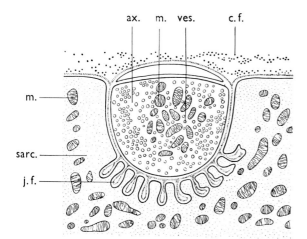

Figure 8-34 Schematic drawing of a motor end-plate on vertebrate striated muscle: m., mitochondrion; ax., axoplasm; ves., vesicle; sarc., sarcoplasm; j.f., junctional folds of muscle plasma membrane; c.f., collagen fibrils. (Courtesy of R. Couteaux, Exp. Cell Res., Suppl. 5, p. 298, 1958.)

muscle, the rate of bifurcation of individual fibers increases and each ultimate branch ends on a single fiber within the muscle (Fig. 8-32). In this way many muscle fibers, sometimes numbering in the hundreds, come to be innervated by a single motor neuron. The motor neuron and the muscle fibers which it innervates constitute a functional and anatomic unit, called the *motor unit*. Each time the motor neuron conducts an impulse, all the muscle fibers it ends upon are stimulated to contract. As the motor fiber nears its terminus, the Schwann cell ends in contact with the sarcolemma. The motor axon usually implants itself near the middle of the muscle fiber. Ultrastructural studies (Fig. 8-34) show that the axon does not penetrate the sarcolemma nor does the axoplasm fuse with the sarcoplasm, as was believed by many before the advent of electron-microscope studies. The naked axon ends in a trough of folded or fluted sarcolemma. The trough may have many branches, each of which contains a division of the axon. The axonal twigs are separated from the sarcolemma by an interval of 400 to 600 Å in vertebrate striated muscle and 50 to 200 Å in certain insect myoneural junctions. The axoplasm contains numerous mitochondria and vesicles (approximately 450 Å in diameter), but neurofilaments are not seen (Fig.

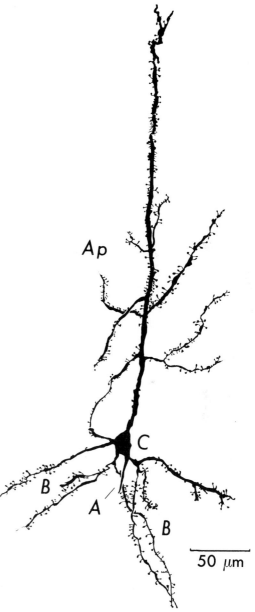

Figure 8-35 Pyramidal neuron in layer V, rat parietal cerebral cortex. Camera lucida drawing. Golgi-Cox preparation. Note apical (Ap) and basal (B) dendrites covered with numerous spines. Axon, A; cell body, C. (Courtesy of I. Kaiserman-Abramoff.)

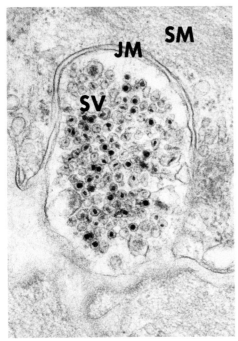

Figure 8-36 Myoneural junction of autonomic fiber on smooth muscle in vas deferens of adult rat: SM, smooth muscle fiber; SV, synaptic vesicles; JM, junctional membranes. Approximately ×50,000. (Courtesy of M. Grillo.)

8-34). Vesicles have also been reported in the subjacent sarcoplasm.

In the light microscope the myoneural junctional region sometimes appears to be elevated. The elevation covers an area of 40 to 60 μm^2 and is

Figure 8-37 Nerve fibers ending around and within an alveolus of the submandibular gland of the cat. Golgi method. ×765. (Rossi and Mocchi.)

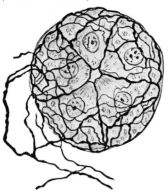

termed the *sole* or *motor plate*. A number of nuclei are concentrated within the sole plate, some of them Schwann nuclei and others nuclei of the muscle fiber. In their gross ramifications the terminal fibers may appear beaded (*terminaisons en grappe*), may be arranged together like a "crow's foot," or may take still other shapes and dispositions. A thin, unmyelinated fiber, believed by some to be sympathetic, has been reported on occasion to join this ending.

Smooth and cardiac muscle and glands receive motor fibers from the autonomic system that are unmyelinated and finer in caliber than the motor fibers of striated muscle. They also show considerable branching and form plexuses from which slender fibers proceed to end in nodular thickenings or loops. In contrast to striated muscle, not all smooth muscle fibers receive nerve endings. This difference reflects the intimate association of cells of smooth and cardiac muscle which allows the propagation of a wave of motility from one cell to the next. The endings in cardiac muscle are more readily identified and may be provided with a small cluster of terminal bodies. Electron-microscope studies show a contact between terminal axons and smooth muscle, without sarcolemmal folds. Axons which supply the smooth muscle of the intestinal wall have terminal end-bulbs which resemble synaptic end-feet separated by a 200-Å space from the muscle fiber and which contain the dense-core synaptic vesicles (Fig. 8-36) found in sympathetic neurons.

Axis cylinders have also been demonstrated within the connective tissue of glands and have been reported to ramify between adjacent gland cells or at the base of cells and to form complicated networks around the secretory portions (Fig. 8-37). Only a few secretory cells are contacted by axons, and in many glands the fibers have been traced only to the blood vessels.

Sensory endings Sensory endings are located in strategic positions throughout the body, often in relation to special receptors which serve as transducers of the energy of stimulation. According to the central connections of the parent neuron, the endings subserve various modalities of sensation such as pain, touch, pressure, heat, cold, proprioception, vision, hearing, equilibrium, taste, and olfaction. The receptors and nerve fiber relations for the special senses of hearing, vision, taste, and olfaction are described in other chapters and will not be touched upon here. For the other receptors, there is some confusion in terminology and description; many types have been listed where distinction rests only upon differences in the way the nerve fiber ramifies within the receptor. It has been suggested in recent literature that the same cutaneous endings may mediate a number of sensory modalities (for example, pain and touch) according to the pattern of stimulation and the number of endings involved. No attempt is made here to detail all the recorded variations in endings or the differences in opinion concerning their functions. Instead, the end organs whose histology in various vertebrates is better known are described with occasional comments on functional significance.

Some sensory fibers unassociated with a special receptor are observed to divide and ramify freely in other tissues and are, therefore, called *free nerve endings* (Figs. 8-38, 8-40, and 8-41). As they terminate, they may lose all their sheaths. These twigs frequently arise from nonmyelinated fibers of fine caliber. Free ramifications are abundant in the skin, particularly in the dermis. They also penetrate as naked fibers into the epidermis, where they may wander for a short distance among the epidermal cells (Figs. 8-38 and 8-41), and they are reported in the stratified epithelium of mucous membranes such as the oral mucosa. In the earliest studies of epithelial innervation, they were observed in

Figure 8-38 Nerve fibers in regenerating epidermis of the salamander. Approximately ×400.

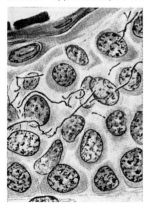

abundance in the cornea, where they were described as penetrating to the outermost layers and even hanging free in the precorneal fluid. They may end as small knobs or as leaf-like flattened enlargements among the epithelial cells. Free nerve endings occur not only in stratified epithelia and in dermis but also in muscle, tendon, connective tissue, and elsewhere (Fig. 8-40). The ultimate branches of termination are so delicate that they are seldom revealed after silver stains; however, they have been demonstrated with the light microscope by the methylene blue method applied to living or fresh tissue (Fig. 8-40). Electron micrographs of corneal epithelium reveal fibers as small as 0.2 μm in diameter running in grooves between epithelial cells.

Free nerve endings are commonly considered to be pain receptors, since they alone are found in tissues where the primary sensation is pain, such as the pulp and dentin of teeth and the cornea. However, some touch reception must also be ascribed to them. Indeed, the free nerve endings of the epidermis are sometimes associated with a modified, disc-shaped cell, the *tactile cell of Merkel,* around which axons terminate in networks (Fig. 8-41). Tactile cells are presumably touch receptors. They have been reported variously in the snout of the pig and other mammals, in the skin of fingertips, and in the sheath of the hair follicle.

Terminal corpuscles are encapsulated endings that are found scattered among the connective tissues of the body. They are sensory receptors in which a nerve fiber or knot of small branches is enclosed in a special connective tissue capsule. The terminal ramifications of the axis cylinder show irregular swellings. Generally, the connective tissue sheath of the entering fibers blends with the capsule, and the myelin-Schwann sheath is lost just within it. Terminal corpuscles have been classified in various ways according to their structure and presumed function. They include, among others, *Meissner's corpuscles, Pacinian and Herbst corpuscles, muscle and tendon spindles*, and *cylindrical end-bulbs.*

Meissner's corpuscles (or tactile corpuscles) subserve the sensation of touch (Fig. 8-43). They are elliptical structures 40 to 100 μm thick containing a core of flattened tactile cells arranged in layers across the long axis of the corpuscle. The

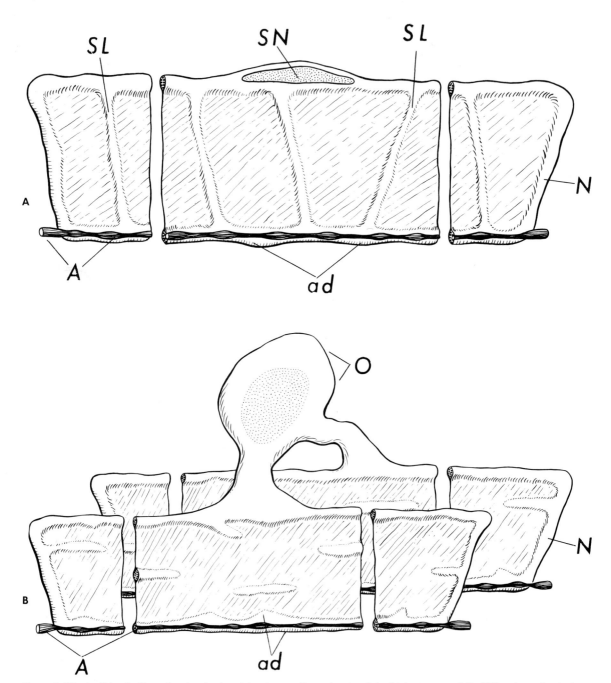

Figure 8-39   A. ''Unrolled'' myelin sheath of peripheral nerve fiber, showing Schmidt-Lanterman clefts (SL), adaxonal cytoplasm (ad), paranodal cytoplasm (N), and Schwann nucleus (SN).   Drawn to scale based on a sheath with 20 turns but exaggerating the diameter of the axon, which should be less than half that shown.   B. ''Unrolled'' myelin sheath of two central nerve fibers formed by one oligodendrocyte (O).   Note absence of Schmidt-Lanterman clefts but presence of a continuous tube of cytoplasm around the rim of the sheath plus occasional wisps of cytoplasm enclosed in the sheet.   Note size of axon, which is somewhat exaggerated, compared to unrolled sheath of about 20 turns around the axon: *ad,* adaxonal layer of oligodendrocyte cytoplasm; N, paranodal cytoplasm.

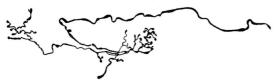

Figure 8-40   Free nerve endings in the pleura pulmonalis of a dog. Methylene blue. (Larsell.)

layers of flattened cells are separated by a ground substance containing collagen fibrils and are situated within a lamellated capsule of connective tissue. Both the flattened and the lamellated cells of the capsule are believed to be derived from connective tissue. From one to five medullated fibers enter the lower end of a tactile corpuscle. They lose their sheaths soon after entering and give off branches which pursue a tight spiral course through the corpuscle, frequently parallel to the tactile cells, making contact with flattened portions of these cells. Thickening of cell membranes, collections of vesicles in both sides of the thickenings, and massive accumulation of mitochondria indicate possible synaptic contacts at these sites. These corpuscles are found in some of the papillae, or connective tissue elevations beneath the epidermis, being especially numerous in those of fingertips,

Figure 8-41 Tactile cell in epidermis of snout of a mole. Nerve fibers form a terminal network around a modified epithelial cell. Underlying dermal connective tissue can be seen in the lower third of the figure. (Courtesy of Penfield, ''Cytology,'' Hoeber, New York, 1932.)

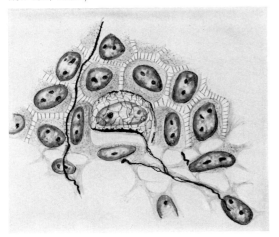

sole, and palm (as many as 23 per mm^2); they occur also in the nipple, border of the eyelids, lips, glans penis, and clitoris. Special techniques are required to visualize the innervation of these touch corpuscles, like most other types of endings.

Hair also serves as an important organ of tactile sensibility, a function which has been greatly elaborated for the vibrissae (whiskers) of animals such as the cat. A complicated innervation which incorporates both free and corpuscular endings has been described around the hair follicle. Rings of nerve fibers surround the follicle and end freely around it. Touch cells resembling Merkel's corpuscles have also been seen in the root sheath.

Cylindrical end-bulbs of Krause contain a single axial nerve fiber, with few or no branches, terminating in a knob-like or rounded extremity consisting of a tangle of intricate convolutions and ramifications of the fiber. The confusing tangle of fibers is surrounded by a semifluid substance, sometimes described as an inner bulb, which is enclosed in a few concentric layers of connective tissue cells that are continuous with the sheath of the nerve fiber. Cylindrical corpuscles are found in the mucous membrane of the mouth, in the connective tissue of muscles and tendons, in genital organs, in skin, and elsewhere. Many variants of Krause end-bulbs have been described and have been given different names, often according to their position in the body. Genital corpuscles of the glans penis and clitoris, articular corpuscles, and others show striking resemblances, although the size, arrangement of connective tissue, and number of nerve fibers of supply may differ (Figs. 8-44 and 8-45, see color insert). Krause end-bulbs have been thought of as cold receptors, and similar structures, such as the genital corpuscles, found throughout the skin are considered receptors for heat. Other authors consider these organs tactile receptors. In subcutaneous tissue near coils of sweat glands and in the fingers *terminal cylinders* (of Ruffini) are sometimes observed with less distinct capsules but with plaques of ramifying nerve fibers. They are said by some authors to be receptors of heat stimuli.

Pacinian (or *Vater-Pacinian*) *corpuscles,* or *lamellar corpuscles,* are macroscopic elliptical pressure receptors 0.5 to 4.5 mm long and 1 to 2 mm wide. They were first observed in dissections and

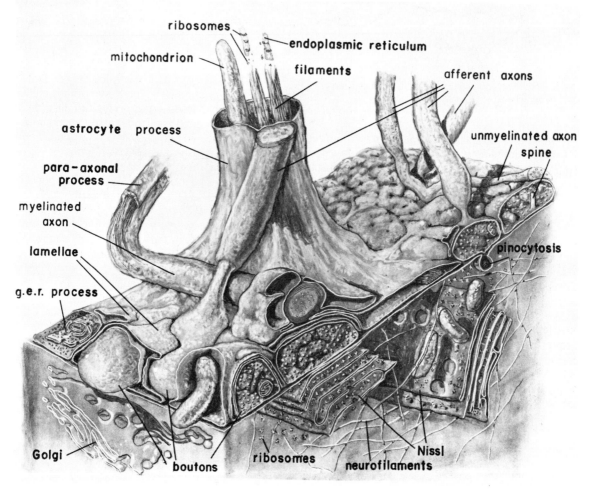

ribosomes

mitochondrion

endoplasmic reticulum

filaments

afferent axons

astrocyte   process

unmyelinated axon
spine

para-axonal
process

myelinated
axon

lamellae

g.e.r. process

pinocytosis

Golgi

boutons

ribosomes

neurofilaments

Nissl

Figure 8-42   Drawing of perikaryon of motor neuron from cat spinal cord showing internal organelle contents and structures in contact with the surface.   Note the large astrocytic process spread over the motor neuron, with granular endoplasmic reticulum (g.e.r.) in one of its extensions.   (Courtesy of R. Poritsky, J. Comp. Neurol., **135:**423, 1969.)

may be seen grossly as minute vesicular bodies along the mesenteries.   They are attached to the terminal branches of nerve fibers.   Microscopically they are striking objects and, except for their nerve fibers, they are easily identified in sections stained with ordinary techniques (Fig. 8-25C, see color insert).   In such sections they resemble the cut surface of a sliced onion bulb.   The axial core of the corpuscle is surrounded by concentric layers, sometimes as many as sixty, which consist of flattened cells enclosing connective tissue.   A large

nerve fiber enters a slender stalk on one end of the corpuscle and loses its myelin-Schwann sheath as it traverses the lamellae (Fig. 8-46).   It extends through the semifluid core as a naked fiber, sometimes flattened and bandlike; it may fork at its far end, form a coil of branches, or end in an enlargement.   It has been observed on occasion to pass out of one corpuscle and then to enter another.   Ordinarily the corpuscles are sectioned obliquely or transversely so that the concentric layers completely encircle the inner core (Fig. 8-25C, see

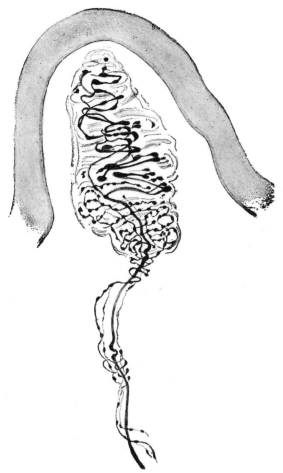

color insert).   Special methods have shown that the axial fiber may possess many short lateral branches ending in knobs and that it may be accompanied and encircled by one or more delicate nerve fibers. A small artery may enter the corpuscle with the nerve fiber to supply the lamellae (Fig. 8-46). Lamellar corpuscles are abundant in the subcutaneous tissue of the hand and foot and occur in deeper regions of the dermis, in the mammary gland and nipple, clitoris, penis, urethra, and in the territory of the pudendal nerve.   They are found near the joints (particularly on the flexor side) and in the periosteum and perimysium, in the connective tissue around large blood vessels and nerves, and in the tendon sheaths.   They are found also in serous membranes, particularly the mesenteries, where they may be quite large.   Pacinian corpuscles appear to be receptors of pressure or of tension, and upon being deformed, presumably stimulate the embedded axon.   *Herbst corpuscles* are much smaller than Pacinian corpuscles but of similar structure.

There are special sensory endings in striated muscle and tendon which report to the central nervous system the state of muscular activity and the tension of tendons.   These, together with the sensory endings of joints, provide information on the position and movements of parts of the body in relation to one another, a modality of sensation which has been termed *proprioception*.   The proprioceptive receptors of striated muscles are specially modified and encapsulated muscle fibers (*intrafusal muscle fibers*) arranged in groups within a muscle (Fig. 8-47) and known, together with their innervation, as *muscle spindles*.   Muscle

Figure 8-43   A Meissner's corpuscle within a dermal papilla of human finger.   The shaded area is epidermis.   Methylene blue. (Dogiel.)

Figure 8-44   An encapsulated nerve apparatus from the outer connective tissue lamina of the prostate of a dog.   A thick and thin myelinated fiber penetrate the structure.   Methylene blue.   (Timofeew.)

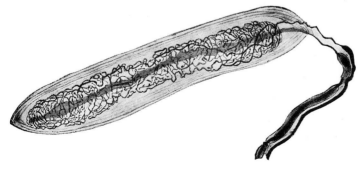

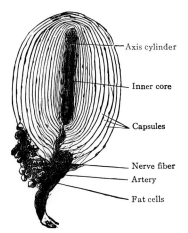

Figure 8-46   Diagrammatic sketch of a small Pacinian corpuscle from the mesentery of a cat. The myelin of the nerve fiber may be traced to the inner core.   ×50.

Labels on Figure 8-46:
- Axis cylinder
- Inner core
- Capsules
- Nerve fiber
- Artery
- Fat cells

spindles are absent in some muscles but are abundant in those of the extremities. A spindle consists of a group of 3 to 20 slender muscle fibers about 1 to 4 mm long and 0.08 to 0.2 mm wide, around which nerve fibers terminate (Fig. 8-48). The spindles are surrounded by a thick connective tissue sheath or capsule, continuous with the perimysium (Fig. 8-47). The muscle fibers of the spindle are poorly differentiated but possess motor terminations and can contract within the sheath. They are distinctly striated toward their tapering, very slender ends, but in their middle portions the sarcoplasm and nuclei are abundant and the striations are ill-

defined. Three or four nerve fibers terminate in each spindle (Fig. 8-48). The nerve fibers branch and lose their sheath as they pass through the perimysial capsule to the muscle cells. The axons that terminate at the middle of the muscle cells spiral around the cell and are closely applied to the muscle fiber (called *annulospiral ending*). They are sensory, recording passive stretching of the muscle; motor fibers run to the slender ends of the muscle cells and terminate in modified motor plates. Other types of sensory endings have been described in the spindle and elsewhere in the muscle. In the smooth musculature of the bronchi of the lungs, muscle spindles are described in which the sensory axon ends in short, knobbed branches on and between the muscle fibers.

Tendons possess two types of sensory endings, *tendon spindles* and *free nerve endings*. The former are small portions of the tendon, about 1 to 3 mm long and 0.2 to 0.3 mm wide, enclosed in sheaths of connective tissue (Fig. 8-49). The few nerve fibers which terminate in a tendon spindle lose their sheaths and branch freely, ending in club-shaped enlargements. They are stimulated during muscle contraction when the tendon is under tension and, in contrast to annulospiral endings, appear to record active contraction of muscle. Electron-microscope studies show a very intimate contact between terminal sensory nerves and the organs innervated. A 200-Å space, without interposed membrane, separates the two elements. The nerve terminals are devoid of sheaths and are characterized by a massive accumulation of mitochondria.

Figure 8-47   Muscle spindle, transverse section.   The nerve fibers form a net.

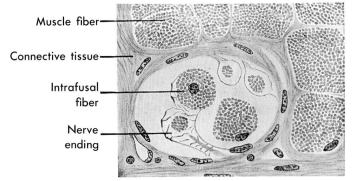

Labels on Figure 8-47:
- Muscle fiber
- Connective tissue
- Intrafusal fiber
- Nerve ending

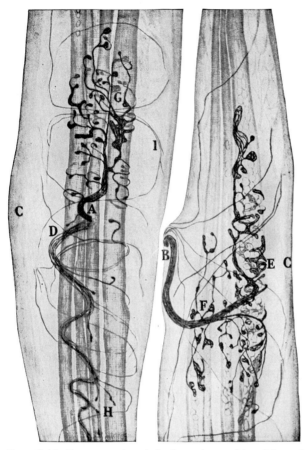

Figure 8-48   Neuromuscular spindles from a human fetus of 6 months, in longitudinal view.   Connective tissue capsule (C) enclosing modified muscle fibers.   Sensory fibers (A and B) enter the capsule, ramify, and entwine muscle fibers.   They terminate in claw- or leaf-like endings (E, F, G).   Other fine sensory fibers (I) are seen within the capsule.   A motor component (D) forms terminations (H) on the muscle fiber. (Tello.)

Figure 8-49   Terminal ramification of tendon spindle of an adult cat.   ×345.

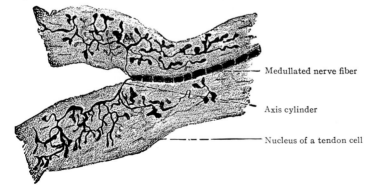

— Medullated nerve fiber

Axis cylinder

Nucleus of a tendon cell

Appearance and identification of nervous tissue in sections

Following the application of light-microscopic techniques which are specific for elements of the nerve fiber, fibers and nerves are readily identified in tissue sections. With specific methods for myelin (for example, osmic acid fixation or oxidative fixatives followed by staining with hematoxylin) the nerve fibers appear in cross section as a series of rings because of staining of the myelin sheath (Fig. 8-50A), with the axis cylinder unstained or only faintly stained. In longitudinal view the myelin sheaths appear as parallel stained bands (Fig. 8-21A). Nonmyelinated fibers are not identifiable after such staining; and when they are numerous, their position in the nerve is represented by local unstained regions (Fig. 8-50A).

In contrast to myelin stains, sections impregnated with silver reveal the axis cylinders as dark circular structures (Fig. 8-50B) whose edges are sometimes more heavily stained. Around the larger myelinated axons in such cross sections is an unstained area marking the position of the myelin sheath. In longitudinal view the axons are arranged in parallel (Figs. 8-8, 8-15, and 8-51). In the scattered smaller nerves seen in tissue sections, the fibers may be cut variously (Fig. 8-38) because of their individual courses. They are frequently seen in both cross and longitudinal view within the same section (Fig. 8-25E, see color insert).

In sections stained with common histologic acid and basic dye combinations such as hematoxylin and eosin, eosin and methylene blue, and the tri-acid dye combinations of Masson or Mallory, single nerve fibers and groups of a few fibers are impossible to identify, and larger nerve units may frequently be difficult to distinguish. In these cases the axis cylinder is stained very faintly or not at all and the myelin-Schwann sheath is hardly visible. However, identification of a nerve may be made from the disposition of Schwann nuclei and connective tissue, particularly the presence of a distinct perineurium, and further confirmed by the recognition of the neurokeratin network remaining after dissolution of the myelin lipid, by suggestions of axis cylinders, and by the position of the nerve in relation to other tissue structures. Drawings of small nerves as they appear ordinarily in a section stained with eosin and hematoxylin are shown in Fig. 8-25E and F; see color insert. The investing sheath of connective

Figure 8-50 Cross sections of the human femoral nerve. A. Stained for myelin with a modified Weigert technique. The unstained patches of A represent localized concentrations of unmyelinated fibers. B. Stained for axis cylinders with the Bodian silver method. In B the fibers are more numerous and the myelin is represented by blank circles around the larger fibers. Note the range in fiber size. Drawn at ×390.

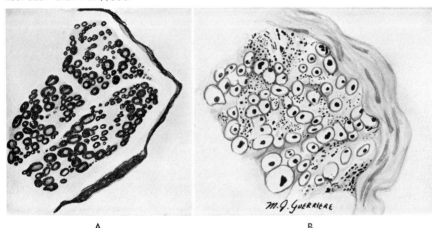

A   B

tissue (perineurium), seen even in small nerves, sets off the nerve from surrounding tissue and appears like a capsule when the nerve is cut in cross section (Fig. 8-25F, see color insert). The sheath nuclei are roughly oriented in a similar direction within the nerve, as though caught in a current of a wandering stream. Since the course of the individual nerve fiber is never straight, some of the Schwann nuclei are oriented at right angles to the plane of section and others lie parallel (observe local regions of Fig. 8-25E and F in color insert). Scattered concentrations of collagenous tissue and smooth muscle are most frequently confused with nerve in tissue sections stained with ordinary dyes, since in both instances the nuclei may be similarly oriented along the length of the structure and may resemble Schwann nuclei. These structures, however, are not in general delimited by an investing sheath; the smooth muscle nuclei may be relatively large and staggered but oriented regularly in the same direction, whereas in connective tissue they are scattered and irregularly disposed, and surrounding substance in which the nuclei are embedded appears more fibrous and often faintly stained. Nevertheless, there are instances where it is difficult to differentiate between the nerve and these other tissues, as in sections of the urethra.

Cell bodies, whether scattered individually, for example along the intestinal tract (Fig. 8-25D, see color insert), or concentrated in discrete ganglia, are generally identifiable after ordinary or special staining. Characteristically, the cell body is large, oval, or round, and the cytoplasm is abundant. The nucleus is invariably central, large, relatively round, and devoid of chromatin but has one or two well-defined nucleoli. Satellite cell nuclei are disposed around the cell body.

The electron microscope makes it possible to visualize all the neural elements with their investing sheaths simultaneously (Figs. 8-11, 8-12, 8-16, 8-23, 8-24, 8-26, 8-30, 8-31, 8-33, 8-36, and 8-42). This method presents new problems in identification but has clarified many aspects of nervous system organization. The nerve cell bodies are easily identified in electron micrographs mainly by their size, shape, and disposition, but also may be identified by their low density and central nuclei with prominent nucleoli. The nuclear envelope is typically double, showing nuclear pores, and the outer membrane of the envelope usually does not have the attached dense granules frequently seen in other cells. The mitochondria are usually small and structurally dense. The cristae are arranged irregularly, often oriented along the long axis of the mitochondrion, especially in the nerve process. Axis cylinders have received most scrutiny. They contain numerous elongated mitochondria, few tubules, some vesicles and are packed with longitudinal filaments 80 to 100 Å in diameter, which may appear beaded. Dendrites can be distinguished from axons or glial processes by numerous longitudinally arrayed tubules 200 to 300 Å in diameter. They also contain dense ribonucleoprotein granules, elongated mitochondria, vesicles 400 to 800 Å in diameter, and occasional filaments. These characteristics are less striking at a great distance from the nerve body, and there the dendrites are distinguished only with uncertainty from glial elements. Another identifying feature of dendrites is the surrounding synaptic end-bulbs with their characteristic fine structure described above.

In many ways the fine structural features of Schwann cells surrounding peripheral axons and of satellite cells surrounding spinal and autonomic ganglia are identical. Their nuclei are relatively dense and fusiform. Prominent nucleoli are not seen. The cytoplasm appears sparse and contains numerous vesicles and thin filaments. Occasional elongated profiles of endoplasmic reticulum are present. Mitochondria are less dense and larger than those of axons or cell bodies. Schwann cells are most easily identified in normal tissue by their position close to the enveloped axis cylinders and their association with myelin. The content of the Schmidt-Lanterman clefts and nodal spirals, unlike that of the Schwann cell body, is sparse and resembles that of the astrocyte process. The adaxonal Schwann layer tends to be granular, variable in thickness, and displays an occasional dark body.

Surrounding the Schwann cell is an amorphous layer, and outside that are thin collagenous fibrils constituting the endoneurium. The distinguishing characteristics of myelin have already been recounted in detail and need not be reiterated here. The identifying features of the neuroglia under the light and electron microscopes are recorded in a later section.

Degeneration and regeneration of neurons

Their extended course exposes peripheral nerve fibers to frequent injury. If the injury cuts the fibers, as in stab or bullet wounds, or crushes the nerve, a series of degenerative changes are observed, later followed by reparative ones, provided the cell body survives the injury. The axis cylinder and the myelin of the sheath distal to the point of destruction degenerate completely, but the Schwann cells persist and form a cellular tube. Moreover, the parent cell body and a portion of the fiber proximal to the wound also show important and characteristic changes. The degenerative changes which the peripheral stump undergoes are called *wallerian degeneration* and are obvious within 2 or 3 days under the light microscope. In electron microscope studies changes may be detected a few hours after injury. There are striking early changes in the axoplasm adjacent to the sheath and in the Schwann cell. The axoplasm shows localized accumulations of glycogen granules and mitochondria. The Schwann cytoplasm burgeons; its adaxonal layer increases and develops numerous densely stained smooth-walled tubules, granules, and lysosomes; and the Schmidt-Lanterman clefts become more prominent. Beginning about 24 hr after transection, the axolemma shows areas of erosion adjacent to the regions of swollen adaxonal Schwann cytoplasm. The rim of axoplasm and the adaxonal cytoplasm become so commingled that it is difficult to distinguish one from the other; the combined region may now be called the *reactive zone*. In subsequent days it takes on the character more of adaxonal cytoplasm than axoplasm, leading to the conclusion that the major destruction of the axon is caused by the Schwann cell. The neurotubules disappear early, then the axolemma, the mitochondria, the vesicles, the granules, and the ground substance of the axoplasm; the neurofilaments persist, sometimes for days, but are compacted into the center of the fiber. Within a week, in most instances, the entire axon is destroyed. Within the first few days, the reactive zone is voluminous and contains many lysosomes and numerous tubules; the incisures multiply, invading the electron-dense lamellae of the myelin wrappings. They contain granules, lysosomes, and tubules; and the Schwann cell body is greatly enlarged. The increased prominence of the clefts in light-microscope sections, sharply delimiting areas of intervening myelin, cause the fibers to appear broken into a series of ovoids encompassing a fragment of the axon. Actually, recent ultrastructural studies show that the myelin-Schwann segment is not broken; rather the electron-dense lines of the myelin are progressively invaded by the growing Schwann cytoplasm until they eventually disappear except for occasional whorls of myelin figures within the cytoplasm. It is commonly stated that Schwann cells phagocytise fragmented myelin. In reality, myelin is never separated from the Schwann cell. It is destroyed within the burgeoning Schwann cell cytoplasm. The axon, reduced to a central remnant, is fragmented and digested by the Schwann cell. What remains is a series of tubes linked end to end, the wall of the tube consisting of Schwann cytoplasm (Fig. 8-51). In ensuing weeks the wall thickens, and the diameter of the tube shrinks progressively until it is less than half of the original; the bore may be obliterated unless regenerating axons invade it. The sheath nuclei multiply during this time, and their staining characteristics are altered. As the sheath thickens and the Schwann cells multiply, the degenerating fiber comes to look more and more like a cord rather than a tube (the so-called *cord of Bünger*). Coinciding with wallerian degeneration of the fibers, the gross appearance of the nerve changes. Instead of its normal white, glistening, ribbon-like appearance, it now appears rounded and condensed, dull gray, somewhat solid, and less flexible and compressible.

Degeneration extends to the very terminations. It has been described as simultaneous, occurring over the length of the fiber at once, or progressive, beginning near the wound and extending rapidly through the rest of the fiber. Within the central nervous system, similar degenerative phenomena occur. In most instances, degeneration does not travel beyond the synapse, a fact which originally was cited as evidence for discontinuity at the synapse. There are important instances where degeneration does not stop at the synapse but proceeds to the next neuron (*transynaptic*, or *transneuronal*, *degeneration*). Transneuronal degeneration is observed particularly in those nuclear centers which receive terminal fibers from a limited source, a classic example being the lateral geniculate body, which receives optic tract fibers.

The reaction of the cell body to injury of its axon is often called *retrograde degeneration;* changes in the stump proximal to the injury are included under retrograde degeneration or are called *traumatic degeneration,* since they occur close to the wound. Degeneration in this region of the fiber is similar to wallerian degeneration, but it is of shorter duration and is said to extend proximally only to the first node of Ranvier above the injury. In addition, there is an outpouring of freed Schwann cells from the cut surface into the wound area. This also occurs from the distal cut surface but is less pronounced. Many connective tissue elements also invade the wound area, mingling with the Schwann cells. The sheath cells reestablish the continuity of the nerve across the wound area, provided the transected ends are close to one another. However, since nerves are under a certain amount of tension, the stumps tend to retract, and establishment of a bridge of Schwann cells may not be accomplished unless the ends are surgically approximated. When the stumps are widely separated, the sheath cells, continuously flowing from the proximal stump and proliferating along with fibroblasts, may grow into a sizable tumor (*schwannoma*) consisting of whorls of Schwann cells. The tumor may be invaded by tangles of regenerating nerve fibers of the proximal stump (Fig. 8-52); such an innervated structure is called a *neuroma* and may be the source of painful and bizarre sensory disturbances.

The response of the cell body to damage of the peripheral process was first described by Nissl in 1892. The most characteristic change is *chromatolysis (chromolysis, tigrolysis),* the "dissolution" of the Nissl substance. Classically, chromatolysis was studied in motor horn cells, in which the reaction is most obvious, but it is also demonstrable elsewhere, varying among nuclear groups in extent and rate. Nissl material breaks up and appears to dissolve into the cytoplasm, beginning near the axon hillock in motor neurons and spreading to other parts of the cell (Fig. 8-53). In addition, the cell body swells and there is an associated shift of the nucleus from its normal central location in the cell body to a peripheral one, but away from the axon

Figure 8-51 Degenerating and regenerating nerve fibers of the sciatic nerve of the rabbit. Frequently branching regenerating axis cylinders of various sizes and irregular degenerating fragments are shown. Bodian silver stain. Drawn at about × 1,000.

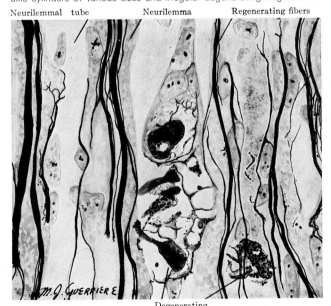

Neurilemmal tube   Neurilemma   Regenerating fibers

Degenerating fibers

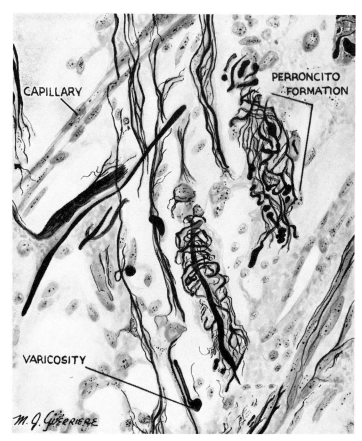

CAPILLARY

PERRONCITO
FORMATION

VARICOSITY

M. J. Guerriere

Figure 8-52   Regenerating fibers in wound area 11 days after transection of sciatic nerve of rabbit.   Note the irregular course of the fibers and the curious tangle sometimes formed (Perroncito formation).   Bodian silver method.   Drawn at about ×500.

hillock.   Retrograde degeneration sets in approximately 1 day after axonal injury and reaches its height within about 2 weeks.   In studies of pathologic material, such changes observed in nuclear centers of the cord and brain constitute evidence of primary neuronal damage.   Experimentation based on the chromatolytic response of cells is frequently done to locate the cell bodies of origin of interrupted tracts or nerves.   In order to evaluate the results properly, one must know the normal pattern of the Nissl substance for any given group of cells, since this is quite variable.   It is important to note that the degree of chromatolysis of motor cells corresponds roughly to the relative amount of cytoplasm in the peripheral processes that is amputated from the neuron.   Amputation of a very distal

process may yield no detectable response, whereas section of the major trunk yields a severe reaction and sometimes death of the neuron.

Retrograde changes, other than dissolution of Nissl substance, include breakup and dispersion of the Golgi apparatus.   There is also an increase in the activity of hydrolytic enzymes, and enzymes such as cytochrome oxidase and succinic dehydrogenase are greatly reduced in activity.   Van Gehuchten, many years ago, described retrograde changes as a return to an embryonic state, since the level of enzyme activity and the morphologic state of the reactive cell body resemble those of the developing neuron.

During retrograde cellular changes, regeneration of the axon is initiated and in time the retrograde response is slowly reversed. There is a reconstitution of the original Golgi and Nissl structure, a return to normal enzyme activities, a decline in the swelling of the cell body, and a return of the nucleus to its typical central position. In contrast to the rate at which chromatolysis sets in, restitution of the cell body is drawn out over several months.

The first signs of axonal regeneration occur within a week after injury. Many sprouts arise from the end of the axon, but abortive sprouting has been observed even after the first day following injury. The sprouts are exceedingly fine and at their advancing ends are enlarged into a swelling called a *growth cone* or *club*. Electron-microscope studies demonstrate the existence of cones containing microvesicles of 20 to 70 nm, elongated mitochondria, and multivesicular bodies 300 to 650 nm in diameter. In their fine structure the regenerating axonal sprouts resemble embryonic ones. They accompany the Schwann cells across the gap between cut ends and enter the tubes of Schwann cells within the peripheral degenerated nerve (Fig. 8-51) where they eventually are enwrapped by the Schwann cells, which show prominent mesaxons and voluminous cytoplasm. Very fine neurofilaments are present in the axoplasm. Large vesicles and tubules having dilated areas are also observed.

Varicosities appear along the length of regenerating fibers, presumably where the fiber in its growth has encountered an obstacle, and the forward-flowing cytoplasm is temporarily dammed up (Fig. 8-52). Before reaching the distal stump, the fibers may form curious tangles, other irregularities in direction of growth, and varicosities (Fig. 8-52) owing to the obstruction of invading connective tissue. If the stumps are separated by a great gap, many sprouts may fail to reach the distal end and, instead, may be confined to the schwannoma of mixed sheath and fibrocellular tissue. Even though axons may be unable to complete their regeneration to the periphery, they apparently retain their capacity for regrowth for many years. If surgical approximation of the cut nerve ends is done after a sufficient lapse of time has permitted the development of solid cords or thick-walled tubes of Schwann cells, the axons grow within or outside of the Schwann cytoplasm to the periphery. The calculated rate of axonal growth through freshly degenerated peripheral mammalian nerve is approximately 3 to 4 mm per day, but there is great variation. The greatest rate of growth has been recorded in the developing antler of the deer—2 cm per day. From this result it may be inferred that the growth potential of axons is much greater than local conditions ordinarily permit. Nevertheless, regeneration is a slow process when one considers the great distance that may be required for regrowth, for months may elapse before the sprouts reach their termination. Once the fibers have reached the periphery, they connect with the end organ and function is restored. Functional return depends in large part upon reestablishment of connections with the periphery. However, the possibility of sprouts of the original innervating neuron reaching the origi-

Figure 8-53 Normal (left) and chromatolytic (right) motor neurons from lumbar cord of same rhesus monkey after section of sciatic nerve. Gallocyanin after acetone fixation. ×400. (Courtesy of D. Bodian and R. C. Mellors, J. Exp. Med., **81**:469, 1945.)

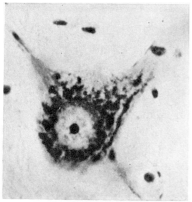
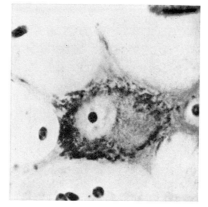

nal termination is substantially diminished, since precise end-to-end alignment of the individual fibers is impossible to achieve when the nerve is spliced surgically, so axons find their way into tubes originally belonging to other neurons. For example, sensory fibers may follow a pathway peripherally which leads to a motor ending, and motor fibers to a sensory ending. Repeated branching of the sprouts tends to increase the chances that the original Schwann tube is entered.

During the months following regeneration of the axis cylinder the myelin sheath is developed anew, the axon enlarges in diameter (Fig. 8-51), and, provided functional connection with the periphery is made, the axon eventually tends to approach its original caliber and the myelin-Schwann sheath returns to its original condition. The magnitude of axoplasm resynthesis in regeneration of the axon is impressive; for example, Bodian and Mellors noted that regeneration of a gastrocnemius motor fiber may involve the formation of axoplasm having a volume 250 times that of the parent cell body.

DEPENDENCE OF MUSCLE AND OTHER END ORGANS UPON THE NERVE

In addition to an obvious functional dependence, many of the receptor and effector end organs require intact nerve fibers to maintain their morphologic integrity. If the nerve is interrupted, degeneration of the end organ may also ensue. An example of this dependence is seen in striated muscle. Following denervation, and therewith paralysis, striated muscle undergoes a sequence of degenerative changes which may be reversed completely upon reinnervation. Within a few hours the sensitivity of the muscle fiber to the chemical mediator acetylcholine is altered, and within a few days metabolic changes are observed. Moreover, the muscle become flaccid, showing little of its original tone. In the ensuing months there is a gradual wasting of the sarcoplasm, and the muscle fiber becomes progressively thinner. Then the striations and the fibrils gradually disappear. Coincident with this loss there is an increase in fibrocellular tissue; eventually the entire muscle may be replaced by fibrous tissue. Reinnervation causes a reversal of these changes, and morphologic and physiologic reconstitution of the muscle.

A receptor which shows a striking morphologic dependence upon the nerve is the taste bud; it degenerates completely when denervated. However, when regenerating fibers reappear in the oral epithelium, taste buds develop anew.

Muscle and taste bud dependence upon the nerve are but two examples of a widespread nervous function known as the *neurotrophic* phenomenon. Axons give off a trophic factor important for maintenance and growth of the structures upon which they end. The most striking evidence of neurotrophic activity is seen in regeneration of body parts in lower vertebrates and invertebrates. For example, salamanders regenerate amputated limbs. If the limb stump is denervated, regeneration does not occur until nerve fibers reinvade the wound area.

Neuroglia, meninges, ventricles, chorioid plexuses, and cerebrospinal fluid of the central nervous system

NEUROGLIA

Neuroglia (*glia*, or ''glue'' of the central nervous system) together with the meninges constitute the supporting and ''connective'' tissue of the brain and spinal cord. Neuroglia are cells with many processes which extend and interlace, forming a framework for support and protection of cell bodies and fibers of the central nervous tissue. Glial cells are also thought to serve in the nutrition of nervous tissue. In addition, they function in repair of lesions of the central nervous system, and their sensitive response to diseases serves as an important criterion for study of neuropathologic events. Moreover, glial cells may be important in other functions, including nervous conduction.

There are four major types of neuroglia: *astrocytes* (*astroglia*), *oligodendroglia* (*oligodendrocytes*), *ependyma*, and *microglia* (*mesoglia*). The first three develop from the ectoderm of the medullary tube. They first appear as differentiated elements at about the third month of human intrauterine development. The term *neuroglia* is sometimes reserved for these neurectodermal derivatives, and the microglia are listed separately. The microglia are not neurectodermal but originate from the pia mater and the cells around blood vessels. They invade the central nervous system in showers at approximately the time of birth. Because of their mesodermal origin they are sometimes called *mesoglia.*

During embryonic development the cells of the medullary or neural tube differentiate in two directions, as *neuroblasts,* which develop into neurons, and as neuroglia other than microglia. The cells destined to become neuroblasts develop neuronal processes after a period of rapid multiplication. The glial derivatives of neurectoderm are differentiated from the remaining cells, which elongate and form a delicate framework within the thickness of the neural tube. Early in development the ependymal processes extend radially to the outer margins of the tube, but this arrangement persists into the adult in only a few regions, as in the median ventral wall of the cord and the retina of the eye. In certain regions of the future brain, as in the chorioid plexuses of the ventricles (Fig. 8-61), the wall of the tube remains thin throughout development and the ependymal cells form a sheet of cuboidal epithelium in direct contact with mesodermal derivatives; together with the pia mater, this forms the *tela chorioidea.* Elsewhere the ependymal processes extend for a short distance in the wall of the tube. The ependymal cells thus come to form the cellular lining of the internal canal system of the brain and spinal cord. Other neuroglial cells lie within the neural tube, and the processes of some (astrocytes) attach to the outer surface, where they are felted into an external limiting membrane.

The body of the neuroglial cell is generally smaller than the neuron cell body and the processes are shorter, although they may be very numerous and highly branched. The processes and cytoplasmic boundaries are difficult to reveal in the light microscope without specialized techniques, but the nuclei stain readily with basic dyes and other nuclear stains.

The best-known and earliest known type of glial cell is the *astrocyte,* so called because processes from its cell body extend in all directions (Fig. 8-54). Methods successfully applied to the dem-

Figure 8-54   Astrocytes: protoplasmic (A) and fibrous (B).   (Hortega.)

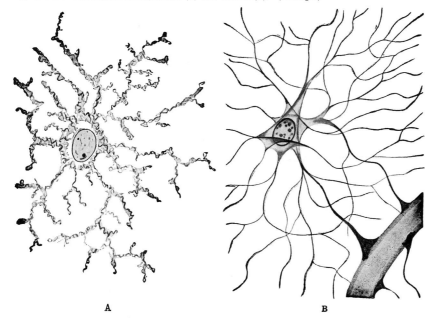

A   B

onstration of astrocytes were the chrome-silver method of Golgi and the later gold chloride sublimate method of Cajal. Two kinds of astrocytes are ordinarily described: protoplasmic (Fig. 8-54A) and *fibrous* (Fig. 8-54B), although a mixed type has been reported on occasion. The fibrous astrocyte has a smaller cell body enclosing an oval or spherical nucleus which is fairly large (yet much smaller than that of a nerve cell), and many long, slender, smooth processes, not much branched. Granules have been described in the cytoplasm of the cell body and processes. The definitive characteristic of fibrous astrocytes is the presence of stiff-looking fibrils within the cell body and processes, although some question has been raised concerning the declared intracellular position of fibrils. The fibrils are only revealed by certain stains, one of which, phosphotungstic acid hematoxylin, also reveals fibroglia and myoglia fibrils, which the neuroglia fibrils closely resemble in form and arrangement. When the fibrils are stained, the finer cytoplasmic processes which accompany them are usually impossible to distinguish. The fibrils form an intricate network, loosely surrounding nerve cells and nerve fibers. An occasional process of each cell reaches and spreads out on the surface of a blood vessel, where it is anchored by a perivascular trumpet-shaped foot which may wrap around the vessel (Fig. 8-54B). The termination around the vessel is supposed to derive nourishment from the blood and has been called the "sucker foot." Other feet of astrocytes may also attach firmly to the pia mater. The processes of these cells vary in length but can be quite extensive. Fibrous astrocytes are most abundant in white matter, where they provide support and binding for tracts of nerve fibers.

The protoplasmic astrocyte is more abundant in gray matter and contains fewer fibrils. The processes are predominantly thicker, more branched, and contain many vacuoles and granules. They have larger, more oval nuclei with many heavy chromatin granules near the membrane. They also have sucker feet.

Recent electron-microscope studies of the central nervous system reveal an apparently empty but voluminous cytoplasm in the astrocyte (Figs. 8-30 and 8-33). Mitochondria are few but larger than those in neurons or oligondendroglia; rough ER is scarce; and the Golgi complex is elaborate. Thin

bundles of very fine, long filaments, 60 to 100 Å thick, have been reported in the cytoplasm, oriented in swirls about the nucleus. Presumably these are the constituents of the larger fibrils seen in the fibrous astrocyte. The nuclei are irregularly ovoid, have well-defined nucleoli, and their chromatin is condensed around the nuclear membrane. Astrocytic processes establish close contact with some neurons, blood capillaries, and pial membranes, with only about 20-nm separations (Figs. 8-30, 8-42, 8-55, and 8-62). The astrocytes fill all the spaces between dendrites and axons in the gray matter and thus occupy much of the space previously believed to be extracellular (Figs. 8-42 and 8-55). Since the astrocytes form bridges between neurons, capillaries, and cerebrospinal fluid via end-feet on the pia, it has been postulated that they constitute water-ion compartments for transport of metabolites (Fig. 8-55). Moreover, they play a role in controlling the substances which enter the nervous tissue from the bloodstream ("blood-brain barrier").

Oligodendroglia ("few dendrites") are found surrounding nerve cell bodies and in rows along the fiber tracts of brain and cord (Figs. 8-55 to 8-58). Their relation to nerve cells resembles that of the satellite cells of ganglia. They also bear the same relation to axons of the central nervous system as do Schwann cells to those of the peripheral system, although their cytology differs (Figs. 8-39B and 8-57). Oligodendrocytes were first distinguished from astrocytes by Cajal in 1913, and their processes were stained specifically with the silver carbonate method introduced by del Rio Hortega in 1919. The cell body of oligodendrocytes is often angular and frequently somewhat square or rectangular. From the angles of the cell body, short, slender, and beaded processes arise which branch at near right angles (Fig. 8-56). Rows of oligodendrocytes surrounding the myelin sheath send long expansions up and down the nerve fiber. Smaller, more delicate processes encircle the myelin and invest it in a lace-like network (Fig. 8-56). It is believed that the central myelin is formed by oligodendroglia, much as peripheral myelin is from Schwann cells (Fig. 8-57).

Seen with the electron microscope, oligodendrocytes are small cells with dense, granulated cytoplasm. Their mitochondria are small and have tu-

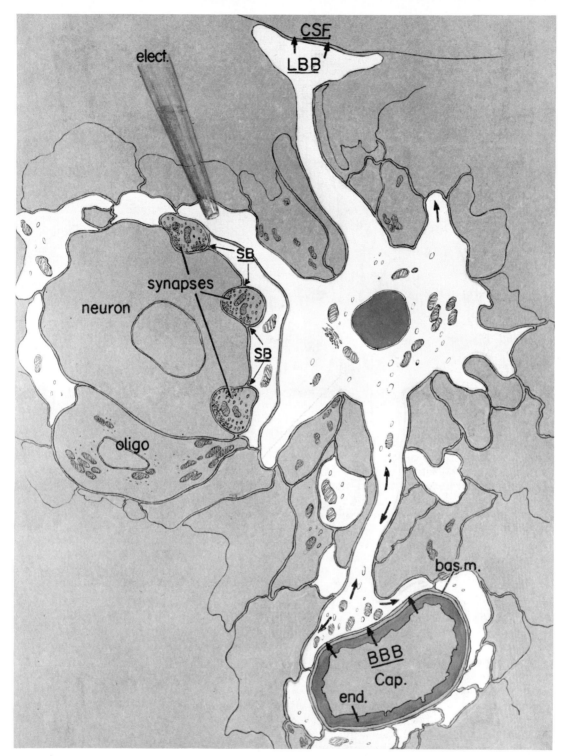

Figure 8-55 Diagram showing the relationships between an astrocyte and other components of the central gray matter. The astrocyte contacts a capillary, the pia-glial membrane, and a nerve cell: Cap, capillary; BBB, blood-brain barrier; end., endothelium; bas. m., basement membrane (basement lamina); oligo, oligodendrocyte; SB, synaptic barriers, LBB, liquor-brain barrier; CSF, cerebrospinal fluid. At ''elect.'' there is an extraneuronal recording microelectrode implanted in the glia. Arrows represent possible movement of fluids and solutes within the cytoplasm. (Courtesy of E. De Robertis and H. M. Gerschenfeld, Int. Rev. Neurobiol., **3:**17, 1961.)

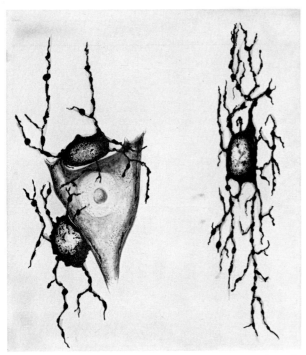

Figure 8-56   Oligodendroglia: on the left, as perineuronal satellites; on the right, stretched along nerve fiber of white matter. Note characteristic swellings (gliosomes) of processes.   (Courtesy of Cowdry, "Special Cytology," Hoeber, New York, 1928.)

bular cristae.   There are densely packed ribosomes, free and attached to endoplasmic reticulum.   Occasionally filaments and a few strands of endoplasmic reticulum are encountered in the cytoplasm. The nuclei are round or oval with clumps of chromatin and occasional small nucleoli.

Microglia are morphologically and developmentally different from other neuroglia (Fig. 8-58). As noted before, they are derived from the mesoderm and appear in the central nervous system toward the end of intrauterine life and during the early days after birth, when the elaboration of the capillary supply of the brain and spinal cord is at its height.   Their major source is the pia mater and the adventitia of blood vessels from whence the cells migrate into the brain and cord by ameboid movements.   Once they reach their final positions, they develop processes which show an increasing affinity for colloidal silver.   The character and arrangement of the processes vary but, in general, are somewhat wavy, gradually thin out distally, and branch one or a few times, with secondary and

further branches.   The processes and the branches are covered with numerous little spines which give them a hairy or thorny appearance.   As in other neuroglia, there is no common stain which reveals both nuclei and processes at the same time.   When nuclear stains are used, the oval, rod-like, or bent nucleus of the microglial cell is more darkly stained and smaller than other glial nuclei.   Until the silver techniques of del Rio Hortega were introduced, the processes and cytoplasm could not be identified in microglia and oligodendroglia, and the nuclei were often spoken of as "naked."   The electron-microscope image of microglia is very distinctive.   Both the nucleus and cytoplasm are exceedingly dense and occasionally phagocytic inclusions can be identified.

Microglia are the "scavengers" or "macrophages" of the central nervous system.   During pathologic states they recover the motility which they originally showed when invading the central nervous system; they retract their processes, become ameboid, and migrate to the site of damage.

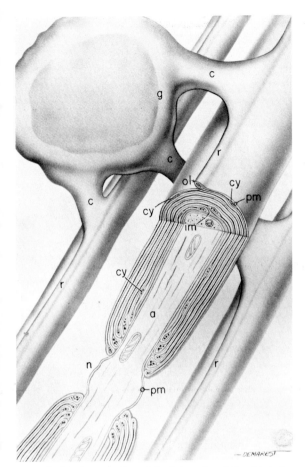

Figure 8-57 Diagram of possible glial-myelin relationship in the central nervous system: g, glial cell; a, axon; n, central node; pm, plasma membrane; im, inner mesaxon; cy, cytoplasm; ol, cytoplasm confined to a loop of plasma membrane, possibly continuous with glial cell by means of connections (c). (Courtesy of M. B. Bunge, R. P. Bunge, and H. Ris, J. Biophys. Biochem. Cytol., **10**:67, 1961.)

In certain circumstances the phagocytic cells and their nuclei are rod-shaped (*Stäbchenzellen*). In intense reactions, such as acute inflammation and hemorrhagic processes, phagocytized leukocytes or erythrocytes and other inclusions can be demonstrated in their cytoplasm.

Ependyma is the epithelium which lines the cavities of the brain and spinal cord. In the early embryo and in adult lower vertebrates, ependymal cells have processes which extend radially to the limiting margin of the neural tube. The processes form a structural network in which other tissues of the nervous system develop. In later embryonic and postembryonic life, the processes do not reach as far. During embryonic development long cilia are formed on the inner ends of the cells. The shapes and processes of ependymal cells vary greatly. Ependyma modified for special functions, for example that of chorioid plexuses, is observed in various localities of the brain. Ependymal cells function in support. Secretory and regenerative functions have also been ascribed to them.

MENINGES

The meninges consist of thin sheets of tissue often containing fibrous connective tissue which completely invest the brain, spinal cord, the optic nerve, and the proximal parts of cranial and spinal nerve roots. They are three in number, the innermost delicate *pia mater,* the overlying cobwebby *arachnoid,* and the outermost dense and thick *dura mater* (Fig. 8-59). Because of their abundant interconnections and basic similarity of structure and origin, the first two (collectively called *leptomeninges*) are sometimes described as a single membrane. The dura mater is mesodermal in origin. The arachnoid and pia are believed to arise from the neural crest and are therefore ectodermal derivatives.

The *dura mater* (*pachymeninx*) is composed predominantly of fibrous connective tissue containing only occasional elastic fibers. It has sensory nerves and blood vessels, but the latter are less abundant than in the leptomeninges. A layer of flat cells constituting a sheet of mesenchymal epithelium forms the inner surface of the dura.

Figure 8-58 Neuroglia cells from brain of rabbit. Microglial cell (above) and oligodendroglia.

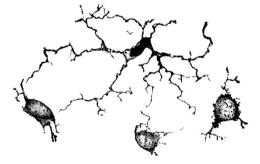

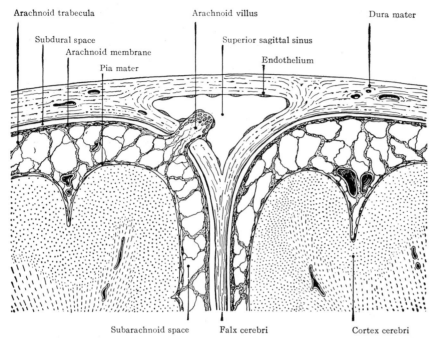

Figure 8-59   Diagram of cross section of dorsomedial region of cerebral hemispheres at the sagittal fissure, showing meninges and the subarachnoid and subdural spaces.   (Courtesy of L. H. Weed, Am. J. Anat., **31:**202, 1923.)

The dura mater, as well as the other meninges, continues over the nerve roots and the sensory ganglia approximately to the origin of the mixed nerve, where it becomes continuous with the connective tissue of the nerve.   The mesothelial surface of the dura is separated from the arachnoid membrane by the subdural space, which contains a thin layer of fluid (Fig. 8-59).

The dura mater of cord and brain is continuous through the foramen magnum, but there is a difference in the dura of these two regions.   The dura of the cord is separated from the internal periosteal lining of the vertebrae by an *epidural space* containing some fat concentrations and blood vessels. The dura of the brain, on the other hand, is inseparably fused with the internal lining of the bones surrounding the cranial cavity, so the epidural space is lacking.   Another point of difference is that here and there the cerebral dura forms reduplications which extend as sheets between the right and left hemispheres (*falx cerebri*), between the cerebrum and cerebellum (*tentorium cerebelli*), and elsewhere.

The term *arachnoid* (following Henle) is commonly applied to the membrane beneath the dura, although by virtue of its numerous filamentous communications with the pia mater it has often in the past been thought of as the outer layer of the pia (Figs. 8-59 and 8-60).   The arachnoid is thin and contains a core of connective tissue which is lined on the inner and outer surface with an epithelium.   Many trabeculae, or pillars, connect the arachnoid and pia, and the cobwebby character which these impart to the arachnoid gives it its name.   The surfaces of the trabeculae are covered with epithelium, and the trabecular cores are filled with connective tissue.   Both the connective tissue and surface epithelium are continuous with those of the arachnoid at one end and the pia at the other.   Between the pia mater and arachnoid is the subarachnoid space, which contains the cerebrospinal fluid.   The subarachnoid space is traversed by the numerous trabeculae which convert it into a swamp-like region through which the cerebrospinal fluid slowly percolates (Fig. 8-60).   The arachnoid follows the contours of the central nervous system more closely than does the dura but much less so than the pia mater, which is intimately applied to the nervous tissue. The arachnoid slips from one prominence to the next, whereas the pia mater faithfully follows the nervous system into each crevice. The subarachnoid space varies considerably in size from one region to another. In regions where it is quite large, the spaces are called *cisterns,* as at the angle between the cerebellum and medulla (*cisterna magna*), where cerebrospinal fluid may be tapped directly with a needle.

The pia mater is a delicate and highly vascular layer through which arteries and veins run to and from the brain and cord. It contains an epithelial surface layer and is bound tightly to the nervous tissue by the numerous feet of astrocytes which attach to it (Fig. 8-55), and therefore it can be separated only with difficulty from the cord and brain. Since the pia mater contains a glial component (the feet of astrocytes), it is sometimes called instead the *pia-glial membrane.* Where arteries dip into the central nervous tissue, they and the perforated nervous tissue are lined for some distance by the pia, which thus encloses a channel around the artery, called the *Virchow-Robin,* or *perivascular, space.* Electron microscopy of the central nervous system has shown a true Virchow-Robin space only around these large blood vessels, not around the smaller blood vessels. Around the latter is a submicroscopic space between the astrocytic end-feet and the vascular wall (Figs. 8-30 and 8-55). The leptomeninges are continuous with the perineural epithelium enclosing peripheral and autonomic nerves.

Another important relation of the meninges of the vascular system is observed for the venous drainage of the brain. Blood is returned by numerous veins which leave the surface of the brain and pour mainly into large venous sinuses located within the dura mater, primarily along the line of its reduplications (for example, along the lines of origin of the falx cerebri and tentorium cerebelli) (Fig. 8-59). The veins open into the sinuses at such an angle that back pressure in the venous system tends to close the orifice between the two and prevent engorgement of the brain with blood. The sinuses drain mainly toward the occipital region of the skull, where they join and finally lead into the internal jugular veins.

In addition to receiving the venous return of the brain, the sinuses of the dura (especially the superior sagittal sinus) also receive cerebrospinal fluid from the subarachnoid space by way of special structures, the *arachnoid villi* (Fig. 8-59). Arachnoid villi are finger-like projections of the subarachnoid space into the venous sinus. They are completely lined by arachnoidal membrane. The dura over the tip of the villi is considerably thinned so that a slight tissue barrier of arachnoid, dura, and venous epithelium separates cerebrospinal fluid and blood; through this barrier cerebrospinal fluid filters into the general circulation. With age, calcium salts are deposited in the connective tissue of the arachnoidal villi. These depositions, called *Pacchio-*

Figure 8-60 Diagram of leptomeninges and cerebral tissue showing the reflection inward of the pia along a blood vessel to form a lining of the perivascular space. Note that the perivascular and subarachnoid spaces are continuous. (Modified from L. H. Weed, Amer. J. Anat., **31**:203, 1923.)

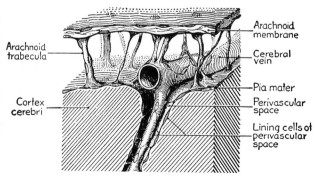

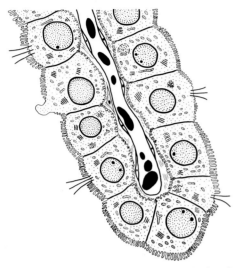

Figure 8-61   Diagram of choroid villus in the choroid plexus of a rabbit.   Cuboidal epithelium surrounds the central capillary separated from it by connective tissue fibrils.   Note cytoplasmic infolding on the basal surface and the brush border of villi and occasional cilia on the ventricular surface.   (From J. W. Millen and G. E. Rogers, J. Biophys. Biochem. Cytol., **2:**408, 1956.)

nian granulations, enlarge greatly and can be readily seen in the dura of the superior sagittal sinus.   As they enlarge, they press against the overlying calvarium, and in response to this pressure, the bone is resorbed and somewhat hollowed.

VENTRICLES AND CHORIOID PLEXUSES

The central nervous system in its development is a tubular structure containing a central cavity (Fig. 8-65).   Although only remnants of the central cavity remain in the adult spinal cord, that of the brain persists and is enlarged in certain regions to form the four *ventricles:* the two *lateral ventricles* within the cerebral hemispheres, the *third ventricle* in the diencephalon, and the *fourth ventricle* of the pons and medulla.   The connections between them are retained in the adult as the *interventricular foramina* (*foramina of Monro*) connecting the lateral ventricles to the third ventricle, and the *aqueduct of Sylvius* (*cerebral aqueduct*) between the third and fourth ventricles.   The ventricles and communicating channels are filled with cerebrospinal fluid. They are lined by ependyma and surrounded by the nervous substance of the brain except in one region

of each ventricle, where there is an absence of nervous tissue so that the ependyma is in direct contact with the pia mater and its blood vessels. This membrane of combined ependyma and pia, the *tela chorioidea,* forms a large part of the roof of the fourth ventricle, where it is somewhat rhomboid in shape.   The lateralmost angle of each side is perforated by an opening, the *foramen of Luschka,* through which cerebrospinal fluid escapes into the subarachnoid space, and some believe that there is a third opening, medially and caudally placed, the *foramen of Magendie.*   The roof of the third ventricle is also formed of a tela, which is continuous anteriorly at the interventricular foramina with the two telae of the lateral ventricles.   The latter telae are thin, pencil-line deficiencies of the medial wall of the cerebral hemispheres, conforming in shape with the ventricles.

In certain regions of the tela chorioidea of each ventricle, the small arteries and capillaries of the pia mater form tufts of vessels which lie within the ventricle, having pushed the tela ahead of them in their development.   The combined invaginated structure of glomerular tufts of vessels and tela chorioidea, called the *chorioid plexus,* produces the cerebrospinal fluid of the ventricles.   The chorioid plexuses of the lateral ventricles are the largest; almost all the tela chorioidea is included in their structure.   The third ventricle has two parallel and inconspicuous plexuses located in its roof.   The plexuses of the fourth ventricle are substantial, located in the lateral recesses of the tela chorioidea near the foramina of Luschka.

The ependymal epithelium of the chorioid plexus is modified (Fig. 8-61); the cells are usually cuboidal and contain fatty droplets, numerous mitochondria, and other inclusions.   The electron microscope shows that the basal surface adjacent to the endothelium is thrown into deep folds; a brush border (Fig. 8-61) consisting of microvilli, containing numerous vesicles and even cilia, has been reported on the ventricular surface.   The cells are active in the transfer of fluid from the blood to the ventricles.   They probably contribute a secretory product of their own, since they have secretory granules and a dense, rough ER.   Nerve fibers have been demonstrated in the chorioid plexus, and endings have been reported on the epithelial cells.

CEREBROSPINAL FLUID

Cerebrospinal fluid is a clear, watery fluid containing some dissolved protein and other organic substances, salt, and a small number of white blood cells. Two major sources have been described for cerebrospinal fluid. A most important one is the contribution from the blood by way of the chorioid plexuses, together with possible secretory contributions from the chorioidal epithelium itself. The cerebrospinal fluid deposited in the ventricles by the chorioid plexuses moves in a definite course. The fluid of the lateral ventricles moves through the interventricular foramina into the third ventricle and, together with the contribution of the chorioid plexus of the third ventricle, through the cerebral aqueduct into the fourth ventricle. The combined contributions from all plexuses leave the brain through the foramina of Luschka, and perhaps Majendie as

Figure 8-62   Drawing of synaptic and glial covering of a motor neuron from spinal cord of cat. Note that the entire somal and dendritic surface and part of the axon at its origin is covered with synaptic end-feet and glial processes. (Courtesy of R. Poritsky, J. Comp. Neurol. **135:**423, 1969.)

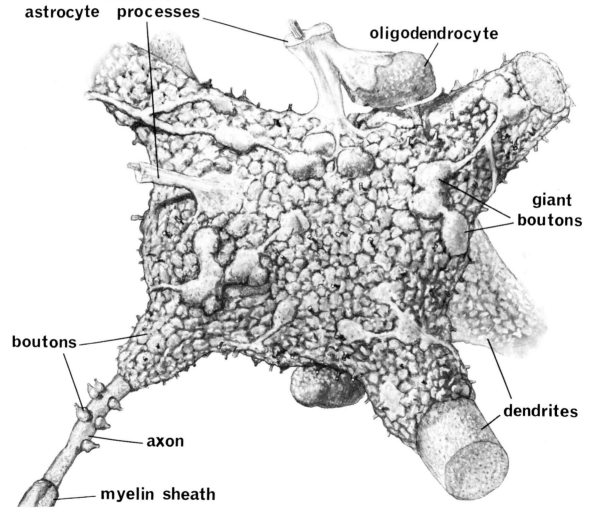

well, and pass into the subarachnoid space. A second source of cerebrospinal fluid is a continuous ooze along the perivascular spaces from the tissue of the brain and the spinal cord directly into the subarachnoid space.

A number of views are held concerning the pathway by which cerebrospinal fluid returns to the general vascular circulation. One means of disposal is through the arachnoid villi into the venous drainage. A supplementary drainage system along the nerve roots into a plexus of veins of this region has been suggested. Communications with the lymphatic system have also been reported, since it is possible to demonstrate by x-ray that material (thorium dioxide) introduced into the subarachnoid spaces of the living animal is transferred rather readily into the cervical lymph nodes. Drainage into the lymphatic system has been suggested to occur also along the endoneurial spaces of the peripheral nerve from the nerve roots. Indeed, as noted above, the leptomeninges and the perineural epithelium are believed to be continuous and to enclose a continuous peripheral flow of cerebrospinal fluid.

BLOOD-BRAIN BARRIER

Certain acid dyes and other compounds bearing negative charge will not penetrate the living brain when injected into the bloodstream, whereas electropositive dyes and other substances will traverse the capillary wall and enter the brain. This selective physiologic barrier, the *blood-brain barrier*, exists in the cerebrum, cerebellum, and medulla. It is not present in the early embryo or in specific areas of the adult brain such as the chorioid plexus itself. In all the areas where there is an active blood-brain barrier, the electron microscope has revealed an intimate contact between astrocytic end-feet and endothelium of blood vessels (Figs. 8-30 and 8-55). Only a 20-nm space that contains a basement membrane but no connective tissue fibrils separates the two elements, whereas in areas with no blood-brain barrier, fibrils are seen in the space around the blood vessels. Coulter suggested that the blood-brain barrier involves a transport mechanism in the astrocytic end-feet which pumps water and certain ions back after they have crossed the capillary wall. Consistent with this hypothesis is the large number of mitochondria concentrated in the astrocyte end-feet that could provide the necessary energy.

Substances that traverse the barrier, including metabolites, are then distributed to the neurons and glia by a pathway which is not yet understood. Some believe the movement is confined to the space between cells; others invoke also transport through glial processes, notably those of the astrocyte. The intercellular spaces in gray and white matter are only about 20 nm wide. Indeed, calculations on the total volume of these extracellular channels shows it to be very small, amounting to about 6 to 10 percent of the total volume.

The autonomic nervous system

The autonomic nervous system, sometimes called the *visceral, interofective,* or *vegetative system,* is concerned with the internal environment and provides a neural mechanism for movements of smooth and cardiac muscle and for glandular secretions. It adjusts internal bodily activities such as blood pressure and flow, cardiac rate, and digestion and maintains a steady state (homeostasis) of the fluids and tissues despite the variability of the demands upon the body. The term *autonomic* is misleading, since it implies autonomous function. Actually a number of centers within the brain and spinal cord govern the activity of this system, and autonomic functions frequently reflect the activity of the highest centers of the brain.

The commonly held conception of the arrangement and connections of the neurons in this system emerged particularly from the physiologic experiments and anatomic descriptions of Langley and Gaskell. Following their views, the autonomic nervous system may be defined as a motor system whose unit of function and structure is a chain of two neurons originating in the central nervous system and extending to involuntary muscle and glands (Fig. 8-64). Although excluded by definition from this system, sensory fibers that mediate visceral sensations accompany the motor fibers in their entire course. The cell body of the first neuron of the motor chain, the *preganglionic neuron* (*general visceral motor* in neuroanatomical literature), is located in a nucleus of the central nervous system where it receives impulses from a variety of sources (Fig. 8-63, see color insert). Its axon, the *preganglionic fiber,* leaves the central nervous system by way of certain cranial nerves and the ventral roots of most spinal nerves and makes its way to internal regions where autonomic ganglia are located. The cell body of the second, or *postganglionic, neuron* is located in an autonomic ganglion where it receives synaptic connections from the first neuron. The axon of the second neuron terminates in an effector organ, such as smooth or cardiac muscle or a gland. The preganglionic axon is invariably larger in diameter than the postganglionic axon and is generally a *white* or myelinated fiber, whereas the postganglionic fiber is a *gray* fiber with little or no myelin.

It should be emphasized here that the preceding description of the arrangement of autonomic neurons is based largely on physiologic evidence. There is ample reason to believe that the true anatomic arrangement is much more complicated and that more neurons may be involved in the chain from the central nervous system to the peripheral organ. In addition, there is evidence for local reflexes that are not mediated through the central nervous system.

There is one notable exception to the rule that the preganglionic fiber synapses with a postganglionic neuron. The adrenal medulla (Fig. 8-63, see

Figure 8-64   Diagramatic section through the spinal cord and a spinal nerve in the thoracic region to illustrate the essential two neuron chains of the autonomic nervous system (in this case, the sympathetic), the system's course to the end organ, and its relation to somatic sensory and motor fibers. (After Ransom-Clark, "Anatomy of the Nervous System," 8th ed. Saunders, Philadelphia, 1947.)

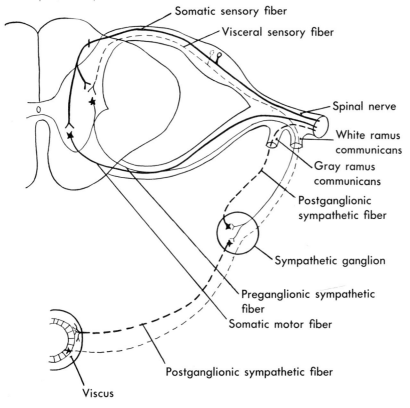

color insert) and other similar *chromaffin tissues* are innervated by sympathetic preganglionic fibers that end directly on secretory cells. By homology, the adrenal medulla and chromaffin tissue constitute a postganglionic segment of the sympathetic system; this homology is based on both embryologic origin and function. Both adrenal medulla cells and sympathetic postganglionic neurons originate in the neural crest or neural tube and migrate to their definitive positions along the outgrowing preganglionic fibers, and both receive the terminations of these fibers. They differ in their specialization, for the sympathetic preganglionic tissue develops nerve processes and the adrenal medulla cells become special secretory cells. Nevertheless, the homology extends even here, to their chemical functions; the postganglionic neurons secrete norepinephrine as their chemical mediator, and the adrenal medulla cells secrete epinephrine, and the two hormones have similar effects on smooth muscle and glands—the one by nervous and the other by hormonal stimulation.

The two divisions of the autonomic system, sympathetic and parasympathetic (Fig. 8-63, see color insert), are distinguished from one another anatomically and physiologically. First, they differ in the locations of the cell bodies and axons of the preganglionic neurons. Parasympathetic preganglionic cell bodies are located in one of four nuclei of the brain stem (*dorsal motor nucleus of nerve X, superior and inferior salivatory nucleus of nerves VII and IX*, and the *Edinger-Westphal nucleus of nerve III*), and in the lateral horn of gray substance of the second, third, and sometimes the fourth sacral segments of the spinal cord; their axons leave via these four cranial and two (or three) sacral spinal nerves, so the parasympathetic system is often called the *craniosacral division* of the autonomic nervous system. In contrast, the sympathetic system is called the thoracolumbar division, because its preganglionic cell bodies are located in the lateral horns of all the thoracic segments of the cord and the upper two or three lumbar segments, and their axons leave via these spinal nerves.

A second difference between these two subdivisions concerns the location of their postganglionic cell bodies. Sympathetic ones are located in ganglionic accumulations of the sympathetic chain (*vertebral ganglia*) and in some ganglia, such as the celiac or superior mesenteric ganglia, located in plexuses close to the organ of innervation (Fig. 8-63, see color insert). There is no chain system for the parasympathetic system, and except in the head region, the ganglia are less discrete and more scattered (Fig. 8-63, see color insert). Indeed, in visceral regions, postganglionic parasympathetic cell bodies are found very close to or within the wall of the organ that is innervated (Fig. 8-25D, see color insert) and may be identified in sections through the intestinal tract, the stomach, the heart, and other visceral structures. The cell bodies, unmistakably characterized by large, round or oval nuclei with prominent nucleoli, lie within a plexus of nerves.

A further difference between the two systems is that sympathetic postganglionic fibers are also distributed to smooth muscles and glands of somatic (nonvisceral) regions; no comparable distribution has been established for the parasympathetic division. There is also the fact that preganglionic sympathetic fibers divide more frequently and thereby tend to synapse with many postganglionic neurons, whereas there is more of a 1:1 ratio between pre- and postganglionic neurons in the parasympathetic system.

Finally, there are a few structures that are innervated by the sympathetics alone (such as the sweat glands and the nictitating membrane of the cat's eye) but none innervated by the parasympathetics alone. In general, structures innervated by the autonomic system receive a dual innervation from the parasympathetics and sympathetics, however, and the two systems tend to oppose each other, one being stimulatory, the other inhibitory. Some examples that may be cited are the influence on the heart, the coronary vessels, and the intestinal tract. Sympathetic activity is reflected in increased heart rate, dilatation of coronary vessels, and decrease in motility of the intestinal tract. These responses reflect the needs of the body during emergency states of high physical or emotional response. In contrast, the parasympathetics decrease the heart rate, increase the motility of the gut, and constrict the coronary vessels, thus initiating rest and conservation of body energy. There are a few instances where the activities of the two divisions appear to be supplementary rather than antagonistic; for example, secretion by the salivary glands is greater with stimulation by both than with either alone.

The sympathetic system evokes a more widespread and generalized response; for example, upon discharge of the sympathetics, increased blood pressure and heart rate and decreased intestinal motility may occur all at once, since each preganglionic fiber synapses with many postganglionic neurons, each of which may control a different end organ. The sympathetic response is also widespread because the synaptic transmitter given off at sympathetic endings, norepinephrine, escapes into the blood and is carried to various regions of the body, and because this effect is supplemented by the simultaneous secretion of epinephrine into the blood by the adrenal medulla.

By contrast, the parasympathetics are more discrete in their action because there is more of a 1 : 1 relation between pre- and postganglionic neurons. Moreover, there is no reinforcing mechanism comparable to that for the sympathetics. Finally, the stimulating substance given off by parasympathetic fibers, acetylcholine, is rapidly destroyed at the synapse and in the blood by an enzyme (cholinesterase) which thus prevents its diffusion elsewhere.

HISTOLOGY OF THE AUTONOMIC NERVOUS SYSTEM

Autonomic ganglia consist chiefly of multipolar nerve cells, smaller than those of the spinal or cranial ganglia, though a few unipolar and bipolar cells are also present. They resemble other nerve cells in the character of their nuclei and cytoplasm and often contain pigment. The neurofibrils are slender and arranged in a fine net, and the Nissl substance consists of small, ill-defined bodies (Fig. 8-25D, see color insert). The endoplasmic reticulum is usually in the form of dispersed vesicles and cisternae. In neurons of autonomic ganglia, dense inclusions, possible secretory, have been described. These have also been described in autonomic nerve fibers, particularly at their efferent endings (Fig. 8-36). Unlike the cells of the spinal ganglia, those of the autonomic are incompletely encapsulated. In some instances the dendrites ramify beneath this capsule, where they form an open network, either uniformly distributed or grouped at one side of the cell. The dendrites mingle with axons from other cells which pierce the capsule, and the mass of interlacing dendrites and fibers is known as a "glomerulus." The axons of these postganglionic neurons, as noted before, are usually unmyelinated. In the plexuses within the walls of visceral organs, the cell bodies are scattered in small groups and may be readily identified after ordinary methods of staining (Fig. 8-25D, see color insert). The axons in such preparations may be visible as fine dots or lines associated with occasional Schwann nuclei.

Electron-microscope studies of postganglionic autonomic fibers show their essential similarity to other peripheral unmyelinated fibers (Fig. 8-24). Numerous axons (usually more than in sensory nerves) share one Schwann cell. The axons are typically enfolded by the Schwann cell cytoplasm, and frequently two or more axons are seen sharing the same mesaxon. Vesicles containing dense granules varying in size (approximately 10 to 100 nm) have been reported within various autonomic fibers in addition to multivesicular bodies and the usual axonal organelles such as neurofilaments, elongated mitochondria, and clear vesicles. These dense granules have also been described in fine-structural studies of autonomic endings on smooth muscles and glands and presynaptic endings in autonomic ganglia (Fig. 8-36).

Autonomic nerve endings on smooth muscles differ from those on striated muscles by the absence of junctional folds of the sarcolemma and an interposed basement membrane (Fig. 8-36). There is an intimate contact between axon and muscle, with a separation sometimes of only 20 nm between the two. The axon divests itself of its schwannian element and its terminal end is swollen; the swelling sits in a shallow pocket formed of the smooth muscle plasma membrane.

CHEMICAL MEDIATION OF THE NERVE IMPULSE

It is now known, through the experiments of Loewi and others, that the nerve impulse is mediated at autonomic synapses and at other terminations by chemical transmitters. In the autonomic synapses and all vertebrate effector endings other than most of the sympathetic ones, the transmitter is acetylcholine. In the sympathetic endings, norepinephrine is the transmitter; in a few exceptions, such as the endings on sweat glands, acetylcholine is secreted instead.   On the basis of such differences, physiologists have classified effector fibers into two groups: *cholinergic* (producing acetylcholine) and *adrenergic* (producing epinephrine).   Associated with the mechanism of acetylcholine production is an enzyme, *cholinesterase,* which rapidly hydrolyses acetylcholine and ensures that prolonged action of the mediator does not occur.   There is no comparable system of rapid destruction for the chemical mediator of adrenergic fibers, which escapes into the blood and is carried elsewhere to stimulate other organs, a fact which accounts in part for the widespread nature of sympathetic stimulation.

Development of the nervous system

The nervous system arises in the young embryo as a thickened region of the dorsal surface ectoderm along the median plane (Fig. 8-65). By continued proliferation and differential growth, beginning anteriorly and proceeding backward, the *neural plate* folds along its median axis into a *neural (medullary) groove* or *furrow,* which is formed in front of the primitive knot and appears in cross section as a median dorsal depression. By coalescence of its dorsal edges, the groove becomes a tube, which gradually becomes completely separated from the epidermal layer of the ectoderm. For a time, the tube opens to the exterior both anteriorly, at the *anterior neuropore,* and posteriorly, at the *posterior neuropore,* but eventually these neuropores close and the tube is then detached from the epidermal layer.

As the tube is formed, a line of cells extending fore-and-aft along the tube at the region of closure of the folds separates from the remaining neurectoderm. The *neural crest,* as it is called, is present dorsally on each side of the tube (Fig. 8-65C). Periodic enlargements along its length, corresponding with body segments, give the crest a fluted appearance. From these enlargements the spinal ganglia, their satellite cells, and the Schwann cells arise (Fig. 8-65). The sympathetic ganglia, the adrenal medulla, and other related chromaffin

Figure 8-65   The development of the nervous system as seen in cross sections of rabbit embryos: A. 7½ days; B. 8½ days; C. 9 days; D. 10½ days; E. 14 days: c.c, central cavity; d.r, dorsal root; d. ra, dorsal ramus; ep., ependymal layer; g.c, ganglion cells; g.l, gray layer; m.g, medullary groove; m.t, medullary tube; o.b, oval bundle; s.g, sympathetic ganglion; sp.g, spinal ganglion; s.ra, sympathetic ramus; v.r, ventral root; v.ra, ventral ramus; w.l, white layer.

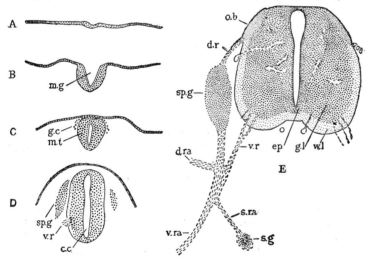

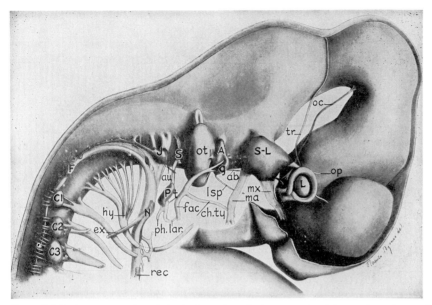

Figure 8-66   A reconstruction of the brain and cerebral nerves of a 12-mm pig embryo.   Olfactory (not shown); optic (fibers in the stalk of the eye, the lens of which is marked L); oculomotor, oc; trochlear, tr; trigeminal, semilunar ganglion, S-L; ophthalmic, op; maxillary, mx; mandibular, ma; abducent, ab; facial, geniculate ganglion, g; large superficial petrosal, lsp; chorda tympani, ch.ty; facial, fac; acoustic, a; supplying the otocyst, ot; glossophayngeal, superior, S, and petrosal, P, ganglia; tympanic, t; lingual, lar; pharyngeal, ph; vagus, jugular, J, and nodose, N, ganglia; auricular, au; laryngeal, rec being the recurrent nerve; the main stem proceeds to the abdomen; accessory, internal ramus joining the vagus and the external ramus, ex; hypoglossal, hy; Froriep's rudimentary hypoglossal ganglion, F, sometimes sends fibers to the hypoglossal nerve. C1, C2, C3: first, second, and third cervical ganglia.   (Reconstruction made by F. T. Lewis.)

tissue also arise from the neural crest; the neural tube itself has been described as a supplementary or alternative source.   In Amphibia the neural crest is also the source of pigment cells.

The anterior part of the neural tube expands to form the brain; the posterior part grows caudally to form the spinal cord (Fig. 8-66).   As development proceeds, the anterior region, by differential enlargement, becomes subdivided into the three primary regions of the brain and later into further divisions.   The detailed morphogenesis of the central nervous system does not fall within the scope of the present chapter.   It is sufficient here to give a brief description of the histogenesis of the central, peripheral, and autonomic nervous systems.

Very early in development the cells of the medullary tube which border upon its lumen or central canal proliferate markedly, causing the tube to thicken.   In the floor and roof of the tube a corresponding thickening fails to take place, as shown in Fig. 8-65E.

The lateral walls of the tube become divisible very early into three layers.   The inner layer consists of germinal, or proliferating, cells and is prominent only in the embryo.   In the adult it becomes reduced to a single layer of cells which lines the central canal like a simple epithelium to constitute the *ependyma*.   The middle, or *mantle, layer* is composed of cells derived from the germinal layer, and in the adult it constitutes the gray substance of the cord.   The outer, or *marginal, layer* is at first entirely free of nuclei; later it contains only a few, belonging to the neuroglia and to the endothelium of vessels which come to penetrate the central nervous system.   In later development, axis cylinders invade this layer in great abundance and form tracts.   The marginal layer becomes the white substance of the cord and brain stem as the tracts are myelinated.   The cells of the middle layer undergo a period of rapid multiplication after which differentiation sets in to form the nuclear centers.   The cells may differentiate in one of two directions, as

axon, which thus appears as the first process of the developing neuron. As the axon continues its growth, the dendritic processes make their appearance. The axonal process appears to advance by formation of a pseudopodia growth cone which spins out the fiber behind it (Fig. 8-68). As a result of the ameboid activity of the growth cone, it extends farther and farther from its cell body. In its advance it forms many sprouts, some of which are resorbed while others persist and enlarge. Coincident with the appearance of the cytoplasmic process and apparently associated with its elaboration is a rapid differentiation of the Nissl material and the nucleolus. There is also an increase in protein synthesis and an enlargement of the nucleus. Fine structural studies reveal numerous tubules about 30 to 500 nm thick, running longitudinally within the developing fibers. Once growth is initiated, the axon elongates at a very rapid rate (Fig. 8-67). Some axons grow toward other developing neurons of the gray substance of the same or opposite side and shortly make connections, at which time electrical activity can be recorded in the nervous system. Other axons enter the marginal layer and ascend or descend in tracts within the forming framework of glial processes. Their destinations are the neurons of developing nuclei at other levels of the nervous system in the brain or the cord. Finally, some axons traverse the marginal layer somewhat obliquely and leave the brain or cord to form one of the motor roots of cranial or spinal nerves (Fig. 8-67). Except for a small number which terminate on ganglion cells of the autonomic nervous system, they form motor endings on developing striated muscle. In all peripheral nerves, Schwann cells travel along the nerve fibers from the neural crest, proliferating as they migrate along the axon and its branches.

In the brain there is a considerable alteration and distortion of the three-layer arrangement described for the cord, owing to the shift of developing nuclear centers. Nuclear concentrations become intermingled with major areas of white substance and, indeed, in the elaboration of the cerebral cortex, they come to lie peripheral to the major fiber tracts.

Neuroblasts which arise from the neural crest and develop into sensory ganglion cells are at first round; then they become bipolar by sending out two

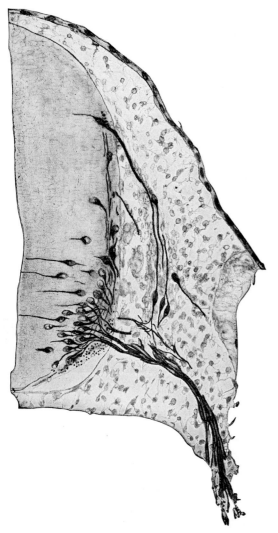

Figure 8-67 A cross section of a 10-mm pig embryo showing the formation of neuroblasts in the medullary tube and adjacent ganglion. (Held.)

neuroglia or as neuroblasts. The neuroglia cells develop processes which initially extend radially from the central cavity of the neural tube to the external limit. Other processes run in various directions and form a meshwork in which the nerve cells are held.

The neuroblasts which appear in the mantle layer become somewhat pear-shaped by the growth of a process usually directed toward the periphery (Fig. 8-67). The process elongates and becomes the

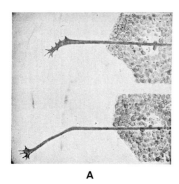 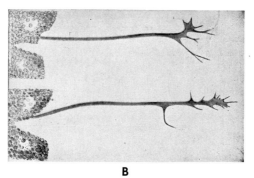

A   B

Figure 8-68   The growth of nerves in tissue cultures.   A. Two views of the same nerve fiber taken 25 min apart, during which time the fiber has grown 20 μm.   B. Two views of another fiber, at lower magnification, taken 50 min apart.   (Harrison.)

processes from opposite ends of the cell, one toward the periphery and the other toward the neural tube (Figs. 8-69 and 8-70).   With further growth, the bipolar condition becomes unipolar in higher vertebrates; the nucleated cell body grows to one side to unite the two processes at their origin into a single slender stalk (Fig. 8-69).   Such T-shaped axons are characteristic of adult spinal and cranial ganglia cells, with the exception of the acoustic ganglion neurons which retain the primitive bipolar condition seen in all sensory ganglia of lower vertebrates.   The process which grows into the neural tube generally divides into an ascending and descending branch.   The descending branch makes connections with nuclei at a lower level, while the ascending branch terminates in a nucleus of a higher level of the cord or brain.   The peripheral fibers of the ganglia grow outward through the mesenchyme and terminate freely or in developing sensory receptors.   In their course they may accompany motor fibers to form the mixed spinal or cranial nerves.   Other cells of the neural crest form

the much smaller satellite cells which come to encapsulate each ganglion cell.

The neuroblasts destined for autonomic ganglia migrate along the outgrowing preganglionic motor fibers to their final position.   They elaborate their (postganglionic) axons, which grow to a terminus in smooth muscle or glands.

Myelination of fibers in man begins in about the fourth or fifth month of intrauterine life, at a time when the major tracts of the central nervous system and the peripheral nerve pattern are well advanced.   It begins on fibers of the ventral roots, first in the medulla and upper cervical region and then elsewhere.   It spreads proximally along the motor roots into the central nervous system and distally along the peripheral nerve.   The dorsal roots are soon involved, then the tracts of the central nervous system.   According to Langworthy (1933), myelination is initiated, with some exceptions, in the oldest systems of the brain and cord, phylogenetically speaking.   Tracts which have evolved most recently, such as those of the cerebral hemispheres, are myelinated last.   Myelination is a slow process and is not completed until approximately the twenty-fifth year or later.

The process of myelination and the relation which Schwann cells bear to it has been observed in vivo by Speidel (1933) in the peripheral nerves of the tail of the tadpole.   Schwann cells accompany the axis cylinder in its peripheral growth and divide to supply the divisions of the main stem. They may pass from one fiber to an adjacent one. Eventually the Schwann cell ceases its movement and divisions, and the myelin-Schwann sheath

Figure 8-69   Spinal ganglion cells.   The upper bipolar forms are from a chick embryo incubated 6 days.   The lower one shows the later monopolar form (T cell).

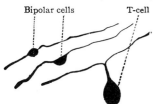

Bipolar cells   T-cell

from one individual to the next are remarkable. Various theories or combinations of them have been advanced to explain the forces which specify the pattern of fiber growth and direct the fiber to its synaptic site. The theories may be grouped in various categories: electrical, chemical, and mechanical. The electrical theory holds that electrical potential differences which guide the fiber exist between the outgrowing fiber and the surrounding tissue. The chemical theory reasons that chemical gradients direct the outgrowing fiber along prescribed lines and that fibers of various chemical specificities respond differently to the chemical milieu of a region. The mechanical theory, in its older sense, arose from the observation that nerves lie in fascial planes between organs, suggesting that structured pathways exist between developing organs to guide growing fibers to their destination. It is more evident in recent years that the advance of the fiber is governed by a number of factors rather than any single one. Weiss (1955) has advanced the principle of ''contact guidance'' on the basis of tissue culture and other experiments, whereby the protein micellae of the submicroscopic structural framework in the ground substance of embryonic tissue provide a physical and chemical pathway to guide the fibers according to their individual specificities. The orientation and other characteristics of the micellae are laid down by an actively growing region and its developing tissues. Weiss observed that growing axons of neuroblasts cultured on a plasma clot ordinarily grow out radially in all directions; but if the plasma is stroked in one direction during clotting so the fibrin molecules are preferentially oriented, the axons of neuroblasts subsequently transplanted to the clot follow the stroke lines in their outwandering. In elaborating this hypothesis further, he speaks of three stages in the development of nerve patterns. There is first the outgrowth of *pioneering* fibers which follow the pattern of the ground substance according to the schema described above. The second phase is that of application, in which the pioneering fibers make appropriate terminations and, once attached, elongate according to the growth of the peripheral structure. Then there is the phase of *appositional growth* by which other and later fibers follow the pioneering fiber. The reason certain fibers will follow preferentially one particular pathway and others

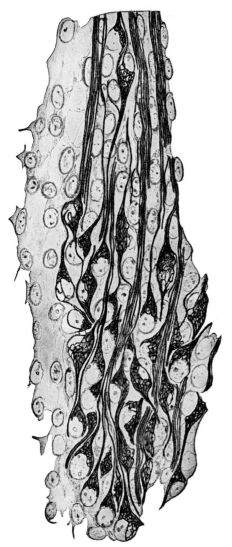

Figure 8-70   A longitudinal section of a spinal ganglion of a 17-mm pig embryo showing the bipolar nature of the early sensory cells.   Note the neurofibrils.   To the left are developing connective tissue cells.   Cajal's silver method.   (Held.)

differentiates.   The sheath spreads in both directions along the fiber to form the internodal segment.

A major neuroembryologic problem as yet unsolved concerns the forces which direct the axis cylinder along a particular pathway and eventually to an appropriate synaptic site. The orderliness and similarity in the pattern of nerves and tracts

another one cannot be explained beyond certain generalities. Nor is there an adequate explanation of the selectivity of termination whereby fibers of particular modalities of sensation find appropriate sensory receptors and motor fibers find a particular muscle. It is known that sensory or motor fibers fail to form endings when caused to grow respectively to motor or sensory end organs.

THE NEURON DOCTRINE

It is now commonly accepted that the cell body and all its cytoplasmic processes develop from and constitute a single cellular unit. This statement, known as the neuron doctrine, was established in the studies of many neurobiologists of the nineteenth and early twentieth centuries and was the center of considerable controversy for many years. Among the alternative views and their variants was the idea that the cytoplasmic processes represent a series of chain-like contributions from cells along the course of the axis cylinder, for example, from sheath cells or mesodermal elements. Another view was that the nervous system is a diffuse network of structurally continuous fibers and not one of individual cells and their processes. One of the critical experiments which resolved the problem in favor of the view that the neuron is a genetic, morphologic, and functional unit was the classical experiment of Harrison (1910) who cultured fragments of the medullary tube of tadpoles in lymph at a stage when the tube consists entirely of round cells. After a day or two he observed the actual outgrowth of the axis cylinder from the cell body (Fig. 8-68), thus confirming what His had long maintained from his studies of the embryo. Harrison's study on the neuron also introduced the method of tissue culture.

References

ADAMS, C. W. M.: "Neurohistochemistry," Elsevier, Amsterdam, 1965.

BARONDES, S. H. (ed.): Cellular Dynamics of the Neuron," vol. 8, Symposia of International Documents for Cell Biology, Academic Press, New York, 1969.

BARRNETT, R. J.: The Fine Structural Localization of Acetylcholinesterase at the Myoneural Junction, *J. Cell. Biol.*, **12**:247 (1962).

BODIAN, D.: The Generalized Vertebrate Neuron, *Science*, **137**:323 (1962).

BODIAN, D.: Cytological Aspects of Synaptic Function, *Physiol. Rev.*, **22**:146 (1942).

BOURNE, G. H.: "The Structure and Function of Nerve Tissue," Academic Press, New York, 3 vols., 1968, 1969.

BUNGE, M. B., R. P. BUNGE, and G. D. PAPPAS: Electron Microscopic Demonstration of Connections between Glia and Myelin Sheaths in the Developing Mammalian Central Nervous System, *J. Cell. Biol.*, **12**:448 (1962).

CAJAL, S. RAMON Y.: "Degeneration and Regeneration of the Nervous System," translated and edited by R. M. May, 2 vols., London, Oxford University Press, 1928.

DE ROBERTIS, E.: "Histophysiology of Synapses and Neurosecretion," Pergamon, New York, 1964.

DE ROBERTIS, E., and H. M. GERSCHENFELD: Submicroscopic Morphology and Function of Glial Cells, *Int. Rev. Neurobiol.*, **3**:1 (1961).

ECCLES, J. C.: "The Physiology of Synapses," Springer-Verlag, Berlin, 1964.

ELFVIN, L. G.: The Ultrastructure of the Nodes of Ranvier in Cat Sympathetic Nerve Fiber, *J. Ultrastruct. Res.*, **5**:374 (1961).

ERLANGER, J., and H. S. GASSER: "Electrical Signs of Nervous Activity," Johnson Foundation Lectures, Philadelphia, 1937.

GEREN, B. B.: Formation from the Schwann Cell Surface of Myelin in the Peripheral Nerves of Chick Embryos, *Exp. Cell Res.*, **7**:323 (1954).

GRAY, E. J.: Tissue of the Central Nervous System, S. M. Kurtz (ed.), "Electron Microscopic Anatomy," Chap. 15, Academic Press, New York, 1964.

GRAY, E. G., and V. P. WHITTAKER: The Isolation of Nerve Endings from Brain: An Electron Microscopic Study of Cell Fragments Derived by Homogenization and Centrifugation, J. Anat., 96:79 (1962).

HARRISON, R. G.: Neuroblast Versus Sheath Cell in the Development of Peripheral Nerves, J. Comp. Neurol., 37:123 (1924).

HARRISON, R. G.: The Outgrowth of the Nerve Fiber as a Mode of Protoplasmic Movement, J. Exp. Zool., 9:787 (1910).

HELLER, H., and R. B. CLARK (eds): "Neurosecretion. A Symposium of Society for Endocrinology," Academic Press, New York, 1962.

HYDÉN, H.: "The Neuron," Elsevier, Amsterdam, 1967.

HYDÉN.: The Neuron, in J. Brachet and A. E. Mirsky (eds.), "The Cell," vol. IV, p. 215, Academic Press, 1960.

KATZ, B.: "The Release of Neural Transmitter Substances," Charles C Thomas, Springfield, Ill., 1969.

KATZ, B.: "Muscle and Synapse," McGraw-Hill, New York, 1966.

LANGWORTHY, O. R.: Development of Behavior Patterns and Myelinization of the Nervous System in the Human Fetus and Infant, Contrib. Embryol., 24(139):1, (1933).

NAKAI, J.: "Morphology of Neuroglia," Charles C Thomas, Springfield, Ill., 1963.

NAUTA, W. J. H., and S. O. E. EBBESON: "Contemporary Research Methods in Neuroanatomy," Springer-Verlag, Berlin, 1970.

PENFIELD, W. (ed.): "Cytology and Cellular Pathology of the Nervous System," 3 vols., Paul B. Hoeber, Inc., New York, 1932.

PETERS, A., S. L. PALAY, and H. DE F. WEBSTER: "The Fine Structure of the Nervous System, the Cells and Their Processes," Harper and Row, New York, 1970.

RODAHL, K., and B. ISSEKUTZ: "Nerve as a Tissue," Harper & Row, New York, 1966.

SCHMITT, F. O., and R. S. BEAR: The Ultrastructure of the Nerve Axon Sheath, Biol. Rev., 14:27 (1939).

SINGER, M., and J. P. SCHADÉ (eds.): Mechanisms in Neural Regeneration, in "Progress in Brain Research," vol. 13, Elsevier, Amsterdam, 1964.

SPEIDEL, C. C.: Studies of Living Nerves: II. Activities of Amoeboid Growth Cones, Sheath Cells, and Myelin Segments, as Revealed by Prolonged Observation of Individual Nerve Fibers in Frog Tadpoles, Amer. J. Anat., 52:1 (1933).

VAN DER LOOS, H.: Fine Structure of Synapses in the Cerebral Cortex, Z. Zellforsch., 60:815 (1963).

WAELSCH, H. (ed.): "Biochemistry of the Developing Nervous System," Academic Press, New York, 1955.

WEDDELL, G., E. PALMER, and W. PALLIE: Nerve Endings in Mammalian Skin, Biol. Rev., 30:159 (1955).

WEISS, P. A.: Nervous System (Neurogenesis), in B. H. Willier, P. A. Weiss, and V. Hamburger (eds.), "Analysis of Development," pp. 346–401, W. B. Saunders, Philadelphia, 1955.

chapter 9

The cardio-vascular system

EDWARD H. BLOCH
AND
ROBERT S.
McCUSKEY

GENERAL CHARACTERISTICS OF THE CARDIOVASCULAR SYSTEM

The structure of the cardiovascular system indicates its functions, which are to circulate the blood, to bring it close to the cells of organs, and to provide a semipermeable membrane for the transit of selected substances between the blood and cells. The cardiac muscle provides the major force for circulating the blood, and this force is supplemented by the elastic tissue in the major arteries. The circulation is maintained in its circuit back to the heart by contraction of the smooth muscle in vessels of the venous system; by valves which assure unidirectional flow; by differences in the intravascular pressures between the arterial and venous systems; and by extravascular forces that affect the circulation, such as the contraction of skeletal muscle in the limbs and of smooth muscle in organs like the intestine, and by pressures produced in the thoracic and abdominal cavities owing to movement of the diaphragm and contraction of the anterior abdominal wall. Close apposition is assured be-

tween the blood and cells of organs by circulating the blood through vessels whose internal diameters are about the size of a single red cell (approximately 8 μm) and these vessels are arranged in a pattern which brings nearly every parenchymatous cell of an organ next to a blood vessel. Moreover, these vessels provide an enormous surface area across which materials may be exchanged with cells. An appreciation may be gained for the area that is available by considering the number of vessels in human skeletal muscle. There are about two thousand capillaries in one square millimeter of muscle, and in a 150-lb man, 6,300 square meters of surface area are available for exchange. (Such a maximum area would be called into play under the most extreme muscular effort.) The exchange is controlled by the response of endothelium, a semipermeable tissue which lines all blood vessels including the heart. In short, endothelium characterizes the cardiovascular system just as the neuron characterizes the nervous system.

The dimensions, contents, and responses of mi-

315

croscopic blood vessels can be examined in most organs in experimental animals and in some sites in man. The most striking difference in the living microvascular system, as compared to histologic sections, is that the vessels are the most noticeable structures since they occupy a much larger area of tissue than postvitally because of the volume, color, and movement of the blood. For example, in the mammalian liver the sinusoids occupy almost half the volume of the organ (Fig. 9-1e), and in the frog lung the capillaries may compose more than two-thirds of an alveolus (Fig. 9-1a and b). In contrast to the lung of the frog, the vascularity and the number of red blood cells in a capillary are considerably less in the mammalian lung (rabbit and rat), as illustrated in Fig. 9-1c and d. Differences in the number of vessels located in endocrine and exocrine glands are also striking. In the pancreas, for example, capillaries abut several sides of each endocrine cell in the islets, whereas in the exocrine tissue only the base of each acinar cell is in contact with a capillary. Furthermore, the dynamic morphology of the flow of the formed elements of the blood and their relationship to the vessel wall and to each other can be determined by in vivo microscopy. For example, in health all the formed elements of the blood exist as individual cells that do not adhere either to each other or to the endothelium (Fig. 9-1a to i). The formed elements are well intermingled with each other so that neither leukocytes nor platelets are preferentially located in a specific part of the flowing bloodstream. (The presence of numerous leukocytes or platelets adjacent to a vessel wall is known as *margination* and indicates pathology.) It has also been established that the shape of erythrocytes and their relationship to each other in the arterial and venous systems are not only complex (Fig. 9-1g to i) but also change rapidly, that is, within a fraction of a second (Fig. 9-1h and i).

The structural characteristics of the cardiovascular system make it both a communicating and an integrating system because the circulating blood ensures that metabolites that are produced by the cells are distributed (communication) at rates that are sufficient to maintain adequate functions (integration); the latter process, of course, is aided by the nervous system. Thus, the cardiovascular and nervous systems are dependent on each other, as both are involved in communication and integration.

For descriptive purposes, morphologically and functionally, the cardiovascular system is divided into a gross and a micro system. The gross system consists of the heart and all the vessels that can be identified by direct inspection; the microvascular system requires magnification for identification of its vessels.

GENERAL FACTS ABOUT THE MICROVASCULAR SYSTEM

Of approximately 1.2×10^9 vessels in the human body, over 99 percent are counted as part of the microvascular system, leaving only about four thousand in the gross vascular system. Most of the

Figure 9-1 Vascular morphology of the living microvascular system. (From E. H. Bloch, 1955 to 1970.) [Unless noted otherwise all figures are single frames from 16-mm motion picture film taken at 16 to 24 frames per second (fps).] Arrows indicate the direction of blood flow. Size markers equal 10 μm. a. Alveolus (frog). The rapidity of flow is indicated by the streak lines (S). Red cell (R) is momentarily caught on the bifurcation of a capillary. E, epithelial cell. b. Alveolus (frog). Although cytoplasmic inclusions (C), nucleus (N), and the plasmalemma (P) of the alveolar epithelial cells can be identified readily, the cytoplasm of the endothelial cells is so thin that it cannot be differentiated from the plasmalemma of the epithelial cells. c. Alveolus (rabbit). The capillaries are considerably wider than the red blood cells, which measure approximately 6.5 μm. In spite of the slow flow, the shapes of the red cells differ (compare with Fig. 9-1 g, h, and i). d. Alveolus (rat). Although the rate of flow was roughly similar to that in the alveolus of the rabbit (Fig. 9-1c), the capillaries are barely wider than the erythrocytes, in contrast to those depicted in the rabbit (Fig. 9-1c). Note the paucity of the red blood cells and the platelets (P). (Both the linear velocity of flow and concentration of red blood cells in the alveolar capillaries vary considerably; the flow can be so rapid that no cells can be distinguished at recording rates of 24 fps or it can appear that the capillary is filled completely with cells.) e. Liver (mouse). (35-mm frame: 1/500 sec.) Each hepatic cell abuts two sinusoids, and each sinusoid (S) is a cylinder with a different diameter. A bile canaliculus (B) lies just above a plate of hepatic cells. f and g. A 30-μm arteriole and derivative capillary in the mesentery of a frog. Part f illustrates the pattern of flow as visualized by the observer or recorded at ordinary motion-picture framing rates. The cellular orientation is determinable when recorded with high-speed cinephotography, in this case at 3,700 fps, Fig. 9-1 g, h, and i. A 12-μm arteriole in the mesentery of a rat. The images were secured at 3,000 fps. Note the orientation of the erythrocytes and the differences in the orientation of the blood cells between the two illustrations; the elapsed time between the two images was less than 0.02 sec.

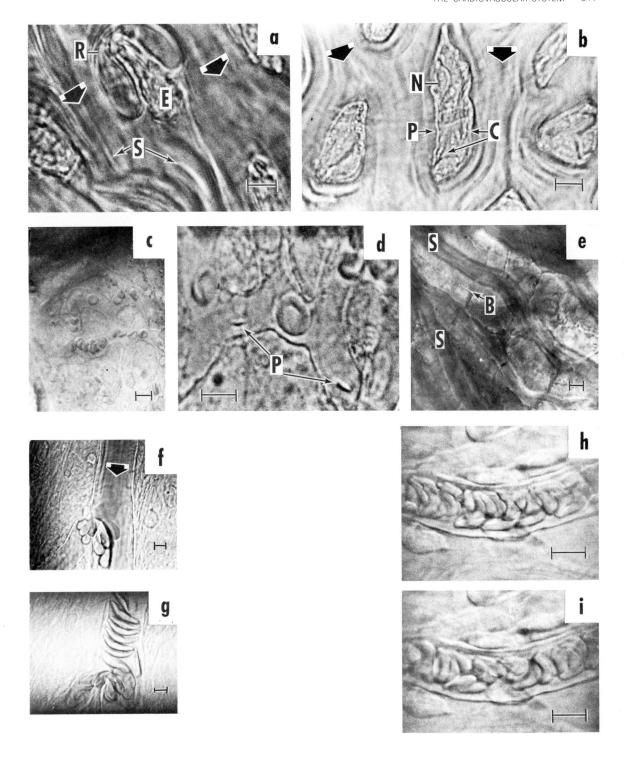

microvasculature consists of *arterioles, capillaries, and venules*. In addition, there are two other types of vessel that shunt blood from arterioles to venules. *The arteriovenous anastomoses* are structurally similar to arterioles, less than 300 μm in diameter, and relatively short. They contain epithelioid cells in their media layers that look like smooth muscle cells but are larger, contain fewer myofibrils, and have more lightly staining nuclei. Furthermore, they are usually open only for short periods. They contrast to the *thoroughfare* or *preferential channels* which are similar to capillaries and function like them but have blood flowing through them continuously. In addition, liver, spleen, and bone marrow contain *sinusoids* which function like capillaries but usually have a larger diameter.

THE GENERAL STRUCTURE OF BLOOD VESSELS

All vessels have four major characteristics: (1) their spatial arrangement in organs and tissues, (2) their longitudinal configuration, (3) their internal structure, and (4) their cellular components. Several of these characteristics are often extensively modified, depending upon the sites of vessels in the body, and because of such modification it is desirable to know both the general structural plan of vessels and the nature of the variations in the major organs. In short, vessels are only "typical" for a specific organ.

The spatial arrangement of vessels in an organ is related to its functions and is reflected in the complexity and density of its vascular pattern. In general, the vascularity of an organ is directly proportional to its metabolic activity. This principle is illustrated by contrasting the liver and mesenteries. The liver has two inflow tracts, the hepatic artery and portal vein, and one outflow tract, the hepatic vein.[1] In this microvascular system, the terminal vessels of the hepatic artery join capillaries (sinusoids) as well as the terminal segments of the portal vein via arteriovenous anastomoses (arterioportal anastomoses), thereby making it possible to perfuse the exchange vessels (sinusoids) with all venous (portal) blood, all arterial blood, or any mixture of the two. In addition each hepatic cell is bounded on at least two sides by sinusoids so it is in intimate contact with the blood. In contrast, the metabolic activity of mesenteries is considerably less, the vascular pattern is simple, and capillaries are separated by many tens of micrometers.

In longitudinal section, the arterial and venous vessels are cone-shaped, with a taper about 1 to 2° per branch toward the capillary vessels, and capillaries are cylindrical. Thus, the greatest resistance to flow is in the arterial system as the blood flows into vessels having an ever-decreasing bore; the opposite occurs in the venous system as their bore increases in the normal direction of flow.

The basic structure of all vessels is similar throughout the cardiovascular system, including the heart. All have three coats or tunics: an internal *tunica intima,* an intermediate *tunica media,* and an external *tunica adventitia.* The ratio of one layer to another varies considerably. Each tunic is characterized by a predominant function and cell type: the intima, by the endothelial cell and exchange with blood; the media, by the smooth muscle cell and control of vessel diameter; and the adventitia, by connective tissue, nerves, and blood vessels that provide protection and nourishment to a vessel (Fig. 9-2).

General features of the tunica intima   The characteristic cell of this tunic is the endothelial cell. When these cells are examined with the light microscope, they exhibit little detail. A prominent nucleus, usually oriented longitudinally, is observed bulging into the lumen. When stained with silver nitrate, the cell borders can be identified but the cytoplasm appears almost structureless and transparent.

The electron microscope reveals the diversity of endothelial structure, which has been used to classify capillaries into several types (Fig. 9-3). (Capillaries are built principally of endothelium. Their media consist of an incomplete sheet of cells called *pericytes,* or Rouget cells, which are considered to be related to smooth muscle cells, and their ad-

---

[1] The type of vascular pattern found in the liver is defined as a "portal system" because blood perfuses *two* capillary systems in series before emptying into a venous system that carries the blood to the heart. Such a portal system exists not only in the liver (mesenteric capillaries to portal vein to sinusoids to hepatic vein to heart) but also in the kidney (afferent arteriole to glomerular capillaries to efferent arteriole to peritubular capillaries to interlobular veins) and in the anterior lobe of the pituitary (internal carotid to superior hypophyseal arteries to capillaries of the pars tuberalis and infundibular stem that drain into venules draining into capillaries in the pars distalis whose blood empties into hypophyseal veins and flows into the cavernous sinus).

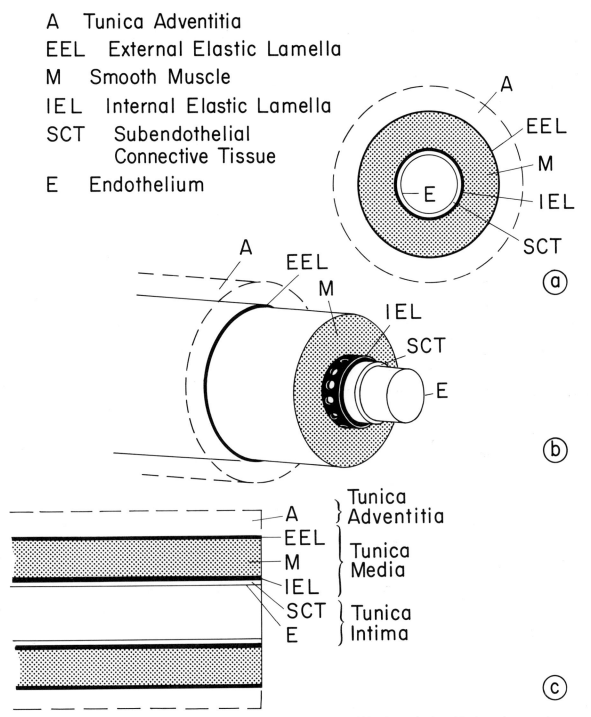

A   Tunica Adventitia
EEL   External Elastic Lamella
M   Smooth Muscle
IEL   Internal Elastic Lamella
SCT   Subendothelial
       Connective Tissue
E   Endothelium

Figure 9-2   Schematic drawing of the basic arrangement of the structure of blood vessels viewed in three planes: a, in cross section; b, tangentially; and c, in longitudinal section.

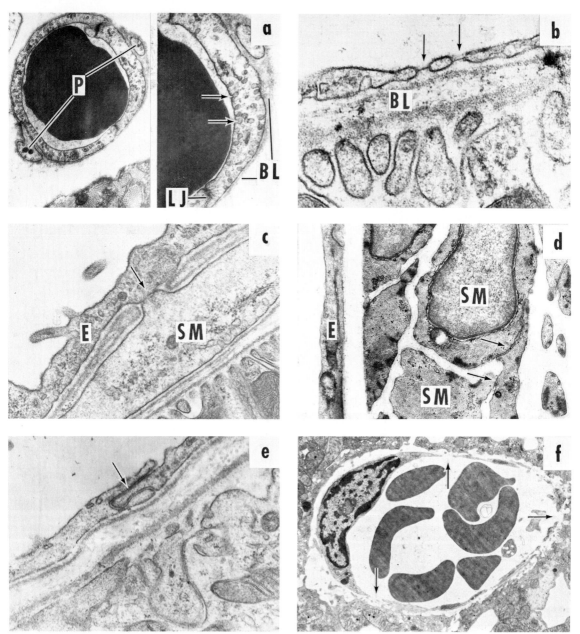

Figure 9-3 Ultrastructure of small blood vessels. a. Capillary in striated muscle (rat). This capillary is an example of a nonfenestrated endothelium with continuous basal lamina (BL), lap joint (LJ), intracytoplasmic vesicles (arrows), and pericytes (P) enveloped by the basal lamina. ×15,000 and ×30,000. (Courtesy of C. R. Basom.) b. Capillary in renal glomerulus (hamster). The endothelium is thin and contains fenestrate covered by a diaphragm (arrows). Note the thick basal lamina (BL). ×40,000. (Courtesy of C. F. Oestermeyer.) c. Myoendothelial junction (arrow) in an arteriole (mouse kidney). Note the intimate contact between the endothelial (E) and smooth muscle cell (SM). At this site basal lamina (BL) is absent. ×36,000. (Courtesy of C. F. Oestermeyer.) d. Myo-myo junctions (arrows) between adjacent smooth muscle cells (SM) in the tunica media. E is the endothelium. ×40,000. (Courtesy of J. A. G. Rhodin and Academic Press.) e. Capillary in renal glomerulus (hamster). A mortis joint (arrow) is illustrated between two endothelial cells. ×36,000. (Courtesy of C. F. Oestermeyer.) f. Sinusoid in liver (mouse). Note the discontinuities in the endothelium (arrows) as well as its very thin wall. Compare with Fig. 9-3a. Also notice the absence of a basal lamina and the space around the sinusoid (perisinusoidal space). ×15,000.

ventitia contains scattered fibroblasts and their fibers.) The cytoplasm of endothelial cells consists of relatively few mitochondria adjacent to the nucleus, a sparse rough ER, a Golgi complex near the nucleus, tonofibrils or microtubules, lysosomes, and vesicles. The greatest mass of cytoplasm is located near the nucleus. In other areas of the cell the cytoplasm may be very thin, and in some vessels it is perforated (fenestrated). Finally, the entire cell is circumscribed by a typical trilaminar (unit) membrane.

The junctions of endothelial cells, when viewed in profile by electron microscopy, reveal their complexity in both general configuration and localized modifications. The junctions may be in the form of a mortis joint (Fig. 9-3e) or a lap joint (Fig. 9-3a), which bring a relatively large area of each cell into contact with its neighbor— about 1 to 2 μm of overlap when viewed *en face*. It is *this* area which is rendered visible as a junction when endothelium is stained with silver nitrate and studied with the light microscope. This area contains the "intercellular cement" described by light microscopists, but it is *not* intercellular, since it consists primarily of the peripheral borders of endothelial cells and the actual intercellular "space" measures about 200 Å.

Like other epithelia (Chap. 3), endothelial cells may form either a zonula occludens (Fig. 9-3a) or a zonula adhaerens at their junctions. The cells may also have unmodified membranes at their junctions, separated by a less electron-dense substance or even by gaps (Fig. 9-3f).

The interfaces of endothelium are different at the luminal and basal surfaces. At the luminal surface there may be some substance(s) attached to the outer layer of the membrane. An endocapillary layer has been described which is irregular in contour after staining with ruthenium red and has been interpreted as mucopolysaccharide or mucoprotein. Whether or not this layer exists, there is no doubt about the presence of a structure at the basal surface of endothelium, the basal lamina, which consists of a moderately electron-dense band, 500 to 700 Å thick, that follows the contour of the bases of the endothelial cells and is separated from them by a less electron-dense zone approximately 400 Å thick consisting of an amorphous collagen matrix in which thin filaments are embedded.

The characteristics of capillary endothelium vary throughout the cardiovascular system. For example, the capillaries of skeletal, smooth, and cardiac muscle, as well as those in the central nervous system, have endothelial cells in which the cytoplasm contains invaginations and vesicles (cavaeolae) (500 to 700 Å) → and which have a continuous basal lamina (Fig. 9-3a). In contrast, capillaries in the renal glomeruli, endocrine glands, and gastrointestinal system have a cytoplasm that is very thin and contain fenestrae (pores) that may or may not be covered with a diaphragm and a central knob . The basal lamina, in renal glomeruli is quite thick and continuous, whereas in the sinusoids of the liver it is incomplete or absent (Fig. 9-3b).

It should be noted that endothelial cells exhibit chemical differences as well. Differences in enzyme activity occur not only between arterioles, capillaries, and venules but also with respect to their location in the body. For example, acid phosphatase activity is found in the cytoplasm of endothelial cells containing vesicles such as those in the lung or skeletal muscle, but not in fenestrated capillaries such as those in the renal glomerulus, whereas alkaline phosphatase activity occurs in capillaries and arterioles but not in venules.

General features of the tunica media The cell that characterizes this tunic is the smooth muscle cell which occurs in all vessels except capillaries. In capillaries the endothelium is embraced, at irregular intervals, by a *pericyte*, a multibranched cell containing numerous pinocytotic vesicles, a few dense bodies adjacent to the cell membrane, abundant rough ER, ribosomes, lysosomes, and a basal lamina that is common with the apposed endothelial cell. Because they have occasional dense bodies and a basal lamina, pericytes are considered to be related to smooth muscle cells.

All other vessels contain smooth muscle in the tunica media, but the orientation of the muscle varies considerably throughout the arterial and venous systems. Vascular smooth muscle consists of discrete cells which are smaller than smooth muscle cells in viscera. They are thin cylinders (approximately 3 to 5 × 30 to 60 μm) with a cytoplasm that contains dense bodies and myofilaments, many of them actin filaments (30 to 100 Å) that are randomly oriented. (Thick or myosin filaments are probably organized during contraction; they are not observed in fixed material.) The thin filaments are intimately related to dense bodies attached to the plasmalemma; they measure 400 to 900 × 2,000 to 5,000 Å. (The plasma membrane and the basal lamina constitute the sarcolemma.) An ellipsoid nucleus is usually located in the center of the cell, and adjacent to it is a Golgi complex. In addition, the cytoplasm contains rough ER, mitochondria, and microtubules parallel to the long axis of the cell but of unknown function.

The attachment is modified between smooth muscle cells (myo-myo junctions) and to endothelial cells (myoendothelial junctions), apparently to facilitate excitation and information transfer respectively (Figs. 9-3c and d). These are tight junctions, and they become more frequent and increase in length as the diameters of vessels *decrease*. (For example, nexus formation is prominent in arterioles but absent in elastic arteries.) Their configuration is often of the peg-and-socket type, thus

In vessels with concentric layers of smooth muscle, the cells are arranged circumferentially and separated by a thick envelope of glycoprotein in which are embedded collagen and reticular and elastic fibers. Furthermore, at the periphery of the media are bands of elastic tissue forming internal and external elastic lamellae. In certain vessels, like the aorta, there are many (about sixty to seventy) fenestrated lamellae throughout the media (Fig. 9-6a). (The aorta contains the greatest number of lamellae.) In each lamella the elastic fibers are oriented in one direction, clockwise or counterclockwise, alternating with each lamella. In muscular arteries, the elastic lamellae are reduced to an internal lamella between the intima and media and an external one between the media and adventitia (Fig. 9-6e). In the media there is abundant ground substance (especially in the aorta) that contains chondroitin sulfate, and the only cell is the smooth muscle cell. This cell is probably responsible for the maintenance and production of the collagen and elastin fibers since it is virtually the only cell type present.

General features of the tunica adventitia This layer may be considered the protective and nutrient component of vessels. It contains three major components: (1) a matrix of loose connective tissue and associated macrophages, (2) nerves, and (3) blood vessels (vasa vasorum).

The connective tissue is often the major obvious component of the adventitia. The fibers are arranged both parallel and tangential to the lumen of the vessel and are part of the complex of connective, elastic, and reticular fibers in the other tunics which add to the physical strength of a vessel and limit its transverse and longitudinal expansions.

Although all vessels except capillaries are innervated, the nerves are essentially limited to the adventitia, the only exception being heart, which has nerves throughout all its layers. Fibers from spinal and cranial nerves are found in the adventitia as a reticulated network. Three types can be distinguished: sensory, postganglionic sympathetic, and pre- and postganglionic parasympathetic fibers. The parasympathetic fibers have a more restricted distribution since they are absent in the vessels of the extremities. Sensory fibers terminate in simple, free endings or in complex convolutions (glomeruli): Some sensory nerves in the adventitia affect the operation of the cardiovascular system much more than others by indirectly affecting the heart. These effects are transmitted by fibers of the IXth cranial nerve (glossopharyngeal) which conducts impulses from the carotid body and sinus (located at the origin of the internal carotid artery) to the central nervous system (medulla). Similar conduction occurs from selected areas in the adventitia of the aorta (aortic bodies) via the Xth cranial (vagus) nerve to the medulla. (In the aorta the nerves are affected by changes in the intravascular pressure, while in the carotid artery they are affected by changes in the carbon dioxide or oxygen content of the blood.) Motor nerves are recognized by the morphology of their vesicles and by their fluorescence due to catecholamines. Finally, the adventitia of certain vessels in the thorax (for example, coronary arteries) and abdomen (for example, celiac and mesenteric arteries) contain pre- and postganglionic parasympathetic fibers as well as ganglia (Fig. 9-4).

The third principal component of adventitia is a segmental network of vessels (vasa vasorum) that nourish both arterial and venous vessels whose

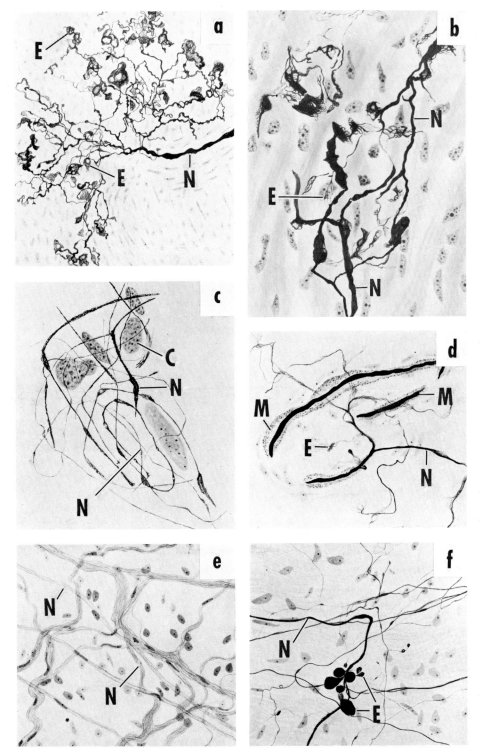

Figure 9-4 Innervation of human cardiovascular system. The illustrations are examples of the extensive innervation of blood vessels. (Courtesy of A. Ábrahám). a. Carotid sinus. Bielschowsky–Gros-Cauna. Sensory nerves (N) and nerve endings (E) in adventitia. ×400. b. Aortic arch. Bielschowsky–Gros. The terminal nerve plexus in the adventitia: N. Nerve fiber; E. nerve ending. ×1,420. c. Carotid body. Bielschowsky–Gros. Nerve fibers (N) coil around chemoreceptor cells (C). ×1,800. d. Great cardiac vein. Bielschowsky–Gros-Cauna. Myelinated (M) and unmyelinated (N) nerve fibers and a termination (E) in the adventitia. ×1,350. e. Cerebral artery. Bielschowsky–Gros. A plexus of nerves (N) in the adventitia. ×600. f. Cerebral vein. Bielschowsky–Gros. Sensory nerves (N) and their endings (E) in the adventitia. ×800.

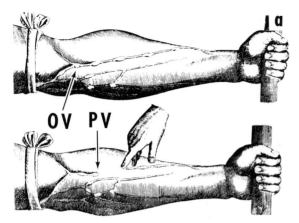

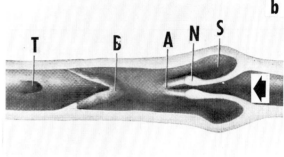

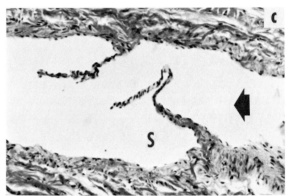

Figure 9-5   Valves in veins.   a. An illustration by William Harvey, 1628, demonstrating the location and function of valves in the cephalic vein of the forearm.   The upper figure illustrates the function of the valves when a tourniquet restricts venous flow, which brings the valves in the subcutaneous veins into prominence.   OV is an ostial valve.   The lower figure illustrates that the vessels are filled from the periphery and a parietal valve (PV) prevents back flow.   b. Reconstruction of segment of the saphenous vein of a 5 to 12 month (186-mm) fetus demonstrating a bicuspid parietal valve (A).   B is a vestigal parietal valve; T is a tributary. N is the nodular thickening of cusps.   S is a sinus. The arrow indicates the direction of blood flow.   (Redrawn, slightly modified after Kampmeier and Birch, courtesy of Wistar Institute).   c. A bicuspid parietal valve of a vein showing sinus (S).   The arrow indicates the direction of blood flow.   ×100. H&E.

diameters are greater than about 200 μm (Fig. 9-6). Each segment contains an arteriole, capillaries, and a venule.   The arteriole is usually derived from adjacent larger arterioles or from small derivative branches of the parent arterial vessel.   The capillaries ramify throughout the adventitia, usually stopping at the external border of the media.   In arteries, the venule of the vasorum leaves the adventitia to join adjacent venules, while in veins the venule may drain directly into the lumen of the vessel it supplies.

Normal vessels exhibit two other general structural features—valves and longitudinal smooth muscle.

Valves occur in many veins that lie below the level of the right atrium and especially those that have little external support and are subjected to considerable hydrostatic pressure, like the subcutaneous veins in the extremities.   The valves are located at the bifurcations of veins (ostial valves) or along the course of such vessels (parietal valves). Usually a valve consists of two cusps, each of which is a core of connective tissue covered with elastic fibers, then in some cusps by smooth muscle, and in all by endothelium.   At the site at which a cusp is attached to a vein, the vein wall is thinner and the circular smooth muscle in the media is partially or wholly replaced by longitudinal smooth muscle (Fig. 9-5).

Longitudinal smooth muscle occurs in numerous arteries and veins that are subjected to repetitive flexion or longitudinal stress.   It is also the product of age and may occur in any one of the tunics (see below).

As an aid in relating blood vessel structure to function, vessels have been classified as *elastic arteries* (aorta, brachiocephalic, common carotid, subclavian, thyrocervical trunk, origin of the common iliac and proximal sections of the internal carotid, vertebral, and internal thoracic arteries) which contain many layers of elastin[2] in their media; *muscular or distributing arteries* whose media consist primarily of smooth muscle (exemplified by the radial, popliteal, and femoral arteries); *hybrid arteries* which exhibit characteristics of elastic and muscular arteries with circular smooth muscle in the inner layers of their media and elastic lamellae in their external layers (for example, vertebral and superior mesenteric arteries); *arterioles* or *resistance vessels; capillaries; sinusoids; venules;* and veins of *small, medium and large caliber,* or *capacitance vessels* (Figs. 9-6 and 9-7). Although this general classification is useful, it is essentially limited to the gross arterial system. To date no generally acceptable terminology exists for the vessels of the microvascular system or for the gross venous system. The problem of communication is illustrated by the term *capillary.* In the clinical literature the term often refers to any small blood vessel (arteriole, capillary, or venule), but in the literature of general physiology it is often used to denote the vessels which participate in the bulk of the exchange between blood and parenchymatous cells—the capillaries and venules. Finally, among investigators who study small blood vessels in living tissues and organs with the microscope, these vessels are often defined differently, as shown by terms such as "true" capillaries, arterial capillaries, and thoroughfare channels.

It is also unrealistic and too simplistic to restrict the description of vessels to a few standard categories, since such classifications often unwittingly tend to deemphasize such factors as the influence of age and the influences of spatial exigencies on the modification of vessels. Therefore such descriptions may not emphasize the structure of the vessels that are most prone to disease. This brings into focus the reasons for studying blood vessel structure. Probably most studies are related to two different concepts and two types of vessels. One type of study involves transvascular exchange and

[2] One reason for elastin formation is apparently the stimulation provided by high pulse pressure, since in its absence elastin production is much reduced. For example, in an acardiac human twin the aorta fails to develop elastic lamellae; it has the structure of a muscular artery. Also, postnatal regression of elastin occurs normally in the main pulmonary artery but persists in the presence of pulmonary hypertension.

therefore concentrates on the structure of capillaries, sinusoids, and venules. The other type of study is related to diseases of blood vessels and is centered on macroscopic vessels such as the aorta, coronary arteries, and major vessels in the brain. This aspect is illustrated by the pathologic process of arteriosclerosis. Different aspects of this disease process affect different vessels of the arterial system. For example, atherosclerosis, which is characterized by fatty streaking, wax-like plaques, ulcers, and calcification, principally involves the intima of "large" arteries such as the aorta, coronaries, and cerebrals. On the other hand the form of the disease called medial sclerosis of Mönckeberg involves the media of muscular arteries such as the radial and superficial temporal arteries. The disease destroys the smooth muscle, which becomes calcified so that these vessels look and feel like miniature tracheae. Finally, in the diffuse hyperplastic sclerosis form of the disease, the intima of small arteries and arterioles, such as the afferent arterioles of the kidney, undergoes an extensive hyperplasia of the subendothelial connective tissue. Thus, to understand disease, one needs both types of information. Hence as the general structure of blood vessels has been described, the modifications of their structure related to normal aging and their spatial distribution in the human body will be considered.

The structures of all blood vessels are affected variously by aging and by their spatial location. These effects are especially notable in the gross vessels, including the heart. Furthermore, the structure of gross vessels is modified by such physical forces as gravity and flexion. These normal effects are reflected by subendothelial changes, by alterations in the structure of elastic lamellae, by developing smooth muscle in the intima or adventitia, by increasing production of acid mucopolysaccharides, and by the deposition of calcium salts and lipids throughout their walls. The aging process is well illustrated by the coronary arteries and aorta. In the fetus almost all the endothelium in the coronary arteries touch the internal elastic lamina, which consists of a single layer of elastic tissue. Occasionally along the lamina's length the layer is duplicated (split) and the intervening space is filled with acid mucopolysaccharide, which represents the earliest evidence for a subendothelial

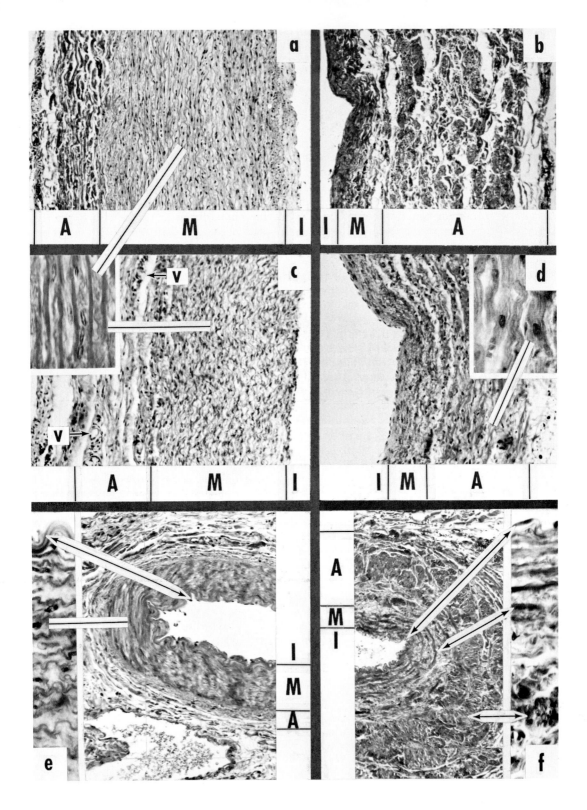

layer—that is, hyperplasia of the intima. This process accelerates in the first year of life, and by early adulthood a well-defined musculoelastic layer with longitudinal smooth muscle exists in the intima.[3] During the third decade of life, the width of the intima may equal or exceed that of the media, and from the fifth decade on, it may grow severalfold. Concurrent with these developments in the intima of the coronary arteries is the deposition of calcium salts and lipoid crystals.

In the media of the coronary arteries, longitudinal smooth muscle appears between the circular smooth muscle as early as the second month of life, and in some areas such muscle may involve the entire media. The development of longitudinal smooth muscle increases so that by the second decade it occurs regularly throughout the media.

The aorta shows similar age-related changes. In the second decade a musculoelastic layer is developed in the intima, containing irregularly oriented smooth muscle and histiocytes. (The subendothelial smooth muscle cells in the intima may become transformed into vesiculated lipoid-containing cells, or *Langhans' cells*.) This type of change is especially pronounced in the abdominal aorta, where a third innermost layer appears in middle age that consists largely of collagen, elastic fibers, and mucopolysaccharides. In subsequent

[3]Subendothelial remodeling in the intima also occurs at the downstream ends at bifurcations of arteries. At these sites longitudinal smooth muscle is arranged in layers that are separated by elastic lamellae, and the total structure has the appearance of a pad.

years the smooth muscle is replaced by collagen.

Functional considerations of blood vessels require information not only about the structure and orientation of vascular smooth muscle but also about their metabolic activities in relation to their position in the body. For example, the metabolism of arterial smooth muscle is predominantly anaerobic as indicated by the marked activity of lactic dehydrogenase. Furthermore, the Q_{O_2} of the aorta is significantly less than the terminal branches of the arterial system, as arterioles 150 μm in diameter or less have a significantly higher Q_{O_2} than vessels with a diameter twice as great (Q_{O_2} of 1.05 as against 0.85).

The veins of the gross vascular system exhibit structural changes related to age and position in the body even more extensively than the vessels of the arterial system. These changes are deviations from the idealized structure of a vessel, either an increase or decrease in structure, depending on the extent of physical forces affecting a vein, such as intravascular pressure and repetitive flexion. With respect to their spatial location, veins can be classified into two classes: The saphenous, femoral, superior mesenteric, portal, renal, and inferior vena cava are *propulsive* veins, which actively propel blood to the heart, whereas the sinuses of the dura mater, cerebral, ophthalmic, jugular, facial, and brachiocephalic veins are *draining* veins, which return blood to the heart by gravity.

As might be anticipated, propulsive veins contain appreciable amounts of smooth muscle and draining veins contain little or no smooth muscle but a

Figure 9-6 A comparison of the structural differences between gross arteries and veins. The arteries are on the left side of the figure and the veins are on the right side. Explanation of symbols: A, tunica adventitia; M, tunica media; I, tunica intima. All large figures are the same magnification. ×63. Inserts, ×250. H&E. a and b. Thoracic aorta and inferior vena cava. The principal structural component of the aorta consists of elastic lamellae between which the smooth muscle cells are sandwiched. In contrast, the major structural component in the inferior vena cava is the bundles of longitudinal smooth muscle in the adventitia. These differences illustrate the relationship between structure and function of these vessels. The blood pressure in the aorta is high during systole, and the elastic tissue stores the potential energy. This energy is released during diastole by elastic recoil, thereby maintaining blood flow to the periphery. In contrast, the blood pressure in the inferior vena cava is low, and the longitudinal smooth muscle in the adventitia provides the force for pumping the blood back to the heart. c and d. Pulmonary artery and pulmonary vein. The root of the pulmonary artery (extrapulmonary portion) is illustrated. This part of the artery has a structure that is similar to the aorta as it contains elastic lamellae in the tunica media. Note vasa vasorum (V). In contrast, the pulmonary vein, in its extrapulmonary course has bundles of longitudinal cardiac muscle in the tunica adventitia. These are not present, however, throughout the course of the vessel in the human lung. e and f. Pancreatic artery. This vessel illustrates the characteristics of a muscular artery by containing a tunica media which is large in comparison to the diameter of the lumen, and the ratio of smooth muscle to elastic lamellae is greater than that of elastic arteries. The intima has little subendothelial connective tissue, and there is a prominent internal elastic lamella. In contrast to the pancreatic artery, the tunica adventitia of the pancreatic vein is the prominent tunic. It contains numerous bundles of longitudinal smooth muscle, whereas the tunica media contains circular smooth muscle whose fibers are separated by considerable connective tissue.

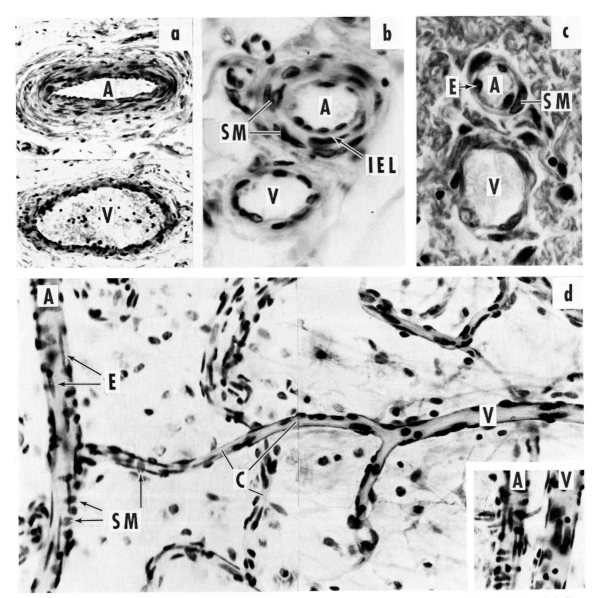

Figure 9-7   Vessels of the microvascular system.   Explanation of symbols: A, arteriole; C, capillary; V, venule; E, endothelium; IEL, internal elastic lamella; SM, smooth muscle: a. ×100.   b. ×400.   c. ×450. H&E.   a, b, c.   The decrease in the tunicas as the microvessels approach capillaries.   There is a progressive reduction of the tunicas adventitia and media.   Compare with d, which illustrates the morphology of a microvascular bed in the mesentery.   d. Note that the endothelial nuclei (E) are parallel to the axis of the vessels and the smooth muscle cells (SM) encircle the vessels and are perpendicular to its axis.   ×250. H&E.

considerable amount of collagenous and elastic tissue, which is often the most prominent feature of the adventitia. (Compare Fig. 9-8a and b.) The entire wall of a vein may be purely fibrous, as in many cerebral veins, or the wall may consist of longitudinal fascicles of smooth muscle composing two-thirds or more of the entire wall, as in the inferior vena cava.

Longitudinal vascular smooth muscle is a result of the remodeling of the initial (fetal) orientation of the smooth muscle in vessels. The smooth muscle from the media apparently migrates into the intima or adventitia where it is reoriented longitudinally or obliquely. The forces responsible for this remodeling are the hydrostatic pressures produced by gravity on the venous blood or the repetitive flexion and extension that occur in organs like the heart and lung or across joints like the knee, affecting both veins and arteries. Longitudinal smooth muscle is absent or very sparse at birth, but becomes quite noticeable during the first and second decades of life and continues to increase during subsequent decades. (Compare Fig. 9-8c and d.) How extensive such changes are in microscopic vessels has not been documented, but apparently the vessels respond to these forces much as gross vessels do.

HISTOPHYSIOLOGY OF BLOOD VESSELS

The function of the vascular system is to store blood and distribute it to the tissues where a transvascular exchange or transport of various materials can occur; this requires a delicate control of blood flow. There is only a sketchy understanding of the structural basis of exchange and control and a very limited understanding of the physical and chemical mechanisms in these processes. Although a great deal of information about blood vessels has been produced by histochemistry, light and electron microscopy, and microscopy of living tissues, the data and interpretations are often contradictory or too fragmentary to warrant the construction of a concept of cardiovascular function that is in accord with gross physiology and dynamic pathology. The problem is not so much to establish the presence of a structure as to determine how the structure operates in the living organism.

Structural elements controlling blood flow   The structures that control blood flow to the vessels engaged in transit (capillaries, sinusoids, and the immediate postcapillary venules) are the heart, which produces the physical force; the elastic arteries, which produce the pulse pressure; the muscular arteries, which distribute the blood; and the smooth muscle and certain endothelial cells of the terminal arterial microvasculature, which control the flow in vessels where transit occurs.

It is generally agreed that the smooth muscle in the media of arterioles can and does contract throughout its length. Also there is general accord that scattered, isolated smooth muscle cells at the junctions of capillaries with arterioles, the precapillary sphincters, control flow into the capillary bed. In addition, endothelial cells have been observed to control blood flow into the capillary bed; this mechanism of control has been observed in the vessels of the liver, spleen, bone marrow, and lung, whereas smooth muscle precapillary sphincters have been observed in the mesentery, skeletal muscle, and kidney.

It is an attractive assumption that the precapillary smooth muscle sphincters would be the most responsive structure in the arterial tree for controlling blood flow into a capillary bed and that when more widespread control of flow is required, the smooth muscle along the entire vessel would be called into play. Evidence obtained by direct inspection of the terminal vasculature in exposed skeletal muscle supports this hypothesis. However, when similar vessels are studied in unexposed skeletal muscle (in transparent chambers), it is found that segmental constriction of the media of arterioles along the vessel or at the bifurcations with larger arterioles controls flow without participation of precapillary sphincters. Furthermore, in organs like the liver, lung, and spleen where some vessels have no smooth muscle, it is the endothelial cell which actively controls flow through the capillaries or sinusoids. Although several structural components of the microvascular system (smooth muscle and endothelial cells) are located at sites which can control blood flow, the basic problem is to determine which of these components participate in each normal physiologic process.

Once blood reaches the vessels where exchange occurs, the exchange is affected by intra- and extravascular physical forces and the chemical environments in the blood and parenchyma as well as by

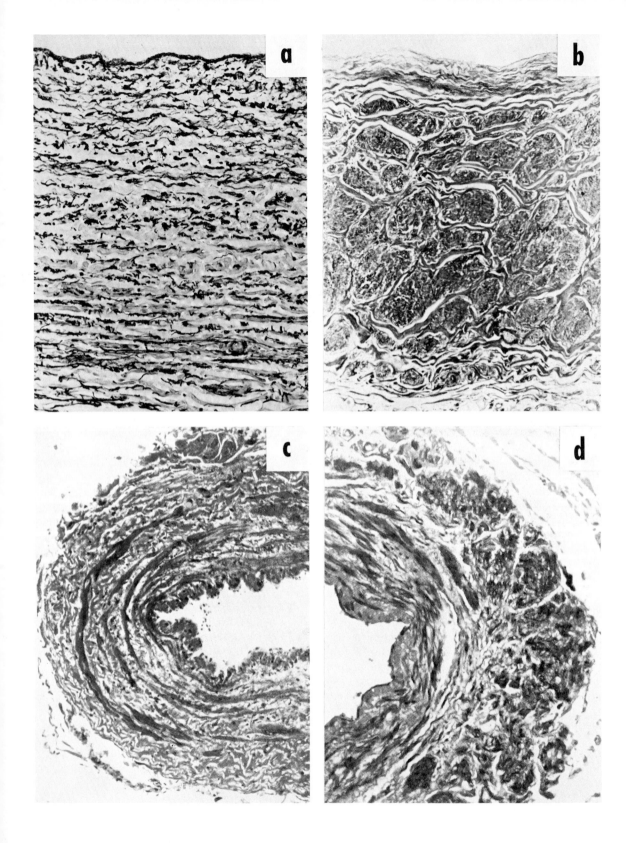

the structure of the vessels and their topology. The complexity of the structure of endothelial cells delineates but one aspect of their morphology, a static one. In life one would expect the structures to be constantly remodeled by the exigencies of function. For example, there are often rapid changes in permeability of capillaries, sinusoids, or immediate postcapillary venules concomitant with an organ's activity, as with exercise or inflammation.

The structural characteristics of the vessels engaged in exchange need to be considered in relation to the size of the substances that move, as their size ranges from 2.98 Å for oxygen to 12 μm for leukocytes. Each substance might be transported through a special site in the endothelium, but there is neither sound experimental evidence for, nor general agreement on, the specific site(s) in a vessel where *any* of these substances pass. For example, indirect evidence suggests that molecules like water and ions pass through the walls of capillaries via "pores," but neither the substances in their passage nor the pores have been identified anatomically. A similar state of uncertainty exists for the transport of proteins as large as or larger than globulin in those vessels that are usually impermeable to the bulk of the plasma proteins. These proteins may be carried via vesicles across the cells, via fenestrae or between endothelial cells, but there is no overwhelming evidence for any one of these sites. Finally, erythrocytes and leukocytes have been observed to pass through *and* between endothelial cells, but it would be dogmatic to state that one or the other was the preferred site for passage. If one is to hazard an opinion about the sites in vessels where transit occurs, it is probably anywhere along the endothelium extending from arterioles that are essentially bare of smooth muscle, throughout capillaries, and through the endothelium of those postcapillary venules that have little or no smooth muscle embracing their walls. Thus the bulk of the movement, from oxygen to cells, probably occurs anywhere along endothelial cells (which,

after all, present more than 95 percent of the surface area in contact with the blood) and the remainder, less than 5 percent, occurs in the areas between endothelial cells. Furthermore, there is no reason to presume that at special sites and for varying periods of time the sites of permeability may be shifted to occur between endothelial cells.

A special and highly important process is the phagocytic removal of particulates from the circulation by endothelial (reticuloendothelial) cells that line the sinusoids of the liver, spleen, and bone marrow. Particulates such as damaged red blood cells, bacteria, and cellular debris disappear with half-times that range from a fraction of a second to minutes or hours. These stationary phagocytes, in contrast to free phagocytic cells like leukocytes, are one of the chief defense mechanisms in the body as they constantly remove and destroy bacteria that enter the bloodstream from such sites as the oral cavity and the gastrointestinal tract.

The story of transvascular exchange must not be considered solely from the structural point of view. Although the morphology of vessels is assumed to influence exchange, the extent of the influence is unknown. More important than their structure may be the chemistry of endothelial cells in conjunction with intra- and extravascular physical factors. Histochemical evidence is accumulating to support the suggestion that enzymes in endothelial cells may play critical roles in transport. For example, the impermeability of cerebral vessels to certain drugs and dyes (the bloodbrain barrier) is apparently due to the presence of monoamine oxidase and dopa decarboxylase. (Other enzymes have been found in vessels, but their role in transvascular exchange is not clear.) Finally, metabolites released during tissue activity, like lactic acid in skeletal muscle, may increase vessel permeability. However, in all these examples it is not known if or how these substances affect the structure of endothelium.

In short, it is no longer tenable to consider endothelium as a relatively inert, semipermeable membrane in which the role of the endothelial cell is

Figure 9-8 Comparison of the structure of veins. a. Superior vena cava. Elastin Hollborn; ×110. b. Inferior vena cava. Mallory-Azan; ×77. The inferior vena cava contains numerous bundles of longitudinal smooth muscle in the tunica adventitia for aiding in the propulsion of blood back to the heart; the superior vena cava lacks such specialization since here venous return is dependent upon gravity. c. Saphenous vein from a 4-year-old. Mallory-Azan; ×180. d. Saphenous vein from a 60-year-old. Note the increased accumulation of longitudinal smooth muscle in the tunica adventitia with increased age. Mallory-Azan; ×160. (Courtesy of L. Bucciante.)

to produce and maintain a hypothetical intercellular cement.   More realistically, transit across endothelium is probably the product of metabolites in the blood and parenchyma that affect the metabolism of endothelial cells, whereupon their structure is remodeled in accordance with the demands.

THE HEART

Since the heart develops from a simple blood vessel, it retains the usual three tunics or coats; an intima, the *endocardium;* a media, the *myocardium;* and an adventitia, the *epicardium* (visceral serous pericardium).   Like other blood vessels, it has valves and a vasa vasorum, the coronary vasculature.   The heart differs from other blood vessels, however, by containing two kinds of striated muscle: cardiac muscle, rather than smooth muscle, that generates the propulsive force for ejecting the blood into the systemic, pulmonary, and coronary circuits; and atypical or modified cardiac muscle that conducts electric impulses in an orderly manner from the right atrium to the left and right ventricles.   It also has a specialized framework, or ''skeleton,'' of collagen for attaching the cardiac muscle and for anchoring the cardiac valves, two of which, the tricuspid and mitral, differ from the valves in veins by having cords (chordae tendineae) that anchor their free margins to the cardiac wall by way of the papillary muscles.   Further differences between the heart and vessels are the presence of nerves throughout all the tunics, rather than being restricted to the adventitia; the presence of lymphatics, which are absent in other vessels; and the heart's enclosure in an essentially indistensible container, the pericardial sac.

Endocardium   All the chambers of the heart, including the valves, are lined with endothelial cells that are contiguous with similar cells lining the vessels that join the organ.   The endothelial cells in the heart are nonfenestrated and have a continuous basal lamina.   Underneath the lamina, there is a subendothelial layer that is thicker in the atria than in the ventricles (Fig. 9-9a and b), a subendocardial conducting system, connective tissue, varying amounts of smooth muscle adjacent to the myocardium, vessels of the coronary vascular system, and sympathetic and parasympathetic nerves as well as sensory nerves.

Myocardium   The bulk of the heart consists of cardiac muscle, which differs from skeletal muscle in having fibers connected to each other by intercalated discs and nuclei that are deeply rather than superficially embedded in the abundant sarcoplasm.   Most of the muscle is contained in the ventricles, where it circumscribes the chambers in a spiral and complex manner so that when it contracts it literally wrings the blood from the chambers.   In the auricles the cardiac muscle is arranged in ridges that resemble a comb (pectinate) and between the ridges of muscle the wall is so thin that the endo- and epicardium are almost in contact with each other.

The muscle is arranged into several layers and fascicles with different functions.   For example, the superficial muscles of the ventricles stabilize the apex and cusps of the AV valves by means of the papillary muscles to prevent the valves from bulging into the atria and help to keep them closed during isometric contraction.   The deep sinospiral muscle which forms the main mass of the right ventricle provides the force for the pulmonary circulation, and the deep bulbospiral muscle empties the left ventricle.

Figure 9-9 The human heart. a. Right atrium. E, endocardium; note its thickness as compared with that of left ventricle. b. There is an artifactual separation between endo and myocardium, M. H & E; ×25. b. Left ventricle. E, endocardium; M, myocardium. H&E. ×25. c. Purkinje fibers in the right ventricular bundle branch. H&E. ×250. d. Representative cardiac muscle fibers. Note the difference between the Purkinje fibers (modified cardiac muscle fibers) and regular cardiac muscle fibers. The Purkinje cells have greater diameter than regular cardiac muscle fibers and have a paucity of myofibrils in their cytoplasm. H&E. ×250. e. Diagram and histologic section of a portion of the cardiac skeleton (annulus fibrosum). The diagram illustrates the complex configuration of the annulus as it circumscribes the four valves of the heart: M, mitral valve; T, tricuspid valve; A, aortic valve; P, pulmonary valve. The adjacent figure is a histologic section of the annulus fibrosum and the base of the posterior cusp of the mitral valve; A, left atrium; V, left ventricle. H&E. ×63. f. Posterior cusp of the tricuspid valve. Note that the thickened endocardium of the atrium (left) continues over the surface of the valve. Compare with a and b. Also, note the core of the cusp consists of dense fibroelastic connective tissue. H&E. ×100.

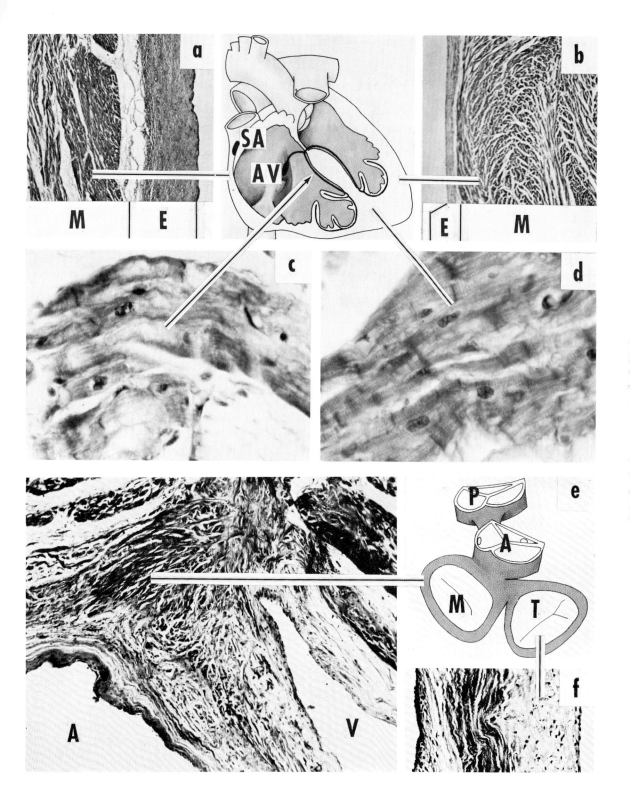

a

M | E

b

E | M

c

d

SA

AV

P

e

A

M | T

f

A

V

Epicardium   This is the external layer of the heart that consists of connective tissue, principally collagen, which intervenes between the myocardium and the external surface of mesothelial cells. Mesothelial cells form the visceral surface of the serous pericardium. In the connective tissue layer underneath the epicardium are lymphatics, nerves, and blood vessels. As the major branches of the coronary blood vessels lie in the sulci that are formed between the chambers of the heart, the epicardium is correspondingly thicker to accommodate these vessels as well as a considerable amount of adipose tissue associated with them.

Pericardium   The heart is enclosed by a sac which consists of two layers, a fibrous and a serous pericardium. The fibrous pericardium is external and consists principally of dense connective tissue which is supplied with blood vessels, nerves, and lymphatics. This sac is essentially indistensible. The thick fibrous pericardium is lined by the thin serous pericardium, whose inner surface consists of mesothelial cells that are contiguous with those of the epicardium. For descriptive purposes, the serous pericardium lining the fibrous pericardium is called the *parietal* serous pericardium, and the part that forms the surface of the heart is called the *visceral* serous pericardium (epicardium). Thus, the mesothelial cells of the serous pericardium provide a smooth lubricated surface for the beating heart.

The conducting system   This system consists of the sinoatrial (SA) and atrioventricular (AV) nodes and the atrioventricular bundle and its branches (Fig. 9-9). In the human heart the system is usually *not* visible on direct inspection as it is in the hearts of large mammals like the horse or cow.

The sinoatrial node (discovered by Keith and Flack) measures about 2 × 6 mm and lies in an area which is indicated superficially by the posterior aspect of the right auricle with its junction to the atrium and superior vena cava. The body of the node occupies the area between the epicardium and the endocardium and is usually pierced by the nodal artery, a branch of the right coronary artery. Strands from the node radiate through the walls of the atrium and reach the atrioventricular node.

The atrioventricular node (discovered by Tawara) is located between the orifice of the coronary sinus and the area just above the septal cusp of the tricuspid valve. Contiguous with the node is the atrioventricular bundle (His, Kent) which lies in the same subendocardial plane as the node. This common bundle, about 15 mm in length and 1 to 3 mm in width, passes into the interventricular septum and wall to terminate in right and left branches. The right branch radiates to the anterior wall of the chamber via the trabecula septomarginalis (moderator band), which lies at the apex of the ventricle. The left branch penetrates the interventricular septum to emerge in the subendocardium of the left ventricle in the area between the right and posterior cusps of the aortic valve and then radiates throughout the walls of the ventricle.

To the above description of the major distribution of the conducting system in the ventricles which lies in the longitudinal plane in the subendocardium there must be added the radial distribution. Radially the fibers pass throughout the myocardium, almost reaching the epicardium.

The two types of cells (fibers) found in this system are both modified cardiac muscle, namely the nodal and Purkinje cells. The nodal fibers are about one-half to two-thirds the diameter of regular cardiac muscle, contain little sarcoplasm, are fusiform in shape, and are arranged in a syncytium. In contrast, the Purkinje fibers, which constitute the atrioventricular bundle and branches, measure from just slightly larger than the regular cardiac fibers up to three times their diameter, and contain abundant sarcoplasm in which the myofibrils are so widely dispersed that the fibers appear pale in contrast to the other cardiac muscle fibers (compare Fig. 9-9c and d).

Innervation of the heart   The heart is richly supplied by nerves. Myelinated and nonmyelinated nerve fibers, as well as ganglion cells, are found in many areas of the organ. The nerve fibers are distributed between and around nodal and Purkinje fibers, regular cardiac muscle, and blood vessels. Nerves and ganglion cells are especially abundant in and around the SA and AV nodes. Sensory nerve fibers from the heart terminate principally in the thoracic region of the spinal cord between the first and fifth vertebral levels, whereas the motor fibers, derived from the sympathetic nerves, originate from cells that are located at a similar level but lie in the intermediolateral cell column of the cord. In the heart these sympathetic fibers are postganglionic, in contrast to the parasympathetic motor fibers that are both pre- and postganglionic. The parasympathetic ganglia and fibers belong to the vagus nerve, and some of the ganglia are located throughout the heart but, as mentioned above, are especially abundant adjacent to the nodes. Sensory fibers from the vagus are undoubtedly present but cannot be distinguished from sensory fibers that accompany the sympathetic nerves. Furthermore the function of the sensory fibers in the vagus nerve is unknown, as pain from the heart is considered to be transmitted by fibers that terminate in the spinal cord.

The intrinsic cardiac vasculature The vascular architecture of the heart is complex and consists of at least four systems: the coronary, myocardial, conducting, and valvular systems. The major histologic features of the coronary vessels have been described above. In brief, the subendothelial layer and elastic lamellae increase with age, and smooth muscle develops in the intima.

The human myocardium is richly endowed with capillaries. It is estimated that there are about three thousand five hundred capillaries per square millimeter, which is almost twice that of skeletal muscle. Although the pattern of the microscopic vessels supplying the atrioventricular bundle and its branches is similar to that in regular cardiac muscle, the number of vessels per square millimeter is less except in the nodes, where the vascularity is greater.

Briefly the pattern of blood flow through the wall of the heart is as follows: Blood from the coronary arteries flows into the arterioles, capillaries, and venules of the wall and then into veins that drain into the coronary sinus or anterior cardiac veins, both of which empty into the right atrium. Venous blood can also return to any one of the four chambers but especially to the ventricular chambers via Thebesian veins. These veins are involved during various phases of the heartbeat. For example, in diastole the aortic and pulmonic valves are closed and the pressure in the coronary system is greater than in any of the chambers. In this condition, blood from the coronary arterial system in the walls of the heart flows into the Thebesian veins, which carry it into the chambers.

Lymphatics The heart is liberally supplied with lymphatic vessels, most of which are microscopic in size. These vessels are arranged in plexuses entwined about the conducting system in the subendocardium, around cardiac muscle fibers in the myocardium (the most extensive plexus), and in the subepicardial connective tissue where the minor and major collecting trunks are also embedded. All the lymph from the plexuses drains into the subepicardial trunks, which in turn flow into the principal trunks (a right and left) that carry the lymph to lymphatic trunks in the anterior mediastinum.

In the endocardium and myocardium the lymphatic vessels are valveless, but valves are present in the collecting trunks of the subepicardium. Also, lymph nodes are absent in the endocardium and myocardium and are present in the subepicardium of the fetus and child, but are sparse in the adult.

The ultrastructure of the lymphatic vessels of the heart is presumed to be similar to that of the lymph vessels in other parts of the body. The endothelial cells may or may not have tight junctions, and the basal lamina may or may not be complete, depending on the internal dimension of the lymph vessel, as in the mesentery, but their structure in the heart has yet to be described.

References

ÁBRAHÁM, A.: ''Microscopic Innervation of the Heart and Blood Vessels in Vertebrates Including Man,'' Pergamon Press, Oxford, 1969.

ABRAMSON, D. I. (ed.): ''Blood Vessels and Lymphatics,'' Academic Press, New York, 1962.

ALTMAN, P. L., and DITTMER, D. S. (eds.): "Respiration and Circulation," Federation of American Societies for Experimental Biology, Bethesda, Md., 1971. (Data, in tabular form, for the vascularity in organs.)

BENNETT, H. S., LUFT, J. H., and HAMPTON, J. C.: Morphological Classifications of Blood Capillaries, *Amer. J. Physiol.*, **196**:381 (1959).

BENNINGHOFF, A.: Blutgefässe und Herz, in W. von Möllendorf (ed.), "Handbuch der mikroskopischen Anatomie des Menschen," vol. 6, Part 1, pp. 1–232, 1939. (A mine of information about the structure of blood vessels as determined by light microscopy.)

BLOCH, E. H.: A Quantitative Study of the Hemodynamics in the Living Microvascular System, *Amer. J. Anat.*, **110**:125 (1962).

BLOCH, E. H.: Microscopic Observations of the Circulating Blood in the Bulbar Conjunctiva in Man in Health and Disease, *Ergebn Anat. Entwicklungsgesch.* **35**:1 (1956).

BRIGHTMAN, M. W., and REESE, T. S.: Junctions between Intimately Apposed Cell Membranes in the Vertebrate Brain, *J. Cell Biol.*, **40**:648 (1969).

BUCCIANTI, L.: "Microscopie Optique de la Paroi Veineuse," Symp. Int. Morphologie Histochimie Paroi Vasculaire (Fribourg, 1963), Part II, pp. 211–308, 1966. S. Karger, New York. (An extensively illustrated work on human veins as they are affected by aging.)

DRINKER, C. K.: "The Lymphatic System," Lane Medical Lectures, University Series, Medical Sciences, **42**:1942, Stanford University Press, Stanford, Calif. (A stimulating description of the interrelationship of small blood vessels and lymphatics.)

FAWCETT, D. H.: "The Cell. An Atlas of Fine Structure," Saunders, Philadelphia, 1966.

FERNANDO, N., and MOVAT, H.: The Fine Structure of the Terminal Vascular Bed, *Exp. Molec. Path.*, **3**:87 (1964).

FLOREY, H., POOLE, J., and MEEK, G.: Endothelial Cells and "Cement" Lines, *J. Path. Bact.*, **77**:625 (1959).

FRANKLIN, K. J.: "A Monograph on Veins," Charles C Thomas, Springfield, Ill., 1937.

GROSS, L., EPSTEIN, E. Z., and KUGEL, M. A.: Histology of the Coronary Arteries and Their Branches in the Human Heart, *Amer. J. Path.*, **10**:253 (1934).

KISCH, B.: "Electron Microscopy of the Cardiovascular System," Charles C Thomas, Springfield, Ill., 1960.

KNISELY, M. H., E. H. BLOCH, and L. WARNER: Selective Phagocytosis (A Study of the Living Frog Liver), *Det Kong. Danske Videnskab. Selskab.*, **4**:1 (1947).

KROGH, A.: "Anatomy and Physiology of Capillaries," Yale University Press, New Haven, 1922, 1929.

LANG, J.: Mikroskopische Anatomie der Arterien, Int. Symp. Morphologie Histochemie, Gefässwand, Fribourg, 1965. *Angiologica* (Teil 1), **22**:225 (1965).

MCCUSKEY, R. S.: Microscopy of the Living Liver *in Situ*. III. Erythropoiesis, *Anat. Rec.*, **161**:267 (1968).

MCCUSKEY, R. S., and T. M. CHAPMAN: Microscopy of the Living Pancreas, *Amer. J. Anat.*, **126**:395 (1969).

MAJNO, G.: Ultrastructure of the Vascular Membrane, in W. F. Hamilton and P. Dow, (eds.), "Handbook of Physiology," Sec. 2, Circulation, vol. 3. pp. 2293–2375, American Physiological Society, Washington, D.C., 1965.

MALL, F. P.: On the Muscular Architecture of the Ventricles of the Human Heart, *Amer. J. Anat.*, **11**:211 (1911).

MEYER, W. W.: Die Lebenswandlungen der Struktur von Arterien und Venen, *Verh. Deutsch. Ges. Kreislaufforsch.*, **24**:15 (1958).

MITCHELL, G. A. G.: "Cardiovascular Innervation," Livingstone, Edinburgh, 1956.

RAMSEY, E. M.: Nutrition of the Blood Vessel Wall: Review of the Literature (Vasa vasorum), *Yale J. Biol. Med.*, **9**:14 (1936–37).

RHODIN, J. A. G.: The Ultrastructure of Mammalian Arterioles and Precapillary Sphincters, *J. Ultrastruct. Res.*, **18**:181 (1967).

RHODIN, J. A. G.: Ultrastructure of Mammalian Venous Capillaries, Venules and Small Collecting Veins, *J. Ultrastruct. Res.*, **25**:452 (1968).

ROBERTS, J. T.: The Conducting System, in A. A. Luisada (ed.), "Development and Structure of the Cardiovascular System," pp. 71–84, McGraw-Hill, New York, 1961.

ROUVIERE, H. "Anatomie des Lymphatiques de l'Homme," Translated and rearranged as a compendium by M. J. Tobias ("Anatomy of the Human Lymphatic System"), Edwards Bros., Ann Arbor, Mich., 1938. (See for cardiac lymphatics.)

STOTLER, W. A., and MCMAHON, R. A.: The Innervation and Structure of the Conductive System of the Human Heart, *J. Comp. Neurol.*, **87**:57, (1947).

TRUEX, R. C., and COPENHAVER, W. M.: Histology of the Moderator Band in Man and Other Mammals with Special Reference to the Conduction System, *Amer. J. Anat.*, **80**:173 (1947).

WEARN, J. T.: The Extent of the Capillary Bed of the Heart, *J. Exp. Med.*, **47**:273 (1928).

WEARN, J. T.: The Nature of the Vascular Communications between the Coronary Arteries and the Chambers of the Heart, *Amer. Heart J.*, **9**:143 (1933).

WEARN, J. T.: Morphological and Functional Alterations of the Coronary Circulation, *Harvey Lectures*, **35**:243 (1940).

chapter 10 Blood

LEON WEISS

The blood is a fluid connective tissue composed of circulating cells and a liquid intercellular substance, the *blood plasma*. The blood is enclosed in blood vessels and flows through the body, propelled by the contraction of the heart, the recoil of the great vessels, the movement of muscles, the excursions of the lungs, and the force of gravity. Blood volume in the normal human adult is approximately five liters.

Freshly drawn human blood is a red fluid of specific gravity 1.052 to 1.064. On standing but a short time it clots into a jelly-like mass, but if clotting is prevented the blood cells gradually settle, leaving the plasma supernatant. This sedimentation may be greatly accelerated by centrifugation. Three layers may be observed in a column of sedimented blood (Fig. 10-1). The lowermost layer, about 45 percent of the total blood volume, is red and consists of packed *erythrocytes*, or *red blood cells*. Above the erythrocytes is a thin gray-white layer, approximately 1 percent of the total blood volume, called the *buffy coat*. It is formed of *platelets* and of *leuckocytes*, or *white blood cells*, of which there are five types in human beings: lymphocytes, monocytes, polymorphonuclear neutrophils, polymorphonuclear eosinophils, and polymorphonuclear basophils. The uppermost layer is the plasma, a slightly alkaline, straw-colored, proteinaceous fluid which constitutes the intercellular substance. The volume of packed blood cells is termed the *hematocrit*, a measurement of clinical value in determining the degree of an anemia and response to therapy.

The structure of blood cells

LIVING BLOOD CELLS

Living blood cells may be studied in hanging drops, in tissue culture, in chambers of special design placed in the ear or other accessible part of an animal, or in such favorable places as the web of the toe, the tongue, or the mesentery in whole animals. Living cells may be studied unstained by phase-contrast microscopy. Certain structures, moreover, may be selectively demonstrated by supravital staining. Our discussion, although applicable to many mammals, is directed specifically to human blood [Figs. 10-2 to 10-5 (color insert) and 10-8].

Unstained blood cells Fresh red cells are orange-yellow in color without intrinsic motion. They are remarkably deformable, reversibly flexing, and twisting. Their biconcavity is striking, and they tend to aggregate into columns of cells similar to stacks of coins, called *rouleaux*. Rouleaux increase in size and frequency in certain diseases, notably those affecting plasma proteins. Their excessive presence may cause the blood to sludge within capillary beds of the body and interfere with efficient flow. Erythrocytes in hypertonic media lose water by osmotic pressure and shrink somewhat. The plasma membrane is thrown into folds, and the cells assume a burr-like or *crenated* appearance. In hypotonic solutions, on the other hand, water enters erythrocytes. Their hemoglobin is leached out and they become enlarged, virtually colorless structures, termed *ghosts*. This process, hemolysis, is used experimentally to obtain red cell membranes. Since leukocytes are relatively resistant, hemolysis may be used to eliminate erythrocytes and obtain leukocyte suspensions.

Living leukocytes may be motile. As they move, they assume a characteristic polarization, with an active anterior end producing pseudopodia, a central portion containing the nucleus and the bulk of the cell, and a passive, trailing, cytoplasmic tail. This pattern is best seen when a leukocyte moves over a flat surface and is obscured as it worms its way through a clot or other three-dimensional matrix. Lymphocytes in motion give the appearance of a hand mirror; they show a round anterior nucleus surrounded by a rim of cytoplasm with the remainder of the cytoplasm trailing like a handle. The pseudopodia are delicate processes projecting forward in advance of the nucleus. The polymorphonuclear cells contain distinctive cytoplasmic granules; many of these can be seen as refractile structures in living cells. Platelets have little or no motility. They tend to aggregate into masses and readily become associated with clot formation. They are found at intersections of fibrin strands making up the clot and are essential in clot retraction.

Figure 10-1 Blood before and after sedimentation. The volume of packed erythrocytes is almost 45 percent of the total blood volume. The leukocytes and platelets form a buffy coat, accounting for about 1 percent of the blood volume. The remainder of the blood is the supernatant plasma.

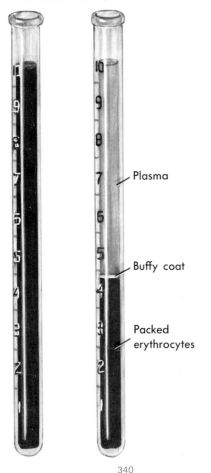

Plasma

Buffy coat

Packed erythrocytes

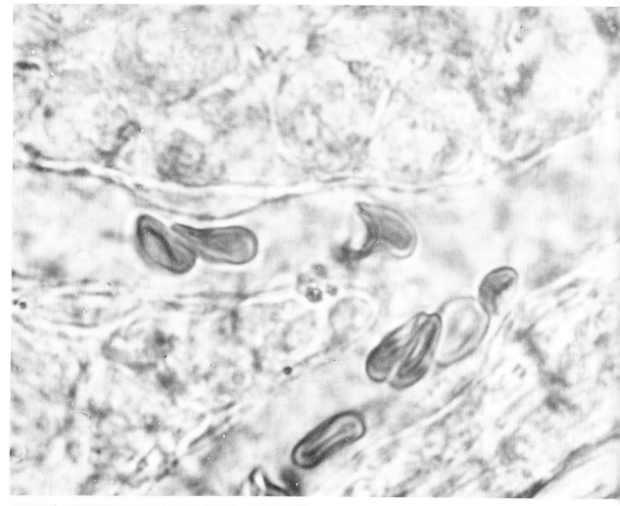

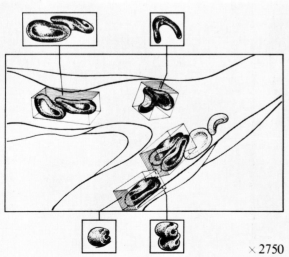

×2750

Figure 10-2 Deformation of erythrocytes in venule with an explanatory diagram illustrating Brånemark's interpretation of the mode in which each red cell has been stretched, bent, and twisted. Intravital photomicrogram of a human microvessel in connective tissue. ×2,750. (From P-I. Brånemark, "Intravascular Anatomy of Blood Cells in Man," S. Karger AG, Basel, Switzerland, 1971.)

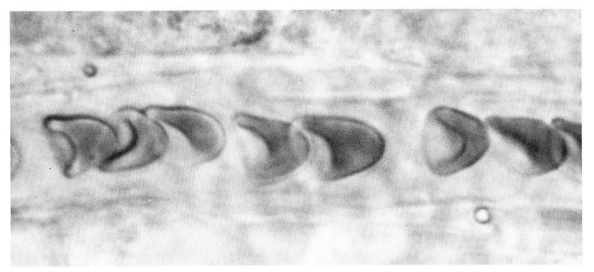

Figure 10-3 Deformation of human erythrocytes flowing in single file in a small venule. Intravital photomicrogram of a human microvessel. ×3,000. (From P-I. Brånemark, "Intravascular Anatomy of Blood Cells in Man," S. Karger AG, Basel, Switzerland, 1971.)

Figure 10-4 Fresh blood with chylomicrons. Right half of the field is under dark field; left half, under light field. (Courtesy of S. H. Gage and P. A. Fish and the Wistar Institute of Anatomy.)

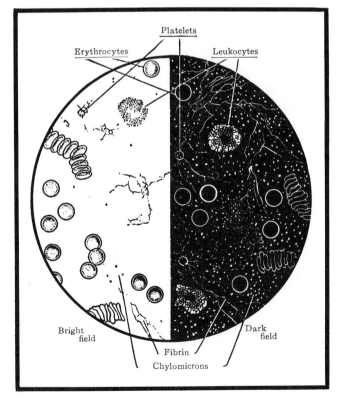

Chylomicrons and hemoconia are visible in fresh blood, especially with phase or dark-field microscopes. Chylomicrons are highly refractile fatty bodies about 1 to 3 μm in diameter. They increase considerably in number after a fatty meal. They are absent in most stained preparations of blood because they are soluble in alcohol, the fixative most commonly used. Hemoconia or blood dust are tiny particles of diverse origin—fragments of blood and endothelial cells, particles of ingested material, etc. Since optimum visualization depends on the Tyndall effect, they are seen best in dark field rather than by transmitted light.

Supravitally stained blood cells It is possible to stain organelles in the living state and to observe them in the surviving cells (Fig. 10-5). Thus, mitochondria are revealed selectively by their ability to maintain *Janus green B* in its oxidized or colored state. The granules of each of the polymorphonuclear leukocyte cell types take up the dye *neutral red*, which is a pH indicator that can differentiate by color the cytoplasmic granules of neutrophils, eosinophils, and basophils. Neutral red may also stain phagocytic and other vacuoles. A rosette of neutral-red-stained vacuoles characteristically surrounds the centrosome in monocytes. Supravital staining, once actively prosecuted by Florence Sabin and her students in an effort at delineating certain lymphatic and hematopoietic cell types, though engrossing morphologically, is now scarcely used. A most important exception, however, is the supravital staining of freshly produced erythrocytes by brilliant cresyl blue, new methylene blue, or other suitable basic dye.

THE STRUCTURE OF BLOOD CELLS IN ROMANOVSKY-STAINED SMEARS

After fixation, blood cells may be studied by light microscopy or by electron microscopy. We shall consider the structure of blood cells in blood smears stained with Romanovsky-type stains. Again, our treatment centers upon human blood.

Blood smears are made quickly and easily (Fig. 10-6) by spreading a drop of blood on a slide or a cover slip in a layer so thin that minute cytologic details may be studied. They obviate many of the artefacts, expense, and consumption of time inherent in sectioned material and are of inestimable

value in clinical and experimental work in determining the cytology and differential proportions of blood cell types. Cover-slip smears are somewhat more difficult to make than slide smears and are more fragile, but they offer the advantage that the leukocytes are randomly distributed, permitting accurate differential counts. In slide smears, in contrast, leukocytes are thrown to the edge and end. The techniques for making cover-slip and slide smears are illustrated in Fig. 10-6. Blood smears are air-dried and may be examined unstained by phase-contrast microscopy or stained with a variety of methods.

Romanovsky-type stains are routinely employed both in the clinical and experimental study of blood smears because they reveal great cytologic detail and are easily applied. These stains are complex dye mixtures designated neutral stains. In addition to ionic dyes—eosin[-], methylene blue[+], and the oxidation products of methylene blue, the azures[+]—these dyes contain neutral dye salts represented by nondissociated eosinates of methylene blue and the azures. Variants of Romanovsky stains, which include the Wright stain (the most commonly used), and Giemsa's, MacNeil's, Leishman's, and May-Grünwald's mixtures, differ in the manner of oxidation of methylene blue to the azures.

The Wright-stained blood smear (Fig. 10-7, color insert) is pink macroscopically because of eosin binding by erythrocytes, by far the most numerous element, numbering about 5 million per ml as compared with 5,000 leukocytes per ml.

Erythrocytes are round or slightly oval in outline. Their diameter is fairly constant for an individual, ranging in man from 6.5 to 8.0 μm and averaging 7.5 μm. They are deeply stained around their thicker periphery but the color gradually becomes very faint in their thin centermost zone.

Polymorphonuclear neutrophils, approximately 12 to 15 μm in diameter, contain a prominent nucleus segmented into three to five lobes joined by thin, sometimes invisible, strands of chromatin. Chromatin is coarse and entirely heterochromatic, and nucleoli are absent. Occasional nuclei may be but barely indented or, on the other end of the range, have five or six nuclear segments. The cytoplasm of these cells is moderately abundant. The hyaloplasm is stained a faint pink and contains

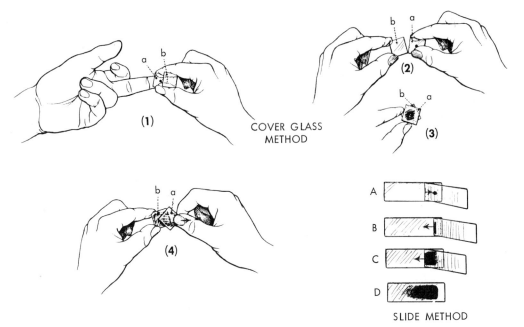

COVER GLASS
METHOD

SLIDE METHOD

Figure 10-6   Techniques of preparing blood smears on cover glass and slide.   *Cover-glass method.*   (1) A drop of blood is placed on one cover glass (a) by touching the surface of the glass to a drop of blood welling from a nick in a fingertip.   (2) A second cover glass (b) is placed directly upon the first.   (3) The drop of blood spreads out by capillary action between the cover slips. (4) As the drop reaches its maximal spread the cover glasses are separated by pulling them apart in a sliding motion in a plane parallel to the surface of the glasses.   In the process each cover slip bears a smear of blood.   *Slide method.*   A. A drop of blood is placed near the edge of a slide lying horizontally.   A short edge of a second slide is placed across the first slide at an angle of about 30° and drawn backward so that the drop of blood is caught in the angle of the two slides.   B. The drop spreads out in the angle.   C. The second slide is drawn over the horizontal one.   D. The blood is pulled over the surface of the horizontal slide and distributed as a smear.

many fine, usually inconspicuous granules. A moderate number are visible as punctate azurophilic structures, but most are barely resolvable, faint, dust-like particles.

Eosinophils, 12 to 15 μm in diameter, often contain a nonnucleolated, trilobed nucleus that typically consists of two large lobes joined by a large strand of chromatin from which a third small lobe hangs. The nucleus may lie near the circumference of the cell, with its lobes extending centrally. The chromatin is coarse, as in neutrophils, and heterochromatic. The cell is dominated by striking eosinophilic granules. These are large, closely packed, circular in outline, uniform in size, and stained a deep bright red or orange. They fill the cytoplasm so that little or no hyaloplasm is evident. They tend not to overlie the nucleus.

Basophils, too, measure 12 to 15 μm in diame-

ter. Their nuclei contain two or three lobes often less distinctly segmented than those in neutrophils or eosinophils. Chromatin is heterochromatic, and no nucleoli are evident. Cytoplasmic granules are most prominent, deeply stained a metachromatic red-violet. When well preserved, the granules are, as are eosinophilic granules, spherical, uniform in size, and tightly packed. But they may be quite variable in size and shape in Wright-stained smears because they are difficult to preserve and some of the granule's contents are extracted during fixation and staining. The granules of basophils overlie and obscure the nucleus.

Monocytes, 12 to 18 μm in diameter, may be among the largest of the white blood cells. The nucleus is often horseshoe-shaped but may show only a slight indentation. A subtle but important identifying characteristic is that the chromatin of monocytes forms a lacy, delicate network, in contrast to the relatively coarse, heterochromatin-rich nuclei of lymphocytes. Nucleoli, as a rule, are not visible. Monocyte cytoplasm is abundant, gray or blue in color. It may contain very many fine particles which impart a "dusty" character. A prominent centrosome lying in the nuclear indentation or *hof* may be present. Both nucleus and cytoplasm of monocytes may show folds.

Lymphocytes vary in size. Although their size distribution falls on a bell-shaped curve, they are often grouped as small, medium, and large. The smallest, 5 to 8 μm in diameter, may be smaller than erythrocytes (Fig. 10-8). In small lymphocytes the nucleus is almost the entire cell. It is round or slightly indented, with coarse chromatin and without visible nucleoli. It is surrounded by a thin rim of basophilic cytoplasm containing a few small azure-colored granules. The cytoplasm is typically stained a deep, clear blue. Larger lymphocytes, up to 15 μm in diameter, have proportionally more cytoplasm. Their nucleus is often flattened or indented, and the chromatin tends to

be less completely heterochromatic than that of smaller cells. Nucleoli may be visible.

Blood platelets are ovoid bodies, 2 to 4 μm in length, that tend to clump, often in groups of two or three, occasionally into large, irregular masses. Platelets contain a central blue granular zone, the *granulomere*, and a lighter peripheral zone clear of granules, the *hyalomere*.

A few dead or dying leukocytes are always present in the blood. Degenerated cells are more fragile than normal ones and, in part because of mechanical stress in preparing the smear, they may extend over a relatively large area and appear reticulated or spongy, often with parts torn. Their capacity to bind dye after fixation is reduced. Their nuclei may be pycnotic. Some dead cells retain their morphology so poorly that they are simply called *smudge cells*.

CYTOCHEMICALLY STAINED BLOOD CELLS

A great deal of chemical information may be inferred about blood cells from their appearance in Romanovsky-type preparations, such as the strongly

Figure 10-8 Lymphocytes of human blood. A. Blood film has been fixed and stained with Wright's stain. Two small lymphocytes are present. B. Small blood lymphocyte is seen in a phase-contrast photomicrograph. ×2,400. (From the work of G. A. Ackerman.)

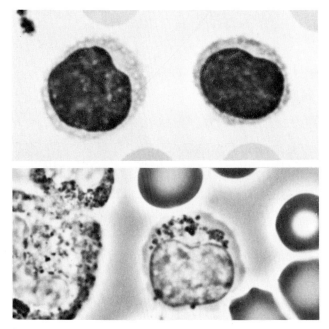

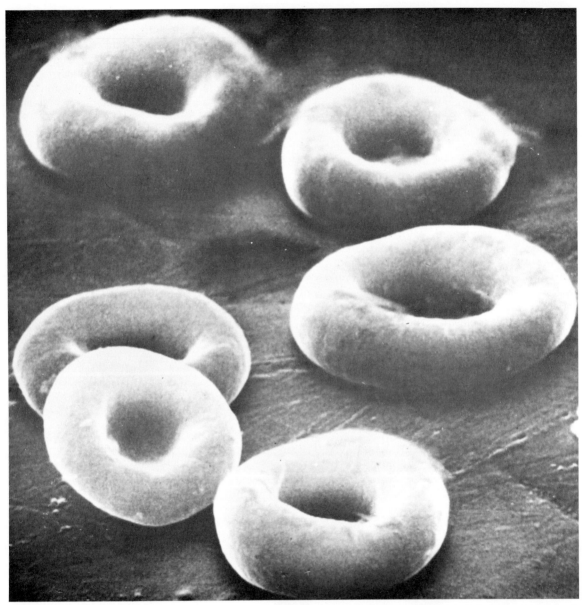

Figure 10-9   Human erythrocytes; scanning electron micrograph.   ×10,000.   (From F. M. M. Morel, R. F. Baker, and H. Wayland, J. Cell Biol., **48**:91, 1971.)

anionic character of eosinophilic granules and the cationic metachromatic nature of basophilic granules.   But this information may be refined and considerably extended by the use of selective or specific cytochemical reagents.   Thus ribonucleic acid may be disclosed in the cytoplasm of lymphocytes, monocytes, platelets, and occasionally in other cell types by showing that their basophilia is abolished by pretreatment of the cells with ribonuclease. Erythrocytes are positive in tests for hemoglobin

Neutrophils contain some granules rich in acid phosphatase and other lysosomal enzymes and other granules rich in alkaline phosphatase. The pronounced eosinophilia of the eosinophilic granule is due to a high concentration of the amino acid arginine, which bears a strongly cationic, terminal guanidinium group ($pK > 11$). The eosinophilic granules also contain lipid, being reactive both with Sudan black B and with methods for phospholipid, and a number of enzymes, a prominent one being myeloperoxidase which can serve as a marker. The intense metachromatic basophilia of the granules of the basophils is due to heparin, a strongly anionic, sulfated mucopolysaccharide. These granules also contain histamine and, in rodents, serotonin. They are positive in the PAS reaction, indicating the presence of 1,2 glycol groups (Chap. 2), which, by inference, are usually associated with carbohydrate moieties.

Basophilic granules, particularly in human beings, are difficult to fix well, since they are soluble in most fixatives; by their staining reactions and, after satisfactory fixation, by their size and shape, they are similar or identical to mast cell granules. Lymphocytes may show no distinctive cytochemical reactions except the presence of cytoplasmic RNA. However, some lymphocytes may produce antibody, and their cytoplasm and plasma membrane may contain antibody as revealed by immunofluorescence or other immunocytochemical reactions. Monocytes contain lysosomes and therefore show reactions for acid phosphatase and other lysosome-related enzymes. Platelets contain a contractile protein, *thrombostenin*, which has been demonstrated cytochemically (Fig. 10-17). They also contain glycogen, RNA, and a number of enzymes which can be demonstrated cytochemically.

ELECTRON MICROSCOPY OF BLOOD CELLS

Blood cells share many features with other cells. The following descriptions are largely confined to distinctive features of human cells.

Erythrocytes contain a uniformly granular density representing hemoglobin. Some ferritin may be present. Ribosomes, mitochondria, ER, Golgi, and lysosomes are absent in mature cells. Clear small vesicles may be present. Peripheral bands of microtubules are consistently present in inframammalian erythrocytes but are absent in human cells.

The plasma membrane is trilaminar by conventional electron microscopy (Fig. 1-24), but contains many discrete structures after freeze-fracture etch (Fig. 1-26). Under the scanning electron microscope their biconcave shape is striking (Fig. 10-9).

The description of granulocytes will be confined to their specific granules. The genesis of these granules and other ultrastructural findings are presented in Chap. 11.

Neutrophils[1] possess two types of granules. Primary, type A granules, corresponding to the azurophilic granules of light microscopy, account for about 20 percent of the granules. They are large (approximately 0.4 μm), dense, and homogeneous when well fixed. Often some extraction occurs during processing, however, leaving less dense, irregular structures. Approximately 80 percent of the granules (the cell contains a total of about 200) are secondary, type B. They are smaller (less than 0.3 μm) and less dense than primary granules and may contain a crystalloid. Both primary and secondary granules are bounded by a unit membrane. Each type of granule varies somewhat in morphology (Fig. 10-10).

Mature eosinophils have large (0.6 to 1.0 μm), spherical, dense, homogeneous granules which contain an angular, very dense, tightly lamellated crystalloid (Figs. 10-11 and 10-12).

When well fixed, the granules of basophils are dense structures about 0.5 μm in diameter (Figs. 10-13 and 12-10) which may contain granular material, myelin figures, lucent zones, and crystalloids. Both eosinophilic and basophilic granules are bounded by a unit membrane.

Lymphocytes (Figs. 10-14 and 10-15) contain a number of lysosomes and small to moderate-sized Golgi complexes. They may contain polyribosomes and some profiles of smooth ER, but unless undergoing transformation, they possess little rough ER.

Monocytes are distinguished by their content of moderate numbers of lysosomes, several prominent

[1]The term *neutrophil* designates the human cell. In rabbits and certain other species the secondary granules are often eosinophilic and relatively large. To distinguish these cells from the true eosinophils, they are termed *pseudoeosinophils*. The generic term, embracing this cell type regardless of species and staining reaction, is *heterophil*. Under the electron microscope heterophils of rabbits (pseudoeosinophils) and human beings (neutrophils) are remarkably alike.

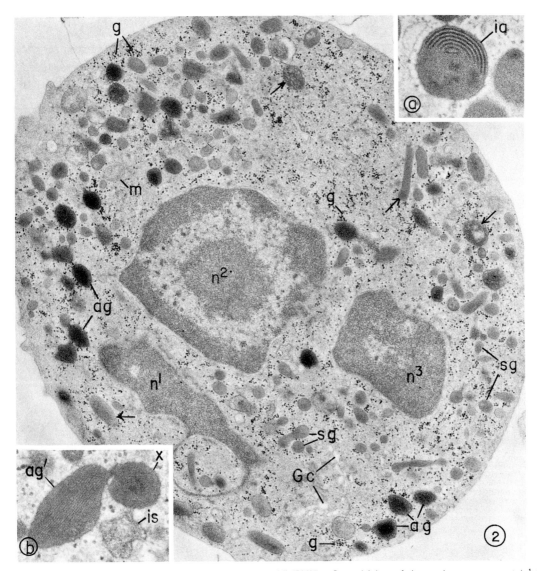

Figure 10-10 Mature human polymorphonuclear neutrophil (PMN). Several lobes of the nucleus are present (n^1 to n^3), and numerous granules, as well as glycogen (g), are scattered throughout the cytoplasm. A few mitochondria (m) and a small Golgi complex (Gc) are also visible. Some of the granules present are large and dense (ag), whereas others are small and less dense (sg). However, many granules are intermediate in size and density. Elongated forms, including football and dumbbell shapes, are also present (arrows). The insets depict internal structure within the large, dense (azurophilic) granules. Inset a shows a spherical granule (ia) containing concentric half-rings. Inset b illustrates the crystalline lattice with periodicity of approximately 100 Å which is commonly seen in football or ellipsoid forms (ag'). A cross section (X) of the ellipsoid form and an immature specific granule (is) are also present in this field taken from a PMN myelocyte. The sequence of development of these cells together with additional electron micrographs (Fig. 11-17) is presented in Chaps. 11 and 12. a. ×45,000; b. ×45,000. (From D. F. Bainton, J. L. Ullyot, and M. G. Farquhar, J. Exp. Med., **134**:907, 1971.)

Golgi complexes, and rough ER. The centrosome is large and may be surrounded by microtubules. The surface of the cell is often thrown into microvilli.

Platelets (Figs. 10-16, 10-17, and 12-11) are limited by a unit plasma membrane with a thin, moderately dense surface coat that probably forms bridges to other platelets (Fig. 10-16). A further distinctive characteristic of the platelet plasma

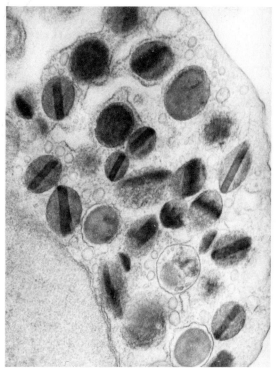

Figure 10-12 Electron micrograph of an eosinophilic leukocyte of the rat. In this species the distinctive granule contains a dense meridional bar which, like the less regular angular bodies in human eosinophils, consists of tightly lamellated dense membranes. ×25,000.

Figure 10-11 Portion of the cytoplasm of an eosinophilic leukocyte from human marrow. A small portion of a neutrophilic leukocyte is at the bottom of the figure. The granules of the eosinophil are bounded by membrane. The clear space about them may be artefactitious. The granules themselves are dense and contain a denser plaque. In the human being this dense plaque, even in mature cells, may be variable in size and shape. In many other animals it is rather regular in appearance and forms a meridional bar (see Fig. 10-12). At higher magnification the denser portion of the eosinophilic granules may be resolved as made of closely lamellated membranes. ×32,000.

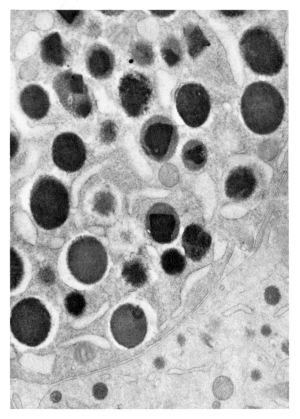

membrane is that it may dip into the cytoplasm to form an extended series of deeply penetrating canaliculi. Thorium dioxide, an electron-dense colloid, and other markers placed in the plasma gain ready access to even the deeper canaliculi. A number of membrane-bounded granules are present. A group 0.5 to 1.5 μm in diameter is very dense, similar to certain synaptic vessels, and appears to contain serotonin. A moderate number of lysosomes may be found. A well-developed microtubular system runs about the platelet beneath the plasma membrane; this may well be a skeletal structure, necessary to maintain the lenticular shape of the platelet. Among the microtubules and extending to the inner surface of the plasma membrane are microfilaments which are probably thrombostenin (Fig. 10-17).

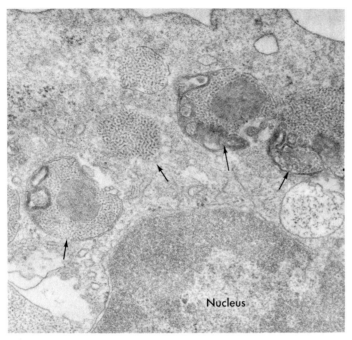

Nucleus

Figure 10-13 Electron micrograph showing part of a human basophilic leukocyte. The granules (arrows), which are membrane bounded, contain particulate material, material which forms myelin figures and sometimes crystals. (From the work of R. Hastie.)

Functions of blood

The blood, carried through virtually every tissue of the body, is one of the great homeostatic forces of the body. Blood distributes heat; carries respiratory gases, nutrients, and wastes; and flows through specific sensors capable of reacting selectively to such factors as osmotic tension, pH, temperature, and the levels of certain hormones in the blood. The blood provides cellular transport among the hematopoietic tissues, the connective tissues, and other tissues and organs. Thus it comprises a pervasive, regulative tissue, the basis of integration, distribution, and exchange among tissues of the body.

Certain functions of the blood directly dependent upon blood cells will be considered.

THE RESPIRATORY FUNCTIONS OF ERYTHROCYTES
Erythrocytes transport the respiratory gases oxygen and carbon dioxide between pulmonary alveoli and the tissues. In alveoli the partial pressure of oxygen exceeds 100 mm Hg, whereas in systemic venous blood coming from the tissues it is approximately 40 mm Hg.

This blood also carries carbon dioxide at a pressure of almost 50 mm Hg, far greater than that of the alveolar air. As a result, oxygen diffuses through the alveolar wall into blood plasma. From the plasma it diffuses into erythrocytes where it is loosely bound by the heme of hemoglobin. At the same time, carbon dioxide leaves the plasma and hemoglobin where it travels as a bicarbonate and carbaminohemoglobin and diffuses into the alveoli. Oxygenated blood has an oxygen tension of about 96 mm Hg, whereas in the tissues the tension is only about 35 mm Hg. When oxygenated blood reaches capillaries, oxygen dissociates from the hemoglobin and diffuses through the blood and capillary wall and out into the surrounding tissues. As it passes through the tissues, the oxygen tension drops from 96 percent in arterial blood to 64 percent in venous blood. Concomitantly carbon dioxide diffuses into the plasma and into erythrocytes from the tissue, the pressure there being greater than in the blood.

The iron of hemoglobin must be maintained in a ferrous form in order to transport oxygen. The oxidized form, *methemoglobin,* is incapable of respiratory functions. Erythrocytes contain an enzyme, methemoglobin reductase, which reverses the oxidation of ferrous hemoglobin into methemoglobin. The energy required for the maintenance of reduced hemoglobin is derived from glycolysis.

Erythrocytes are highly differentiated, considerably simplified cells. They may be viewed as sacs, bounded by plasma membranes, containing

Figure 10-14   Lymphocytes of a rat. These cells have been isolated from the spleen. Many of them contain nucleoli.   ×5,000. (From L-T. Chen, A. Eden, V. Nussenzweig, and L. Weiss, Cell Immun., **4**:279, 1972.)

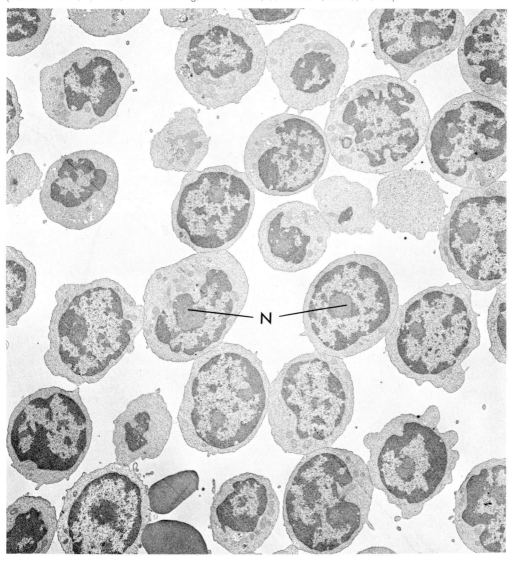

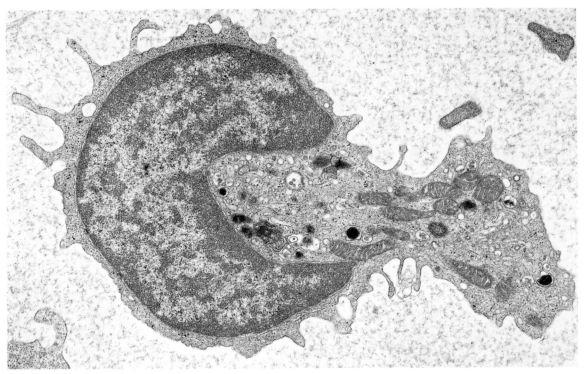

Figure 10-15   Human lymphocyte.   A motile lymphocyte contains a moderate number of membrane-bounded granules.   Note the microvilli on the cell surface.   ×9,200.   (From the work of G. A. Ackerman.)

hemoglobin in so concentrated a solution that it approaches the crystalline.   Indeed, hemoglobin is in a paracrystalline state, constituting about 33 percent of the weight of the cell.   Mature erythrocytes, without nucleus, ribosomes, and mitochondria, have lost their capacities for protein synthesis and aerobic metabolism.   They depend upon glycolysis for energy, most of which is used to maintain hemoglobin in the reduced state and maintain proper internal ion concentration.   Erythrocytes have even lost the capacity to synthesize new membrane.   Within the circulation and in passage through the spleen, erythrocytes lose portions of their plasma membrane and hence their biconcave shape, becoming more nearly spherical and therefore less deformable and more fragile. Hemoglobin also becomes irreversibly oxidized with age.   The cell, after a life of about 120 days in man, finally deteriorates to a point where it is removed from circulation, probably by the spleen.

The parceling of hemoglobin into small anucleate corpuscles is a mammalian characteristic representing an efficient evolutionary change.   Hemoglobin occurs in some invertebrates, typically as a high-molecular-weight plasma protein.   As a result the blood is quite viscous.   In inframammalian vertebrates and certain invertebrates hemoglobin occurs within cells which are nucleated and rather large.   The bulk of each of these erythrocytes requires relatively large capillaries.   Moreover, the large corpuscular size and shape of erythrocytes of lower vertebrates relative to anucleate mammalian corpuscles are less efficient for gaseous exchange between cellular hemoglobin and the plasma.   The small size and biconcave shape of mammalian erythrocytes make the interior of the cell quite accessible to oxygen and carbon dioxide.   (Because a spherical cell affords least surface per volume, its center is far from the surface.)   The biconcave shape also permits a considerable degree of flexibility and contributes to the cell's capacity to squeeze and twist through capillaries and spaces smaller than itself. Under certain common conditions of flow, moreover, the central biconcavity is drawn out and the erythrocyte circulates in the shape of a cone, apex forward (Fig. 10-13).

THE FUNCTIONS OF LEUKOCYTES

Inflammation is a complex, common reactive phenomenon in which leukocytes play a central role. Indeed, many of the functions of leukocytes, such as motility, chemotropism, and phagocytosis, are exhibited during inflammation. We shall, therefore, use the phenomenon of inflammation as a basis for considering certain fundamental properties of leukocytes.

If certain stimuli, often foreign substances such as chemical irritants or bacteria, are applied to the body or enter it, a series of reactions is initiated which constitute inflammation. Inflammation is largely a connective tissue phenomenon. The ground substance is depolymerized and becomes more liquid. Capillaries supplying the affected area become dilated, increasing the blood supply to the part and hence its temperature. The permeability of the capillary wall is increased, and plasma pours into the surrounding connective tissue, causing swelling and increased pressure on local nerve endings. Macrophages, eosinophils, mast cells, and other connective tissue cells in the locale respond. Circulating polymorphonuclear leukocytes, monocytes, and lymphocytes escape through the capil-

Figure 10-16   Platelet enmeshed in a fibrin clot from human blood. The platelet has a peripheral clear area, the hyalomere, and a central area containing mitochondria, ribosomes, and lysosomes, the granulomere. The platelet contains some glycogen, which is here selectively stained with lead, as minute granules. The fibrin forms an interlacing network which is in intimate contact with the platelet plasma membrane. ×32,000. Compare with Figs. 10-17 and 12-11.

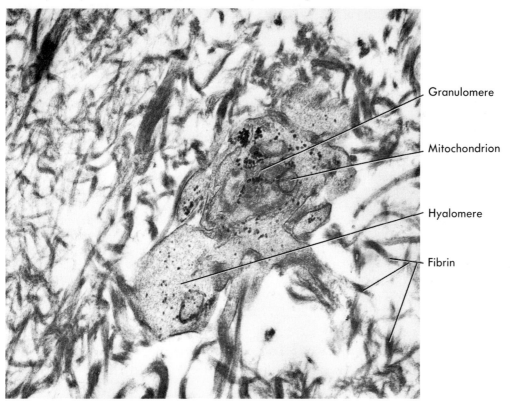

Granulomere

Mitochondrion

Hyalomere

Fibrin

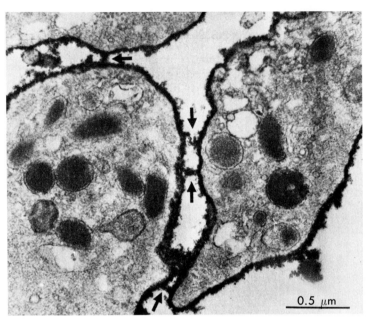

0.5 μm

Figure 10-17 Platelets of human blood. Immunohistochemical localization of thrombostenin on the platelet surface and inter-platelet bonds (arrows). (From F. M. Booyse and M. E. Rafelson, Jr., Series Haematologica, **4**:152, 1971.)

lary and postcapillary venular wall in great numbers and move into the site. If the irritants are bacteria they are phagocytized—to a degree dependent upon their virulence and the resistance of the host. Leukocytes, largely neutrophils, die after a short time as a result of bacterial action, change in environmental pH, and an inherently limited life-span. Dead and dying leukocytes, in aggregate yellowish in color and often creamy or somewhat granular in consistency, are called *pus*. These are the events that underlie the swelling, redness, pain, and warmth of a boil or carbuncle.

The ancients recognized these characteristics of inflammation: *tumor, rubor, dolor*, and *calor*. They constitute the cardinal clinical features of the process. As the acute phase of inflammation subsides, macrophages come on the affected zone and clear some of the cellular remnants and persisting irritants by phagocytosis and the release of lytic enzymes. Although local macrophages participate in these reactions, in most instances of inflammation of any intensity, most of the macrophages come from circulating monocytes that leave blood vessels, move to the site of inflammation and, as they

do, undergo transformation into macrophages which quickly become indistinguishable from resident macrophages of the connective tissues. These incoming phagocytes, at the outset smaller than some of the resident cells, have been termed *polyblasts*. Macrophages may, in some instances, accumulate and form nodules or *granulomata*. Indeed, there is a group of diseases, which includes tuberculosis and brucellosis, characterized by such accumulations of macrophages and identified as granulomatous diseases.

Eosinophils and basophils, like the neutrophils, are phagocytic. They appear, in addition, to play a more selective role in inflammation, especially in relation to immune reactions.

In addition to the cells outlined above, there are serum factors that are significant in at least some forms of inflammation. These include antibodies which facilitate phagocytosis, termed *opsonins*, polypeptides and proteins termed *kinins*, which affect vascular dilatation and permeability, and the proteins of the complement and coagulation systems.

We shall now examine certain leukocytic phenomena exhibited in inflammation: motility, chemotropism, endocytosis, and the release of mediator substances. Chemotropism is the directed movement of cells, specifically leukocytes or phagocytes, toward a substance (Fig. 10-18). It is clear that chemotropism in inflammation is due, at least in part, to complement and other serum factors which leak into the inflammatory zone from capillaries and venules whose permeability has been increased. It is likely, moreover, that some bacteria release polypeptides or small protein molecules which attract leukocytes. Having reached the inflammatory site, leukocytes exhibit *endocytosis*. This is a generic term which includes phenomena such as pinocytosis, phagocytosis, and emperipolesis, wherein materials are taken into a cell enclosed within membrane derived from the plasma membrane.

The essence of phagocytosis is the ingestion of particulate material that is carried in within a vacuole formed by invaginated plasma membrane. Thus any specific receptors or other chemical or physical properties of the membrane, as a glycoprotein coat, probably remain, coating the internal surface of the phagocytic vacuole or *phagosome*. Within the cytoplasm of the cell, however, the phagosome is subject to change. The vacuolar membrane is semipermeable, and water and salts may be transported across it. The pH within the vacuole typically drops into the acid range, in contrast to the slightly alkaline surrounding cytoplasm. As a result of such changes and of the activation of enzymes in the phagosome membrane, the phagocytized material may begin to undergo alteration. A critical and more fundamental change initiated soon after the formation of the phagosome, however, is its fusion with specific granules. The specific granules in the mature heterophil are membrane-bounded structures of at least two types (see above). Perhaps 10 to 20 percent of the granules are of the A, or primary, type which are lysosomes. They contain acid phosphatase and other acid hydrolytic enzymes that are the signature of the lysosome. In addition, in heterophils they carry sulfated mucopolysaccharide, basic proteins, and peroxidase. But approximately 80 percent of the granules are the smaller secondary, or B, granules rich in alkaline phosphatase and lysozyme which are not lysosomal. When the phagosome enters the cell, granules move toward it, the membranes of the phago-

some and the granule fuse and break down, and the phagosome and granule contents mix in a common vacuole (Fig. 10-19), thereby initiating the action of the granule contents upon the phagocytized material.

Several substances in leukocytes possess antimicrobial action. Protein or polypeptide antibacterial compounds have been extracted from leukocytes or their granules. These vary in their stability to heat, pH optima, amino acid composition, and other physical characteristics. They include *phagocytin*, bacteriocidal at acid pH and inactivated by moderate heating, and *leukin*, rich in arginine, stable to heat, and active against gram-negative bacteria. An iron-binding compound, *lactoferrin*, in secondary granules is bacteriocidal when not saturated with iron. The acid hydrolytic enzymes in the primary granules may lyse bacteria. The lysozymes of the secondary granules destroy the cell walls of bacteria and are thereby markedly bacteriocidal. The high concentrations of peroxidase, also present in the primary granules, have a powerful antimicrobial action. In addition to such specific factors, there are other compounds, resulting from the metabolic consequences of phagocytosis, which are bacteriocidal. The drop in vacuolar pH due to lactic acid is not only directly bacteriocidal; it provides an appropriate pH for the action of the lysosomal enzymes and such antibacterial compounds as phagocytin. Peroxides accumulate and are toxic to bacteria. Fatty acids and lecithins turn over and damage microbes.

Phagocytosis is associated with a spurt-like output of energy, dependent in large part upon the utilization of glycogen, glucose, and the hexose monophosphate shunt. ATP (adenosine triphosphate) is rapidly depleted by phagocytosis; it is regenerated by glycolysis. Oxygen consumption is increased. In addition to this metabolic burst, lipid turnover is increased in phagocytosis. This lipid may be involved in synthesis of new plasma (and vacuolar) membrane and in the constituents of the specific granules. Some lipids (see above) are bacteriocidal.

The events outlined above reveal that leukocytes are remarkably effective bacteriocidal cells. They should be visualized as a large circulating pool freely exchanging with an intravascular marginal pool, and supported by a large reserve of mature and near

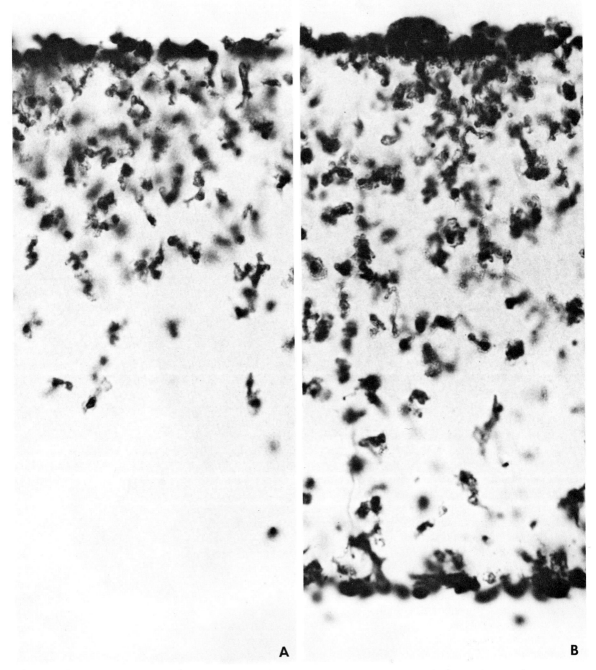

Figure 10-18   Chemotropism of neutrophilic leukocytes of the rabbit.   Sagittal section of a millipore filter whose top surface has been layered with neutrophils.   The bottom surface of A has been covered with serum alone.   In B, however, a chemotropic substance has been applied to the bottom surface and the cells have migrated from the upper surface, through the filter, to the bottom surface.   (From R. Snyderman, H. Gewurz, and S. E. Mergenlagen, J. Exp. Med., **128**:259, 1968.)

mature cells in the bone marrow which can be quickly released. The leukocytes circulate for a short time, having a half-life of but 8 hr after release from the marrow. In human beings they leave the bloodstream for the connective tissue spaces, where they die. Within that life-span they are capable of responding chemotactically to microbial invasion, pouring across the walls of capillaries and postcapillary venules in large numbers, reaching the site of microbes, and phagocytizing avidly. These cells, in distinction to macrophages, form the *microphage system*. They differ from macrophages in several important respects. These include the inability of microphages to regenerate and modify their lysosomes in relationship to material endocytized, considerably shorter life-spans than macrophages, and the absence of a complex life cycle. Heterophils are short-lived, nonadaptable, efficiently antimicrobial cells. To a certain extent, eosinophils and basophils partake of heterophil functions, but these cells have certain distinctive properties (see below).

Figure 10-19 Phagocytic polymorphonuclear heterophil of the rabbit. This cell, harvested from the peritoneal cavity, has ingested zymosan particles (Z). The specific granules of the heterophil are lysosomal in character and discharge their content of hydrolytic enzymes into the phagocytic vacuole. The granule moves toward the phagocytic vacuole; its membrane fuses with the membrane of the vacuole (arrows); and the contents of the granule enters the phagocytic vacuole. ×30,000. (D. Zucker-Franklin.)

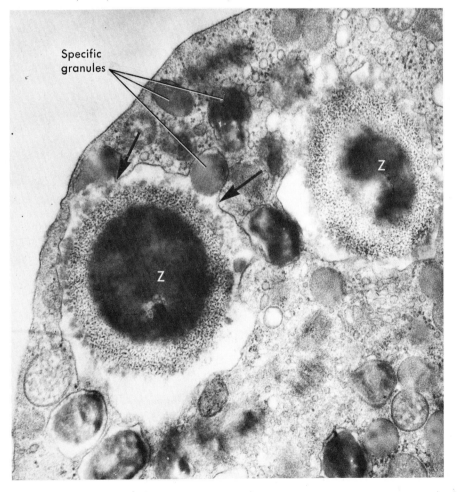

Phagocytosis has been emphasized as central to the antimicrobial activity of granulocytes. Their antimicrobial effects may be augmented without phagocytosis. Through the release of granules, akin to secretion, or the dissolution of the whole granulocyte, many powerful compounds are released and, where many granulocytes infiltrate and lyse, host tissue, as well as bacteria, may be damaged.

There are a number of syndromes in which heterophil granule formation or release is impaired. These conditions—which include chronic granulomatous disease of childhood, Chediak-Higashi syndrome, myeloperoxidase deficiency—interfere with the individual's ability to handle microorganisms and may be so severe as to result in death by uncontested infection.

BASOPHILS AND IMMUNOGLOBULIN E

Basophils are phagocytic and, having within their granules the lysosomal constituents of primary heterophil granules, they undoubtedly share some of the antimicrobial features of heterophils. In addition, the granules of basophils contain the anticoagulant and lipid-dispersant *heparin,* a sulfated mucopolysaccharide responsible for the metachromatic basophilia of the granules. The granules also contain histamine, a decarboxylation product of the amino acid histidine. Histamine is a powerful mediator causing muscular constriction and then dilation and increased vascular permeability. Serotonin, a vasoactive peptide mediator, occurs in rodent basophil granules. Slow reacting substance (SRS) is a vasodilating agent inducing increased vascular permeability. It is probably a constituent of the basophil's granules. Unlike histamine, whose effects are prompt and transient, SRS acts in a more sustained fashion following a latent period. SRS is an uncharacterized lipid, possibly related to the fatty acid hormones known as prostaglandins. Thus the granules of basophils contain certain very powerful vasoactive mediators which, on abrupt release, can induce widespread effects so severe as to induce vascular collapse. The granules of mast cells are similar to those of basophils and the two cell types may be considered part of the same system. These granules may well be discharged following a variety of stimuli. But a most important type of degranulation occurs by a specific immunologic reaction. Certain antigens,

for reasons unknown, induce the production of a distinctive antibody class, immunoglobulin E (IgE), by plasma cells. Relatively little IgE is found circulating in the plasma because soon after production it becomes fixed to the surface of basophils and mast cells. So charged with IgE, the basophils and mast cells remain, apparently undisturbed. But when the antigen which induced the formation of IgE reenters the body it specifically combines with the cell surface-bound IgE, acute degranulation is induced, and histamine and the other mediators are released. The reaction may be localized to certain shock organs such as the skin (the so-called Prausnitz-Küstner reagenic response) and the lungs (as bronchial asthma)—or the reaction may be severe, systemic, and lethal as in the anaphylactic response following a bee sting or an injection of penicillin in allergic individuals.

Thus, by their content of pharmacologically powerful mediators, their selective capacity to bind IgE, and their degranulation with release of mediators on the specific complexing of antigen with IgE, basophils and mast cells have a distinctive role in inflammation.

EOSINOPHILS AND ALLERGY

Eosinophils, like heterophils, are motile phagocytic cells containing lysosome-like specific granules. Like heterophils, therefore, they must possess antimicrobial properties. The basic proteins and the considerable peroxidase in eosinophilic granules contribute additional bacteriocidal properties. Eosinophils have been described as having an affinity for antigen-antibody complexes.[1] They are attracted to these complexes and engulf them. Antigen-antibody complexes, though themselves inactive, are capable of initiating a train of events with far-reaching effects. For example, antigen-antibody complexes bind complement, a series of serum proteins, and as a result induce cellular lysis. The whole spectrum of inflammation may result. Eosinophils, by phagocytizing and inactivating antigen-antibody complexes, may suppress or dampen the response set in motion by such complexes.

In the horse, moreover, eosinophils are charac-

[1] The antigen-antibody complexes considered here are free, not cell-bound as in the IgE system. The antibody involved here, moreover, is IgG or IgM, not IgE (see p. 384).

teristically attracted to mast cells and basophils or, specifically, to the histamine these cells release. There may be a type of balance or pairing off of eosinophils which mute allergic inflammatory responses and basophils and mast cells which excite them.

Certain processes drive the percentage of circulating eosinophils to more than 90 percent of the circulating leukocytes. These are parasitic infestations of muscle of which *trichinosis* is the paradigm. Evidence exists that extracts of trichina worms induce a class of lymphocyte to stimulate the marrow to produce eosinophils. Eosinophils accumulate in allergic reactions, perhaps called there by the action of histamine and other mediators. In the pulmonary tissues in bronchial asthma, where eosinophils collect in great number, characteristic crystals—Charcot-Leyden crystals—occur. These are probably derived from the dense core or crystalloid in the eosinophilic granule.

Eosinophils thus constitute circulating, phagocytic cells capable of antimicrobial activity. They phagocytize antigen-antibody complexes and, at least in a limited number of species, they can antagonize the actions of basophils. The eosinophils reduce the intensity of allergic reactions.

LYMPHOCYTES IN IMMUNOLOGIC RESPONSES AND AS STEM CELLS

Since comprehension of the role of lymphocytes and of hematopoietic and lymphatic tissue depends upon knowledge of elements of immunology, we shall consider this subject here and in Chaps. 11, 13, 14, and 15.

Immunologic mechanisms, themselves genetically determined, constitute a means of recognizing genetic relatedness. Thus, if foreign skin is grafted, a host will reject it. However, if an animal's own skin—or skin from a genetically identical animal—is grafted it will be accepted. If a foreign virus or protein is injected into a host, it will react against it. But if an animal's own cells or serum protein is injected, it will accept them without reaction. One root of a body's ability to distinguish ''self'' from ''nonself'' is its immunologic competence.

Immunologic mechanisms consist of an interrelated series of cellular and humoral phenomena initiated in response to foreign substances and having the broad functions of limiting and destroying foreign materials entering the body. Under certain circumstances these mechanisms can become deranged and directed at the body's own tissues, with dire results to health and life. The plasma and certain leukocytes are intimately associated with immunologic mechanisms. Before considering these associations, it is necessary to define the terms *antigen* and *antibody*. Antigens are large molecules of protein or carbohydrate, usually foreign to the host, which, on introduction into that host, are capable of eliciting the large-scale production of a highly specific gamma globulin or *immunoglobulin* which is sterically complementary to the antigen and may combine with it. This immunoglobulin is produced in lymphatic tissue by plasma cells and lymphocytes and is termed *antibody*. Antibody circulates in blood and lymph as a component of serum and is capable of combining with reintroduced antigen. Combination of antibody with antigen may itself have little effect. But the subsequent binding of *complement* and other serum factors by the antigen-antibody complex may set in motion an inflammatory response and other mechanisms which may have the salutory effect of limiting the penetration of antigen. For example, invading bacteria, met by antibody, may be agglutinated and their phagocytosis by polymorphonuclear leukocytes facilitated. In certain instances, however, the inflammatory response of the body to an antigen is exaggerated. Massive swelling extending beyond the initially affected area, extensive tissue death, severe smooth muscle spasm, and drop in blood pressure are among the exaggerated responses which may occur with explosive suddenness. Depending upon its extent, such a reaction may result in a slight transient swelling hardly distinguishable from simple inflammation, or it may lead to serious illness or death.

In the presence of adequate titers of circulating or humoral antibody, an antigen elicits a rapid response. Hence immunologic responses mediated by humoral antibody are designated as types of *immediate hypersensitivity*. Being dependent upon circulating antibody, they can be transferred from sensitized to nonsensitized host by passage of serum. *Delayed hypersensitivity* is a second fundamental immunologic response which may well have evolved before the capacity to produce circulating antibodies. Delayed hypersensitivity embraces a variety of immunologic phenomena having in common a latent period of hours or days before becoming manifest. Delayed hypersensitivity is mediated by cells. It does not depend upon the presence of humoral or serum-borne antibody and thus, in contrast to immediate hypersensitivity, cannot be transferred by serum from one subject to another It can be transferred only by the passage of sensitized cells. In delayed hypersensitive responses an antigen, on first entrance into the body, induces sensitivity by drainage into a local lymph node or by reaching the blood, which then enters the spleen. Thus the antigen must reach a lymphatic tissue. On second entrance of the antigen, or if the antigen persists, lymphoid cells of the sensitized host move toward it, surround it, and may, by their own direct action or by the elaboration of factors which induce actions in other cells, destroy the antigen. Tubercle bacilli induce a delayed hypersensitive reaction. Here foci of tubercle bacilli in a delayed hypersensitive animal are surrounded by a cluster of host cells, including many lymphocytes and macrophages, and may be either contained or destroyed. A second major example is a skin graft genetically different from that of the host in the H_2 locus; that genetic locus which most strongly determines if a graft persists. The graft, in its early phase, attracts little reaction but in this period graft proteins and H_2-determined structures are reaching lymph nodes or spleen and inducing a reaction. In about two weeks, in the case of foreign grafts, the bed of the graft becomes infiltrated by the host cell types characteristic of delayed hypersensitive reactions, primarily lymphocytes and macrophages. Soon thereafter, by action against the vasculature of the graft or the graft itself, the viability of the graft is compromised and it is rejected as a largely necrotic tissue.

A significant but paradoxical immune response is the development of tolerance, a state in which the body does not exhibit sensitivity to antigens which would be expected to elicit such a response. The mechanisms of tolerance, although the hypotheses intended to explain it are intriguing, have not been well worked out.

The development of immunologic competence At birth most mammals are immunologically inactive, both because their capacities to produce antibody and to participate in delayed hypersensitivity are not fully developed and because the placental barrier has shielded them, at least in part, from foreign material. In this period the newborn is protected against many infectious diseases by maternal antibodies, which cross the placental barrier and circulate in his body. Such transplacental transfer of antibody is a passive type of immunization. Within a few days of birth, however, the newborn's own immunologic mechanism becomes active. It is a matter of great theoretical significance that if a foreign substance is introduced into an animal before it is immunologically competent, that is, before the concept of "self" develops, and that substance persists, it becomes a part of "self" and antibodies are not produced against it. It thus is possible to give neonatal rabbits a powerful antigen, bovine serum albumin, and these animals will not elaborate antibody against this antigen if it persists in the body, despite the fact that they become immunologically competent. This phenomenon is of clinical significance in some cases of twinning, where fraternal twins of different blood types are tolerant of one another's blood because of some prenatal mixing.

A type of immunologic unresponsiveness may be induced in mature individuals by damaging the lymphatic tissue with x-ray or radiomimetic drugs. Advantage is taken of this phenomenon in the treatment of patients requiring transplants of kidneys or other tissue. To facilitate the acceptance of the graft, the patient is subjected to whole-body radiation or radiomimetic drugs at doses calculated to suppress immunologic competence temporarily.

Lymphocytes are central to all the immune responses: antibody production, delayed hypersensitivity, and tolerance. So complex and inextricably bound to their life cycle are these lymphatic functions that their consideration will be deferred to the treatment of sites of hematopoiesis and life cycles of the blood cells in Chaps. 11, 13, 14, and 15.

Monocytes may be essential in immune responses as precursors of macrophages. Macrophages are an early and consistent cell type in delayed hypersensitivity. Their behavior, for example, their capacity to migrate, is influenced by factors elaborated by lymphocytes. Antibody production to cellular or particulate antigen, moreover, often requires macrophages. The role of the macrophage may simply be to break down large masses to an appropriate size. Thus antibody production to whole erythrocytes requires that they be phagocytized, but ultrasonic fragmentation of erythrocytes is a satisfactory substitute for macrophage action. It is possible, in some instances, however, that a distinctive modification of a substance by macrophages is necessary for immunogenicity. Whatever the macrophage action, those antigens which are phagocytized tend to be better antigens, that is, induce a greater antibody response, than those which are not phagocytized. Eosinophils and basophils have immunologic roles which were considered earlier.

Lymphocytes have been cast as hematopoietic stem cells by the monophyletic school of blood formation. The evidence for the existence of stem cells and their possible lymphocytic nature is presented in Chap. 11.

References

See reference list at the end of Chap. 11.

chapter 11

The life cycle of blood cells

LEON WEISS

Origin and development of blood cells

This chapter treats the development, distribution, life-span, and destruction of blood cells. Blood cells are produced in specialized centers called *hematopoietic tissues*. Erythrocytes and granulocytes evolve from precursor cells by a series of profound cytologic transformations. The changes associated with lymphocytes and monocytes are less marked. Blood cells normally are released to the circulation only when sufficiently mature. They circulate within blood vessels but they may be withdrawn from the circulation and remain pooled within certain vascular beds. They may leave blood vessels and enter the connective tissues, where they function, undergo transformation into other cell types, or are destroyed. Or, apparently unchanged, they may reenter the circulation, often via lymphatic vessels. Blood cells have a predictable life-span, and when they die some of their components are reutilized in the manufacture of new cells.

SITES OF PRODUCTION OF BLOOD CELLS

The major postnatal hematopoietic organs are bone marrow, spleen, lymph nodes, and thymus. In the embryo the major phases of hematopoiesis occur in the yolk sac, liver, bone marrow, and thymus. The spleen and lymph nodes are also hematopoietic. The hematopoietic tissues not only produce blood cells but destroy them. They produce antibodies and possess most functions of connective tissues.

With the exception of the thymus, which has both epithelial and mesenchymal components, the major hematopoietic organs in mammals consist of specialized reticular connective tissues of mesenchymal origin. They contain a stroma made of reticular cells and fibers, and blood and lymphatic vessels, nerves, capsule, and trabeculae. Free cells include the blood cells and their precursors, macrophages, plasma cells, and other cells of the connective tissues.

HEMATOPOIESIS IN THE EMBRYO

Hematopoiesis in the human embryo begins in the second week of life, extraembryonically, in the wall of the yolk sac. Small nests of hematopoietic cells, largely erythroblastic (that is, productive of erythrocytes), lie in the mesenchyme. Most of these nests are surrounded by incomplete or isolated segments of developing blood vessels. These foci constitute blood islands. Later the segments of vessels enlarge and coalesce, form a confluent network within the wall of the yolk sac, connect to the systemic intraembryonic vessels by means of the vitelline vasculature, and become part of the circulation. Most hematopoietic foci in the yok sac are enclosed by endothelium, but some hematopoiesis is extravascular. By conveyance through the circulation or by direct migration of cells, hematopoietic cells of yolk-sac origin become distribted through the embryo.

Figure 11-1 Liver of a fetal mouse. A light micrograph of 1-μm section of epon-embedded 11-day fetal mouse liver (gestation 21 days, 057B1/6J strain). Sinuses (S), endothelium of sinuses (En), and cords of hepatic parenchymal epithelium and differentiating erythroid cells (HP) are noted. Within the sinuses circulate nucleated red cells of the yolk-sac series. They are darkly stained because of their high hemoglobin content. Within the parenchymal cords the erythroblasts of the definitive erythroid lineage are observed as relatively distinct, rounded cell types. Between them, often vacuolated, are processes of the hepatocytes. ×780. (From the work of R. A. Rifkind.)

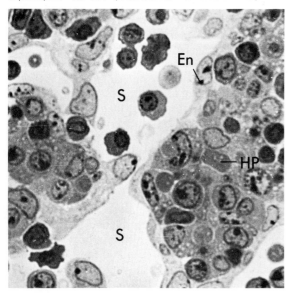

By the sixth week of embryonic life in human beings, hematopoietic foci appear in the liver; by the twelfth week, the hematopoietic activity on the yolk sac having dwindled, the liver is established as the major hematopoietic center (Figs. 11-1 and 11-2). Again erythropoiesis dominates. Myelopoiesis (the production of granulocytes) is minor, but there is moderate production of platelets and macrophages.

Two types of erythroblasts, *primitive* and *definitive* are produced in embryonic life. There is a shift from the first to the second during the hematopoietic shift from yolk sac to liver. The pattern of shift is species-dependent. In the mouse, only primitive erythroblasts are produced in the yolk sac and then turned off. Definitive erythroblast production is initiated with the initiation of hepatic hematopoiesis. In rabbits, guinea pigs, and cats great numbers of definitive erythroblasts are produced in the yolk sac but in man only moderate numbers. Primitive erythroblasts are relatively large cells with a large nucleus having little heterochromatin. Definitive erythroblasts are smaller cells, with a small, heterochromatic nucleus. Unlike primitive erythroblasts, definitive erythroblasts extrude their nuclei near the end of their maturation cycle and become anucleate discs. It is likely that the definitive erythroblast is responsive to the hormone erythropoietin and the primitive erythroblast is not. Associated with the shift from the earlier to the later erythroblast is a shift in the chain structure of hemoglobin: from fetal (HbF) to adult type (HbA and HbA$_2$).

Virtually all hepatic hematopoiesis is extravascular, occurring amidst the hepatic parenchymal cells. Hematopoiesis in man subsides in the liver at about the fifth month of gestation, at the time the marrow becomes hematopoietic, but some erythroblastosis may continue into the early postpartum weeks.

On a minor level, hematopoiesis goes on in the spleen parallel to that in the liver. Hematopoiesis, largely erythropoietic, becomes established in the spleen in the third fetal month and, in human beings, fades in the fifth. In mice splenic erythropoiesis occurs throughout life.

Bone marrow appears in the clavicle in the second month of human fetal life and, with the increased ossification of cartilage and membranes,

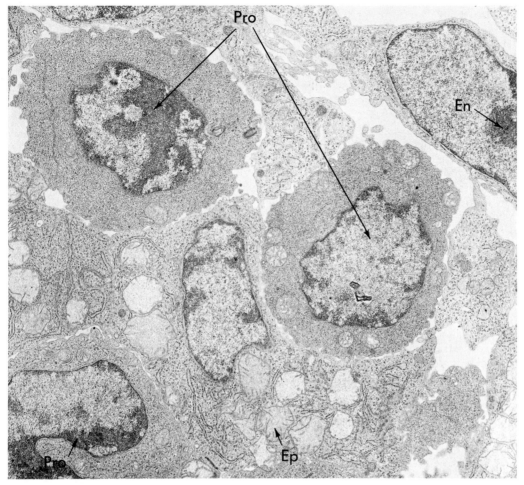

Figure 11-2   Electron micrograph from a preparation similar to that in Fig. 11-1.   A sinus endothelial cell is seen (top right, En). Three early erythroblasts are seen within the cord (Pro).   Hepatocytes (Ep) are distinguished by their content of endoplasmic reticulum and extended contours.   The erythroblasts show minimal ER, many free ribosomes, few mitochondria, and a rounded, compact contour.   Hematopoiesis (definitive cell line) is predominantly, if not exclusively, an extravascular event.   By day 12 reticulocytes may be observed which then pass across the endothelial border and enter the circulation.   ×5,000.   (From the work of R. A. Rifkind.)

becomes more extensive. It is heir to hepatic hematopoiesis. It becomes the dominant hematopoietic organ in the latter half of gestation and throughout postnatal life, the site where definitive erythropoiesis continues, myelopoiesis assumes major proportions, and platelets, monocytes, and lymphocytes are produced. A relatively high concentration of hematopoietic stem cells is maintained here. Streams of cells emanate from the marrow to circulate and populate lymphatic and other tissues.

Although the main hematopoietic sequence is from yolk sac to liver to marrow, a more restricted lymphatic type of hematopoiesis occurs in thymus, lymph nodes, and splenic white pulp. The thymus, an active lymphopoietic organ in the second month of gestation, becomes the largest lymphopoietic organ and remains so well into postnatal life. It yields this status only after a large-scale involution in adolescence. The spleen, most of whose pulp is erythroblastic (see above) develops a lymphocytic collar about its major arterial vessels. These sheaths, largely derived from lymphocytes (T cells) emigrated from the thymus, begin to appear in the second fetal month and increase in size through gestation and the first few months of postnatal life. In the postnatal period these sheaths are augmented by different lymphocytes (B cells) derived directly from cells leaving the marrow. Such bone-marrow-derived lymphocytes typically also form nodules within the lymphatic sheaths. Lymph nodes contain lymphocytes between the second and third fetal months. As with splenic white pulp, they hold, and permit the proliferation of, lymphocytes from both thymus and bone marrow.

The maintenance of hematopoiesis and its movement from the liver to the marrow depend upon the movements of hematopoietic cells, particularly the movements of stem cells. Thus, in the definitive layout of hematopoiesis which emerges in the late weeks of fetal life and becomes established in the weeks after birth, the bone marrow is the central hematopoietic organ. In human beings it produces all the erythrocytes, granulocytes, and platelets; it produces the monocytes, the source of the macrophages of the body, and the stem cells or lymphocytes which circulate to the thymus and upon which the lymphopoietic capacity of the thymus depends. It supplies lymphocytes to the spleen, lymph nodes, and other lymphatic tissues and is the source of antibody-producing cells. The thymus is an active lymphopoietic center that receives cells from the marrow, induces their proliferation, and releases relatively few with a thymic imprimatur, the T cells which circulate and stock specific sites in the spleen and lymph nodes. The latter structures constitute tissues which—although supporting considerable cellular proliferation, especially in an antibody response—are primarily traps wherein cells and materials from the blood and lymph are sequestered and permitted to interact. Thus spleen and lymph nodes trap monocytes released from the marrow and lymphocytes released from both marrow and thymus and, with antigens trapped from the blood (spleen) and lymph (lymph node), permit the sequential cellular interactions which result in an immune response.

The liver is inactive hematopoietically in man after birth. It reserves its potential for hematopoiesis, however, and in cases of failure of the marrow, hematopoiesis may be resumed in the liver, a phenomenon termed *extramedullary hematopoiesis.*

CYTOLOGIC CHANGES IN THE DEVELOPMENT OF BLOOD CELLS

Each of the circulating blood cells may be identified by specific morphologic criteria. Thus erythrocytes are anucleate cells which contain the pigment hemoglobin. Granulocytes contain specific cytoplasmic granulation and polymorphous nuclei. These morphologic characteristics, representing a highly differentiated status, gradually evolve in hematopoietic cells. Early hematopoietic cells are free cells which contain a spherical nucleus, nucleoli, and basophilic cytoplasm. They lack cytoplasmic granulation, pigment, or other evidence of belonging to a specific cell line. They closely resemble large or medium-sized lymphocytes.

SCHOOLS OF HEMATOPOIESIS

Sharply divergent views have been held regarding the earliest of the hematopoietic cells. These views have been codified in the *monophyletic* and *polyphyletic schools of blood formation.*

The monophyletic school considers the earliest recognizable precursor of blood cells, termed *hemocytoblasts,* capable of differentiating into any blood cell type. Further, it holds that the lymphocyte and the hemocytoblast are equivalent cells. In other words, the lymphocyte is considered a multipotential stem cell.

The complete polyphyletists recognize a separate stem cell for each of the blood cell types, that is, a stem cell for erythrocytes, another for granulocytes, another for lymphocytes, and another for monocytes. The most strongly presented polyphyletic position evolved into a "dualist" position in which two precursor cell types are recognized: a primitive white cell that can produce granulocytes, lymphocytes, and monocytes, and an endothelial cell, lining a collapsed sinusoid or an intersinusoidal capillary, that can produce erythrocytes and megakaryocytes.

But the essence of the struggle between monophyletists and polyphyletists has revolved around the capacity for differentiation of lymphocytes. The polyphyletists regard these cells as an end stage incapable of further differentiation. The monophyletists regard them as capable of differentiating into the other blood cells.

HEMATOPOIETIC STEM CELLS

The monophyletic and polyphyletic positions outlined above were developed almost a half century ago. We must now consider whether, by more recent evidence, a hematopoietic stem cell, defined as a cell capable both of differentiating into any of the blood cells and of maintaining itself by mitotic division, exists. If it exists, moreover, what is its relationship to lymphocytes?

Experiments within the past 15 years by Ford, Barnes, and their associates and by Till and McCulloch and their associates strongly indicate that a hematopoietic stem cell exists (Figs. 11-3 to 11-5). Their work depends upon observations of cells which bear distinctive chromosomal markers (revealed in the metaphase karyotype) and are injected into irradiated hosts. Their data and conclusions result from the following type of experimental model.

After lethal irradiation (that is, more than 900 rads) a mouse dies with a profound depletion of all its blood cells (pancytopenia). Death may be averted if such an irradiated mouse is given a suspension of bone marrow cells. Animals so treated survive and in early stages of recovery show in their spleen, against a background of radiation-induced devastation, grossly visible nodules which represent small colonies of proliferating hematopoietic cells. The cellular composition of these colonies varies but significant numbers contain erythroblasts, myeloblasts, megakaryocytoblasts, and cells of lymphoid character—in short, precursors of all the blood cells. There is direct and indirect evidence that each of these colonies, including those with multiple cell types, is a clone, that is, is derived from a single cell. Such a cell, termed a CFU or CFC (colony-forming unit or colony-forming cell) by Till and McCulloch, would clearly fit the definition of a stem cell.

The direct evidence for the existence of stem cells is obtained by irradiating the donor marrow cells referred to above severely, *but not lethally,* to induce chromosomal damage. This chromosomal

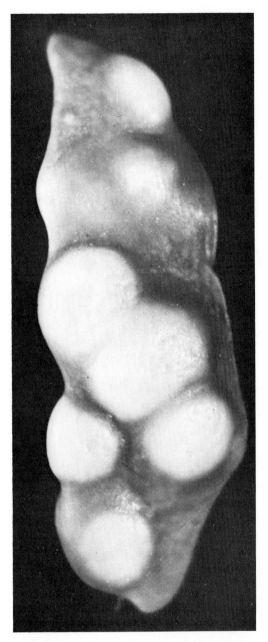

Figure 11-3 Splenic nodules. This spleen was removed from an animal given lethal irradiation and then a ''rescuing'' injection of bone marrow cells. The marrow cells circulated to the irradiated spleen where they remained, proliferated, and formed these macroscopic colonies. It is likely that each of these colonies is a clone (see text). (From the work of J. Till and E. McCulloch.)

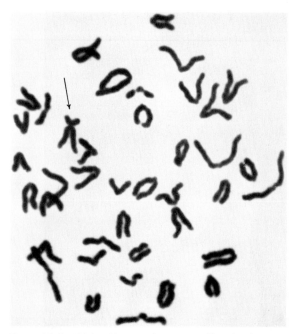

Figure 11-4 ''Unique'' mouse karyotype. The clonal nature of the splenic colonies exemplified in Fig. 11-3 is revealed by distinctive or unique karyotypes in the donor marrow cells. These karyotypes are induced by lightly irradiating the donor cells (see text). Arrow points to the distinctively damaged chromosomes which serve as a marker. (From the work of W. T. Wu, J. Till, and E. McCulloch.)

Figure 11-5 Splenic nodule. A number of splenic nodules have a diverse hematopoietic population including virtually all hematopoietic cell types. This light-microscopic field is from such a nodule. (From the work of W. T. Wu, J. Becker, J. Till, and E. McCulloch.)

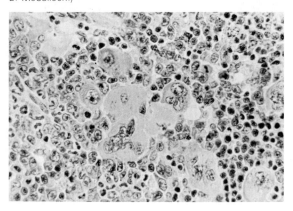

damage, induced in a widespread, unpredictable way, typically results in unique or highly distinctive abnormal karyotypes. When such irradiated donor cells, containing uniquely damaged karyotypes, form splenic colonies in lethally irradiated recipients, it can be found that different hematopoietic cell types within a given colony bear the same distinctive karyotype. This reveals that different blood cell lines, such as erythrocytes, granulocytes, and platelets, can originate from the same cell. Indirect evidence supporting the clonal nature of splenic colonies includes the existence of a linear relationship between the number of nucleated donor cells and the number of splenic colonies without an initial threshold and the resemblance of the radiation survival curve of colony-forming cells to that of single cells in tissue culture or tumor transplants.

In addition to the experimental work of the Till and McCulloch group, the occurrence in human myelogenous leukemia of the Philadelphia chromosome, an abnormal chromosome revealed in karyotype analysis, suggests the presence of a stem cell because this abnormal marker may be found not only in myelocytes but in every other blood cell type in this disease.

More differentiated cell types derive from the CFC. These include the precursor of erythroblasts, a cell sensitive to the action of erythropoietin (the hormone stimulating erythropoiesis) and known as the erythropoietin responsive cell (ERC). There is, in addition, a myelopoietic stem cell.

What of the morphology of the stem cell? What of the claims that lymphocytes are stem cells? We now recognize that lymphocytes, though morphologically similar, may be functionally dissimilar in terms of immunologic roles. Clearly, many lymphocytes are not stem cells, but some lymphocytes may be, and some indirect evidence suggests lymphocytes as stem cells. Thus the number of stem cells in certain experimental models has been correlated with the number of lymphocytes. But no direct evidence on the structure of the stem cell exists. We may infer the presence of stem cells by the presence of a clone containing several cell types. But regarding the appearance of the stem cell as it moved into the spleen and undertook colony formation, we have no information. It is a paradox that the question whether hematopoietic stem cells exist, a question that preoccupied morphologists for more than half a century and constituted their exclusive preserve, has been resolved without reference to the morphology of the stem cell.

The greatest concentration of stem cells in the adult, as determined by splenic colony assay, is in the bone marrow. The total CFC in the marrow of the mouse may be 40,000 cells. In contrast, the mouse spleen may have but 2,000. The vastly greater capacity of the marrow to restore an irradiated recipient relative to that of the spleen is explicable by its twentyfold superiority in stem cell content. Even its relatively high content of stem cells does not represent, for the marrow, a high concentration; in the mouse only about 1 in 10,000 nucleated cells is a CFU.

In the mouse, approximately 10 CFU are present in each cubic centimeter of blood; this is a concentration of approximately 1 CFU per 1,000,000 nucleated blood cells. This is one one-hundredth the concentration in the marrow. It is likely that the CFU in blood represent stem cells released from the marrow and traveling to lymphatic tissues where they are destined for lymphoid differentiation.

CFU circulate in the fetus and occur in fetal liver and marrow. At the time of the decline in hepatic hematopoiesis the number of circulating CFU is unusually high, suggesting large-scale hematopoietic movement to the marrow. It is unlikely that CFU similar to those in liver and marrow are present in yolk sac.

Erythrocytes

DEVELOPMENT

The formation of an erythrocyte requires profound progressive changes in the nucleus and cytoplasm of its precursor cell. The nucleus becomes smaller and increasingly heterochromatic and is finally extruded. The cytoplasm, after becoming rich in polyribosomes, synthesizes and accumulates hemoglobin and then loses its ribosomes and other organelles. There is thus a transformation of a nucleated cell endowed with most organelles into a biconcave, anucleate disc containing hemoglobin in concentrations so high as to be paracrystalline, specialized enzymes necessary for the maintenance of hemoglobin as a respiratory pigment, and an anaerobic source of energy.

ERYTHROPOIETIN

Erythropoiesis is initiated and regulated by erythropoietin, a glycoprotein hormone of molecular weight 70,000. It appears to be produced by the interaction of factors produced in the kidney. It circulates in the plasma and acts on the bone marrow, driving erythropoietin-sensitive cells to differentiate into erythroblasts. In the fetus it is active in the hepatic phase of hematopoiesis but not on the yolk sac. Erythropoietin is not entirely dependent upon the kidney for its production; its production continues after nephrectomy.

CYTOLOGY OF ERYTHROCYTIC DIFFERENTIATION

Basophilic erythroblasts, the first of the cells in the erythroid line recognizable as erythroblasts, are free cells approximately 15 μm in diameter. Under the light microscope they are identified by the presence of ribonucleoprotein and little hemoglobin in the cytoplasm and a relatively small nucleus with densely stained, coarse chromatin. In Romanovsky preparations, hemoglobin binds the anionic dye eosin, since its protein globin is strongly cationic. The phosphate ion of RNA binds the cationic dyes methylene blue and the azures.[1] Accordingly, in erythroblasts of the early stages, with little hemoglobin, the cytoplasm is stained deeply with basic dyes. In late stages of development with little ribonucleoprotein and abundant hemoglobin, the cytoplasm is stained deeply with anionic or acid dyes. Therefore, early erythroblasts are termed *basophilic erythroblasts,* and late erythroblasts are called *orthochromatic erythroblasts.* The latter cells are often designated *normoblasts.* In stages intermediate between these extremes of development, the hue of the cytoplasm represents a combi-

[1] Cationic dyes are termed *basic dyes* by histologists. Tissue components binding basic dyes are termed *basophilic.* See Chap. 2.

nation of the colors of the acid and basic dyes. Such intermediate forms are *polychromatophilic erythroblasts* (Figs. 11-6 and 11-7, see color inserts).

By electron microscopy (Figs. 11-2, 11-8, 11-9, and 12-7) the cytoplasm of erythroblasts is noteworthy for the presence of polyribosomes, for a density due to hemoglobin, for ferritin, and for the scanty development of endoplasmic reticulum (ER). Polyribosomes are most abundant and con-

Figure 11-8   Polychromatophilic erythroblasts, bone marrow, of the rat.   Two polychromatophilic erythroblasts press against different points of the endothelium (end) of vascular sinuses of the marrow.   The erythroblasts are marked polarized.   The cytoplasm, at one pole, contains ribosomes and mitochondria as well as hemoglobin.   The nuclear pole is surrounded by a thin rim of hemoglobinized cytoplasm.   The nuclear pole will be detached and phagocytized, and the cytoplasmic pole will become a reticulocyte. ×40,000.   Consult Chap. 12 and Figs. 12-4, 12-7, and 12-8.   (From L. Weiss, J. Morph., **117:**467, 1965.)

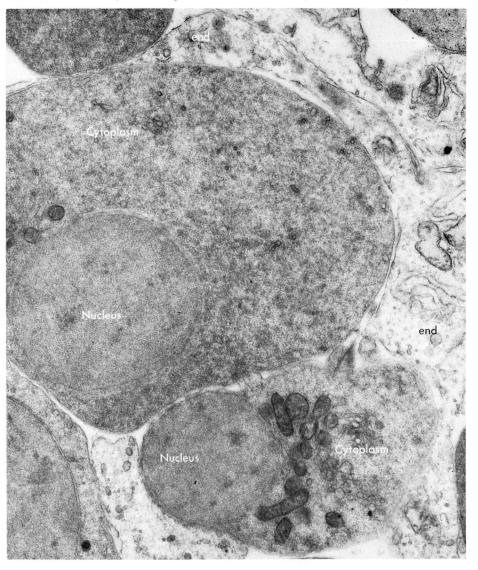

tain the largest number of ribosomes in basophilic and early polychromatophilic erythroblasts. By the orthochromatic stage the polyribosomes are considerably reduced both in concentration and ribosomal number. The density of the cytoplasm, due to hemoglobin, increases throughout maturation. Ferritin is present in these cells at every stage, and its presence in certain cells without evidence of hemoglobin may mark those cells as erythropoietin-sensitive erythroblast precursors (ERC). Ferritin is a storage form of iron, a protein linked to micellar iron and capable of holding as many as 2,500 iron atoms. It may be scattered as single molecules that have a characteristic structure under the electron microscope or collected in large, membrane-bounded aggregates termed *siderosomes*. Erythroblasts may often display ferritin at their surface, sometimes in invaginations suggesting pinocytosis. It has been stated that ferritin passes into erythroblasts as a source of iron directly used in hemoglobin formation. But a clearly defined form of utilizable iron is transported by a special iron-binding globulin, *transferrin,* and ferritin in erythroblasts may, instead, simply represent excess or storage iron. In basophilic erythroblasts a slight to moderate amount of rough ER is present, but this rapidly becomes scanty. One or more Golgi complexes occur in basophilic erythroblasts, but again these become quite small and disappear by the orthochromatic phase. Mitochondria diminish in number and size in polychromatophilic cells. A few remain in orthochromatic erythroblasts and are absent in mature erythrocytes. Few lysosomes are present in erythroblasts.

The nucleus of basophilic erythroblasts, relative to other hematopoietic cells, is small and heterochromatic. It contains several nucleoli and conspicuous nuclear pores. With maturation, the nucleus becomes smaller, anucleolate, more pronouncedly heterochromatic, and more nearly spherical. At the time of nuclear loss, erythroblasts become markedly polarized, with the nucleus at one pole of the cell and the bulk of cytoplasm at the other. The cells break in two, and the nuclear-containing fragment is often rapidly phagocytized. A *free* nucleus is not released; it is surrounded by a very thin rim of hemoglobinized cytoplasm.

The loss of a nucleus converts an erythro*blast* to an erythro*cyte*. Nuclear loss occurs near the end of erythroblast maturation, near the orthochromatic stage. The nucleus may be lost at earlier stages, resulting in polychromatophilic or even basophilic *erythrocytes*. Then further maturation may proceed in the anucleate cell. In fact, even in orthochromatic erythroblasts some ribosomes are present. (See discussion of reticulocytes below.)

The cell diameter decreases as erythroblasts mature into erythrocytes. Basophilic erythroblasts may measure about 15 μm in diameter. The diameter of erythrocytes is about 7.5 μm. The relatively constant size of erythrocytes makes them useful in gauging the size of other structures in histologic sections.

Reticulocytes A freshly produced erythrocyte, that is, one which has just lost its nucleus (Fig. 11-6, see color insert), always contains some ribosomes. Less than 1 percent of human erythrocytes have enough ribosomes to be classed as *polychromatophilic* or *basophilic* as determined by their appearance in a blood film stained with a Romanovsky-type stain. A more sensitive method for revealing ribonucleoprotein in such newly produced erythrocytes is *supravital staining*. The technique consists of mixing a drop of freshly drawn blood with a drop of brilliant cresyl blue or other suitable dye and making a smear of the mixture. The residual ribonucleoprotein appears as a striking blue web or reticulum. These smears may be counterstained with a Romanovsky stain in the usual manner and the blue web will be superimposed on a pink erythrocyte. Such supravitally stained cells, termed *reticulocytes*, constitute about 2 percent of circulating erythrocytes. The enhanced sensitivity of supravital staining over conventional Romanovsky staining in demonstrating the small amount of ribonucleoprotein of freshly produced erythrocytes lies in the dispersion of ribonucleoprotein. In supravital staining, ribosomes are clumped into masses (the reticulum) visible by light microscopy. In the air-dried, methanol-fixed material of Romanovsky staining, the ribonucleoprotein of new erythrocytes remains, in some cells, so finely dispersed that it is below the limit of resolution of the light microscope.

ERYTHROKINETICS

The erythroid cells in man may be divided into four categories: nucleated cells of the marrow, marrow reticulocytes, circulating reticulocytes, and circulating mature erythrocytes. The size of each of these classifications, as determined by Donahue, Gabrio, and Finch (1958), is as follows:

Erythroid cells	Number of cells per kilogram of body weight
Erythroblasts	5.59×10^9
Marrow reticulocytes	5.73×10^9
Circulating reticulocytes	3.22×10^9
Circulating mature erythrocytes	$309.0 \ \times 10^9$

The bulk of this population circulates. The marrow, moreover, has a population of reticulocytes as a ready reserve somewhat greater than the number in the blood, and equal to the number of erythroblasts.

It is possible to calculate the turnover rate of circulating erythrocytes since the number of erythrocytes in the blood is constant and known and the life-span of erythrocytes (see below) is about 120 days. In a 70-kg man, the turnover rate being 0.83 to 1.0 percent daily, 17.9 to 21.6×10^{10} erythrocytes are produced each day and the same number destroyed. Further, the mean life-span of marrow reticulocytes is 36 to 44 hr and that of the circulating reticulocytes approximately 25 hr. The time required for erythroblasts to double by mitotic division is 36 to 44 hr. Thus the total marrow turnover time is about 72 to 88 hr from erythroblast to mature erythrocyte.

THE LIFE-SPAN OF ERYTHROCYTES

Erythrocytes display no clear morphologic changes as they age, but they gradually become more mechanically fragile; they become unable to maintain their hemoglobin in a reduced, functional state; and the activity of certain enzymes, such as glucose 6-phosphate dehydrogenase, declines. The change that triggers the destruction of an erythrocyte is not known. Relatively few erythrocytes are destroyed at random; instead, about 120 days after a human red cell is released into the bloodstream, it is withdrawn from the circulation and destroyed.

The life-span of erythrocytes may be determined by several methods. Radioactive chromium tagging of erythrocytes, using ^{51}Cr, is now most commonly employed. A few microliters of washed red cells are mixed with a solution of $Na_2{}^{51}CrO_7$ and then reinjected into the subject from whom the blood was taken. The ^{51}Cr adheres tenaciously to hemoglobin without appreciably damaging the cells. Life-span is estimated by the persistence of circulating radioactivity.

THE DESTRUCTION OF ERYTHROCYTES

The reticuloendothelial system, notably in the spleen, liver, and bone marrow, plays a major part in the destruction of aged or damaged erythrocytes. Erythrocytes destined for destruction are withdrawn from the circulation, sequestered for short but variable periods, and then phagocytized. The hemoglobin is quickly degraded. The iron enters a labile pool from which it may be transferred by *transferrin* to the marrow, where it is reutilized in the production of new hemoglobin for new erythrocytes. Iron is stored as ferritin or hemosiderin, as discussed above. The labile iron pool exchanges with ferritin, which is present in erythroclastic tissues. The non-iron-containing portion of hemoglobin undergoes alteration to the bile pigment *bilirubin*.

Polymorphonuclear leukocytes

DEVELOPMENT

In the formation of granulocytes from myeloblasts, the cytoplasm progressively acquires granules of a specific type and the nucleus becomes flattened, indented, and then lobulated [Figs. 11-6 and 11-7 (color insert), and 11-9 to 11-17]. A granulocyte precursor more differentiated than the CFU exists,

demonstrable by plating marrow suspensions in soft agar. Clones, predominantly of granulocytic cells, form in 7 to 10 days. Although its presence is suspected, a *leukopoietin,* the counterpart to erythropoietin, has not been characterized.

The first recognizable precursor of the granulocytes is the myeloblast, a relatively small cell (ap-

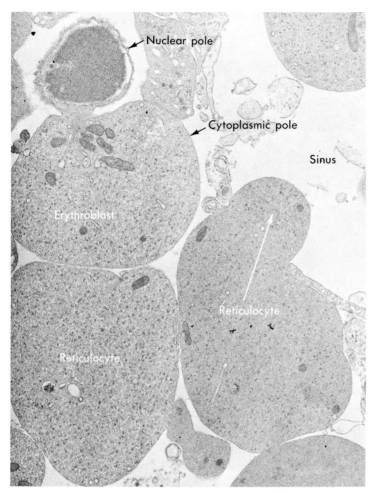

Nuclear pole

Cytoplasmic pole

Sinus

Erythroblast

Reticulocyte

Reticulocyte

Figure 11-9   Bone marrow from a mouse.   A reticulocyte is apparently passing across the wall of a sinus, through an aperture (arrow).   An erythroblast is sharply polarized.   Its nucleus, surrounded by a thin rim of cytoplasm, at the upper pole; its cytoplasm at the lower pole.   The poles will probably separate with the formation of a reticulocyte.   This process typically occurs at the wall of a vascular sinus.   Reticulocytes contain some polyribosomes and, often, a few mitochondria, in addition to hemoglobin. ×12,000.   (From the work of J. Chamberlain, R. Weed, and L. Weiss.)

proximately 10 μm in diameter) containing, in Romanovsky-stained smears, a large nucleus rich in euchromatin, three to five nucleoli, and a granule-free basophilic cytoplasm.

In the cytoplasm the first clear evidence of differentiation in Romanovsky preparations is the appearance of a few granules in the cytoplasm. This marks the *promyelocyte* stage. Gradually cytoplasmic basophilia decreases and more and more granules accumulate until the full complement is attained. Granules destined to become neutrophilic are large and azurophilic when first formed. These are the primary granules. (See discussion of electron microscopy below.) By the time the cell is mature most of the granules are small, definitive, or secondary granules, barely resolvable by light microscopy. Basophilic and eosinophilic granules may usually be definitively recognized soon after they appear, although initially the latter may be somewhat basophilic or fail to bind eosin avidly.

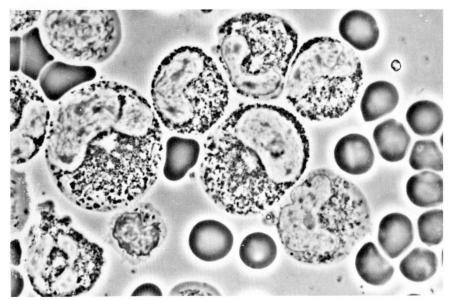

Figure 11-10 Human bone marrow cells. This field contains myelocytes together with erythrocytes. ×1,300. (From the work of G. A. Ackerman.)

Figure 11-11 Human bone marrow cells. Myelocytes are present in this electron micrograph. Cells 1 to 4 are early myelocytes; 5 and 6, late. ×9,200. (From the work of G. A. Ackerman.)

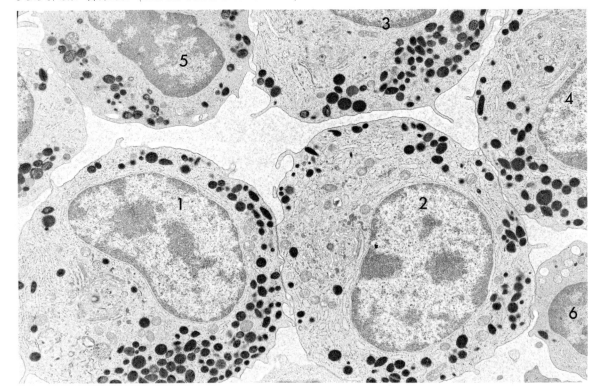

MARROW (development, 14 days)

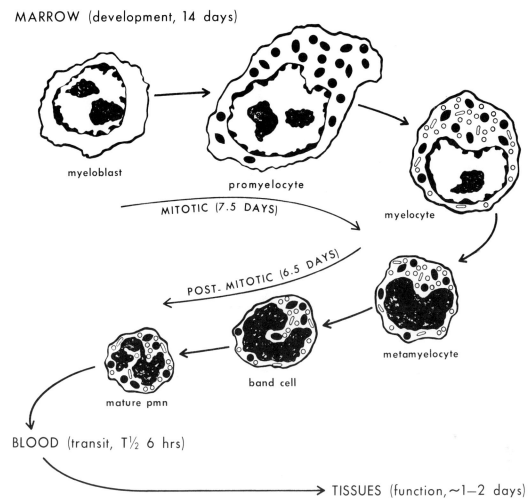

Figure 11-12   Diagrammatic representation of the polymorphonuclear neutrophil (PMN) life cycle and stages of PMN maturation. The myeloblast has a large oval nucleus, large nucleoli, and cytoplasm lacking granules.   It is followed by two granule-producing stages: the promyelocyte and the myelocyte.   During each of these stages a distinct type of granule is produced: azurophils (solid black), formed only during the promyelocyte stage, and specific granules (light forms) produced during the myelocyte stage.   The metamyelocyte and band forms are nonproliferating, non-granule-producing stages which develop into the mature PMN.   The latter is characterized by a multilobulated nucleus and cytoplasm containing primarily glycogen and granules.   The times indicated for the various compartments were determined by isotope-labeling techniques.   (From D. F. Bainton, J. L. Ullyot, and M. G. Farquhar, J. Exp. Med., **134**:907, 1971.)

In adult neutrophils the hyaloplasm is usually slightly acidophilic.   The hyaloplasm of circulating basophils and eosinophils may be slightly basophilic or appear to bind no dye.

The first nuclear changes are subtle, consisting of condensation of chromatin and some loss in its fine texture.   Shortly before cytoplasmic granules reach their maximal number, the nucleus begins to flatten on one side and then becomes more and more deeply indented until it is markedly lobulated, the lobes connected only by slender threads of nuclear material.   Two- to five-lobed nuclei are produced.   Nuclear configuration in the circulation ranges from slight indentation to marked lobula-

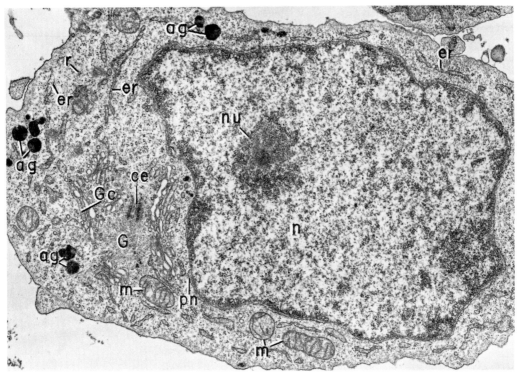

Figure 11-13   Human polymorphonuclear neutrophil (PMN); early myelocyte reacted for peroxidase.   The nucleus (n) with its prominent nucleolus (nu) occupies the bulk of this very immature cell.   The surrounding cytoplasm contains a few azurophilic granules (ag), a large Golgi complex (G), several mitochondria (m), scanty rough endoplasmic reticulum (er), many free polysomes (r), and a centriole (ce).   All the azurophilic granules (ag) appear dense, since they are strongly reactive for peroxidase.   The granule-producing apparatus [the perinuclear cisterna (pn), rough endoplasmic reticulum (er), and some of the Golgi cisternae (Gc)] is also reactive, although less so than the granules.   ×21,000.   (Legend and figure from D. F. Bainton, J. L. Ullyot, and M. G. Farquhar, J. Exp. Med., **134**:907, 1971.)

tion.   A cell with a flattened or indented nucleus and many granules is a *myelocyte*.   When nuclear indentation becomes sufficiently advanced to give the nucleus a U, V, or T shape the cells are called *metamyelocytes* or *juvenile cells*.   Further indentation results in nuclear lobes, the early stages of which have been termed *band forms*.   Finally, when nuclear segmentation is marked and clear lobes formed, mature granulocytes exist.   Metamyelocytes and more mature forms may be normally present in human circulating blood.   Nuclei of eosinophils are often bilobed but may show a small median lobe.   Nuclear polymorphism of basophils is not pronounced.   Nuclei of neutrophils usually have three to five lobes.   The degree of nuclear polymorphism appears directly related to the age of the cell; hypermature polymorphonuclear leukocytes may contain six or more nuclear lobes, whereas juvenile cells show only nuclear indentation.   Certain diseases, as pernicious anemia, are characterized by hypersegmented nuclei.   In the Pelger-Huet anomaly, on the other hand, nuclear segmentation is deficient.   With increasing nuclear polymorphism the chromatin becomes progressively coarse and thick, that is, increasingly heterochromatic.   In mature granulocytes it is clumped and almost glassy in appearance.   Nucleoli persist in granulocytes for only a very short time following nuclear indentation.

In living cells nuclear changes other than those affecting shape are difficult to visualize with phase-contrast microscopy or by supravital methods (Figs.

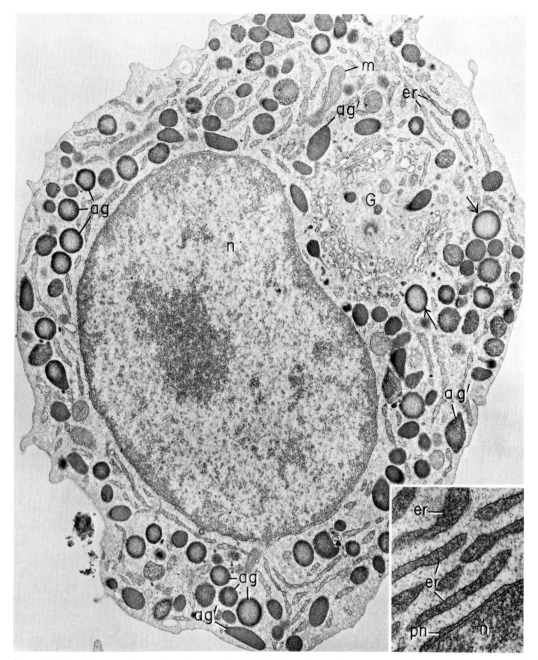

Figure 11-14   Human polymorphonuclear neutrophil (PMN); early myelocyte, reacted for peroxidase.   This cell is the largest (approximately 15μm) of the neutrophilic series.   It has a sizable, slightly indented nucleus (n), a prominent Golgi region (G), and cytoplasm packed with peroxidase-positive azurophilic granules (ag).   Note the two general shapes of azurophilic granules, spherical (ag) or ellipsoid (ag').   The majority are spherical, with a homogeneous matrix, but a few ellipsoid forms containing crystalloids are also present.   Many of the spherical forms (arrows) have a dense periphery and a lighter core, owing presumably to incomplete penetration of substrate into the centers of granules.   Peroxidase reaction product is visible in less concentrated form within all compartments of the granule-producing apparatus [endoplasmic reticulum (er), perinuclear cisterna (pn), and Golgi cisternae].   No reaction product is seen in the cytoplasmic matrix, mitochondria (m), or nucleus (n).   The inset depicts a portion of another promyelocyte at higher magnification, showing to better advantage flocculent deposits of peroxidase reaction product in the rough ER (er) including the perinuclear cisterna (pn).   ×15,000; inset, ×34,000.   (From D. F. Bainton, J. L. Ullyot, and M. G. Farquhar, J. Exp. Med., **134**:907, 1971.)

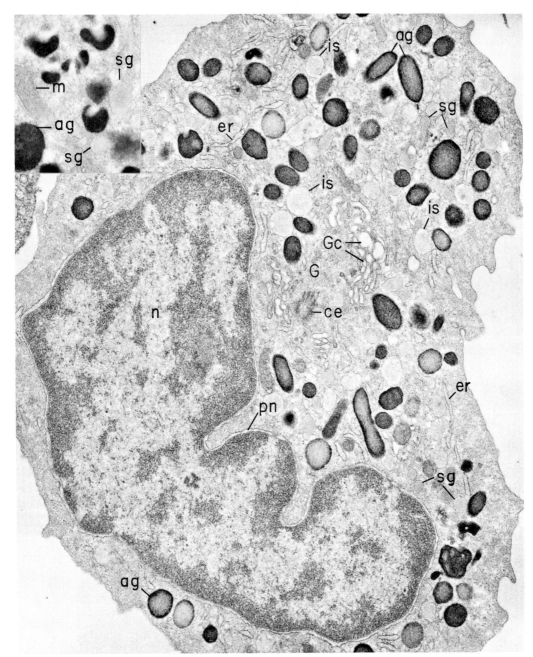

Figure 11-15 Polymorphonuclear neutrophilic (PMN) myelocyte, human peroxidase reaction. At this stage the cell is smaller (approximately 10 μm) than the promyelocyte (see Fig. 11-14), the nucleus is more indented, and the cytoplasm contains two different types of granules: (1) large, peroxidase-positive azurophils (ag) and (2) the generally smaller specific granules (sg), which do not stain for peroxidase. A number of immature specifics (is), which are larger, less compact, and more irregular in contour than mature granules, are seen in the Golgi region (G). The inset, a portion of a myelocyte, depicts a cluster of peroxidase-positive granules, most of which are smaller and more pleomorphic than the surrounding specifics (sg) and azurophils (ag). These are presumed to represent azurophil variants, since they appear during the promyelocyte stage. ×20,000; inset ×41,000. (From D. F. Bainton, J. L. Ullyot, and M. G. Farquhar, J. Exp. Med., **134**:907, 1971.)

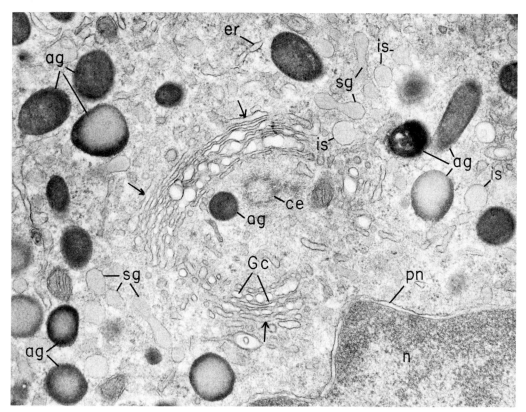

Figure 11-16   Higher-power view of the Golgi region of PMN myelocyte similar to the cell shown in Fig. 11-15.   As in the preceding figure, peroxidase reaction is seen in azurophils (ag) but not in specific granules (sg).   The stacked, smooth-surfaced Golgi cisternae (Gc) are oriented around the centriole (ce).   Note that the outer cisternae have a content of intermediate density (arrows) which is similar to the content of the specific granules.   The images are less suggestive than in the rabbit, but they are compatible with the view that specific granules arise from the convex face of the Golgi complex in both species.   ×33,000.   (From D. F. Bainton, J. L. Ullyot, and M. G. Farquhar, J. Exp. Med., **134**:907, 1971.)

11-9 and 11-10).   Pinacyanol may be used as a supravital nuclear stain, but nuclear detail is not rich.   Cytoplasmic granules are stained with neutral red, and the earliest granules, often masked by cytoplasmic basophilia in Romanovsky-type stains, are visible.   The character of the granules may be told by their staining reaction, size, and distribution.   Mitochondria, present in the myeloblast in considerable number, become reduced in number and size until, in the mature cell, few are present, and they are not readily visible.   Ameboid movement, activity of the plasma membrane, and movement of cytoplasmic granules are present only in mature granulocytes.   The 50-Å-thick actin-like cytoplasmic filaments appear to develop only near

maturity.   The inability of granulocytes to move until they are mature favors the release of only mature cells to the circulation.

Knowledge of granule production has been provided by the electron-microscope studies of Bainton, Ullyot, and Farquhar (1971) and of G. A. Ackerman (Figs. 11-12 to 11-17).   As in the red cell series, the maturation of granulocytes is a continuous process.   The human *myeloblast*, the first recognizable cell in the sequence of maturation, is a relatively small cell (approximately 10 μm) without granules.   The cytoplasm has many free polyribosomes and mitochondria.   Annulate lamellae may be seen.

The *promyelocyte* in man is larger (approximately

15 μm) than the myeloblast and contains peroxidase-positive granules which correspond to the azurophilic granules of light microscopy. A large Golgi complex and moderate amounts of rough ER

Figure 11-17 Human polymorphonuclear neutrophil (PMN), reacted for peroxidase. The cytoplasm is filled with granules; the smaller peroxidase-negative specifics (sg) are more numerous, azurophils (ag) having been reduced in number by cell divisions after the promyelocyte stage. Some small, irregularly shaped azurophilic granule variants are also present (arrow). The nucleus is condensed and lobulated (n¹ to n⁴), the Golgi region (G) is small and lacks forming granules, the ER (er) scanty, and mitochondria (m) few. Note that the cytoplasm of this cell has a rather ragged, moth-eaten appearance due to the fact that the glycogen, which is normally present, has been extracted. The insets depict portions of the cytoplasm of mature PMN reacted for peroxidase. Inset a demonstrates that the peroxidase-positive azurophils (ag) can be easily distinguished from the unreactive specifics (sg). Note that one of the specifics is quite elongated (approximately 1,000 μm). Inset b illustrates the narrow connection between two lobes (n₁ and n₂) of the PMN nucleus. Inset, specimen preparation as in Fig. 11-15. Figure 11-17, ×21,000; inset a, ×36,000; inset b, ×14,000. (From D. F. Bainton, J. L. Ullyot, and M. G. Farquhar, J. Exp. Med., **134**:907, 1971.)

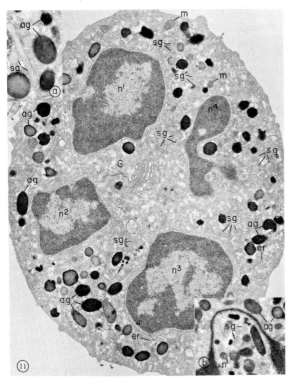

are present. The granules are of two main shapes. The majority are round, approximately 500 nm in diameter, and contain flocculent material at first and dense, homogeneous material on maturation. Less common are football-shaped forms, approximately 300×900 nm, which frequently contain crystalline inclusions. The Golgi cisternae, the perinuclear space, and the rough ER—which constitute the secretory apparatus of the promyelocyte—often contain peroxidase-positive material. It is this material, of course, which is membrane-bounded to form the azurophilic granules. Promyelocytes actively divide.

The *myelocyte* is smaller than the promyelocyte (approximately 10 μm). The nucleus in this stage flattens and indents. The cell has a prominent Golgi complex and mixed population of granules, including newly produced peroxidase-negative granules as well as the peroxidase-positive azurophilic granules of the promyelocyte. The new granules are the specific ones; they are spheres, approximately 200 nm in diameter, or rods, approximately $130 \times 1,000$ nm, with homogeneous low-density content. These granules appear to form at the outer convex surface of the Golgi, in distinction to the azurophilic granules which probably are produced at the inner concave surface. Myelocytes actively divide.

The *metamyelocyte* (juvenile cell), band form, and mature neutrophil are nondividing cells which no longer produce granules. The Golgi is small and inactive. The nucleus is lobulated or segmented, and a mixed population of granules is present, numbering approximately 200 to 300 per cell. The ratio of definitive to primary granules is approximately $2:1$.

The polymorphonuclear leukocytes of the blood are similar to the later marrow stages.

The primary or azurophilic granules are lysosomal; they contain myeloperoxidase, as indicated above, acid phosphatase, β-galactosidase, 5'-nucleotidase, and other enzymes characteristic of lysosomes. The secondary or definitive granules lack these acid hydrolytic enzymes. They contain alkaline phosphatase and a variety of compounds (see Chap. 10) many of which are known to have bacteriocidal properties.

Eosinophilic granules show little change on maturation, save that an increasing number of granules develop a crystalloid element. These granules are unusually rich in arginine, containing the strongly cationic guanidinium group which accounts for the marked eosinophilia of the granule. They contain a myeloperoxidase, which is somewhat different from that of the heterophil's primary granule; some acid phosphatase activity, on a reduced level relative to heterophil granules; and some alkaline phosphatase activity. They are, thus, complex granules with a limited amount of lysosomal character.

Basophilic granules show virtually no change on development.

Important physical and functional changes are associated with the maturation of neutrophils. Some are schematized in Fig. 11-18.

KINETICS OF GRANULOCYTE PRODUCTION AND DISTRIBUTION

Although the bulk of the erythroid complex is in the circulation, as Donahue, Gabrio, and Finch (1958) have also shown, granulocytic forms in the bone marrow far outnumber those in active circulation. The table below indicates the numbers of different granulocytes.

Granulocyte	Number per kilogram of body weight
Circulating	0.3×10^9
Total marrow granulocytes	11.4×10^9
Segmented forms	1.6×10^9
Band forms	3.6×10^9
Myelocytes	2.6×10^9
Metamyelocytes	2.7×10^9
Adult granulocytes	2.5×10^9

A ready reserve of adult granulocytes and metamyelocytes of about 5×10^9 cells per kg body weight is in marrow. This represents more than 16 times the number of circulating cells. Counting all marrow granulocytes, the ratio of cells in marrow to those of the blood is 38:1. The blood normally contains some metamyelocytes.

Studies of the distribution and kinetics of leukocytes have been carried out with radioactive tags. A useful one is diisopropyl fluorophosphate, the phosphate being radioactive ($DF^{32}P$). $DF^{32}P$ couples irreversibly with esterases. Experiments with this tracer have shown that there are two pools of

granulocytes in blood vessels. The first is a circulating pool; the second, a marginating pool. The latter consists of cells within blood vessels lying out of flow or marginated against the walls. The marginated pool may be mobilized very quickly. The concept of an extravascular pool of granulocytes appears untenable. Indeed, it is likely that granulocytes leaving the bloodstream do not return. The two major sources of ready-reserve granulocytes, therefore, are those in the marrow and those in marginated pools.

Granulocytes remain in the circulation for only hours, in the neighborhood of 8 to 12 hr in man. They appear, moreover, to leave the circulation at random, without regard to age. In an acute *leukocytosis*, that is, a sudden increase in the number of circulating granulocytes as may be seen in infectious diseases, a greater percentage of young cells are present in the blood. The term "shift to the left" is employed in clinical medicine to refer to a population of circulating granulocytes having a large portion of young cells. The term "shift to the right" signifies that a larger than normal portion of the circulating granulocytes are hypermature.

The model shown below, modified from the work of Mauer, Athens, Warner, Ashenbrucker, Cartwright, and Wintrobe, indicates the relationship of the several granulocyte components.

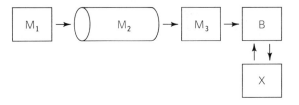

M_1 = pool of mitotically active cells in the marrow, including myeloblasts and myelocytes

M_2 = maturation phase, from which cells are not normally released until mature

M_3 = storage pool of mature granulocytes in marrow

B = granulocytic pool in blood

X = marginating cells in equilibrium with B

THE FATE OF GRANULOCYTES

Mature granulocytes are end forms, incapable of further differentiation or of mitotic division. Their

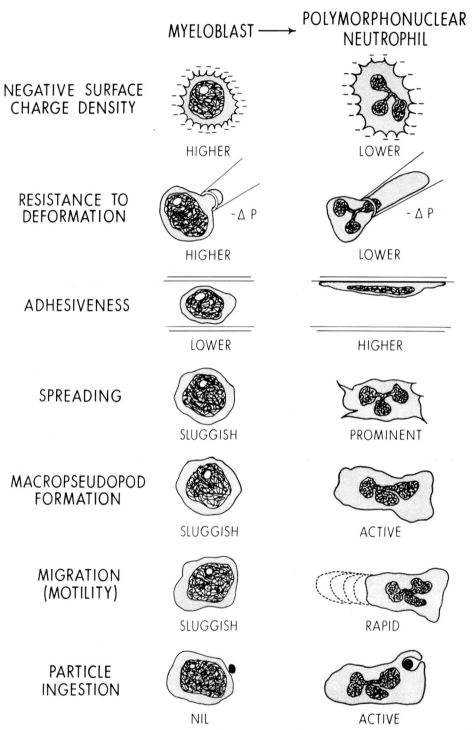

Figure 11-18 Physical and functional changes in polymorphonuclear neutrophils during maturation. (From M. Lichtman and R. Weed, Blood, **39**:301, 1972.)

brief sojourn in the blood is but a fraction of their potential life-span. In tissue culture, for example, neutrophils may survive for more than a week. Since extravascular granulocytes fail to return to the blood, we may conclude that 8 to 12 hr after release to the blood from the marrow, granulocytes enter the connective tissue spaces. They die there or leave the body. A small number of granulocytes die in the bloodstream, as indicated by their reaction to supravital dyes; that is, they are nonselectively stained throughout.

MONOCYTES

Monocytes are a major cell in a life cycle which constitutes the cellular sequence *promonocyte, monocyte, macrophage, epithelioid cell,* and *multinucleate giant cell.* Except for the last type, these cells may look remarkably alike. Moreover, they show a fair amount of variation of form. They each may range from 10 to 20 μm in size. The nuclear configuration may be oval, reniform, or horseshoe-shaped. The cytoplasm, usually ample, is finely granulated and vacuolated. The cell surface is subject to variation: It may be smooth or thrown into projections of several sorts.

The promonocyte is somewhat larger than a monocyte, with a larger Golgi. It is a cell of the bone marrow, rather actively dividing and in relatively small numbers. Within 6 hr of labeling in mice, these cells are in the circulation, suggesting but a brief marrow sojourn.

Monocytes are released to the blood and remain in the circulation or marginal pools about 8 to 12 hr in mice. They are the source of the macrophages of the body, undergoing the transformation within the circulation in places of sluggish blood flow, in the peritoneum or related visceral cavities, or in connective tissue spaces.

The transformation of monocytes to macrophages usually results in a cell, the macrophage, with increased phagocytic capacity; more voluminous cytoplasm; an increased number of lysosomes, heterolysosomes, microtubules, and microfilaments; a large cell center, including Golgi membranes; and changes in nuclear shape with the appearance of one or two prominent nucleoli. Macrophages live several weeks. They actually enjoy a circulation which includes a bloodstream phase, although they are not commonly recognized as blood cells. They collect in large numbers, for example, in the peritoneal and other serous cavities. They emigrate from these cavities through lymphatics in small but regular numbers and thus reach the blood and are distributed throughout the body, reaching such beds of macrophages as the splenic red pulp and the lymph nodal medulla.

It is likely that "fixed" macrophages, constituting parts of the reticulum or endothelium, such as Kupffer cells (Chap. 19), come from circulating monocytes or macrophages. Certain "fixed" macrophages, moreover, such as the Kupffer cells, may detach from their endothelial position and circulate once again.

Epithelioid cells are polygonal, rather like epithelium in appearance because of their shape and tendency to lie together in cellular sheets with little intercellular material. They may be very much like macrophages, lacking evidence of phagocytized material. Often the microtubular element in these cells is well developed, forming branching bands which encircle the Golgi, endoplasm, and nucleus. Lysosomes may be quite numerous.

Giant cells, representing fused epithelioid cells, constitute a strikingly different cell type from those earlier in the sequence. Their features include a large fused cytocentrum containing many centrioles; a ring of nuclei, varied in size, shape, and ploidy; an ample endoplasm particularly rich in mitochondria; and a broad, undulating membrane. Giant cells, closely resembling osteoclasts, may range from binucleate to cells containing more than 100 nuclei. Giant cells, in turn, may fuse to form vast syncytial sheets. Consult Chap. 4 for further discussion of these cells.

The full cell cycle from promonocyte to syncytia need not unfold; it often goes no further than the macrophage phase. However, in certain granulomatous diseases of which tuberculosis is an example, epithelioid cell and giant cell development is favored.

Certain cytochemical changes are significant in this life cycle. Promonocytes in mice have peroxidase-containing granules which do not occur in monocytes. With the massive development of lysosomes in macrophages, the activity of acid phosphatase and of other acid-hydrolytic, lysosomal enzymes considerably increases. Giant cell formation is heralded by the decrease in lysosome enzymes and an increase in mitochondrial-associated respiratory enzymes, such as cytochrome oxidase, as shown in avian cells.

LYMPHOCYTES

Lymphocytes have resisted efforts to establish their life cycles. Without such markers as pigment, specific granules, or polymorphous nuclei, and with only intimations of their function, it has been possible only recently, with such sophisticated and modern techniques as light- and electron-microscopic autoradiography and cytochemistry, thymectomy and other ablation procedures and sensitive immunologic techniques, to lay out the elements of lymphocytic life cycles. The emergent pattern appears to be as follows (see also Chap. 10).

Lymphocytes originate in the bone marrow. One group of marrow cells leaves the marrow either as lymphocytes or stem cells (whose morphology is not yet known) and enters the thymus. Within the thymus these cells, recognizable as lymphocytes, proliferate, and bear, only when in the thymus, a marker antigen, TL, on the cell surface. More than 90 percent of them die and a small percentage is released. These released lymphocytes are long-lived, small lymphocytes, capable of years of life in man and months or even years in rodents. They recirculate through blood, lymphatic tissue, and lymphatics (Chaps. 13 to 15). They bear a characteristic antigen on their surface, known as theta (θ), which becomes apparent on their leaving the thymus. They have been designated T cells. They play a primary role in delayed hypersensitivity, a class of immunologic response exemplified by graft rejection and mediated by cells rather than by circulating antibody. They are, moreover, capable of reacting with antigen and of interacting with B cells (see below) to induce antibody formation. The T cells do not themselves produce antibody. B cells are antibody producers, but the T cell is often necessary, in a way not yet understood, for antibody production by the B cells. This interaction, resulting in antibody production, appears to be a close physical one, as observed in both tissue culture and in histologic section, exhibiting clusters of 20 to 100 cells. In the case of antibody production to foreign erythrocytes, these clusters include macrophages, lymphocytes, and plasma cells. If the clusters are

disrupted, antibody production ceases. If dispersed cells are permitted to reaggregate, antibody production resumes. T cells account for most of the small lymphocytes in thoracic duct lymph and in the blood. They populate specific loci within spleen, lymph nodes, and other lymphatic tissues.

The lymphocytes designated B cells originate from the marrow and are released to the blood. In addition to circulating, they congregate in certain sites in spleen, lymph nodes, and other lymphatic tissues capable of producing antibody. B lymphocytes are small cells which have a remarkable important characteristic: Antibody molecules of a single specificity are attached to their surface. The surface antibody molecules are probably synthesized by the B lymphocytes and serve as receptors or combining sites for antigen. B cells are thus antibody producers, although in unstimulated cells the production is probably at a low level, sufficient only to provide surface antibody. When antigen combines with this surface antibody under appropriate circumstances (which, for some antigens at least, includes the involvement of T cells) B cells are stimulated to proliferate and differentiate, forming a clone of antibody-producing cells. If they produce large amounts of immunoglobulin G (a highly evolved, efficient, small-molecular-weight antibody) the B cells probably undergo transformation into *plasma cells*. This transformation is associated with the enlargement of the small lymphocytic B cell to a larger lymphocytic or blast-like cell, its proliferation, and development of rough ER and other features that characterize plasma cells (Fig. 11-19). Plasma cells are short-lived cells, having a life-span of but a week or two. Exceptionally, some plasma cells may survive for much longer periods. If the antibody produced is immunoglobulin M (a large-molecular-weight, relatively "primitive" type of antibody) the B cells may remain lymphocytes.

The presence of cells with immunoglobulin "spots" on their surface capable of being stimulated to clone formation and massive immunoglobulin synthesis is a matter of enormous theoretical significance. A conceptual dichotomy, not unlike the monophyletic-polyphyletic schism, has arisen in cellular immunology: Does an antigen instruct a multipotential cell to produce antibody complementary to that antigen, or does an antigen move

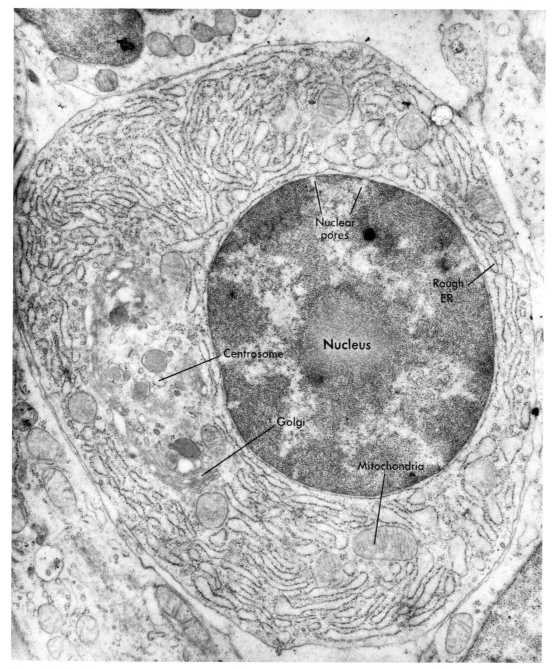

Figure 11-19 Plasma cell. Note the clumped chromatin, eccentric nucleus, prominent cytocentrum, and granular endoplasmic reticulum. Compare with light micrograph, Fig. 11-7.

through the circulation and lymphatic tissue until it reaches a cell already producing the appropriate antibody, in fact, having that antibody studded on its surface and functioning as a receptor? More succinctly stated, does antibody formation depend upon instruction or selection? A number of cogent lines of evidence, a major one being the single-specificity antibody "spots" on a given B cell, offer strong support to selection. There seems little doubt that some form of selection underlies antibody formation.

The small lymphocytes of the blood are made up of lymphocytes of the B and T types. They include, of course, not only cells directly released from the bone marrow and the thymus but cells which have passed through spleen and lymph nodes or proliferated there, and, not being stimulated, continue to circulate and recirculate. The distribution of B and T cells, as determined for the mouse by Raff and his colleagues, is presented in Table 11-1.

What is the significance of lymphocyte size? A number of large lymphocytes of the blood may result from antigenic stimulation of small lymphocytes and constitute the early stages in an immune response. There are undoubtedly lymphocytes stimulated in the wall of the gastrointestinal tract, for example, which are carried by lymphatics into the blood. The response to this stimulation may be both mitosis and heightened immunologic activity, with the development of medium or large lymphocytes. These cells will reach a lymphatic tissue within a short time after stimulation and remain there to continue their reactions. In addition, a lymphocyte may enlarge, preparatory to mitosis, without immunologic stimulation, and such large and medium-sized lymphocytes may run in the cir-

culation. Agents exist, such as phytohemagglutinin and pokeweed, which have mitogenic effects, although their mechanism of action is not understood.

In summary, we may visualize the lymphocytes as being of several types, but all having an immunologic role. The lymphocytes circulate, in some instances at least, for long periods of time, passing not only through the blood but also the lymph and lymphatic tissues. At one point in this cycle the lymphocytes meet antigen. In a meeting that produces antibody, the antigen and T and B lymphocytes interact. The interaction typically occurs or continues in the spleen, lymph nodes, bone marrow, or other effector lymphatic tissue, but not in the thymus, resulting in a cluster of cells, of which the B cells produce antibody. Interactions of a different sort occur in delayed hypersensitivity. Here T cells appear to play the major effector role. Lymphocytes also play a role in the development of tolerance, but their actions have not yet been defined. Consult Chaps. 10, 13, and 14 for further discussion.

PLATELETS

Platelets are small units of cytoplasm separated from giant cells, *megakaryocytes*. In man, megakaryocytes are restricted to the marrow. In many other mammals they may also be found in the spleen.

Figure 11-20   Megakaryocyte from the bone marrow of a kitten, showing pseudopodia extending into a blood vessel (V) and giving rise to blood platelets (bp). (From J. H. Wright, J. Morph., 21:263, 1910.)

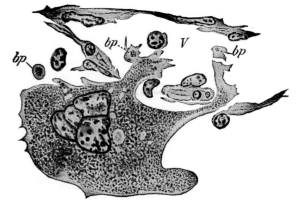

Table 11-1   Small lymphocytes of the mouse

Tissue	Percentage of theta (θ) cells	Percentage of B cells
Thymus	100	0
Thoracic duct	85	15
Blood	70	30
Lymph nodes	65	35
Spleen	35	65
Peritoneal cavity	35	65
Peyer's patches	30	70

A megakaryocyte may measure more than 100 μm in diameter. Its nucleus is a large, twisted, lobulated structure. It is polyploid, degrees of ploidy up to 64N being regular. Although claims for multinucleate cells have been made, a single large, polymorphous, polyploid nucleus is the rule. (See Chap. 1 for a consideration of the value of polyploidy.)

The abundant cytoplasm is divisible into three zones. The perinuclear zone contains Golgi, rough ER, polyribosomes, and some granules—in short, most of the organelles associated with a cell in large-scale protein and membrane synthesis. The intermediate zone consists of putative platelets demarcated to varying degrees of completeness by smooth ER. The outermost zone resembles ectoplasm; it is finely granular and contains packets of microfilaments but is largely free of organelles [Figs. 11-7 (color insert), 11-20, 11-21, 12-3 to 12-5, and 12-11].

A megakaryocyte forms platelets by the confluence of the vesicles or channels of ER which demarcate them. Either individual platelets or large portions of megakaryocytic cytoplasm may be separated in this manner. In the latter case, subsequent confluence of the demarcating ER can produce individual platelets. Megakaryocytes sit astride vascular sinuses in the marrow, delivering

Figure 11-21 Electron micrograph of a megakaryocyte in human bone marrow. The nucleus is large and polymorphous. The cytoplasm contains lysosomes of varying density and small mitochondria. The arresting cytoplasmic characteristic is the extensive smooth-surfaced endoplasmic reticulum which loculates platelet zones in the peripheral cytoplasm. Later the platelets will separate completely and become free circulating structures. ×9,300. (From the work of I. Berman.)

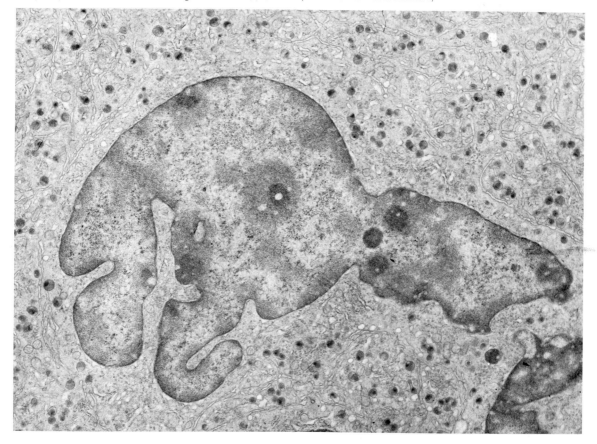

their platelets through mural apertures directly into the vascular lumen.

Although the three zones of megakaryocyte cytoplasm are typical, megakaryocytes may be found in which virutally the whole mass of cytoplasm is demarcated into platelets (lower cell, Fig. 11-7).

Megakaryocytes originate from stem cells. The first morphologically identifiable precursor of megakaryocytes is a large cell 25 to 40 μm in diameter with a large oval or spherical nucleus and a cytoplasm containing ribosomes and other organelles, but without hint of platelet formation. This cell may be designated a *megakaryocytoblast*. It undergoes DNA replication to its final level of ploidy before the nucleus becomes polymorphous. In a population of megakaryoblasts, dependent somewhat on the species, ploidy varies from 2N to 64N. In general, both the nuclear and cytoplasmic sizes of the megakaryocyte are proportional to the degree of ploidy. On cessation of DNA replication the megakaryocytoblast undergoes nuclear polymorphism and cytoplasmic differentiation.

Circulating platelets, in man, have a life-span up to about 10 days, determined in labeling experiments. The curve of labeled platelets decreases considerably in 6 to 8 days and tails off in about 10. It is likely that platelets are utilized randomly, that is, without reference to age.

It is quite likely that the number and size of circulating platelets are regulated by a hormone, *thrombopoietin*. The site of production and the nature of the hormone are not known. Its presence is inferred from the thrombopoietic activity of serum from individuals with low blood platelet levels (*thrombocytopenia*). Thrombopoietin may stimulate the conversion of certain stem cells into the megakaryocytic line and may, as well, induce an acceleration in maturation of megakaryocytes. As a result of such maturation, the number and size of megakaryocytes, and the size of platelets, are increased.

References

ARCHER, G. T.: Motion Picture Studies on Degranulation of Horse Eosinophils during Phagocytosis, *J. Exp. Med.*, **118:**276 (1963).

ASHBY, W.: Determination of Length of Life of Transfused Blood Corpuscles in Man, *Blood,* **3:**486 (1948).

BAINTON, DOROTHY FORD, JOAN L. ULLYOT, and MARILYN G. FARQUHAR: The Development of Neutrophilic Polymorphonuclear Leukocytes in Human Bone Marrow. Origin and Content of Azurophil and Specific Granules, *J. Exp. Med.*, **134:**907 (1971).

BLOOM, W., and G. W. BARTELMEZ: Hematopoiesis in Young Human Embryos, *Amer. J. Anat.*, **67:**21 (1940).

COHN, Z. A., and J. G. HIRSCH: The Isolation and Properties of the Specific Cytoplasmic Granules of Rabbit Polymorphonuclear Leukocytes, *J. Exp. Med.*, **112:**983 (1960).

CRADDOCK, C. G., JR., S. PERRY, L. E. VENTZKE, and J. S. LAWRENCE: Evaluation of Marrow Granulocytic Reserves in Normal and Disease States, *Blood,* **15:**840 (1960).

DE BRUYN, P. P. H.: Locomotion of Blood Cells in Tissue Culture, *Anat. Rec.*, **89:**43 (1944); **95:**177 (1946).

DONAHUE, D. M., B. W. GABRIO, and C. A. FINCH: Quantitative Measurements of Hematopoietic Cells of the Marrow, *J. Clin. Invest.*, **37:**1564 (1958).

EBERT, R. H., A. B. SANDERS, and H. W. FLOREY: Observations of Lymphocytes in Chambers in the Rabbit's Ear, *Brit. J. Exp. Path.*, **21:**212 (1940).

FOWLER, J. H., A. M. WU, J. E. TILL, E. A. MC CULLOCH, and L. SIMINOVITCH: The Cellular Composition of Hemopoietic Spleen Colonies, *J. Cell Physiol.*, **69:**65 (1967).

GILMOUR, J. R.: Normal Haemopoiesis in Intrauterine and Neonatal Life, *J. Path. Bact.*, **52**:25 (1941).

HIRSCH, J. G., and Z. A. COHN: Degranulation of Polymorphonuclear Leukocytes Following Phagocytosis of Microorganisms, *J. Exp. Med.*, **118**:1005 (1960).

HOWELL, W. H.: The Life History of the Formed Elements of the Blood: Especially the Red Corpuscles, *J. Morph.*, **4**:57 (1890).

ISAACS, R.: The Physiologic Histology of Bone Marrow, *Folia Haemat.*, **40**:395 (1930).

JOFFE, R. H.: The Reticuloendothelial System, in H. Downey (ed.), "Handbook of Hematology," vol. 2, Paul B. Hoeber, Inc., New York, 1938.

JORDAN, H. E.: The Evolution of Blood-forming Tissues, *Quart. Rev. Biol.*, **8**:58 (1933).

KINDRED, J. E.: A Quantitative Study of the Hematopoietic Organs of Young Adult Albino Rats, *Amer. J. Anat.*, **71**:207 (1942).

MAXIMOW, A. A.: The Lymphocytes and Plasma Cells, in E. V. Cowdry (ed.), "Special Cytology," vol. 2, Paul B. Hoeber, Inc., New York, 1932.

MIKLEM, H. S., C. E. FORD, E. P. EVANS, and J. GAR: Interrelationships of Myeloid and Lymphoid Cells: Studies with Chromosome-marked Cells Transfused into Lethally Irradiated Mice, *Proc. Roy. Soc. (London), Ser. B.*, **165**:78 (1966).

SABIN, F. R.: Bone Marrow, *Physiol. Rev.*, **8**:191 (1928).

SABIN, F. R.: Studies of Living Human Blood Cells, *Bull. Hopkins Hosp.*, **34**:277 (1923).

SIMINOVITCH, L., E. A. MC CULLOCH, and J. E. TILL: The Distribution of Colony-forming Cells Among Spleen Colonies. *J. Cell Comp. Physiol.*, **62**:327 (1963).

WRIGHT, J. H.: The Histogenesis of Blood Platelets, *J. Morph.*, **21**:263 (1910).

WU, A. M., J. E. TILL, L. SIMINOVITCH, and E. A. MC CULLOCH: Cytological Evidence for a Relationship between Normal Hematopoietic Colony-forming Cells and Cells of the Lymphoid System, *J. Exp. Med.*, **127**:455 (1968).

WU, A. M., J. E. TILL, L. SIMINOVITCH, and E. A. MC CULLOCH: A Cytological Study of the Capacity for Differentiation of Normal Hematopoietic Colony-forming Cells, *J. Cell Physiol.*, **69**:177 (1967).

COMPREHENSIVE REFERENCES

DOWNEY, H. (ed.): "Handbook of Hematology," 4 vols., Paul B. Hoeber, Inc., New York, 1938; reprinted by Hafner Publishing Company, Inc., New York, 1966.

This is a major source of hematological information up to the late 1930s.

GORDON, A. S.: "Regulation of Hematopoiesis," 2 vols., Appleton Century Crofts, New York, 1970.

A recent source of basic hematological studies.

STOHLMAN, F.: "Symposium on Hemopoietic Cellular Proliferation," Grune & Stratton, Inc., New York, 1970.

WEISS, L.: "The Cells and Tissues of the Immune System," Prentice-Hall, Inc., Englewood Cliffs, N.J., 1972.

WINTROBE, M. M.: "Clinical Hematology," 5th ed., Lea & Febiger, Philadelphia, 1961.

YOFFEY, J. M., and F. C. COURTRICE: "Lymphatics, Lymph and Lymphoid Tissue," Harvard University Press, Cambridge, Mass., 1960.

chapter 12   Bone marrow   LEON WEISS

Contained within the bones of the body, marrow tissue is a specialized, richly cellular portion of the connective tissues. In human beings it originates in the second month of intrauterine life within the clavicles, the first bones to ossify, and it expands with the maturation of the remaining bones (Fig. 12-1). The scapulae, innominate bones, occipital bones, ribs, and vertebrae contain marrow in the third fetal month. When it first appears, the marrow is concerned with the growth and modeling of bone, and it maintains its osteogenic functions throughout life. Secondarily, it assumes hematopoietic functions, and so active does it become in the production of blood cells that in the latter half of fetal development and throughout postnatal life the bone marrow is the major hematopoietic tissue. Like other hematopoietic tissues, the bone marrow plays a part in the destruction of blood cells. It also has major immunologic functions, is hemoclastic (that is, active in blood-cell destruction), and has the general functions of a connective tissue.

Structure of bone marrow

GROSS CHARACTERISTICS

On gross examination, bone marrow may be red or yellow. The color of red marrow is due to erythrocytes and their pigmented precursors and is usually indicative of a hematopoietic marrow. The major cell type in yellow marrow is fat cells, which impart a yellow color. This marrow has little hematopoiesis. Both the fat and hematopoietic elements are in a labile state and under certain conditions may rapidly displace one another (Fig. 12-2).

In neonatal human beings all the marrow is red. Fat begins to appear in the shaft of the long bones

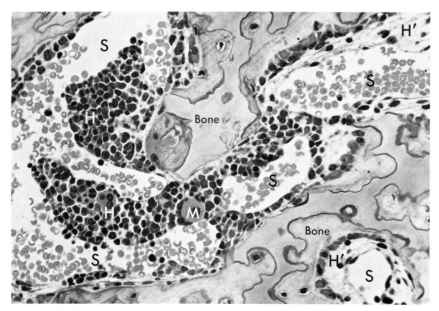

Figure 12-1   Bone marrow from central femur of human fetus, 200 mm crown rump length (22 weeks gestational age).   The marrow tissue occurs in the spaces within bone.   In the adult the bone will be removed from much of the center of the shaft of the femur, remaining only to form a cortical shell.   The marrow will therefore become a solid cylindrical plug of tissue.   The marrow contains large thin-walled vascular sinuses (S) containing blood.   Outside the sinuses lie the hematopoietic compartments. Some of these (H) are filled with hematopoietic cells.   Note the large megakaryocyte (M) characteristically set on the outside wall of the sinus (see text).   In some sites, the hematopoietic compartments have not yet filled with hematopoietic cells but contain a primitive fibrous connective tissue (H').   ×1,000.   (From L-T. Chen and L. Weiss.)

Figure 12-2   Normal adult human bone marrow.   A. Red marrow rich in hematopoietic cells.   B. Yellow marrow rich in fat cells. (The fat has been extracted by embedding reagents and is represented by clear oval spaces.)   C. Marrow intermediate to A and B in the proportion of hematopoietic and fat cells.   ×400.

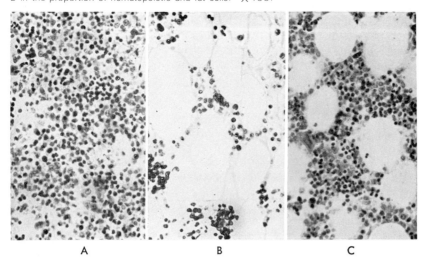

A   B   C

in the fifth to seventh years, and by the eighteenth year almost all the marrow of the limbs is yellow. Patches of red marrow persist about the joints. Hematopoietic marrow in adult human beings is virtually restricted to the bones of the skull, clavicles, vertebrae, ribs, sternebrae, and bones of the pelvis. The bone marrow accounts for 3.5 to 5.9 percent of adult body weight, or about 1,600 to 3,700 gm.

THE HISTOLOGIC ORGANIZATION OF BONE MARROW

The marrow lies entirely within bone, reached by blood vessels and nerves which pierce its bony housing. The internal surface of bone is typically ridged with shelves and spicules of bone, the *trabeculae,* which protrude into the marrow cavity. Endosteum, composed of osteoblasts and osteoclasts, lines this surface of bone. The marrow contains fixed and free cells and extracellular connective tissue. The fixed cells include fat cells and cells which are primarily associated with blood vessels, nerves, and endosteum. The free cells occupy the remaining space.

The organization of the marrow may be understood through the layout of its vasculature.

ARTERIAL VESSELS

Arteries reach the marrow by penetrating the bony shell. Depending upon both the species and the location of the bone, there may be multiple small arterial twigs which enter the marrow or there may be a major vessel, the *nutrient artery,* that enters the marrow at about midshaft in a long bone. The nutrient artery bifurcates, and each of its branches and any of their major branches run to opposite diaphyses in the central longitudinal axis as *nutrient or central longitudinal arteries.* In addition, arterial branches enter the marrow from the epiphyseal end. The central longitudinal arteries send out many radial branches which run through the marrow toward the encasing bone. They break into capillaries near the periphery of the marrow and communicate with venous sinuses (see below). Many arterial capillaries actually enter the bone, where they may become part of osteones that supply the bone; but some of these capillaries may curve back toward the marrow and, either in the bone or again in the marrow, communicate with the vascular sinus system of the marrow.

VENOUS VESSELS

The vascular sinuses of marrow, the first vessels in the venous system, are thin-walled vessels 50 to 75 μm in diameter. At the periphery of the marrow they typically form richly anastomatic systems. They run radially toward the central longitudinal axis where they empty into the *central longitudinal vein,* which runs in company with the major arterial vessels.

Thus in a cross section of marrow large or medium-sized arteries are present in cross section near the center. They distribute radial branches which extend to the periphery of marrow. There the vascular sinuses originate and converge on the center, where they drain into a large, thin-walled vein (Figs. 12-3 and 12-4).

Studies on the living circulation in the rabbit femur indicate that there is continuity of arterial capillary with venous sinus: the circulation is closed. In the fastidious experiments yielding these results Brånemark (1959) immobilized the thigh of an anesthetized rabbit, exposed the femur, and planed down the bony cortex until it was reduced to coverslip thickness, while leaving the marrow intact and little disturbed. He was then able to carry out high-power light-microscopic studies of the underlying marrow vasculature, with the light coming from above and passing through the planed-down bone.

THE ORGANIZATION OF THE MARROW

The large, prominent radial system of sinuses, together with the far less evident arteries, constitutes the *vascular compartment* of the marrow. The remainder of the marrow lies between these vessels as irregular columns and constitutes the *hematopoietic compartment* (Figs. 12-3 to 12-6). In red marrow this compartment is filled with hematopoietic cells. Hematopoiesis is most active in the periphery of the marrow. Some fat occurs near the center about the great vessels. In yellow marrow, virtually all the hematopoietic compartment is fatty. Some megakaryocytes may be present. Vascular sinuses, moreover, are reduced in number and diameter.

THE STRUCTURE OF VASCULAR SINUSES

The vascular sinus is the principal avenue of cellular exchange between the marrow and the circulation. The sinus wall is regularly and frequently crossed

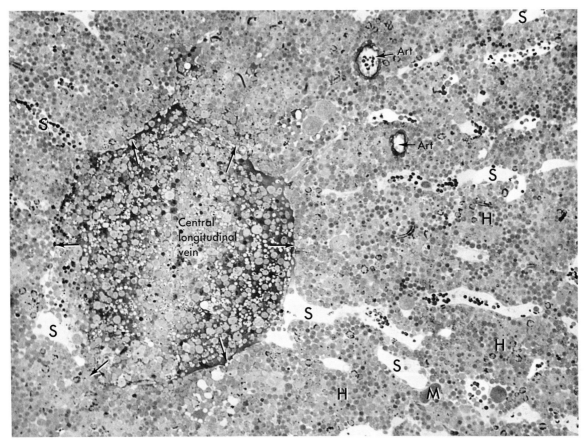

Figure 12-3   Rat bone marrow. This is a cross section of the marrow showing the relationships of major structural elements. The central longitudinal vein and branches of the nutrient artery (ART) are cut in cross section. The lumen of the vein is filled with cells: its wall is indicated by arrows. The sinuses (S) constitute a thin-walled radial system of venous vessels running into the vein. They are cut in longitudinal section. They are separated by hematopoietic compartments (H) containing the developing blood cells packed together. Megakaryocytes (M) lie characteristically against the outside wall of a sinus. ×750. (From L. Weiss, J. Morph. **117**:481, 1965.)

by cells in transit. It is a responsive wall which has three layers in fullest development: endothelium, ground substance constituting a basement membrane, and an adventitial layer (Fig. 12-7). The endothelium is, however, the only layer whose presence is consistent.

The endothelium is a thin, simple layer which may show adherent junctional complexes (adhesion belts). The cell type composing the endothelium appears to be the reticular connective tissue cell modified to assume endothelial form. It contains many small vesicles, some ribosomes and

lysosomes, and small Golgi complexes. It may contain microfilaments and microtubules and it may be phagocytic. The endothelium may be very thin. Hematopoietic and blood cells usually pass through the endothelial cells. The endothelium may be the only mural element, especially where hematopoietic cell passage is active (Figs. 12-8 to 12-10), but adventitial cells normally coat a large portion of its outside surface. Thus in the rat, more than 60 percent of the outside surface of the femoral vascular sinuses is covered by adventitial cells. When the level of cell passage is heightened experi-

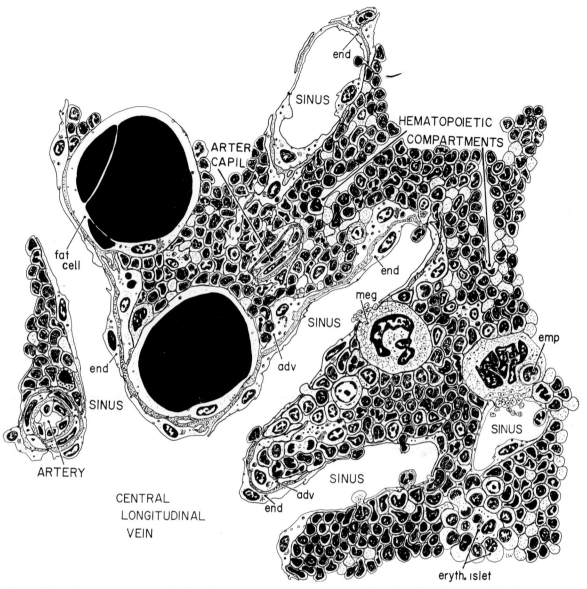

Figure 12-4   Bone marrow, schematic view of cross section near central longitudinal vein.   Several sinuses drain into the central longitudinal vein.   The sinuses are cut along their long axis, the vein, in cross section.   A portion of the nutrient artery (ART) is present as is an arterial capillary.   Hematopoietic cells lie between the sinuses, constituting the hematopoietic compartment. Where hematopoiesis is relatively quiet, the wall of the sinus and of the central longitudinal vein is trilaminar consisting of endothelium (end), a basement membrane, and adventitial cell (adv).   The adventitial cell may become volumnous, encroaching upon the hematopoietic space and thereby displacing hematopoietic cells.   The increased volume of the adventitial cell may be due to a gelatinous change wherein its cytoplasm becomes rarefied, presumably due to hydration.   If this change is widespread, the marrow may become grossly white and gelatinous.   A second and more common basis for large bulk of adventitial cells is fatty change, where they become fat cells.   Contrariwise, when hematopoiesis is active the hematopoietic compartment is large and packed with myelocytes, erythroblasts, and megakaryocytes.   The sinus wall becomes thin, reduced to an endothelial layer alone as the adventitial cells are displaced or lifted from the wall by infiltrating hematopoietic cells.   Apertures appear in the endothelium, moreover, as maturing hematopoietic cells cross the sinus wall and enter the sinus lumen.   Megakaryocytes characteristically lie against the outside of the sinus wall, discharging platelets into the lumen through an aperture.   Occasionally the cytoplasm of megakaryocytes is entered by other cell types which remain visible and later leave the megakaryocyte.   The phenomenom is known as emperipolesis (emp).   Erythroblasts tend to be present in clusters near the sinus wall.   Erythroblastic islets (see text) may be present.   Granulocytes usually develop near the center of the hematopoietic space.   Lymphocytes occur throughout the marrow. Macrophages are common, and mast cells, plasma cells, and other connective tissue cells are also present.

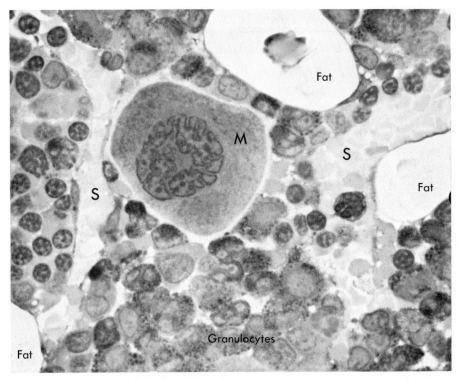

Figure 12-5   Rabbit bone marrow.   Two sinuses (S), each having very thin walls, are present in this light-micrographic field. A megakaryocyte (M) lies against the outside wall of one of the sinuses.   Portions of three fat cells (fat) are present; the one on the right lies against the wall of a sinus in an adventitial position.   The hematopoietic compartment contains many granulocytes along the lower margin of the field.   ×1,200.

mentally, however, the percentage of adventitial cover may be reduced to 20 percent or less. Adventitial cells may be similar in appearance to endothelial cells, but they tend to be more varied. They are more phagocytic.   They may be quite voluminous and "empty" in appearance, probably owing to marked water uptake.   They may contain fat and constitute fat cells.   Adventitial cells commonly extend processes into the perivascular hematopoietic tissue that may be quite long and stout, and constitute spurs or partitions that incompletely compartmentalize the perivascular tissue.   The adventitial cell, although less consistently present than the endothelial cell, affects the general character of the marrow.   If adventitial cells become voluminous and hydrated, they may impart a gelatinous consistency to the marrow.   If their fatty change is large scale, affecting many cells, the

marrow is yellow or fatty.   By their phagocytic capacity they may prevent impaired cells from reaching the circulation.   A layer of ground substance may lie between adventitial and endothelial cells; it is inconstant, difficult to preserve, and seldom reaches the development and extent that would constitute a basement membrane.

The central vein has a structure similar to that of the vascular sinuses.   The marrow lacks lymphatic vessels.   Indeed, lymphatic vessels are absent from sites in the spleen, liver lobule, and other places served by blood vascular sinuses.   Nerves in the marrow are associated with large vessels and are vasomotor.

THE HEMATOPOIETIC COMPARTMENT

The hematopoietic tissue lying between the vascular sinuses consists, in hematopoietic marrow, primarily of hematopoietic cells. It may contain any of the connective tissue cells, however, and mast cells, plasma cells, and macrophages are always present, sometimes in great number. The relative numbers of nucleated marrow cells, as determined in smear preparations, are given in Table 12-1. Although their distribution may, on first view, appear random, there is a pattern to the arrangement of hematopoietic cells.

Megakaryocytes occupy a consistent and prominent place tight against the adventitial surface of the wall of vascular sinuses (Figs. 12-3–12-5 and 12-11). They lie over an aperture in the wall, moreover, and discharge platelets through the aperture into the lumen. Platelets may be discharged singly or as larger cytoplasmic fragments requiring further maturation. The large size of the megakaryocyte is ideal for providing a vast cytoplasmic mass capable of large-scale platelet production. Further, by lying over an aperture in the sinus wall, the megakaryocyte efficiently delivers platelets to the circulation and by its large size both resists being swept into the circulation and prevents vascular leakage from the aperture.

Erythrocytes are produced near the sinuses. As erythroblasts mature to the point where nuclear polarization is marked, the cells press against the

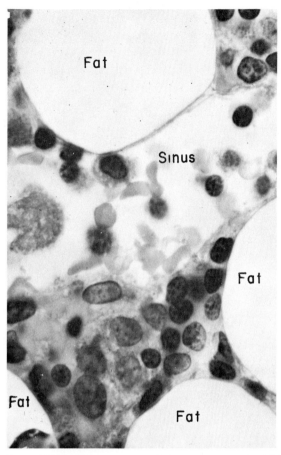

Figure 12-6 Rat bone marrow. A sinus runs across the field. It is surrounded by hematopoietic cells except with the occurrence of fat cells, which lie against the wall of the sinus in an adventitial position. The fat cells displace the hematopoietic cells. ×1,200. (From L. Weiss., J. Morph. **117**:467, 1965.)

Table 12-1. Relative number of nucleated cells in normal human bone marrow

	Range	Average
Myeloblasts	0.3– 5.0	2.0
Promyelocytes	1.0– 8.0	5.0
Myelocytes		
Neutrophilic	5.0–19.0	12.0
Eosinophilic	0.5– 3.0	1.5
Basophilic	0.0– 0.5	0.3
Metamyelocytes ("juvenile" forms)	13.0–32.0	22.0
Polymorphonuclear neutrophils	7.0–30.0	20.0
Polymorphonuclear eosinophils	0.5– 4.0	2.0
Polymorphonuclear basophils	0.0– 0.7	0.2
Lymphocytes	3.0–17.0	10.0
Plasma cells	0.0– 2.0	0.4
Monocytes	0.5– 5.0	2.0
Reticular cells	0.1– 2.0	0.2
Megakaryocytes	0.03– 3.0	0.4
Pronormoblasts	1.0– 8.0	4.0
Erythroblasts (basophilic, polychromatophilic, and acidophilic)	7.0–32.0	18.0

sinus wall. The cytoplasmic pole typically pushes into the adventitial surface of the wall, whereas the nuclear pole is directed away. Nuclear and cytoplasmic poles separate, and the cytoplasmic portion, now a reticulocyte, remains at the wall preparatory to passing through the endothelial cytoplasm and into the lumen of the sinus.

Granulocytes are typically produced in nests somewhat away from the vascular sinus. On maturation, at the metamyelocyte stage, they become motile and capable of moving to the sinus.

Lymphocytes, monocytes, their precursors, mast

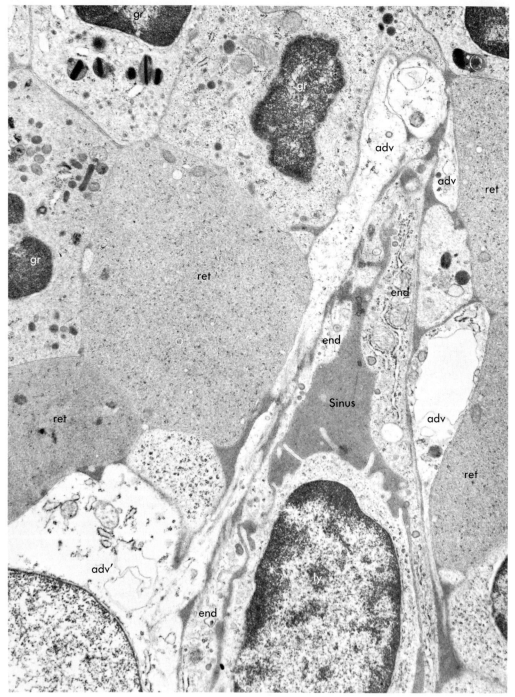

Figure 12-7   Rat bone marrow.   A sinus is present, closely surrounded by hematopoietic cells.   The lumen of the sinus contains a lymphocyte (ly).   Its wall consists of endothelial (end) and adventitial (adv) layers.   At the lower left corner of the field, the cytoplasm of an adventitial cell (adv') is voluminous and extends into the surrounding hematopoietic space.   Reticulocytes (ret) and granulocytes (gr) surround the sinus.   ×15,200.   (From L. Weiss, Blood **36**:189, 1970.)

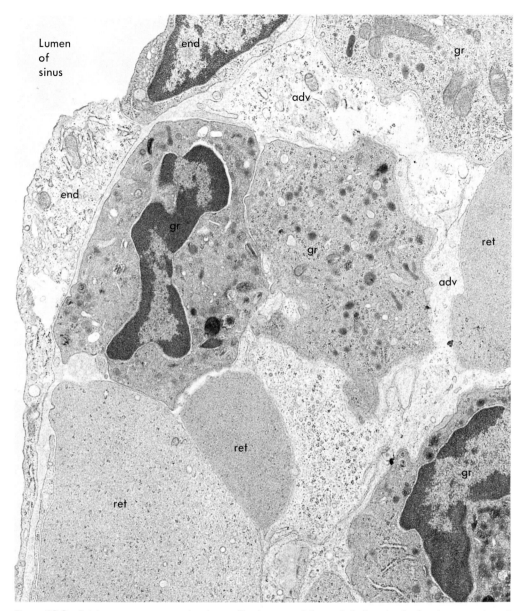

Figure 12-8   Rat bone marrow, vascular sinus. The lumen and the endothelium (end) of a sinus run along the left margin of the field. An adventitial cell (adv) is displaced from the wall by two granulocytes (gr) and two reticulocytes (ret). Thus the endothelium and its subjacent basement membrane are the only elements separating the late-stage hematopoietic cells from the lumen. The field also contains other reticulocytes and granulocytes. ×15,000. (From L. Weiss, Blood **36**:189, 1970.)

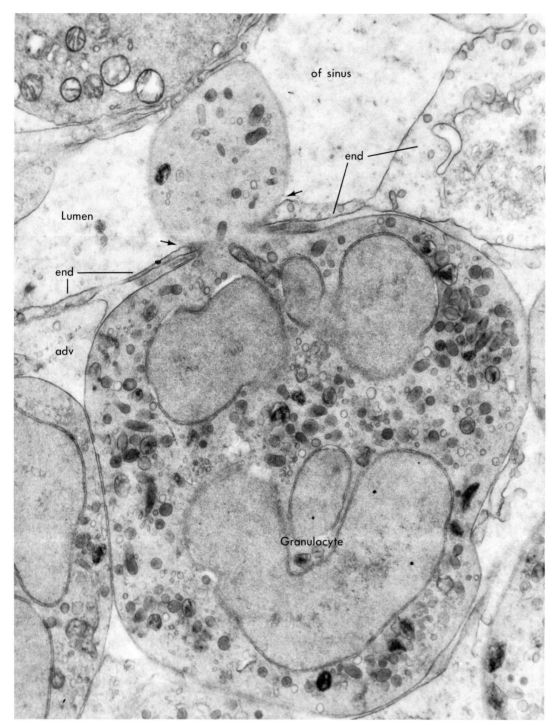

Figure 12-9 Rat bone marrow. A portion of a sinus, its lumen labeled, is at the top of the field. The wall of the sinus consists of endothelium (end), or lining cells, and adventitial cells (adv). A large granulocyte occupies most of the field. It lies almost entirely outside the sinus in the hematopoietic space and extends a process through an aperture (arrows) in the wall of the sinus and into the lumen. This granulocyte is crossing the wall of the sinus and will enter the circulation in the sinus. ×29,000. (From L. Weiss, J. Morph. 117:467, 1965.)

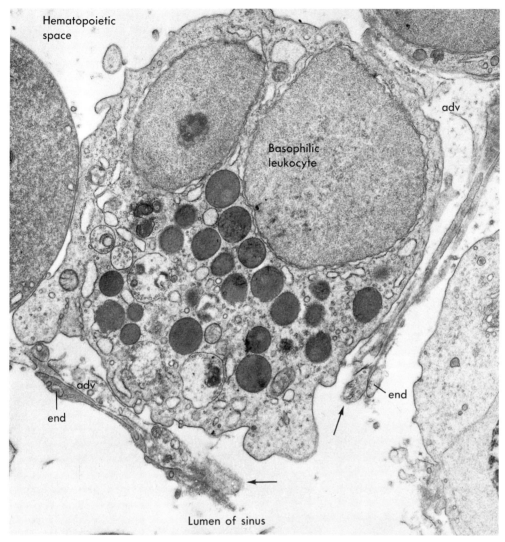

Figure 12-10   Rat bone marrow.   A mature basophilic leukocyte is crossing from the hematopoietic space across the wall of sinus into the lumen.   The wall of the sinus shows both endothelial cells (end) and adventitial cells (adv).   The leukocyte is passing into an aperture whose limits are indicated by arrows.   ×27,000.   (From L. Weiss, J. Morph. **117:**467, 1965.)

cells, and plasma cells have not as yet had their characteristic place in the hematopoietic compartment defined.

Hematopoiesis in the marrow is almost entirely extravascular.   Yet even in unstimulated marrow, erythroblasts, myelocytes, and masses of platelets and other hematopoietic elements may be present in the lumen of sinuses.   The occurrence is vastly magnified in erythroblastic or myeloblastic mar-row.   It is likely, therefore, that some hemato-poietic maturation does occur intravascularly.   In addition, however, such immature forms may be carried to the spleen or other sites where they will form hematopoietic colonies.   It must be empha-sized that a few cells not commonly considered as mature blood cells normally circulate.   Thus mega-karyocytes, myelocytes, and erythroblasts are found in blood in small numbers, as are stem cells.

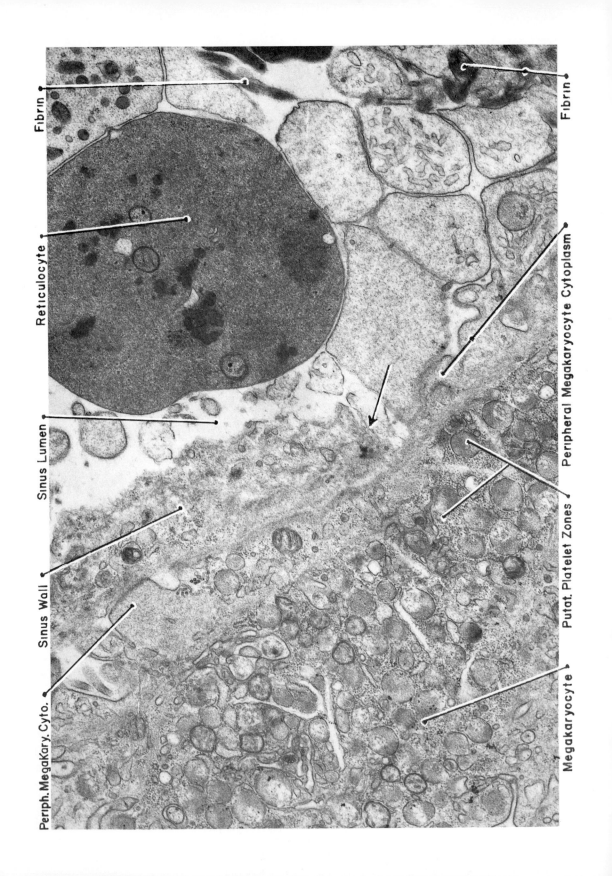

Fibrin

Fibrin

Reticulocyte

Peripheral Megakaryocyte Cytoplasm

Sinus Lumen

Sinus Wall

Putat. Platelet Zones

Periph. Megakary. Cyto.

Megakaryocyte

Principal methods for the study of bone marrow

The marrow is a fragile gelatinous tissue within a rigid capsule. In making microscopic preparations, care must be taken to avoid rupturing fat cells or stretching such delicate structures as sinuses. Marrow may be studied in decalcified bone by standard histologic methods of fixation, embedding, and sectioning, but the use of celloidin or plastic embedding material to minimize distortion is recommended. Such preparations permit study of the architectural relationships of marrow but do not yield the cytologic detail found in smears. Methods of vascular injection have been of great value, exemplified by Doan's studies of pigeon marrow and, more recently, by electron-microscopic studies. Blood flow in the marrow has been studied vitally by the methods of Brånemark (1959) (see above). The size of the marrow cavity and the size and distribution of trabeculae may be determined by x-ray examination of the marrow.

Two methods have been valuable in the clinical study of bone marrow in living patients: bone marrow biopsy and bone marrow aspiration. Biopsy is a surgical procedure involving removal of a small portion of bone with the associated marrow tissue. The specimen obtained may be decalcified and subsequently embedded and sectioned. Marrow aspiration is accomplished by thrusting a specially designed needle of fairly large gauge through the cortex of sternum or ilium prepared by infiltration with local anesthetic. A few drops of marrow tissue are drawn through a syringe attached to the needle and spread on a slide. This preparation yields excellent cytologic information but little on the histology of marrow.

Factors affecting the cellular composition of bone marrow

The normal pattern of red and yellow bone marrow is affected by age, disease, and experimental conditions. Heat enhances hematopoiesis and cold depresses it. Huggins and Blocksom (1936) found yellow marrow replaced by red marrow in rats maintained at an environmental temperature of 33 to 36°C. In another group of animals kept at environmental temperatures of about 20°C, the distal portion of the tail was denuded of skin, brought forward, and surgically inserted and fastened into the warmer abdominal cavity. This portion of the tail, whose vertebrae characteristically housed yellow marrow, developed red marrow, while the portion outside the abdominal cavity kept its yellow marrow.

In pathologic states yellow marrow may be replaced by hematopoietic tissue and normal hematopoietic tissue replaced by abnormal tissue. After severe hemorrhage yellow marrow may quickly give way to red. In *leukemia,* abnormal leukocytes may be produced to the exclusion of normal red and white cells and may crowd the normal cells out. In *polycythemia,* there is a hypertrophy of the erythroblastic mass, but here the number of leukocytes and megakaryocytes may also be markedly increased, and the fat is displaced from the marrow. So intense may erythropoiesis be in certain anemias that the internal surface of the bone is eroded and the trabeculae become reduced in size and number. Despite this considerable increase in erythro-

---

Figure 12-11   Rat bone marrow. This field shows the typical relationship of a megakaryocyte to a sinus. The peripheral cytoplasm of the megakaryocyte, incompletely segmented into putative platelets by ER, is on the left. The peripheral cytoplasm may be granular or swollen and relatively free of organelles. The megakaryocyte abuts the outside surface of a sinus wall, which consists only of endothelium. The wall is defective with an aperture present in the lower third of the field, beginning at the arrow. The megakaryocyte cytoplasm protrudes through this aperture into the sinus lumen. Here incipient platelets, fully formed except for an attachment to the megakaryocyte, as well as detached platelets, may be seen. These platelets are somewhat swollen and lack lysosomes and ribosomes. Several do contain a complex branching system of ER, the canaliculi (see text). The platelets lie upon strands of fibrin and show the changes associated with platelets in clots. A reticulocyte also lies within the lumen of the sinus.   ×20,000.   (From L. Weiss, J. Morph. **112:**467, 1965.)

poiesis, the number of circulating erythrocytes is quite severely reduced since the erythrocytes are markedly defective cells with considerably short-ened life-spans. Moreover, there is a possible inter-ference with the release of cells from the marrow to the blood. The cortex and trabeculae of bone may be so thinned by the expansion and erosion of marrow in these anemias and in leukemia that fractures of bone commonly occur after slight trauma.

Contrarily, hematopoietic marrows may become inactive. Doan (1922) studied avian marrow re-duced to a fatty state by starvation. He observed the rapid resumption of hematopoiesis after feed-ing. Many chemicals are toxic to marrow. Lead and benzene are industrial hazards capable of pro-ducing a severe depression of bone marrow termed *aplastic anemia*. Certain toxins are selective or may be controlled; for example, the *nitrogen mus-tards,* derivatives of the ill-reputed mustard gas, are used therapeutically to suppress or destroy an ab-normal bone marrow. Hormonal imbalance due to unchecked production of calcitonin may result in bony overgrowth and reduction in the volume of the marrow cavity. Malignant tumors may metastasize to bone marrow and create aplastic marrows by suppressing or displacing normal marrow tissue. In some instances vascular sinuses may become widely dilated with blood, encroaching upon hemato-poietic tissue and, paradoxically, conferring a bril-liant red color upon a tissue which is inactive hema-topoietically.

The functions of bone marrow

Although the marrow is a hematopoietic tissue, it does have other connective tissue and osteogenic functions. Its activities may be listed as follows:

THE PRODUCTION OF BLOOD CELLS AND THEIR RELEASE TO THE CIRCULATION

In human beings, all erythrocytes, granulocytes, platelets, and monocytes and a portion of lympho-cytes are produced in the bone marrow. The kinet-ics of hematopoiesis are described in Chapter 11. The mature human marrow contains 5.6×10^9 erythroid precursors per kilogram of body weight and 11.4×10^9 neutrophilic precursors. The rel-ative numbers of nucleated cells in normal human bone marrow are given in Table 12-1. Approxi-mately 1.5 percent of the cells are in mitotic divi-sion, the number of dividing erythroblasts slightly exceeding the number of leukocytes. Almost all the dividing leukocytes are myelocytes. Almost all the dividing erythroblasts are polychromatophilic.

HEMATOCLASIA

The marrow and the spleen not only produce blood cells but also destroy imperfectly produced, aged, or damaged cells. The process, termed *hemato-clasia* (or hemoclasia), requires the discrimination of defective cells, their sequestration, and phago-cytosis. Hematoclasia also occurs in the spleen.

RETICULOENDOTHELIAL FUNCTIONS

The bone marrow has a population of free macro-phages whose concentration increases after hemol-ysis of erythrocytes and other events requiring phagocytosis. The marrow therefore is capable of phagocytosis, inactivation of toxins, and other func-tions of the reticuloendothelial system. Moreover, the marrow is the source of the macrophages of the body through its production of monocytes.

IMMUNOLOGIC FUNCTIONS

The marrow supplies lymphocytes or stem cells to the thymus which are necessary to maintain its store of thymic lymphocytes, or T cells, that are essential in certain immunologic reactions. The bone marrow, moreover, produces and releases lymphocytes with immunoglobulin molecules on their surface, the B cells, that are probably ances-tral to the plasma cells which synthesize antibody on a large scale. Macrophages which, as indicated above, come from the marrow, have important immunologic roles. They are, for example, neces-sary to make certain antigens immunogenic.

Moreover, the marrow in human beings and cer-tain other species is capable of producing anti-body. The marrow contains a larger number of hematopoietic stem cells than any other tissue. For this reason, suspensions of marrow cells are capable of restoring the structure and functions of the entire hematopoietic system after lethal irradiation. Spleen, thymus, or lymph node suspensions cannot.

OSSEOUS FUNCTIONS
The marrow contains osteoclasts and osteoblasts, and supplies blood vessels to the bone.

GENERAL CONNECTIVE TISSUE FUNCTIONS
By its content of reticular cells, mast cells, macrophages, foreign-body giant cells, and other connective tissue elements, the marrow partakes of general connective tissue functions.

References

BLOOM, W., and G. W. BARTELMEZ: Hematopoiesis in Young Human Embryos, *Amer. J. Anat.*, **67**:21 (1940).

BRÅNEMARK, P. I.: Vital Microscopy of Bone Marrow in Rabbit, *Scand. J. Clin. Lab. Invest.* (Suppl. 38), **11**:1 (1959).

DOAN, C. A.: The Capillaries of the Bone Marrow of the Adult Pigeon, *Bull. Johns Hopkins Hosp.*, **33**:222 (1922).

DONAHUE, D. M., B. W. GABRIO, and C. A. FINCH: Quantitative Measurement of Hematopoietic Cells of the Marrow, *J. Clin. Invest.*, **37**:1564 (1958).

FLEIDNER, T. M.: Research on the Architecture of the Vascular Bed of the Bone Marrow of Rats, *Z. Zellforsch.*, **45**:328 (1956).

FLEIDNER, T. M., W. CALVO, et al.: Morphological and Cytokinetic Aspects of Bone Marrow Stroma, in F. Stohlman (ed.), "Hematopoietic Cell Proliferation," Grune and Stratton, New York, 1970.

GILMOUR, J. R.: Normal Haemopoiesis in Intrauterine and Neonatal Life, *J. Path. Bact.*, **52**:25 (1941).

HUGGINS, C., and B. H. BLOCKSOM: Changes in Outlying Bone Marrow Accompanying a Local Increase of Temperature within Physiological Limits, *J. Exp. Med.*, **64**:253 (1936).

WEISS, L.: "The Cells and Tissues of the Immune System," Prentice-Hall, Englewood Cliffs, N.J., 1972.

WEISS, L.: The Histology of the Bone Marrow, in A. S. Gordon (ed.), "Regulation of Hematopoiesis," vol. I, p. 79, Appleton-Century-Crofts, New York, 1970.

WEISS, L.: Transmural Cellular Passage in Vascular Sinuses of Rat Bone Marrow, *Blood*, **36**:189 (1970).

WEISS, L.: The Structure of Bone Marrow. Functional Interrelationships of Vascular and Hematopoietic Compartments in Experimental Hemolytic Anemia, *J. Morph.*, **117**:467 (1965).

ZAMBONI, L., and D. C. PEASE: The Vascular Bed of Red Bone Marrow, *J. Ultrastruct. Res.*, **5**:65 (1961).

chapter 13　　　The thymus　　LEON WEISS

The human thymus is a lymphatic organ, pyramidal in shape, located in the superior mediastinum dorsal to the sternum. It achieves its greatest absolute weight, approximately 40 gm, at puberty. The base of the thymus rests upon the pericardium; the pulmonary vessels, aorta, and trachea are dorsal to it. It is bilaterally symmetric, consisting of halves which meet in the midline except at the apex, which extends into the neck and diverges about the trachea. The thymus is derived from the epithelium of the third branchial pouch. Lymphocytes enter the epithelial rudiment, and the definitive thymus is a *lymphoepithlial* organ.

Two major functions of the lymphatic system are to supply lymphocytes and to produce antibodies. The thymus occupies a position of control over each of these functions. It is required for a normal concentration of certain lymphocytes, T cells, in blood, spleen, and lymph nodes. The immunologic competence of animals, as determined by their ability to reject grafts of foreign tissue and their capacity to produce certain antibodies, is dependent upon the presence of the thymus. Thymic influences upon lymphocytes and immunologic competences are marked in neonatal animals and are present, but less evident, in adults. The thymus is also required for the development of lymphatic leukemia in certain strains of mice and other animals. The thymus is sensitive to the effects of hormones, notably cortisone and related hormones of the adrenal cortex, which cause a marked depletion in thymic lymphocytes.

The thymus displays remarkable atrophy or involution on aging. It develops precociously, unlike the spleen and lymph nodes, and is well developed at birth. Before puberty the thymus is a rounded, fleshy organ of some prominence. After puberty it begins to involute, its parenchyma being replaced by fatty and fibrous tissue until in old age it may be a shriveled fibrous cord lying, barely recognizable, in the fat of the superior mediastinum. Despite postpubertal involution, the thymus remains a functional organ well into adulthood.

The thymus is divided into lobes and lobules by

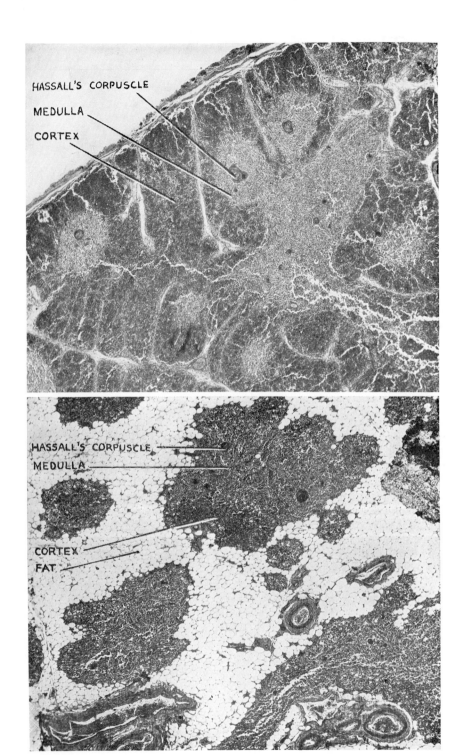

septa which extend into the organ from the surrounding connective tissues.   The lobules are
broad, roughly rectangular in outline, and are 0.5
to 2.0 mm in length.   Each lobule is divided into
a peripheral zone relatively rich in lymphocytes, the
cortex, and a central zone relatively rich in epithelial
cells, the *medulla* (Figs. 13-1 to 13-4).

Structure of the thymus

MAJOR CELL TYPES
Before proceeding to a discussion of the structure
of the capsule, cortex, and medulla of the thymus,
its major cell types will be considered.

Epithelial cells   Epithelial cells in the thymus may
assume several forms.   They line the walls of cysts
or other unmistakably epithelial structures.   This
epithelium is cuboidal or columnar and contains
mucous cells and ciliated cells.   These epithelial
structures probably represent remnants of branchial
epithelium.   They may be present in the human
thymus but are quite conspicuous in that of dogs,
guinea pigs, and certain other animals.

A major group of thymic epithelial cells is that
in intimate association with lymphocytes.   Fundamentally this epithelium is similar to other epithelia,
with cells attached to one another by desmosomes.   Lymphocytes in masses move in and separate these epithelial cells, but the latter still maintain contact with · one another by slender
cytoplasmic processes joined by desmosomes, and
so they may assume a branched or stellate appearance.   They thereby superficially resemble the mesenchymal reticular cells of the cords of spleen and
lymph nodes and have been called *reticular cells.*
Here these epithelial cells will be designated *epithelial-reticular* cells (Figs. 13-2, 13-4, and 13-5).
They form a meshwork in whose interstices lie the
lymphocytes that separate them.   This meshwork
is a cytoreticulum, free of reticular fibers and of the
intercellular substance associated with mesenchymal reticulum.

The epithelial-reticular cells are large, branched
cells with large nuclei, prominent nucleoli, and voluminous eosinophilic cytoplasm.   By light microscopy their epithelial nature may be suspected but
not ascertained.   In electron micrographs, these
cells show tonofilaments, desmosomes, and cytoplasmic inclusions, some suggesting a secretory
function.   In addition, they contain moderate but
variable concentrations of ribonucleoprotein, moderate numbers of mitochondria, and a well-developed endoplasmic reticulum and Golgi apparatus.

Another major group of epithelial cells form thymic corpuscles.   Here the epithelial cells may be
swollen or flattened and tightly wound upon one
another.

Lymphocytes   Lymphocytes in the thymus are
small, medium, and large (Figs. 13-2 to 13-5).
Like lymphocytes elsewhere, thymic lymphocytes
are spherical cells with basophilic cytoplasm containing free ribosomes but scanty endoplasmic reticulum.   Small thymic lymphocytes are somewhat
smaller than small lymphocytes of other lymphatic
organs, and while in the thymus they may bear a
distinctive surface antigen, the TL antigen, which
may serve as a marker.

**Macrophages, fat cells, mast cells, and plasma
cells**   Macrophages are invariably present in large
numbers within the thymus, scattered among the
lymphocytes and epithelial cells of cortex and
medulla.   There is considerable lymphatic death in
the thymus, and many macrophages are there in

Figure 13-1   Human thymus before and after involution.   The tissue in the upper micrograph is from a 4-year-old individual; the
lower, from a 72-year-old person.   Note the lobular pattern in the upper micrograph.   The medulla is a branching structure.   The
cortex surrounds the lobular projections of the medulla.   A thin fibrous capsule is present.   Artefactitious cracks are present in
the section.   Involutional changes are evident in the lower micrograph.   The cortex is markedly diminished, and the organ is fatty.
The blood vessels display thickened sclerotic walls.   Note, however, that the medulla has suffered relatively little change.   ×30.
(Preparations provided by B. Castleman.)

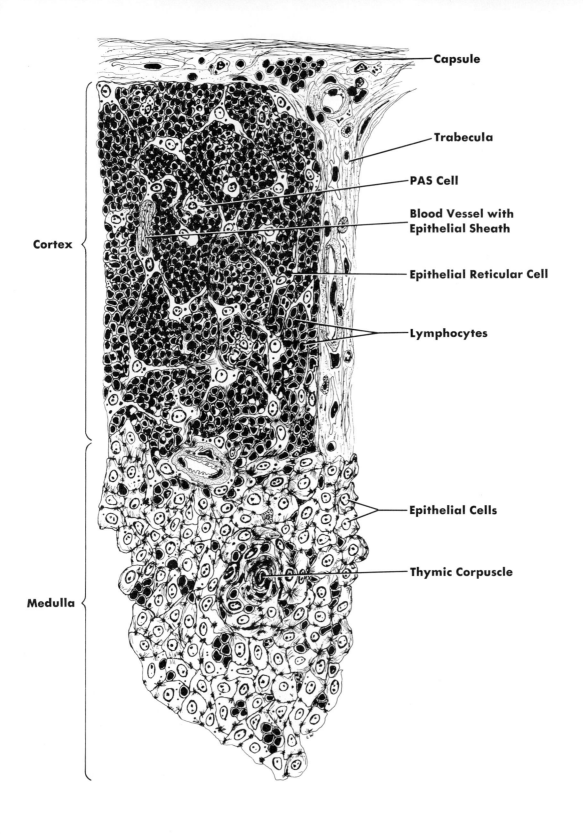

Capsule

Trabecula

PAS Cell

Blood Vessel with
Epithelial Sheath

Epithelial Reticular Cell

Lymphocytes

Epithelial Cells

Thymic Corpuscle

Cortex

Medulla

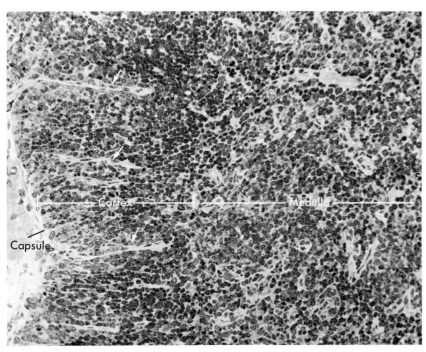

Figure 13-3   Thymus of a mouse.   Both cortex and medulla are infiltrated with lymphocytes.   The deeper parts of the cortex are particularly heavily infiltrated.   The deep connective tissue ingrowths which cross the cortex (arrows) carry blood vessels. Toluidine blue stain.   ×300.

response.   Fat cells are particularly prominent in aged thymus.   Mast cells are always present in the capsule and septa and occasionally in the parenchyma of the organ; involuted thymuses may contain great numbers of them.   A few plasma cells may be found scattered in the thymus.

Other blood cells and connective tissue cells may be found in fluctuating but usually small numbers.

CAPSULE

The thymus is enclosed by a thin, well-defined capsule of dense white connective tissue variably rich in macrophages, plasma cells, granular leukocytes, mast cells, and fat cells (Figs. 13-1 to 13-3). Connective tissue continuous with the capsule dips into the organ separating the lobes and lobules and forms *septa* (Fig. 13-6) or *trabeculae*.   Large blood vessels, lymphatic vessels, and nerves run in the capsule and septa.

MEDULLA

The medulla is a broad, branched mass of tissue which forms the central part of the thymus (Figs. 13-1 to 13-3).   The branches of the medulla provide the lobar and lobular patterns of the organ. The medulla is rich in epithelial cells.   These cells may line cysts but most are present as *cytoreticulum*.   Although there are many lymphocytes in the medulla, there are far fewer than in the cortex, and so the epithelial cells are not as widely separated

Figure 13-2   Portion of lobule of the thymus.   The cortex is heavily infiltrated with lymphocytes.   As a result, the epithelial cells become stellate and remain attached to one another by desmosomes.   The medulla is closer to a pure epithelium, although it too is commonly infiltrated by lymphocytes.   A large thymic corpuscle, consisting of concentrically arranged epithelial cells, is figured.   The capsule and trabeculae are rich in connective tissue fibers (mainly collagen) and contain blood vessels and variable numbers of plasma cells, granulocytes, and lymphocytes.   (From L. Weiss, "The Cells and Tissues of the Immune System," Prentice-Hall, Inc., Englewood Cliffs, N.J., 1972.)

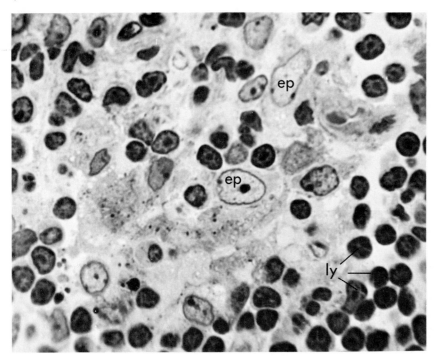

Figure 13-4   Thymus of a mouse, medulla. Several large epithelial cells are present. Their cytoplasm contains deeply stained inclusions. Many lymphocytes closely surround the epithelial cells. Compare with Fig. 13-5. PAS-hematoxylin stain. ×1,300.

as in the cortex, not as markedly branched, and more typically epithelial than cortical epithelial-reticular cells. Indeed, they may be polygonal and lie next to one another in sheetlike formations.

The medulla contains many large blood vessels, from which collagenous and reticular fibers radiate and thread between epithelial cells.

Variable numbers of plasma cells, mast cells, eosinophils, and melanocytes are present in the medulla, usually near blood vessels.

Thymic corpuscles   Thymic corpuscles, or *Hassall's corpuscles,* are organizations of epithelial cells unique to the thymus (Figs. 13-6 to 13-8). They consist of epithelial cells rather tightly wound about one another in a concentric pattern. The central

cells in these arrangements are prone to become swollen, keratinized, calcified, and necrotic and may undergo lysis, leaving a cystic structure. The peripheral epithelial cells in a thymic corpuscle blend into the cytoreticulum of the medulla. Thymic corpuscles may be well over 100 μm in diameter and are subject to considerable specific variation. They are well developed in human beings and guinea pigs but poorly developed in mice.

The essential changes in epithelial cells which signify a conversion to thymic corpuscles are hyalinization of cytoplasm and swelling of nucleus and cytoplasm. In electron micrographs the tonofilaments of epithelial cells in thymic corpuscles are markedly developed and the density and complexity of desmosomes are marked. Small corpuscles may

Figure 13-5   Electron micrograph of the cortex of rat thymus, showing a characteristic relationship of lymphocytes and epithelial-reticular cells. The lymphocytes are present in clusters. Their nucleus is spherical, their cytoplasm scanty and rich in ribonucleoprotein but poor in endoplasmic reticulum and mitochondria. The epithelial-reticular cells are larger cells. The nucleus is less dense and may contain a moderately sized nucleolus. The cytoplasm is voluminous, extending between lymphocytes as slender cytoplasmic processes, and contains distinctive multivesicular vacuoles, some ribonucleoprotein, and some endoplasmic reticulum. In other species these epithelial cells may contain cytoplasmic filaments.

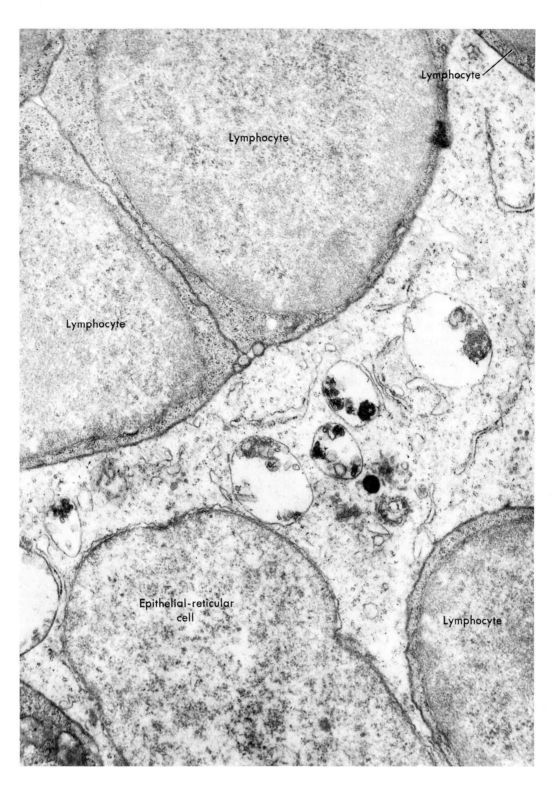

Lymphocyte

Lymphocyte

Lymphocyte

Epithelial-reticular
cell

Lymphocyte

consist of a few cells or only one cell. As more cells contribute to a corpuscle, its concentric pattern evolves. Thymic corpuscles become larger with age. They may eventually become huge, multiform structures.

The function of thymic corpuscles is unknown. They may have immunologic functions or may simply be degenerated structures.

CORTEX

The cortex is a thick layer of lymphocytes and epithelial cells which follows the contour of the medulla and therefore assumes a lobular pattern. In the preinvolutional thymus numerous lymphocytes lie between epithelial cells, separating them. The epithelial-reticular cells are highly branched and form a cellular meshwork (Figs. 13-1 to 13-3 and 13-6).

The lymphocytes separating epithelial cells may be so plentiful as to obscure even the large branches of epithelial cells, allowing one to observe only the perikaryon in most light-microscopic preparations. Unlike the cortex of lymph nodes or the white pulp of the spleen, the thymic cortex normally contains no germinal centers.

BLOOD VESSELS OF THE THYMUS

The major arterial vessels of the thymus, branches of the subclavian artery, enter the medulla through septa. There are numerous arterial branches in the medulla. The blood supply of the cortex is derived from arterioles which run along the junction of cortex and medulla. From these vessels, arterial capillaries run outward to the capsule. They return as venous capillaries to drain into venules running in company with the arterioles in the corticomedullary junction. The venules drain into medullary veins, which receive tributaries from the medulla as well. Most medullary veins empty into the innominate vein.

Capillary blood vessels in the thymus may be only 4 to 6 μm in outside diameter and are thick-

Figure 13-6 Thymus of a human being 20 years of age. Lymphocytes are concentrated in the cortex. They are present in the medulla as well but are scattered loosely among epithelial-reticular cells. A large, multicentric thymic corpuscle is present in the medulla. The interlobular septum is slender and contains lymphatic vessels, blood vessels, and nerves. ×200. (Preparation from B. Castleman.)

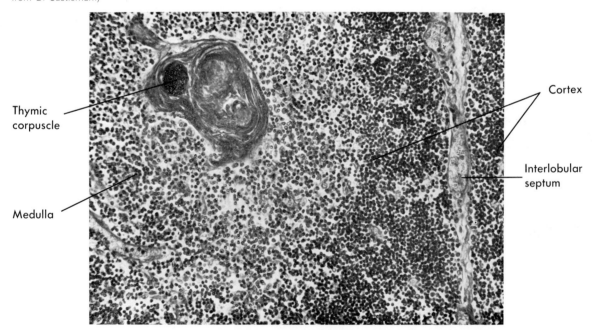

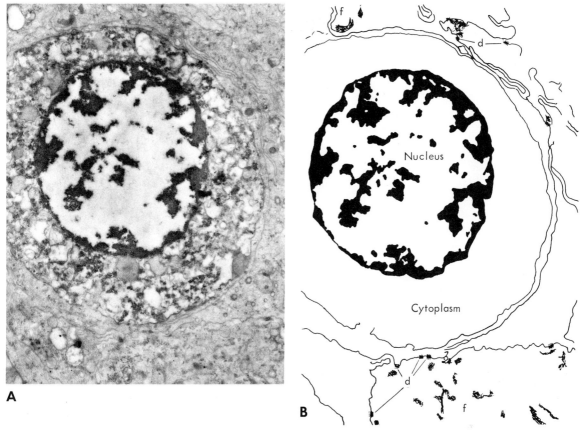

Figure 13-7 Thymus of a mouse. A. Electron micrograph of a small corpuscle. By light microscopy this would probably appear as a unicellular corpuscle. Note the large swollen nucleus and the similarly degenerated cytoplasm. The epithelial cells surrounding the large central cell are arranged circumferentially, with desmosomes present at their cell membrane. (From Fig. 5, P. Kohnen and L. Weiss, Anat. Rec., **148**:29, 1964.) B. Tracing of the corpuscle shown in A. Desmosomes are at d; cytoplasmic filaments at f. ×4,000.

walled. The endothelium forms a complete layer, and subendothelial extracellular substance, including a basement membrane, is thick. Epithelial-reticular cells envelop capillaries and larger vessels, particularly in the cortex of the thymus, thereby constituting the most peripheral cell of the vessel wall. These cells also extend cytoplasmic processes outward between perivascular lymphocytes. Epithelial-reticular cells in thymic vessels thus occupy a position similar to that of the glial cells investing blood vessels in the central nervous system. They constitute an element in the *blood-thymus barrier* (Figs. 13-2 and 13-9) just as glial

cells contribute to the *blood-brain barrier*. The epithelial envelopment of thymic blood vessels, however, is typically incomplete.

LYMPHATIC VESSELS
There appear to be no afferent lymphatic vessels. Several groups of efferent vessels leave from the medulla, in septa, and drain into mediastinal lymph nodes.

NERVOUS SUPPLY
The capsule of the thymus is moderately rich in small myelinated and unmyelinated nerves from the

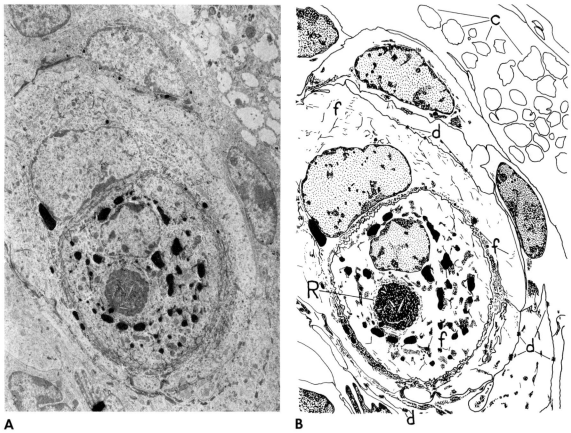

A   **B**

Figure 13-8 Thymus of a guinea pig. A. Electron micrograph of a thymic corpuscle. There is a small compressed central cell (labeled R in the accompanying tracing). Note the concentrate pattern of the cells. The inner cells have droplets, probably keratohyaline droplets. Cytoplasmic filaments and desmosomes contribute to this corpuscle. A portion of an epithelial cell in the cytoreticulum in the right upper corner contains intracytoplasmic vacuoles. (From Fig. 1, P. Kohnen and L. Weiss, Anat. Rec., **148:**29, 1964.) B. Tracing of the corpuscle shown in A. Desmosomes are at d; cytoplasmic filaments at f, and intracytoplasmic vacuoles at c. R is degenerated nucleus ✕5,000.

vagus, cardiac plexus, first thoracic ganglion, and ansa hypoglossi. Unmyelinated vasomotor fibers enter the organ with blood vessels.

DEVELOPMENT

The human thymus develops from the outer portion of the third branchial pouch. There may be a small contribution from the fourth. The thymic rudiment in embryos of 10-mm crown-rump length is a slender, tubular prolongation which extends caudad and mediad. It reaches into the mediastinum just caudal to the thyroid and parathyroid rudiments. The tip of the prolongation proliferates, becoming

bulbous. The intermediate portion, constituting the connection to the pharynx, vanishes, leaving the proliferating terminal bulb free in the mediastinum at the 35-mm crown-rump stage. The process is bilateral.

The epithelial thymic rudiment becomes surrounded by a layer of mesenchyme. Soon after, lymphocytes are found in the midst of the epithelium. Lymphocytes and epithelial cells proliferate, and when the embryo is 40 mm in length, the lobular pattern is achieved. Thymic corpuscles begin to appear at 60 to 70 mm.

The development of the thymus outstrips that of

the remaining lymphatic organs, as the thymus is fully developed prenatally. Only in the postnatal period do the spleen and lymph nodes attain full development.

INVOLUTION OF THE THYMUS

Involution, the process of atrophy and depletion of the thymus, is accelerated after puberty and consists primarily of a decrease in weight, a conspic-

Figure 13-9   Thymus of a rat.   Electron micrograph of a capillary at the junction of cortex and medulla.   The vessel displays a complete endothelium, a broad basement membrane rich in collagenous fibers, and surrounding epithelial cells, which form a complete vascular investment.   Thorotrast, a colloidal material consisting of thorium dioxide (ThO_2) stabilized in suspension by dextrins, was injected shortly before thymectomy.   Some ThO_2 is present within the vessel and some is localized in a small vacuole in one of the investing epithelial cells.   The epithelial cell contains highly characteristic vacuoles.   Note the lymphocytes; their cytoplasm is rich in RNP but lacking endoplasmic reticulum, separated from the lumen by three layers: epithelial cell, basement membrane, and endothelium.   ×22,000.

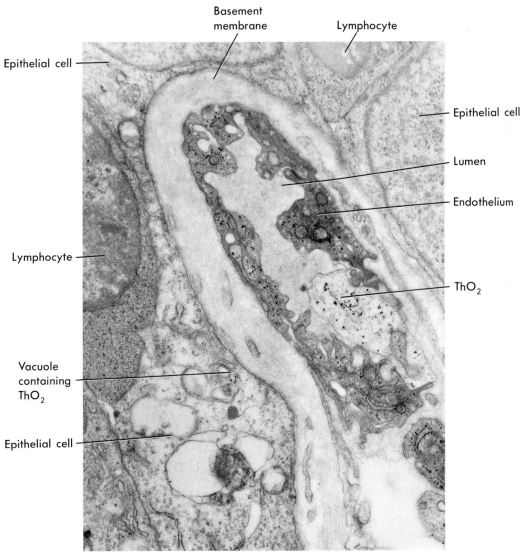

Table 13-1   Age and thymus weight

Age, years	Weight, grams
Newborn	13.26
1–5	22.98
6–10	26.10
11–15	37.52
16–20	25.58
21–25	24.73
26–35	19.87
36–45	16.27
46–55	12.85
56–65	16.08
66–75	6.00

uous loss of cortical lymphocytes and their replacement by fat, and an increase in size and a slight increase in number of thymic corpuscles. The septa show a proportionate increase in width as the lobules atrophy (Fig. 13-1). But the age-associated wasting of the organ has been perhaps unduly stressed, since it remains substantive and functional in adulthood. The normal pattern of involution is complicated by a precipitous involution associated with disease, so-called *accidental involution.* The thymus in infants dying suddenly and for no apparent reason is occasionally very large and has been considered causative in their death, a condition designated *status thymicolymphaticus,* but it is likely that this state represents simply a normal organ undiminished by accidental involution.

The thymus is at its greatest relative size at birth and at its greatest absolute size at puberty. The figures in Table 13-1, taken from Hammar's work, represent average weights of the thymus at different ages in human beings. Note that the weight of the organ diminishes in adulthood. Lymphatic tissue throughout the body suffers a decrease in the process of aging, but in the thymus the process is more marked.

COMPARATIVE ANATOMY OF THE THYMUS
The thymus is present in every vertebrate. The organs in all mammals are remarkably alike, although such variations as differences in development of thymic corpuscles exist.

BURSA OF FABRICIUS
The bursa of Fabricius is a lymphoepithelial organ in birds which originates as a dorsal epithelial diverticulum of the cloaca. It becomes infiltrated by lymphocytes and, in being a gut-derived epithelial structure intimately associated with lymphocytes, it resembles the thymus. In the bursa, however, unlike the thymus, the epithelial diverticulum retains connection with the cloaca, the lymphocytes are organized about epithelial follicles, and many plasma cells are present. The bursa involutes markedly on sexual maturation; indeed its development may be entirely suppressed by applying male sex hormones to the shell of embryonated eggs.

Birds possess a pharyngeal thymus and exhibit a division of labor between bursa and thymus which is of great theoretical importance. The cells released from the thymus (T cells) are primarily concerned with delayed hypersensitivity, although they may have an essential auxiliary role in antibody production against some antigens. However, cells released from the bursa (B cells) are humoral antibody producers. The thymus in mammals has similar functions to that of birds. As yet, however, no mammalian counterpart to the bursa has been discovered. Both the thymus and the bursa depend upon the bone marrow for a supply of stem cells.

Functions of the thymus

LYMPHOCYTIC TURNOVER
The mitotic rate of thymic lymphocytes is greater than that of lymphocytes in spleen, lymph nodes, and Peyer's patches by a factor of 3 to 5. This ratio, however, is an overall one. Foci of proliferation (that is, germinal centers) occur in spleen or lymph nodes, mounting antibody responses in which the mitotic rate equals that of the thymus. Despite its high mitotic rate, the thymus normally contains no germinal centers. Germinal centers, originally regarded primarily as foci of lymphocytic proliferation, are now recognized as primarily foci of antibody production. The thymus produces little or no antibody.

Despite the high rate of proliferation of its lymphocytes, the thymus depends upon outside sources for lymphocytes. Indeed, it is startling to consider that more than 90 percent of the lymphocytes within the thymus die within a few days. In fetal life the thymus is supplied by cells produced and released into the circulation by the liver. When hematopoiesis moves to the marrow, that tissue becomes the source of thymic lymphocytes, a function it maintains throughout life.

The lymphocytes released from the thymus are distinctive in having a specific surface antigen, the theta (θ) antigen. These T cells may enjoy a long life—months or years in rodents and years in man. They circulate and recirculate in distinctive pathways through lymphatic tissues (excluding the thymus), blood, and lymph. They occupy distinctive sites in spleen and lymph nodes. See Chaps. 12, 14, and 15.

The development of the spleen, lymph nodes, and other lymphatic tissue is dependent upon the thymus. Without it these organs are considerably diminished in size owing to a lack of small T-type lymphocytes. The periarterial sheaths of spleen and infranodular or deep cortex of lymph nodes is specifically depleted. The level of small lymphocytes in the blood may be reduced 60 percent or more and that in the lymph to an even lower level. Associated with this lymphocytic depletion after thymectomy are immunologic deficiencies.

THYMIC HUMORAL FACTOR

There is evidence that the thymus elaborates a humoral factor which stimulates the production of lymphocytes. This evidence depends heavily upon neonatal thymectomy. Thus a newborn mouse thymectomized at birth becomes deficient in both lymphocytes (Fig. 13-10) and immunologic capacity. By grafting with a thymus from a litter mate, however, such deficiencies are averted. If a thymectomized newborn mouse is supplied with a thymus grafted into his peritoneal cavity, but wrapped in a cell-tight envelope fabricated of a millipore filter, the treated animal will have a partial restoration of his lymphocytes and suffer no immunologic deficiencies. In short, a factor which stimulates lymphocytic production sufficiently to allow normal immunological function appears to be escaping the millipore envelope: This preparation has largely substituted for the thymus. Further support for a thymic humoral factor comes from experiments in which thymectomized immunologically deficient female mice, on becoming pregnant, are found to have their immunologic competence restored, even though the genetic patterns and placental arrangements preclude cellular transfer from fetus to mother. There is some suggestion that epithelial cells in the thymus elaborate a secretory product. But the existence of a thymic humoral factor must remain uncertain until it is isolated or a clear assay system is devised.

IMMUNOLOGIC FUNCTIONS

The thymus possesses a fundamental immunologic role, best revealed after neonatal thymectomy. The lymphocytic depletions which follow this procedure are associated with major immunologic deficiencies. Most consistently there is an impairment in delayed hypersensitivity or cellular immunity, namely, those immunologic reactions which depend upon the physical presence of lymphoid cells at the site of antigen. Thus after thymectomy in the newborn, homografts (a graft from a genetically different animal but one within the same species, as mouse to mouse but not within the same inbred mouse line), instead of being rejected, may persist indefinitely. In addition, there is spotty interference with antibody production. Those antigens (as foreign erythrocytes) that require the cooperation of T cells for a response fail to elicit an antibody response. These deficiencies can be fully corrected by thymic grafts.

Thymectomy in adults is attended by no such clear-cut change because the extrathymic tissues and circulation are already stocked with T cells. A significant reduction in splenic and lymph nodal weight occurs after thymectomy in adult rats, for example, although 6 to 8 weeks are required for the change. If, however, adults are thymectomized and then irradiated enough to deplete the stores of T cells in their lymphatic tissue, a neonatal picture emerges.

ROLE OF THE THYMUS IN LEUKEMIA

In certain strains of mice and other animals, the incidence of leukemia is high. For example, 60 to 80 percent of mice of the AKR strain develop leukemia by their second year. In addition to this

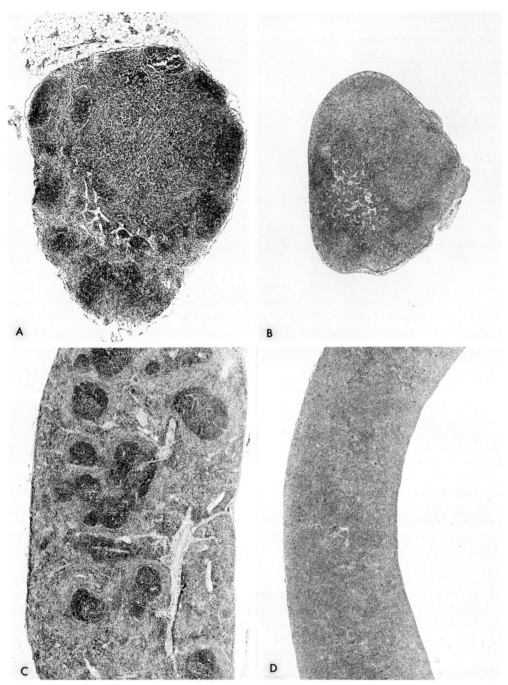

Figure 13-10   This plate illustrates the dependence of the lymph nodes and spleen upon the thymus.   The tissues are taken from C57BL mice. A. Lymph node of 8-week-old mouse sham-operated at birth.   ×32.   B. Lymph node of 8-week-old mouse thymectomized at birth.   ×32.   C. Spleen of 7-week-old mouse sham-operated at birth.   ×32.   D. Spleen of 7-week-old mouse thymectomized at birth.   ×32.   Thymectomy is followed by a decrease in size of the lymph nodes and spleen, due primarily to depletion of small lymphocytes (T cells).   (From J. F. A. P. Miller.)

genetic predisposition, the presence of a virus and of the thymus is required for the appearance of leukemia. In high-leukemia strains of mice, the virus is transmitted transplacentally with the result that it is distributed in virtually every tissue of every individual. Thymectomy prevents the occurrence of the disease. The role of the thymus is unknown. Normally the mitotic rate of thymic lymphocytes is three to five times that of lymphocytes elsewhere. In leukemic strains, the mitotic rate in the preleukemic period may exceed that of nonthymic lymphocytes by a factor of 7 to 10.

THE INFLUENCE OF HORMONES
Following the administration of certain adrenocortical hormones, the thymus undergoes massive involution. The process primarily affects the cortex, as large numbers of lymphocytes are damaged and die. Macrophages in great numbers become mobilized and ingest these lymphocytes. These events resemble those of acute involution. Indeed, it is possible that acute involution is mediated by adrenocortical secretion. Other lymphatic organs undergo involution after adrenocortical hormones but the effects are not so marked as in the thymus. Sex hormones may elicit similar responses in the lymphatic system but they are not so pronounced as those of the adrenal cortex. Adrenocorticotropic hormone of the pars distalis influences the lymphatic system through the adrenal cortex. Growth hormones stimulate the thymus.

References

ARNASON, B. G., and C. WENNERSTEN: Role of the Thymus in Immune Reaction in Rats. II. Suppressive Effect of Thymectomy at Birth on Reactions of Delayed (Cellular) Hypersensitivity and the Circulating Small Lymphocyte, *J. Exp. Med.*, **116**:177 (1962).

DEFENDI, V., and D. METCALF (eds.): "The Thymus," Wistar Institute Press, Philadelphia, 1964.

DOWNEY, H.: Cytology of Rabbit Thymus and Regeneration of Its Thymocytes after Irradiation; with Some Notes on the Human Thymus, *Blood,* **3**:1315 (1948).

GOOD, R. A., and A. E. GABRIELSEN (eds.): "The Thymus in Immunobiology: Structure, Function, and Role in Disease," Paul B. Hoeber, Inc., New York, 1964.

GOOD, R. A., and B. W. PAPERMASTER: Phylogeny of the Immune Response, *Fed. Proc.,* **20**:26 (1961).

HARRIS, J. E., and C. E. FORD: Cellular Traffic of the Thymus: Experiments with Chromosome Markers. I. Evidence That the Thymus Plays an Instructional Part, *Nature* (*London*), **201**:884 (1964).

HARRIS, J. E., C. E. FORD, D. W. H. BARNES, and E. P. EVANS: Cellular Traffic of the Thymus: Experiments with Chromosome Markers. II. Evidence from Parabiosis for an Afferent Stream of Cells, *Nature* (*London*), **201**:886 (1964).

JANKOVIC, B., B. H. WAKSMAN, and B. G. ARNASON: Role of the Thymus in Immune Reactions in Rats. I. The Immunologic Response to Bovine Serum Albumin (Antibody Formation, Arthus Reactivity and Delayed Hypersensitivity) in Rats Thymectomized or Splenectomized at Various Times after Birth, *J. Exp. Med.,* **116**:159 (1962).

JOLLY, J.: La Bourse de Fabricius et les organes lympho-épithéliaux, *Arch. Anat. Micr.,* **16**:363 (1915).

KINDRED, J. E.: A Quantitative Study of the Hematopoietic Organs of Young Albino Rats, *Amer. J. Anat.,* **67**:99 (1940).

KOHNEN, P., and L. WEISS: An Electron Microscopic Study of Thymic Corpuscles in the Guinea Pig and the Mouse, *Anat. Rec.,* **148:**29 (1964).

LEVEY, R. H., N. TRAININ, and L. W. LAW: Evidence for Function of Thymic Tissue in Diffusion Chambers Implanted in Neonatally Thymectomized Mice, *J. Nat. Cancer Inst.,* **31:**199 (1963).

LINNA, J., and J. STILLSTRÖM: Migration of Cells from the Thymus to the Spleen in Young Guinea Pigs, *Acta Path. Microbiol. Scand.,* **68:**465 (1966).

METCALF, D.: The Thymus: Its Role in Immune Responses, Leukaemia Development and Carcinogenesis, in "Recent Results in Cancer Research," no. 5, Springer-Verlag OHG, Berlin, 1966.

MILLER, J. F. A. P.: Effect of Neonatal Thymectomy on the Immunological Responsiveness of the Mouse, *Proc. Roy. Soc., Ser. B.,* **156:**415 (1962).

MILLER, J. F. A. P., A. H. E. MARSHALL, and R. G. WHITE: The Immunological Significance of the Thymus, *Advances Immun.,* **2:**111 (1962).

MOORE, M. A. S., and J. J. T. OWEN: Experimental Studies on the Development of the Bursa of Fabricius, *Develop. Biol.,* **14:**40 (1966).

OSOBA, D., and J. F. A. P. MILLER: The Lymphoid Tissues and Immune Responses of Neonatally Thymectomized Mice Bearing Thymic Tissues in Millipore Diffusion Chambers, *J. Exp. Med.,* **119:**177 (1964).

PARROTT, D. M. V., M. A. B. DE SOUSA, and J. EAST: Thymus-dependent Areas in the Lymphoid Areas of Neonatally Thymectomized Mice, *J. Exp. Med.,* **123:**191 (1966).

SAINTE-MARIE, G., and C. P. LEBLOND: Thymus-cell Population Dynamics, in R. A. Good and A. E. Gabrielsen (eds.), "The Thymus in Immunobiology," p. 207, Paul B. Hoeber, Inc., New York, 1964.

WAKSMAN, B. G., B. G. ARNASON, and B. D. JANKOVIC: Role of the Thymus in Immune Reactions in Rats. III. Changes in the Lymphoid Organs of Thymectomized Rats, *J. Exp. Med.,* **116:**187 (1962).

WEISS, L.: "The Cells and Tissues of the Immune System," Prentice-Hall, Inc., Englewood Cliffs, N.J., 1972.

WEISSMAN, I. L.: Thymus Cell Migration, *J. Exp. Med.,* **126:**291 (1967).

WOLSTENHOLME, G. E. W., and R. PORTER (eds.): "The Thymus: Experimental and Clinical Studies," A Ciba Foundation Symposium, Little, Brown and Company, Boston, 1966.

chapter 14 Lymphatic vessels and lymph nodes

LEON WEISS

Lymphatic vessels

Lymphatic vessels make up a network of channels which originate in connective tissue spaces as blindly ending or anastomosing capillaries. The capillaries flow into larger collecting vessels, and the largest and most proximal lymphatic vessels empty into systemic veins in the base of the neck. Like blood vessels, lymphatic vessels are a system of endothelium-lined tubes of varying diameter which carry cellular elements suspended in a fluid intercellular substance. Unlike blood vessels, they do not form a continuous circular system but originate in the connective tissue spaces and carry their contents, called *lymph,* in only one direction, toward the base of the neck. The major function of lymphatic vessels is to recover fluids that escape into the connective tissue spaces from blood capillaries and return these fluids to the blood. In amphibians the lymphatic wall is thickened in certain places by muscle to form lymph hearts which help to propel lymph. In mammals, dense collections of lymphocytes develop, often in sites corresponding to lymph hearts. The propulsive function is lost and the lymph now percolates through these collections, called *lymph nodes,* as it moves toward the veins. Lymph nodes filter the lymph, add lymphocytes to the efferent lymph, and produce antibodies.

Lymphatic vessels from all the body except the right side of the head, neck, and thorax drain into the *thoracic duct,* the main lymphatic vessel of the body, which empties into the *left innominate vein.* Lymphatic vessels draining the upper right portion of the body form several trunks which separately enter the great veins at the right side of the base of the neck. These trunks may join into the *right lymphatic duct.*

DISTRIBUTION
Lymphatic capillaries are most numerous in the connective tissues beneath body surfaces. The

423

skin; the mucous membranes of the gastrointestinal, respiratory, and genitourinary tracts; and subserous tissues are rich in lymphatics. Beneath the skin and mucous membranes lymphatic capillaries are often arranged in superficial and deep plexuses (Figs. 14-1 to 14-3), both of which tend to be more deeply placed than blood capillaries. Large areas in the body, however, are not supplied with lymphatics. The central nervous system contains none. The spleen has lymphatic vessels in its capsule, trabeculae, and white pulp, but not in red pulp. The bone marrow contains no lymphatic vessels. Fascial planes within striated muscle may contain lymphatic vessels in the perimysium. The structures within the globus oculi are without lymphatic drainage. Within the liver, lymphatic capillaries reach only into the perilobular spaces and do not extend into the liver lobule. In the liver, spleen, and bone marrow and those tissues supplied by reticuloendothelial sinuses, where such sinuses exist, lymphatic capillaries are absent, and the sinuses subserve lymphatic functions.

STRUCTURE

Lymphatic capillaries are frail, tubular structures, up to 100 μm in diameter, whose walls are made of a single layer of flattened endothelial cells (Figs. 14-4 to 14-6). Collagenous fibers and ground

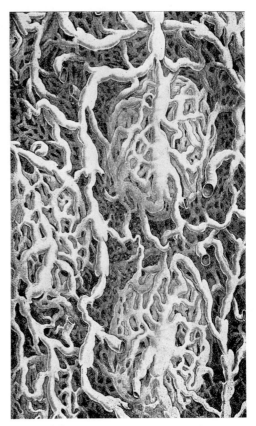

Figure 14-2 Lymphatic network in the human appendix as viewed from the surface. Note the enlargement of vessels over the lymphoid nodules and in the valves in the larger vessels. ×40. (From Teichmann.)

Figure 14-1 Lymphatic vessels of a dog. Superficial and deep vessels in the wall of the stomach as viewed from the surface. ×30. (From Teichmann.)

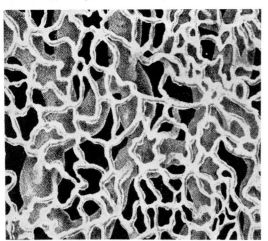

substance surround the vessels, and fine anchoring filaments run from the collagen and attach to the outer surface of the endothelium. In inflammatory states, in which the tissue pressure surrounding these vessels may build up considerably with the accumulation of inflammatory fluids, these filaments, or anchoring filaments (Fig. 14-6), pull on the vessel wall, like a guy rope on a tent, and help to keep lymphatic channels open. From a surface view, the individual endothelial cells tend to be roughly equal in extent along their transverse and longitudinal axes. In contrast, endothelial cells of blood capillaries tend to be elongated. By light microscopy the existence of a lymphatic vessel may be recognized only by the characteristic disposition

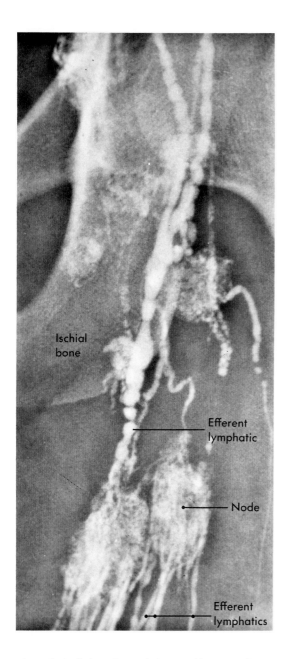

Ischial
bone

Efferent
lymphatic

Node

Efferent
lymphatics

Figure 14-3 Lymphogram of human inguinal lymph nodes and lymphatics. A radiopaque dye was injected into the lymphatic vessels in the thigh. It is carried by afferent lymphatic vessels into the draining lymph nodes of the inguinal region. The dye flows through the nodes and enters its efferent lymphatic vessels. The dye will continue centrally through the lymphatic system and eventually flow into the veins at the base of the neck. This lymphogram is an x-ray of the inguinal region some minutes after the injection of dye. Against the background of the soft tissues of the thigh and the pelvic bones, the lymphatic vessels and nodes are visualized. Note the large number of slender afferent lymphatics. The nodes are oval, the dark zones within them representing lymphocytes and other cells around which the dye flows. The efferent lymphatics have a wide caliber. The beaded appearance of the largest vessel is due to the presence of valves.

Figure 14-4 Skin of guinea pig. A lymphatic capillary is present in the dermis. A small blood-filled venule is nearby. (From D. Chou and L. Weiss, in L. Weiss, ''Cells and Tissues of the Immune System'' Prentice-Hall, Inc., Englewood Cliffs, N.J., 1972.)

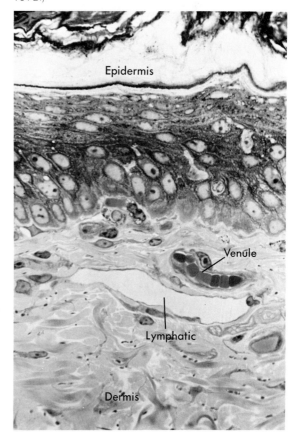

Epidermis

Venule

Lymphatic

Dermis

of endothelial cell nuclei, so thin are the cytoplasmic structures.

Unlike blood capillaries, lymphatic capillaries have no basement lamina or very poorly developed ones. The endothelium forms a complex layer in most sites. In some instances—for example, the

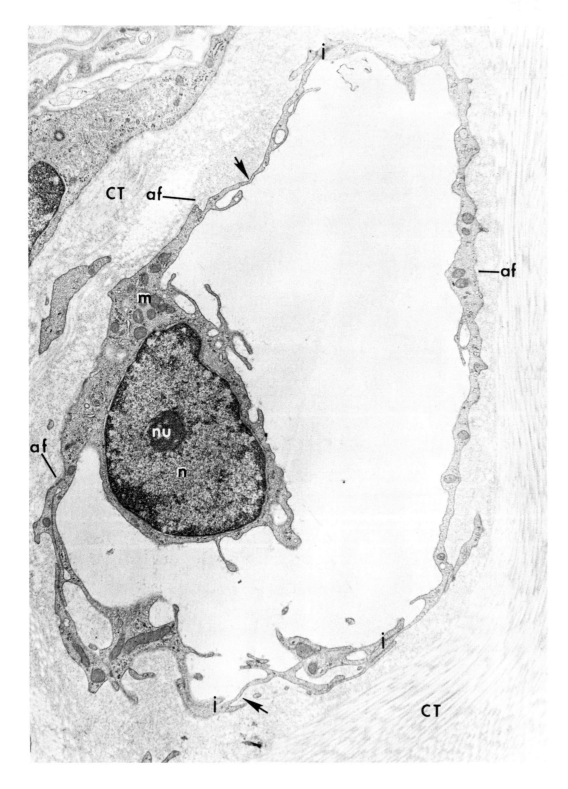

lacteals, the lymphatic capillaries in the villi of the intestine—small apertures are present.

Lymphatic capillaries lead into collecting vessels. These are slender, thin-walled vessels structurally similar to veins but without clearly defined mural layers. Lymphatic vessels frequently anastomose with one another and tend to travel in company with veins. Veins may be girdled in a web of lymphatic channeling. A characteristic of collecting channels is that lymph nodes are inserted along their course in the path of lymph flow. Lymph must pass through the lymph node and is then once again channeled by a lymphatic vessel. It is likely that no lymph reaches the venous system without flowing through at least one node.

Collagenous fibers, reticular fibers, elastic fibers, fibroblasts, and smooth muscle invest the endothelial walls of collecting vessels in varying proportions and dispositions, depending on the size of the vessel and its location. Three coats, or tunics, are present, in conformity to the pattern seen in arteries and veins: *tunica intima, tunica media,* and *tunica adventitia* (Figs. 14-7 and 14-8). Even in the thoracic duct, however, it is difficult to delineate these layers as clearly as in veins. The fibers of the intima and adventitia run longitudinally; those of the media are circular. Nerves are present in larger vessels (Fig. 14-9).

The thoracic duct, largest of the lymphatic vessels, is 4 to 6 mm in diameter. Its wall is stouter than those of other lymphatic channels, especially in its most dependent portion. An *internal elastic membrane* is present. The thoracic duct is supplied by blood vessels and nerves which penetrate the adventitia and the media, disposed much as the vasa vasorum and nerves of blood vessels.

Valves are a conspicuous feature of collecting vessels (Figs. 14-3 and 14-7). Valves consist of paired projections which originate from opposite endothelial surfaces and extend into the lumen. The base of a single valve cusp takes up approximately 180° of circumference so that the entire circumference of the vessel wall provides attachment for a valve. Occasional tricuspid valves are found. The cusps are formed as folds of the endothelium. A few connective tissue fibers and even muscle fibers extend between the folded endothelial surfaces of the cusps from the subendothelial tissue. The cusps project into the lumen in the direction of lymph flow and appear to be the most important factors in controlling the direction of flow. A valve in each of the great lymphatic channels at its junction with the systemic veins prevents the gurgitation of blood into the lymphatic system. Valves are also responsible for the beaded appearance of lymphatic vessels.

ORIGIN AND REPAIR

Lymphatic channels appear in the human embryo at the age of 6 weeks. It is likely that lymphatics originate independently of veins, connecting to them secondarily (Fig. 14-10).

Lymphatic capillaries can regenerate by proliferation of endothelium of the remaining viable lymphatics. The process is similar to but slower than that of blood capillaries. Visualizing lymphatics by intradermal injection of dyestuffs, McMaster observed the regeneration of lymphatics across an incision in the skin of the rabbit in 7 to 10 days (Fig. 14-11).

FUNCTION

The primary function of the lymphatic vessels is the return to the blood of material that has escaped from the blood across the walls of capillaries and venules, which function as semipermeable membranes. They permit the diffusion of small-molecular-weight materials through their walls and retain larger molecules (proteins, certain fatty complexes, etc.) and the cellular elements of the blood. A considerable amount of protein does escape blood vessels, however, and this protein in the extravascular, extracellular spaces is, at least in part, absorbed into lymphatic capillaries and returned to the

Figure 14-5   Cross section of lymphatic capillary. A close association of the surrounding interstitial elements (CT) with the capillary wall is maintained by numerous anchoring filaments (af) which appear as a network of small filaments in this low-power micrograph. The extreme attenuations (arrow) achieved by the endothelium is illustrated in various regions of the capillary wall. The nucleus (N) with its nucleolus (nu) protrudes into the lumen, and several intercellular junctions (j) are observed. Mitochondria (m) occur in the perinuclear regions and also throughout the thin cytoplasmic rim of the endothelial wall; × 11,000. (From the work of L. Leak and J. Burke.)

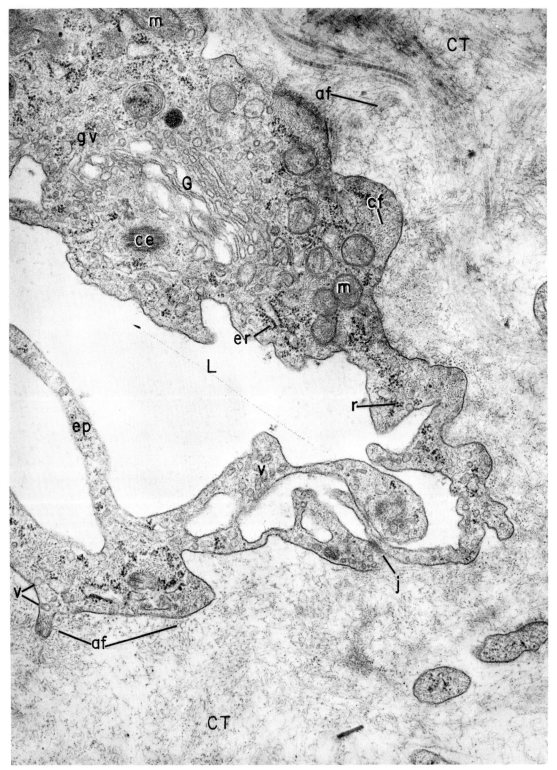

Figure 14-6 Lymphatic capillary. In this electron micrograph, the wall of a lymphatic capillary lies in its connective tissue bed. The lymphatic endothelium contains mitochondria (m), a Golgi complex (G), Golgi vesicles (gv), ribosomes (r), rough ER (er), a centriole (ce), luminal endothelial processes (ep), and pinocytotic vesicles (V). (From the work of L. Leak and J. Burke.

after this ligation, the patient had cramps after eating, but she gained 16 lb in a month and was discharged free of complaints. The concentration of protein in the lymph ranged from 3.19 to 5.28 gm per 100 ml.

Lymphatic vessels absorb fat, especially neutral fat, from the intestine. The patient reported in the above case history was given olive oil stained with Sudan IV. Approximately $1\frac{1}{2}$ hr after the ingestion of the labeled olive oil, the dye appeared in the thoracic duct lymph.

In the resting state, probably 95 percent of the volume of thoracic duct lymph comes from the liver and intestine. The greater portion of protein in thoracic duct lymph, moreover, originates in the liver. Within the liver, lymphatic vessels accompany the hepatic artery, portal vein, and bile ducts in their branchings. The hepatic lobule, however, is not supplied with lymphatic capillaries; lymphatic

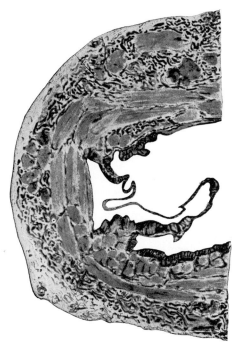

Figure 14-7 Lumbar lymphatic trunk of a human adult. A valve is present. Weigert's resorcinfuchsin and picro-indigo carmine. (From the work of Kajava.)

Figure 14-8 Portion of the wall from the upper part of the thoracic duct of a human adult. Weigert's resorcinfuchsin and picro-indigo carmine. (From the work of Kajava.)

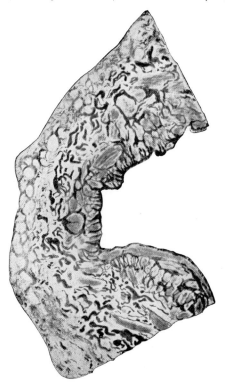

bloodstream. The importance of the conservation of extravascular protein is shown by the following case report from Crandall, Barker, and Graham (1943):

A 30-year-old woman was shot in the left side of the neck, 1 hr before admission to the hospital. The left internal jugular vein was ligated 2 days after admission. During the operation straw-colored fluid steadily welled up in the wound so that the skin was not closed. After the operation the dressings were rapidly saturated with this fluid and, for the next 6 weeks, a ceaseless leakage of what was unquestionably thoracic duct lymph continued. The patient at once took the regular hospital diet and, after she had eaten, the leaking fluid became milky. But she lost weight at the rate of 5 lb a week, and her plasma protein fell to 3.5 gm per 100 ml in just a month. A diet high in protein brought this to 4.6 gm per 100 ml in 13 days, but weight loss continued. Accordingly, in a second operation the thoracic duct was ligated and the wound closed. For 2 weeks

protein carried away from the liver by lymphatic vessels must be protein released directly into extravascular tissues by liver parenchymal cells and thence absorbed into lymphatics, without having escaped blood vessels.

The lymphatic supply to the intestine is notable

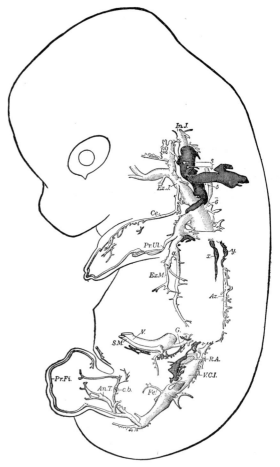

Figure 14-10   Lymphatic vessels and veins in a rabbit of 14 days, 18 hr. 14.5 mm.   The lymphatics are heavily shaded; x, a vessel along the left vagus nerve; y, along the aorta.   The large jugular lymph sac is in contact with the internal jugular vein.   In J, it passes to the junction of the external jugular (Ex J) and subclavian veins, the latter being formed by the union of the primitive ulnar (Pr UI) and external mammary veins (Ex M).   The mesenteric sac is in front of the vena cava inferior (VCI) and below the renal anastomosis (RA).   Other veins include Az, azygos; V, vitelline; G, gastric; SM, superior mesenteric; etc.   The figures indicate the position of the corresponding cervical nerves.   ×11.5.   (Lewis.)

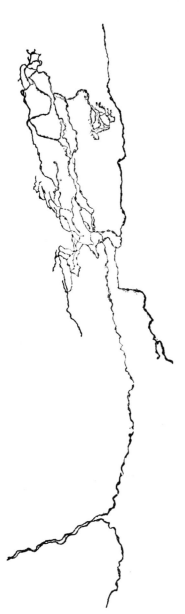

Figure 14-9   Nerve fibers in the adventitia of the thoracic duct of a dog.   Methylene blue.   (From the work of Kytmanof.)

vessels reach only to the perilobular spaces.   These vessels capture materials carried into the liver by the portal veins or hepatic artery.   Particulate material injected into blood vessels can be recovered from lymphatics draining the liver.   A portion of the

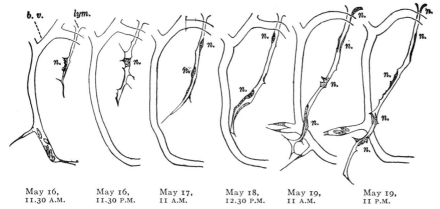

May 16,   May 16,   May 17,   May 18,   May 19,   May 19,
11.30 A.M.   11.30 P.M.   11 A.M.   12.30 P.M.   11 A.M.   11 P.M.

Figure 14-11   Successive stages in the growth of a lymphatic vessel (lym) in the tail of a tadpole (*Rana palustris*).   bv; blood vessel; n, nucleus of the lymphatic vessel.   ×135.   (From the work of E. Clark.)

for the *lacteal,* a large lymphatic capillary which runs in the connective tissue core of each villus, extending the length of the papillary part of the villus.   Its contents flow through mesenteric lymphatics to the thoracic duct.   Small apertures have been described in the lacteal wall.

FACTORS CONTROLLING ABSORPTION INTO LYMPHATIC CAPILLARIES

Lymphatics in the skin are permeable to highly diffusible dyes.   After intradermal injection such dyes are taken up and transported from the site by lymphatics.   The permeability of lymphatic vessels increases greatly under certain mild conditions. Pressure sufficient to obstruct the flow of lymph results in an increase in permeability before visible dilation of the lymphatic.   Stroking with a blunt wire or scratching the skin without breaking the epidermis causes an immediate great increase in lymphatic permeability.   Warming the ears of mice to 43°C increases permeability.   Similar reactions have been observed in the lymphatics in the skin of human beings.   Histamine causes an increase in lymphatic permeability.

Since the permeability of lymphatic endothelium may be greatly enhanced by phenomena which occur normally or, at most, represent but a slight departure from the normal, such increased permeability may commonly permit the entrance of large-sized materials into lymphatic capillaries.

Pinocytotic vesicles appear active in the trans-port of particles across the lymphatic endothelium. Cells in passage may cross through endothelial cells or, more often, pass between them.

MOVEMENT OF LYMPH

Although larger lymphatic vessels respond to certain drugs, there is no evidence that the caliber of lymphatic capillaries is directly affected by the administration of such powerful vasoconstrictor agents as epinephrine or pituitrin.   Lymphatic capillaries are highly elastic structures, however, and have been distended by one-third without rupture. Collecting vessels contract rhythmically; the circular muscle in the walls of lymphatic collecting vessels reduces the diameter of the lumen whereas the longitudinal muscle widens the lumen.   Coordinated contraction of the smooth muscle of the lymphatic wall produces effective propulsive movements.

Remitting compression of lymphatic vessels by surrounding structures (particularly muscles and pulsating blood vessels), respiratory movements, propulsive actions of the lymphatic walls, and the force of gravity (in the lymphatic vessels superior to the entrance of vessels into great veins) are the major forces promoting lymph flow.   The direction of flow is controlled primarily by lymphatic valves.

The rate of lymph flow varies considerably, depending upon the location and structure of lymph vessels, the volume of lymph, the permeability of the vessels, and other factors.   A small amount of a trypan blue solution injected into the hind foot of a dog reaches thoracic duct lymph in seconds.

The volume of lymph poured into the bloodstream is considerable. In a resting human patient, the subject of the case described earlier, Crandall, Barker, and Graham (1943) reported an average lymph flow rate from the thoracic duct of 0.93 ml per min, or 1.38 ml per kg per hr. The range of flow was 3.9 to 0.38 ml per min. Flow was increased by the ingestion of food or water or by abdominal massage.

Lymph nodes

Lymph nodes are encapsulated structures ranging in size from a few millimeters to more than a centimeter in their largest dimension, and varying but generally ovoid in shape (Figs. 14-2, 14-3, and 14-12 to 14-14). They are present in the path of collecting lymphatic vessels, and through them lymph flows toward the junctions of lymphatics and veins. Lymph nodes reach their highest level of development in mammals. In birds they may be seen in their most primitive form consisting of loosely organized lymphoid tissue which lies alongside rather than in the lymph stream. In fishes, amphibians, and reptiles there are lymph hearts but no lymph nodes. In mammals, lymph hearts appear transiently in the embryo but disappear with the development of nodes.

Lymph nodes are grouped in great numbers in certain areas of the body; the bases of the extremities, the neck, retroperitoneal areas in the pelvis and abdomen, and the mediastinum are sites especially rich in nodes.

STRUCTURE
A lymph node consists of capsule, reticulum, lymphocytes, other free cells, blood and lymphatic vessels, and nerves (Figs. 14-12 to 14-14).

Figure 14-12   Lymph node of a human being.   Giemsa stain.   ×30.

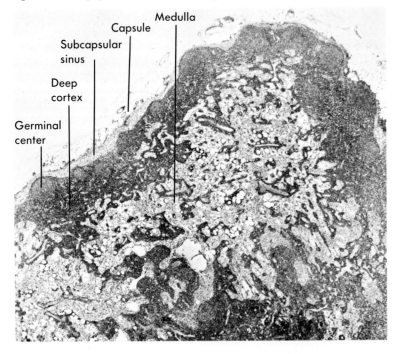

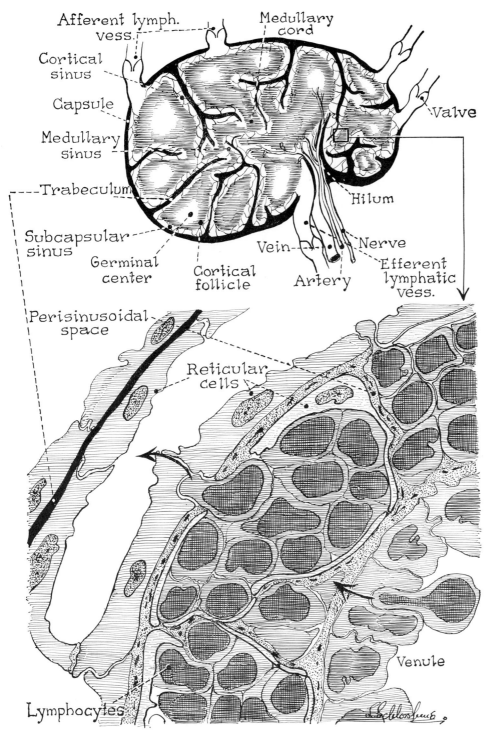

Figure 14-13 Schematic depiction of a lymph node is in the upper portion of the plate. In the boxed area, presented in the enlargement below, a sinus, a zone of lymphocytes, and a postcapillary venule are shown. The sinus is lined by reticular cells. Note that processes of the reticular cells extend into and cross the lumen of the sinus. Reticular cells also extend away from the sinus and, together with extracellular reticulum (stippled), from a meshwork within which free lymphocytes lie. The postcapillary venule has a high endothelium. Lymphocytes pass from the blood into the lymph node through its endothelium. The lympho-cytes in the node then gain the efferent lymph by passing into the lymph sinus as shown.

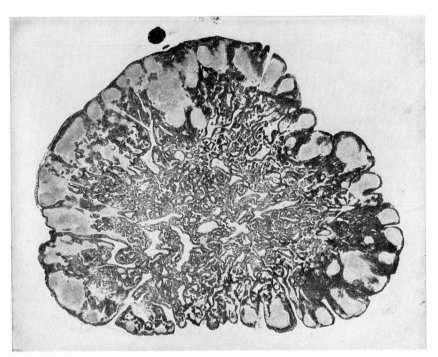

Figure 14-14   Lymph node injected with india ink. The sinus system is well outlined. ×10.

The *capsule* is composed of dense collagenous connective tissue with some muscle. It presents a broad convex surface and, at one aspect, a deep indentation, the *hilus* or *hilum*. Afferent lymphatic vessels pierce the convex surface of the capsule and empty into the node. Lymphatic vessels leave at the hilus, and blood vessels enter and leave there. The inner capsular surface is irregular. A number of *trabeculae* project into the node.

The *reticulum* of a lymph node is a delicate meshwork, occupying the space enclosed by the capsule and trabeculae (Fig. 14-15), where the lymphocytes and other free cells of the node lie and where the fine blood vessels and lymphatic sinuses run. The reticulum, as in the spleen, consists of two elements: extracellular reticulum and cellular reticulum. The extracellular reticulum consists of reticular fibers which, in turn, contain two elements: collagenous filaments and a ground substance. The proportion of filaments to ground substance varies from place to place in the node. The ground substance is usually the major element, and its reactivity accounts for the argyrophilia of the reticulum and its capacity to stain in the PAS reaction. The cellular reticulum consists of branching reticular cells whose cytoplasm ensheaths the reticular fibers, thereby forming a meshwork coincident with that of the extracellular reticulum. In

Figure 14-15   Schema of reticular meshwork. This is a simple meshwork with an artery above and a vascular sinus below. The meshwork consists of reticular cells and reticular fibers (stippled). The fibers form a branching meshwork, the extracellular reticulum or fibrous reticulum. It may be impregnated with silver or stained with the PAS reaction. Reticular cells branch and cover reticular fibers. They thus form a cellular reticulum coincident with the extracellular reticulum. Reticular cells probably synthesize and maintain reticular fibers. They may, in certain sites, be phagocytes. On the right the reticulum is empty. On the left, it is crowded with a variety of free cells. The types of free cells depend upon the tissue. In lymph nodes they consist primarily of lymphocytes, macrophages, and plasma cells. In the spleen, other cell types may be present. Note that the vascular sinus is similar in structure to the reticulum and may, in fact, represent a differentiated portion of reticulum. (From L. Weiss, ''The Cells and Tissues of the Immune System,'' Prentice-Hall, Inc., Englewood Cliffs, N.J., 1972.)

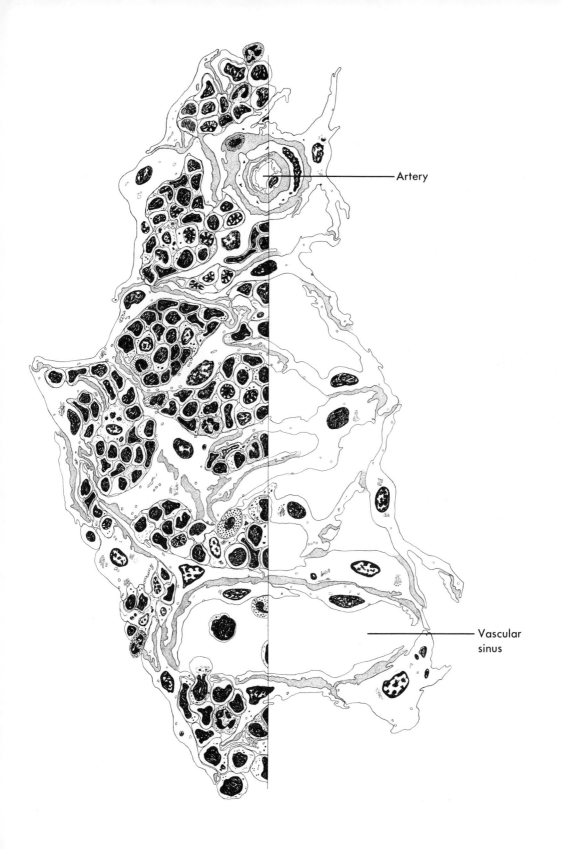

Artery

Vascular
sinus

most light-microscopic preparations, the nuclei of reticular cells are the only parts clearly visible.

In certain sites reticular cells are somewhat modified and provide the lining surface of sinuses (see below).

Lymphocytes are the most conspicuous of the free cells lying within the reticular meshwork. In the peripheral parts of a node they are tightly packed, form a blanket of cells, and thereby create the cortex of the node. Central to the cortex and extending to the hilus is the medulla where lymphocytes are grouped in branching cords, the *medullary cords* (Figs. 14-12, 14-14, and 14-16).

Within the cortex there are dense, uniform spherical nodules of lymphocytes, the *primary nodules* or *primary follicles*. Within a spherule may be found a smaller spherical or oval mass, the *germinal center*, consisting of larger cells with more voluminous cytoplasm and less heterochromatin, as a result of which the germinal center is relatively lightly stained (Fig. 14-12). Nodules containing germinal centers are termed *secondary nodules*. Nodules occur at the periphery of the cortex. Their presence establishes two other zones: (1) internodular cortical tissue and (2) a deep part of the cortex between the nodules and medulla. The deep cortex has been termed *tertiary nodules* or the *tertiary cortex* (Fig. 14-12).

Figure 14-16   Medulla of a lymph node of an ox.

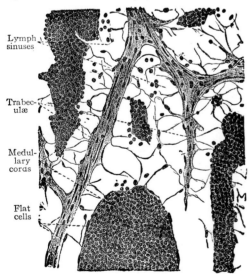

Lymph sinuses

Trabec-ulæ

Medul-lary cords

Flat cells

Most of the cells in the cortex and medulla (except the germinal center) are small lymphocytes. Mixed among them are many macrophages, large and medium-sized lymphocytes, and some plasma cells, eosinophils, and other blood cells. Germinal centers are exceptional in consisting primarily of large lymphoid cells. Many macrophages are present there, as are variable numbers of plasma cells. A conspicuous number of mitoses usually occur there. These centers, also termed *reaction centers* in emphasizing their phagocytic character, produce antibodies.

The medullary cords are rich in plasma cells, macrophages, and lymphocytes.

VASCULAR SUPPLY

Lymphatic vessels   Collecting lymphatic vessels pierce the capsule. They are afferent vessels carrying lymph from the connective tissue spaces or from a more peripheral lymph node. They empty into a large *subcapsular sinus,* which lies directly beneath the capsule and is coextensive with it. *Cortical sinuses* run radially from the subcapsular sinus, passing between cortical lymphocytes, often along trabeculae. These become the *medullary sinuses* as they pass between the medullary cords and converge toward the hilus, where they become confluent with the *efferent lymphatic channels* leaving the node (Fig. 14-13).

The sinuses within a node are lined by flattened reticular cells, which provide a rather irregular surface. Indeed, processes of these cells crisscross the lumen, undoubtedly causing retardation and turbulence in lymph flow.

Blood vessels   Blood vessels enter the node at the hilus. Arterioles reach the follicles of the cortex through the trabeculae and break up into a rich capillary plexus. These vessels group into venules, tributaries of veins which run from cortex to medulla and then leave the node via the hilus. Postcapillary venules lie in the parafollicular and tertiary cortex. These are distinguished by a high endothelium, cuboidal or even columnar, and a broad layer of subendothelial, extracellular connective tissue. The wall of these vessels is often infiltrated with small lymphocytes (Figs. 14-13 and 14-16 to 14-18). As shown by Gowans, Marchesi, and

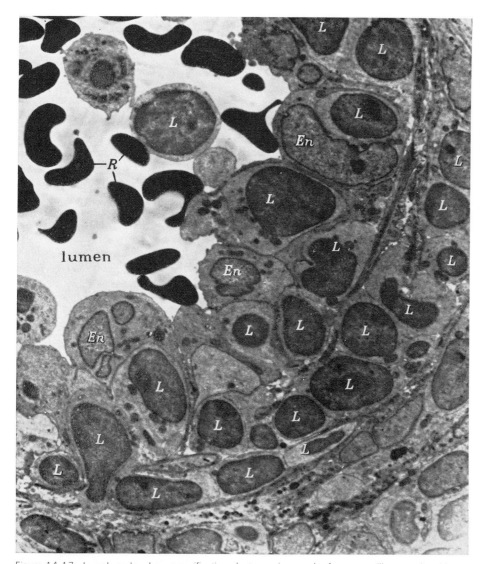

Figure 14-17 Lymph node. Low-magnification electron micrograph of a postcapillary venule. Many lymphocytes (L) are present in the vessel wall. Most of the lymphocytes are outside the endothelium (En, nuclei of the endothelial cells) but are retained within the wall of the vessel by the various layers of the periendothelial sheath. Red blood cells (R) are seen in the lumen of the vessel. ×2,700. (From V. T. Marchesi and J. L. Gowans, Proc. Roy. Soc. (London), Ser. B, **159**:283, 1964.)

Knight, using radioactively labeled cells and autoradiography, these lymphocytes pass from the blood into the parenchyma of the node. They are found in the lumen, within the endothelial cells as well as between them, and in the subendothelial connective tissue. Germinal centers and medullary cords are supplied by arterial twigs.

A few small blood vessels enter the node from the convex surface of the capsule. Some unmyelinated nerves enter the node at the hilus. They run with blood vessels and are probably vasomotor.

Other lymphatic tissues In addition to such discretely organized tissue as lymph nodes and spleen,

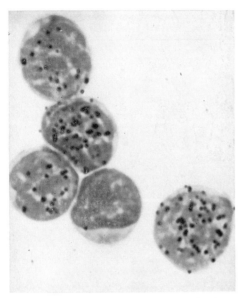

Figure 14-18 Autoradiographs of thoracic duct cells which had been incubated in vitro with tritiated adenosine for 1 hr at 37°C. Exposure, 14 days. Leishman stain. ×2,250. (From J. L. Gowans and E. J. Knight, Proc. Roy Soc. (London), Ser. B., **159:**257, 1964.)

other lymphatic tissue exists; the wall of the alimentary tract is infiltrated with it. Some tissue, as Peyer's patches in the lamina propria of the small intestine and the tonsils in the pharynx, is well organized (Fig. 14-19) whereas in the appendix and, indeed, the remainder of the gut, lymphatic tissue infiltrates the lamina propria and extends into other layers without clear limits. The respiratory and urinary tracts are often less markedly infiltrated, and, with appropriate stimulation, loci of lymphatic tissue may readily develop in virtually any site.

DEVELOPMENT AND DECLINE OF LYMPH NODES

Lymph nodes appear in the human embryo during the third month of life (Figs. 14-20 and 14-21) along the course of lymphatic channels. At sites of lymph node development lymphatic vessels display a richly plexiform character and are termed *lymphatic sacs*. Lymphocytes aggregate about the network of vessels. The complete development of lymph nodes is not realized until some weeks postpartum, for not until this time do cortex and medulla clearly differentiate and germinal centers appear.

Lymphatic tissue undergoes decline or involution with age. The thymus begins a dramatic involution at about the time of puberty; the aging of lymph nodes and spleen is more gradual and the changes are subtle.

Regression in lymph nodes begins shortly after puberty, the period during which they reach their maximal development. Hellman found that the lymph node mass of rabbits decreased in size after puberty but that certain nodes underwent a transient secondary growth period in adulthood. In old rabbits lymph nodes were reduced to approximately one-half size. Lymph nodes, however, retain the capacity to enlarge in response to appropriate stimuli throughout life. The histologic picture in aging lymph nodes consists of absence of germinal centers and reduction in the numbers of lymphocytes with thinning of cortex and medullary cords. Fat appears under the capsule, especially at the hilus and in the septa. In man, even moderate degrees of fatty or connective tissue replacement of lymphatic tissue are seen only in advanced age. In-

Figure 14-19 Postcapillary venule in a mesenteric lymph node 15 min after the initiation of a transfusion. Labeled cells have penetrated the endothelium of the vessel but have not yet migrated into the node. L, lumen of the vessel. Exposure, 28 days. Methyl green–pyronin stain. ×1,200. (J. L. Gowans are E. J. Knight, Proc. Roy Soc. (London), Ser. B., **159:**257, 1964.)

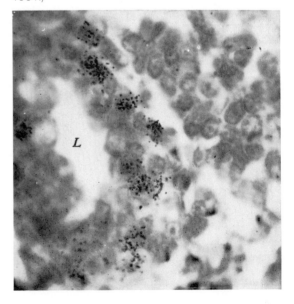

deed, Krumbhaar states that most nodes go on to 60 years with but little atrophy.

FUNCTIONS OF LYMPH NODES

Filtration and phagocytosis Lymph nodes constitute extensive filtration beds which prevent the systemic distribution of infectious and other agents. Thus popliteal lymph nodes receive and filter lymph from the sole of the foot and dorsum of the leg. The reticular meshwork crisscrossing the sinuses and the parenchyma constitutes a mechanical

Figure 14-20 Lymph node of a human fetus, 57-mm crown-rump length (12 weeks gestational age). Lymph nodes develop in relationship to a plexus of lymphatic vessels, the lymph sacs. The lymph node consists of a loose connective tissue which becomes infiltrated by lymphocytes. At this stage, the ovoid shape of the node, its moderate content of lymphocytes, and its relationship to lymphatic vessels are evident. Toluidine blue. ×250. (From the work of R. P. Bailey.)

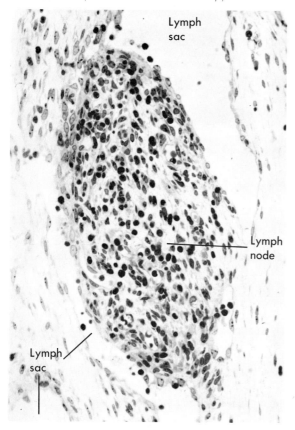

filter. Flow in these large vascular spaces is quite slow, and the tremendous surface of phagocytic reticular cells and large population of macrophages not only are phagocytic, but by their bulk they further impede flow. Lymph nodes produce antibodies and other substances which help to immobilize and agglutinate bacteria and cells, facilitating filtration and phagocytosis. The filtration power of lymph nodes has been demonstrated by Drinker, Field, and Ward (1934): 5 ml of a serum-broth culture containing 600 million colonies per ml of hemolytic streptococci were perfused through a lymph node and collected at the efferent lymphatic vessels. Cultures of effluent lymph contained 4.5 million colonies per ml, indicating 99 percent filtration.

Thus both mechanically, by the arrangement of reticulum, and biologically, by action of its phagocytes and production of antibodies and other factors, lymph nodes constitute very effective filters. The efficiency of this system makes lymph nodes vulnerable to disturbances in the regions they drain. Thus a focus of infection frequently infects the vessels and nodes which drain it. With them as new foci, the infection may spread into the blood stream and throughout the body. Malignant tumors, after invading the lymphatic system, may be disseminated widely.

Immunologic functions The lymph node is an immunologic structure highly specialized in the production of antibodies to antigen coming from the region it drains. Thus antigen introduced into the foot pad elicits an antibody response in a popliteal lymph node. This responsiveness of the lymph node to regional influences complements that of the spleen, which produces antibodies to blood-borne antigen.

That lymphatic tissue produces antibody was shown by McMaster and Hudack (1935), who injected antigen into the ears of rats and recovered antibody from the draining lymph nodes before it could be detected elsewhere. Two antigens were injected, one in each ear, and the antibody to each of the antigens was first detected in the node draining the ear in which homologous antigen had been injected.

On initial administration of antigen a primary immune response follows which varies with the

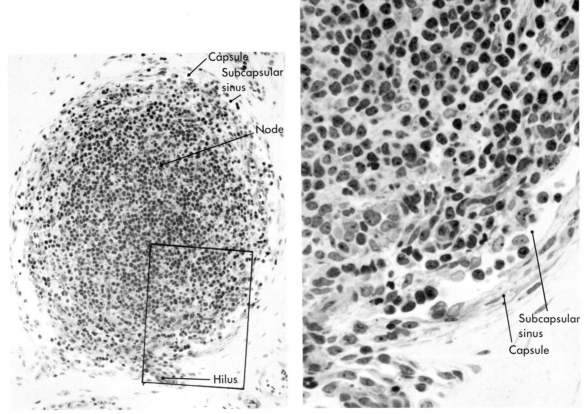

Figure 14-21 Lymph node of a human fetus, 200-mm crown-rump length (22 weeks gestational age). A (left). The node is an oval structure, considerably infiltrated by lymphocytes. The capsule and subcapsular sinus are well defined. Cortex and medulla have not yet differentiated, however. B (right). An enlargement of the boxed area in A. Toluidine blue. ×450. (From the work of R. P. Bailey.)

character of antigen, dose, and route of administration. With particulate antigens, phagocytosis is one of the earliest responses. The antigen is engulfed in the sinuses, and in the medullary regions most conspicuously. Later some antigen is visible in the parafollicular cortical regions, and somewhat later some antigen is held or trapped on the surface of reticular cells in the cortex, particularly in and near the nodules.

Antibody-producing cells appear first in the cortex and then in the medulla, where they tend to accumulate in large numbers ranged within the cords. After the initial response, as a rule, antibody production occurs in germinal centers. As determined histochemically and by assay of isolated portions of lymphatic tissue, antibody production here is intense.

On subsequent exposure to antigen (the secondary response) germinal centers dominate the response. They are large, synthesize antibody very actively, and may expand at such a rate as to blur their margins. Over a period of weeks the cells synthesizing antibody in the germinal center die or are dispersed and the titer of antibody begins to fall. Relative to a primary response, a secondary response is much more rapid, more intense, and more prolonged. The basis of the secondary response lies in cells with "immunologic memory" which may well reside in or circulate into germinal centers. It has been noted that reticular cells in the nodules trap antigen on their surface. They may hold it for long periods of time and by this capacity efficiently concentrate antigen and present it to the immunologically competent cells which are closely held in the reticulum. Indeed, the proliferation of immunologically competent cells stimulated by antigen trapped by reticular cells may be the basis of germinal center formation. The germinal center contains many cells rich in antibody, presumably manufacturing it. Macrophages are always plentiful in a germinal center.

The cell types producing antibody, both in germinal centers and elsewhere in lymph nodes, are of two types morphologically: lymphocytes and plasma cells. Intermediate forms are often found, suggesting the evolution of plasma cells from a lymphocyte-like precursor.

We shall, at this point, consider some of the major cytologic techniques for identifying antibody-producing cells.

Antibody may be located within cells by the use of a fluorescent marker and examination of a tissue under the fluorescent microscope. An example of this technique is as follows: A rabbit is given bovine serum albumin (BSA) as an antigen. The rabbit's lymphatic tissue is removed at an appropriate time, fixed and sectioned, and treated with BSA. As a result, wherever antibody to BSA is present, it links to the BSA which was used as a reagent. Next, the tissue is covered with a complex consisting of an antibody to BSA conjugated to a fluorescent dye. The anti-BSA-fluorescein will couple to those sites where BSA is affixed to antibody. Under the fluorescent microscope these sites can be identified. See Chaps. 1, 2, and 15 for examples of fluorescent immunocytochemistry.

Electron-microscopic techniques depend upon attaching electron-dense groups as markers, fluorescent compounds not being electron-opaque. Ferritin has been successfully used. More recently horseradish peroxidase, whose presence is revealed by a dense product of the peroxidase reaction, has been valuable. Consult Chap. 2 for further discussion.

Methods for isolating antibody-producing cells have become increasingly useful. We will consider three examples: (1) Antibody-producing tissues have been reduced to cell suspensions by sieving or mincing. The cells may be passed through a column coated with antigen. The antibody-producing cells stick; the other cells pass through. (2) Cells may be induced to produce antibody to flagella of bacteria, and single cells suspected of antibody production may be held in a microdrop with some motile bacteria. If the bacterial flagella are clumped and the organisms thereby rendered nonmotile, the cell is revealed as an antibody producer. (3) Cells may be induced to produce antibody against foreign erythrocytes. Then by their capacity to lyse the erythrocytes or to agglutinate them the antibody-producing cells may be identified.

Antibody-producing cells, subject to light- and electron-microscopic analysis, are found to be lymphocytic or plasmacytic in type. The plasma cells are visible in a variety of forms, their common feature being the presence of rough ER that may be vesicular, flat, or irregular and contains antibody. The perinuclear space is often rich in antibody. Those cells which produce a great deal of antibody, particularly immunoglobulin G (IgG), are usually plasma cells. (IgG is the definitive type of immunoglobulin or antibody produced in the latter phase of a primary reaction and throughout the secondary reactions. It is the immunoglobulin of immunologic memory.) Lymphocytes may also be antibody producers. Here it may be emphasized again that lymphocytes are a diverse group of cells functionally different though morphologically alike. All lymphocytes are not capable of antibody production. Lymphocytes tend to be associated with production of immunoglobulin M (IgM), although they can produce IgG. (IgM is a relatively primitive antibody produced only at the outset of an immune response. It has less affinity for antigen than IgG.) In addition, lymphocytes tend to be the cell type found where relatively little antibody is produced; where antibody is produced in large volume, plasma cells are probably the producers.

Antibody-producing cells appear to be B cells, circulating lymphocytes derived from bone marrow with immunoglobulin on their surface. One may visualize that a cell producing antibody to BSA, for example, is derived from a precursor B cell producing just enough antibody to BSA (anti-BSA) to cover the cell surface. This precursor is itself specified through genetic mechanisms *in the absence of antigen*. When the antigen enters the body it *se-*

lects the cell already producing antibody to it, recognizing it by the antibody on its surface. The antigen then complexes with this surface antibody and induces the cell to divide and produce antibody in far greater amount. Thus antigen does not induce a cell to initiate antibody production; it recognizes a cell already producing its antibody at a low level and stimulates it to produce antibody much more actively. This stimulation may require the presence of T cells and other factors in a manner as yet not understood. Plasma cells derive from a certain group of lymphocytes. Indeed, the development of a significant amount of rough ER in plasma cells is simply the morphologic adaptation to large-scale antibody secretion, rough ER being characteristic of cells secreting protein. We recognize, therefore, that some lymphocytes engaged in antibody production may be cells on their way to becoming plasma cells, whereas others may well remain lymphocytes.

THE PRODUCTION AND RECIRCULATION OF LYMPHOCYTES

The lymphocytes within lymphatic tissue are both circulating lymphocytes and lymphocytes which are produced in the node. The proportion of newly produced lymphocytes to those in the recirculation pool varies from species to species but recirculating cells in antigenically unstimulated animals are preponderant.

Recirculating lymphocytes are small. They enter the node through its arterial vessels, pass through capillaries, and reach the postcapillary venules. They then pass through these venules and lie in the parafollicular cortex, particularly the tertiary or deep cortex (Figs. 14-17 to 14-19). They remain there for variable periods of time and then migrate to the medulla. They leave the node through efferent lymphatics and reach the veins at the base of the neck through the system of lymphatic vessels. Once in the bloodstream they circulate and, in time, again reach a lymph node and repeat the cycle. Most recirculating lymphocytes are T cells from the thymus, as can be shown by a number of experiments, including the observation of a drastic decrease in the number of these cells after thymectomy. The deep cortex (tertiary cortex) where T cells aggregate is characterized as *thymic-dependent*. Following prolonged thoracic duct cannulation, moreover, depletion of recirculating lymphocytes and tertiary cortex occurs. It is of interest that the thymus is excluded from the pathway of recirculation. Gowans and his associates (1964) have traced the pathway described above in the rat by the use of small lymphocytes obtained from the thoracic duct, labeled with tritiated adenosine, and injected intravenously. At different times after the injection of lymphocytes, tissues were fixed and embedded, and sections and autoradiographs prepared. Passage of lymphocytes across the postcapillary venule was documented by electron microscopy (Figs. 14-17 to 14-19).

Large lymphocytes do not recirculate. Most injected large lymphocytes migrate from the blood into the wall of the gut.

References

CLARK, S.: The Reticulum of Lymph Nodes in Mice Studied with the Electron Microscope, *Amer. J. Anat.*, **110**:217 (1962).

COONS, A. H., E. H. LEDUC, and J. M. CONNOLLY: Studies on Antibody Production. I. A Method for the Histochemical Demonstration of Specific Antibody and Its Application to a Study of the Hyperimmune Rabbit, *J. Exp. Med.*, **102**:49 (1955).

CRANDALL, L. A., S. B. BARKER, and D. G. GRAHAM: A Study of the Lymph Flow from a Patient with Thoracic Duct Fistula, *Gastroenterology*, **1**:1040 (1943).

DOWNEY, H.: The Structure and Origin of the Lymph Sinuses of Mammalian Lymph Nodes and Their Relations to Endothelium and Recticulum, *Hematologica*, **3**:31 (1922).

DRINKER, C. K., M. E. FIELD, and H. K. WARD: The Filtering Capacity of Lymph Nodes, *J. Exp. Med.,* **59:**393 (1934).

DRINKER, C. K., G. B. WISLOCKI, and M. E. FIELD: The Structure of the Sinuses in the Lymph Nodes, *Anat. Rec.,* **56:**261 (1933).

GOWANS, J. L., and E. J. KNIGHT: The Route of Recirculation of Lymphocytes in the Rat, *Proc. Roy. Soc. (London), Ser. B,* **159:**257 (1964).

GOWANS, J. L., D. MC GREGOR, and D. COWEN: Initiation of Immune Responses by Small Lymphocytes, *Nature (London),* **196:**651 (1962).

HAN, S.: The Ultrastructure of the Mesenteric Lymph Node of the Rat, *Amer. J. Anat.,* **109:**183 (1961).

LEAK, L. V., and J. F. BURKE: Ultrastructural Studies on the Lymphatic Anchoring Filaments, *J. Cell Biol.,* **36:**129 (1968).

LEAK, L. V., and J. F. BURKE: Fine Structure of the Lymphatic Capillary and the Adjoining Connective Tissue Area, *Amer. J. Anat.,* **118:**785 (1966).

LEAK, L. V., and J. F. BURKE: Studies on the Permeability of Lymphatic Capillaries during Inflammation, *Anat. Rec.,* **151:**489 (1965).

MARCHESI, V. T., and J. L. GOWANS: The Migration of Lymphocytes through the Endothelium of Venules in Lymph Nodes: an Electron Microscope Study, *Proc. Roy. Soc. (London), Ser. B,* **159:**283 (1964).

MC MASTER, P. D., and S. HUDACK: The Formation of Agglutinins within Lymph Nodes, *J. Exp. Med.,* **61:**783 (1935).

MOE, R.: Electron Microscopic Appearance of the Parenchyma of Lymph Nodes, *Amer. J. Anat.,* **114:**341 (1964).

MOE, R.: Fine Structure of the Reticulum and Sinuses of Lymph Nodes, *Amer. J. Anat.,* **112:**311 (1963).

ORTEGA, L., and R. MELLORS: Cellular Sites of Formation of Gamma Globulin, *J. Exp. Med.,* **106:**627 (1957).

PARROTT, D. M. V., M. A. B. DE SOUSA, and J. EAST: Thymic Dependent Areas in the Lymphoid Organs of Neonatally Thymectomized Mice, *J. Exp. Med.,* **123:**191 (1966).

PECK, H. M., and N. L. HOERR: The Effect of Environment Temperature Changes on the Circulation of the Mouse Spleen, *Anat. Rec.,* **109:**479 (1951).

WEISS, L.: "The Cells and Tissues of the Immune System," Prentice-Hall, Inc., Englewood Cliffs, N.J., 1972.

YOFFEY, J., and F. COURTICE: "Lymphatics, Lymph and Lymphoid Tissue," Harvard University Press, Cambridge, Mass., 1956.

chapter 15   The spleen   LEON WEISS

The human spleen is a highly vascular hemato-poietic organ located in the left upper quadrant of the abdomen and weighing approximately 150 gm in adults. It receives blood from the splenic artery and drains into the portal venous system. The spleen may be best understood as a discriminatory filter, consisting of specialized vascular spaces through which blood flows. There is no element of the blood, cellular or plasmal, which the spleen may not affect. It clears the blood of damaged blood cells and of foreign substances in plasma It provides a site and the stimulation for the trans-formation of lymphocytes and monocytes into plasma cells and macrophages. It reacts vigorously to blood-borne antigen with the production of anti-body. It sequesters certain circulating cells from the blood for varying periods of time. It normally contributes new lymphocytes to the blood and, in some pathologic states of failure of bone marrow, even erythrocytes and granulocytes. The adult spleen is not essential to life; in fact, it may some-times eliminate circulating cells with such avidity that it must be removed to save life.

Structure of the spleen

CAPSULE AND TRABECULAE

The spleen in man is enclosed by a capsule of dense, white connective tissue, a few millimeters in thickness. From the internal capsular surface, a rich branching network of trabeculae subdivides the organ into communicating compartments sev-eral millimeters in each dimension (Fig. 15-1). The capsule contains relatively little muscle and is therefore incapable of the profound contraction exhibited by the muscular capsule of the spleen in dogs and cats. Over the spleen the mesothelium of the peritoneum may be cuboidal and possess

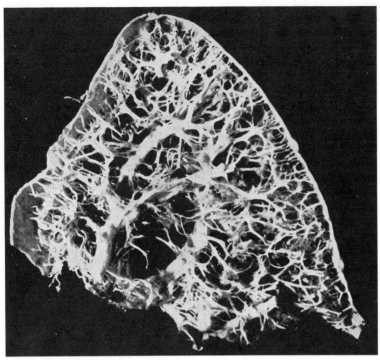

Figure 15-1 Human spleen. The trabecular framework and capsule remain after the pulp has been digested away by 1 percent sodium carbonate. ×4. (From the work of Schleicher.)

microvilli. The capsule is deeply indented at the medial aspect of the organ where it is penetrated by blood vessels, lymphatic vessels, and nerves. Arterial vessels branch into the trabeculae and from there enter the pulp or parenchyma of the organ. Veins and lymphatics also run in the trabeculae, entering from the pulp.

SPLENIC PULP

The tissue enclosed within the capsule, the splenic pulp, is a reticular connective tissue (Figs. 15-2 to 15-7). Most of the pulp is red, due to blood, and is designated the *red pulp*. The red pulp is made up almost entirely of two kinds of structure: large, branching, thin-walled blood vessels, *splenic sinuses* (or *splenic sinusoids*), and thin plates or partitions of tissue which lie between the sinuses, *splenic cords*. Scattered in the red pulp are compact white nodules, variable in size but typically a few millimeters in diameter. In aggregate these nodules in human spleen are the major components

of the *white pulp*. They are collections of lymphocytes and related free cells lying in a meshwork of reticular cells and fibers. The zone separating white pulp and red pulp is designated the *marginal zone*.

BLOOD FLOW

The pattern of blood flow in the spleen will be outlined as a preliminary to consideration of the structure of white pulp, marginal zone, and red pulp. Blood enters the spleen by way of splenic arteries, passing through the hilus. The splenic artery branches into the trabeculae as *trabecular arteries* which turn out of the trabeculae and enter the white pulp, where they are known as *central arteries*. Most branches of the central arteries end in the marginal zone and the red pulp. In the red pulp and in the marginal zone the blood reaches the *splenic sinuses*, which are tributaries of *veins of the pulp*. These veins enter the trabeculae as *trabecular veins*. At the hilus the trabecular veins are continuous with

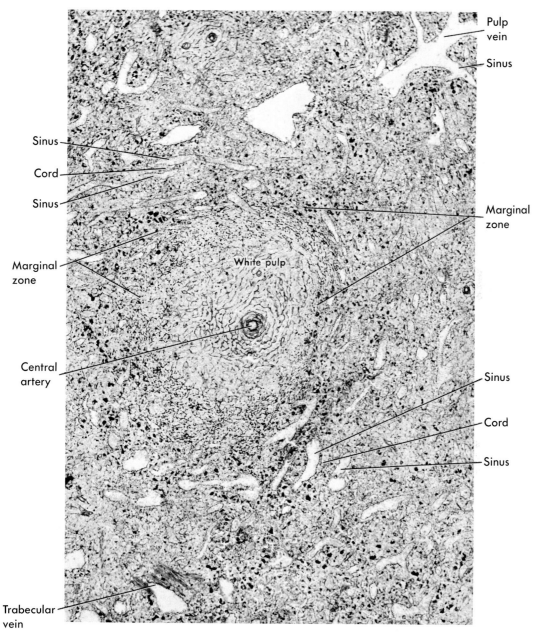

Figure 15-2 Spleen of a rat. The extracellular reticulum is stained by the PAS reaction. The white pulp contains a darkly outlined central artery. Note the circumferential pattern of the reticulum of white pulp. A marginal zone surrounds the white pulp and contains a relatively dense meshwork of reticulum and many darkly stained cells. Beyond the white pulp and marginal zone lies the red pulp, accounting for the greater part of the splenic volume. The clear spaces represent splenic sinuses, for the most part, but also pulp veins and trabecular veins. The splenic cords constitute the relatively solid tissue lying between the sinuses. ×225. (From L. Weiss. J. Anat., **93:**465, 1959.)

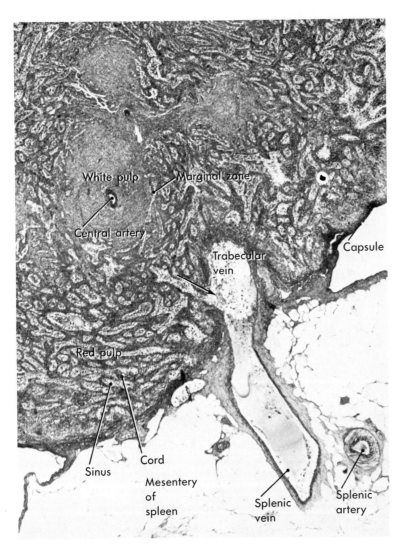

Figure 15-3 Spleen of a hedgehog. In this low-power field, the white pulp, red pulp, blood outflow tract, and splenic mesentery are shown. The white pulp, occupying a relatively small volume, is nodular. In one of the nodules a central artery has been cut in cross section. The red pulp occupies most of the field. It is made up almost entirely of relatively clear spaces, the splenic sinuses, which form an anastomosing system of venous vessels. The splenic cords, darkly stained tissue lying between the sinuses, consist of a reticular meshwork which contains blood cells and macrophages and receives arterial terminations. Blood is carried out of the spleen through trabecular veins which drain into the splenic vein. Splenic veins leave the spleen at the hilus and enter the splenic mesentery. At the arrow, splenic sinuses empty into a pulp vein which drains into a trabecular vein. The marginal zone lies between white pulp and red pulp. The mesentery contains a branch of the splenic artery which will enter the spleen at the hilus. ×150. (From V. Janout and L. Weiss, Anat. Rec., **172**:197, 1972.)

the splenic veins which lie outside the organ. The nature of the vascular connections between the arterial terminations and splenic sinuses, the so-called *intermediate circulation* of the spleen, is difficult to analyze. Further consideration of blood flow will be deferred until the structure of the spleen is presented.

LYMPH FLOW

Lymphatic vessels are associated with a fluid flow through the spleen counter to blood flow. The fluid wave originates at the venular end of the red pulp, sweeps across the red pulp, marginal zone, and white pulp, and enters lymphatic vessels which lie in white pulp and trabeculae (Fig. 15-6).

Figure 15-4 Schematic view of the organization of the human spleen. The white pulp has two components: a periarterial lymphatic sheath and a lymphatic follicle. The latter is made up of a germinal center and a surrounding mantle zone. The white pulp is surrounded by a marginal zone. The remainder of the tissue depicted is the red pulp, which consists primarily of splenic sinuses separated by splenic cords. The pattern of blood flow is as follows: A trabecular artery enters the white pulp and becomes the central artery. The central artery passes through white pulp and gives rise to many branches. A few end within white pulp; some supply the germinal center and mantle zone of the secondary nodule. Most terminate at the periphery of the white pulp, emptying in or near the marginal zone. A number of arterial vessels emerge from the white pulp, pass into the marginal zone, reach the red pulp, and curve back to empty into the marginal zone. Some arterial branches, in addition to the main stem of the central artery, run into the red pulp. Almost all terminate in the cords. Here, too, variation exists. Some arterial vessels terminate in a cord close against a sinus wall whereas others terminate in the midst of a cord, away from any sinus. Arterial vessels may terminate as capillaries or as somewhat larger vessels. Some arterial vessels may bear sheaths shortly before termination. The sinuses drain into pulp veins which, in turn, drain into trabecular veins. A sinus may abut the white pulp and receive lymphocytes or other free cells which migrate from white pulp across its wall and into its lumen. See text.

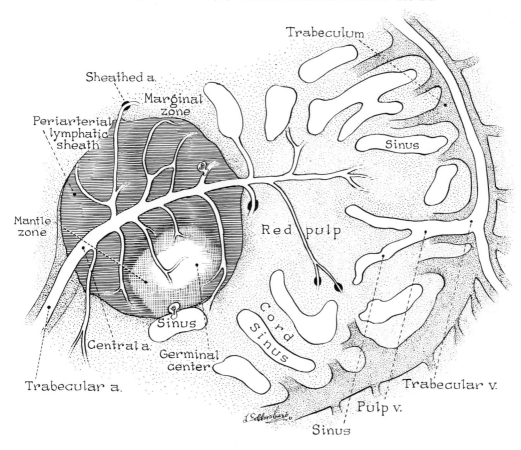

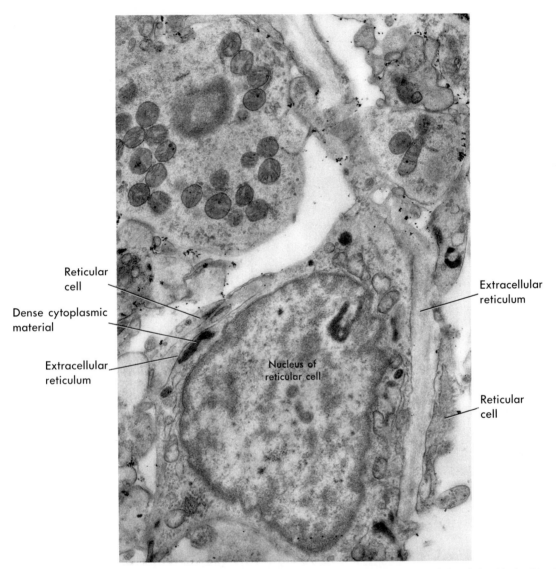

Figure 15-5   Spleen of a rabbit.   Reticular cells and reticular fibers are shown in characteristic relationship in this electron micrograph.   The reticular fibers are clothed by the cytoplasm of reticular cells.   The cytoplasmic cover may be quite thin, as on the right.   Reticular fibers form a branching network, the extracellular reticulum, which is modified in different parts of the spleen as described in the text.   The reticular cells, since they cover the fibers, form a corresponding reticulum, the cellular reticulum. Reticular cells contain certain distinctive cytoplasmic structures including a dense cytoplasmic material made of closely packed microfilaments.   See discussion of reticulum under lymph nodes. $\times 22,400$.   (From L. Weiss, Bull. Hopkins Hosp., **115**:99, 1964.)

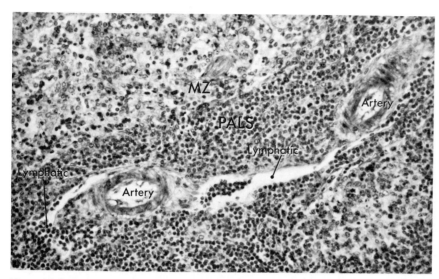

Figure 15-6 Spleen of a hedgehog. Lymphatic vessels are shown in this field. They lie within the periarterial lymphatic sheath (PALS) of white pulp in relationship to the central artery, two branches of which are shown (Art). The PALS consists of a reticular meshwork obscured by many lymphocytes crowded together. Outside the PALS is the marginal zone. ×950. (From V. Janout and L. Weiss, Anat. Rec., **172:**197, 1972.)

WHITE PULP

The white pulp of the spleen is a lymphatic tissue consisting of lymphocytes, plasma cells, macrophages, and other free cells lying in a reticular meshwork and surrounding the major arterial vessels of the spleen. The white pulp is divisible into two components: *periarterial lymphatic sheaths* and *lymphatic nodules* (Figs. 15-7 to 15-9). The periarterial lymphatic sheaths are cylinders which coaxially surround the central artery; for this reason the term *central artery* is used. About the periphery of the lymphatic sheath, the reticular elements tend to follow a circumferential pathway and form a rim to the white pulp (Fig. 15-12). Lymphocytes are the most numerous of the free cells in these sheaths, and most of them are small. Large but variable numbers of macrophages and some plasma cells are present and contribute to the population of free cells. The reticulum is not notably phagocytic. Periarterial lymphatic sheaths persist about arterial vessels until the vessels become small arterioles, although beyond the larger arterioles the sheaths are quite attenuated. Lymphatic nodules, spherical or ovoid structures resembling the nodules

of the cortex of lymph nodes, lie here and there within periarterial lymphatic sheath, often at arterial bifurcations. These nodules, like those of lymph nodes, may contain germinal centers. In a nodule which contains a germinal center, the peripheral zone of small lymphocytes may be termed the *mantle* (Fig. 15-7). The nodules in the human spleen may be several millimeters in diameter and may be grossly visible on the cut surface of the spleen. They constitute *malpighian corpuscles.* The nodules push the central artery aside, forcing it to assume an eccentric position in the periarterial lymphatic sheath.

There is a marked species variation in the development of the two components of white pulp. In the rabbit and rat the periarterial lymphatic sheaths are well developed, and the lymphatic nodules, although often present, are not large. In the cat and dog, however, nodules are large and the periarterial lymphatic sheaths are not.

Vascular supply of white pulp The central artery is a medium-sized muscular artery which gives off many branches as it courses through the periarterial

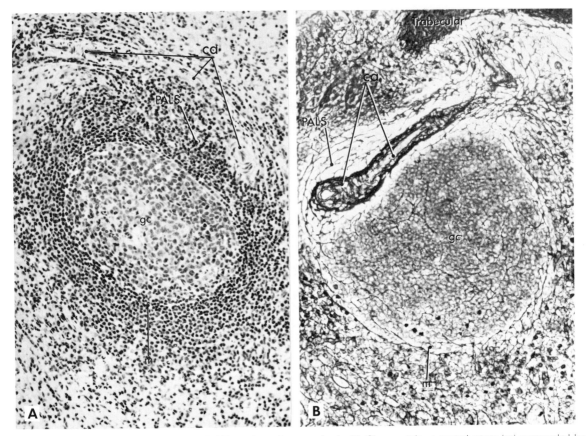

Figure 15-7 Human spleen, white pulp. A. Where the cells are stained with Giemsa stain, a central artery (ca) surrounded by the small lymphocyte-rich periarterial lymphatic sheath (PALS) curves into the field from the left. At the left leader it is cut in longitudinal section; at the right leader, in cross section. Hanging from the lower border of the PALS is a large lymphatic nodule, consisting of a large germinal center surrounded by a dense mantle (m) of small lymphocytes. B. In a reticulum preparation, in which the extracellular reticulum is blackened by silver, a similar field is shown. A central artery (ca) curves in from the right. It probably comes from the nearby trabecula (trab). The central artery is surrounded by a PALS. Note the circumferential pattern of the reticulum of the PALS around the central artery. Again, a large lymphatic nodule hangs from the PALS. The periphery of the nodule, constituting the mantle (m) of small lymphocytes, actually represents the PALS which has been carried out by the presence of the large germinal center (gc). ×450. (From the work of K. Richardson.)

lymphatic sheath (Figs. 15-10 and 15-11). The branches tend to follow a radial pattern, often coming off at right angles to the principal stem and running toward the periphery of the white pulp. A few run only a short distance and terminate as capillaries within white pulp. Many run beyond the periphery of the white pulp and empty into the marginal zone. A moderate number pass out of the white pulp, penetrate variable distances into the red pulp, and terminate as described below.

Lymphatic nodules may be well supplied with blood by way of arterioles which enter a nodule, reach its center, and then divide into smaller radicals which run to its periphery. Other branches of the central artery run to the surface of the nodules and supply their peripheral region.

MARGINAL ZONE
The marginal zone consists of an unusually fine meshwork of branched reticular cells associated

Reticular cell

Capillary

Reticular fiber

Cytoplasm of reticular cell

Capillary

Reticular cell

Branch of central artery

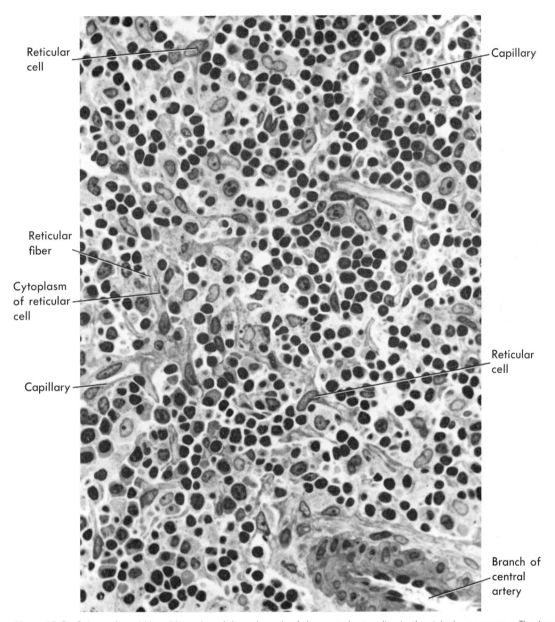

Figure 15-8   Spleen of a rabbit, white pulp.   A large branch of the central artery lies in the right lower corner.   The larger part of the field consists of a reticular meshwork within which lies the small, densely stained round lymphocytes and related free cells. The meshwork is made of branching reticular cells and reticular fibers.   The reticular cells ensheath the more lightly stained reticular fibers.   Small blood vessels are present in places in this field.   Their adventitial layers are continous with the reticular meshwork, as are the adventitial layers of the branch of the central artery in the right lower corner.   ×600.   (From L. Weiss, Bull. Hopkins Hosp., 115:99, 1964.)

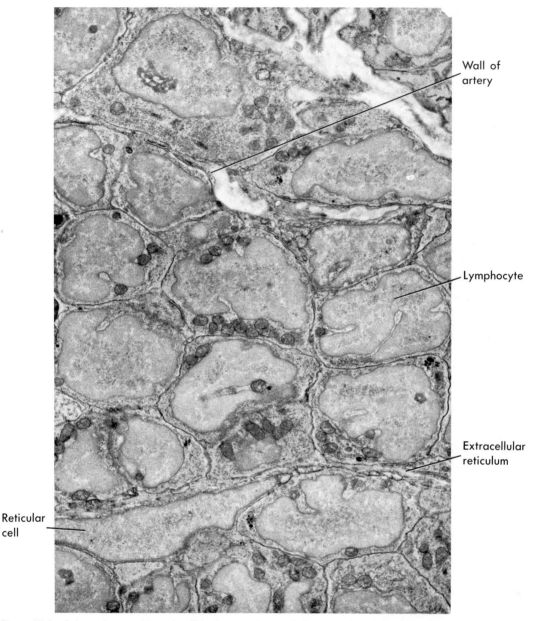

Wall of
artery

Lymphocyte

Extracellular
reticulum

Reticular
cell

Figure 15-9   Spleen of a rat, white pulp.   This electron micrograph illustrates the relationships of an arterial vessel, lymphocytes, and the reticular meshwork.   The adventitia of a large branch of the central artery is in the upper part of the field.   Small lymphocytes are present, tightly packed together.   Note that their scanty cytoplasm is rich in ribonucleoprotein and in mitochondria but lacks endoplasmic reticulum.   A reticular cell in the lower part of the field is associated with a small segment of extracellular reticulum. ×15,000.   (From L. Weiss, Bull. Hopkins Hosp., **115**:99, 1964.)

Endothelium

Lumen

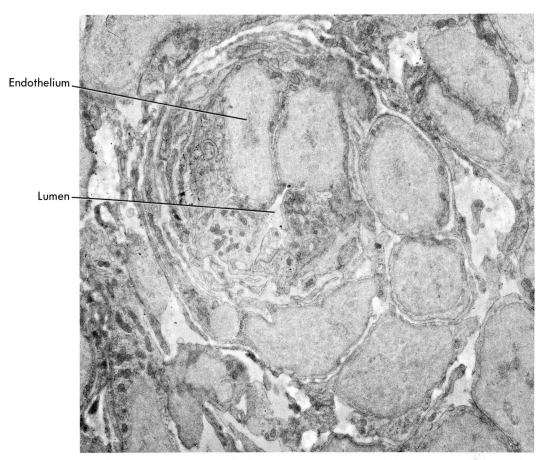

Figure 15-10 Spleen of a rat. An arteriolar branch of the central artery in the outer third of white pulp is present in this electron micrograph, demonstrating two distinctive characteristics often present in the central artery and its branches. They are (1) a high endothelium which effaces the lumen in whole or in part and (2) slender cytoplasmic projections from the base of the endothelial cells which extend into the subendothelial extracellular connective tissue and wind about the vessel, meeting corresponding processes of adventitial cells. Thus a lamellated pattern of cytoplasm and extracellular connective tissue results, best seen here at the left. ×17,000. (From L. Weiss, Bull. Hopkins Hosp., **115:**99, 1964.)

with extracellular reticulum, into which many arterial vessels open (Figs. 15-4, 15-12, and 15-13). The arterial vessels opening into the marginal zone may have a funnel-shaped orifice and often bifurcate just before ending. A number of arterial vessels run through the marginal zone, reach the red pulp, and curve back to empty into the marginal zone. Sinuses regularly come into the marginal zone. Infrequently, a terminating arterial vessel may open directly into such a sinus. The cords of the red pulp are directly continuous with the marginal zone and have a similar structure.

RED PULP
The red pulp is supplied by arteries and drained by sinuses and veins. The sinuses and the tissue between them, the cords, constitute most of the red pulp. After distributing many branches to the white pulp and marginal zone (Figs. 15-2 to 15-4), the attenuated main stem of the central artery, together

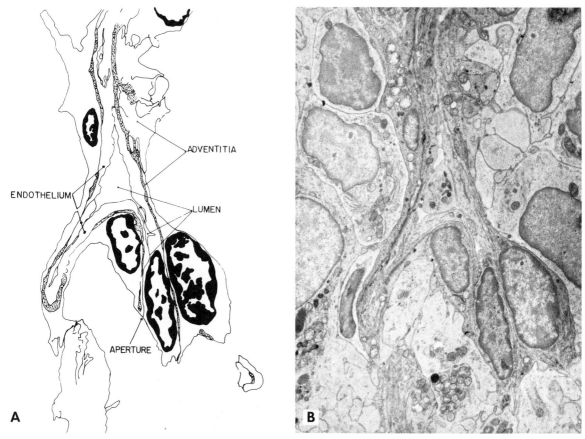

Figure 15-11   Spleen of a rat, white pulp.   An arterial vessel enters the field at the top and bifurcates into two vessels of capillary size.   Such a vessel has three components to its wall: an endothelium, a basement membrane (stippled in tracing), and an adventitial cell layer.   In the branch on the right the lumen, although effaced by the endothelium, may be followed to its aperture into the white pulp.   The vessel is surrounded by lymphocytes, macrophages, and other elements of white pulp.   ×22,000.   (From L. Weiss, Bull. Hopkins Hosp., 115:99, 1964.)

with some branches, runs on into the red pulp for a variable distance, and branches into straight, non-anastomosing slender vessels, about 25 μm in out-side diameter, called *penicilli*.   They display a well-developed basement membrane, adventitial cells, and occasionally some strands of smooth muscle. The penicilli may terminate as such or may go on to become finer *arterial capillaries*.   Some arterial capillaries in human spleen are sheathed (see below).   Each vessel in this system has a high endothelium, although that in arterial capillaries is some-times flat.

Splenic cords   Splenic cords (Figs. 15-14 to 15-24) are continuous partitions of tissue of varia-ble thickness lying between splenic sinuses.   The continuous nature of the cords and their position between sinuses may be understood if they are regarded as a mass of tissue honeycombed by si-nuses.   The cords merge with the marginal zone. The cords constitute a vascular space crisscrossed by reticulum, like the sinuses of lymph nodes.   The cords contain blood, and arterial vessels (see below) empty into them.   In addition to blood, the cords contain free connective tissue cells.   They are no-

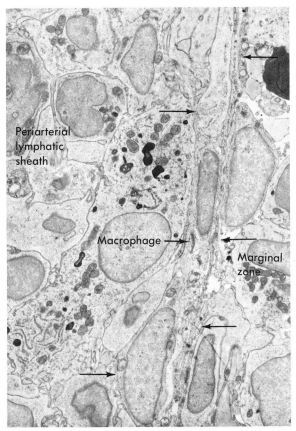

Figure 15-12 Spleen of a rat. In this field, the periphery of white pulp (the periarterial lymphatic sheath, PALS) is present. On the left are the closely packed cells of the PALS. A large macrophage may be seen. Its location at the periphery of white pulp is characteristic. The PALS has a well-defined rim of concentric strands of reticulum, running from top to bottom of this field (between arrows). This rim is well shown in silver preparations in which the extracellular reticulum is stained (see Fig. 15-7). The marginal zone is on the right. ×19,000. (From L. Weiss, Bull. Hopkins Hosp., **115**:99, 1964.)

tably rich in macrophages and typically contain large numbers of plasma cells. Hematopoietic cells, probably emigrated from the marrow or produced in the cords, are also present.

Splenic sinuses Splenic sinuses (Figs. 15-14 to 15-25) are long vascular channels 35 to 40 μm in diameter, made up of two elements: endothelium and a basement membrane. The endothelial cells are elongate with tapered ends which lie parallel to the long axis of the vessel. In cross sections of sinuses, therefore, the endothelial cells are cut in cross section and present a cuboidal shape. They lie side by side, without desmosomes, or other attachments, and so they may be easily separated from one another. Blood cells traverse the wall of a splenic sinus between endothelial cells (Fig. 15-24). In the basal portion of these lining cells are concentrations of microtubules and microfilaments, as determined by electron microscopy. These structures are disposed in rows, running parallel with the lining cells; some account for "basal striations" of light microscopy and may have a contractile function or provide cytoskeletal support

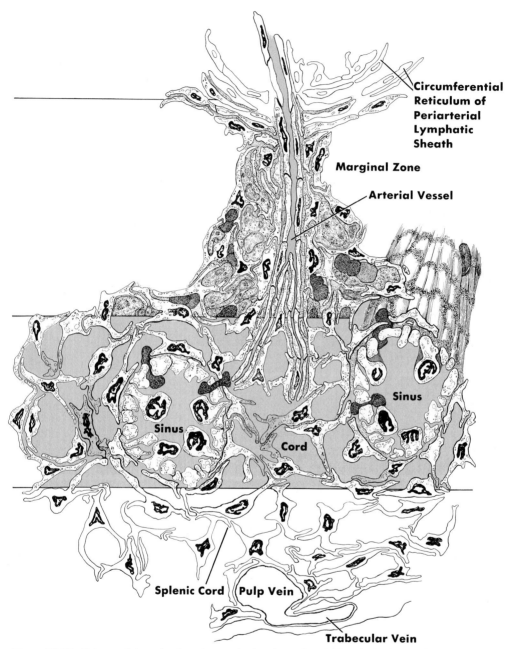

Circumferential Reticulum of Periarterial Lymphatic Sheath

Marginal Zone

Arterial Vessel

Sinus

Sinus

Cord

Splenic Cord   **Pulp Vein**

Trabecular Vein

Figure 15-13   Spleen.   Schematic view of artery leaving the periarterial lymphatic sheath of white pulp and entering red pulp. It enters a splenic cord and bifurcates between two sinuses.   (From L. Weiss, ''The Cells and Tissues of the Immune System,'' Prentice-Hall, Inc., Englewood Cliffs, N.J., 1971.)

to the endothelial cells. The endothelium is normally only slightly phagocytic (Fig. 15-25).

The endothelium lies upon a basement membrane, which may be deeply stained in the PAS reaction and may be impregnated by silver. The arresting feature of the membrane is that it is perforated by large fenestrae arranged almost as regularly as the squares on a checkerboard, so that the little material that remains of the basement membrane is reduced to slender strands separating and outlining the openings, and the picture it presents on surface view is that of an almost rectilinear net or of chicken wire. In man the transverse component of the basement membrane is heavy and the longitudinal links relatively slight. In section the membrane appears as a succession of points or short lines of PAS-reactive, or silver-impregnable, substance. In electron micrographs, the basement membrane in the human spleen, like the extracellular reticulum elsewhere, consists of both collagenous fibers and ground substance, the latter usually markedly predominant.

The luminal contents of sinuses are subject to considerable variation. They may contain blood, like systemic vessels. Some sinuses contain a disproportionate volume of plasma, whereas others are packed with lymphocytes. Macrophages are found in sinuses, as are plasma cells.

Splenic veins (Figs. 15-3 and 15-4) Sinuses are tributaries of the *veins of the pulp* and these in turn drain into the *trabecular veins*. The transition of splenic sinus into pulp vein is almost insensible, the latter being somewhat larger. Before these veins join the trabecular veins, the lining cells become typical squamous endothelium, the basement membrane becomes an unperforated sheet, and the medial and adventitial tunics become represented by a few strands of muscle and some fibroblasts.

Splenic vein blood is often rich in macrophages and other elements not usually thought of as blood cells. Undoubtedly many of these cells are filtered from the circulation by the liver and, should they pass the liver, by the lung.

Figure 15-14 Human spleen, reticulum stain. The periarterial lymphatic sheath (PALS) of the white pulp, demarcated by a well-defined rim of reticulum, is at the upper left. The rest of the field consists of red pulp. Clear spaces represent sinuses (S). The reticular tissue between sinuses constitutes the cords. Two arteries are present (see Fig. 15-15). ×600. (From the work of K. Richardson.)

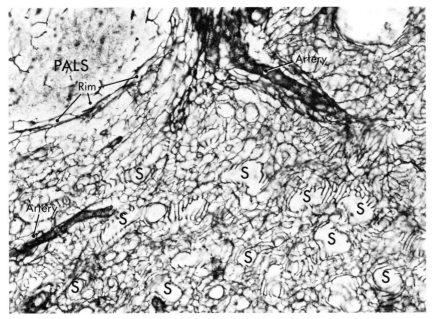

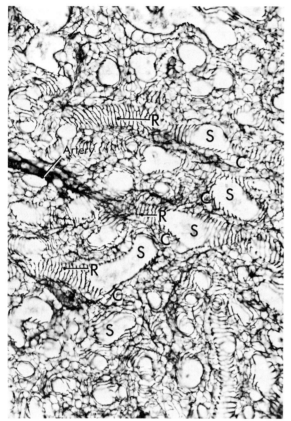

Figure 15-15   Red pulp of human spleen, reticulum stain. Sinuses are present as clear spaces. Their basement membrane is exposed as consisting primarily of "ring fibers" (R), deeply stained. This membrane is continuous with the reticular fibers of the cords (C). An artery (art) entering from the left appears to open into the cord. Compare with Fig. 15-14.   ×600. (From the work of K. Richardson.)

Relationship of splenic cords and splenic sinuses
The cords may be regarded as cavernous vascular spaces, inasmuch as they receive blood from arterial vessels. The cords differ from the sinuses primarily in that reticular cells of the cords branch, dividing the cordal space into communicating compartments, like the sinuses of lymph nodes.

Free cells and other materials in the cords enter sinuses by passing between sinus endothelial cells. This passage may be no more difficult than that through arterial vessels which have a high endothelium (Fig. 15-25).

Sheathed capillaries   Terminal arterial capillaries may be modified by a striking spherical, elliptical, or cylindrical sheath of closely packed phagocytic cells and reticular fibers (Figs. 15-26 and 15-27). The sheathed capillary, moreover, may branch within its sheath. In the dog and cat these sheaths are very prominent. Rabbits have no sheathed capillaries. The sheaths in human spleen are relatively small, and not every arterial capillary bears one. The endothelium contains microfilaments and may be contractile. The basement membrane may be incomplete or absent, so that the phagocytic cells of the sheath may lie directly subjacent to the endothelium. The exceptional phagocytic capacity of the sheath may be demonstrated by its concentration of india ink or other particulate matter injected intravascularly.

Termination of arterial vessels in red pulp   In the red pulp most terminal vessels end in the cords (Figs. 15-23 and 15-28). They may open into the cords by a funnel-shaped orifice or by a cylindrical opening and may bifurcate just before ending. They may communicate with the cords first by the development of a slit-like aperture in their wall. They may terminate lying close to the wall of a sinus, or they may lie in the center of the cord, not directly next to sinuses. A few arterial vessels terminate in sinuses.

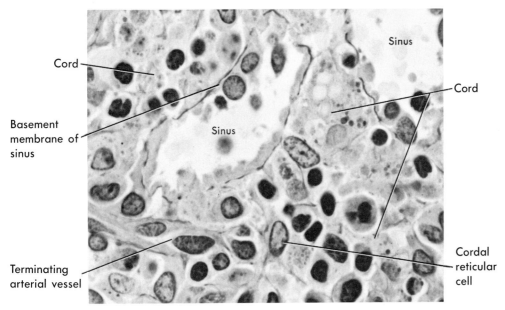

Cord

Basement membrane of sinus

Terminating arterial vessel

Sinus

Sinus

Cord

Cordal reticular cell

Figure 15-16   Spleen of a rabbit, red pulp.   Sections of two sinuses with intervening cords are present in this light micrograph. The basement membrane, stained deeply with the PAS reaction, is interrupted (see Fig. 15-13 to 15-15) in this section because of its fenestrated character.   The cords are crowded with macrophages.   Reticular cells and PAS-stained reticular fibers are present in the cords.   An arterial vessel which opens into a cord is also present.   PAS-hematoxylin stain.   ×1,200.   (From L. Weiss, J. Anat., **93**:465, 1959.)

Figure 15-17   Spleen of a rabbit, red pulp.   A sinus and contiguous cords are present in this light micrograph.   An arterial vessel enters the field at the lower left margin and bifurcates.   Each branch quickly terminates, opening into a cord.   PAS-hematoxylin stain.   ×1,200.   (From L. Weiss, J. Anat., **93**:465, 1959.)

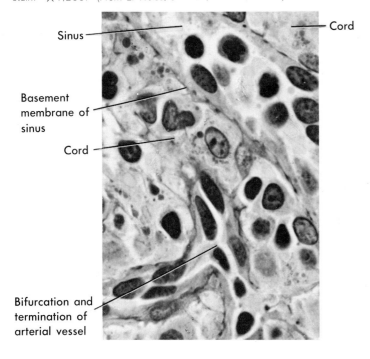

Sinus

Cord

Basement membrane of sinus

Cord

Bifurcation and termination of arterial vessel

The circulation of blood through the spleen

Several pathways of blood flow exist in the spleen, since arterial vessels may terminate in various ways in several places, namely, white pulp, marginal zone, and cords, and in different relations to sinuses.

Rate studies of erythrocytes tagged with radioactive chromium indicate that circulation through the spleen may be both fast and slow. Normal red cells flow through normal spleens as rapidly as they pass through other organs, but abnormal red cells or normal red cells in certain abnormal spleens have a retarded flow.

Histologic study of the sections of fixed human and rabbit spleen indicate that most of the arterial endings open into the vascular spaces of marginal zone and cords, whereas only a few open into si-

Figure 15-18 Spleen of a rabbit, red pulp. These fields demonstrate the nature of the fenestrated basement membrane of splenic sinuses. A. A splenic sinus runs from top to bottom in the right half of the field. The section exposes the basal surface of the endothelium or lining cells at the top of the field and cuts into the lumen in the lower half. A cord is present to the left of the sinus, and to the left of the cord is a second sinus. B. The field is the same but the fine adjustment of the microscope has been turned a bit, bringing the plane of focus somewhat above that of A. Along the sinus the basement membrane now comes into focus where, in A, lining cells were exposed. The basement membrane may be viewed as a cylinder of extracellular connective tissue sheathing the endothelium or lining cells of the vessels. It is regularly fenestrated; hence little of its substance remains, and on surface view, as here, it looks like chicken wire. A labeled macrophage appears in both planes of focus. PAS-hematoxylin stain. ×900. (From L. Weiss, J. Anat., **93:**465, 1959.)

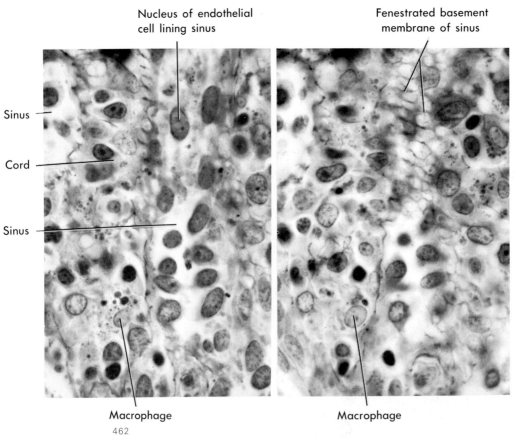

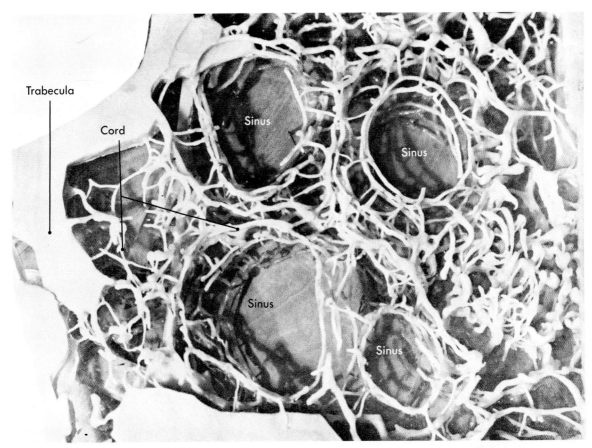

Figure 15-19 Human spleen. Reconstruction of extracellular reticulum of red pulp. Four sinuses are present in this field, outlined by the "ring fibers" of the basement membrane. The reticular fibers in the cords form a meshwork. In the human spleen the reticular fibers of the cords, as seen well between the upper two sinuses, form a collar or circlet about the sinus. The reader is referred to Koboth's work for additional valuable reconstructions of red pulp. (From E. Koboth, Beitr. Path. Anat., **103:**11, 1939.)

nuses. The cords and marginal zone are criss-crossed by reticular cells and extracellular reticulum, and in some cordal areas the interstices of the reticular meshwork are plugged with macrophages and other sequestered cells. Such areas would not permit direct and rapid flow of blood. In other places the reticular meshwork is empty and may even have a tubular conformation, making possible the same kind of flow that exists in direct vascular connections.

An effort to determine the pathway of blood by direct observation of the living circulation was made by Knisely (1936). The spleen of several animals,

among them the mouse and the kitten, was partially exposed in a lightly anesthetized animal and trans-illuminated by a quartz rod placed beneath the organ. Through water-immersion lenses, magnifications of 600 were possible. Knisely's conclusions are that blood flow in the spleen is through preformed channels, from arterial vessels directly into cucumber-shaped vascular channels, which appeared to be sinuses. He observed, moreover, that blood cells could be retained in sinuses, held by sphincter action at the distal end of the vessel, and that the plasma associated with these cells leaves the sinus through its wall. As a result, the

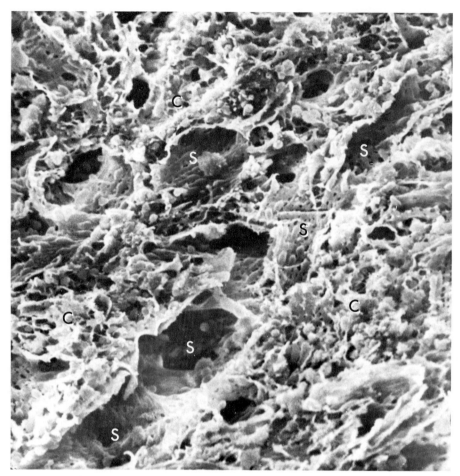

Figure 15-20 Spleen of a rabbit. Low-power scanning electron micrograph of a cut surface of red pulp. Winding furrows or caves with their wall of a lattice-like appearance are sinuses cut open (S), among which the cords (C) show a spongy profile (see Fig. 15-21). ×360. (From M. Miyoshi, T. Fujita, and J. Tokunaga, Arch. Histol. Jap., **32**:289, 1970.)

blood cells become a pasty mass, which nonetheless may be released after many hours into splenic veins, apparently undamaged. Knisely's work has been confirmed by several investigators, including Peck and Hoerr, and, although there has been some dissent, his findings are generally accepted. It is difficult to relate observations on living spleen with those on fixed histologic sections, but despite the fact that few direct artery-to-sinus connections are found in sections of the spleen, there need be no inconsistency with transilluminated studies in which passage through apparently preformed channels is observed, for an arterial vessel which terminates in a cord may terminate close to the wall of a sinus. Blood passing through this vessel may pass readily through the fenestrated basement membrane of the sinus and between its lining cells, and thus enter the lumen of the sinus. Such flow in the living spleen may appear to be through continuous vessels and be as efficient as through such vessels.

Embryology

The primitive disposition of hematopoietic elements is in the wall of the gastrointestinal tract. The spleen originates in the dorsal mesogastrium at about 5-mm crown-rump length (CRL) in human embryos. At 40 mm CRL the spleen consists of an encapsulated vascular spongework (Figs. 15-29 and 15-30). By 55 mm primitive sinuses are evident and the spongework is much more open. It contains many free blood cells and macrophages (Fig. 15-31). There soon develops a rich vascular supply in a mesenchymal matrix. By 100 mm reticular cells tend to lay out the plan of the spleen and assume a circumferential pattern around arteries, defining the periarterial lymphatic sheaths and

Figure 15-21 Spleen of a rabbit, red pulp. Scanning electron micrograph. A large branching sinus (S) is present surrounded by cordal tissue (C). The nuclei (N) of the sinus endothelial cells are seen as spindle-shaped protrusions over the inner surface of the sinus wall. (The orifices in the sinus wall may result from the perfusion techniques used in preparing the material or from other technical procedures. They are not present in such sectioned material as in Fig. 15-22. They may well indicate paths of communication between cords and sinuses which open readily.) ×1,100. (From M. Miyoshi, T. Fujita, and J. Tokunaga, Arch. Histol. Jap., **32**:289, 1970.)

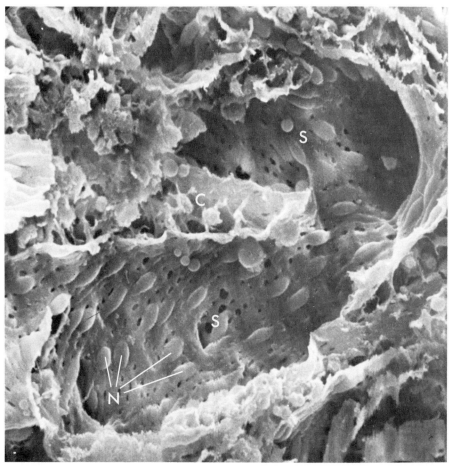

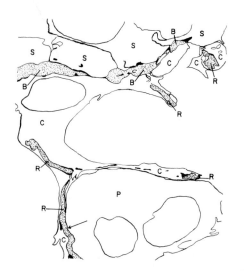

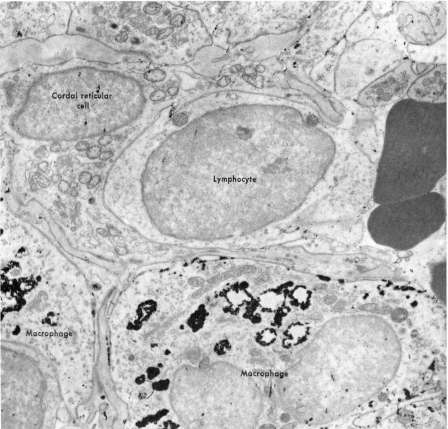

Figure 15-22 Spleen of a rabbit, red pulp. In this electron micrograph, the characteristic relationship of splenic cord and contiguous splenic sinus is shown. The sinus is at the top, its lining cells (S in the tracing) cut in cross section. The basement membrane of the sinus (B), lies directly subjacent to the sinal lining cells and is shown stippled. Reticular cells (C) of the cords lie upon the reverse surface of the basement membrane of the sinus and extend processes into the space of the cords. One such cell just left of center has extended its processes in association with extracellular reticulum (R), which is continuous with the basement membrane of the sinus. Crowded between the processes of the cordal reticular cells are portions of two phagocytes (containing a colloidal material, Thorotrast, which had been administered 20 min before splenectomy) and a lymphocyte. Erythrocytes are also present in the cordal space. ×20,000. (From L. Weiss, Amer. J. Anat., 113:51, 1963.)

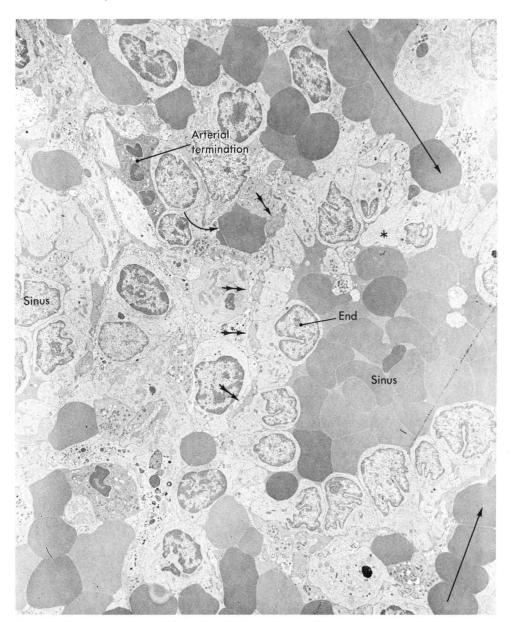

Figure 15-23 Human spleen, red pulp. Two sinuses and surrounding cords are present in this low-power electron micrograph. The sinus on the right is filled with erythrocytes. Its wall is cut in cross section. The endothelium consists of tapered rod-shaped cells lying longitudinally and is, therefore, cut in cross section. Nucleated sections of the endothelium protrude into the lumen. Cells are present in passage across the wall (*) between endothelial cells. The basement membrane (double-headed arrows) is present as segments. The sinus on the left is almost collapsed. The cords contain lymphocytes, platelets, erythrocytes, and other free cells. Two columns of erythrocytes are present (arrows) which may represent paths of flow through cords, across the sinus wall, and into the sinus lumen. An arterial capillary is present. It is completely surrounded by a basement membrane except at one point where it opens into a cord. In fact, a cell (arrow) is passing through the aperture of the capillary and into the cord A granulocyte occupies the capillary lumen. ×2,500. (From L-T. Chen and L. Weiss, Amer. J. Anat., **134**:425, 1972.)

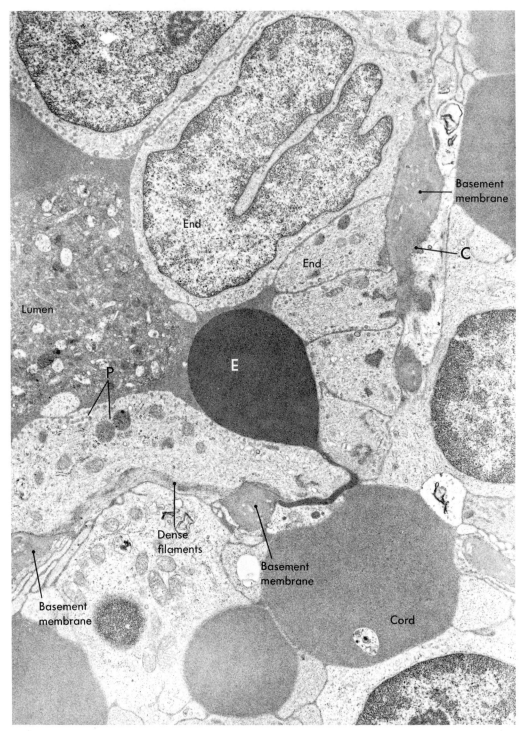

Figure 15-24 Human spleen, red pulp. An erythrocyte passes from a cord and through the sinus wall between endothelial cells (end) into the lumen of the sinus. The erythrocyte is drawn into a thin strand as it passes through the mural slit. The endothelial cells contain many pinocytotic vesicles (P) at the luminal surface and dense filaments in the basal cytoplasm which arches across the fenestrae of the basement membrane (BM). Small portions of cordal reticular cells applied to the abluminal surface of the basement membrane are present. The cord is filled with erythrocytes and other free cells. ×10,000. (From L-T. Chen and L. Weiss, Amer. J. Anat., 134:425, 1972.)

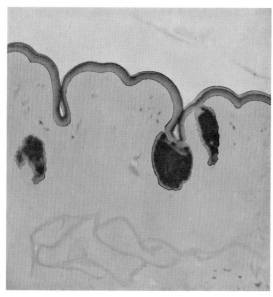

Figure 2-13 Villus of small intestine stained by the periodic acid–Schiff procedure, counterstained with fast green. Tissue fixed in OsO$_4$, embedded in methacrylate, and sectioned at 1 µm. The mucus in the goblet cells as well as that covering the striated border of the epithelial cells ("fuzz") reacts intensely. ×1,700. (Micrograph courtesy of S. Ito).

Figure 2-17 Mucosa of stomach stained to demonstrate the activity of thiamine pyrophosphatase (nucleoside diphosphatase) by a modified Gomori metal-salt method. Note the color of the lead sulfide, the final reaction product. This enzyme resides in the Golgi apparatus of the surface epithelial cells, as well as in capillary walls. ×800. (Courtesy of H. Ragins.)

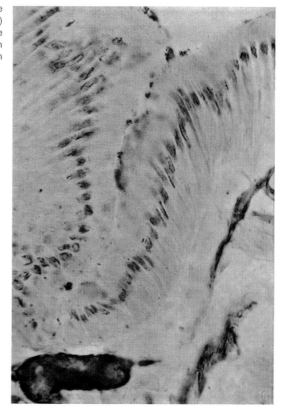

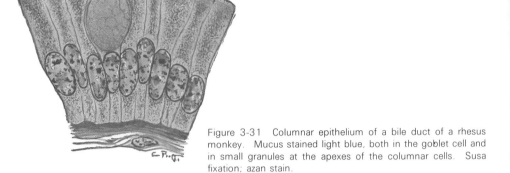

Figure 3-31 Columnar epithelium of a bile duct of a rhesus monkey. Mucus stained light blue, both in the goblet cell and in small granules at the apexes of the columnar cells. Susa fixation; azan stain.

Figure 4-5 Development of reticular fibers in 20-day tissue culture. The delicate network of argyrophilic fibers is closely associated with fibroblasts shown in color. (Drawn from Maximow, Z. Mikr. Anat. Forsch., **17**, 1929.)

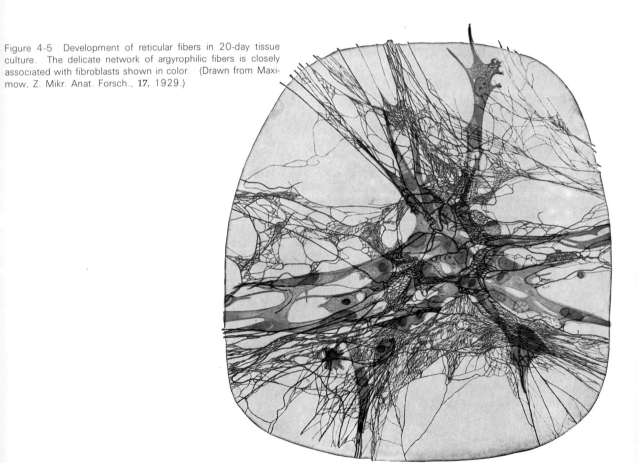

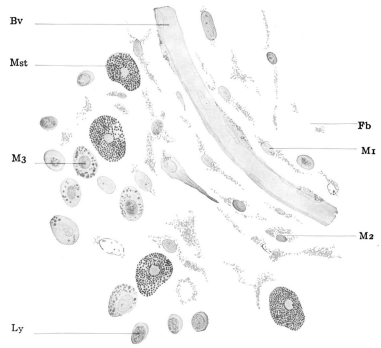

Bv

Mst

Fb

M₃

Mɪ

M₂

Ly

Figure 4-15   Mesentery of a rat stained vitally with pyrrole blue.
The macrophages (M_1,M_2,M_3) have ingested much of the dye.
Other cells are not as phagocytic: lymphocytes (ly) or mast cells
(mst) have ingested none of the particulate and the fibroblasts
(fb) have taken relatively small amounts only.

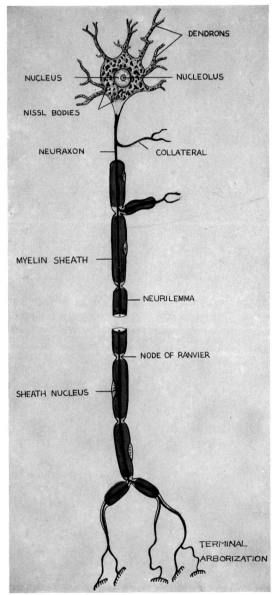

Figure 8-3 A motor nerve cell and investing membranes.

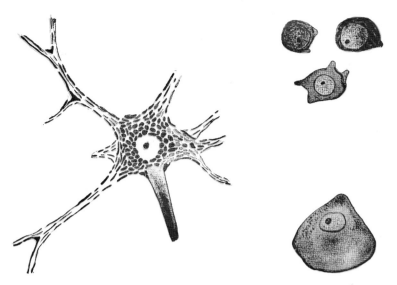

Figure 8-10 Nerve cells, Nissl strain. Motor from spinal cord; sympathetic (upper right); sensory (lower right). (von Mollendorff and Malone.)

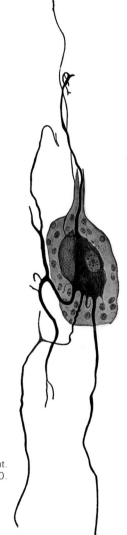

Figure 8-18 Autonomic nerve cell (superior cervical ganglion) containing yellow pigment. Observe the syncytium which encapsulates the cell body. Bielschowsky method. ×500. (Courtesy of P. Stohr, Jr.)

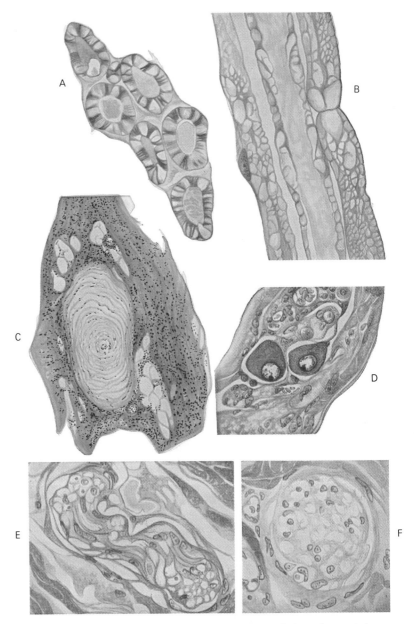

Figure 8-25   A and B. Neurokeratin networks and axis cylinders of cat sciatic nerve. Stained with methylene blue (pH 6.5) after alcoholic fixation.   A. Cross section.   ×975. B. Longitudinal view.   ×650.   C. A Pacinian (lamellar) corpuscle in the connective tissue of the female urethra of a monkey.   The core which contains the sensory fiber is cut transversely, and the nuclei of the capsule cells are visible. Azan technique.   ×65. D. Two autonomic ganglion cell bodies (presumably postganglionic parasympathetic) in the submucosa of the human duodenum. HE.   ×325.   E. Semilongitudinal section of human breast demonstrating small nerves.   F. Cross section of human breast demonstrating small nerves. HE.   ×325.

Figure 8-45 End-bulb from the glans penis. Methylene blue. (Dogiel.)

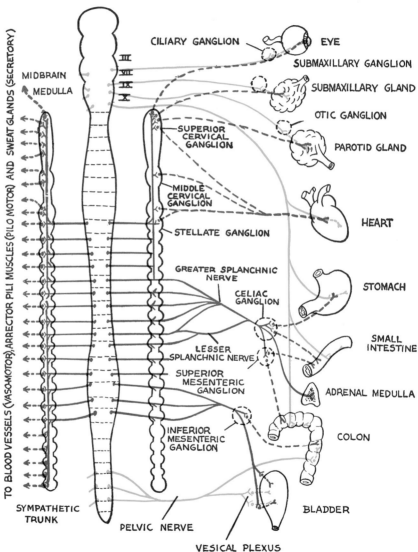

TO BLOOD VESSELS (VASO-MOTOR),ARRECTOR PILI MUSCLES (PILO MOTOR) AND SWEAT GLANDS (SECRETORY)

MIDBRAIN
MEDULLA

CILIARY GANGLION
EYE
SUBMAXILLARY GANGLION
SUBMAXILLARY GLAND
OTIC GANGLION
PAROTID GLAND

III
VII
IX
X

SUPERIOR
CERVICAL
GANGLION

MIDDLE
CERVICAL
GANGLION

STELLATE GANGLION

HEART

GREATER SPLANCHNIC
NERVE

CELIAC
GANGLION

STOMACH

LESSER
SPLANCHNIC NERVE

SMALL
INTESTINE

SUPERIOR
MESENTERIC
GANGLION

ADRENAL MEDULLA

INFERIOR
MESENTERIC
GANGLION

COLON

BLADDER

SYMPATHETIC
TRUNK

PELVIC NERVE

VESICAL PLEXUS

Figure 8-63 Diagram of the arrangement of the autonomic nervous system: sympathetics in red; parasympathetics in blue; postganglionic fibers, broken lines; preganglionic, solid lines. Sympathetic postganglionic distribution to somatic regions of the body shown on left. (After Strong and Elwyn, "Human Neuroanatomy," 2d ed., Williams & Wilkins, Baltimore, 1948.)

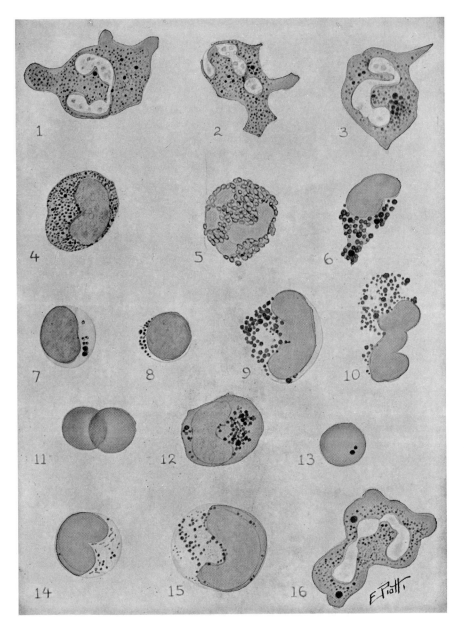

Figure 10-5 Human blood cells stained supravitally. All cells are from the same individual and are drawn the same scale. Cells 1−13 are stained with neutral red only (granules and phagocytic vacuoles). Cells 14−16 are stained with neutral red and Janus green (mitochondria). Legend on facing page. (Preparation Courtesy of E. Tompkins.)

Figure 10-5

BLOOD

1. Polymorphonuclear neutrophil stained for 20 min at 37°C. The small dots are the specific, refractive granules, which appear brown-red or gray, depending on focus. Unlike phagocytic vacuoles, these do not change with time. The pseudopodia are usually free of the streaming granules. The larger droplets represent the phagocytic vacuoles. There are few of these in a normal neutrophil within this period of time.

2. A neutrophil from the same field after the film has been at room temperature for 1 hr. Phagocytosis is slight at the lower temperature, and there is little change in the vacuoles.

3. The same cells as in 2 after the film has been at room temperature for 2 hr. The number of lobes of the nucleus has changed somewhat as the result of ameboid movements. The cell has become toxically injured after long exposure and is phagocytosing abnormally.

4. Myelocyte film stained at 37°C for 1 hr. There are no ameboid movements and little phagocytosis. The specific granules are more refractive and stain more on the acid side than the granules of polymorphonuclear neutrophils. This type of staining is considered an indication of youth when it occurs in the latter cells.

5. Polymorphonuclear eosinophil from the same film as 4. The granules are highly refractive, and the intensity of their color consequently varies with focus. They are large, rice-shaped, and fairly uniform in size. They are straw-colored when freshly stained but gradually take on an apricot tint with exposure. Eosinophils rarely contain phagocytic vacuoles.

6. Polymorphonuclear basophil. The granules are large, round, very uniform, and highly refractive; the intensity of staining therefore varies with focus. The granules stain a deeper crimson than phagocytic vacuoles or than the granules of any other cells of the blood. The nucleus rarely shows lobing, and the cells are practically never phagocytic.

7. Intermediate-sized lymphocyte from same film as 4 after the film stood at room temperature for 1 hr. The cytoplasm is very clear and contains few phagocytic vacuoles. These are much fewer than in monocytes and are arranged indiscriminately. Lymphocytes should rarely be confused with monocytes. Double staining with Janus green also serves to differentiate the two types (see 13 and 14).

8. Small lymphocyte from same film as 7 after the film has stood at room temperature for 2 hr.

9. 10. Monocytes from the same film after it has stained for 5 min at 37°C, and 1 hr and 2 hr, respectively, at room temperature. Monocytes vary constantly in shape and degree of phagocytosis, depending upon ameboid movement. They have the greatest number of phagocytic vacuoles of all blood cells and no granules. The vacuoles vary in size and change position constantly. They increase in both size and number with time of exposure.

11. Two normal erythrocytes. They do not stain. Their color is due entirely to their content of hemoglobin.

12. Monocyte from same film as 9 and 10. The cell is somewhat younger than those, less ameboid, and tends to aggregate the phagocytic vacuoles into rosette formation.

13. Erythrocyte from same film as 12. The cell is younger than those in 11 and contains reticulum, which was stained with neutral red.

14. Lymphocyte stained with neutral red and Janus green (compare with 7). Janus green inhibits phagocytosis somewhat. The mitochondria stain blue-green, are definitely rod-shaped, and tend to cluster toward the nucleus. They are larger than the mitochondria of monocytes.

15. Monocyte stained with neutral red and Janus green. Phagocytosis has been inhibited somewhat. The mitochondria are smaller than those in lymphocytes and more scattered (compare with 14).

16. Polymorphonuclear neutrophil stained with neutral red and Janus green. The mitochondria are the size of those in monocytes but are less abundant. Janus green is soon toxic to cells, and this cell shows the toxic action in the form of unusual phagocytic vacuoles.

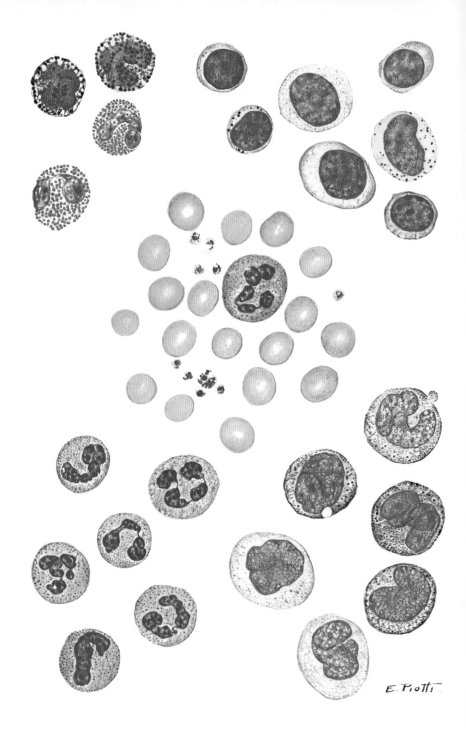

Figure 10-7 Cells from a smear preparation of normal human blood, Wright's stain. In the center, adult red corpuscles, blood platelets, and a polymorphonuclear neutrophil. At left above, two polymorphonuclear basophils and two polymorphonuclear eosinophils. At right above, three large and four small lymphocytes. At left below, polymorphonuclear neutrophils. At right below, six monocytes.

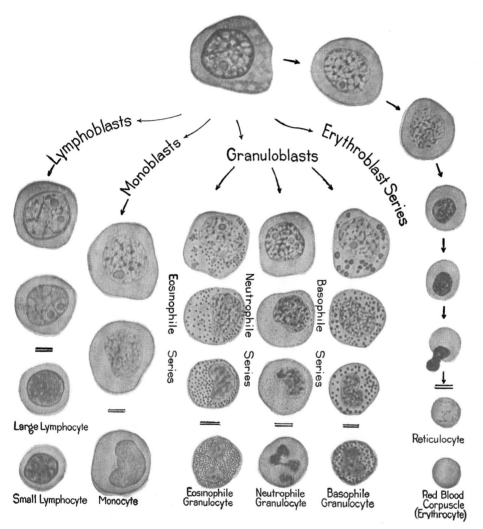

Figure 11-6 Stages in cytogenesis of blood cells, arranged in developmental sequences. (Courtesy of B. M. Patten, "Human Embryology," 2d ed., McGraw-Hill Book Company, New York, 1953.)

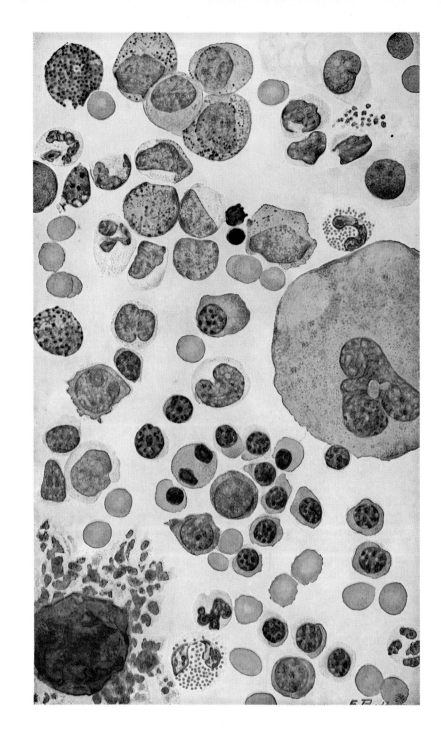

Figure 11-7   A and B.   Composite plate of blood cells.   A, eosinophilic myelocyte; B, myelocyte; D, blast form; E, basophilic leukocyte; F, small lymphocyte; G, medium-sized lymphocyte; H, large lymphocyte; I, blast form; J, basophilic erythroblast; K, megakaryocyte; L, eosinophilic leukocyte; M, neutrophilic leukocyte; O, polychromatophilic erythroblast; P, platelets; Q, reticulum cell; R, monocyte; S, plasma cell.

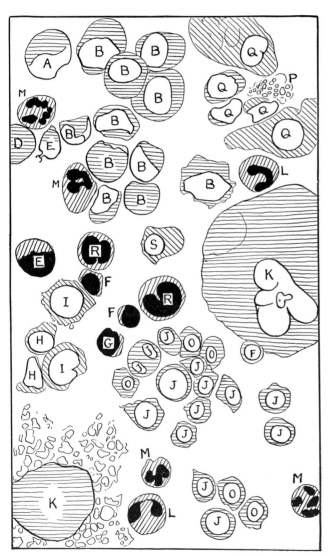

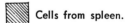 Cells from bone marrow.

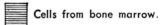 Cells from spleen.

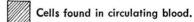 Cells found in circulating blood.

B

Figure 17-5 A. Stellate reticulum of enamel organ of human fetus (130-mm C-R length). Fixed in basic lead acetate and stained with 0.5% toluidine blue solution. The ground substance is intensely metachromatic. B. Odontoblasts and subjacent dental pulp of human fetus (130-mm C-R length). The small cells of the pulp are surrounded by metachromatic ground substance (toluidine blue). C. Gingiva of a young child, clinically·normal, showing metachromasia of the ground substance and numerous mast cells. ×7 ocular; ×40 objective. D. Enamel from the growing portion of an incisor tooth of a 4-day-old rat, stained by the Prussian blue method for sulfhydryl and disulfide groups. The interprismatic areas stain brownish-red by the carmine counterstain. A well-defined greenish-blue reaction has taken place in the organic substance of the enamel prisms. ×7 ocular; ×90 objective. E. Enamel from the calcifying portion of an incisor tooth of a rat 1½ months of age. Longitudinal ground section. Fixation in a 4% solution of basic lead acetate. Stained for ½ hr in 0.5% solution of toluidine blue. Note the metachromatic staining of the prism sheaths and the prism cross striations. ×10 ocular; ×40 objective. F. Enamel from an erupted human premolar tooth. Longitudinal ground section. Fixed in basic lead acetate and stained in toluidine blue. Note the metachromatic reaction of the alternating Hunter-Schreger's bands, which are relatively less calcified. ×10 ocular; ×20 objective. G. Dentin of an adult rhesus monkey's tooth, stained with Masson's connective tissue stain. Undecalcified section cut transversely. The dentinal matrix is stained green and the odontoblastic processes red by this mixture of acid dyes. The green staining of the matrix is due to collagen. H. Dentin of an adult human tooth. Fixed in Rossman's fluid and stained by McManus's periodic acid-Schiff technique. Undecalcified ground section. Observe that the dentinal matrix and odontoblastic processes are stained. I. Dentin of an adult rhesus monkey's tooth. Fixed in basic lead acetate and stained in methylene blue for 24 hr at pH 2.9. Undecalcified ground section. The only objects stained at this pH are the areas located around the odontoblastic processes, indicating that these peritubular structures are strongly basophilic. J. Dentin of an adult human tooth. Fixed in basic lead acetate and stained with toluidine blue. Undecalcified ground section cut obliquely. The calcified dentinal matrix is unstained. Observe the metachromatic staining of the peritubular dentin. (Sections marked A, B, G, H, I, J courtesy of G. B. Wislocki, M. Singer, and C. M. Waldo, Anat. Rec., **101**:487, 1948; C, D, E, F, courtesy G. B. Wislocki and R. F. Sognnaes, Amer. J. Anat., **87**:239, 1950.)

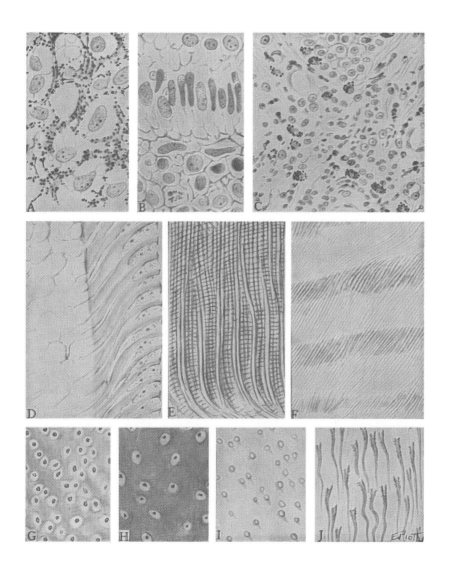

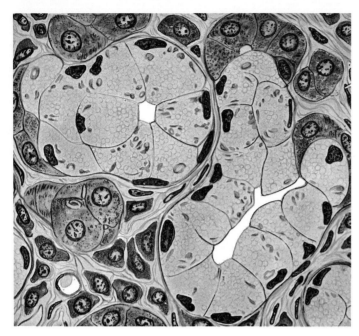

Figure 18-16   Section of the sublingual gland of a 30-year-old executed man.   The mucus-secreting cells are stained blue; the serous cells are gray.   Zenker fixation; iron-hematoxylin and Mallory's connective tissue stain.   (Clara.)

Figure 18-34 Drawing of two gastric glands of the adult human stomach. Four cell types are evident in the epithelium: the surface mucous cell (extending down into the pits), the neck mucous cell, the acidophilic parietal (or oxyntic) cell, and the basophilic chief (or zymogenic) cell. The epithelium has shrunk away from the underlying basement membrane and connective tissue. Zenker fixation; eosin and methylene blue.

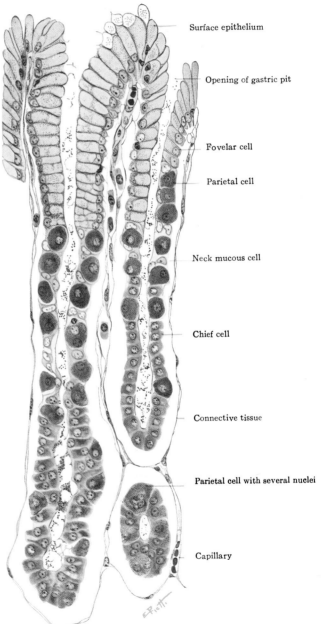

Surface epithelium

Opening of gastric pit

Fovelar cell

Parietal cell

Neck mucous cell

Chief cell

Connective tissue

Parietal cell with several nuclei

Capillary

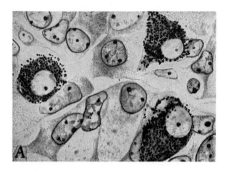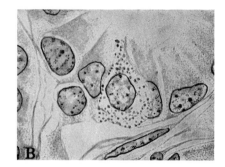

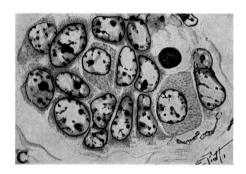

Figure 18-39   Reactions of granules in argentaffin cells from the small intestine of a pig.   A. Fixed in alcohol-formalin-acetic acid; stained by Bodian silver method.   B. Fixed in acetone; stained by Gomori method for acid phosphatase.   C. Fixed in Zenker-formalin; stained with eosin and methylene blue.   ×1,200.   (Courtesy of G. B. Wislocki and E. W. Dempsey.)

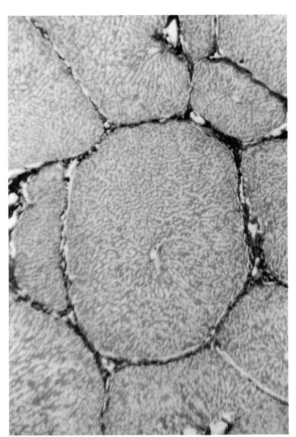

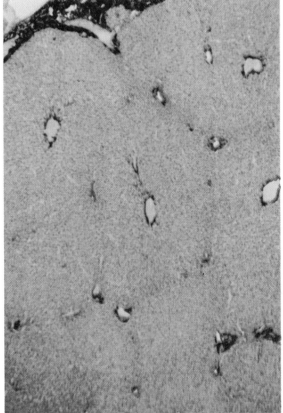

Figure 19-9 Low-power photomicrograph of a section of pig liver, showing a classic lobule. Mallory-Azan.

Figure 19-10 Low-power photomicrograph of a section of human liver, illustrating boundaries of a classic lobule. Mallory-Azan.

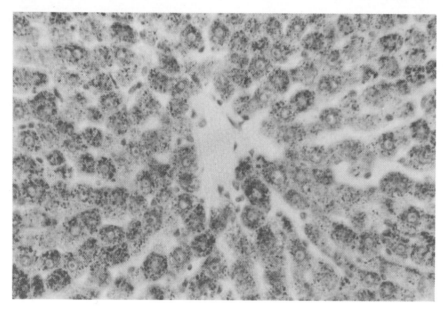

Figure 19-13 Glycogen deposits within the parenchymal cells are stained red by Best's carmine. The quantity of glycogen within the cells varies with the time interval after the last meal and the position of the cell in the lobule. Glycogen is not preserved in routine histologic preparations. Rat liver. Carnoy's fixative. Hematoxylin and Best's carmine.

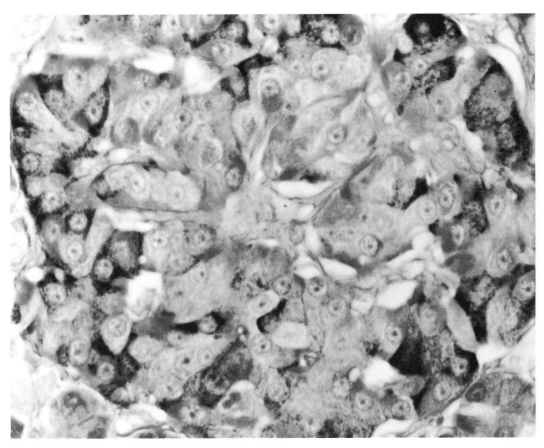

Figure 20-8   A photomicrograph of a human pancreatic islet stained with aldehyde fuchsin and light-green counterstain. The granular nature of the islet cell cytoplasm is evident at this magnification.   The alpha cell granules are a deep purple, the beta cell granules are red, and connective tissue fibers are green ×800.   (Courtesy of A. Like.)

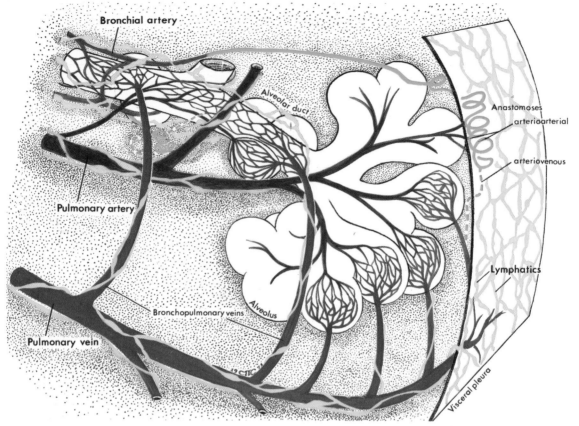

Figure 21-41 Diagram showing the interrelationships among the airways, the vascular systems, and the lymphatic networks of the lung. (After diagrams of W. S. Miller and J. Lauweryns.)

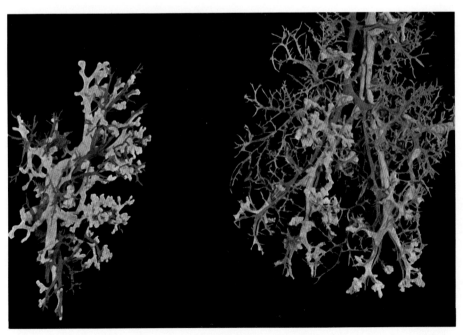

Figure 21-42 Cast of the peripheral airway, showing the actual relationships presented in Fig. 21-41. Airway, green, pulmonary artery, red, pulmonary vein, blue. (Courtesy of J. Lauweryns; from ''De Longvated,'' pp. 1–302, copyright Ed. Arscia, Brussels, 1962.)

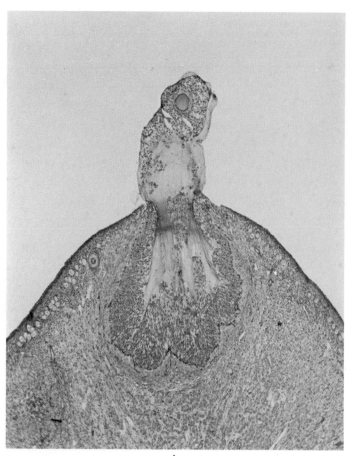

A

Figure 23-14   A. Photomicrograph of an ovulation observed in situ in a living anesthetized rabbit. Immediately after ovulation the ovary was fixed, removed, and cut in sections.   PAS stain.   B. A thick section of a rat ovary in which the blood vessels were perfused with carmine-gelatin. Notice also the rich vasculature of the corpora lutea.

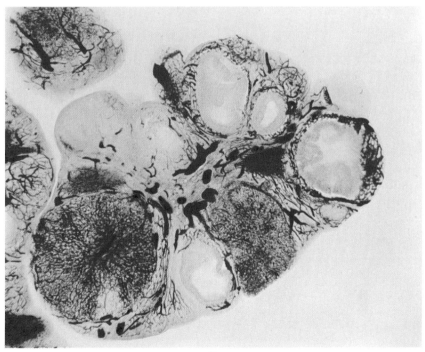

B

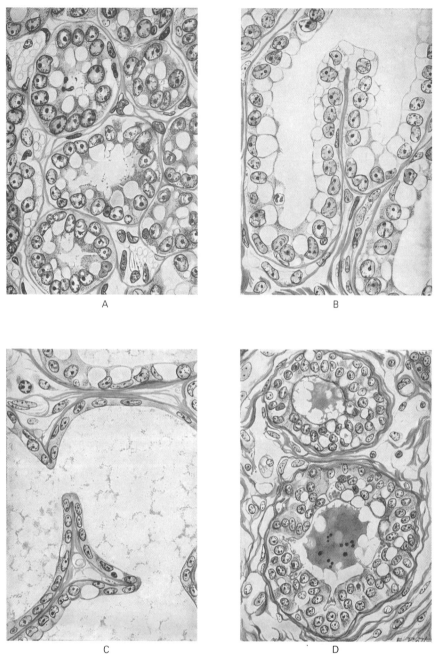

Figure 24-5 Human mammary gland in different functional states. A. Late pregnancy. B. Lactation, active phase. C. Alveoli distended with secretion. D. Regression of mammary gland during the secretory phase. The alveolar cells are tall and often contain large fat globules, which may equal the size of the nuclei.

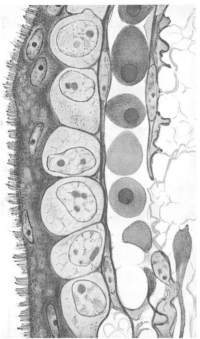

Figure 25-14 Drawing illustrating the structure of the human placental villus at 3 months of gestation. The trophoblast consists of an internal layer of large, clear, chromophobic Langhans' cells and a superficial layer of darkly stained syncytial trophoblast. The free surface of the syncytium, bordering the intervillous space, possesses a brush or microvillous border. The Langhans' cells rest upon a basement membrane. Note the difference in the size of the nuclei of the cellular and syncytial trophoblast. A capillary, containing nucleated fetal erythrocytes and lined by endothelial cells, is closely applied to the trophoblast. The distance between the intervillous space and the lumen of the capillary constitutes the "placental barrier" through which transfer of substances between mother and fetus takes place. Mallory's connective tissue stain. ×1,520. (Courtesy of G. B. Wislocki and H. S. Bennett.)

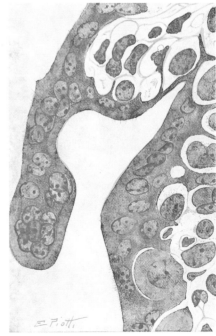

Figure 25-16 Drawing of a section of a human placental villus at 13 weeks. On the left, a tag composed exclusively of syncytium protrudes from the surface of the villus. There is marked cytoplasmic basophilia in the syncytium at the level of the nuclei, which indicates a high content of ribonucleoprotein, since this staining is eliminated by prior treatment with ribonuclease. In the cytoplasm of the Langhans' cells, there are only traces of basophilia. Methylene blue. ×1,140. (Courtesy of E. W. Dempsey and G. B. Wislocki.)

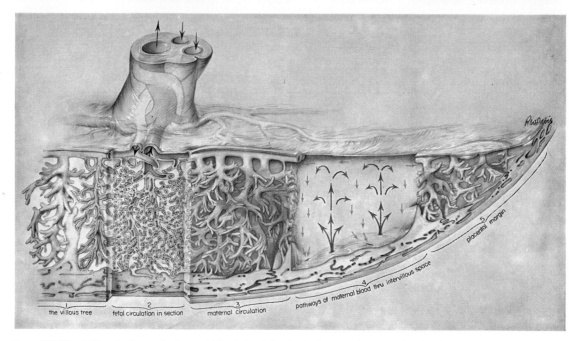

Figure 25-22   A. Structural organization and blood circulation in the human placenta.   Panel 1 illustrates the form of a stem villus, its origin at the chorionic plate, its branches in the intervillous space, and its anchorage to the basal plate.   Panel 2 shows the CO_2-rich blood of the umbilical arteries entering the villous tree and being returned to the fetus in oxygenated form via the umbilical vein.   In panels 3 and 4 maternal blood is shown entering the intervillous space through open-ended utero-placental arteries.   It enters in spurts and is driven toward the chorionic plate; then, as maternal pressure lessens, lateral dispersion occurs.   Maternal blood drains into numerous venous openings along the basal plate.   Panel 5 illustrates the peripheral portion of the intervillous space, which consists of a series of interrupted pools or lakes.   (E. M. Ramsey and J. W. S. Harris, 1966.)

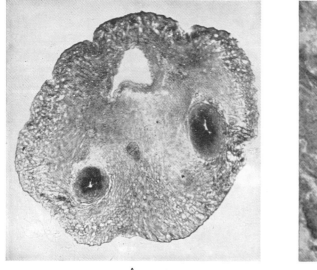

A

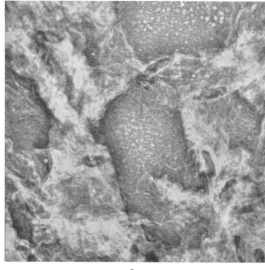

B

Figure 25-30   Human umbilical cord at full term stained with toluidine blue.   A. The umbilical vein is the upper, single vessel with a relatively thin wall and large lumen.   The two lower vessels are the umbilical arteries with their thick walls and constricted lumina.   The intense metachromasia of the ground substance of the mucous connective tissue is evident.   ×6. B. Higher power view of A.   Lakes of metachromatic mucous ground substance fill the interstitial spaces among the unstained collagenous framework.   Only the nuclei of the fibroblasts are evident; they are stained an orthochromatic blue. ×500   Frozen dried section fixed with Formalin-ether vapor.   (Courtesy of E. H. Leduc and G. F. Odland.)

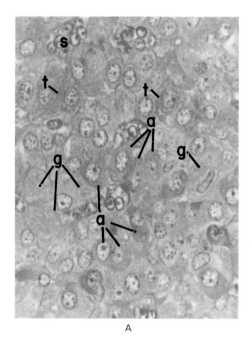

A

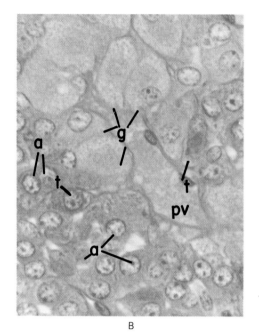

B

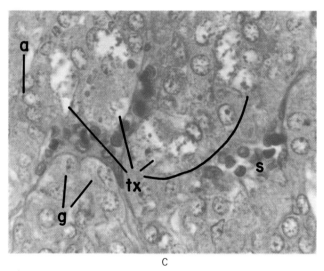

C

Figure 27-8 Rat anterior lobes. A. Normal male. Note acidophils (a), angular thyrotropic cells (t), and rounded gonadotropic cells (g). B. Male rat 30 days after castration. Acidophils (a) and thyrotropic cells (t) are unchanged, gonadotropic cells (g) are hypertrophic and hyperplastic. A portal vessel (pv) is shown. C. Male rat 30 days after thyroidectomy. Gonadotropic cells (g) are slightly smaller; only a few acidophils (a) have remained somewhat granulated; thyrotropic cells have lost their granules and given rise to large, multi-vacuolated ''thyroidectomy cells'' (tx). The capillaries (s) are engorged. Aldehyde fuchsin-trichrome.

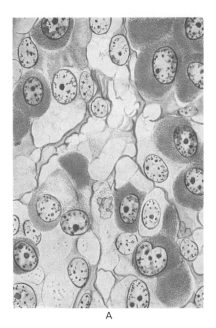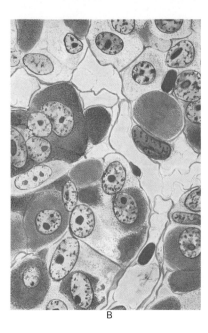

A

B

Figure 27-9 Anterior lobe of the cat hypophysis. A. Anestrous female. Orange acidophils, basophils (blue), and chromophobes (light blue) can be seen. B. Last week of pregnancy. Note presence of numerous red carmine cells. Modified azan stain. (Drawn from preparations of A. B. Dawson.)

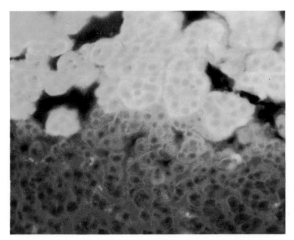

Figure 31-15 Fluorescence photomicrograph of a section of the adrenal medulla of the rat. Chromaffin cells have a characteristic yellow-green fluorescence whereas cortical cells (bottom) are dark green. The capillaries are filled with a dye which appears red by this technique. ×100. (Courtesy of Dr. Donald McDonald.)

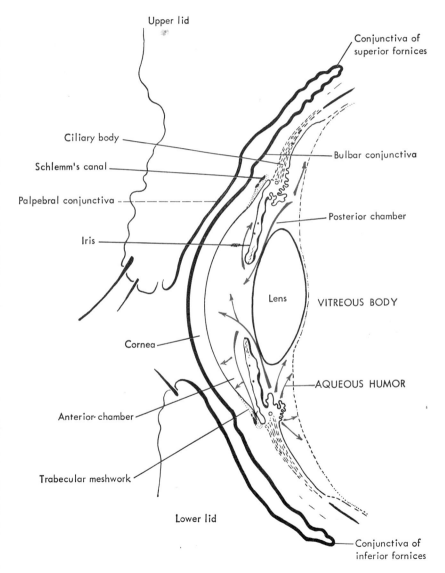

Upper lid

Conjunctiva of
superior fornices

Ciliary body

Schlemm's canal

Palpebral conjunctiva

Iris

Bulbar conjunctiva

Posterior chamber

Lens

VITREOUS BODY

Cornea

AQUEOUS HUMOR

Anterior chamber

Trabecular meshwork

Lower lid

Conjunctiva of
inferior fornices

Figure 32-18 Diagram of the anterior segment of the eye and lids, showing circulation within the eye. Aqueous humor is formed chiefly at the ciliary processes. From the posterior chamber it passes, for the most part, through the pupil into the anterior chamber and thence out of the eye by way of the trabecular meshwork and Schlemm's canal.

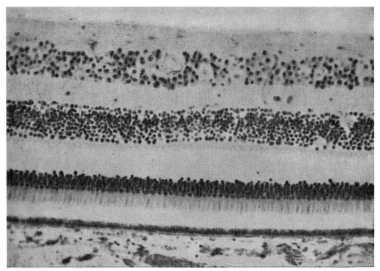

A

Figure 32-43 Cross section of the retina,
showing thick ganglion cell layer. A. Near
the macula. B. Some distance from the
macula. (From Amer. J. Ophthal.,
54:347, 1962.)

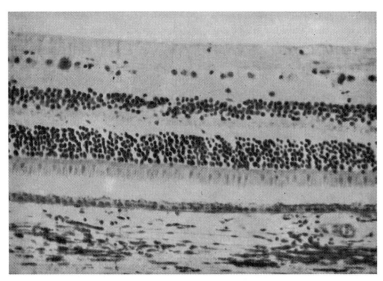

B

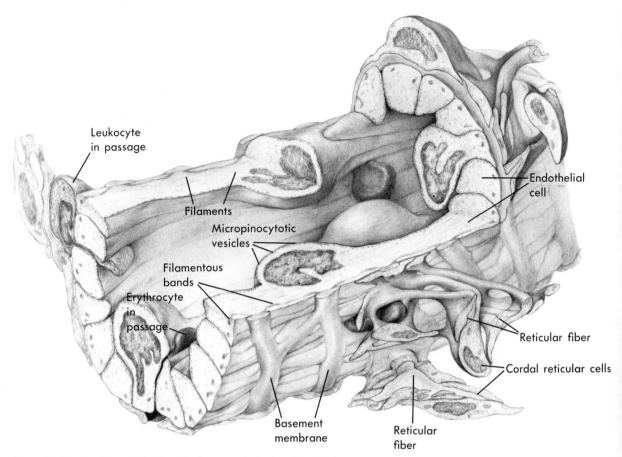

Figure 15-25   A schematic drawing of a human splenic sinus in red pulp.

The endothelial cells are tapered rods which lie side by side with their long axis parallel to the long axis of the vessel. Virtually all arterial vessels end in the surrounding cords without direct connection to the sinuses. Accordingly, blood entering the vascular sinus must enter from the surrounding cord, squeezing through the slit-like spaces between sinus endothelial cells. Note that several blood cells in passage across the sinus wall are shown. The endothelial cells show several distinctive cytological features. These include a row of pinocytotic vesicles just beneath the plasma membrane on the luminal and lateral surfaces, and two sets of cytoplasmic filaments. One set of filaments, rather loosely organized, runs longitudinally through the cytoplasm. The other set is tightly organized into dense bands in the basal cytoplasm. These bands arch between strands of the basement membrane. They appear to insert into the plasma membrane where it overlies the basement membrane and then continue through the plasma membrane into the substance of the basement membrane. These filaments are likely part of the cytoskeletal system which stiffens the basal cytoplasm and maintains the shape of endothelial cells and the slit-like interendothelial space. They or the other set of filaments, may be contractile. They play an important role in the spleen's capacity to recognize damaged blood cells and destroy or modify them (see text).

The basement membrane is fenestrated leaving heavy strand-like transverse "ring" components and lighter longitudinal strands joining the rings. The large fenestrae or apertures in the basement membrane leave ample unimpeded space for blood cell passage through the sinus wall. The cordal surface of the basement membrane is covered by cordal reticular cells which branch into the surrounding cord and is continuous with reticular cells which ensheath them, form the reticular meshwork of the cords (see text). (From L-T. Chen and L. Weiss, Amer. J. Anat., **134:**425, 1972.)

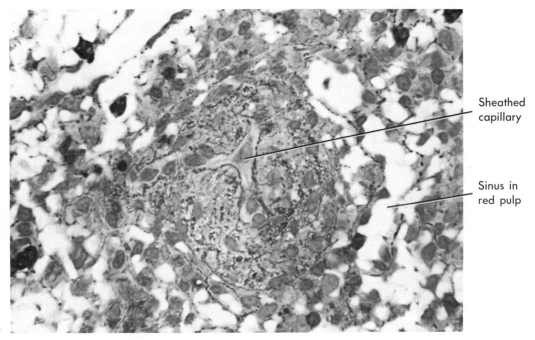

Sheathed
capillary

Sinus in
red pulp

Figure 15-26 Spleen of a dog, red pulp. In this light micrograph, an arterial vessel, which is actually a capillary, bifurcates within the sheath. Its endothelium is high, effacing the lumen. The sheath consists of phagocytes with strands of extracellular reticulum running between them (see Fig. 15-26). The sheath is about 75 μm in diameter. The surrounding red pulp contains sinuses. The darkly stained free cells in the red pulp are granulocytes. One, in the left upper corner of the field, is crossing the wall of a sinus. Erythrocytes, which abound in red pulp, are unstained in this preparation. PAS-hematoxylin stain. ×650. (From L. Weiss, Amer. J. Anat., **111**:131, 1962.)

marginal zone. Soon thereafter lymphocytes move into the periarterial sheaths. By the end of the first half of gestation the periarterial lymphatic sheaths are well developed. In the latter half of gestation (by 200 mm) sinuses are present but the full development of their basement membrane and endothelium does not occur until after birth.

In the first trimester of pregnancy, the fetal spleen is erythropoietic and myelopoietic. These functions are preempted successively by the liver and the marrow. In mice, however, they may remain splenic, on a reduced level, through life, supplementing a fully hematopoietic marrow. In man, splenic erythropoiesis fades after the fifth prenatal month.

Comparative anatomy

Many differences exist between spleens of different species. The dog's spleen is a large organ, weighing more than 100 gm in a small dog. In a big rabbit the spleen may weigh only a few grams. In dogs and men the spleen is an ovoid structure in the left upper abdominal quadrant. In rabbits, rats, and mice it is a ribbon-like organ lying upon the greater curvature of the stomach. The capsule in the spleen of dogs, oxen, and armadillos is rich in muscle, whereas in man and rabbits little muscle is present. Vascular arrangements in the red pulp may be quite different from spleen to spleen. The

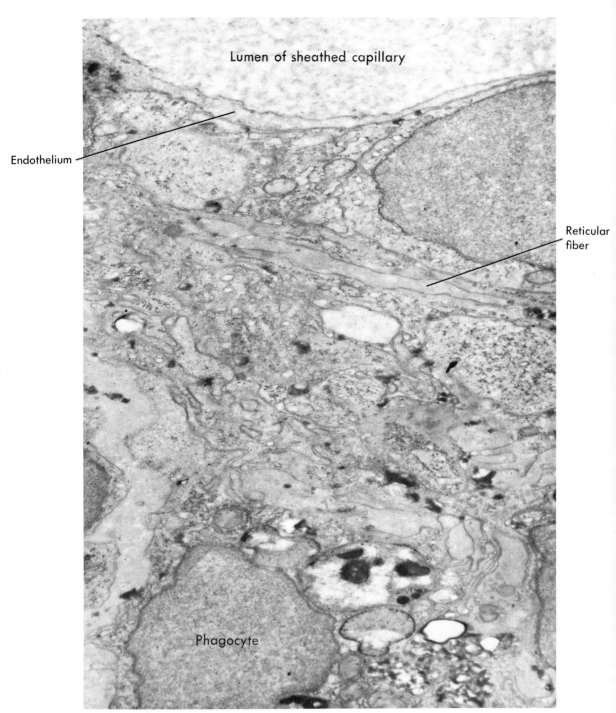

Lumen of sheathed capillary

Endothelium

Reticular fiber

Phagocyte

Figure 15-27 Spleen of a dog, sheathed capillary. In this electron micrograph, the endothelium is quite low. The surrounding cells constituting the sheath are enmeshed in extracellular reticulum. They are phagocytes and contain diverse phagocytic vacuoles. ×22,500. (From L. Weiss, Amer. J. Anat., **111:**131, 1962.)

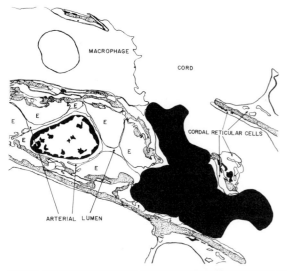

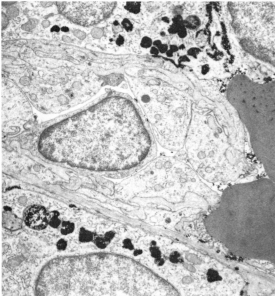

Figure 15-28   Spleen of a rabbit, red pulp.   An arterial vessel ends in a cord.   This vessel is typical of many terminating arterial vessels in red pulp.   It is a small arteriole.   Its endothelium (E in tracing) is high.   Its lumen and the surrounding red pulp contain Thorotrast, which was injected intravenously several minutes before splenectomy.   About two layers of extracellular reticulum (stippled in tracing) are present in the vessel wall.   The inner one underlies the endothelium and constitutes a basement membrane.   Portions of two macrophages lie above and below the vessel.   The vessel opens to the right, and several erythrocytes lie just outside the orifice.   ×18,000.   (From L. Weiss, Amer. J. Anat., **113**:51, 1963.)

sinuses of the spleen are well developed in man, rabbits, and dogs but not in cats and mice.   The spleen of dogs has large and well-developed ellipsoidal sheaths about terminal arterial capillaries. Rabbits have none.   Lymphatics are well developed and extensive in hedgehogs and men but not in rats.   Megakaryocytes are normally present in the spleen of mice but are absent in man.   The white pulp consists primarily of periarterial lymphatic sheaths in rabbits and rats, whereas in cats secondary lymphatic nodules are the major element of white pulp.   Any generalization about the circulation or function of the spleen is severely circumscribed by such species differences.

Figure 15-29   Spleen of human fetus, 42-mm crown-rump length (approximately 9 weeks gestational age).   The spleen at this stage consists primarily of a spongework of reticular cells containing vessels (a vein crosses this field).   See Figs. 15-30 and 15-31.   ×1,000.

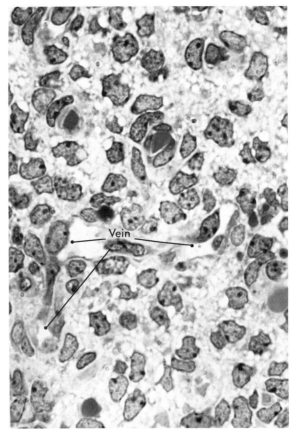

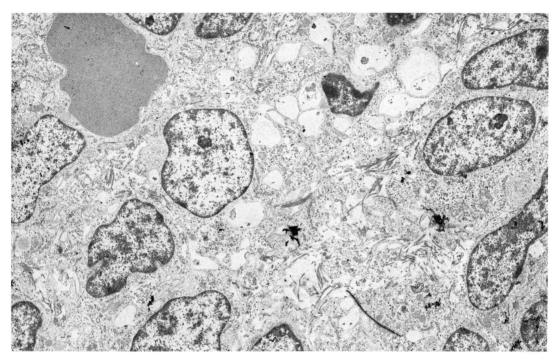

Figure 15-30   Spleen of human fetus, 42-mm crown rump length.   The primary reticulum is present as a relatively closed spongework of primitive reticular cells at this fetal stage.   Collagen fibrils lie between the reticular cells.   Free erythrocytes may be present in the reticular meshwork.   ×9,500.

Functions of the spleen

SEPARATION OF BLOOD CELLS AND PLASMA

Plasma is separated from cells in the splenic circulation, and so blood cells are unusually concentrated in the red pulp, as determined both by direct puncture of the spleen and by microscopic study of the living circulation.

The mechanism of separation depends upon muscular constriction of the splenic vein following sympathetic stimulation, and so plasma is forced out of sinuses and cords and picked up by the lymphatics. The lymphatics carry the plasma out of the spleen to the thoracic duct. Barcroft and Poole (1927) abolished the spleen's capacity to remove plasma by cutting its nerve supply.

Concentration of blood cells in the spleen enhances its storage function. In those animals having a heavily muscular capsule, such as dogs, a reserve mass of blood cells may be rapidly reintroduced into the circulation by adrenergic stimulation, which is followed by massive capsular contraction.

CLEARANCE OF BLOOD

The removal of certain elements of the blood and their consequent storage, phagocytosis, or transformation are major functions of the spleen.

Aged or damaged erythrocytes are sequestered or trapped in the vascular bed of the spleen. These erythrocytes are then phagocytized and, presumably within the macrophage, the ferrous and pigment portions of hemoglobin are separated. The iron is converted to a transport form, complexed to a plasma protein *transferrin,* and sent to bone marrow for reutilization in erythropoiesis. The pigment is ultimately converted to bile pigments.

Lymphocytes released from the marrow (B cells) and from the thymus (T cells) are received in the spleen and, with antigen that is also held in the spleen, interact to mount an immune response. Recirculating small lymphocytes (T cells) take a distinctive pathway through the spleen. They enter the periarterial lymphatic sheaths through venous sinuses of the marginal zone that abut the sheath. If not involved in an immune response, they pass through the sheath and probably leave the spleen through deep lymphatics. The periarterial sheath is quite rich in T cells and is, accordingly, recognized as a *thymic-dependent zone*.

Monocytes are sequestered in the white pulp, the marginal zone, or cords. They rapidly undergo conversion into macrophages. In traumatic shock, the circulating leukocytes may fall from a concentration of 10,000 per ml^3 of blood to 700 or fewer per ml^3. Many of these cells are removed from the circulation and are stored in the vascular spaces of the spleen. Perhaps 25 percent of the platelet

population is normally stored in the spleen. Under certain conditions, however, platelets may be trapped in the spleen with such avidity that there are too few in the circulation and hemorrhage results. Similarly, the spleen may remove slightly damaged but functionally competent erythrocytes with such zeal that an anemic crisis is precipitated.

In addition to the entrapment and subsequent processing of blood cells, the spleen removes particulate material from the blood. Thus, if carbon is injected intravenously, it is rapidly removed from the circulation by the spleen. The material is phagocytized in the sluggishly flowing blood in the cords or marginal zone. The capacity of the spleen to clear materials from the blood may be estimated by tagging such materials with radioactive isotopes, injecting them intravascularly, and determining the rate of accumulation of the isotope in the left upper quadrant of the abdomen by linear counters moved

Figure 15-31 Spleen of human fetus, 57-mm crown-rump length (approximately 10.5 weeks gestational age). The primary reticular meshwork has become much more open. A primitive sinus (S) is present. A granulocyte (gr) lies in the meshwork. ×9,000.

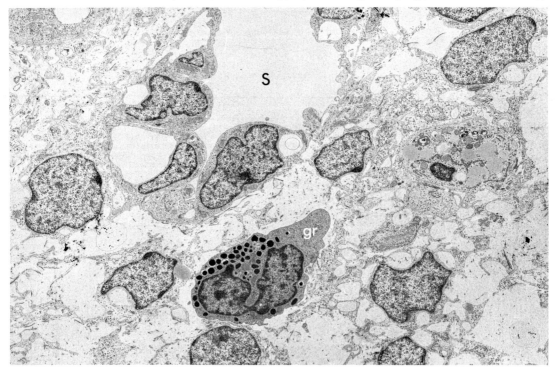

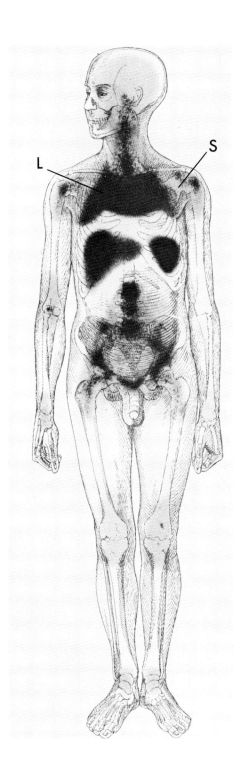

slowly over the surface of the body (Fig. 15-32).

The clearance of cells and particulate materials from blood is a function shared with the spleen by the lungs, liver, bone marrow, and other reticuloendothelial tissues. It is likely, however, that the capacity of the spleen for clearance, per gram of tissue, is greatest.

ANTIBODY PRODUCTION

The spleen is specialized for trapping blood-borne antigen and subsequent large-scale antibody production. It will, however, respond to antigen introduced by routes other than the blood since such antigen usually finds its way rapidly into the circulation.

Antigen is first trapped and then phagocytized by macrophages in the marginal zone. Subsequently it is held in and around the lymphatic nodules of white pulp. Within the nodules the antigen is trapped on the surface of cells which appear to be related to reticular cells.

In a primary response, antibody-producing cells, responding to certain "strong" antigens, appear first within the periarterial lymphatic sheath. They move to the periphery of the sheath and then, either through blood or lymph, are probably carried out of the spleen into the circulation. They rapidly find their way back to the spleen, however, and accumulate in marginal zone and red pulp cords. Thus, although red pulp is not the primary site of antibody formation, it may accumulate large numbers of plasma cells.

Somewhat after the periarterial response, the tempo varying with species, antigen, dose, and route of administration, large-scale antibody production by germinal centers begins and may dominate the picture. In secondary responses, as in lymph nodes, the germinal center response is almost immediate and large-scale. The germinal center houses "memory cells" primed for a secondary response. The cytology of antibody-producing cells is discussed in Chap. 14.

Figure 15-32 Reticuloendothelial system (RES). The RES has been imaged in a living patient by administering a radioactive colloid which is taken up by the phagocytes of this system. The liver (L), spleen (S), axial bones, and proximal parts of humeri and femora are visualized. (From P. McIntyre, Hosp. Pract., **6:**77, 1971.)

References

BARCROFT, J., and H. W. FLOREY: Some Factors Involved in the Concentration of Blood by the Spleen, *J. Physiol. (London)*, **66**:231 (1928).

BARCROFT, J., and L. T. POOLE: The Blood in the Spleen Pulp, *J. Physiol. (London)*, **64**:23 (1927).

BJÖRKMAN, S. E.: The Splenic Circulation. With Special Reference to the Function of the Spleen Sinus Wall, *Acta Med. Scand.*, (Suppl. 191) **128**:1 (1947).

GALINDO, B., and T. IMAEDA: Electron Microscope Study of the White Pulp of the Mouse Spleen, *Anat. Rec.*, **143**:399 (1962).

JANOUT, V., and L. WEISS: Deep Splenic Lymphatics in the Marmot: an Electron Microscopic Study, *Anat. Rec.*, **172**:197 (1972).

KLEMPERER, P.: The Spleen, in H. Downey (ed.), "Handbook of Hematology," vol. 3, Paul B. Hoeber, Inc., New York, 1938.

KNISELY, M. H.: Spleen Studies. I. Microscopic Observations of the Circulatory System of Living Unstimulated Mammalian Spleens, *Anat. Rec.*, **65**:23 (1936).

KOBOTH, I.: Über das Gitterfasergeriist der roten Milzpulpa mit einem Bertrag Zu ihrer Gefässtruktur und Blutdurchströmung, *Beitr. Path. Anat.*, **103**:11 (1939).

MALL, F. P.: On the Circulation through the Pulp of the Dog's Spleen, *Amer. J. Anat.*, **2**:315 (1902).

MILLS, E. S.: The Vascular Arrangements of the Mammalian Spleen, *Quart. J. Exp. Physiol.*, **16**:301 (1926).

SNOOK, T.: The Histology of Vascular Terminations in the Rabbit's Spleen, *Anat. Rec.*, **130**:711 (1958).

SNOOK, T.: A Comprehensive Study of the Vascular Arrangements in Mammalian Spleens, *Amer. J. Anat.*, **87**:31 (1950).

WEISS, L.: "The Cells and Tissues of the Immune System," Prentice-Hall, Inc., Englewood Cliffs, N.J., (1972).

WEISS, L.: The White Pulp of the Spleen: The Relationships of Arterial Vessels, Reticulum and Free Cells in the Periarterial Lymphatic Sheath, *Bull. Hopkins Hosp.*, **115**:99 (1964).

WEISS, L.: The Structure of Intermediate Vascular Pathways in the Spleen of Rabbits, *Amer. J. Anat.*, **113**:51 (1963).

WEISS, L.: The Structure of Fine Splenic Arterial Vessels in Relation to Hemoconcentration and Red Cell Destruction, *Amer. J. Anat.*, **111**:131 (1962).

chapter 16   Skin

JOHN S. STRAUSS
AND
A. GEDEON
MATOLTSY

The skin is an organ consisting of an epidermis and a dermis (Fig. 16-1). The former is of ectodermal and the latter is of mesodermal origin. The cutaneous appendages such as hair, nails, and sebaceous and sweat glands develop from germinative cells of the epidermis. The dermis primarily consists of collagen and elastic fibers, along with fibroblasts and other mesenchymal cells, blood vessels, lymphatics, and nerves. The pigment cells, which come from the neural crest, are primarily found in the epidermis and the hair. The primary function of the skin is to separate and protect the body from the environment. Most important is the protection that the skin provides against the loss of body fluids and the penetration of noxious agents into the body.

Epidermis

The epidermis is a protective tissue noted for its high structural stability and chemical resistance. It extends over the body as a continuous sheet about 0.1-mm thick. On the surface, horny ridges and valleys form characteristic patterns which are best seen on the palms and soles. At the base, numerous ridges interdigitate with dermal papillae. The epidermis consists of epithelial cells arranged in tightly bound layers (Figs. 16-2 and 16-3) along with scattered pigment cells and nerve endings, but no capillaries; the epidermis receives its nutrients by diffusion from the dermis.

With light microscopy, the epidermis can be divided into four cell layers, called (proceeding from the deepest layer to the surface) the strata basale, spinosum, granulosum, and corneum (Fig. 16-3). The stratum basale consists of a single row of basal cells which rest on the underlying dermis and have

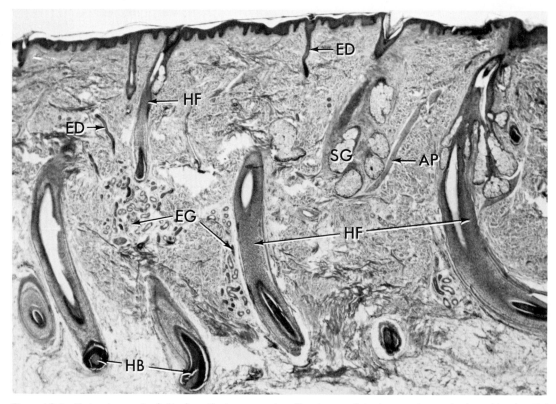

Figure 16-1   Photomicrograph of skin from the human scalp.   The dense cellular layer at the top is the epidermis.   Below this is the thick and compact connective tissue layer, the dermis.   At the bottom of the section some of the subcutaneous tissue is shown.   Several hair follicles (HF) are present.   In the larger follicles, the hair bulb (HB) with its dermal papilla is in the sub-cutaneous tissue.   An arrector pili (AP) muscle is present.   There are several sebaceous glands (SG).   Eccrine sweat glands (EG) and their ducts (ED) are also present.   ×30.

Figure 16-2   Photomicrograph of human skin from the interdigital space of the foot.   The epidermis (E) is relatively thick.   The portion of the dermis (D) that is shown is not compact and represents the pars papillaris.   Dermal papillae (DP) and their capillary loops (CL) are well developed.   ×220.

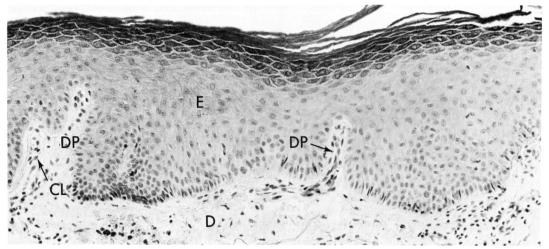

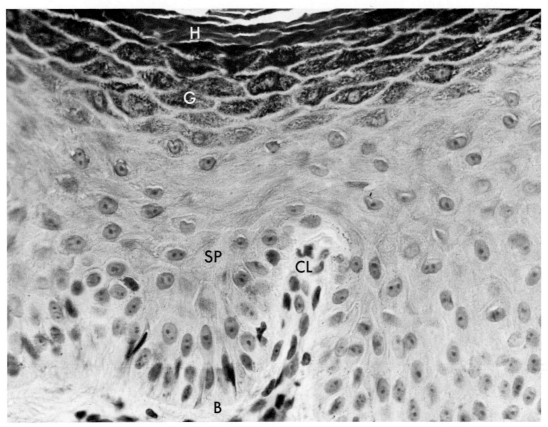

Figure 16-3   Higher magnification of Fig. 16-2, showing the basal (B), spinous (SP), granular (G), and horny (H) layers of the epidermis.   Note "prickles" between spinous cells.   Tonofibrils can be seen in both basal and spinous cells.   ×750.

large nuclei and relatively scant cytoplasm containing many tonofibrils.   The stratum spinosum is several layers of polyhedral spinous cells that become flattened as they approach the surface.   The spinous cells appear to be connected to one another by numerous intercellular bridges, the "prickles." The thickness of the stratum granulosum varies. The cells are flattened but larger than the spinous cells.   They contain the irregular granular material keratohyalin in their cytoplasm.   The stratum corneum is made up of a series of tightly packed, flat, amorphous-appearing cells.   On examination with a polarizing microscope, the stratum corneum shows positive double refraction with reference to the surface plane, indicating the presence of an ordered molecular structure in the horny material.

The tonofibrils also show double refraction, but keratohyalin granules are not birefringent.

In the electron microscope, the epidermis is seen separated from the dermis by a 50 to 70 nm thick basal lamina (Figs. 16-4 and 16-5) which is bound to the dermis by relatively short anchoring fibrils having a repeating band pattern of 70 to 120 nm (Fig. 16-5).   All the cells of the epidermis, except those of the stratum corneum, are limited by an ordinary trilaminar plasma membrane, which is usually straight and forms specialized structures, the desmosomes, at the attachment sites between adjacent epidermal cells (Fig. 16-6).   Each desmosome is composed of two dense plaques on opposing plasma membranes, intersected by a thin intracellular lamella.   Filaments converge upon the

Stratum
basale

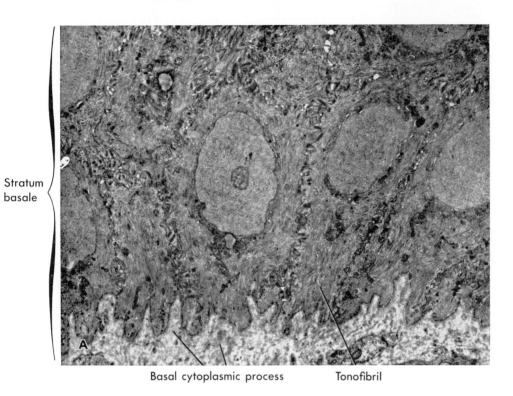

Basal cytoplasmic process   Tonofibril

Stratum
corneum

Stratum
granu-
losum

Stratum
spinosum

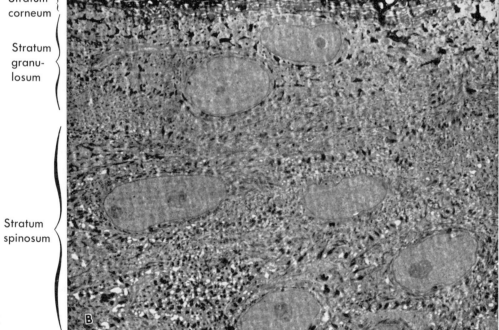

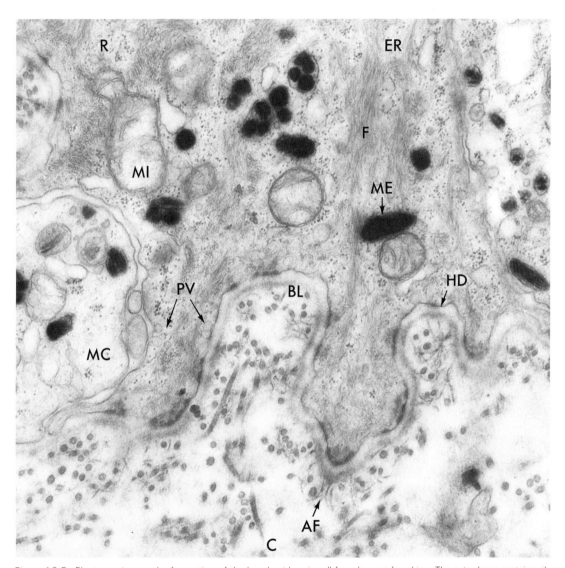

Figure 16-5 Electron micrograph of a portion of the basal epidermis cell from human foreskin. The cytoplasm contains ribosomes (R), endoplasmic reticulum (ER), mitochondria (MI), melanin granules (ME), abundant filaments (F), and pinocytotic vesicles (PV). The basal cell is attached to the basal lamina (BL) by half-desmosomes (HD). The basal lamina is bound to the dermis by anchor filaments (AF). Collagen fibrils (C) appear scattered in the dermis. On the left, a small portion of a melanocyte (MC) is shown with melanosomes, revealing different stages of maturation. ×37,000. (Courtesy of Dr. T. Huszar, Boston University School of Medicine.)

Figure 16-4 Electron micrographs from specimens of skin of man showing, in A, basal epidermal cells and, in B, the stratum spinosum, stratum granulosum, and stratum corneum. Tonofibrils are particularly apparent in the cytoplasm of the basal cells. Irregular basal cytoplasmic processes of basal epidermal cells are directed toward dermal connective tissue in the region of basement lamina. ×3,300.

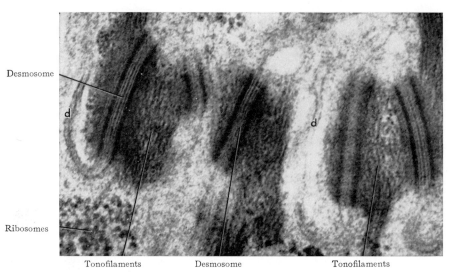

Desmosome

Ribosomes

Tonofilaments   Desmosome   Tonofilaments

Figure 16-6   Electron micrograph of the interface between two adjacent human epidermal cells showing details of demosomes. ×52,000.

dense plaques of desmosomes, but they do not cross between cells, as was once assumed from light microscopy. The desmosomes are numerous between adjacent epidermal cells and play an important role in the cohesiveness of the epidermis. Basal cells have many hemidesmosomes at their base, which provide a firm attachment to the basal lamina (Fig. 16-5).

The cytoplasmic matrix of the basal cells is relatively dense and contains many 60 to 80 Å filaments, either singly or in bundles scattered throughout the cytoplasm. Ribosomes are numerous and clustered; mitochondria are present in moderate numbers; and there are few Golgi vesicles and rough ER membranes. Pinocytotic vesicles are occasionally seen at the base of these cells (Fig. 16-5).

The spinous cells contain the same complement of organelles and inclusions as basal cells, along with new cytoplasmic components called lamellated granules or membrane-coating granules (Fig. 16-7). These ovoid granules vary in size from 0.1 to 0.5 μm. They are covered by a double-layered membrane and are filled with parallel lamellae

about 20 Å thick oriented along the short axis of the granule. Lamellated granules usually appear first in the vicinity of Golgi vesicles but later are seen throughout the cytoplasm.

Granular cells contain synthetic organelles and numerous filament bundles, lamellated and keratohyalin granules (Fig. 16-7), and occasional lysosomes. In these cells, the lamellated granules have migrated to the cell periphery or are discharged into the intercellular space with their lamellae spreading between the cells (Figs. 16-8 and 16-9). The keratohyalin granules, which are the distinguishing characteristic of the granular cells, may be round or irregularly shaped, and vary in size from submicroscopic to microscopic dimensions (Fig. 16-10). They are not membrane-bound, and their bulk consists of closely packed, amorphous, 20-Å particles. Filament bundles may pass across the entire length of the keratohyalin granules or be blended into their peripheral parts.

The horny cells are enveloped by a modified plasma membrane 150 to 200 Å thick (Fig. 16-8) whose outer layer is somewhat thickened, and whose inner layer is considerably widened by the

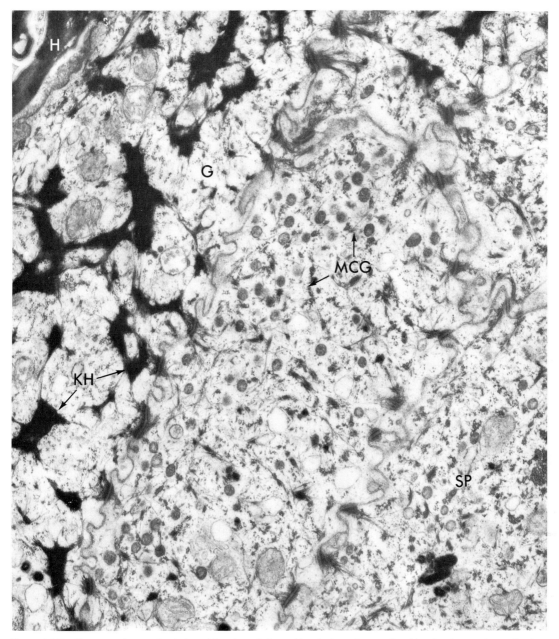

Figure 16-7   Electron micrograph of the midportion of the epidermis from human foreskin showing portions of spinous (SP), granular (G), and horny (H) cells. The rounded granules in the spinous cell are membrane-coating granules (MCG). The irregular bodies in the granular cell are keratohyalin granules (KH).   ×23,000.   (Courtesy of Dr. T. Huszar, Dept. of Dermatology, Boston University School of Medicine.)

deposition of an amorphous material. This modified membrane is highly convoluted and interdigitates with the membranes of adjacent cells. Desmosomes are present in a more or less preserved form. There are relatively few remnants of cell organelles in horny cells; they are mainly filled by 60 to 80 Å filaments embedded in an amorphous matrix (Fig. 16-11).

Functionally, basal cells correspond to reproductive cells, spinous and granular cells to differen-

Figure 16-8   Electron micrograph of mouse oral epithelium showing attachment of a membrane-coating granule to the plasma membrane prior to discharge (D) of its content into the intercellular space.   Discharged lamellae (L) appear in the intercellular space between adjacent granular and horny cells.   Note that the plasma membrane of the horny cell (TPM) is thickened, whereas that of the granular cell (PM) is normal.   ×18,000.   (Courtesy of A. G. Matoltsy and P. F. Parakkal, J. Cell Biol., 301:24, 1965.)

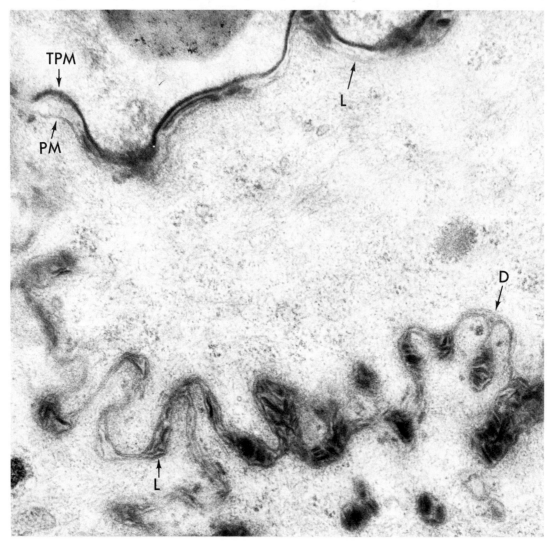

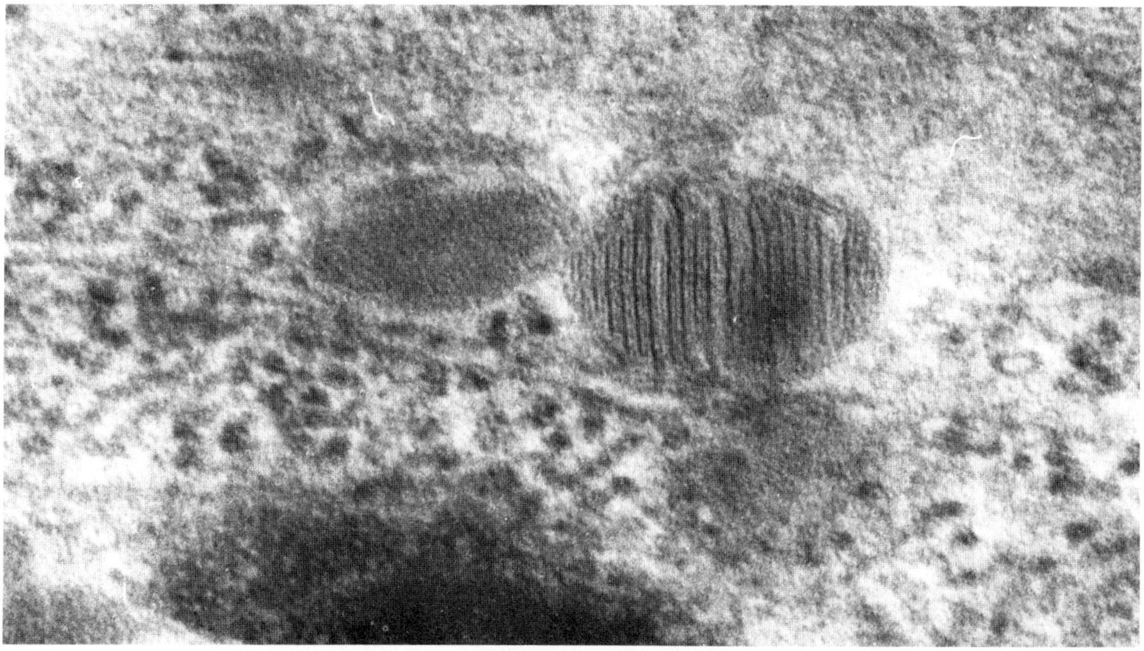

Figure 16-9   Electron micrograph of a membrane-coating granule showing the lamellar structure. ✕ 236,000. (Courtesy of A. G. Matoltsy and P. F. Parakkal, in A. G. Zelickson (ed.), ''Ultrastructure of Normal and Abnormal Skin,'' Lea & Febiger, Philadelphia, 1967.)

tiating cells, and horny cells to differentiated cells— that is, to the terminal products of the epidermis. The basal cells maintain the epidermis by mitosis, and for each division, a basal cell enters the course of differentiation. The differentiating cells abandon mitotic activity and form new products. They are constrained to a specific pathway, and subsequent events run their courses irreversibly. The differentiated cells are retained in the horny layer until they are lost into the environment by shedding. Thus, the life history of the cells shows that the epidermis is continuously self-renewing; mitotic reproduction below and desquamation at the surface are balanced to achieve a steady state. Renewal time varies among different species and within various body regions. In general, epidermal renewal takes 3 to 4 weeks in man.

Keratinization may be regarded as a form of epithelial cell differentiation consisting of a synthetic phase and a degradative stage. After mito-

sis, epidermal cells pass through these stages more or less independently (Fig. 16-12). During the synthetic stage, cytoplasmic components such as filaments, keratohyalin granules, and lamellated granules are formed in large numbers. These are largely proteins synthesized by ribosomes, and the Golgi system is probably involved in the formation of lamellated granules. After the differentiating cells become filled with such products, the lamellated granules are discharged into the intercellular space, and their remnants coat the surface of the cells. Subsequently, lysosomal enzymes degrade the synthetic organelles, but the filaments and keratohyalin remain unaffected. Concomitant changes in the plasma membrane result in the loss of degraded materials into the intercellular space. Ultimately, the remaining cell content, composed mainly of filaments and keratohyalin masses, consolidates into a fibrous-amorphous material and becomes encased by a thickened cell envelope.

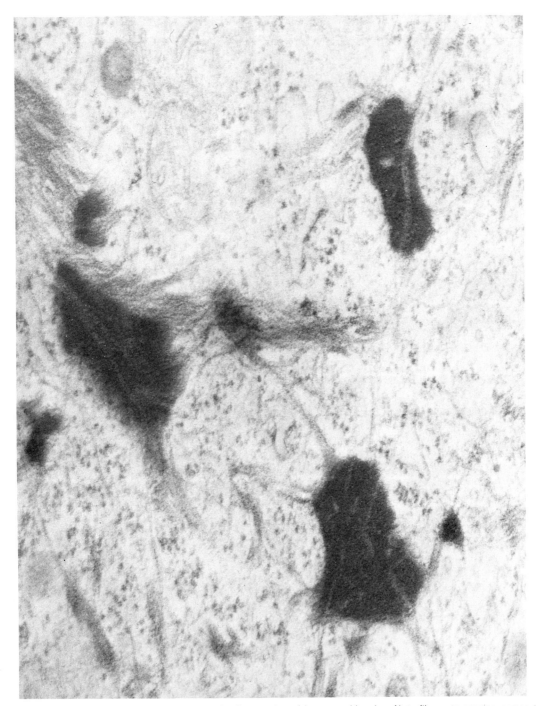

Figure 16-10 Electron micrograph of keratohyalin granules of human epidermis. Note filaments passing across the granules and attached to their surfaces. ×83,600 (Courtesy of R. M. Lavker and A. G. Matoltsy, J. Ultrastruct Res., **35**:575, 1971.)

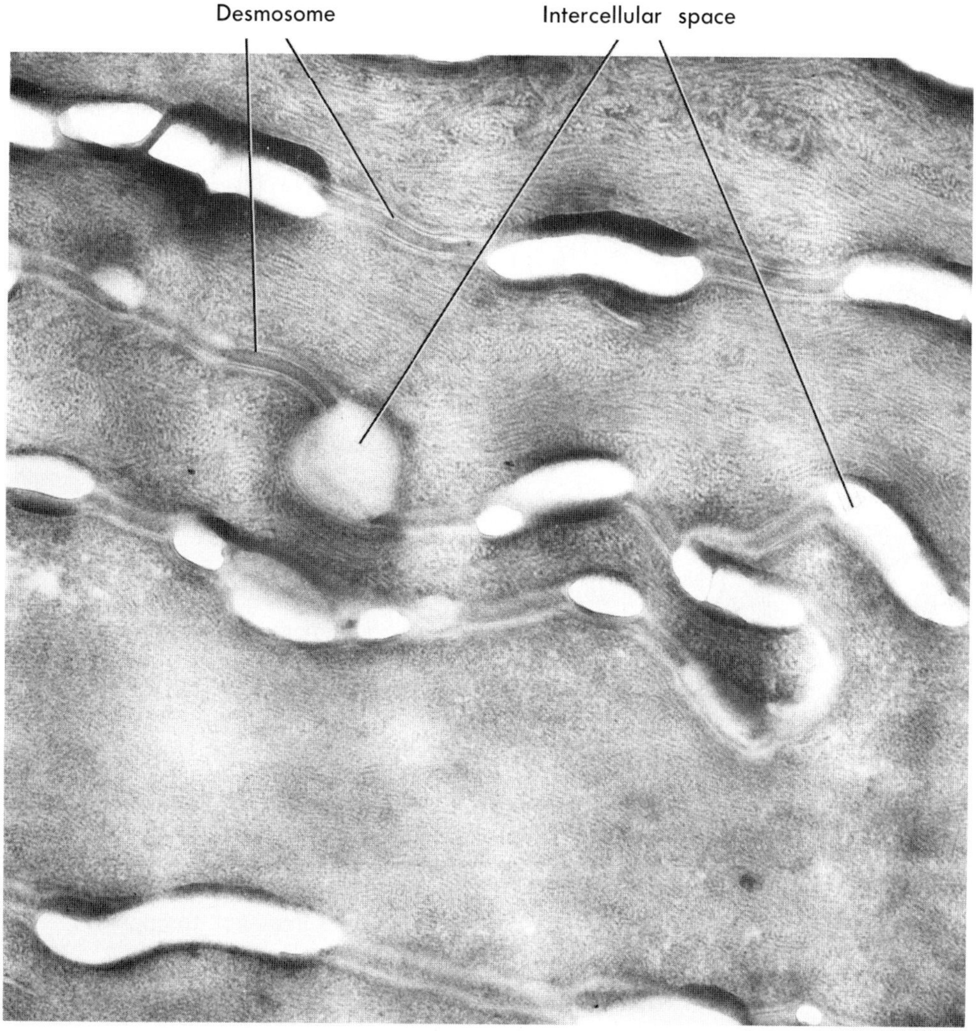

Figure 16-11   Portions of five cells of the stratum corneum of human epidermis.   In the cytoplasm there is a dense continuum enclosing low-density filaments.   The wide intercellular spaces represent artifacts.   ×65,000.

Thus, keratinization is a complex process, and the protective material formed may be regarded as being composed of three basic structural units: (1) 60 to 80 Å filaments (2) an amorphous horny matrix, and (3) a thickened cell envelope.

The structural stability and chemical resistance of the protective layer is primarily assured by large amounts of proteins containing sulfur, which are made relatively insoluble by covalent bonds between the polypeptide chains, such as disulfide cross-linkages between cysteine residues.   The filaments are a fibrous protein with a comparatively small amount of sulfur.   Segments of polypeptide chains forming this protein have a helical structure and are responsible for the α-keratin x-ray diffraction pattern given by the horny layer.   The matrix of the horny cells is composed of sulfur-rich amorphous proteins, including that originally contained by keratohyalin granules.   The association of sulfur-poor fibrous, and sulfur-rich amorphous, proteins in the

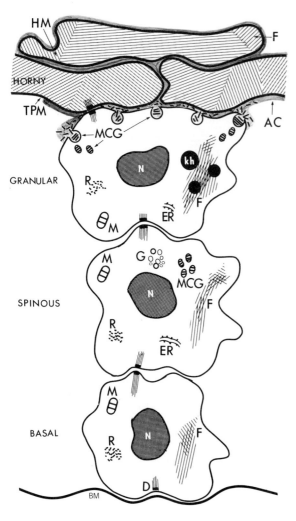

Figure 16-12 Schematic illustration of ultrastructural changes of a keratinizing epithelial cell: basement membrane (BM); desmosome (D); filament (F); ribosome (R); nucleus (N); mitochondrion (M); endoplasmic reticulum (ER); membrane-coating granule (MCG); Golgi complex (G); keratohyalin granule (KH), thickened plasma membrane (TPM); amorphous coat (AC); horny matrix (HM). (Courtesy of A. G. Matoltsy and P. F. Parakkal, in A. S. Zelickson (ed.), "Ultrastructure of Normal and Abnormal Skin," Lea & Febiger, Philadelphia, 1967.)

horny cell afford flexibility, elastic recovery, and structural stability of the protective layer. This protein complex is generally referred to as *keratin*. The most chemically resistant components of the horny layer are the thickened envelopes of horny cells which are in direct contact with the environment. These envelopes contain a sulfur-rich amorphous protein, lipids, and some carbohydrate. The protection offered by the epidermis is provided by the tightly packed and highly resistant horny layer formed by the keratinization process, but the stratum corneum as a whole acts as a barrier to the movement of material through the skin. There is no special portion of the stratum corneum which acts selectively as the barrier.

Nail

The nail is a rather rectangular horny plate which is attached to the nail bed, with its proximal end continuous with the nail matrix. Proximally and laterally, cutaneous folds cover the edges of the nail, with the underlying soft epithelial mass merging with the living part of the epidermis. The distal end of the nail plate extends over the dorsum of the distal phalanx of the fingers and toes. Between the epidermis and the distal end of the nail bed, a boundary called the *hyponychium* is formed. The nail is semitransparent and shows the color of the underlying blood vessel-rich tissues. Near the

proximal cutaneous fold is the whitish, semicircular portion of the nail called the lunula, which is the matrix of tightly packed epithelial cells from which the nail grows (Fig. 16-13). At the base of the matrix, deep ridges interdigitate with the dermal papillae. The cells of the deepest layer of the matrix are cylindrical; above them are several layers of polyhedral cells. Both cell types have a relatively large nucleus, and the cytoplasm contains tonofibrils. As the cells approach the surface, they become somewhat larger and flattened and contain more tonofibrils. A distinguishing characteristic of cellular differentiation in the nail is the absence of keratohyalin. The horny cells are flat and filled with a homogeneous-appearing material. The tonofibrils are birefringent, and the nail plate shows double refraction perpendicular to the direction of growth.

In the electron microscope, the nail matrix is seen separated from the dermis by a basal lamina similar to that separating the epidermis from the dermis. The fine structure of cylindrical and polyhedral matrix cells is comparable to that of basal cells of the epidermis. The cells of the higher layers do not contain lamellated granules or keratohyalin granules; instead, they possess abundant 60 to 80 Å filaments assembled into heavy bundles. The horny cells are enveloped by a thickened plasma membrane and filled with filaments embedded in an amorphous matrix. Desmosomes appear between all the cells of the matrix and horny cells of the nail plate.

The cylindrical matrix cells are reproductive cells which divide frequently and are responsible for continuous growth of the nail. The polyhedral and flattened matrix cells are differentiating cells which become filled with the fibrous-amorphous mass of insoluble proteins known as *nail keratin*. Nail keratin has a higher sulfur content than epidermal keratin, which probably explains its higher structural stability and chemical resistance.

The nail bed is continuous with the lower part of the matrix and is formed by layers containing cylindrical and polyhedral cells. Ridges of the nail bed penetrate deeply into the dermis and interdigitate with dermal papillae rich in blood vessels. The polyhedral cells do not reveal structural manifestations of differentiation; they appear as "resting" cells providing attachment and support for the growing nail plate.

Figure 16-13   Longitudinal section through distal digit of squirrel monkey showing characteristic nail structures: matrix (M); nail bed (NB); nail plate (NP); and, hyponychium (HN).   (Courtesy of Dr. N. Zaias, University of Miami, School of Medicine.)

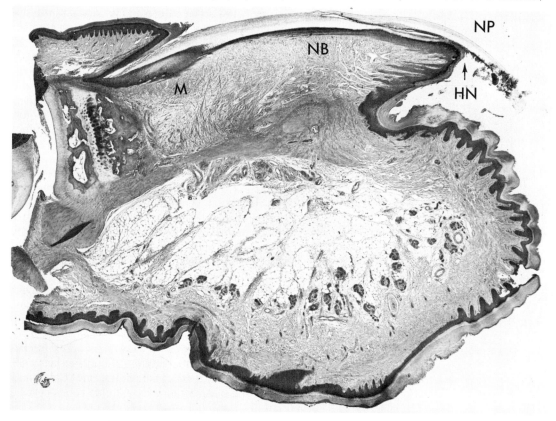

Hair

In man there are two basic types of hairs, the small, lightly pigmented *vellus hairs* which cover the entire body, and the larger, pigmented *terminal hairs.* Hairs are hardened epithelial fibers of various lengths and thicknesses emerging from a soft, bulb-shaped *follicle* residing in the dermis, although the bottoms of large hairs may be in the subcutaneous tissue. The neck of the follicle joins the epidermis, and its bottom is invaginated and filled with a dermal papilla rich in blood vessels (Fig. 16-14). The lower bulb-shaped portion, called the *matrix,* is the germinative center of the hair. Above the matrix, the emerging hair and concentric epithelial sheaths, such as the outer and inner root sheaths, appear (Fig. 16-15). The hair itself is composed of a cuticle, cortex, and medulla. The entire follicle is encased by a connective tissue sheath which is attached by one end to the papillary layer of the dermis by a band of smooth muscle fibers known as the *arrector pili muscle,* which can move the hair into a more vertical position (Fig. 16-1). The development of this muscle varies greatly. The sebaceous gland is connected to the upper part of the follicle by a short duct through which sebum is delivered into the follicular canal. In areas in which apocrine glands are found, they also are attached to the upper portion of the follicle.

The outer root sheath is continuous with the epidermis. At the junction it resembles the epidermis in structure but is distinguished from it by formation of glycogen, as glycogen normally is not seen in epidermal cells. Deeper in the follicle, the outer root sheath thins out and terminates as a single layer when it reaches the matrix area of the follicle. A horny layer is not normally formed by the outer root sheath; it consists only of layers comparable to the basal and spinous cell layers of the epidermis. In the electron microscope, the entire hair follicle is seen separated from the surrounding connective tissue sheath by a basal lamina which is continuous with the basal lamina of the epidermis. Matrix cells and outer root sheath cells are attached to this lamina by hemidesmosomes.

The matrix cells have a comparatively large nucleus which occupies most of the cell. The cytoplasm contains numerous ribosomes and a moderate number of mitochondria. Rough-surfaced ER is scanty, and there are relatively few Golgi vesicles. The plasma membranes of adjacent cells lie

Figure 16-14 Photomicrograph of a hair follicle from human scalp: papilla (P); matrix (MA); connective tissue sheath (CTS); inner root sheath (IRS); cuticle (CU); cortex (CO); medulla (ME); outer root sheath (ORS). ×160.

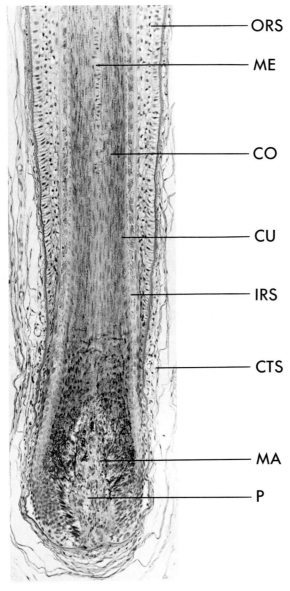

ORS

ME

CO

CU

IRS

CTS

MA

P

close and, at scattered points, are attached by desmosomes. There are only a few short filaments; they occur mainly near the desmosomes. The matrix cells divide more frequently than basal epidermal cells and produce four types of differentiating cells (Fig. 16-16). Those appearing in the periphery of the matrix form a circular multilayered *inner root sheath,* which desquamates as it reaches the skin surface. The more centrally located differentiating cells produce the cuticular, cortical, and medullary layers of the emerging hair. The medulla is poorly developed in man; human hairs essentially consist of a thin cuticle and a thick cortex.

Within the cytoplasm of various types of differentiating cells emerging from the matrix, various products are formed. The columnar inner root sheath cells first develop many 60 to 80 Å filaments which are packaged into tonofibrils. Later, small amorphous particles appear in the vicinity of the filament bundles; these are early forms of trichohyalin granules. The fully formed trichohyalin granules are comparable to keratohyalin granules of epidermal cells. After inner root sheath cells become filled with filaments and trichohyalin granules, the synthetic organelles disintegrate and the trichohyalin granules disperse. The remaining cell contents become condensed, and a filament-matrix complex is formed. The cell envelope thickens, and the widened intercellular spaces are filled with an amorphous substance.

The cuticular cells contain only a few filaments; their cytoplasm is filled with 300 to 400 Å granules

Figure 16-15 Photomicrograph of midportion of the hair follicle from human scalp: medulla (ME); cortex with melanin granules (CO); cuticle (CU); inner root sheath (IRS); outer root sheath (ORS). ×750.

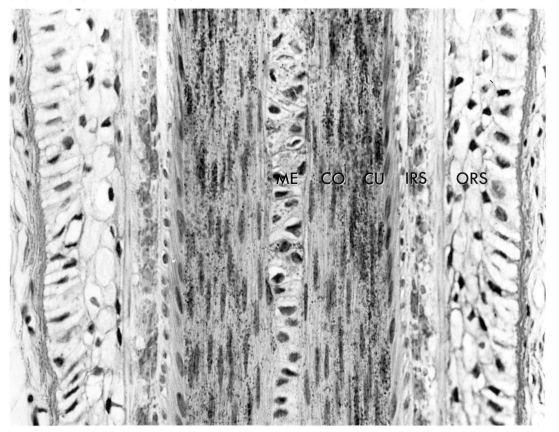

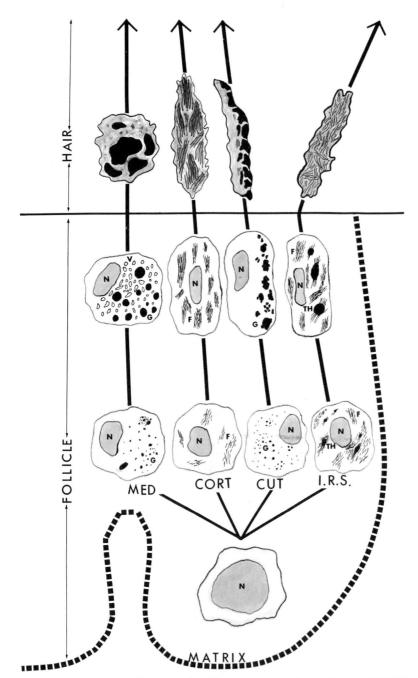

Figure 16-16 Schematic illustration of cell lines arising from the matrix of the hair follicle. Differentiation products, observable in the electron microscope, are shown. Medulla cells (MED) form abundant amorphous granules (G) and vesicles (V), which are ultimately filled with large masses of amorphous material. Cortical cells (CORT) develop many filaments (F) and terminally contain a filament-amorphous matrix complex. Cuticular cells (CUT) contain small amorphous granules (G) which coalesce and accumulate at the cell periphery facing the hair surface. Inner root sheath cells (IRS) form both filaments (F) and trichohyalin granules (TH). Terminally, the horny cells are filled with a filament-amorphous matrix complex.

which are not observable in the light microscope. The granules are not limited by a membrane, and they grow both by continuous deposition of an amorphous material and by coalescence. Cuticular cells are mainly filled with this amorphous material when they elongate, overlap, and form the outer layer of the hardening hair fiber.

The differentiating cortical cells, which are the structural cells of the hair, develop many 60 to 80 Å filaments which are assembled into heavy bundles. As these cells assume a spindle shape and form the cortex of the emerging hair fiber, they become filled with filaments between which an amorphous matrix is deposited.

The medullary cells, which are few in number, develop spherical granules 300 to 500 Å in diameter. These granules grow extensively and may reach dimensions of several micrometers. The granules eventually coalesce, and an amorphous mass fills the cell in the medulla of the hair.

As in the epidermis, the keratinization process may be divided into a synthetic phase and a degradative stage. Keratinization of the hair, however, is more complicated than in the epidermis, since the matrix forms four different cell types, each of which ultimately changes into a structurally and chemically different horny cell. The factors which induce and direct the various differentiative pathways are not understood. Chemical studies indicate that the keratinized inner root sheath cells and cortical cells are filled with a sulfur-poor fibrous protein and a sulfur-rich amorphous protein. The fibrous protein makes these cells birefringent and produces the α-keratin x-ray diffraction pattern given

by the hair fiber. Cornified cuticular cells contain a sulfur-rich amorphous protein, and medullary cells an amorphous protein with little or no sulfur.

The hair does not grow continuously as the nail does; it is lost and renewed periodically. Hair loss begins when matrix cells cease dividing, so that new cells no longer start to differentiate, and the differentiation process runs its course within cells which have already started. Soon all cells which have left the matrix undergo keratinization in situ and form a club-like mass attached to the hair. Such *club* or *telogen hairs* (Fig. 16–17) lack firm anchorage to the scalp and can be easily plucked from the follicle. These are the hairs that form the normal defluvium of the scalp. Normally about 5 percent of the scalp hairs are in telogen. During the rest period, many matrix cells become atrophic, and the follicle is rebuilt by a relatively small number of matrix cells. The growing hair, known as an *anagen hair* (Figs. 16-1 and 16-14), is firmly attached to the follicle by the root sheaths and is not easily dislodged. The thickness at the bulb determines hair thickness—the larger the bulb, the more mitotic activity there is and the thicker the hair produced. The length of the growth period determines the ultimate length of the hair. Thus, scalp hairs have a very long anagen phase, whereas the vellus hairs have a short anagen phase. Growth and rest progress in cycles, and in man each hair follicle has a different growth and rest period, so the follicles are independent of each other. In rodents, hair grows in successive waves over the body, and the duration of growth and rest is remarkably constant.

Melanocytes

In ordinary histologic sections the melanocytes appear as somewhat shrunken, clear cells intermixed among the basal cells. The best way to identify the melanocytes is to incubate the skin in the precursor of melanin, dopa (dihydroxyphenylalanine) (Fig. 16-18). This method demonstrates the enzyme tyrosinase which is necessary for the formation of melanin. The morphologic characteristics of the melanocytes are best seen in whole mounts of the epidermis stripped from the underlying dermis. Under these circumstances they appear as

a network of dendritic cells (Fig. 16-19) whose processes fan out in all directions.

On electron-microscopic examination the melanocytes are easily distinguished by the absence of filaments or desmosomes, and the presence of large amounts of rough ER, prominent Golgi zones, and melanosomes in various stages of development (Fig. 16-20). Melanosomes first appear near the Golgi membranes as tyrosinase-positive vesicles, which then develop into elliptical membrane-limited organelles measuring approximately 0.7 × 0.3

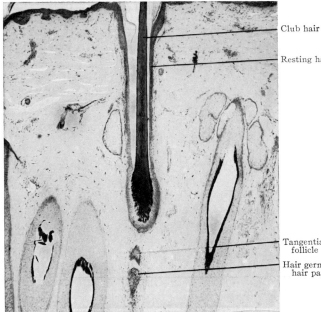

Club hair

Resting hair follicle

Tangential section of active follicle

Hair germ and its potential hair papilla

Figure 16-17   Club hair in resting follicle in human scalp.   Compare this with active growing follicles shown in Figs 16-1 and 16-14.   ×40.

μm. (The size and shape vary somewhat in various genotypes.)   They have a characteristic internal structure consisting of concentrically arranged dense sheets oriented along the long axis of the organelles. The melanosomes gradually fill up with melanin and protein and migrate into the dendritic processes of the melanocytes, from which they can then be transferred to the neighboring epidermal cells.

The combination of a melanocyte and its adjoining epidermal cells is called an *epidermal melanin unit*. The melanocyte is the factory which provides the epidermal cells with their melanin. This melanin is carried up to the surface and desquamates with the horny cells. The melanocytes are always in the basal layer, but some clear cells may be seen higher in the epidermis. These cells, called *Langerhans' cells*, used to be considered effete melanocytes which eventually are desquamated with the cells of the stratum corneum, but since they have also been found in hystiocytic tumors, their origin and function are still not well understood.

The melanocytes are distributed throughout the skin, although there are great regional variations. There may be as many as 2,000 melanocytes per mm² in the face but only half as many on the trunk. The genital skin also contains a large number of melanocytes. The melanocytes come from the neural crest; they migrate to the dermis during embryonic life and invade the epidermis, so some melanocytes may be found in the dermis.

The epidermal melanin unit is responsible for skin color and plays a major role in the protection of the body from ultraviolet radiation. When darkening of the skin occurs after ultraviolet exposure, there is an increase in the degree of melanization of the melanosomes and an increase in the number of melanosomes that are transferred to the epidermal cells. Racial differences in color are also due to the degree of melanization of the melanosomes and the degree of transfer of these melanosomes to epidermal cells, rather than to the number of melanocytes that are present. The grouping of the melanosome complexes may also be responsible for some of the color differences. In Cauca-

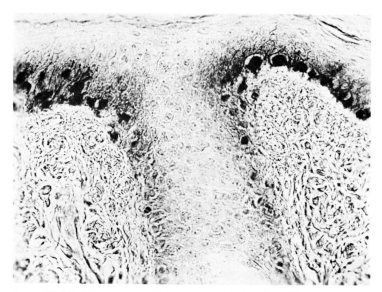

Figure 16-18   Thick section of human retroauricular skin.   The darkly stained, dendritic melanocytes in the basal layer are demonstrated in this dopa-treated section.   The melanocytes are somewhat shrunken and surrounded by a clear halo.   × 330. (Courtesy of Dr. G. Szabó, Harvard University.)

soids and Mongoloids the melanosomes may be grouped, although in others, such as in Negroids and Australoids, they are usually dispersed in the epidermal cells.

Melanocytes are present in the hair matrix. Their activity varies with the hair cycle. During telogen the melanocytes are hard to recognize because they are present as "clear" cells, but soon after anagen starts, they become demonstrable with the dopa reaction. They are strongly dopa-positive and become filled with melanized melanosomes. Toward the end of the anagen period, they transfer their pigment to the cortical cells.

Hair color is determined by both the number of melanosomes present in the cells of the hair shaft (black or blond hair) and by chemical alterations of the black melanin pigment, eumelanin, to sulfur-containing, reddish pheomelanin.

Dermis

The dermis, or corium, is the thick, dense connective tissue layer which extends from the epidermis to the fatty, areolar subcutaneous tissue (Fig. 16-1). It is in this connective tissue stroma that the cutaneous appendages as well as the blood vessels, lymphatics, and nerves are embedded. The dermis can be subdivided into the upper part which is in contact with the epidermis (the *pars papillaris*) and the thicker, denser *pars reticularis*. The papillary layer extends up into the spaces between the epidermal rete ridges (Fig. 16-2). These are the dermal papillae, which are best developed on the palms and soles. Along the border between

the epidermis and the dermis there is a PAS-positive layer generally referred to as the *basement membrane*. The collagen fibers of the papillary dermis are arranged in thin bundles in a loose network. In contrast, the collagen of the reticular dermis is arranged in much thicker bundles. Below, the reticular dermis merges along a rather indistinct border with the subcutaneous tissue, an areolar area containing considerable fatty tissue. The connective tissue of the subcutaneous area merges with, and is continuous with, that of underlying tissues.

In addition to collagen fibers the dermis contains a dense network of elastic fibers (Figs. 16-21 and

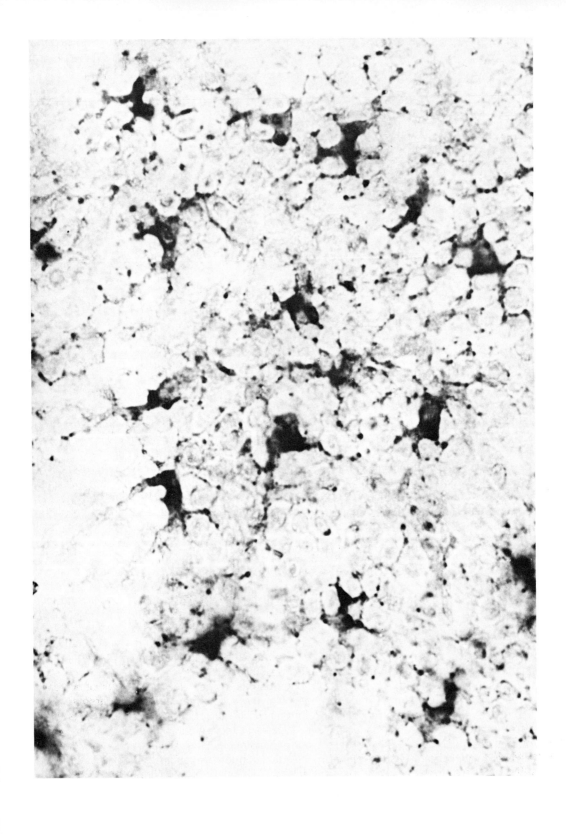

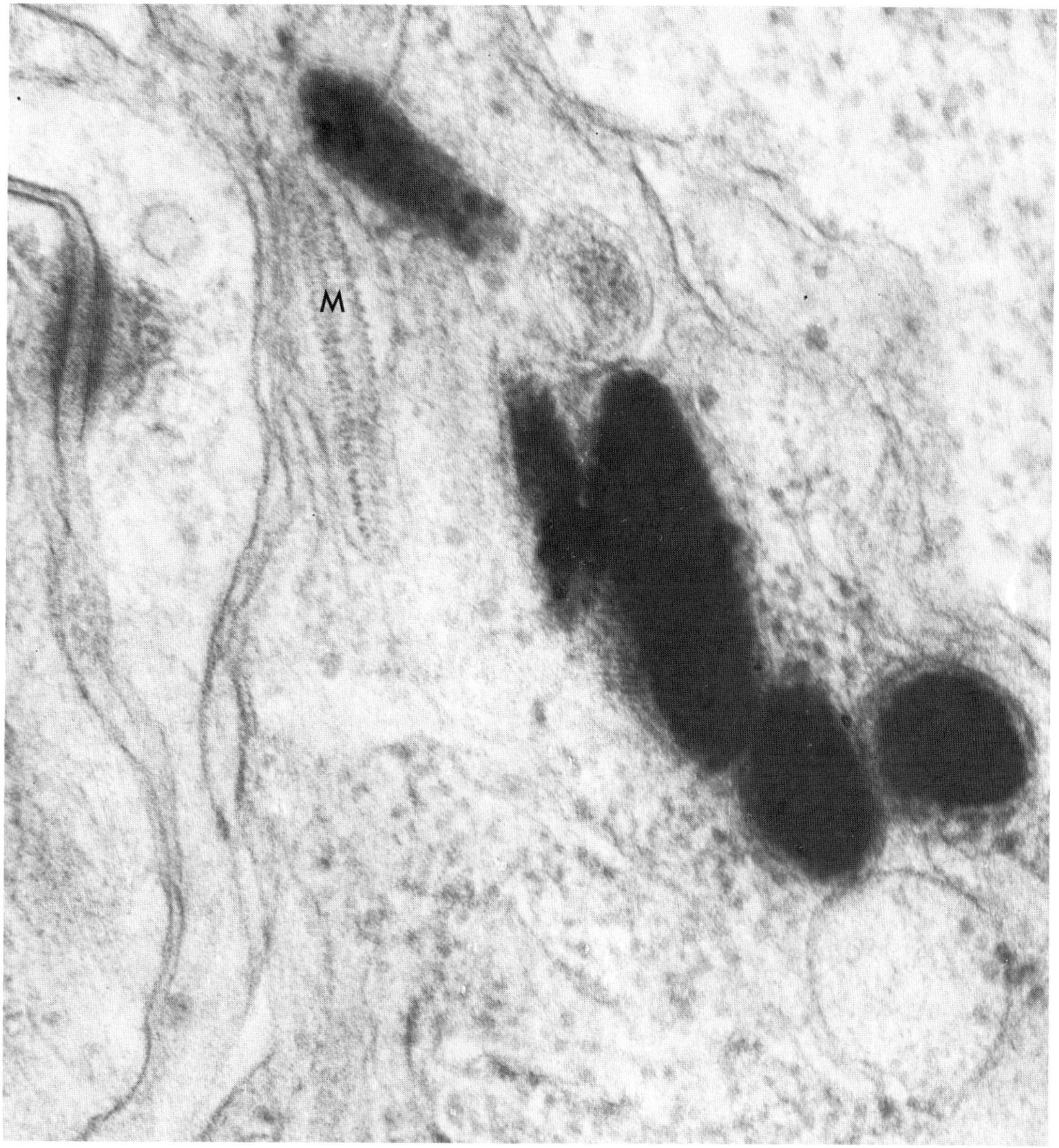

Figure 16-20   Electron micrograph of a portion of a human melanocyte and the adjacent epidermal cells.   In addition to the fully melanized, dark-staining melanosomes, a fully formed unmelanized melanosome is present (M).   The internal structure is well illustrated.   ×105,000.   (Courtesy of Dr. G. Szabó, Harvard University.)

Figure 16-19   Epidermal sheet from human thigh skin, prepared by treating the exised skin with trypsin.   The epidermal sheet was incubated in dopa.   The melanocytes, with many dendritic processes which project between the basal cells of the epidermis, are easily seen.   The melanocyte density in this location is $720 \pm 45/mm^2$.   ×1,000.   (Courtesy of Dr. G. Szabó, Harvard University.)

deep network supply the fat lobules, the sweat glands, some of the deep sebaceous glands, and the hair bulbs, which are surrounded by a rich network of capillaries. A capillary loop ascends into the dermal papilla of the hair. The capillary bed around the sweat glands is also very well developed. Vessels from the superficial plexus supply vessels for the more superficial portion of the cutaneous appendages. From this same plexus, numerous small vessels ascend into each of the dermal papillae to provide the blood supply for the epidermis (Fig. 16-3), although no vessels actually enter the epidermis.

The venous side of the cutaneous vascular tree is like the arterial supply, with two anastomosing arcades in the superficial and deep dermis. Furthermore, in certain areas such as the tips of the fingers and toes, there are direct arterial-venous shunts which help to regulate temperature by shunting blood away from the peripheral capillary

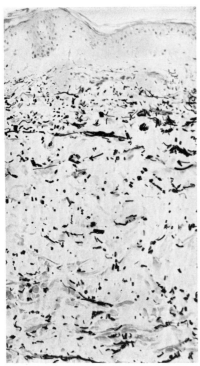

Figure 16-21 Verhoeff stain of human abdominal skin. The elastic fibers are darkly stained. The elastic fibers in the pars papillaris are thinner. ×120.

16-22) that are thinner in the region of the PAS-positive basement membrane (Fig. 16-22). Interspersed between the fibrous components of dermis is the ground substance which contains acidic glycosaminoglycans (hyaluronic acid and chondroitin sulfate). The metachomasia of the glycosaminoglycans is most prominent in the papillary layer near the basement membrane. There are numerous mast cells in the dermis, as well as connective tissue cells such as macrophages and fibroblasts. These cellular components also are more numerous in the papillary dermis.

The blood vessels of the skin are restricted to the dermis. The larger vessels lead to a deep anastomosing network, the cutaneous plexus, from which vessels ascend to the upper dermis where there is another anastomosing network, the sub-papillary plexus (Fig. 16-23). Vessels from the

Figure 16-22 Verhoeff stain of human skin of the sole. The thin elastic fibers of the pars papillaris are well illustrated. × 350.

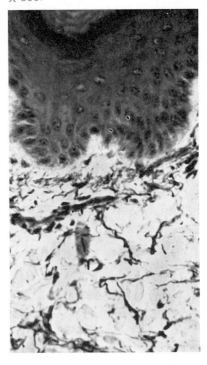

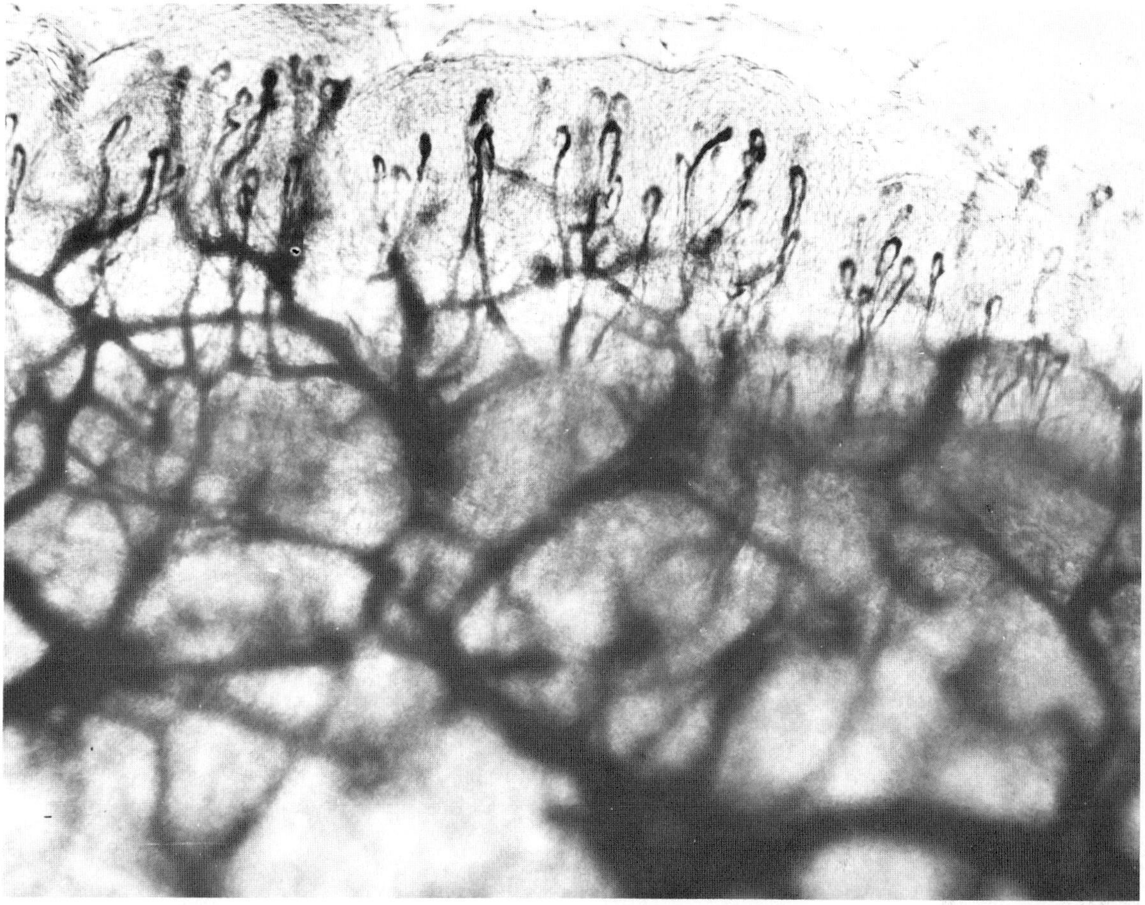

Figure 16-23 Oblique section of the dorsum of the human toe prepared after India ink injection, demonstrating the subpapillary venous plexus together with some of its tributory capillaries. ×110. (Courtesy of R. K. Winkelmann, S. R. Scheen, R. A. Pyka, and M. B. Coventry, in W. Montagna and R. A. Ellis (eds.), "Blood vessels and Circulation," Advances in Biology of Skin, vol. 2, Pergamon, New York, 1961.)

bed where heat loss occurs through radiation and convection. The condition of the vascular bed, as well as the oxygenation of its contained hemoglobin, is an important determinant of skin color.

The dermis also contains a lymphatic collection system which drains to the regional lymph nodes. It, too, is arranged in a superficial and a deep plexus, corresponding with those of the vascular tree.

The skin, which is richly provided with nerve fibers, is an important sensory organ. Studies based upon comparative anatomy would indicate that there are specialized nerve endings for touch, pain, and pressure, but the function of such specialized organs in the human being is open to question, and all sensation may depend upon the distribution of free nerve endings, some of which penetrate into the epidermis. Nerve networks are also found around the various cutaneous appendages and the blood vessels. The capillary loops do not contain any nerves, but the nerves of the arteriovenous anastomosis are well developed and obviously extremely important.

The glands of the skin

The human skin contains three glandular structures. The *sebaceous glands* produce a lipid end product through a process of holocrine secretion in which the entire differentiated cell, after undergoing lipid differentiation, is discharged into the excretory stream. These glands, as well as the apocrine sweat glands, are an integral part of the pilosebaceous apparatus. *Apocrine sweat glands,* found in specialized areas, secrete a milky material. Although the development of these glands is restricted in man, phylogenetically they are extremely important glands which produce territorial marking substances and sexual attractants. In contrast, the third type of gland, the *eccrine sweat gland,* is found in only limited areas in lower animals but is distributed over almost the entire body in man. As man has lost his hair overcoat, they have assumed an important thermoregulatory role. The eccrine sweat glands develop independently of the other epidermal appendages, all of which are grouped together in the *pilosebaceous unit.*

THE SEBACEOUS GLANDS

In man, sebaceous glands are found over the entire body surface, except for the palms, soles, and dorsum of the feet. The sebaceous glands are an integral part of the pilosebaceous apparatus and empty into the follicular canal through a short duct. However, in the mucous membranes, they open directly to the surface. Sebaceous glands not associated with hairs may also be found at the mucocutaneous junction. In the eyelids, large sebaceous glands, the *meibomian glands,* are found.

The sebaceous glands are relatively small over most of the body and usually are found in a density of less than 100 per cm^2 of body surface. The glands of certain areas such as the face and scalp are much larger and more numerous, with a density of up to 800 glands per cm^2. These large glands are hormone-dependent, being stimulated by androgens, so they make their appearance at the time of puberty, and in elderly individuals they may atrophy. There is no relationship between sebaceous gland size and hair size. The largest glands occur in specialized pilosebaceous units called *sebaceous follicles* which have a small vellus hair

and a widely dilated follicular canal. The orifice of such follicles is visible as the ''pore'' seen on the face.

Regardless of size, all sebaceous glands have the same structure (Fig. 16-24). The duct is a transitional zone between the follicular canal and the lipid-producing cells of the individual sebaceous acinus. Therefore, although a granular layer is present at the junction with the follicular canal, it disappears below, and there is an abrupt transformation to lipid-producing cells. The outermost cells of the acinus, the basal cells, rest on a basal lamina comparable to that of the epidermis. The basal cells are the germinative cells of the gland. They are small, flattened or cuboidal, and densely basophilic. Usually there is only one layer of basal cells. It may be thrown into folds so that there are invaginations into the center of the acinus. As the cells proceed toward the center of the acinus, there is a progressive accumulation of lipid. The cells become ladened with lipid droplets so their basophilic cytoplasm becomes compressed into a fine reticulated pattern. The cells enlarge greatly, their nuclei become distorted and disintegrate, and eventually the cells rupture, thus forming sebum, the lipid product of the glands.

In the electron microscope three types of cells are demonstrated. The peripheral (basal) cells contain abundant smooth and rough ER, free ribosomes, glycogen particles, mitochondria, and 60 to 80 Å filaments (Fig. 16-25). Filaments are most prominent in the desmosomal regions. A Golgi zone is present, but there are very few lipid droplets in the basal cells. The partially differentiated cell may have a highly convoluted plasma membrane. Its cytoplasm contains more smooth endoplasmic reticulum, and there are membrane-limited lipid droplets of various sizes (Fig. 16-25). It is believed that both the Golgi apparatus and the smooth ER contribute to the formation of lipid droplets.

In the fully differentiated cell the nucleus is irregular in shape, with clumped chromatin, and the nucleolus becomes dispersed (Fig. 16-26). The entire cell is occupied by large lipid droplets which compress the cellular remnants into thin strands that seem to surround the droplets.

Sebum is a complex mixture of lipids, including

a large proportion of triglycerides which undergo lipolysis in the follicular canal and liberate free fatty acids. Wax esters and squalene are also prominent in sebum, but there is very little, if any, sterol. However, the lipid recovered from the surface of the skin consists of sebum plus lipids formed by the epidermal cells. Sterols are present in the surface film and they are believed to be of epidermal origin. Lipid collected from the surface of the face, where the glands are large, is predominantly from

Figure 16-24   Sebaceous acinus from the human face. The basal cells (BC) appear as small, dark-staining peripheral cells. As lipid differentiation occurs, the cells enlarge and become foamy. Ruptured cellular remnants appear in the secretory stream (SS) in the region of the sebaceous duct (SD). Dark-staining areas in the center of the acinus are fibrous tissue trabelculae (FT). ×180.   (Courtesy of J. S. Strauss and P. E. Pochi, in O. Gans and G. K. Steigleder (eds.), "Normale und Pathologische Anatomie der Haut I," Springer-Verlag, Berlin, 1967.)

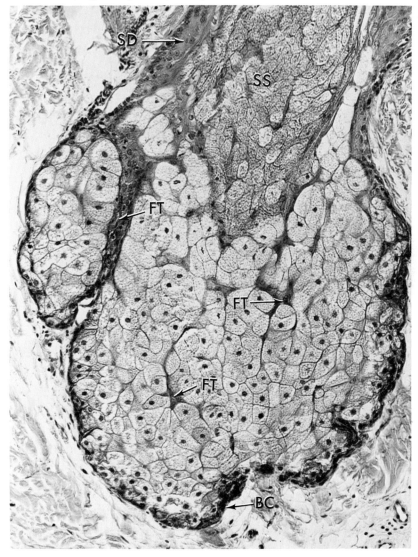

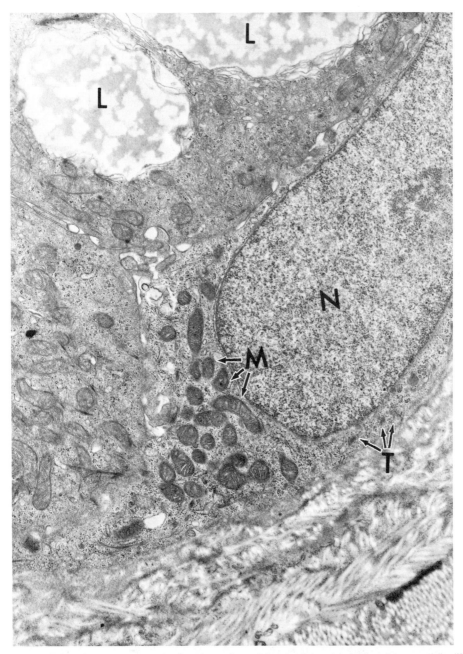

Figure 16-25 Electron micrograph of portions of a peripheral cell (on the right) and two partially differentiated sebaceous cells (on the left and above). A portion of the dermis is present in the lower portion of the picture. The peripheral cell has a large nucleus (N) and scant cytoplasm. The cytoplasm contains endoplasmic reticulum, ribonucleoprotein particles, glycogen, tonofilament (T), and mitochondria (M). Microvilli are prominent at the cellular junctions. Lipid droplets (L) are present in the partially differentiated cells.   ×10,600.   (Courtesy of J. S. Strauss and P. E. Pochi, in O. Gans and G. K. Steigleder (eds.), "Normale und Pathologische Anatomie der Haut I," Springer-Verlag, Berlin, 1967.)

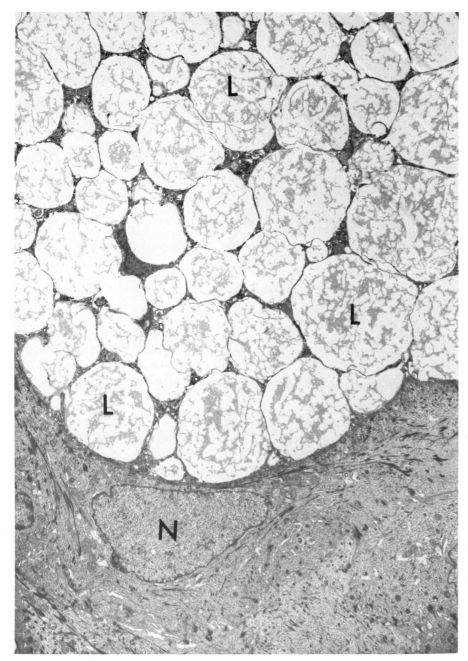

Figure 16-26 Electron micrograph of a fully differentiated sebaceous cell in the region of the sebaceous duct. The duct cell is darkly stained with a prominent nucleus (N). Lipid droplets (L) completely fill the differentiated cell. ×3,400. (Courtesy of J. S. Strauss and P. E. Pochi, in O. Gans and G. K. Steigleder (eds.), "Normale und Pathologische Anatomie der Haut I," Springer-Verlag, Berlin, 1967.)

sebaceous glands, whereas that derived from other areas has a greater percentage of epidermal lipid.

The functions of sebum are not well understood. It has not been shown to be a part of the skin barrier, nor to have any significant role in keeping the skin soft and supple. Although it has some antibacterial and antifungal activity, these effects do not appear to be very significant.

APOCRINE SWEAT GLANDS

Apocrine sweat glands are found over the entire skin surface of many lower animals, but in man they are restricted to certain areas such as the axilla, the anogenital region, the mammary areola, the ear canal (ceruminous glands), and the eyelid (glands of Moll), with scattered single glands found elsewhere on the body. Apocrine sweat glands are simulated by sexual hormones, and therefore appear at puberty, as do the sebaceous glands.

The apocrine glands are large, branched, tubular structures which open into the upper portion of the follicular canal by a relatively straight duct (Fig. 16-27). In sections containing both eccrine and apocrine glands, the differences are easily recognized. The apocrine glands are large enough to be seen without magnification in excised specimens from gland-rich areas such as the axilla. Their tubules have a single type of eosinophilic secretory cell which may be either cuboidal or columnar and whose nucleus, which is round and contains a prominent nucleolus, is located in the basilar portion of the cell. Secretory droplets accumulate in the more columnar cells and are probably discharged directly into the widely dilated canal. These secretory droplets have been seen by electron microscopy. In the past it has been assumed that the luminal portion of the cell was actually pinched off and discharged ("apocrine secretion"), but this is probably an erroneous concept resulting from a fixation artifact. Myoepithelial cells surround the secretory cells. The duct of these glands is straight and empties into the follicular canal. The ductal portion of the apocrine sweat gland is difficult to distinguish from the eccrine sweat gland duct.

The secretory product of the apocrine sweat gland is a milky product which may contain chromogens. In contrast to eccrine sweat, the secretory product contains protein. The apocrine glands respond to stimuli such as fright and pain, but not

Figure 16-27   Apocrine glands from the axilla of adult human being. In addition to the large secretory acini (a) containing cells of varying height, a portion of the small duct (b) is included. The elongated nuclei (c) of the myoepithelial cells can be visualized along the periphery of the secretory cells.   ×200.

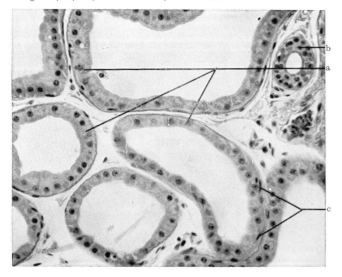

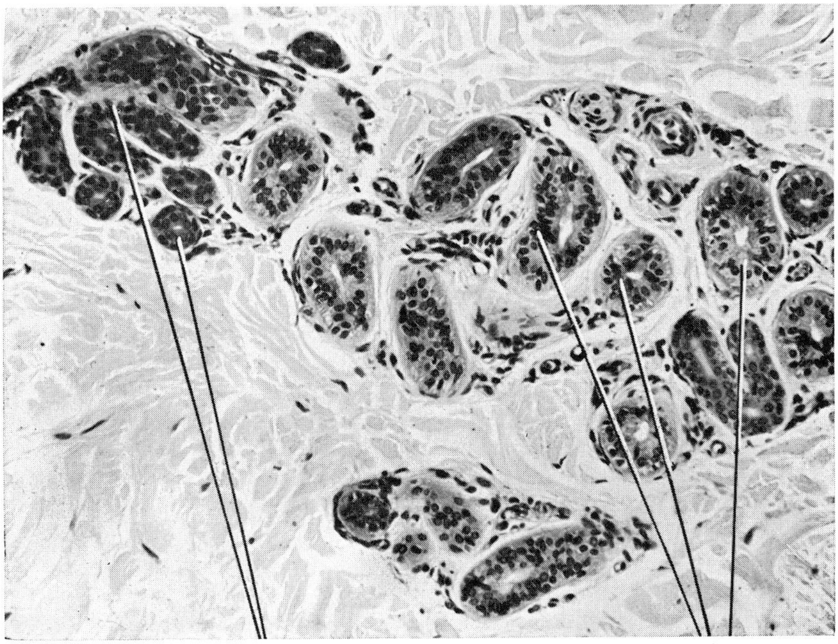

Figure 16-28 Human sweat gland from the abdominal skin. Both the coiled portion of the sweat duct (a) and the secretory portion (b) are present. The secretory portion is much smaller than that of the apocrine sweat gland shown in the same magnification in Fig. 16-27. ×200.

to heat. Apocrine sweating is a two-phase process. The secretory cells secrete their product into the tubular canal, which has a relatively large storage capacity. Then upon adrenergic stimulation, the myoepithelium contracts and forces the contents of the tubule to the surface. There then follows a refractory period of up to 48 hr until enough sweat can accumulate for the myoepithelium to force to the surface. Apocrine sweat is odorless on secretion but becomes odoriferous when acted upon by cutaneous bacteria. Although modern society has attached an undesirable quality to this odor, apocrine sweat was extremely important in lower animals as a sex attractor and territorial marker.

ECCRINE SWEAT GLANDS

The eccrine sweat glands are the most important cutaneous glands and the only ones with a known function in man. They are not connected with the pilosebaceous apparatus, but empty directly into the skin surface by a corkscrew-like duct. The eccrine sweat glands are distributed over the entire body surface except for the lips, the glans penis, the inner surface of the prepuce, the clitoris, and the labia minora. They are most dense on the palms and soles, where their tiny ducts are visible under low magnification on the peaks of the dermatoglyphic ridges. The sweat ducts enter the epidermis at the base of the rete ridges. Sweat gland density is less in the adult than in the child because there is no neogenesis after birth, and as the skin expands, the glands are spread farther apart. Estimates of the number of sweat glands range from 2 to 5 million per person.

The secretory tubule of the eccrine sweat gland is usually unbranched and has a relatively narrow lumen (Fig. 16-28). There are three types of cells in the sweat gland tubule. Around the periphery of the secretory tubule is a layer of myoepithelial cells which rests on the basement lamella. These are spindle-shaped cells which are arranged parallel to the tubule and do not form a complete envelope for the sweat coil. The secretory cells of the eccrine glands are of two types. Most obvious are the large *clear cells* which appear to rest both upon the myoepithelial cells and directly on the basement lamella between these cells. The broad base of the clear cells is on the outside of the tubule and their luminal border is narrow. These cells have an acidophilic cytoplasm. Interspersed between these clear cells are the smaller *dark cells* which have basophilic cytoplasm and an inverted pyramidal shape with the broad base on the luminal surface.

Electron microscopy has clarified the functional properties of these two cell types. The clear cells contain abundant mitochondria, glycogen particles, and considerable smooth ER (Fig. 16-29). Between adjacent clear cells there are well-developed canaliculi which open into the lumen of the tubule. These cells resemble other types of serous secretory cells, such as those found in lacrimal or salivary glands, and are therefore probably responsible for the watery sweat. Indirect evidence for such a function is provided by the depletion of glycogen particles in the clear cells on prolonged sweating, as well as by the observation of eccrine sweating in species that contain no dark cells.

Electron microscopy of the dark cells shows that they are filled with electron-dense vacuoles which are believed to be made up of mucin, and these cells are assumed to secrete mucopolysaccharide. They have fewer mitochondria than the clear cells, whereas the rough ER is comparable. Their luminal surface is made up of a large number of microvilli. The secretory tubule forms approximately half of the sweat gland unit. The duct is easily distinguished from the secretory portion of the ductal coil by its double row of cells, the lack of a myoepithelium, and the acidophilic luminal coating material, which may be the mucopolysaccharide produced by the dark cells.

Eccrine sweat glands are innervated by postganglionic sympathetic nerve fibers, but under physiologic conditions the glands primarily respond to cholinergic stimuli. Eccrine sweating can also be stimulated by adrenergic drugs, but this sweat has a different composition from sweat resulting from thermal stimulation. The sweat glands play a significant role in thermal regulation. Heat prostration or heat stroke is prone to occur in an individual with a congenital lack of sweat glands or blockage of the sweat glands through disease. Whenever convection and radiation heat loss, due to vascular changes, are inadequate to maintain thermal homeostasis, the sweat glands are recruited to produce sweat for evaporative heat loss.

There are many factors that influence the composition of sweat, so no absolute composition can be easily defined. Sweat is a hypotonic solution derived from plasma. Its major cation, sodium, is transported into the canaliculi between the clear cells by an active sodium pump, and water is then passively transferred to restore the isotonicity of sweat. Sweat becomes hypotonic due to the reabsorption of sodium in the sweat duct. Sweat also contains chloride, potassium, urea, and lactate. Its composition may change profoundly in disease states. For instance, the increase in sodium concentration in cystic fibrosis is a reliable test for the disease, and sweat-sodium studies have been an important tool in family studies. Drugs such as desoxycorticosterone or corticotropin will influence sweat composition, and as an adaptive measure, the sweat sodium decreases during protracted heat exposure, a phenomenon called *acclimatization*. It is thus obvious that the sweat gland is well adapted for its role in maintaining the body temperature within normal limits on heat exposure. Man, with his large number of eccrine glands, makes use of the evaporative water loss from a large area of nonhairy skin. In contrast, animals such as dogs have eccrine sweat glands restricted to the paw pads. Since their skin is well insulated by fur, and eccrine glands are restricted to an area from which evaporative water loss is difficult, their thermal regulation depends upon respiratory heat loss, and they pant when they are hot.

Figure 16-29 Electron micrograph of a portion of the secretory coil of an eccrine sweat gland. Three types of cells are present: myoepithelial (M), clear (C), and dark (D). The myoepithelial cells rest on the basement membrane (BM). Intercellular canaliculi (IC) are prominent between clear cells, and several of the clear cells have lipid inclusions (L). The dark cells contain dense secretory granules. ×48,000. (Courtesy of R. E. Ellis, in A. S. Zelickson (ed.), "Ultrastructure of Normal and Abnormal Skin," Lea & Febiger, Philadelphia, 1967.)

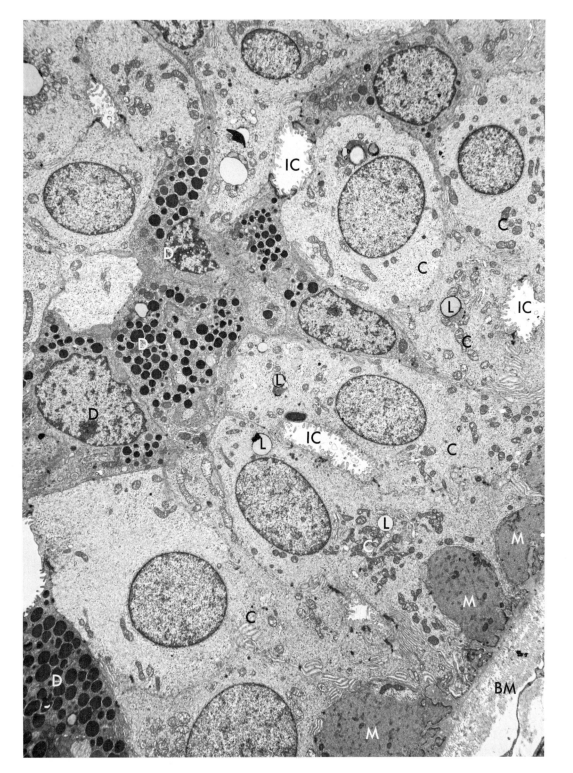

References

GENERAL

BUTCHER, E. O., and R. F. SOGNNAES (eds.): ''Fundamentals of Keratinization,'' American Association for Advancement of Science, Washington, D.C. Publ. 70, 1962.

GANS, O., and G. K. STEIGLEDER (eds.): ''Normale und Pathologische Anatomie der Haut I,'' Springer-Verlag, Berlin, 1969.

LYNE, A. G., and B. F. SHORT (eds.): ''Biology of the Skin and Hair Growth,'' Angus and Robertson, Sydney, 1965.

MONTAGNA, W.: ''The Structure and Function of Skin,'' 2d ed., Academic Press, New York, 1962.

MONTAGNA, W., and W. C. LOBITZ, JR. (eds.): ''The Epidermis,'' Academic Press, New York, 1964.

ZELICKSON, A. S. (ed.): ''Ultrastructure of Normal and Abnormal Skin,'' Lea & Febiger, Philadelphia, 1967.

EPIDERMIS

LAVKER, R. M., and A. G. MATOLTSY: Formation of Horny Cells, *J. Cell Biol.*, **44**:501 (1970).

MATOLTSY, A. G.: Soluble Prekeratin, in A. G. Lyne and B. F. Short (eds.), ''Biology of the Skin and Hair Growth,'' Angus and Robertson, Sydney, 1965.

MATOLTSY, A. G., and M. N. MATOLTSY: The Chemical Nature of Keratohyalin Granules of the Epidermis, *J. Cell Biol.*, **47**:593 (1970).

MATOLTSY, A. G., and P. F. PARAKKAL: Keratinization, in A. S. Zelickson (ed.), ''Ultrastructure of Normal and Abnormal Skin,'' Lea & Febiger, Philadelphia, 1967.

ODLAND, G. F., and T. H. REED: Epidermis, in A. S. Zelickson (ed.), ''Ultrastructure of Normal and Abnormal Skin,'' Lea & Febiger, Philadelphia, 1967.

NAIL

ZAIAS, N., and J. ALVAREZ: The Formation of the Primate Nail Plate, *J. Invest. Derm.*, **51**:120 (1968).

HAIR

RHODIN, J. A. G., and E. J. REITH: Ultrastructure of Keratin in Oral Mucosa, Skin, Esophagus, Claw and Hair, in E. O. Butcher and R. F. Sognnaes (eds.), ''Fundamentals of Keratinization,'' American Association for the Advancement of Science, Washington, D.C. Publ. 70, 1962.

ROGERS, G. E.: Newer Findings on the Enzymes and Proteins of Hair Follicles, *Ann. N.Y. Acad. Sci.*, **83**:408 (1959).

MELANOCYTES

MONTAGNA, W., and F. HU (eds.): ''The Pigmentary System,'' Advances in Biology of Skin, vol. 8, Pergamon Press, Oxford, 1967.

SEIJI, M.: Melanogenesis, in A. S. Zelickson (ed.), ''Ultrastructure of Normal and Abnormal Skin,'' Lea & Febiger, Philadelphia, 1967.

SEIJI, M. K., K. SHIMAO, M. S. C. BIRBECK, and T. B. FITZPATRICK: Subcellular Localization of Melanin Biosynthesis, *Ann. N.Y. Acad. Sci.*, **100**:497 (1963).

SZABÓ, G.: The Biology of the Pigment Cell, in E. B. Bittar and N. Bittar (eds.), "The Biological Basis of Medicine," vol. 6, Academic Press, New York, 1969.

ZELICKSON, A. S.: Melanocyte, Melanin Granule, and Langerhans Cell, in A. S. Zelickson (ed.), "Ultrastructure of Normal and Abnormal Skin," Lea & Febiger, Philadelphia, 1967.

DERMIS

MONTAGNA, W., J. P. BENTLEY, and R. L. DOBSON (eds.): "The Dermis," Advances in Biology of Skin, vol. 10, Appleton-Century-Crofts, New York, 1970.

BLOOD VESSELS

MONTAGNA, W., and R. A. ELLIS (eds.): "Blood Vessels and Circulation," Advances in Biology of Skin, vol. 2, Pergamon Press, New York, 1961.

MORETTI, G.: The Blood Vessels of the Skin, in O. Gans and G. K. Steigleder (eds.), "Normale und Pathologische Anatomie der Haut I," Springer-Verlag, Berlin, 1969.

NERVES

MONTAGNA, W. (ed.): "Cutaneous Innervation," Advances in Biology of Skin, vol. 1, Pergamon Press, New York, 1960.

SEBACEOUS GLANDS

ELLIS, R. A.: Eccrine, Sebaceous and Apocrine Glands, in A. S. Zelickson (ed.), "Ultrastructure of Normal and Abnormal Skin," Lea & Febiger, Philadelphia, 1967.

MONTAGNA, W., R. A. ELLIS, and A. F. SILVER (eds.): "The Sebaceous Glands," Advances in Biology of Skin, vol. 4, Pergamon Press, Oxford, 1963.

STRAUSS, J. S., and P. E. POCHI: Histology, Histochemistry, and Electron Microscopy of Sebaceous Glands in Man, in O. Gans and G. K. Steigleder (eds.), "Normale und Pathologische Anatomie der Haut I," Springer-Verlag, Berlin, 1969.

APOCRINE SWEAT GLANDS

ELLIS, R. A.: Eccrine, Sebaceous and Apocrine Glands, in A. S. Zelickson (ed.), "Ultrastructure of Normal and Abnormal Skin," Lea & Febiger, Philadelphia, 1967.

HURLEY, H. J., and W. B. SHELLEY: "The Human Apocrine Sweat Gland in Health and Disease," Charles C Thomas, Springfield, Ill., 1960.

ECCRINE SWEAT GLANDS

ELLIS, R. A.: Eccrine, Sebaceous and Apocrine Glands, in A. S. Zelickson (ed.), "Ultrastructure of Normal and Abnormal Skin," Lea & Febiger, Philadelphia, 1967.

ELLIS, R. A.: Eccrine Sweat Glands: Electron Microscopy, Cytochemistry and Anatomy in O. Gans and G. K. Steigleder (eds.), "Normale und Pathologische Anatomie der Haut I," Springer-Verlag, Berlin, 1969.

KUNO, Y.: "Human Perspiration," Charles C Thomas, Springfield, Ill., 1956.

MONTAGNA, W., R. A. ELLIS, and A. F. SILVER (eds.): "Eccrine Sweat Glands and Eccrine Sweating," Advances in Biology of Skin, vol. 3, Pergamon Press, New York, 1962.

WEINER, J. S., and K. HELLMAN: The Sweat Glands, *Biol. Rev.*, **35:**141 (1960).

chapter 17   Teeth

ROBERT M. FRANK
AND
REIDAR F.
SOGNNAES

The whole tooth

A tooth consists of three parts: crown, neck, and root, seated in bone (Fig. 17-1). The clinical *crown* is the portion that projects above the *gingiva* (or gum); the *root* is the part inserted in the alveolus or socket in the bone of the jaw; and the *neck* is the point of junction between the root and the crown. These hard portions surround a dental chamber which contains the *pulp,* a jelly-like type of connective tissue. The chamber extends through the root canal to the root apex, where it opens to the exterior of the tooth at the apical foramen. The solid portion of the tooth consists of three calcified substances: the *dentin* (or ivory), the *enamel,* and the *cementum.* Of these, the dentin is the most abundant. It forms a broad layer around the pulp chamber and root canal and it is interrupted only at the apical foramen. Nowhere does the dentin reach the outer surface. In the crown it is cov-

ered with enamel; in the root it is enclosed by cementum. The enamel is thickest at the cusp tips, whereas the cementum is thickest at the root apex. Both tissues thin toward the neck where they join in a variable manner. The cementum, and with it the tooth, is attached to the bony socket by the *periodontal "membrane,"* a connective tissue ligament, which is continuous with the connective tissue of the gingiva. Together these three structures—the cementum, periodontal ligament, and gingiva—serve as the supporting tissues of the tooth. The dental hard tissues, like bone, consist of a densely mineralized organic matrix. Embryologically, the dentin, cementum, pulp, and periodontal ligament of the teeth come from the mesoderm, like bone and other connective tissues, whereas the enamel is a highly specialized ectodermal structure.

Beginning tooth development

Tooth development involves a long process of growth and calcification before the teeth erupt to function in the mouth. The first indication of tooth development is a thickening of the oral epithelium, which has been observed in 6- to 7-week-old human embryos. At this stage the tongue is well developed, but the upper and lower lips are not yet separated by depressions from the structures within the mouth. Although the oral plate, which marks the boundary between oral ectoderm and pharyngeal entoderm, has wholly disappeared, it is evident that this thickening takes place in the oral ectoderm. Soon after its formation, this epithelially derived plate grows into the subjacent mesenchymal tissues following the parabolic curvature of each jaw. The invaginated epithelium undergoes the same type of transformation in both the maxilla and mandible, and the following description of the conditions in the mandible is therefore applicable to both. As the plate descends into the mesenchyme, it divides into two parts. In front, the *labial lamina* separates the lip from the gum. Behind, the *dental lamina* (Fig. 17-2) produces the teeth. Taken as a whole, the dental lamina is a crescentic plate of cells following the line of the gingiva, along which the teeth will later appear. In Fig. 17-2A to D each drawing represents diagrammatically a part of the oral epithelium above and dental lamina below, free from the surrounding mesenchyme.

Figure 17-1 Section of a tooth with its supporting tissues in position in the jaw bone.

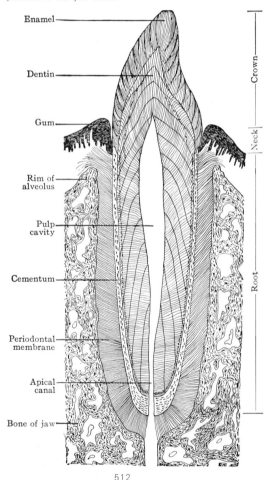

Figure 17-2 The dental lamina (A) and the early development of three teeth (B–D). The anterior tooth is shown in vertical section.

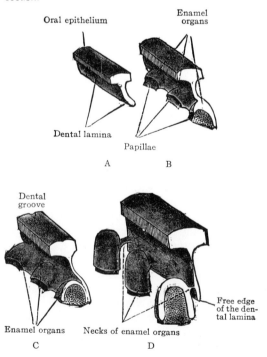

The labial side is toward the left and the lingual side toward the right. Almost as soon as the dental lamina has formed, it produces a series of inverted cup-shaped enlargements along the labial surface (Fig. 17-2B). These become the *enamel organs* (Fig. 17-3).

Enamel organs of deciduous and permanent teeth

There is a separate enamel organ for each of the 10 *deciduous,* or *milk, teeth* in each jaw, and they are all present in embryos of $2\frac{1}{2}$ months. The enamel organs not only produce the enamel but subsequently extend over the roots as an epithelial sheath (Hertwig's sheath). The tissue enclosed by the enamel organ is a denser mesenchyme, constituting the dental papilla (Fig. 17-3). This is the primordium of the pulp of the tooth, and it produces at its periphery the bulk of the tooth substance, the layer of *dentin.* As the tooth develops, the connec-tion between its enamel organ and the dental lamina becomes reduced to a flattened strand of epithelial tissue, which subsequently disintegrates.

The *permanent teeth,* 16 in each jaw, develop similarly. The dental lamina grows backward to produce enamel organs for the three permanent molars, which develop behind the deciduous teeth on each side of the jaws. The enamel organ for the first permanent molar forms at about the seven-teenth week of fetal life; the enamel organ for the second molar forms about half a year after birth,

Figure 17-3   The enamel organ.   This projection drawing (× 50) of parasagittal section passes through the primordium of a lower incisor of a fourteenth-week human embryo.   On the lower left the small sketch indicates the jaw relations of the area represented. (From B. M. Pattern, "Human Embryology"; embryo of 104-mm C-R length, University of Michigan Collection.)

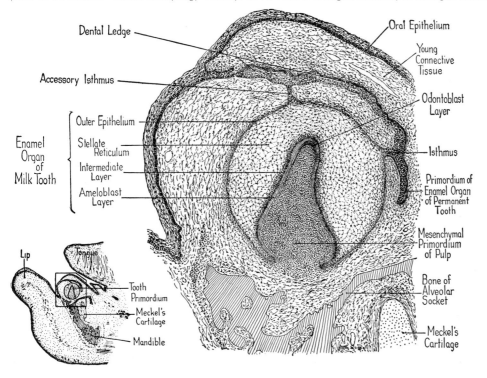

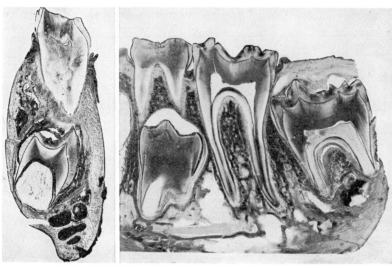

Figure 17-4 Sagittal section (left) and longitudinal section (right) of the mandible of a 2-year-old rhesus monkey. A permanent premolar is developing within the jaw below the second deciduous molar; the first permanent molar (''6-year'' molar in man) is in function, and the second molar (''12-year'' molar) is about to emerge into the mouth. Plastic-embedded ground sections.

and that for the third molar (wisdom tooth) at 5 years.

The permanent teeth anterior to the permanent molars (that is, *incisors, canines,* and *premolars*) develop from enamel organs of the deep portion of the dental lamina. Owing to the obliquity of the lamina, the permanent teeth are on the lingual side of the deciduous teeth. The enamel organs for the incisors develop slightly before those for the canines, but all these are discernible in a fetus of 24 weeks. Between the canines and molars there are two premolars in each quadrant of the jaw. The enamel organs for the first premolars develop in the eighth month. Each permanent tooth anterior to the molars undergoes a complicated series of spatial changes during its development. Be-

tween 6 and 12 years, when the deciduous teeth are being shed one after another, the bony partitions are resorbed together with the roots of the deciduous teeth (Fig. 17-4). It is interesting that the resorption of all the dental hard tissues is accompanied, as in bone, by the appearance of osteoclast-like cells in Howship's lacunae. After the deciduous teeth are shed, entirely new alveolar bone and other investing tissues are produced for the support of the permanent teeth (Fig. 17-4).

The portion of the dental lamina not used in producing enamel organs normally disintegrates, but epithelial remnants may occasionally develop abnormally, forming cysts and tumors (ameloblastomas).

Formation and structure of dental tissues

Tooth formation is initiated by the inner development of a thin layer of coronal dentin, followed by outer deposition of enamel. The extracellular formation of the organic matrices of both tissues is under the control of cellular secretion. The odontoblasts, of mesenchymal origin, will secrete a col-

lageneous matrix, called the *predentin,* which undergoes calcification secondarily. Dentin formation is the result of rhythmic incremental development. The epithelial ameloblasts secrete an organic matrix with special biochemical properties which begins to calcify as soon as it is deposited extracellularly.

However, odontogenesis is not a simultaneous event throughout the tooth. The first dentin and enamel formation begins at the tips of cusps of multicusped teeth or the uppermost portions of unicusped teeth. Following completion of the crown, root formation begins. Here the epithelial root sheath induces radicular pulpal cells to become odontoblasts: following root dentin formation, the adjacent mesodermal connective tissue cells are induced to become cementoblasts and to form cementum.

ENAMEL

The internal cells of the enamel organ (see Fig. 17-3) are at first in close contact, like those of ordinary epithelium; after further differentiation and through an accumulation of viscous intercellular substance, they constitute a reticulum which resembles mesenchyme and is known as the *stellate reticulum* (Figs. 17-3 and 17-5A, see color insert). Toward the oral cavity the stellate reticulum is bounded by the outer enamel epithelium, a single layer of cuboidal cells; toward the dental papilla it is bounded by the inner enamel epithelium, the cells of which elongate and become the enamel-producing ameloblasts. These tall cells are separated from the stellate cells by a layer of flattened cells, the *stratum intermedium* (Fig. 17-6). A basement membrane limits the outer and inner enamel epithelium from the surrounding mesenchymal tissues.

Histochemical reactions reveal that the enamel epithelium first secretes a mucopolysaccharide, forming the ground substance of the stellate reticulum (Fig. 17-5A, see color insert); later, after reversing the polarity of its cells, the inner enamel epithelium, transformed into ameloblasts, will secrete the organic matrix of enamel which gives reaction for sulfhydryl groups (Fig. 17-5D, see color insert). The cells of the stellate reticulum are rich in glycogen and alkaline phosphatase, and the ground substance between them is markedly metachromatic, but is not stained by the periodic acid–Schiff procedure. It is destroyed by hyaluronidase and has no metachromatic antecedent visible in its constituent cells. An intense alkaline phosphatase reaction has been demonstrated in the stratum intermedium as well as in the ameloblasts.

The ameloblasts produce enamel along their distal surfaces (Figs. 17-7 and 17-8). These tall cells, which are directed toward the dental papilla, have their nuclei nearer the stellate reticulum. The Golgi apparatus, which was originally on the side of the nucleus toward the stellate reticulum, shifts to the opposite position. At the stage of active matrix formation, the Golgi apparatus becomes highly developed, as does the rough endoplasmic reticulum. The cytoplasm is rich in ribosomes, microfilaments, and microtubules. The ameloblasts are initially separated from the odontoblasts by a basement membrane, but as soon as the first layer of dentin has calcified, this membrane disappears.

At the apical surface of each ameloblast, a tapering projection known as the *Tomes' process* develops. A great concentration of round secretory granules accumulate within the Tomes' process. These secretory granules are elaborated in the Golgi apparatus and migrate to the distal end of the cell. Electron-microscopic autoradiography suggests that the material in the secretory granules is released in the extracellular space without any discontinuity of the cell membrane and that an important part of the enamel matrix precursors are secreted through these granules. These precursors contain proteins and glycoproteins and may also transport inorganic elements, but experimental evidence for the latter is presently missing.

During the different phases of enamel development, the ameloblasts assume multiple functions of secretion, absorption, and transfer. Biochemically the organic matrix of developing enamel undergoes marked changes, notably a loss in proteins and a change in the amino acid composition. Histochemical studies have indicated the presence in the ameloblast of several lysosomal enzymes and have suggested the presence of an acid phosphatase activity in the highly developed Golgi complex and perhaps in the secretory granules.

The enamel is built up layer by layer. Its formation begins at the top of the crown of each tooth and spreads downward over its sides. If the tooth has several cusps, a cap of enamel forms over each, and these caps coalesce. As soon as the enamel matrix is deposited extracellularly, it starts to calcify, forming enamel rods or prisms approximately 5 μm thick, bounded by zones classically described as rod or prism sheaths (Fig. 17-5E, see color insert) and interrod or interprismatic substance

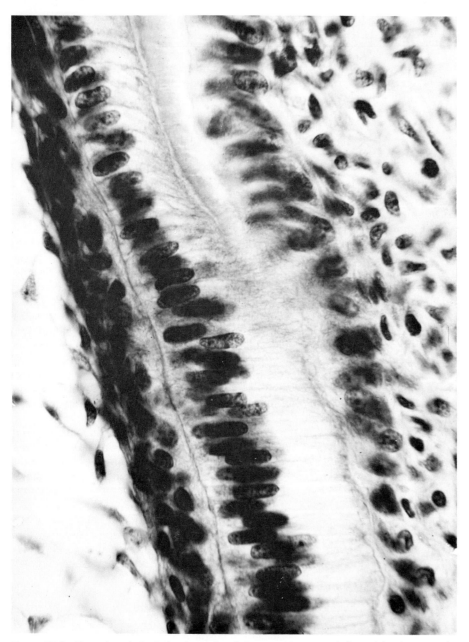

Figure 17-6 Enamel- and dentin-forming cells of the enamel organ. Left to right there are the stellate reticulum, stratum intermedium, inner enamel epithelium, odontoblasts, and pulpal cells. Note the cytomorphologic changes in functionally maturing ameloblasts (left) and odontoblasts (right): The ameloblasts decrease in height, while the odontoblasts become columnar as dentin and enamel formation begins at the upper half of the figure.

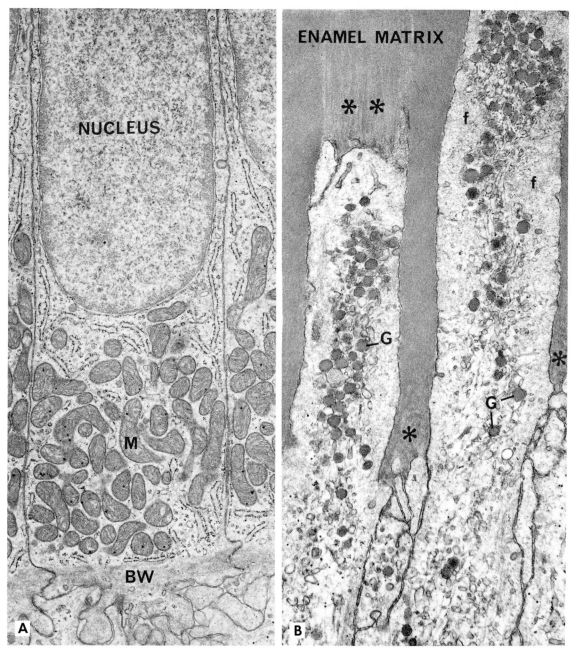

Figure 17-7 A. The infranuclear region of a secretory ameloblast from a rat incisor as seen in the electron microscope. Mitochondria (M) with dense matrices, characteristic of this cell type, abound within the infranuclear cytoplasm. Also present are scattered elements of rough endoplasmic reticulum, the flattened profiles of which may be seen distributed between the mitochondria and adjacent to the lateral cell membrane. A prominent basal web (BW) composed of densely packed microfilaments is located at the base of the cell. ×15,000. (Courtesy of Alfred Weinstock, University of California, Los Angeles). B. An electron micrograph of the apical (Tomes') processes of two ameloblasts from a rat incisor showing their architecture and relationship to the enamel matrix. Each process is limited by a plasma membrane which is closely applied to the matrix. The *distal* portion (upper two-thirds of micrograph) is embedded within the matrix. Secretory granules (G), each delimited by a unit membrane, abound within the central core of cytoplasm in association with microtubules and smooth vesicular or tubular elements. This core is usually ensheathed by a feltwork of fine filaments (f) which extends to the plasma membrane. The *proximal* portion of each process (lower one-third of micrograph) is not embedded in matrix and contains scattered secretory granules. Although the enamel matrix appears relatively homogeneous at this magnification, it shows an arrangement of parallel lines in two regions: (1) the matrix abutting the distal end of each process (**, upper left), and (2) at the proximal ends of the prongs of matrix (*) projecting between the processes. This striated matrix, lying opposite the secretory zones, represents the most recently deposited matrix and corresponds to the so-called "growth regions" of enamel. ×21,000. (From A. Weinstock, and C. P. Leblond, J. Cell Biol., **51**:26, 1971.)

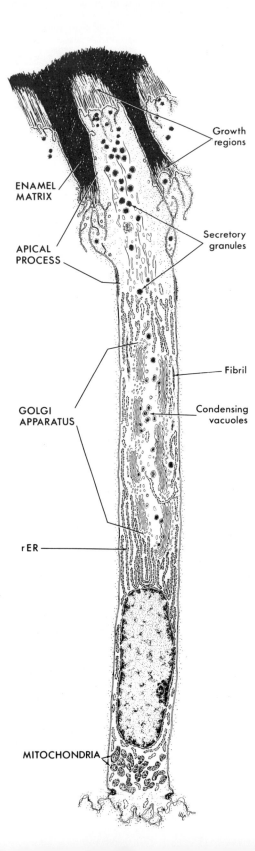

Growth
regions

ENAMEL
MATRIX

Secretory
granules

APICAL
PROCESS

GOLGI
APPARATUS

Fibril

Condensing
vacuoles

rER

MITOCHONDRIA

(Figs. 17-9 and 17-10). Initially, the prism sheath appears as a thin, noncalcified area filled with organic material and limited by apatite crystals of the prism and the interprismatic substance. With advancing calcification, the prism sheath shrinks, and in the adult enamel, it is practically reduced to a submicroscopic space recognizable by the fact that the limiting apatite crystals on both sides have a different orientation. As enamel increases in thickness, the ameloblasts migrate outward. To accommodate themselves to the greater area of the outer surface of the enamel, the prisms become slightly broader as they develop radially. By the time the tooth is ready to erupt, the enamel organ has ceased to function and is a much reduced structure. When the tooth is functioning, the worn surfaces of enamel become covered by a thin organic layer called the *acquired pellicle*, which comes from saliva.

The fully calcified enamel is the hardest substance in the body. Both the prisms and the interprismatic substance are calcified and contain from 96 to 98 percent inorganic material, 90 percent of which is hydroxyapatite. Amorphous calcium phosphates have also been observed. Traces of calcium carbonate, acid magnesium phosphate, calcium fluoride, and other salts form the remainder. Enamel contains no cells or other cytoplasmic structures (see Table 17-1).

The enamel apatite crystals, the largest of all found in human calcified tissues, are elongated cylinders which, in transverse section, are sometimes flattened hexagons but more frequently are irregular and more or less circular. Their dimensions in human enamel vary from 400 to 1200 Å

Figure 17-8 Diagramatic representation of the structure of a whole secretory ameloblast (combining Fig. 17-7A and B), from the region of enamel matrix secretion in a rat maxillary incisor. Mitochondria are grouped in the infranuclear region between the basal web and the nucleus. The supranuclear region contains the elongated, tubular-shaped Golgi apparatus which is surrounded on all sides by the rough endoplasmic reticulum (rER). Within the central core of cytoplasm demarcated by the Golgi saccules are condensing vacuoles and a few secretory granules. The apical (Tomes') process extends apically from the terminal web, and its distal portion is embedded in the enamel matrix. Secretory granules abound within its central core. The "growth regions" represent the most recently deposited matrix. (From A. Weinstock and C. P. Leblond, 51:26, 1971).

Table 17-1   Comparison of hard tissues

Main components	Bone	Cementum	Dentin	Enamel
Inorganic crystals	Calcium phosphate	Calcium phosphate	Calcium phosphate	Calcium phosphate
Amorphous ground substance	Glycoprotein	Glycoprotein	Glycoprotein	Glycoprotein and special protein
Principal organic component	Collagen	Collagen	Collagen	
Internal cells	Osteocytes	Cementocytes	Cell processes	Absent
Adjacent cells	Osteoblasts, osteoclasts	Cementoblasts	Odontoblasts	Absent
Blood vessels	Present	Absent	Absent	Absent
Adjacent fluid	Connective tissue fluid	Connective tissue fluid	Connective tissue fluid	Saliva

in width and from 2000 to 10,000 Å in length in bright-field electron microscopy. When observed in dark-field electron microscopy, the crystals appeared rectangular with a mean length of 321 Å. In the prisms and the interprismatic substance, the crystals are closely packed and the intercrystalline spaces are about 20 to 30 Å in width. The organic fraction of enamel has a characteristic amino acid composition that is different from both collagen and keratin and contains small amounts of glycoprotein and lipid.

In the prisms, the apatite crystals have their long

Figure 17-9   Transverse section through human fetal enamel rods (R). Note the arcade-shaped form of the peripheral rod sheath areas (S). The rods are continuous with the interrod substance (IP) on one side. ×14,000.

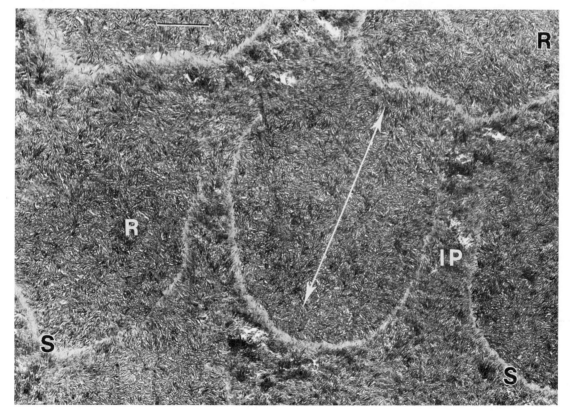

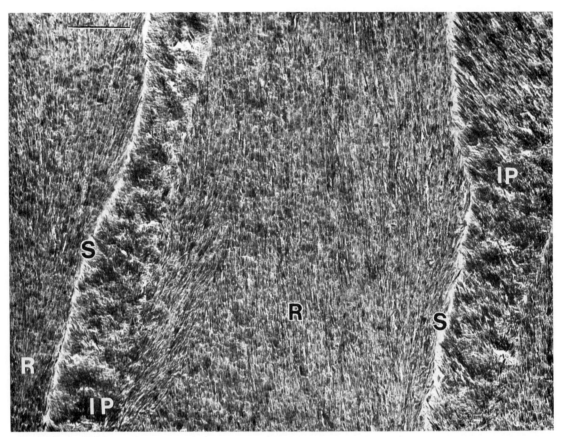

Figure 17-10   Longitudinal section through arcade-formed human fetal enamel rods in a plane indicated by the white arrow on Fig. 17-9.   The divergent orientation of the apatite crystals in the rods (R) versus the interrod substance (IP) is apparent.   The central rod is separated on the right from the interrod substance by a sheath (S), whereas on its left side, it is continuous with the interrod substance.   This configuration is accounted for by examining the longitudinal plane of the section indicated by the arrow on Fig. 17-9.   (The upper right part on Fig. 17-9 corresponds to the left part of Fig. 17-10.)   ×17,000.

axis (c axis) approximately parallel to the longitudinal axis of the prism, whereas in the interprismatic substance the long axis of the crystals forms an angle of more than 40° with that of the prisms. On cross sections of human enamel, it has been shown that the relationships between prism, interprismatic substance, and prism sheath can be variable. Traditionally, the most frequent type has been described as ''arcade-formed'' enamel, because the prism profile has an arcade shape (Fig. 17-9). Other studies suggest a keyhole configuration in which the cross-cut prisms have a head and a tail. In the head, the long axis of the apatite

crystals is approximately parallel to that of the prism whereas, toward the tail, the crystal axis diverges progressively from that of the prism.

Various markings can be seen on the enamel surface or in ground sections. The outer surface of the enamel, especially of young permanent teeth, presents a succession of circular ridges and grooves which may be seen with a hand lens (Fig. 17-11). These ripple marks, or *perikymata* as they are now called, were discovered by Leeuwenhoek in 1687. When a tooth is split in two and the exposed enamel examined with a hand lens, a set of lines or bands can be seen to cross the enamel radially, taking the

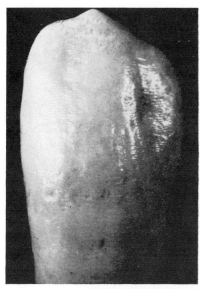

Figure 17-11   Intact enamel surface. The appositional growth pattern of the enamel is reflected in the circular ridges and depressions.

shortest course from the dentin toward the free surface. These radial lines are said to be due to the arrangement of the enamel prisms, and fractures of the enamel tend to follow them. It is also suggested that they may reflect differences in composition. Seen in reflected light under low magnification, they appear as alternating light and dark zones called *lines of Hunter-Schreger* (Fig. 17-12). The bundles of prisms, in crossing the enamel, are bent so that in a radial section they appear as alternating zones of oblique and longitudinal sections. These zones also differ in degree of calcification, as evidenced by the affinity for stain in alternating areas (see also Fig. 17-5F, color insert). The enamel shows other striations, which are broadest and most distinct toward the free surface. Apparently these striations indicate the shape of the entire enamel at successive stages in its development (see Fig. 17-1), and for this reason they are called *growth lines* or *lines of Retzius*. These lines may also represent differences in structure and composition of the enamel. They tend to obstruct transmitted light when viewed in both decalcified and ground sections (Fig. 17-13).

Metabolic disturbances occurring during the development of the teeth often accentuate these lines and are permanently recorded. Similarly, the physiologic change in metabolism at birth stamps an imprint on the teeth known as the *neonatal line.*

In the internal enamel, near the dentin-enamel border, structures called *enamel tufts* often appear and extend various distances between the enamel prisms (Fig. 17-13A). Heavy organic bands derived from saliva and elsewhere, known as *enamel lamellae,* are frequently found along cracks between the enamel prisms (Fig. 17-14). Other structures extend for short distances into the enamel at an angle to the prisms; these are called *enamel spindles* (Fig. 17-15) and are thought to represent extensions of dentinal tubules.

Individual enamel prisms, when seen lengthwise, exhibit transverse markings usually, but not always, aligned to form continuous striations across many prisms (Fig. 17-5E, see color insert). It is apparent that the prismatic striations reflect a periodic rhythm of incremental activity.

For a summary of the characteristic differences between enamel and other hard tissues refer to Table 17-1.

Figure 17-12   Ground section of a tooth photographed in reflected light. The light enamel layer with the alternating dark and light bands of Hunter-Schreger is clearly distinguishable from the dentin. (Meyer-Churchill.)

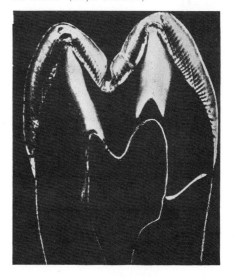

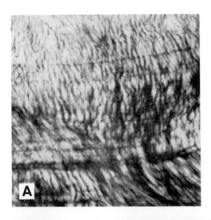

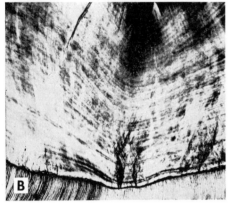

Figure 17-13   A. Paraffin section of decalcified enamel of deciduous molar. The several incremental (Retzius') lines and one accentuated birth line correspond to areas with relatively thicker interprismatic organic matter. B. Undecalcified ground section of enamel and dentin of permanent molar. The enamel shows several incremental lines running parallel and a few tufts extending into enamel from underlying dentin.

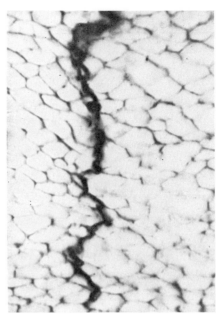

Figure 17-14   Enamel lamella ending blindly between enamel prisms. Paraffin section of decalcified enamel.

Figure 17-15   Enamel spindle running from dentin surface at an angle to the enamel prisms and ending blindly in the enamel. Ground section.

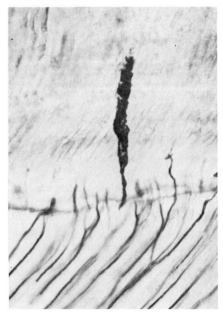

DENTIN

Following the differentiation of the ameloblasts of the enamel organ, the outermost cells of the dental papilla become elongated and arranged in an epithelioid layer and are called *odontoblasts* (Fig. 17-6). They are tall columnar cells, with one or more thin processes directed toward the enamel. As dentin matrix is formed, the odontoblasts recede centripetally, narrowing the pulpal chamber. The cells leave behind an apical extension, the odontoblastic process (*Tomes' fiber*), surrounded by a canalicular structure termed the *dentinal tubule* (Fig. 17-16). The odontoblastic processes should not be confused with the previously described Tomes' processes of the ameloblasts. The thin outermost layer of dentin is the mantle dentin, characterized by an arborescent pattern of dentinal tubules. The bulk of the dentin, the circumpulpar dentin, contains essentially straight tubules that branch dichotomously at the tips and bear smaller side branches. Each process occupies a canaliculus in the dentinal matrix, but the odontoblasts remain always at the inner border of the dentin, receding centripetally, and unlike osteoblasts, do not become buried. They are in contact with adjacent cells and with cells more central in the pulp.

The odontoblast, with an oval-shaped nucleus, contains a well-developed Golgi zone located near the nucleus, on the side facing the enamel, as well as endoplasmic reticulum, mitochondria, ribosomes, microtubules, and microfilaments. Laterally the odontoblasts can be attached by tight, intermediary junctions and desmosomes. Along the predentin, a complex junctional attachment can be seen. The odontoblastic process is limited by the cell plasmalemma and contains a cytoplasmic mass rich in microtubules and microfilaments (Fig. 17-16).

It was thought that during the early stages of dentinogenesis the first fibrils to be formed in mantle dentin originated in mesenchymal pulpal cells and fanned out in the predentin, passing between odontoblasts. With the light microscope these fine argyrophilic fibers, known as Korff's fibers, have been described in the mantle dentin. With the

Figure 17-16   The odontoblastic process (O) of cat dentin (D) is separated from the wall of the tubule by a periodontoblastic organic space (S), containing some collagen fibrils and ground substance.   P = predentin.   ×32,000.

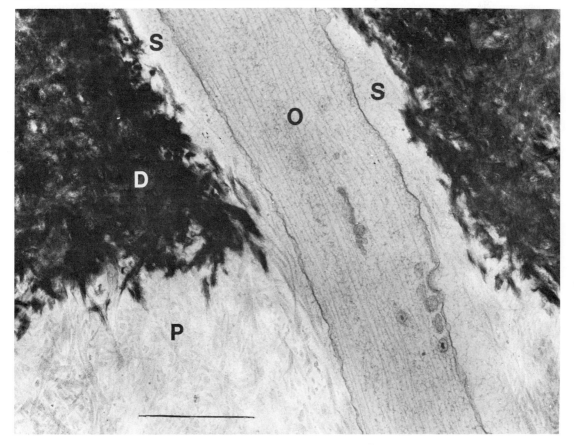

electron microscope, these fibrils show the classical periodic cross-striations typical of collagen, and the main bulk of the dentinal organic matrix, known as *predentin,* is mainly composed of collagen fibrils embedded in a ground substance (Fig. 17-17). Through electron-microscope autoradiography, it has been shown that the secretion of collagen precursors of predentin is mainly under the control of the odontoblast, and it must be noted that only a few collagen bundles could be observed in the lateral extracellular space between odontoblasts. During active dentinogenesis, different types of dense elongated granules and coated vesicles are found in the odontoblast process. An important part of the collagen precursors migrate through the odontoblast in these granules (Fig. 17-17), which are formed within the Golgi zone, as could be demonstrated with ultrastructural autoradiography after injection of tritiated proline.

Even though the odontoblasts differentiate later than the ameloblasts, the dentin matrix is first laid down as a thin layer of predentin below the row of ameloblasts (Fig. 17-6). Calcification is induced through hydroxyapatite growth in this collageneous matrix. The mature apatite crystal in dentin has been described as a needle- or plate-like crystal.

If the inorganic crystals are removed, it is found that the organic matrix of decalcified dentin has a greater electron density than the predentin precursor (Fig. 17-18). Dentin is elaborated through

Figure 17-17   Longitudinal section of an odontoblastic process (O) in the predentin of a newborn cat 1 hr after intravenous injection of tritiated proline. Numerous silver grains are visible in the odontoblastic process containing dense elongated granules (G), some of which are labeled. The collagen fibrils surrounding the process are only slightly labeled at this stage. However, 24 hr after the intravenous injection of tritiated proline, the collagenous matrix is labeled almost exclusively, whereas the odontoblastic process is free of silver grains.   ×28,000.

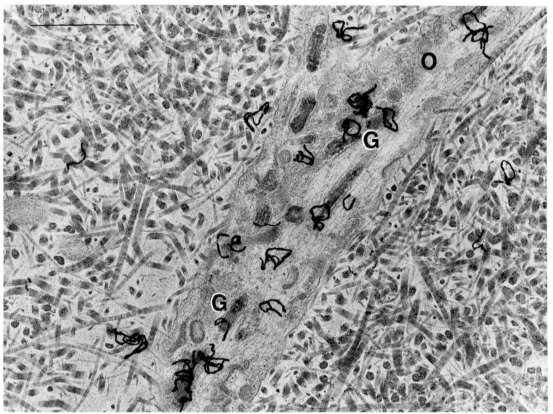

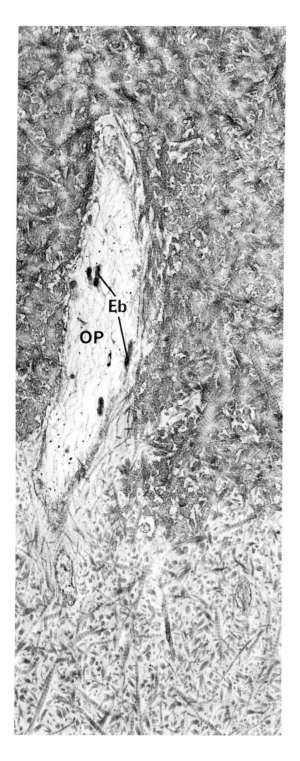

Figure 17-18 An electron micrograph demonstrating the dentin (upper two-thirds of micrograph) and the predentin (lower one-third of micrograph) from an EDTA-demineralized rat incisor. The dentin proper is composed of compact bundles of collagen fibers which, after demineralization, appear to be associated with an electron-dense material. In contrast, the collagen bundles in the predentin lack this dense material. A portion of an odontoblastic process (OP) may be seen penetrating the dentin from the predentin. This process contains elongated granules (Eb), mictrotubules, and microfilaments. ×15,000. [From A. Weinstock, in G. H. Bourne (ed.), "Elaboration of Enamel and Dentin Matrix Glycoproteins," p. 121, Academic Press, New York, 1972.]

incremental deposition of predentin layers followed by either homogeneous or globular calcified masses. Here, as in the young enamel, one can observe a very marked phosphorus uptake in ^{32}P-injected animals accompanied by an intensive alkaline phosphatase activity in the adjacent tooth-forming cells of the dental papilla and enamel organ (Figs. 17-19 and 17-20).

When fully calcified, dentin is not so hard as enamel, since it contains much more organic matter (approximately 30 percent, roughly similar to bone). When the inorganic substances are removed from enamel, the remaining organic framework scarcely holds together, whereas the demineralization of dentin and bone leaves a coherent matrix which preserves the form of the original object.

Figure 17-19 Radioautograph of the jaw of ^{32}P-injected rhesus monkey. Note intense activity in the internal dentin.

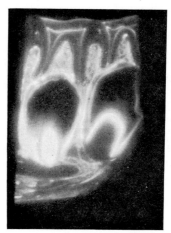

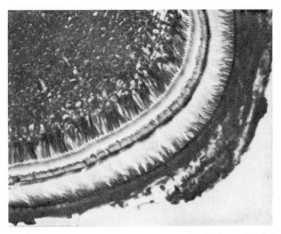

Figure 17-20   Alkaline phosphatase activity in the cells of the enamel organ and dental papilla of developing rat incisor. Paraffin section of the uncalcified growing part of tooth.

The dentinal tubules pass radially through the dentin, often following a somewhat S-shaped course (Fig. 17-21), sometimes with spiral twists and secondary curves. As the tubules penetrate the dentin, they give off many slender lateral branches, some of which seem to anastomose with those from adjacent tubules. They finally become very slender and end blindly.

The tubules of the inner third of calcified dentin are permeated by portions of odontoblastic process (Fig. 17-5G and H, see color insert) that do not completely fill the tubule but leave an organic periodontoblastic space, containing some uncalcified collagen fibrils and ground substance, between the process and the calcified tubule wall (Fig. 17-16). In the peripheral parts of the odontoblastic process, an accumulation of large vacuoles has been observed. On cross sections, the process

Figure 17-21   Ground section of human molar. Several accentuated growth lines in concurrently developed dentin and enamel form V-shaped patterns with the apex at the dentin-enamel junction.

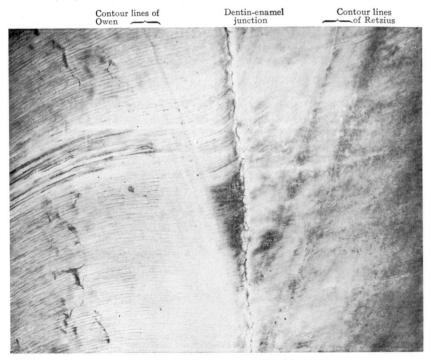

appears as an annular condensation of hyaline cytoplasm with a central vacuole (Fig. 17-22).

In the inner layer of dentin, near the predentin, the dentinal tubules are directly bordered by intertubular dentin consisting of a calcified collageneous matrix (Fig. 17-16). In more peripheral layers are found hypercalcified tubular walls known as peritubular dentin (Fig. 17-22). The peritubular dentin, which is continuous with intertubular dentin, is rich in closely packed inorganic crystals. The exact nature of the scarce organic matrix of the peritubular dentin is still a matter of debate.

Histochemical techniques have revealed basophilic and metachromatic reactions in the areas surrounding the processes of the odontoblasts (Fig. 17-5I and J, see color insert). Besides the collagenous framework (Fig. 17-5G, color insert), a PAS-positive component is interspersed in the ground substance of the dentin (Fig. 17-5H, color insert).

Investigations with the light microscope have alternatively confirmed and denied the presence of nerve fibrils in adult predentin and dentin stained by silver impregnations. A few unmyelinated nerve fibrils in close contact with the odontoblastic processes have been identified with the electron microscope, in predentin as well as in some tubules of the inner dentin (Fig. 17-23). In contrast to the odontoblastic process, they contain many mito-

Figure 17-22   Transverse section through a dentinal tubule located in the middle third of adult human coronal dentin. The odontoblastic process contains a centrally located vacuole (v) with peripheral condensation of hyaline cytoplasm (c). Highly calcified peritubular dentin (Pd) surrounds the tubular lumen. Id = Intertubular dentin.   ×35,000.

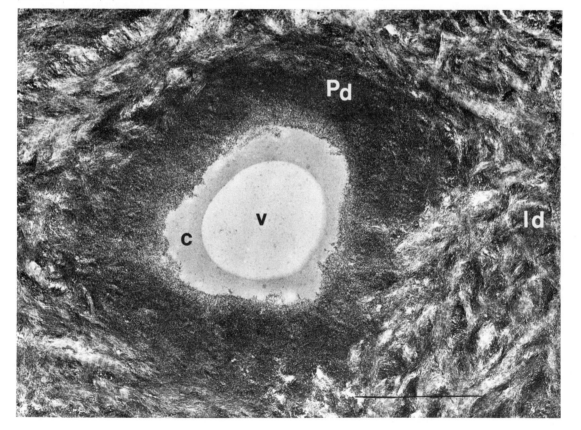

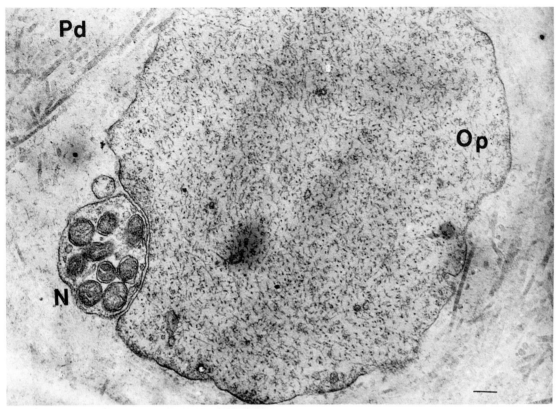

Figures 17-23 Transverse section through an odontoblastic process (Op) in predentin layer of adult human premolar. An unmyelinated nerve fiber (N) can be seen in close association with the process. The axoplasm contains numerous mitochondria and some vesicles. Pd = noncalcified predentinal collagenous matrix. ×61,000.

chondria, as well as some vesicles and neuro-tubules.

The juncture between dentin and enamel is slightly scalloped. Toward the root of the tooth, where the dentin is in contact with the cementum, it exhibits a more or less continuous layer of especially small interglobular spaces known as Tomes' granular layer. According to its appositional pattern, dentin shows parallel incremental lines (of Ebner), and sometimes even broader contour lines of Owen (see Fig. 17-21) corresponding to the lines of Retzius in the enamel (compare with Fig. 17-13).

In human teeth, the dentin matrix is often incompletely calcified, leaving interglobular dentin spaces which appear black in ground sections (Fig.

17-22). They are usually located in the peripheral coronal dentin and are parallel to the dentin-enamel junction.

Dentin continues to be formed slowly throughout life, so that the pulp cavity becomes reduced in size with age. Injury causes an increased deposit of new or secondary dentin. In response to wear and tear, the lumen of the dentinal tubules can be totally occluded by calcification, and this age change produces what is referred to as transparent, or sclerotic, dentin.

PULP

The pulp originates from the dental papilla (see Fig. 17-3), which is composed of condensed mesenchyme. It is enclosed and probably molded by the enamel organ. The young papilla is very cellular. The cells are round or polyhedral and moderately large, with pale, almost unstained cytoplasm and large nuclei. In man and monkey, these round cells have been encountered only in the pulp of fetal teeth. They appear to have no counterpart in other connective tissues, unless it be some resemblance to cartilage cells. The round cells are surrounded by the ground substance of the dental papilla, which in fetal teeth and in the growing incisors of rodents exhibits marked metachromasia (Fig. 17-5B, color insert). As the pulp matures, the round cells of the dental papilla become spindle-shaped and their metachromasia diminishes, whereas an intense alkaline phosphatase reaction persists. Glycogen is plentiful in the pulp cells of growing teeth, and a multitude of sudanophilic particles which are presumably mitochondria has been observed in their cytoplasm.

Besides the odontoblastic layer already described, it appears that the predominant cells of the adult pulp are fibrocytes and fibroblasts (Figs. 17-24 and 17-25). The intercellular spaces are filled with ground substance and a few bundles of collagen fibrils. With the electron microscope it is possible to identify some scarce bundles of small unstriated filaments about 150 Å in diameter. These bundles are ultrastructurally close to elastic fibers and similar to other microfilaments observed in the supporting tissues of the teeth.

The pulp is very vascular. Small arteries enter the apical foramina, then branch and divide into numerous capillaries which may pass between the odontoblasts, but normally do not enter the pre-dentin. The pulpal capillaries can have continuous walls with endothelial cells lined by pericytes and a basement membrane, but fenestrated capillaries with pores in their walls have been observed with the electron microscope (Fig. 17-25). Similar structures are found elsewhere such as in endocrine glands and kidneys, where fast and important liquid exchanges occur. The pulpal blood capillaries empty into very thin-walled veins which are larger in diameter than the arteries. These vessels become smaller and leave the pulp in company with the entering arteries. Whether or not lymphatic

Figure 17-24   Normal pulp of adult human tooth.   Dentin and a light zone of predentin are seen at left adjacent to the row of odontoblasts along the periphery of the pulp.   Centrally, note the delicate walls of the blood vessels of the pulp.   Decalcified section; H&E;   ×100.

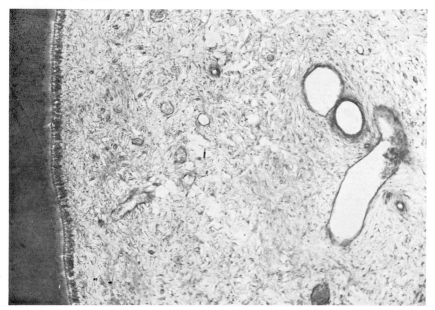

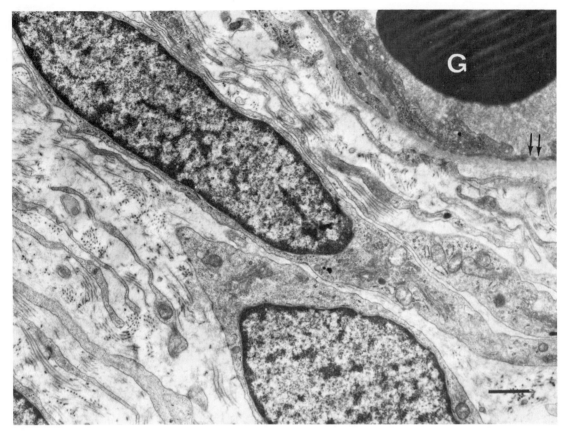

Figure 17-25   Human dental pulp with numerous elongated fibrocytes separated by intercellular spaces filled with some collagen bundles.   A blood capillary, with fenestrated walls (see arrows), contains an erythrocyte.   ×11,000.

vessels are present in the pulp has not been proved. Attempts to inject lymphatics either directly or indirectly sometimes show the injected mass within the pulp, but no conclusive evidence for the presence of such vessels has been presented to date.

The nerves of the pulp are either myelinated or unmyelinated and often twist spirally around the vessels. Myelinated nerve fibrils consist of a central axon, surrounded by a lamellated myelin sheath and a Schwann cell, limited by a basement membrane. The unmyelinated nerve fibrils are covered by a Schwann cell with typical mesaxons. They are also circumscribed by a basement membrane. These unmyelinated nerve fibrils are prominent in

the subodontoblastic layer. Some of the unmyelinated nerve fibrils can be followed with the electron microscope in the predentin (Fig. 17-23) and the inner third of dentin, where they end along the odontoblastic process.

DENTAL SUPPORTING TISSUES
The cells of the inner and outer enamel epithelium together form the *epithelial sheath* of the root, generally referred to as *Hertwig's sheath*. This sheath determines the extent and shape of the downward growth of the root. Each tooth germ, consisting of its enamel organ and papilla (see Fig. 17-3), is completely surrounded by mesenchyme, forming the *dental sac*. After the dentin of the root is

formed, the ectodermal layers degenerate, at first in the region of the neck, leaving the outer surface of the dentin exposed to the surrounding mesenchyme. The mesenchymal cells become similar to osteoblasts. These cells, the cementoblasts, form a modified appositional bone on the dentinal surface, the so-called *cementum*.

Cementum   A thin layer of cementum is deposited before the tooth erupts. This is noncellular, since none of the cementoblasts becomes embedded, and is designated *primary cementum*. After eruption a new layer of cementum forms against the external root surface, and this time the *secondary cementum* becomes much thicker and contains

several layers of cells (Fig. 17-26A). These cells, the *cementocytes*, seem to have their largest and most numerous processes directed away from the dentin, a condition that is reflected in the shape of the lacunae and canaliculi (Fig. 17-26B).

Besides supplying cementoblasts to form the secondary cementum, the mesenchyme of the dental sac also produces the thick collagenous fibers of the periodontal ligament which become embedded in the bone-like cementum matrix. These are called *Sharpey's fibers,* as are comparable structures in bone.

Periodontal ligament   The connective tissue lying in the narrow space between the cementum and

Figure 17-26   Longitudinal ground section of root of human tooth.   A. Left to right: Dentin, Tomes' granular layer, and cementum, largely acellular.   B. A higher magnification of A, showing three cementocytes, granular layer, and dentin with ramifying dentinal tubules.

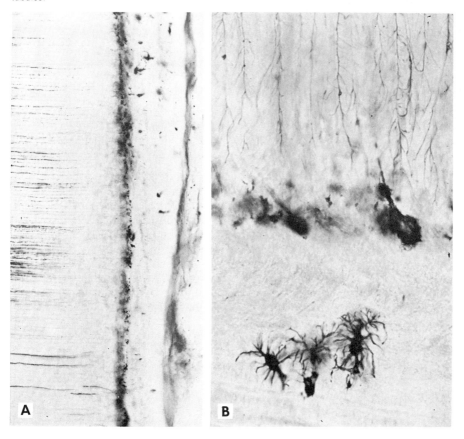

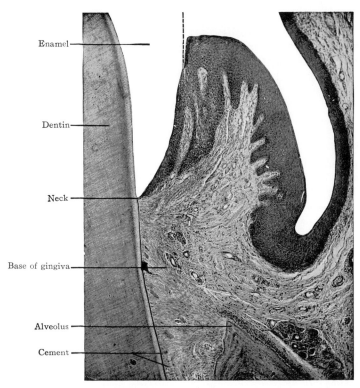

Enamel—

Dentin—

Neck—

Base of gingiva—

Alveolus—

Cement—

Figure 17-27   Tooth, periodontal ligament, and gingiva.   Decalcified section.   The enamel has been dissolved, but it once occupied the wedge-shaped space between dentin, gingiva, and the dotted line.

the bony alveolar process is referred to as the *periodontal ligament*.   Aside from the ground substance and the cellular elements, among which the fibrocytes and fibroblasts are prominent, the periodontal ligament is essentially a ligament made of bundles of collagen fibrils, with some few bundles of small unstriated microfilaments, ultrastructurally reminiscent of elastic fibers.

Some of the collagen bundles, embedded at one end in cementum known as *Sharpey's fibers*, extend from the cementum across the periodontal space and are inserted into the bone of the alveolar process, which forms the tooth socket.   They support the tooth while allowing a certain amount of motion in order to withstand the shock of biting and chewing.   The fiber direction varies at different regions of the tooth (see the diagram in Fig. 17-1).   From the root end to the rim of the alveolar process the

fiber bundles may be grouped into apical, oblique, horizontal, and alveolar crest fibers, according to their directions and attachments.   Above the alveolar processes, the transseptal fibers run between adjacent teeth, and the gingival fibers are attached to the dense connective tissue of the gum.

In addition to the cementoblasts and Sharpey's fibers, the periodontal structures include not only the usual constituents of dense collagenous connective tissue, but, importantly, also occasional epithelial nests or cords.   These are remnants of Hertwig's epithelial sheath, and proliferation of this epithelium is significant in certain diseases.

The blood vessels in the periodontal ligament pass parallel to the tooth, communicating with intralveolar and gingival vessels.   They form fine capillary loops toward the tooth.   The lymphatic vessels also form loops toward the tooth but they are more tortuous. The periodontal ligament is richly innervated, having an extremely wide range of sensitivity.

Gingiva The gum, or gingiva, forms a collar of soft tissue around the neck of each tooth (see diagram in Fig. 17-1). The gum tissue that separates adjacent teeth is called the interdental papilla. A narrow sulcus, normally less than 2 mm deep, separates the gingival margin from the tooth surface (Fig. 17-27). At the base of this sulcus, the gingiva is in contact with the tooth surfaces by a region known as the *epithelial attachment*. Two different situations have been described between the superficial epithelial cells and the enamel surface. In unerupted and in functioning erupted teeth, the plasmalemmas of the epithelial cells exhibit numerous hemidesmosomes and are separated from the enamel apatite crystals by an extracellular space containing an amorphous and granular material (Fig. 17-28, left). Histochemical methods revealed polysaccharides and proteins in this space. The second situation has been observed exclusively in erupted teeth and consists of a cuticular structure, directly in contact with the enamel apatite crystals, which is separated by a small extracellular space from the epithelial cell membranes which contain hemidesmosomes (Fig.

Figure 17-28 Junctions between the superficial cells of the epithelial attachment and the enamel surface (e) of adult human erupted tooth. On the left, an intercellular space (i), filled with granular and amorphous material, separates the cell membrane, which is coated with hemidesmosomes (see arrows), from the enamel apatite crystals (e). On the right, a cuticle (C), the so-called acquired endogenous pellicle, is interposed between the enamel apatite crystals (e) and the intercellular space (i). The epithelial cell membrane is also coated by hemidesmosomes (see arrows). ×44,000.

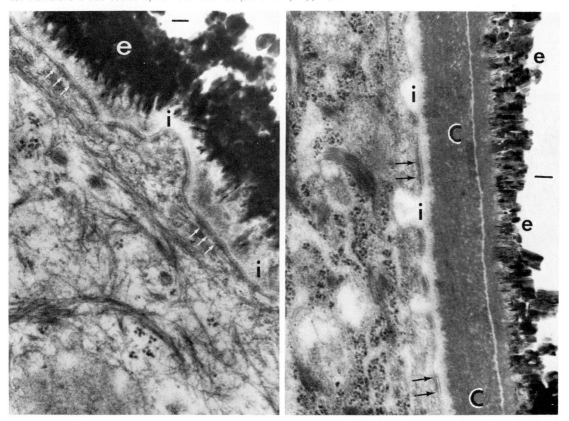

17-28, right).   This cuticle is elaborated after eruption by either epithelial or connective tissue.

In normal conditions, a certain number of lymphocytes and polymorphonuclear leukocytes cross the epithelial attachment and the sulcular epithelium and penetrate into the oral cavity.

Histologically the gingival tissue resembles the epidermis of the skin in many respects, even to the point of cornification.   It is capped by a thick layer of stratified squamous epithelium, but unlike skin, this is indented by many long, basal, connective tissue papillae.   The cell layers and the papillae become fewer as the gum dips to enclose the enamel.   The degree of cornification varies a good deal from person to person and in time, but cornification is absent within the gingival sulcus.   The gingiva contains bundles of collagen in the form of transseptal and gingival fibers.   These are so firmly attached to the neck and root surface of the tooth that they have been referred to as a circular ligament.   In the gingival lamina propria, special bundles of small unstriated filaments can be observed among the collagen fibrils (Fig. 17-29).   Elongated loops of blood and lymphatic capillaries are found in the tall connective tissue papillae under the epithelium.   The gingiva is richly innervated and has several different types of encapsulated and nonencapsulated terminal bulbs and coils in addition to free endings, some of which pass into the epithelium between the cells.

Delicate sudanophilic staining is visible in the intercellular bridges of the cells of the stratum spinosum of the Malpighian layer of the gingival epithelium.   The ground substance of the gingival connective tissue and periodontal ligament is quite perceptibly metachromatic. The stroma of the gingival tissue varies considerably in this regard, but in places it is deeply metachromatic and contains exceptionally large numbers of mast cells (see Fig. 17-5C, color insert), surpassing in this respect most other normal connective tissues.   Glycogen is present in the stratified epithelium of the gingival

Figure 17-29   Intercellular spaces of the lamina propria of the human gingiva contain typical collagen fibrils as well as bundles of small nonstriated filaments (arrows), seen in a longitudinal section on the left ($\times$38,000) and in a transverse section on the right ($\times$29,000).

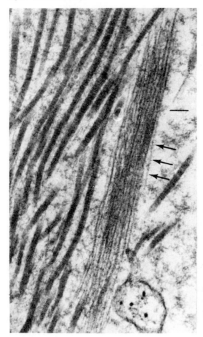
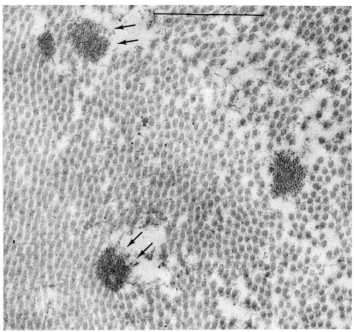

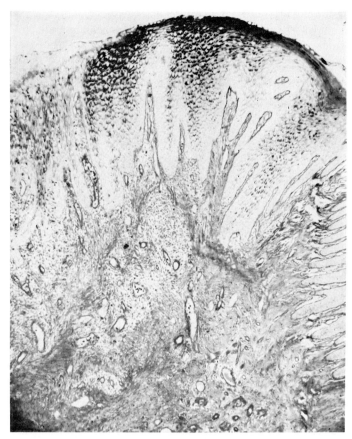

Figure 17-30 Gingival tissue from adult man. Note the tall, slender connective tissue papilla. Stained with the periodic acid–Schiff method, the darkest areas indicate that glycogen is especially abundant in the stratum spinosum of the squamous epithelium. ×90.

mucous membrane, especially in the prickle cell layer (Fig. 17-30). The supporting structures of growing and adult teeth also give a marked reaction for alkaline phosphatase. The lamina propria of the gingiva contains variable quantities of this enzyme, the reaction involving, to various degrees, the cells, fibers, ground substance, and walls of the arterioles.

The continuing persistence of metachromatic ground substance (acid mucopolysaccharide) and alkaline phosphatase in the periodontal membrane and especially in the tunica propria of the gingiva may suggest that the tissues involved are permanently in a state of elevated metabolic activity. The excess of these substances in the gingival tissue may be a response to constant friction, irritation, and abrasion to which the supporting structures of the teeth are continuously subjected.

Alveolar bone The alveolar bone is part of the tooth-supporting tissues, closely associated to the periodontal ligament and the gingiva. Anatomically the alveolar bone can be defined as the part of the mandible or the maxilla surrounding the dental roots. The alveolar bone is continuous with the body of the upper or lower jaw without distinct boundary.

Alveolar bone consists of a thin layer of lamellar bone, the lamina dura or cribriform plate, limiting the socket, and a cortical plate of compact lamellar bone. A small amount of spongy bone, with medullary spaces, is found between the two plates of lamellar bone. The principal fibers of the periodontal ligament penetrate the alveolar bone as Sharpey's fibers. Along the lamina dura, osteoblasts and some osteoclasts can be found in the periodontal ligament. Communicating with the marrow spaces, the lamina dura is perforated by many openings, through which nerves and blood vessels can pass into the periodontal ligament.

References

ANDERSON, D. J., A. G. HANNAM, and B. MATTHEWS: Sensory Mechanisms in Mammalian Teeth and Their Supporting Structures, *Physiol. Rev.*, **50:**171 (1970).

BOYDE, A.: The Development of Enamel Structure, *Proc. Roy. Soc. Med.*, **60:**923 (1967).

BRODIE, A. G.: On the Growth Pattern of the Human Head from the Third Month to the Eighth Year of Life, *Amer. J. Anat.*, **68:**209 (1941).

CARMICHAEL, G. G., and H. M. FULLMER: The Fine Structure of the Oxytalan Fiber, *J. Cell Biol.*, **28:**33 (1966).

CRABB, H. S. M., and A. I. DARLING: The Pattern of Progressive Mineralization in Human Dental Enamel, in "International Series of Monographs on Oral Biology," vol. 2, Pergamon Press, New York, 1962.

EASTOE, J. E.: The Amino-acid Composition of Proteins from the Oral Tissues: II. The Matrix Proteins in Dentine and Enamel from Developing Human Deciduous Teeth, *Arch. Oral Biol.*, **8:**633 (1963).

ENGEL, M. B.: Glycogen and Carbohydrate-protein Complex in Developing Teeth of the Rat, *J. Dent. Res.*, **27:**681 (1948).

FINN, S. B.: "Biology of the Dental Pulp Organ: A Symposium," University of Alabama Press, University, Ala., 1968.

FRANK, R. M.: Autoradiographie Quantitative de l'Amélogenèse en Microscopie Electronique à l'Aide de la Proline Tritiée Chez le Chat, *Arch Oral Biol.*, **15:**569 (1970).

FRANK, R. M.: Étude Autoradiographique de la Dentinogenèse en Microscopie Électronique à l'Aide de la Pronine Tritiée Chez le Chat, *Arch Oral Biol.*, **15:**583 (1970).

FRANK, R. M., and G. CIMASONI: Ultrastructure de l'Epithèlium Cliniquement Normal du Sillon et de la Jonction Gingivo-dentaires, *Z. Zellforsch.*, **103:**356 (1970).

FRANK, R. M., and P. FRANK: Autoradiographie Quantitative de l'Ostéogenèse en Microscopie Electronique à l'Aide de la Proline Tritièe, *Z. Zellforsch.*, **99:**121 (1969).

GARANT, P. R., G. SZABÓ, and J. NALBANDIAN: The Fine Structure of the Mouse Odontoblast, *Arch. Oral Biol.*, **13:**857 (1968).

GLIMCHER, J. M., E. J. DANIEL, D. F. TRAVIS, and S. KAMHI: Electron Optical and X-ray Diffraction Studies of the Organization of the Inorganic Crystals in Embryonic Bovine Enamel, *J. Ultrastruct. Res.* (suppl. 1), **7:**77 (1965).

GREEP, R. O. (ed.): Recent Advances in the Study of the Structure, Composition and Growth of Mineralized Tissues, *Ann. N.Y. Acad. Sci.*, **60:**541 (1955).

GREEP, R. O., C. J. FISCHER, and A. MORSE: Alkaline Phosphatase in Odontogenesis and Osteogenesis and Its Histochemical Demonstration after Demineralization, *J. Amer. Dent. Ass.*, **36:**427 (1948).

GREGORY, W. K.: "The Origin and Evolutions of the Human Dentition," Williams & Wilkins, Baltimore, 1922.

GROVE, C. A., G. C. JUDD, and G. S. ANSELL: Determination of Hydroxyapatite Crystallite Size in Human Dental Enamel by Dark-field Electron Microscopy, *J. Dent. Res.*, **51**:22 (1972).

KALLENBACH, E.: Fine Structure of Rat Incisor Ameloblasts during Enamel Maturation, *J. Ultrastruct. Res.*, **22**:90 (1968).

KATCHBURIAN, E., and S. J. HOLT: Role of Lysosomes in Amelogenesis, *Nature,* **223**:1367 (1969).

LEBLOND, C. P., L. F. BELANGER, and R. C. GREULICH: Formation of Bones and Teeth as Visualized by Radioautography, *Ann. N.Y. Acad Sci.*, **60**:629 (1955).

LEHNER, J., and H. PLENK: Die Zähne, in W. von Möllendorf (ed.), "Handbuch mikroskop. Anat. Menschen," vol. 5, pt. 3, Springer-Verlag, Berlin, 1936.

LISTGARTEN, M. A.: Electron Microscopic Study of the Gingivodental Junction of Man, *Amer. J. Anat.*, **119**:147 (1966).

LORBER, M.: A Study of the Histochemical Reactions of the Dental Cementum and Alveolar Bone, *Anat. Rec.*, **111**:129 (1951).

MECKEL, A. H., W. J. GRIEBSTEIN, and R. J. NEAL: Structure of Mature Dental Enamel as Observed by Electron Microscopy, *Arch. Oral Biol.*, **10**:775 (1965).

MILES, A. E. W.: "Structural and Chemical Organization of Teeth," vol. II, Academic Press, New York, 1967.

NYLEN, M. U. and D. B. SCOTT: An Electron Microscopic Study of the Early Stages of Dentinogenesis, *U.S. Public Health Service Publ.* 613, 1958.

REITAN, K.: Tissue Behavior during Orthodontic Tooth Movement, *Amer. J. Orthodont.*, **46**:881 (1960).

REITH, E. J.: The Ultrastructure of Ameloblasts during Early Stages of Maturation of Enamel, *J. Cell Biol.*, **18**:691 (1963).

REITH, E. J.: The Ultrastructure of Ameloblasts from the Growing End of Rat Incisors, *Arch. Oral Biol.*, **2**:253 (1960).

RÖNNHOLM, E.: The Structure of the Organic Stroma of Human Enamel during Amelogenesis, *J. Ultrastruct. Res.*, **3**:368 (1962).

SCHROEDER, H. E., and J. THEILADE: Electron Microscopy of Normal Human Gingival Epithelium, *J. Periodont. Res.*, **1**:95 (1966).

SELVIG, K. A.: An Ultrastructural Study of Cementum Formation, *Acta Odont. Scand.*, **22**:105 (1964).

SOGNNAES, R. F.: Dental Aspects of the Structure and Metabolism of Mineralized Tissues, in Comar and Bronner, (eds.), "Mineral Metabolism—An Advanced Treatise," vol. I, Part B, p. 677, Academic Press, New York, 1961.

SOGNNAES, R. F. (ed.): Calcification in Biological Systems, Publ. 64, American Association for the Advancement of Science, Washington, D.C., 1960.

SOGNNAES, R. F.: Microstructure and Histochemical Characteristics of the Mineralized Tissues, in "Recent Advances in the Study of the Structure, Composition, and Growth of Mineralized Tissues," *Ann. N.Y. Acad. Sci.,* **60**:541 (1955).

SQUIER, C. A., and J. P. WATERHOUSE: Lysosomes in Oral Epithelium: The Ultrastructural Localization of Acid Phosphatase and Non-specific Esterase in Keratinized Oral Epithelium in Man and Rat, *Arch. Oral Biol.*, **15**:153 (1970).

STACK, M. V., and R. W. FEARNHEAD: "Tooth Enamel: Its Composition, Properties and Fundamental Structure," John Wright & Sons, Bristol, England, 1965.

SYMONS, N. B. B. (ed.): "Dentine and Pulp: Their Structure and Reactions," E. & S. Livingstone, Edinburgh, 1968.

TRAVIS, D. F.: Comparative Ultrastructure and Organization of Inorganic Crystals and Organic Matrices of Mineralized Tissues, in P. Person (ed.), "Biology of the Mouth," Publ. 89, p. 236, American Association for the Advancement of Science, Washington, D.C., 1968.

WAERHAUG, J.: The Gingival Pocket: Anatomy, Pathology, Deepening and Elimination, *Odont. T.* (Suppl. 1), **60**:5 (1952).

WARSHAWSKY, H.: The Fine Structure of Secretory Ameloblasts in Rat Incisors, *Anat. Rec.*, **161**:211 (1968).

WATSON, M. L.: The Extracellular Nature of Enamel in the Rat, *J. Biophys. Biochem. Cytol.*, **7**:489 (1960).

WEIDENREICH, R.: Über den Bau und die Entwicklung des Zahnbeines in der Reihe der Wirbeltiere, *Z. Anat. Entwicklungsgesch,* **76**:218 (1925).

WEINSTOCK, A.: Elaboration of Enamel and Dentin Matrix Glycoproteins, in G. H. Bourne (ed.), "The Biochemistry and Physiology of Bone," 2d ed., vol. II, Academic Press, New York, 1972, p. 121.

WEINSTOCK, A., and J. T. ALBRIGHT: The Fine Structure of Mast Cells in Normal Human Gingiva, *J. Ultrastruct. Res.*, **17**:245 (1967).

WEINSTOCK, A., and C. P. LEBLOND: Elaboration of the Matrix Glycoprotein of Enamel by the Secretory Ameloblasts of the Rat Incisor as Revealed by Radioautography after ³H-Galactose Injection, *J. Cell Biol.*, **51**:26 (1971).

WEINSTOCK, A., M. WEINSTOCK, and C. P. LEBLOND: Autoradiographic Detection of ³H-fucose Incorporation into Glycoprotein by Odontoblasts and Its Deposition at the Site of the Calcification Front in Dentin, *Calcif. Tissue Res.*, **8**:181 (1972).

WISLOCKI, G. B., and R. F. SOGNNAES: Histochemical Reactions of Normal Teeth, *Amer. J. Anat.*, **87**:239 (1950).

YOUNG, R. W., and R. C. GREULICH: Distinctive Autoradiographic Patterns of Glycine Incorporation in Rat Enamel and Dentine Matrices, *Arch. Oral Biol.*, **8**:509 (1963).

chapter 18 The digestive tract

HELEN A. PADYKULA

The digestive tract performs two principal functions: the *propulsion* of foodstuffs from the mouth toward the anus, which is accomplished by waves of contraction (peristalsis) in its muscular layers, and the *digestion* and *absorption* of the usable components of food. The changing functions of the digestive tract are reflected, along its length, by distinct gross, histologic, and cellular variations. After the oral cavity, the hollow digestive tube is differentiated into four major organs: *esophagus, stomach, small intestine,* and *large intestine.* Grossly the organs are separated by muscular valves or sphincters (G. *sphinkter,* that which binds tight); these control the passage of contents from one organ to the next. At these junctions, the nature of the lining layer, the *mucous membrane* or *mucosa,* also changes abruptly. The digestion of carbohydrates is initiated in the oral cavity, but most of the digestion and absorption is accomplished by the mucosae of the stomach and small intestine in coordination with the secretions of the pancreas and

liver. The undigested materials form a semisolid mass in the large intestine for *egestion* from the body. To a lesser degree, the alimentary tract also serves as an avenue of *excretion,* eliminating a number of waste products, some of which are secreted by the liver and carried in the bile to the duodenum, and some of which are secreted by the large intestine. Although it has long been known that lymphatic tissue occurs in abundance in the digestive tube, its participation as a *local immune system* in the body's defense mechanisms has only recently begun to be appreciated. We now know that, in response to the presence of living microorganisms in the lumen, the mucosae produce antibodies, especially immunoglobulin A.

Except for the oral cavity, the histologic organization of the digestive tube has a common plan which is evident throughout its length. This plan will be presented after the description of the principal features of the human oral cavity and of the major salivary glands.

Oral cavity

The initial processing of food occurs in the mouth by chewing. This is assisted by the movements of the tongue which also "tastes" the ingested food through specialized receptors. The digestion of carbohydrates commences through the action of salivary amylase. In addition, defense mechanisms, represented by salivary immunoglobulins and lactoperoxidase, control microbial growth.

In the oral cavity, stratified squamous epithelium covers the red border of the *lip,* the *oral mucosa,* the *tongue,* and the *tonsils.* Embryologically, the oral epithelium also gives rise to a variety of *oral glands.* Additionally, the densely calcified outer enamel layer of the *teeth* originates from the oral epithelium, through a complex process of invagination, growth, differentiation, and calcification.

The mouth is lined by a mucous membrane (*mucosa*) which has two components, a *stratified squamous epithelium* that is smooth-surfaced and an underlying layer of reticular connective tissue called the *lamina propria* which often has accumulations of lymphoid cells (Figs. 18-1 to 18-4). The epitheliostromal interface is usually distinctly scalloped to varying degrees by stromal *papillae* ("pegs") that carry blood, lymphatic, and neural systems into close association with the thick epithelium. In some regions, such as the soft palate and cheeks, a deeper layer of connective tissue called the *submucosa* occurs. No smooth muscle intervenes, however, between these two layers of connective tissue. The submucosa in the oral cavity contains adipose cells and the secretory portions of glands. Wherever the submucosa is well developed, the mucosa can be moved, as, for example, in the cheeks.

KERATINIZED SURFACES
In regions subject to the mechanical forces related to mastication, the stratified squamous epithelium is keratinized and closely resembles the epidermis, even at the ultrastructural level (Schroeder and Theilade, 1966). It has the strata, the basalis, spinosum, granulosum, and corneum (Figs. 18-1 and 18-4A). Such cornified epithelia occur in the *gingiva* (oral mucosa that surrounds the teeth and the external surfaces of the alveolar processes, that is, the gums), *hard palate,* and *dorsal surface* of

the *tongue.* As in the epidermis, there is a labyrinthine intercellular space in the epithelium which is sealed at the free surface by tight junctions and is open toward the basal lamina. A dense material is present in the intercellular spaces associated with the upper layers of the stratum granulosum. Hemidesmosomes occur along the surface of the basal cells associated with the basal lamina. This keratinized mucosa differs from the epidermis in that glycogen may be stored in the cells of the upper spinosum and stratum granulosum. The keratinized epithelia of the gingiva and hard palate are associated with a dense fibrous lamina propria that is firmly attached to cementum of the tooth or to bone.

The gingiva has been intensively studied because of its involvement in dental disease. Investigators have long tried to determine the mode of attachment of the gingival stratified squamous epithelium to the tooth. Ultrastructural evidence indicates that this epithelium is attached directly to the enamel and "cuticles" of the teeth by an apparatus consisting of a basal lamina and hemidesmosomes (Listgarten, 1966). This adhesion is similar to that occurring between any epithelium and its underlying connective tissue; however, it should be pointed out that enamel is not of connective tissue origin. The gingival epithelium, like the epidermis, contains melanocytes. It is renewed every 1 to 2 weeks (monkey); this renewal here and elsewhere in the oral mucosa is subject to diurnal variations.

NONKERATINIZED SURFACES
Nonkeratinized surfaces occur in regions of lower mechanical stress, such as the vestibule, floor of the mouth, cheeks, soft palate, and ventral surface of the tongue (Fig. 18-3). This stratified squamous epithelium differs from that of the gingiva and hard palate in that it lacks a stratum granulosum and stratum corneum. Above the strata germinativum and spinosum, there are desquamating layers of flattened, nucleated cells (stratum disjunctum) that are held together loosely and are easily scraped off. High glycogen content is a characteristic of the nonkeratinized epithelium; during epithelial migration, glycogen accumulates gradually, and peak storage occurs in the upper squamous layers. The

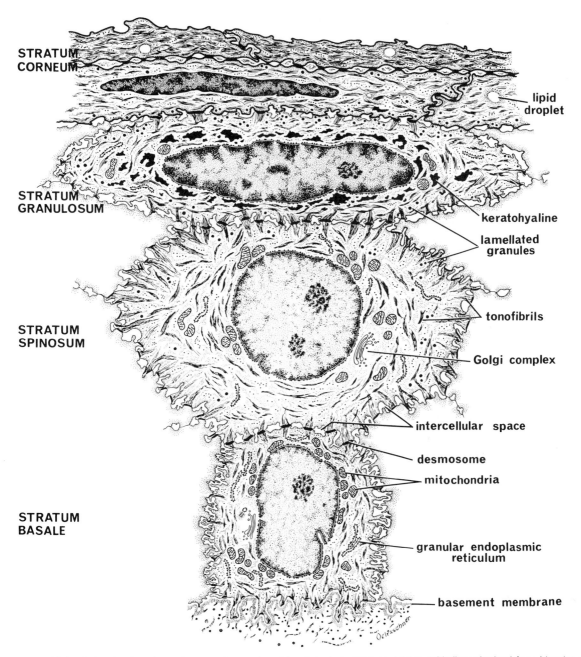

STRATUM CORNEUM

STRATUM GRANULOSUM

STRATUM SPINOSUM

STRATUM BASALE

lipid droplet

keratohyaline

lamellated granules

tonofibrils

Golgi complex

intercellular space

desmosome

mitochondria

granular endoplasmic reticulum

basement membrane

Figure 18-1   A drawing based on electron micrographs of keratinized stratified squamous epithelium obtained from biopsies of the human hard palate.   Each cell is representative of the cells usually found in the four successive cell layers indicated on the left.   Characteristic features are the basement membrane separating the cells of the basal layer from the underlying connective tissue; the desmosomes joining one cell to another; tonofibrils composed of tightly packed tonofilaments; keratohyaline granules in the cells of the stratum granulosum; and the keratin of the stratum coreum.   (Courtesy of Dr. Alfred Weinstock, University of California, Los Angeles.)

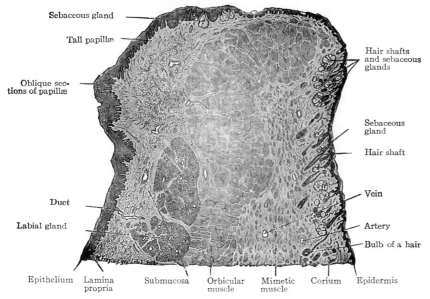

Figure 18-2 Vertical section through the lower lip of a man 19 years of age. Epidermis and corium constitute the skin; epithelium, lamina propria, and submucosa form the oral mucous membrane. ×10.

Figure 18-3 Nonkeratinized oral mucosa. Vertical section from the undersurface of the tongue. Zenker fixation; H&E. (Drawing by E. Piotti.)

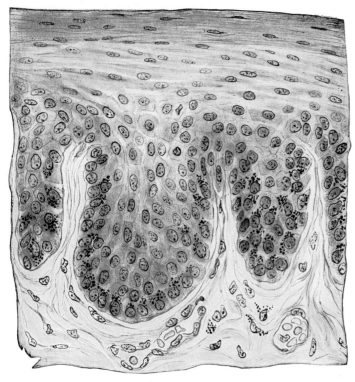

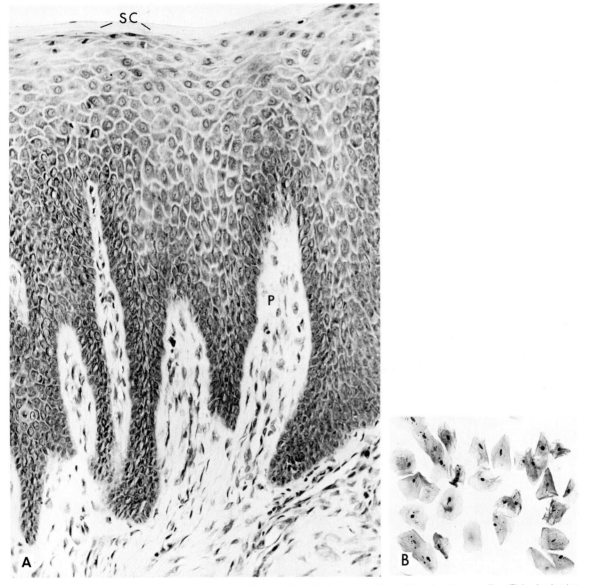

Figure 18-4 A. Keratinized stratified squamous epithelium of the adult human gingiva. Note the deep papillae (P) in the lamina propria. SC, stratum corneum. Toluidine blue. B. Desquamated cells in the normal human oral cavity. (Courtesy of Dr. G. Shklar.)

shed cells occur in large numbers in the saliva (Fig. 18-4B).

An ultrastructural investigation of the human posterior buccal mucosa has revealed that it is remarkably similar to embryonic skin (Hashimoto et al., 1966). Progressive thickening of the plasma membranes occurs during cytomorphosis in the absence of obvious keratinization, and tonofilaments are relatively few in number. Active melanocytes occur here also. In addition, lymphocytes have been observed in migration through the epithelium.

LIPS

The red border occurs only in man and is a transitional zone between the external skin and the internal oral mucosa (Fig. 18-2). Here the stratified squamous epithelium has a well-developed stratum lucidum and a thin corneum. This transparent epithelium is associated with deep stromal papillae that are richly vascularized, creating the red ap-

pearance. The lips and oral mucosa are the most accessible parts of the digestive canal and hence are usually examined as an index of health or disease.

MINOR SALIVARY GLANDS

Minor salivary glands occur throughout the oral mucosa, except in the gingiva and portions of the hard palate. They are either pure mucous glands or mixed glands that have more mucous than serous cells (see section on major salivary glands for definitions). They serve to moisten the lips (*labial,* mixed type), cheeks (*buccal,* mixed type), palate (*palatine,* pure mucous type), and the floor of the mouth (*minor sublinguals,* mixed type).

TONGUE

The adult human tongue has an anterior and a posterior region, each with a different embryonic origin; the boundary between the two regions is V-shaped and is the location of the principal gusta-

Figure 18-5   Dorsum of the human tongue, showing papillae and the palatine tonsils.   (Sappey.)

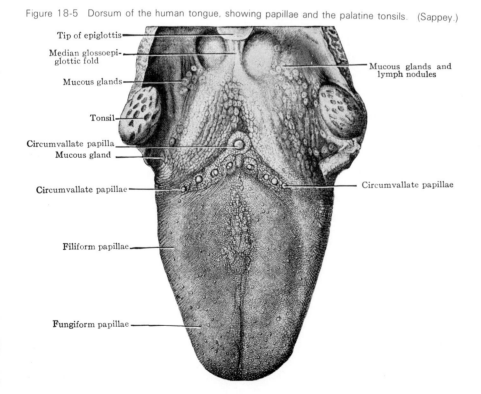

Tip of epiglottis

Median glossoepi-glottic fold

Mucous glands

Tonsil

Circumvallate papilla

Mucous gland

Circumvallate papillae

Filiform papillae

Fungiform papillae

Mucous glands and lymph nodules

Circumvallate papillae

tory receptors, the circumvallate (vallate) papillae (Fig. 18-5). In the adult the dorsal surface of the anterior region of the tongue is rough because of several types of elevations or *papillae* whereas the ventral surface is smooth. The *lingual tonsils* are located on the posterior part behind the circumvallate papillae.

The core of this highly muscular organ consists of interwoven bundles of skeletal muscle fibers that constitute the various intrinsic and extrinsic *lingual muscles*. Some of the muscle bundles are oblique in orientation, whereas others cross at right angles in either horizontal or vertical planes. These muscles are innervated by lingual branches of the hypoglossal nerve which supply all the lingual muscles except the palatoglossus; the latter is supplied by fibers from the vagus nerve. The intricate arrangement of the muscle bundles forms the mechanical basis for the highly varied and delicate voluntary movements that are possible with the tongue.

This muscular mass is covered by a highly specialized mucous membrane that consists of a keratinized stratified squamous epithelium and a dense lamina propria that is continuous with the connective tissue partitions among the lingual muscles. A submucosa occurs only on the ventral surface beneath a typical nonkeratinized oral mucosa. Lingual glands occur in the connective tissue layers, including the stromal partitions among the muscle bundles. The *anterior lingual gland* contains mixed secretory tubules with demilunes and, in some portions, tubules with only seromucous cells (see below). The circumvallate papillae are surrounded by a deep trench which is a circular invagination of the mucosa (Figs. 18-7 and 18-11). This trench is irrigated by pure serous secretion from the *glands of von Ebner*. The *posterior lingual glands* are the pure mucous type.

The velvety appearance of most of the dorsal surface of the tongue is created by mucosal projections called *lingual papillae* (Figs. 18-6 to 18-8), all of which have a stratified squamous epithelial cover. The most numerous, slender, and smallest are the *filiform papillae* that are arranged approximately in rows aligned in relation to the V-shaped gustatory region. The cornified squamous cells are oriented toward the tip of the papilla and are stacked like superimposed hollow cones. The underlying connective tissue core (the *primary papilla*) is thrown into *secondary papillae,* a device for increasing epitheliostromal interaction. Scattered among the filiform projections are the fungiform papillae which are conspicuous elevations that have flattened domelike surfaces (Fig. 18-6). Their epithelium is thinner because of less cornification and thus the underlying high vascularity of the secondary papillae is manifested as redness. The *circumvallate papillae,* generally 6 to 12 in number, occur along the V-shaped boundary of the anterior and posterior parts of the tongue. These broad papillae (1 to 3 mm wide and 1 to 1.5 mm tall) do not protrude beyond the lingual surface but rather each is surrounded by circular invagination of the surface (*papillary crypt*) that forms a moat around it (Figs. 18-7, 18-10, and 18-11). Taste buds are located within the epithelial cover along the lateral walls of the papillae. The upper surface is covered by a smooth thin epithelium that is ridged by the underlying secondary papillae (Fig. 18-7). A fourth type, the *foliate papilla,* is a leaflike mucosal fold that occurs on the lateral surface of the tongue (Fig. 18-8). These papillae are less pronounced in man than in other mammals, such as the rabbit, where they constitute the principal organ of taste. Although taste buds in man occur primarily on the circumvallate and foliate papillae, they occur also to some extent on the fungiform papillae, soft palate, and laryngeal surface of the epiglottis. The gustatory nerves are the chorda tympani, glossopharyngeal, and vagus.

TASTE BUDS

Taste buds are oval groups of elongate epithelial cells that extend from the basal lamina toward the *taste pore,* which is a small opening in the surrounding epithelium (Fig. 18-9). Thus the gustatory receptors are protected by their enclosure within the stratified squamous epithelium from any injury by friction. Taste buds are conspicuous in histochemical preparations that demonstrate membrane ATPase activity (Fig. 18-10A). Light microscopists have generally identified two types of cells in the taste bud: (1) sensory *taste cells* (neuroepithelial taste cells) which have a *taste hair* on their free surface and occupy a central location in the taste bud and (2) *supporting cells* that occur mainly on the periphery. Autoradiographic study of the renewal of cells in the rat taste bud indicates that

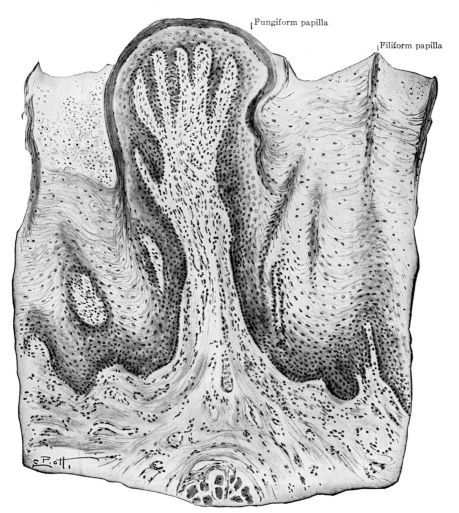

Fungiform papilla

Filiform papilla

Figure 18-6 Fungiform and filiform papillae on the human tongue. Note the primary and secondary papillae. Zenker fixation; H&E.

germinal cells occur in the periphery of the taste bud and that certain daughter cells move in and migrate toward the center (Beidler and Smallman, 1965). It was determined that about one cell enters the taste bud every 10 hr and that the lifespan of an average cell is about 250 hr. There is evidence also of cell death within the taste bud. It is thus a differentiating system of sensory receptor cells that establish contact with intraepithelial gustatory nerve endings. The existence of taste buds is dependent on intact innervation (Fig. 18-10B).

Ultrastructural studies of rabbit taste buds have identified three types of cells, only one of which is extensively associated with nerve endings in a synaptic association and thus may be the gustatory receptor (Murray et al., 1969). Naked nerve terminals occur in an intraepithelial position and are closely apposed to the surface of the neuroepithelial taste cells; vesicles, some with dense cores, are numerous on the "presynaptic side." Ultrastructural interpretation is complicated by the fact that the cells of the taste bud constitute a dynamic

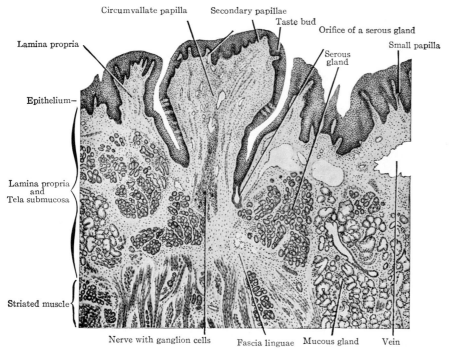

Circumvallate papilla Secondary papillae
Taste bud
Orifice of a serous gland
Lamina propria
Small papilla
Serous
gland
Epithelium—
Lamina propria
and
Tela submucosa
Striated muscle
Nerve with ganglion cells Fascia linguae Mucous gland Vein

Figure 18-7   Vertical section of a human circumvallate papilla. ×25.

differentiating system in which the cells have a relatively short life-span.   Interesting functional speculations have been made about the possibility that sensitivity to different taste stimuli may change during the life-span of a gustatory receptor (Beidler and Smallman, 1965).

Ciliated cells have been recently identified near the floor of the papillary crypt of human circumval-late papillae (Mattern et al., 1970).   These mitochondria-rich cells are located 0.25 to 0.5 mm below the taste buds and somewhat above the openings of the ducts of von Ebner's glands (Fig. 18-11).   Thus, the ciliated cells are equipped, by their cellular machinery and their position, to be a microcirculatory system in the crypt for the movement of gustatory stimuli.

Major salivary glands

The parotid, submandibular (formerly submaxillary), and sublingual glands elaborate a major portion of the saliva.   These compound tubuloacinar glands secrete proteins, glycoproteins, electrolytes, and water into the oral cavity.   This secretory activity is controlled almost entirely by the autonomic nervous system.   The best known protein of saliva is the enzyme salivary amylase, which initiates the digestion of carbohydrate.   The average daily output of saliva in man is about 750 to 1,000 ml; saliva is a dilute aqueous fluid which is not an ultrafiltrate of the blood since it differs in the concentration of hydrogen ions, chloride ions, glucose, proteins, and in other constituents as well.   Within minutes after an intravenous injection of iodide, the concentration of this ion in the saliva is at least 20 times greater than in the serum.   This distinctive composition indicates that the secretion of saliva

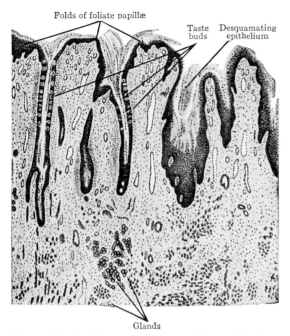

Folds of foliate papillæ

Taste buds   Desquamating epithelium

Glands

Figure 18-8   Vertical section of a human foliate papilla.   Zenker fixation; H&E.   (Sobotta.)

is an energy-requiring process.   Furthermore, it has recently become known that saliva contains gamma globulins, the predominant one being immuno-globulin A (IgA).   Lactoperoxidase has also been recently identified as a component of saliva; this enzyme, along with IgA, may be part of a salivary antibacterial system.

From this brief physiologic introduction, it should be evident that the histologic-cytologic organization of these exocrine glands reflect mechanisms for protein and glycoprotein synthesis and transport, as well as mechanisms related to the transport of water and electrolytes.   It should be noted that among different mammals there is considerable morphologic variation in these glands, which is probably related primarily to dietary differences (carnivores as against herbivores).

These exocrine glands are organized around a branching duct system that carries the secretion to the oral cavity.   The secretory cells are arranged as *acini* or secretory end pieces around the smallest branches of the duct system to form many individual lobules which may be viewed as secretory units (Figs. 18-12 and 18-13).   Each acinus is limited

Figure 18-9   Section on the side (left) and through the center (right) of taste buds of a camel's tongue.   Methylene blue and eosin stain.

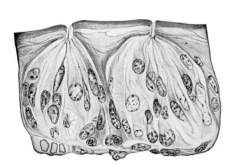

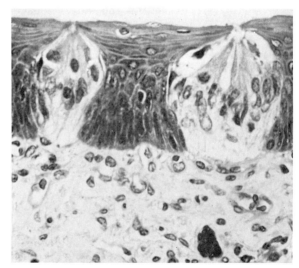

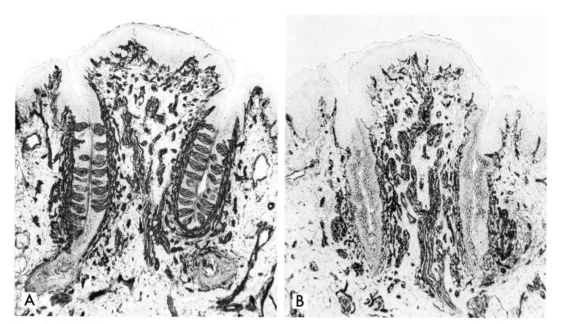

Figure 18-10 ATPase activity in the taste buds of circumvallate papillae (rat).   ×70.   A. Normal papilla.   Note the intense ATPase activity in the numerous taste buds in the epithelium that lines the trench.   B. Papilla 2 weeks after denervation.   The taste buds have disappeared.   (From A. A. Zalewski, Exp. Neurol., **30:**510, 1971.)

by a distinct basement membrane, and two types of secretory cells occur in the acinar epithelium, the *serous cells* and the *mucous cells*.   The parotid gland of most species is composed entirely of serous acini (Fig. 18-14) whereas the submandibular and sublingual glands contain both (Figs. 18-15 and 18-16, see color insert).   In the submandibular gland of man, serous cells outnumber the mucous cells, whereas the opposite is true for the sublingual gland.

The cytology of the serous cells can be most easily comprehended by envisioning them as variations of the pancreatic acinar cells, an enzyme-producing cell that has been so thoroughly investigated by Palade and his associates that it serves as a model cellular system (see Chap. 20).   At the light-microscopic level, the serous cells are pyramidal in shape, their nuclei are basal, cell boundaries are indistinct, the basal and perinuclear cytoplasm are basophilic (Fig. 18-14), and the apical cytoplasm contains secretory granules which vary in number according to functional state.   There are two major variants that can be distinguished by the presence

or absence of histochemically demonstrable carbohydrate polymer in the cytoplasmic granules.   According to this classification (Munger, 1964), the pancreatic acinar cells and the gastric chief cells

Figure 18-11 Circumvallate papilla (human).   Schematic drawing.   Ciliated cells are located in the lining at the base of the crypt just below the taste buds and immediately above the opening of the ducts of the glands of von Ebner.   (Mattern et al.)

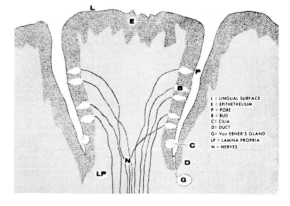

L = LINGUAL SURFACE
E = EPITHETHELIUM
P = PORE
B = BUD
C = CILIA
D = DUCT
G = Von EBNER'S GLAND
LP = LAMINA PROPRIA
N = NERVES

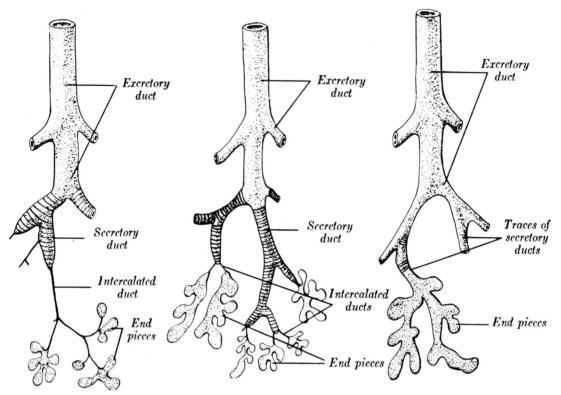

Figure 18-12   Diagram of the salivary glands.   Parotid gland is at the left, submandibular gland in the middle, and sublingual gland at the right.   (From E. V. Cowdry, "A Textbook of Histology," Lea & Febiger, Philadelphia, 1950.)

are termed *serous cells* on the basis of the relative absence of such carbohydrate whereas in the human submandibular gland, where the granules contain sialomucin and sulfomucin, the cells are called *seromucous* cells (Leblond).

At the ultrastructural level, the cytoplasmic basophilia of the serous cells corresponds to an abundant rough endoplasmic reticulum (ER); and the secretory granules occur within the membranes of the supranuclear Golgi complex (Fig. 18-17). These features are typical of cells that produce protein for export. In addition, ultrastructural variations occur that may be related to the secretion of saliva in particular. For example, the serous cells of the human submandibular gland possess numerous slender basal projections that extend beyond the lateral margins as radiating foot processes that interdigitate with adjacent cells.

This device increases surface area directed toward the vascular pole by at least sixtyfold and may be a specialization for transport of electrolytes and water into the primary secretion that enters the acinar lumen. Amylase is probably produced by serous cells because their ultrastructural features are compatible with this function; the parotid gland, which has a high content of amylase, possesses only serous cells. Peroxidase has been localized in the secretory granules of serous cells in the salivary glands of several species.

The mucous cells of the salivary glands may be viewed as variations of the intestinal goblet cell which has been the subject of considerable ultrastructural and analytic interpretation (see below). In the fresh condition, the cytoplasm may be filled with numerous droplets of mucigen; in routine preparations these droplets are usually dissolved out and the cytoplasm assumes an empty or vacuolated appearance (Figs. 18-15 and 18-16, see color insert). The mucous droplets are intensely reactive in the periodic acid–Schiff (PAS) procedure, since they contain neutral glycoproteins and acid mucosubstances, such as sulfomucins or sialomucins (containing hexosamine and sialic acid in combination with protein) (see Leppi and Spicer, 1966). Some mucous cells produce sulfomucin (for example, most acini of the human sublingual) whereas others produce sialomucin or mixtures of the two (human submandibular). When the acid mucosub-

stances are preserved in a tissue section, the droplets are strongly basophilic. In a fully laden cell, the nucleus is basal and appears to be compressed by the accumulated secretion. The ultrastructure of the mucous cell is essentially similar to that of the goblet cell; that is, most of the supranuclear cytoplasm is filled with secretory droplets that have been derived from the large central supranuclear Golgi complex. As secretion accumulates, the mitochondria and rough ER are relegated to the lateral and basal cytoplasm.

A secretory end piece or acinus may be com-

Figure 18-13   Reconstruction of the secretory end piece and intralobular ducts of the submandibular gland. D, demilune composed of serous cells; M, mucous cells; My, myoepithelial cells; SC, secretory capillaries in a serous acinus; ID, intercalated duct; SD, striated duct. A. Cross section through the striated duct. B. Cross section through the intercalated duct. C. Cross section through a mucous acinus. D. Cross section through a serous acinus. (From H. Braus, "Anatomie der Menschen," Springer-Verlag OHG, Berlin, 1924.)

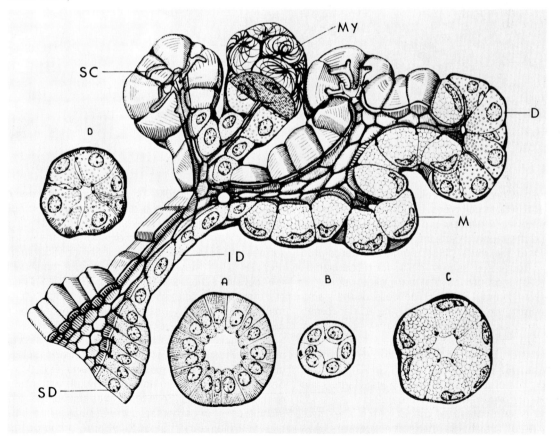

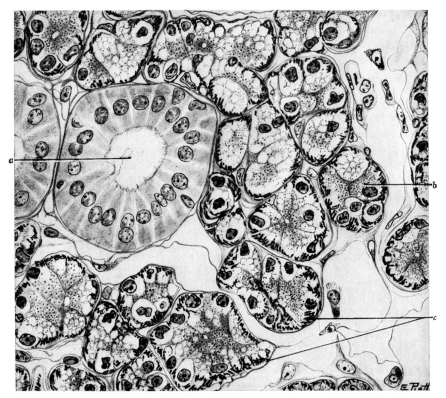

Figure 18-14 Section of a human parotid gland. A. Section of a salivary duct. B. Secretory cell. C. Basal striations. Zenker fixation; methylene blue and eosin.

posed entirely of serous cells or mucous cells or may contain both cell types.   In the latter situation, the serous cells occupy the fundus of the acinar sac, and the mucous cells are located closer to the opening to the initial duct segment (intercalated duct).   Thus the serous cells form basophilic crescent-shaped groups that are called *demilunes* (Figs. 18-13 and 18-15).   The cells of the demilune seem to be separated from the acinar lumen by the mucous cells, but actually they are directly connected by the *secretory capillaries* which are extensions of the acinar lumen that may penetrate deeply between serous cells (Fig. 18-13).   Microvilli occur along these secretory capillaries and thereby increase free-surface area.

Another component of the acinus is the *myoepithelial cell* which, as the name suggests, has

generally been regarded as a contractile element. Myoepithelial cells have a distinctive form and occupy a unique position; they are flat cells with long cytoplasmic processes which extend over the outer surface of the acinus in a basket-like configuration (Fig. 18-13).   They are located between the secretory cells and the basal lamina (Fig. 18-17).   Their stellate form is difficult to discern in routine light-microscopic preparations because usually only their nuclear regions are recognizable in a given section.   Since these cells possess relatively strong alkaline phosphatase activity, their form is better observed in histochemical preparations that demonstrate this enzymatic activity.   The ultrastructure of the myoepithelial cells resembles that of smooth muscle cells; in particular, there are numerous parallel fine filaments that occupy large areas of the cytoplasm. The surface of the myoepithelial cell is smooth and is closely apposed to the secretory cell surface, with occasional desmosomal associations. The geometry and arrangement of the myoepithelial cells, as well as their ultrastructural features, suggest a role in moving the primary secretion.

The primary secretion is most likely modified during its passage through the branching duct system, since certain cytologic features, especially those of the striated ducts, suggest participation in transport activities. The first two segments, the *intercalated duct* and the *striated duct*, also called *secretory* or *salivary duct*, are intralobular (Fig. 18-13). The secretion first enters the intercalated ducts which have a low cuboidal epithelium (Fig. 18-20A) and also have associated myoepithelial cells. Then it moves into the larger striated ducts which are lined by a tall columnar epithelium that is distinctly acidophilic. This segment derives its name from the light-microscopic appearance of the basal cytoplasm of the columnar cells; parallel striations are created by the vertical orientation of mitochondria within numerous slender cytoplasmic compartments that are outlined by deep infoldings of the basal plasma membrane (Fig. 18-18). These basal cytoplasmic compartments represent interdigitating foot processes of adjacent cells, similar to those which occur in the distal tubule of the nephron. This specialization, which creates a vast basal surface area and associates it closely with energy-producing mitochondria (Fig. 18-19), is characteristic of other epithelia known to be involved in rapid transport of ions and water. Myoepithelial cells are absent from the striated ducts. Larger ducts, known as *interlobular ducts,* course through the stroma, become progressively larger, and finally join the primary duct that leads into the oral cavity. The interlobular ducts are initially simple columnar and then pseudostratified columnar with occasional goblet cells. The largest ducts are lined by stratified epithelia, which may be stratified columnar (Fig. 18-20B), and those near the orifice are usually stratified squamous in form.

The salivary glands differ in the extent to which the intralobular ducts are developed (Fig. 18-12). The intercalated ducts are longest in the parotid, and the striated ducts are best developed in the

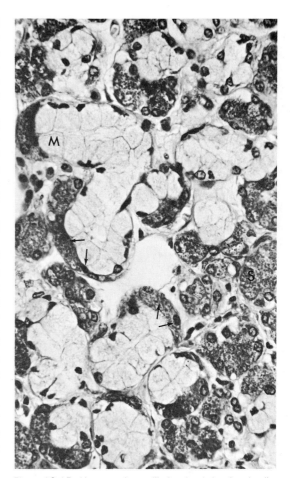

Figure 18-15   Human submandibular gland showing demilunes (arrows) of the mixed acini.   M, mucous cells; S, serous cells.

submandibular gland. Both types of intralobular ducts are quite inconspicuous in the sublingual gland. The varying proportions of striated ducts among the glands should have considerable functional significance.

It has long been known that the connective tissue among the acini of the salivary glands is a reticular connective tissue that contains many plasma cells and some small lymphocytes, as well as the usual stromal cells and fibers. In 1965, in an amazing discovery, Dr. Tomasi and his associates demonstrated the presence of IgA in most of the plasma cells in the interstitium of the human

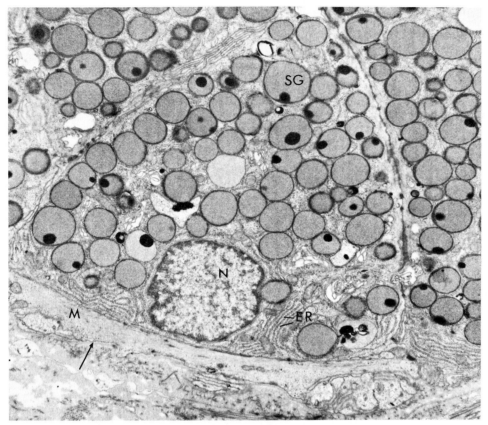

Figure 18-17   Human submandibular gland, serous cell, electron micrograph.   Rough endoplasmic reticulum (ER) occurs in the basal cytoplasm.   Secretory granules (SG) occupy most of the cell.   A process of a myoepithelial cell (M) occurs between the serous cell and the basal lamina (arrow).   ×9,000.   (Courtesy of Dr. Bernard Tandler.)

parotid gland (via the fluorescent antibody technique).   Also, plasma cells containing IgG and IgM occur in the periacinar stroma but in fewer numbers.   Further work led to the following hypothesis: IgA is produced in local plasma cells, it combines with a unique protein called the *secretory piece* which is believed to be produced by the acinar epithelial cells, and then it is released into the secretion as *secretory IgA* which is resistant to proteolysis.   It is likely that secretory IgA plays an important role in the oral cavity in defense against pathogens.

The major blood vessels course through the connective tissue, following the route of the large branching ducts.   Within the lobules, some arteries form rich capillary networks around the intralobular ducts whereas other arterial branches continue to create capillary plexuses around the acini.   The periductal capillaries are denser than the periacinar ones (Leeson).   The venous drainage retraces the arterial pathway.   Arteriovenous anastomoses have been reported to occur.   An extensive system of lymphatic drainage follows the course of the duct system.

Each of the major salivary glands is innervated by both the parasympathetic and sympathetic divisions of the autonomic nervous system, and it is generally agreed that secretory activity is entirely under neural control and that the parasympathetic fibers are secretory whereas sympathetic fibers are

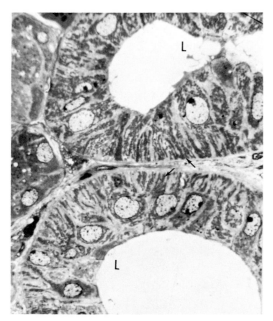

Figure 18-18 Human submandibular gland. Portions of two striated ducts are shown. The basal striations (arrows) created by parallel alignment of mitochondria are evident. L, lumen. Toluidine blue; 1-μm section. ×1,300. (Courtesy of Dr. Bernard Tandler.)

surface. A 20-nm space separates the surfaces of the neuronal and epithelial cells. The nerve fibers have small enlargements that contain many axoplasmic vesicles and mitochondria, ultrastructural features that typify nerve terminals. Acetylcholinesterase activity has been demonstrated in these regions of close apposition. In addition, light-microscopic observations indicate that the autonomic nerve fibers form networks around the intralobular ducts (Leeson).

Figure 18-19 Human submandibular gland. A horizontal section through the base of the striated duct reveals the close association of mitochondria (M) with infoldings of basal plasma membrane (arrows). Electron micrograph. ×17,000. (Courtesy of Dr. Bernard Tandler.)

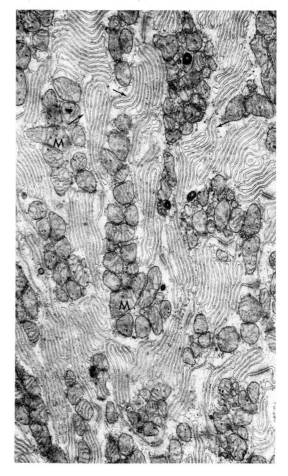

vasoconstrictor in effect. Other neural effects have been noted but species variation complicates interpretation. For example, evidence suggests that in the rat submaxillary gland a single secretory cell of the acinus is dually innervated and the duct cells receive only parasympathetic fibers. Recent ultrastructural observations on the cat submandibular gland indicate that terminations of both sympathetic and parasympathetic fibers are associated with the surface of one acinar cell (Hand, 1970). For the gross aspects of this innervation the reader should consult a textbook of gross anatomy.

Recent electron-microscopic observations have established that autonomic nerve fibers penetrate the acinar basal lamina and assume an intraepithelial position (Fig. 18-21). Within the acinar epithelium, the axons are naked and come into close association with both the secretory and myoepithelial cells. The axons may penetrate deeply between acinar cells or within invaginations of the acinar cell

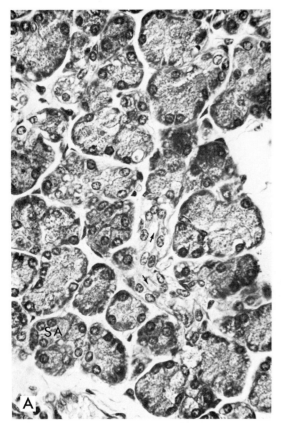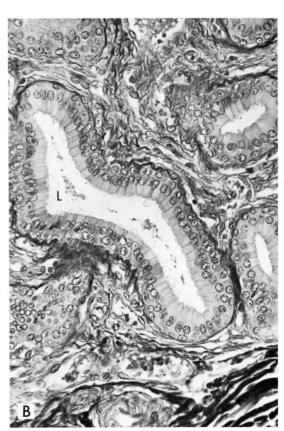

Figure 18-20 Portions of the duct system of salivary glands.   A. The intercalated duct of the human parotid with a flattened simple epithelium.   The arrows are within the lumen of the duct.   B. A large excretory duct of the human sublingual lined with a two-layered stratified columnar epithelium.

SUMMARY OF THE MAJOR FEATURES OF HUMAN SALIVARY GLANDS (Fig. 18-12)

The *parotid gland* is an almost purely seromucous gland (Figs. 18-14 and 18-20A). The secretory granules are PAS-positive, indicating that they are a carbohydrate-protein polymer. The intercalated ducts are long and abundant, whereas the striated ducts are less elaborate.

The *submandibular*[1] (formerly called submaxillary) gland (Fig. 18-15) is a mixed gland with seromucous acini and demilunes predominating over the purely mucous acini. However, lobules vary somewhat in this proportion, with some having a predominance of mucous acini (Leppi and Spicer, 1966). The secretory granules of the seromucous cells are PAS-positive; they are rich in sialomucin although some cells contain sulfomucin. The mucous cells contain either sialomucin or sulfomucin or a mixture of both. The striated ducts are best developed in the submandibular gland; the intercalated ducts are present but less conspicuous.

The sublingual gland[1] is a mixed gland composed mainly of mucous acini although there may be considerable variation in the proportion of mucous to seromucous acini and demilunes in different regions of the gland (Fig. 18-16, see color insert). Sulfomucin is the major component of the abundant mucous secretion. The seromucous cells are rich

[1] Portions of the human submandibular and sublingual glands intermingle in a manner that constitutes a gross submandibular sublingual complex (Leppi, 1967). This intermingling can create a sampling problem in microscopic study.

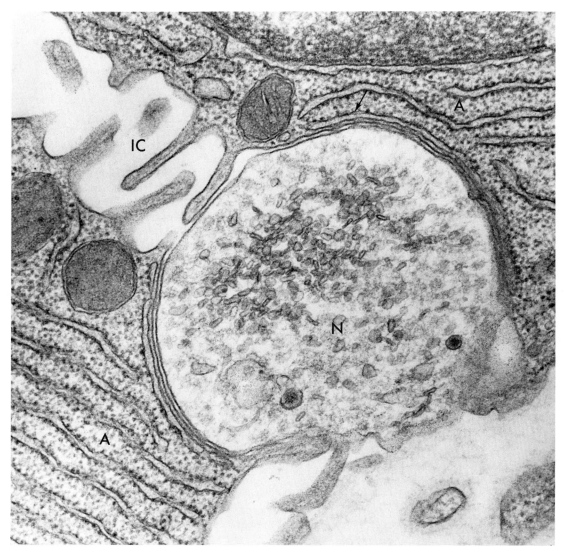

Figure 18-21   Intraepithelial autonomic nerve terminal (N) between two acinar cells (A) of the rat parotid gland.   Note regions of close apposition between the surfaces of the nerve fiber and the secretory cells. A cisterna of endoplasmic reticulum (arrows) parallels the apposed surfaces.   IC, intercellular space.   ×57,000.   (From Hand, 1970.)

in sialomucin.   Both segments (intercalated and striated ducts) of the intralobular duct system are poorly developed.

The *pharynx* is a component of both the digestive and respiratory systems; it is here that the pathways for the passage of gases and food merge and cross.   In its upper regions, the histologic organization follows that of the respiratory system whereas the lower part resembles that of the oral cavity.

The remainder of the digestive tract is organized around a common histologic plan.   The following description of the general structural plan pertains to the remainder of the digestive tube.   Also, essential terminology that is needed to analyze the microscopic anatomy of these organs is presented.

General structural plan for the esophagus, stomach, and intestines

LAYERS

The alimentary canal is made up of four concentric layers which exhibit considerable regularity. Named in order from the lumen outward, these are the *mucosa,* the *submucosa,* the *muscularis,* and the *adventitia* or *serosa* (Fig. 18-22). The *mucosa,* or mucous membrane, has three components: (1) a superficial *epithelium;* (2) an underlying stroma composed of a vascularized, highly cellular, reticular connective tissue (*lamina propria*); and (3) a relatively thin layer of smooth muscle (*muscularis mucosae*). Typically, the fibers in the muscularis mucosae are subdivided into an inner circular and an outer longitudinal layer. Large accumulations of typical lymphatic tissue are often present in the stroma. Furthermore, because of the abundance of plasma cells and lymphocytes, the entire lamina propria of much of the gut might properly be termed *modified lymphatic tissue.* It participates in the immune response.

The lining epithelium may form glands that extend into the lamina propria (*mucosal glands*) or submucosa (*submucosal glands*), or ducts that lead from the wall of the tract to glands situated outside the tube proper (*liver, pancreas*). In other instances the entire mucosa bulges into the lumen as folds (*plicae* and *rugae*) or fingers (*villi*). These invaginations and evaginations of the lining of the gut enlarge its effective surface tremendously. For example, Wood calculated for the small intestine of the cat that the villi expand the surface of the lumen by as much as fiftyfold; the factor is probably still greater in man.

The mucosa, which differs considerably from segment to segment of the alimentary tract, reflects specific functions by characteristic morphology. The surrounding supportive and muscular layers change relatively little, and only their distinctive features will be noted.

The *submucosa* is a fibrous, rather than a highly cellular, connective tissue layer, often containing accumulations of lymphatic tissue, as well as glands that extend from the mucosa in some of the organs. In a sense, the submucosa is a vascular service area containing large blood vessels that send finer vessels into the layers that embody the specific organ functions, the mucosa and muscularis.

The *muscularis* contains at least two layers of muscle. The muscle is smooth in all parts except the upper esophagus and the anal sphincter, where it is composed of skeletal muscle fibers. The fibers of the inner layers are disposed in a roughly circular fashion around the tube (*circular layer*), and those of the outer layer are disposed lengthwise along the tube (*longitudinal layer*). Contractions of the circular layer constrict the lumen; contractions of the longitudinal layer shorten the tube. At the various sphincters and valves along the tube (pharyngoesophageal, esophagogastric, pyloric, ileocecal, and anal), the layer of circular muscle is greatly thickened. Careful dissection of the muscle layers has shown that the fibers are actually disposed in a helical fashion, those in the circular layer forming a tight helix and those in the longitudinal layer an elongated one. The connective tissue fibers in the submucosa and adventitia are likewise oriented helically.

Figure 18-22 Diagrammatic cross section to illustrate the histologic organization of the wall of the digestive tube. (From W. M. Copenhaver, "Bailey's Textbook of Histology," 15th ed., The Williams & Wilkins Company, Baltimore, 1964.)

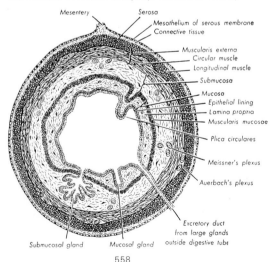

Mesentery
Serosa
Mesothelium of serous membrane
Connective tissue
Muscularis externa
Circular muscle
Longitudinal muscle
Submucosa
Mucosa
Epithelial lining
Lamina propria
Muscularis mucosae
Plica circulares
Meissner's plexus
Auerbach's plexus
Excretory duct from large glands outside digestive tube
Submucosal gland
Mucosal gland

The *adventitia* of the tract is composed of several layers of loose connective tissue, alternately collagenous and elastic. Where the tract is suspended by a peritoneal fold, it is covered by a mesothelium continuous with that of the peritoneum (see later section). Wherever a mesothelial covering occurs, the adventitial layer is customarily termed a *serosa*.

BLOOD VESSELS

At intervals, blood and lymphatic vessels and nerves enter the tract from the surrounding tissues or via the supporting peritoneal fold. The largest arteries are disposed longitudinally in the submucosa, and smaller branches also run in the adventitia (Fig. 18-23A). From these two sets of vessels, branches ramify perpendicularly to both the mucosa and the muscularis. In the latter, the capillaries run parallel with the muscle fibers. In the mucosa, the arteries supply an irregular capillary plexus around the glands and, in the small intestine, send terminal branches into the villi. The small capillaries associated with the gut epithelium typically have fenestrated endothelial cells and a distinct basal lamina.

The veins arising in the mucosa anastomose in the submucosa and pass out of the intestine beside the arteries. The muscularis mucosae has been described as forming a sphincter for the veins penetrating it. Valves are found in the larger veins only in the adventitia or serosa; they disappear again in the mesentery where these veins form the branches of the portal vein leading to the liver.

LYMPHATIC VESSELS

The alimentary tract is richly supplied with lymphatic vessels, which arise as blind tubes in the mucosa. In the small intestine, each villus usually contains a single central lymphatic vessel known as a *lacteal* (Fig. 18-23B). In some stages of digestion, the distention of these lymphatics is great and they are easily recognized in sections. When the vessels are collapsed, their walls are difficult to distinguish from the surrounding reticular connective tissue. Viewed at the ultrastructural level,

Figure 18-23 Diagrams of blood vessels (A), lymphatic vessels (B), and nerves (C) of the alimentary tract, as seen in the small intestine. The layers of the tract are m, mucosa; mm, muscularis mucosae; sm, submucosa; cm, circular muscle layer; ic, intermuscular connective tissue; lm, longitudinal muscle; s, serosa. In A, arteries are shown as coarse black lines, capillaries as fine black lines, and veins shaded. In B, lymphatic vessels are shown as open channels. In C, neurons and nerve fibers are shown. Additional abbreviations: n, lymphatic nodule; s pl, submucosal plexus; m pl, myenteric plexus.

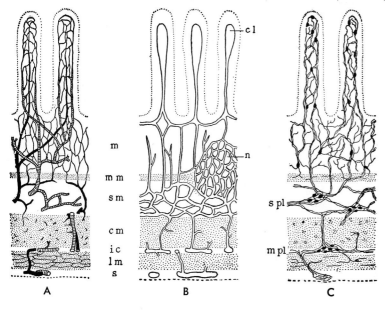

these lymphatic capillaries lack endothelial pores—thus differing from the local blood capillaries—but have little or no basal lamina.

In the submucosa, the larger lymphatic vessels branch freely and have numerous valves (Fig. 18-59). They cross the muscle layers, spreading in the intermuscular tissue and serosa, and pass through the mesentery. Unlike lymphatic vessels in many other parts of the body, those in the mesentery possess muscular walls and are thus able to propel their contents.

LYMPHATIC TISSUE

The lymphatic tissue of the alimentary tract occurs primarily in the lamina propria and assumes three forms: diffuse lymphatic tissue, solitary lymphatic nodules (Figs. 18-41 and 18-57), and aggregate nodules (Fig. 18-58). Large lymphatic masses may break through the muscularis mucosae and spread into the submucosa, as shown in Fig. 18-57. The superficial lymphatic vessels form a plexus as they pass through the nodule (Figs. 18-23B and 18-59). Blood vessels also form a net in the lymphatic tissue.

Diffuse lymphatic tissue occurs under the simple epithelia of the intestines. The degree of cellularity has been related to the bacterial count in the lumen. This layer constitutes the second barrier to foreign organisms and large molecules. The cells found most abundantly are macrophages, plasma cells, and eosinophils.

Solitary nodules are found in the esophagus, in the pylorus of the stomach, and along the entire length of the small and large intestines.

Aggregate nodules (Peyer's patches) occur in the small intestine and in the appendix. They are oval bodies, usually from 1 to 4 cm long but occasionally much larger, composed of 10 to 60 nodules in close contact. These patches distort and push aside the nearby glands, and immediately above the nodules villi are largely effaced. There are 15 to 30 such patches in the human intestine, principally in the lower part of the ileum on the side opposite the mesenteric attachment. A few occur in the jejunum and lower duodenum. Aggregate nodules are always present in the vermiform appendix (Fig. 18-58) but do not occur elsewhere in the large intestine.

This tissue is part of the local immune system that responds to antigenic stimuli by producing secretory immunoglobulin and other antibodies.

NERVES

The nerves consist of both autonomic motor and sensory fibers. (At the two extremes of the tract there is, of course, voluntary innervation of the skeletal muscle fibers.) The motor fibers are both parasympathetic and sympathetic. The fibers of both ramify in the wall of the tract as shown in Fig. 18-23C, forming plexuses in each of the layers. The ganglia of the sympathetic nerves are external to the gut wall, lying in the celiac plexus and in the superior and inferior mesenteric plexuses. The parasympathetic nerves are derived from the vagus and the sacral outflow.

The neurons of the intramural parasympathetic ganglia occur in two locations: (1) in nodes of the *submucosal plexus* (of Meissner) and (2) between the two layers of the muscularis, in the *myenteric plexus* (of Auerbach). The ganglia and the associated fibers form an irregular rectilinear pattern when viewed from the surface (Fig. 18-24). The autonomic ganglion cells, surrounded by the usual satellite cells, possess many dendrites and have eccentrically located nuclei (Fig. 18-25). All axons within the gut wall appear to be C fibers, that is, unmyelinated. They lack Schwann-cell investment in the vicinity of the ganglion cells (Fig. 18-26). Sympathetic fibers ramify through the wall of the tube along with the parasympathetic fibers to innervate the muscularis and the blood vessels.

Minute sensory fibers have been described in the epithelial lining, the muscle fibers, and the blood vessel walls. However, electron microscopists have so far failed to find fibers penetrating the basement membrane of the epithelium. The nature of these putative sensory fibers is not understood. They are activated by different stimuli than sensory fibers elsewhere in the body and are poorly represented in the sensorium. Neurophysiologists claim that sensory fibers participate in local reflex arcs, so that the muscles contract in response to irritation of the epithelium.

Stimulation of the parasympathetic nerves to the intestinal tract, generally speaking, increases muscular activity, circulation, and secretion, whereas these activities are decreased by stimulation of the sympathetic nerves. Since the postganglionic

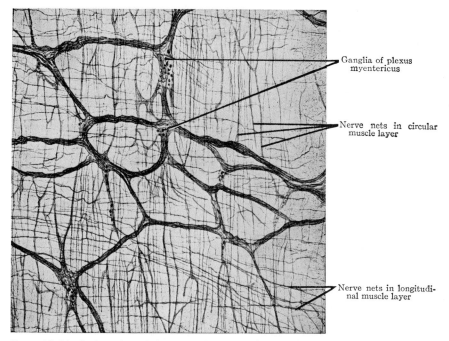

Ganglia of plexus
myentericus

Nerve nets in circular
muscle layer

Nerve nets in longitudi-
nal muscle layer

Figure 18-24 Surface view of the myenteric plexus, showing the distribution of nerves in the circular and longitudinal muscle layers. The neurons occur in ganglia within the plexus. Jejunum of monkey; supravital staining with methylene blue. (After von Mollendorff.)

Figure 18-25 Parasympathetic ganglion in the submucosa of the human stomach wall. N, nerve fibers; GC, large ganglion cell, surrounded by satellite cells. H&E. ×300.

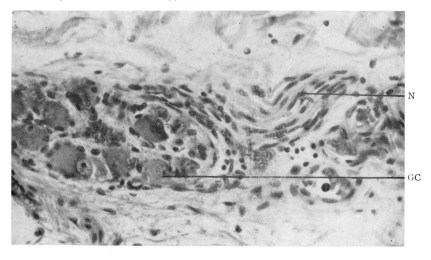

N

GC

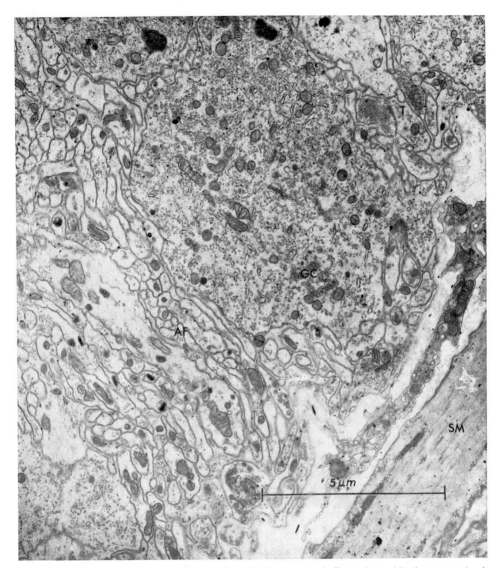

Figure 18-26 Electron micrograph of a ganglion cell plus autonomic fibers situated in the myenteric plexus of a mouse. AF, tuft of autonomic fibers; GC, portion of a ganglion cell; T, fiber terminals containing abundant synaptic vesicles; SM, smooth muscle fiber. ×10,000.

parasympathetic fibers arise locally, their influence may be limited to a fairly short length of the tube. Postganglionic fibers of the sympathetics, however, arise from ganglia external to the gut and possess much wider distribution. Sympathetic activity is reinforced, moreover, by the concomitant release of catecholamines from the adrenal medulla.

SUSPENSORY FOLDS

The esophagus runs through the thorax within the superior and posterior mediastina and lacks any special support. The stomach and intestines are mostly supported by suspensory folds from the peritoneal wall known as the *omenta* and *mesenteries*, respectively. However, the duodenum and the

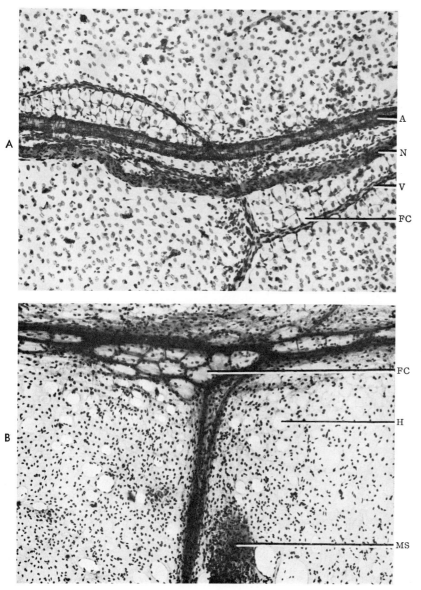

Figure 18-27 A. Spread of mesentery. ×150. B. Spread of omentum. ×75. In these suspensory folds, groups of blood vessels, lymphatic vessels, and nerves travel together in an insulating coating of adipose tissue. The mesentery is a solid sheet, whereas the omenta have holes (H) and frequent "milky spots" (MS), or clusters of monocytes. A, small artery; FC, fat cell; N, autonomic nerve; V, venule. The large pale nuclei in A belong to the flattened mesothelial cells, and the cells with denser nuclei are various connective tissue elements. (Courtesy of D. W. Fawcett.)

ascending and descending limbs of the colon adhere to the posterior wall of the abdominal cavity and are thus considered *secondarily retroperitoneal.*

Suspensory folds are composed of a serous membrane covering the "ventral" surface and sides of the tube and a double-layered suspending membrane, continuous on each side with the peritoneal lining of the cavity. The *peritoneum* thus forms a closed sac and is divisible into the *visceral peritoneum,* covering the viscera, and the *parietal peritoneum,* which lines the body walls. In all cases, its free surface is covered with a single layer of closely packed, polygonal cells, the *mesothelium* (Fig. 18-27). Although very flat, these cells have scattered microvilli on the free surface and may be somewhat phagocytic.

A thin layer of connective tissue, with cells, elastic networks, and interwoven bundles of collagenous fibers, occupies the interval between the two epithelial layers. It is here that the lymphatic vessels, blood vessels, and nerves that supply the various alimentary organs are to be found running together (Fig. 18-27). Mast cells are common, and eosinophils, monocytes, lymphocytes, macrophages, and adipose tissue also occur. Mesothelial cells and the various wandering cells are frequently found free in the peritoneal fluid.

The stomach is peculiar in that it retains a ventral suspensory fold and thus possesses both a *dorsal* (greater) *omentum* and a *ventral* (lesser) *omentum.* The omenta differ from the mesenteries proper in that they are perforated (Fig. 18-27). Especially numerous in these sheets, and also in the peritoneum covering the diaphragm, are "milky spots," which consist of aggregations of blast cells, monocytes, and macrophages. These aggregations apparently play an important role in combating infection in the peritoneal cavity.

Esophagus

The esophagus is a tube about 25 cm long in the adult, its several tunics being continuous superiorly with those of the pharynx and inferiorly with those of the stomach. Because of the tonus of the circular muscle layer, its mucous membrane is thrown into many folds (Fig. 18-28) except during the passage of a bolus.

The epithelium of the mucosa is stratified squamous (Fig. 18-29) and extremely thick (about 300 μm). In man, complete keratinization of the epithelium is rare unless the esophagus is subject to an unusual degree of trauma. Such keratinization occurs normally in some mammalian species, especially rodents and herbivores.

The lamina propria of the esophagus is less cellular than that of lower parts of the digestive tube. Lymphatic nodules occur occasionally, especially around the ducts of glands. The muscularis mucosae is broad, being 200 to 400 μm thick. It is unusual in that it consists of longitudinally directed fibers only. It replaces the elastic layer of the pharynx at the level of the cricoid cartilage.

The submucosa is thick (300 to 700 μm) and is characterized by abundant, coarse elastic fibers, which permit distention.

The muscularis (0.5 to 2 mm) comprises an inner circular layer and outer bundles of longitudinal fibers, arising at the level of the cricoid cartilage. At its upper extremity, there is the *superior esophageal* (pharyngoesophageal) *sphincter,* consisting of a thickened layer of circular (oblique) muscles. In the upper quarter of the tube the fibers are skeletal rather than smooth. Striated and smooth muscle fibers intermingle in the second quarter of the tube (Fig. 18-29). Only smooth muscle fibers occur in the lower half.

The adventitia is loose connective tissue containing many longitudinally directed blood vessels, lymphatic vessels, and nerves. For 2 to 3 cm above the stomach, elastic fibers are numerous and attach the esophagus to the diaphragm.

The orifice between the esophagus and stomach is bounded by a broad band of circular muscles, the *inferior esophageal* (esophagogastric) *sphincter.* There is generally an abrupt change at the esophageal-cardiac junction from stratified epithelium to the simple columnar epithelium that characterizes the stomach (Fig. 18-32).

Glands are isolated in the esophagus and are only of the mucous type. By position, they are

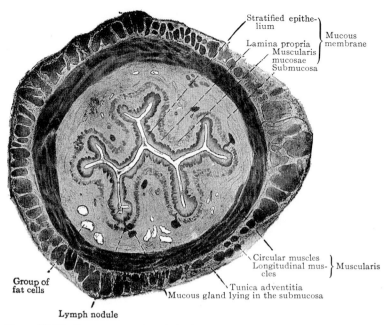

Stratified epithe-
lium

Mucous
membrane

Lamina propria
Muscularis
mucosae
Submucosa

Circular muscles
Longitudinal mus-
cles

Muscularis

Group of
fat cells

Tunica adventitia
Mucous gland lying in the submucosa

Lymph nodule

Figure 18-28   Transverse section of the human esophagus, illustrating the typical arrangement of the tissue layers in the wall of the alimentary tract.   ×5.

classified as superficial (mucosal) and deep (submucosal). The *mucosal glands* are limited to narrow zones near the two ends of the esophagus, between the level of the cricoid cartilage and the fifth tracheal ring and again near the entrance of the stomach (Fig. 18-32). The mucus formed by these superficial glands does not stain metachromatically, as does that of the deep glands. Because of the resemblance of the mucosal glands to those occurring at the cardiac end of the stomach, an alternative name for them is *cardiac glands.*

The *submucosal glands* are scattered, tubular downgrowths that pass through the lamina propria and muscularis mucosae into the submucosa (Fig. 18-30). The cells have the typical cytologic characteristics of mucous cells. The smallest ducts are lined with simple columnar epithelium; the main ducts that enter the mucosa are lined with stratified epithelium. The number of deep glands varies greatly in different individuals. They usually predominate in the upper half of the esophagus.

Stomach

The opening through which the esophagus connects with the stomach is the *cardiac orifice,* and the opening from the stomach to the intestine is the *pyloric orifice* (G. *pyloros,* gatekeeper). The lining of the stomach is thrown into major longitudinal folds, or *rugae,* when the organ is not distended with food (Fig. 18-31).

HISTOLOGIC ORGANIZATION

In man, the *gastric epithelium* is simple columnar throughout. At the cardiac opening, the cells are continuous with the basal layer of the stratified epithelium of the esophagus (Fig. 18-32). The lining of the organ is indented by multitudinous pits (foveolae), leading from *branched, tubular glands.*

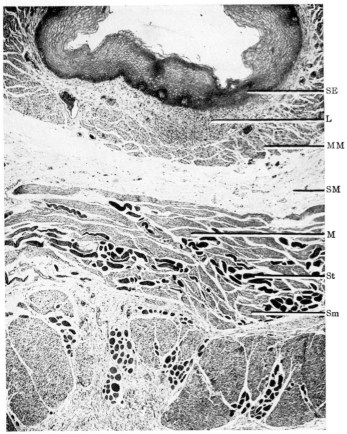

SE

L

MM

SM

M

St

Sm

Figure 18-29 Midregion of the human esophagus, cross section. At this level, the muscularis contains skeletal muscle fibers in addition to smooth muscle fibers. SE, stratified squamous epithelium; L, lymphatic tissue in lamina propria; MM, muscularis mucosae; SM, submucosa; M, muscularis; St, striated (skeletal) muscle fiber; Sm, smooth muscle fibers. Eosin and methylene blue. ×45.

Figure 18-30 The end of a submucosal gland, esophagus of a child. The secretory end pieces produce mucus. H&E.

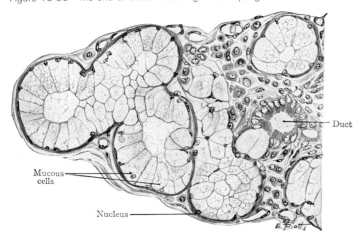

Duct

Mucous cells

Nucleus

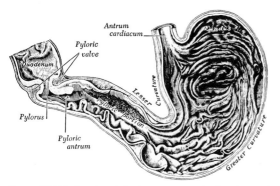

Figure 18-31   Interior of the human stomach showing regional differences and the internal folds or rugae. (From H. Gray and C. M. Goss, "Gray's Anatomy," 28th ed., Lea & Febiger, Philadelphia, 1966.)

There are about 3.5 million foveolae on the stomach wall, serving some 15 million glands. All the glands are restricted to the mucosa.

The glands of the stomach are divided into three categories: The *cardiac glands* occur in the first 5 to 40 mm from the cardiac orifice; the *pyloric glands* occur along the 4 cm from the pyloric vestibule to the pyloric sphincter; between these two extremities lie the *gastric* (or, erroneously, fundic) *glands*. The cells of the cardiac and pyloric glands are primarily mucous. The epithelium of the gastric glands is more diversified, containing enzyme- and acid-secreting cells as well as mucous cells. The cardiac and pyloric glands are conspicuously coiled (Fig. 18-33), whereas the gastric glands are relatively straight (Fig. 18-33A). The pyloric region is distinguished by foveolae that occupy nearly one-half the depth of the mucosa; in the cardia and body of the organ, the pits occupy only one-fourth the thickness of the mucosa.

The *mucous membrane* of the stomach measures 0.3 to 1.5 mm in width, being thinnest in the cardiac region. Underlying the epithelium is a richly vascularized lamina propria, which is often quite cellular, especially in the pylorus (Fig. 18-33B). Occasionally lymphatic nodules occur. Smooth muscle fibers extend upward from the

Figure 18-32   Longitudinal section through the junction of the human esophagus and stomach. Note the sharp transition from stratified epithelium of the esophagus (left) to the simple columnar epithelium of the stomach (right). The simple epithelium is continuous with the basal layer of the stratified epithelium. a. Duct of a mucosal esophageal gland. b. Esophageal epithelium. c. Gastric epithelium. d. Tubule of mucosal gland. e. Lymphatic nodule. f. Lymphatic vessel. g. Muscularis mucosae.

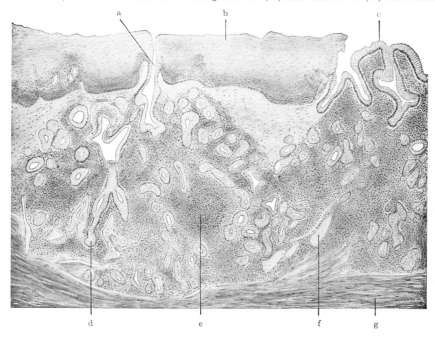

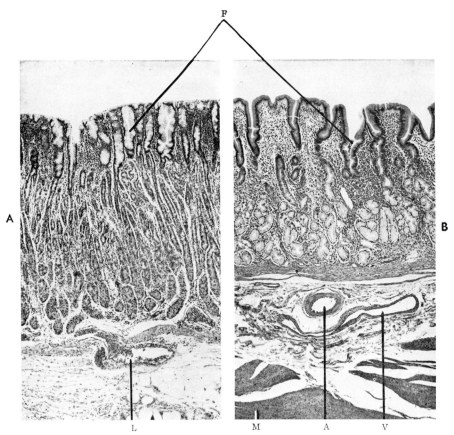

Figure 18-33   Lining in different regions of the human stomach.   A. Mucosa and submucosa, illustrating the low-power appearance of gastric glands from the body of the stomach.   B. Mucosa, submucosa, and a portion of the muscularis in the pyloric stomach. Contrast the straightness of the gastric glands with the coiled nature of the pyloric glands.   Also note the relatively deep pits, or foveolae, in the pylorus.   F, foveolae; L, lymphatic vessel penetrating the muscularis mucosae; M, sphincteric muscle bundles of the pyloric vestibule; A, artery; V, vein in the submucosa.   H&E.   ×50.

muscularis mucosae around the glands, and their shortening may aid in the expulsion of secretory products.

The *submucosa* consists of coarse collagenous bundles and many elastic fibers, plus blood and lymphatic vessels (Figs. 18-33 and 18-41) and the submucous nerve plexus (Fig. 18-25). Clusters of fat cells are common in older people.

The *muscularis* is composed of three primary layers: an inner oblique, a middle circular, and an outer longitudinal layer. The oblique layer is best developed at the cardiac end and in the body of the organ. The circular bundles are thickened at both ends in the regions of the sphincters. The myenteric nerve plexus occurs in the connective tissue lamina separating the circular from the longitudinal muscle layer. The extensive muscle coat produces the churning and homogenization of ingested food as gastric juices are added to it.

The *serosa,* consisting of connective tissue plus mesothelium, is continuous, via the omenta, with the peritoneum.

CYTOLOGY OF GASTRIC EPITHELIAL CELLS

The entire gastric surface and the glands are lined by simple columnar epithelium. Cells of four major types occur: (1) *surface mucous cells,* (2) *neck* mucous cells, (3) parietal or oxyntic cells, and (4) peptic, or chief, cells (Fig. 18-34, see color insert). In addition to these, there are enterochromaffin cells, which contain granules that may be blackened by silver methods or oxidized by chromates or osmium tetroxide.

The surface mucous cells, which cover the entire surface and line the pits (foveolae), are high columnar cells, with basal nuclei. The apical cytoplasm usually appears empty or foamy because the mucous droplets are not preserved in routine preparations. The mucus may, however, be stained by mucicarmine or the PAS procedure. The staining characteristics suggest that the mucus represents the neutral polysaccharide of the stomach. In electron-microscopic preparations, the surface and foveolar cells of the bat exhibit clusters of somewhat elliptical, dense secretory granules in the apical region of the cell (Fig. 18-35A) which first appear in the Golgi zone. Endoplasmic reticulum is sparse, but mitochondria are quite abundant both below and above the nucleus.

In the gastric glands the neck mucous cells lie in the upper ends of the gland proper (as distinguished from the foveola), interspersed among parietal cells. Apparently similar cells line the entire lengths of the cardiac and pyloric glands. The neck mucous cells are smaller than the surface cells and they generally contain fewer droplets. The mucous droplets stain intensely with mucicarmine and by the PAS procedure and also with basic dyes. These properties indicate the presence of acid mucopolysaccharides.

Neck mucous cells exhibit more cytoplasmic basophilia in light-microscopic preparations and more rough ER in electron-microscopic preparations than do the surface mucous cells (Fig. 18-35B). The Golgi complex is exceptionally well developed. The droplets are not dense in electron micrographs and are larger and more spherical than those of the surface cells; mucous droplets often lie deep in the cell as well as near the apex.

The parietal or oxyntic cells are the acid-secreting cells. They are large and intensely acidophilic (Fig. 18-34). They often bulge from the lateral surface of the gland into the lamina propria, hence the name parietal. They lie principally in the neck region of gastric glands proper, but they occur throughout the glands of the pyloric vestibule.

They are essentially absent from cardiac and pyloric glands proper (Fig. 18-37).

The apical surface of the cell indents the cytoplasm, as the so-called intracellular secretory canaliculus, or, more properly, trench (Figs. 18-35C and 18-36). Electron micrographs show that the surface of the trench is further expanded by abundant microvilli. The other remarkable feature of this cell type is the great number of large mitochondria, which contain abundant cristae. It appears that these mitochondria are responsible for the acidophilia of the cytoplasm. A distinctive feature of the oxyntic cell is an abundance of smooth-surfaced tubules in the apical cytoplasm. It has been demonstrated that the membrane of these tubules is continuous with the apical plasma membrane that lines the canaliculi and microvilli. During secretion of gastric acid, there is an increase in apical surface area; it is currently believed that the apical smooth tubules may represent a membrane reserve that is translocated to the surface during acid secretion.

The secretory product of the oxyntic cells is hydrochloric acid. Demonstration of this fact was first provided by Linderstrøm-Lang and Holter. They froze pieces of stomach freshly removed from an animal, punched out a cylinder of tissue with a cork borer, and then cut frozen sections parallel to the mucosal surface. One series of sections was titrated, individually, with alkali; alternate ones were stained for histologic examination. The greatest acidity occurred at levels in which parietal cells were the most numerous.

There are several theories of the mechanism of the hydrogen ion secretion. At the very least it is clear that such secretion depends on the supply of high-energy phosphate bonds derived from oxidative metabolism (in the mitochondria) and on aerobic glycolysis. The chloride ions are transported actively from the blood plasma, as is water, perhaps via the endoplasmic reticulum. Only at the surface of the cell is free acid detectable with indicator dyes.

Oxyntic cells release their acid not only on vagal stimulation, but also when activated by histamine, gastrin, insulin, or alcohol. The latter observation perhaps explains the frequency of gastritis associated with alcoholism.

The chief or peptic cells line the lower portions of the gastric glands, being most numerous in the

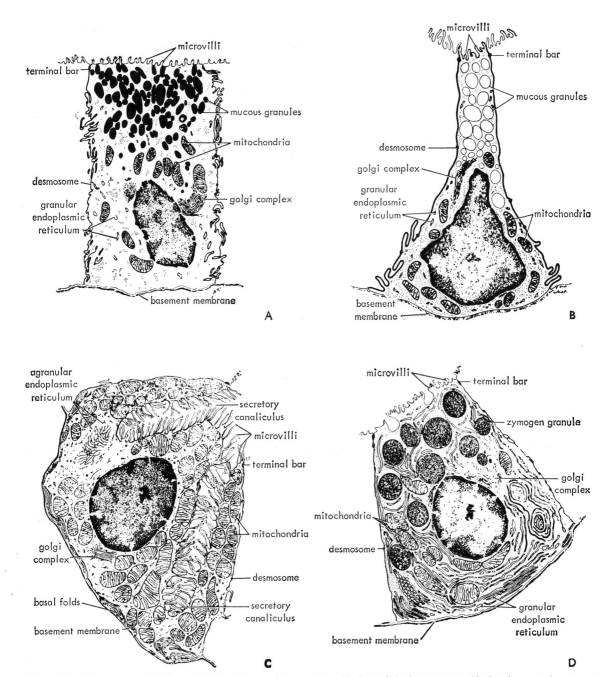

Figure 18-35 Diagrams of the four principal cell types of the gastric epithelium of the bat as seen with the electron microscope. A. Surface mucous cell, with an accumulation of electron-opaque mucous droplets.   B. Neck mucous cell, with less dense droplets. C. Parietal or oxyntic cell, exhibiting the secretory canaliculus, or trench, plus abundant mitochondria.   D. Chief, or zymogenic, cell, with a rich complement of rough endoplasmic reticulum and other characteristics of a protein-secreting exocrine cell.   (Courtesy of S. Ito and R. J. Winchester, J. Cell Biol., **16**:541, 1963.)

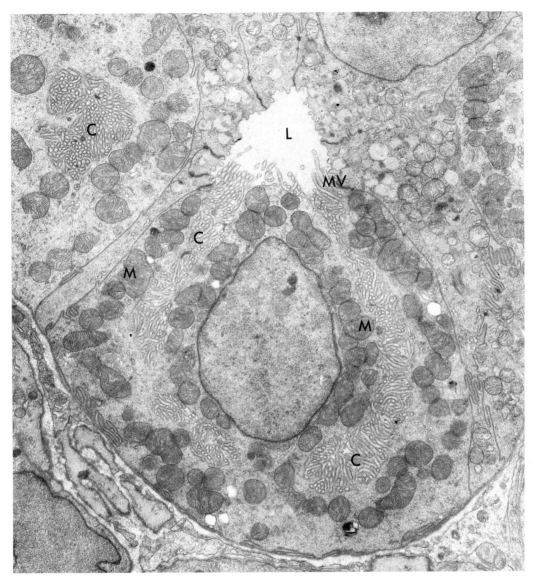

Figure 18-36   Gastric gland of a bat, cross section; electron micrograph.   Portions of oxyntic (parietal) cells are shown.   This stomach has been stimulated in vitro to produce hydrochloric acid.   The secretory canaliculi (C) are occluded, and their lumens are filled with numerous microvilli (MV).   Mitochondria (M) are numerous.   L, Lumen of gland.   (From Ito, 1967.)

glands toward the cardiac end of the organ (Fig. 18-38).   They are typical serous zymogenic cells, resembling the pancreatic acinar cell.   The cell contains an extensive basal rough ER with highly oriented cisternae (Fig. 18-35D).   The secretory droplets are quite basophilic.   Electron microscopy indicates that these droplets form in Golgi vesicles and pass to the apex of the cell, where they are released in the same manner as the droplets of pancreatic acinar cells.

Linderstrom-Lang and Holter also made pioneer quantitative histochemical studies, in which they

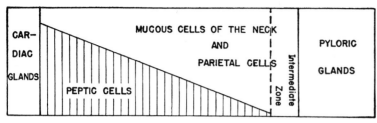

Figure 18-37   Distribution of the various types of epithelial cells along the length of the stomach.   (Modified from B. P. Babkin, "Secretory Mechanisms of the Digestive Glands," 2d ed., Paul B. Hoeber, Inc., New York, 1950.)

showed that these cells contain *pepsinogen,* a precursor of the enzyme *pepsin* which hydrolyzes proteins to smaller fragments.   Their method involved incubating sections of mucosa with protein and a constant quantity of hydrochloric acid; they demonstrated that it was in the layers in which the peptic cells were most numerous that digestion of the protein proceeded rapidly.   Normally, the pepsinogen is converted into active enzyme by hydrochloric acid after its release into the lumen; pepsin then requires an acidic environment for optimal activity. Another proteolytic enzyme, *rennin,* which digests milk proteins, is also secreted in the stomach, presumably by the peptic cells.   The enzymes are released on vagal stimulation.

Gastric intrinsic (*anti-pernicious anemia factor*) is probably also produced by the chief cell.

Considerable current interest centers around recent ultrastructural studies of a group of endocrine-like cells that are widely distributed throughout the gastrointestinal tract.   It has long been known that small cells with minute acidophilic granules (Fig. 18-39, see color insert) occur in the epithelium of the stomach, small and large intestine, appendix, and even in the ducts of the pancreas and liver. The cells rest on the basal lamina but most do not reach the lumen (Fig. 18-40).   Typically the granules are concentrated in the basal cytoplasm.   At the light-microscopic level, several reactions identify the granules of these cells.   They are colored by osmic acid or with potassium dichromate, for which reason they are called *enterochromaffin cells.*

The granules of most of these cells precipitate silver when treated with ammoniacal silver nitrate (Fig. 18-39, see color insert), thus the name *argentaffin cells.*   A minority of the enterochromaffin cells are impregnated by silver only when a reducer is employed.   With the light microscope it could not be ascertained whether one or more cell types were responsible for these reactions.   This system of cells was first associated with the secretion of 5-hydroxytryptamine (serotonin) by the gastrointestinal mucosa.   In their ultrastructure, the enterochromaffin cells as a group resemble peptide-synthesizing endocrine cells.   The granules are enclosed in smooth membranes, and the rough ER and Golgi membranes are well developed.   Free ribosomes and lysosomal derivatives occur quite regularly.   The general polarization of most of these cells suggests that they secrete into the surrounding tissues and bloodstream rather than into the lumen.   Recent ultrastructural analysis has identified five types of enterochromaffin cells which differ morphologically and by characteristic location in the gastrointestinal tract (Forssman et al., 1969). Although all five variants can synthesize serotonin (Rubin et al., 1971), it seems likely that these cells may be involved in the synthesis of catecholamines, gastrin, secretin, glucagon, or other hormones. The secretory and muscular activities of the gastrointestinal tract itself, and of the pancreas and gallbladder, are controlled to a considerable degree by hormones secreted by the gut wall in response to changing properties of the substances in the lumen.

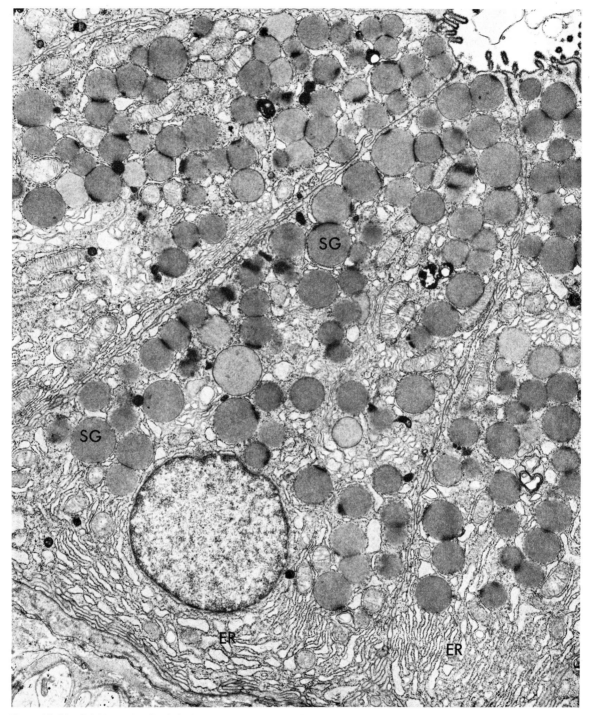

Figure 18-38 Chief (peptic) cells of the human gastric glands. Electron micrograph. The characteristics of zymogenic cells are evident in the abundant basal rough cisternal endoplasmic reticulum (ER) and the numerous secretory granules (SG). ×11,000. (From Rubin et al., 1968).

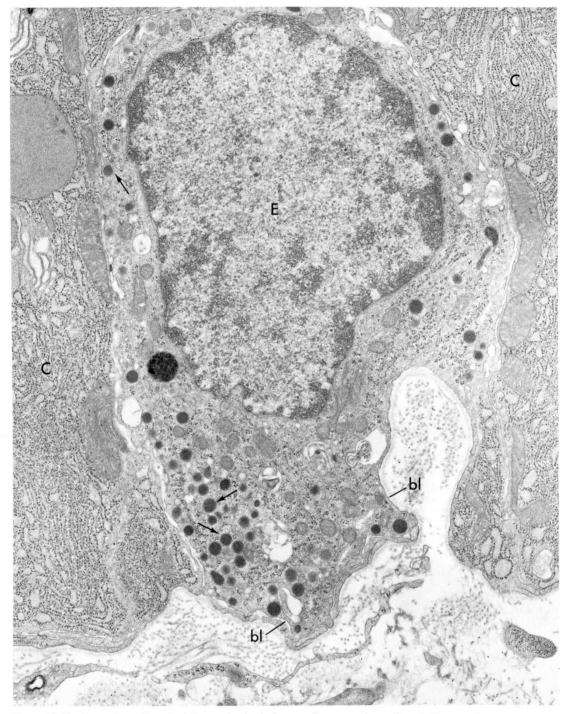

Figure 18-40 Enterochromaffin cell of the gastric gland of a rat. The enterochromaffin cell (E) occurs between two chief cells (C). Its basal surface rests against the basal lamina (bl), and its cytoplasm contains small round dense granules (arrows) that are membrane-limited. ×18,000. (Courtesy of Dr. Susumo Ito.)

Replacement of gastric epithelial cells

In the gastric glands proper, mitotic activity occurs principally at the base of the pits and the uppermost portions (neck) of the glands. Undifferentiated epithelial cells with prominent nucleoli and numerous free polysomes occur in this region. Labeling this dividing population with [^{3}H]thymidine has established that most of these cells migrate upward along the pit to replace the surface epithelium. Thus the surface mucous cells are continually replaced, and in man the gastric surface epithelium is replaced every 4 to 5 days. At the base of the foveolae, undifferentiated precursors of the neck mucous, peptic, and oxyntic cells occur in a region known as the *isthmus*. From here the three cell types migrate deeper into the gland. The neck mucous cells continue to proliferate in the neck where they are recognizable in PAS preparations. Recent evidence indicates that the chief and oxyntic cells are renewed at a slow rate.

Studies made on the regeneration of the epithelium in the body of the stomach over areas denuded either by mechanical means or by treatment with alcohol have revealed that cells in the pit and neck divide and migrate out from the edges of the wound to cover the lesion. Then new pits and glands form, and in them the specialized cells of the glands differentiate.

Small intestine

The human small intestine is a thin-walled tube about 4 meters in length, extending from the pylorus of the stomach to the colon. At the pylorus, the smooth-surfaced gastric mucosa changes abruptly to a rough-surfaced intestinal mucosa composed of numerous projections (villi) (Fig. 18-41). The intestine consists of three portions: the duodenum, jejunum, and ileum. The duodenal-jejunal junction is marked externally by the suspensory ligament of Treitz, a thickening of the mesentery. Otherwise, no definite structural landmarks distinguish the three segments, although certain distinctive histologic features characterize their mucosae (see below). In addition, functional differences in absorptive activities have been demonstrated along the length of the small intestine.

HISTOLOGIC ORGANIZATION

The lining of the small intestine possesses gross and microscopic devices for increasing the surface area available for digestive and absorptive activities. The lining is thrown into large elevations that include the submucosa as well as the mucosa. These are the circularly arranged folds (*plicae circulares*, or *valves of Kerckring*), which are relatively permanent structures. The plicae are highly developed in the jejunum, forming its most conspicuous feature (Fig. 18-42). In the duodenum and ileum they are less conspicuous, and they generally end 2 ft above the entrance to the colon.

The surface of the small intestine is studded with innumerable *villi*, or mucosal projections, that give it a velvety appearance grossly. They are the absorptive units, which are unique to this segment of the adult alimentary tract. At their bases are simple tubular invaginations or pits that extend to the muscularis mucosae but do not penetrate it; these are the *intestinal glands*, or crypts of Lieberkühn (Fig. 18-43). The crypts have generative and secretory functions, as will be described later.

The villi are essentially evaginations or folds of the mucosa; they have a simple columnar epithelial cover and a core of highly cellular reticular connective tissue (lamina propria). The villi vary in height and form in different regions of the human small intestine. Each villus contains an artery, a capillary network, a vein, and a central lymphatic or lacteal (Fig. 18-23). A rich network of blood capillaries ramifies through the lamina propria and is closely apposed to the basement membrane of the absorptive epithelium (Figs. 18-44, 18-45, and 18-46). The vascularity of the villi is considerably greater than that of the tissue around the crypts (Fig. 18-44).

Narrow strands of smooth muscle fibers extend from the muscularis mucosae into the villi, render-

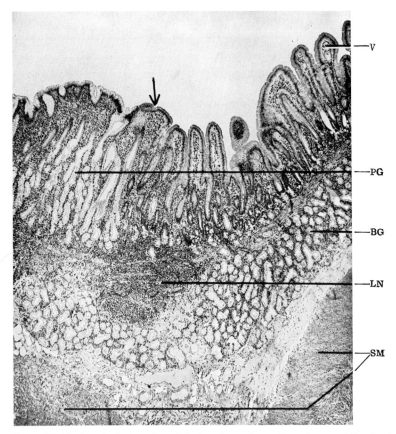

V

PG

BG

LN

SM

Figure 18-41   Longitudinal section of the junction between the pylorus and the duodenum of a monkey.   In the epithelium, the junction occurs approximately at the arrow.   V, villus; PG, pyloric gland; BG, Brunner's (duodenal) gland in the submucosa; LN, diffuse lymphatic nodule; SM, sphincteric (circular) muscles.   Bouin fixation; H&E.   ×50.

ing them contractile.   The villi can change in length and exhibit wavelike motions.   These muscle fibers, arranged lengthwise in the villus, may also aid circulation through the lymphatic vessels.   With the electron microscope, small bundles of unmyelinated nerves have been observed in the lamina propria in association with blood vessels and smooth muscle fibers.

The intestinal mucosa is divided into two histologically distinct regions, the germinative crypts and the absorptive villi.   The simple columnar epithelium that lines the crypts and covers the villi is a continuous sheet, which is constantly being renewed.   It is composed of at least five distinct types of epithelial cells.   In the crypt, the principal cell type is the relatively *undifferentiated columnar*

cell; this cell has a basophilic cytoplasm and divides frequently.   On the villus, the *absorptive cell* is the principal cell type (Figs. 18-45 and 18-46).   It has a moderately basophilic cytoplasm and a conspicuous microvillous surface, the *striated border*.   Interspersed among these major cell types, both in the crypts and on the villi, are mucus-secreting *goblet cells* and *argentaffin cells*.   (See enterochromaffin cells under Stomach.)   The bottom of the crypt is lined with a cluster of *Paneth cells,* which have the cytologic characteristics of zymogenic cells (Figs. 18-47 and 18-48).   These different cell types will be described in greater detail below.   Lymphocytes occur frequently between the epithelial cells (Fig. 18-45).

The epithelial cells rest on a well-defined but

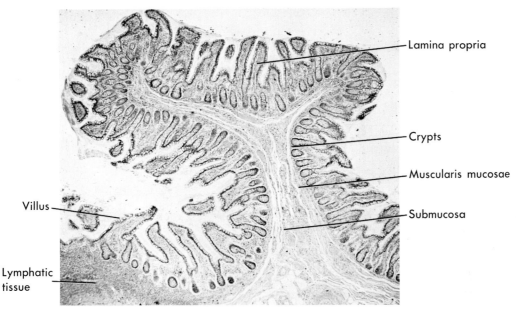

Figure 18-42   Plica circularis of the human jejunum.   The isolated bodies lying near the villi are sections of villi that were bent so that their ends appear in the plane of the section.   H&E.   ×40.

delicate basement membrane.   The connective tissue that forms the core of the villi and surrounds the glands is highly cellular reticular connective tissue typical of the alimentary tract.   Lymphatic nodules and aggregates are common.   The submucosa and muscularis follow the common pattern described earlier in this chapter.

The distribution of blood and lymphatic vessels and nerves in the small intestine has been described earlier (Fig. 18-23).

CYTOLOGY OF THE INTESTINAL EPITHELIUM

The *absorptive cells* of the villi are tall columnar, approximately 25 μm high and 8 μm wide, with oval nuclei located in the lower half of the cell.   The absorptive cells of mammals have a common design, and the following description refers to the well-described cells in the intestinal villi of the (fasted) rat.

Light microscopy shows that the free surface of these cells is a specialized *striated border* (Fig. 18-45) which consists of minute rodlike projections or *microvilli* in a uniform, parallel array (Figs. 18-49 and 18-50).   These numerous surface projections

tremendously increase the cellular surface area presented to the intestinal contents.   (They are about 1.4 μm long and 0.08 μm in diameter in human jejunal cells.)   The border is highly PAS-positive due to a *surface coat* over the microvilli of

Figure 18-43   Spatial scheme of the intestinal epithelium.   The epithelium of the crypts is continuous with that covering the villi.   Epithelial cells originate in the crypt of Lieberkühn; they differentiate and migrate along the villus to its apex, where they are shed at the extrusion zone.   (From Quastler and Sherman.)

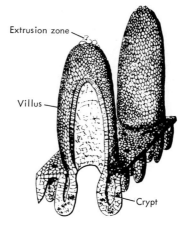

Villus   Crypt

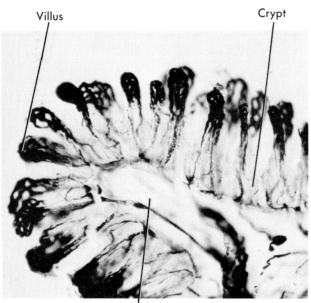

Submucosa

Figure 18-44   Human jejunal mucosa.   India-ink injection of a branch of the mesenteric artery within 1 to 2 hr postmortem. A profuse capillary network exists at the tip of the villus.   Note the lower vascularity in the remainder of the mucosa.   (Courtesy of W. T. Cooke, G. I. Nicholson, and A. Ayres.)

Figure 18-45   Longitudinal section of an intestinal villus of a monkey duodenum.   SB, striated border on absorptive cell; L, lymphocyte migrating through epithelium; BM, basement membrane; GC, goblet cell.   Bouin's fixation; H&E.   ×500.

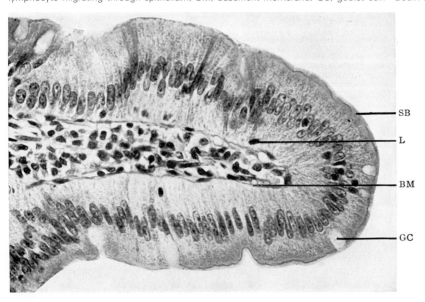

SB

L

BM

GC

Lymphocytes   Venule

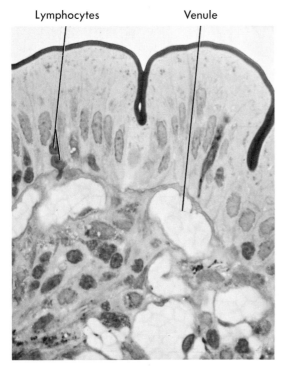

Figure 18-46   Normal human absorptive epithelium. This specimen was obtained with an intraluminal biopsy capsule. The striated border of this simple columnar epithelium is strongly PAS-positive, indicating the presence of a carbohydrate-protein polymer. Note also the fine PAS-positive droplets in the apical cytoplasm of the absorptive cells. Lymphocytes are migrating into the epithelium. Note venules in the lamina propria. Plastic section; osmium tetroxide fixation; periodic acid-Schiff procedure. × 1,000. (Courtesy of H. A. Padykula, E. W. Strauss, A. J. Ladman, and F. H. Gardner.)

fine filaments or fuzz (Fig. 3-23) made of glycoprotein that is rich in acid residues. The surface coat is prominent in man but is developed in varying degrees among other species. Recent radioautographic evidence indicates that the carbohydrate portion of this glycoprotein is synthesized in the Golgi complex and linked to the protein moiety; this secretion migrates through the cytoplasm and is added to the cell coat (Bennett, 1970).

Each microvillus contains a core of longitudinal filaments which merge just beneath the microvillous border with the *terminal web,* a dense meshwork of filaments that lie mostly in a plane parallel to the free surface of the cell and insert into the lateral surfaces of the cell at junctional complexes (Figs. 18-49 and 18-50). The rigid apical ectoplasm composed of the striated border and the terminal web can be readily isolated from homogenates of intestinal mucosa as a morphologically distinct entity (Fig. 18-51). The surface plasma membrane invaginates into the cytoplasm between the bases of the microvilli to form tubules (Fig. 18-56).

The apical cytoplasm immediately beneath the terminal web contains vesicles and tubules of the labyrinthine smooth ER. This dense, tubular network is continuous below, nearer the nucleus, with the rough ER whose anastomosing membranes are oriented in the long axis of the cell. Immediately above the nucleus, the Golgi complex can be selectively demonstrated by metallic impregnation methods or by the cytochemical localization of nucleoside diphosphatase activity. It has the typical configuration of stacked cisternae and associated small and large vesicles. Absorptive cells are characterized by numerous typical mitochondria, generally filamentous, although they may also be branched or spherical (Fig. 18-49). They occur mainly in the apical cytoplasm where they are oriented parallel to the long axis of the cell; the infranuclear mitochondria are oriented more randomly. Thus the absorptive cell is highly polarized, with a characteristic arrangement of membrane systems and mitochondria.

The lateral surfaces of absorptive cells form a well-developed junctional complex, as described and illustrated in Chap. 3, that binds the various cells to each other throughout the intestinal epithelium. Near the free surface, the cells are attached by conspicuous terminal bars which are light-microscopic manifestations of apical intercellular adhesion. Below the junctional complex, the lateral cell surfaces are plicated; near the base of the cell, small footlike processes abut against adjacent cells. The intercellular space is approximately 10 nm wide, although intercellular dilations as great as 200 nm occur in the basal regions of the epithelium (Figs. 18-49 and 18-56A). The basal surface of the cell is flattened on a thin basal lamina.

The villous epithelium is coated by a protective layer of mucus produced by goblet cells located in

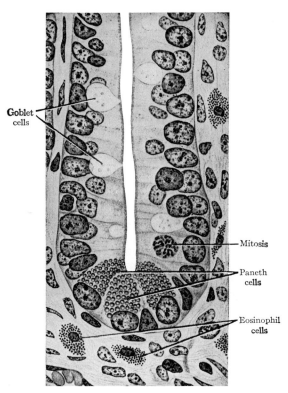

Goblet
cells

—Mitosis

—Paneth
cells

—Eosinophil
cells

Figure 18-47   Cell types at the base of an intestinal gland of human jejunum. In addition to Paneth cells and goblet cells, there are the relatively undifferentiated cells destined to become various epithelial cells. Mitoses occur characteristically in these cells. Zenker fixation; H&E. ×1,000. (Von Möllendorff.)

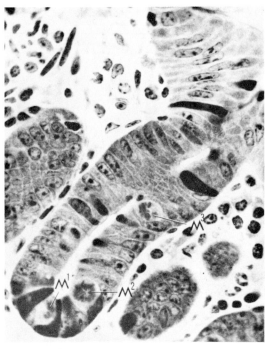

Figure 18-48   Longitudinal section through a crypt in the small intestine (mouse). Several mitotic figures are shown. M^1 and M^2 occur among the Paneth cells at the bottom of the crypt. Undifferentiated columnar cells are evident in the upper crypt. (From Hampton.)

the crypts and on the villi (Fig. 18-49). This mucus lies outside the surface coat of the microvilli (Fig. 3-13). Active goblet cells can easily be recognized by their secretory product, which is strongly basophilic, metachromatic, and PAS-positive. This sulfate-containing mucoprotein material appears as small droplets in the immediately supranuclear region of the goblet cell where the Golgi apparatus is located. As the mucoid store increases, it begins to fill the entire supranuclear cytoplasm; the cell acquires the rounded contours of the goblet, and the basal nucleus becomes somewhat flattened. The cytoplasm of goblet cells is basophilic, being rich in ribonucleoprotein.

With the electron microscope, many additional cytologic features of the production and release of

Figure 18-49   Intestinal epithelium of the villus of a fasted rat. Several absorptive cells and a portion of a goblet cell are shown. The polarity of the absorptive cells is evident in structural differences between the free and attached surfaces and also in the distribution of the organelles. The luminal surface is composed of closely packed, regularly arranged microvilli (MV); the subjacent cytoplasm, which is relatively free of organelles, is the region of the terminal web (TW). Below the terminal web the cytoplasm contains smooth endoplasmic reticulum (SER), whereas somewhat deeper the rough form (RER) occurs. The Golgi complex (G) occurs immediately above the nucleus. Mitochondria are widely distributed and here are heavily concentrated in the infranuclear cytoplasm. The lateral cell surfaces on the supranuclear region are closely apposed and sometimes folded (arrows), whereas below the nucleus (N) the lateral surfaces form interdigitating processes (P) and the intercellular space is wider (*). BL, basal lamina; LP, lamina propria. ×6,000. (R. R. Cardell, S. Badenhausen, and K. R. Porter, J. Cell Biol., **34**:123, 1967.)

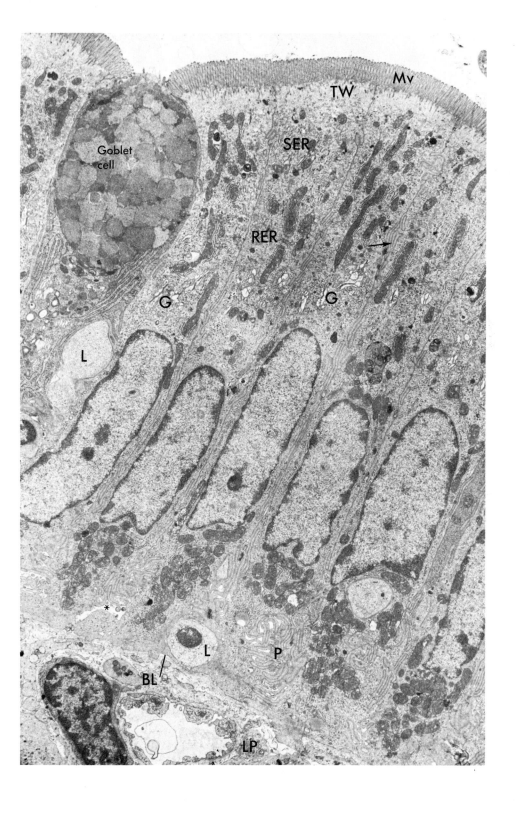

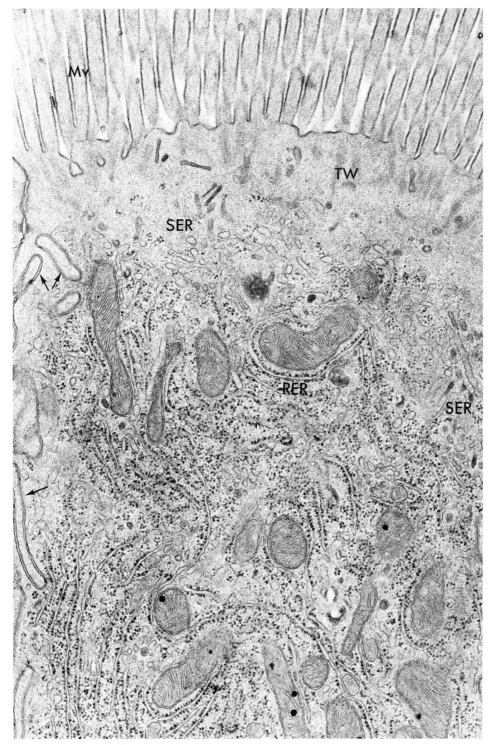

Figure 18-50 Supranuclear cytoplasm of an intestinal absorptive cell in a fasted rat. The smooth endoplasmic reticulum (SER) occurs beneath the terminal web (TW), while the rough endoplasmic reticulum (RER) occupies a deeper location. The interdigitating lateral cell surfaces are indicated by arrows. Mv, microvilli. ×37,800. (H. I. Friedman and R. D. Cardell, Jr., J. Cell Biol., **52:**15, 1972.)

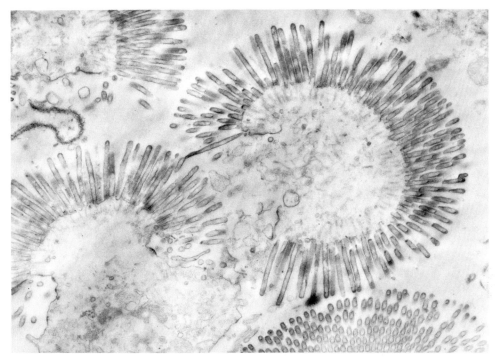

Figure 18-51   Isolated microvillous borders of the hamster small intestine. The ultrastructure of isolated intestinal microvillous borders is illustrated. In addition to the microvillous border, these preparations include the cellular components of the immediately subjacent cytoplasm. Approximately ×9,000. (Courtesy of Overton, Crane, and Eichholz.)

the secretory product are revealed. The ultrastructural changes that occur during the secretory cycle of the goblet cell have been described in detail for the rat jejunum (Fig. 18-52). At the onset of secretion the membrane systems begin to proliferate. The cytoplasm becomes filled with large, branching rough ER cisternae that are longitudinally oriented and contain a dense material. The supranuclear Golgi apparatus expands and increases in complexity, and secretory material accumulates in its vesicles.

Radioautographic studies have demonstrated that the protein moiety of mucus glycoprotein is synthesized in the rough ER whereas the carbohydrate moiety is produced and linked to protein in the Golgi membranes (Neutra and Leblond, 1966). The final product is collected and segregated in the Golgi membranes. As secretory material begins to crowd the supranuclear cytoplasm, the mitochondria and the ER sacs are displaced to

the peripheral cytoplasm, the lateral folds of the cell surface become ironed out, and the microvilli are flattened. The droplets of mucus coalesce, to some extent, and begin to lose their surrounding membranes. Finally, the secretion is released in an apocrine manner by the bursting of the plasma membrane at the apex of the cell, and the contents of the Golgi membranes flow into the intestinal lumen (Fig. 18-53). Radioautographic evidence indicates that synthesis and release of mucus occur continually during the 2 to 3 days of the goblet cell's life.

Protein-producing *Paneth cells* line the bottoms of the intestinal crypts (Figs. 18-47 and 18-48). They are pyramidal in shape and have cytologic characteristics typical of serozymogenic cells. The basal cytoplasm is strongly basophilic, being rich in ribonucleoprotein; in the supranuclear Golgi region there are conspicuous, large, refractile, acidophilic granules. These granules have been

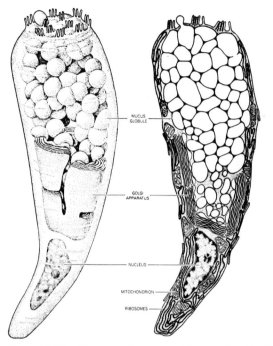

MUCUS GLOBULE

GOLGI APPARATUS

NUCLEUS

MITOCHONDRION

RIBOSOMES

Figure 18-52 Diagrammatic representations of the intestinal goblet cell. (Neutra and Leblond.)

shown to contain a mucopolysaccharide-protein complex. The ultrastructural features resemble those of the pancreatic acinar cell. The secretory granules accumulate during fasting and are released after the ingestion of food. Although the function of these cells has not been established, these various characteristics suggest that they may be involved in the production of proteins, possibly intestinal enzymes.

REGIONAL DIFFERENCES

The three regions of the small intestine, the duodenum, jejunum, and ileum, can be distinguished to some extent by histologic criteria. The upper duodenum is characterized by *Brunner's glands,* which are submucosal in position (Fig. 18-41). These mucus-producing glands are branched and tubuloalveolar in form; they empty into the intestinal crypts. The secretory cells possess tiny supranuclear droplets, rather than the large masses found in goblet cells. This mucus does not stain metachromatically. It probably lubricates the enter-

ing gastric contents and possibly separates and suspends solid food particles.

Plicae circulares occur in all three regions but are best developed in the jejunum (Fig. 18-42). Form differences in the villi occur in the three regions of the human small intestine. In the duodenum they are short, leaflike folds (0.2 to 0.5 mm high) that may be branched; in the jejunum they are rounded, fingerlike projections, whereas in the ileum they tend to have a clublike form. These differences are not easily recognized in sections. In the jejunum and ileum, the villi are 0.2 to 1.0 mm in height, standing 10 to 40 to the square millimeter; they are taller and more numerous in the jejunum than in the ileum. They disappear in the region of the ileocecal valve. The number of goblet cells in the villous epithelium increases progressively from the duodenum to the ileocecal valve, and the basophilia of the mucus likewise increases steadily. Thus the villous epithelium of the ileum has a high percentage of goblet cells. Solitary lymphoid nodules may occur along the entire intestine, but they also tend to be more numerous in the ileum.

Functional differences in absorptive activity have been described along the length of the small intestine. For example, maximal absorption of triglycerides occurs in the proximal small intestine, whereas bile salts and vitamin B_{12} are absorbed by the distal segment. A gradient in the alkaline phosphatase activity along the length of the small intestine of the mature mouse has been demonstrated biochemically; the activity of homogenates is highest in the duodenum, falls sharply to a lower level in the jejunum, and remains low in the ileum. This enzyme is heavily concentrated in the microvilli.

EPITHELIAL REPLACEMENT

The histologic concept of the continuous replacement of the intestinal epithelium in the adult has been developed since 1948, largely through radioautographic studies of Leblond and his associates. It has long been known that there is intensive mitotic activity in the undifferentiated cells in the crypts of Lieberkühn and that mitosis occurs rarely in the normal villous epithelium. It has been established that the absorptive cells and goblet cells originate in the crypts, migrate onto the villus, and move toward its apex, where they are extruded at a

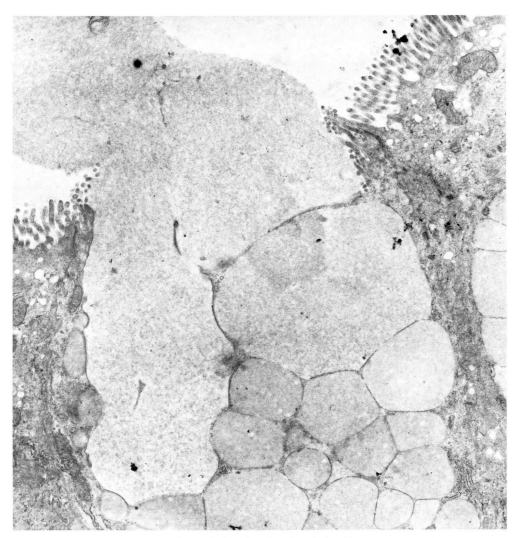

Figure 18-53 Electron micrograph of the apical portion of an intestinal goblet cell in the act of releasing its mucus. ✕13,000.

specific site called the *extrusion zone* (Fig. 18-43).

The most convincing evidence for this epithelial migration is derived from the tagging of dividing cells with tritiated thymidine. This precursor of DNA is incorporated into the dividing cells in the crypt (Fig. 18-54), and then the radioactive tag is carried by the daughter cells during their migration. The radioactive label is picked up by undifferentiated columnar cells (Fig. 18-48) that become absorptive cells and also by *oligomucous cells* that are precursors of goblet cells. The dividing oligomucous cell has been most likely derived from an undifferentiated columnar cell. Such isotopic labeling reveals that the life-span of the cells of the villous epithelium is very short; in experimental animals there is a complete replacement within 2 or 3 days. In man there is likewise evidence that the whole epithelial lining of the gastrointestinal tract, from stomach to rectum, is completely renewed every 2 to 4 days.

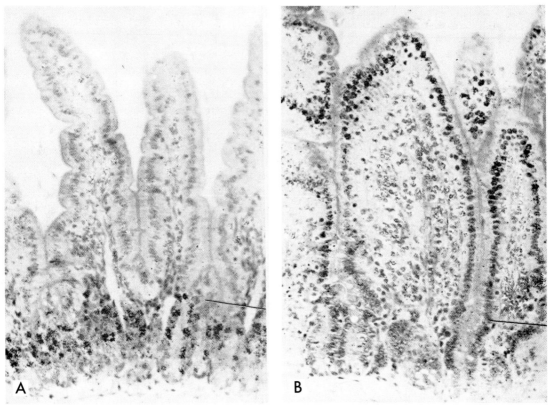

Figure 18-54 Radioautographs of mouse jejunum 8 hr (A) and 72 hr (B) after injection of tritiated thymidine. The horizontal marker indicates the approximate junction of the crypt and villus. At 8 hr, radioactivity is limited to the upper crypts whereas by 72 hr it is located in the surface epithelium of the upper third of the villus. (From Leblond and Messier.)

Mitosis in Paneth cells has not been observed. However, these cells are slowly replaced by progenitors that proliferate at the bottom of the crypt (Fig. 18-48). In the mouse the turnover time for the Paneth cells is about 3 weeks. The argentaffin and other "endocrine" cells of the mouse intestine originate from precursors in the lower half of the crypt and migrate to the villus. Their turnover time is about 4 days.

The extrusion zone at the apex of the villus is marked by a distinct cleft in the epithelium, and the emerging cells round off somewhat as they are shed into the intestinal lumen. Leblond and Walker have presented the interesting concept that the normal histologic appearance of the intestinal mucosa is a result of the balance between cell proliferation in the crypts and cell loss at the extrusion zones. Irradiation upsets this balance by interfering with cell division in the crypts; cell loss at the extrusion zones continues, and the result is atrophy of the villi.

A variety of evidence suggests that during the migration of the absorptive cells toward the apex of the villus they differentiate progressively. For example, the microvilli of the absorptive cells become longer, narrower, and more numerous. This progressive differentiation results in a great increase in the surface area of the plasma membrane at the crest of the villus. There is evidence that in the human jejunum the absorptive cells at the tip of the villus may have a lower RNA content than those at the base. Histophysiologic experiments have demonstrated that the absorptive cells at the villous crest can concentrate lipids, sugars, and amino acids to a greater degree than the younger, more basal absorptive cells. The evidence supports the hypothesis that the differentiation of the intestinal epithelium culminates in the formation of a highly specialized digestive and absorptive surface at the apex of the villus (Fig. 18-55).

MORPHOLOGIC ASPECTS OF DIGESTIVE AND ABSORPTIVE FUNCTIONS

Locus of digestive activity Extracellular digestion is characteristic of the intestines of higher animals, including mammals. Complex molecules are degraded by enzymes secreted into the lumen by glands associated with the digestive tract. The resulting smaller molecules are taken in by the absorptive cells of the small intestine. In addition, recent evidence indicates that certain large molecules can be absorbed directly.

The cellular origin of the intestinal enzymes of mammals is an unresolved problem. Some of the intestinal enzymes are secreted in the crypts or glands of Lieberkühn, presumably by the Paneth cells. Most, of course, come from the pancreas. In addition, a considerable but unknown quantity is derived from desquamated absorptive cells.

The intestinal juice has a low enzymic content that increases with increasing cellular content. When the shed epithelial cells in the intestinal juice are broken up by homogenization, the enzymatic activity increases. Furthermore, digestive activity of the human small intestine toward disaccharides is greater than can be accounted for by the enzymic content of the juice. This evidence led to the suggestion that the terminal hydrolytic digestion in the small intestine may occur on or in absorptive cells rather than in the intestinal lumen.

Although there is virtually no phosphatase in the lumen, phosphate esters are rapidly hydrolyzed by the small intestine. Histochemists have long been aware that the striated border is rich in phosphatases active in the neutral and alkaline range of pH. Recent ultrastructural identification of phosphatase activity localizes it in (or near) the plasma membrane. The isolated microvillous border contains practically all the invertase and maltase activities of the total mucosal homogenate. Furthermore, 75 percent of all the aminopeptidase and

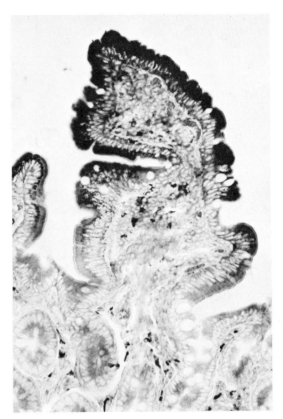

Figure 18-55 Normal human jejunal mucosa biopsied 20 min after ingestion of corn oil. Lipid droplets have accumulated principally in the absorptive epithelium of the upper half of the villus. Epithelial cells at the base of the villus and in the crypt are free of lipid droplets. Heavily sudanophilic cells in the lamina propria are tissue eosinophils. Formalin-fixed; frozen section stained with Sudan black. ×200. (Courtesy of A. J. Ladman, H. A. Padykula, and E. W. Strauss.)

alkaline phosphatase activities of whole intestinal homogenates is recovered in the isolated microvillous border. From in vitro experiments it has been suggested that the hydrolysis of disaccharides, peptides, and sugar phosphates occurs within the microvillous border at an intracellular locus. From this evidence it seems highly probable that the striated border, in addition to providing abundant surface area for absorption, is a locus of hydrolysis and active transport.

Morphologic aspects of absorption In a morphologic study of absorption, it is necessary that the substance being transported be identifiable by some visible tag in tissue sections. The absorption of fats has lent itself to such study because the lipid droplets are sudanophilic and osmiophilic. This process has been analyzed in considerable detail by histochemical identification of lipids with Sudan dyes and with the electron microscope. Some information concerning the absorption of proteins, such as antibodies, has been derived from the use of proteins carrying fluorescent or other labels. Only fragmentary information exists concerning morphologic aspects of the absorption of carbohydrates.

Although the morphologic aspects of lipid absorption have long been studied in laboratory animals, it is only in recent years that it has been possible to study this problem in the normal human being. Intraluminal biopsy procedures have permitted study of the normal and abnormal intestinal mucosa. Within 20 min after a fasted normal human being (or other mammal) ingests fat, such as corn oil, lipid droplets appear within the absorptive epithelium of the proximal small intestine. The absorbed lipid is restricted to the villus, and a conspicuous gradient in the amount of intraepithelial lipid is evident (Fig. 18-55). Most of the droplets are concentrated at the upper half of the villus, and the amount of lipid diminishes progressively from the tip of the villus to its base. Cytologic study with the light microscope reveals that in the absorptive cells nearest the tip of the villus the droplets occur throughout the apical endoplasm; the droplets in the supranuclear Golgi region are generally larger.

Observations with the electron microscope have added greatly to our knowledge of the pathway followed by lipid in the intestinal absorptive cell. However, the exact nature of the mechanism of absorption remains controversial. Soon after instillation of an oil into the stomach of a fasted animal, small lipid droplets (65 nm in maximal diameter) are found lodged in the spaces among the microvilli of the jejunal absorptive cells; no droplets are observed within the microvilli (Fig. 18-56). Droplets are then seen within small vesicles which, beneath the terminal web, join the smooth ER. Here the lipid droplets are generally larger (50 to 240 nm). The labyrinthine network of smooth-surfaced tubules is continuous with the rough ER; lipid droplets may therefore also appear enclosed by membranes studded with ribosomes. Lipid accumulates in the

Golgi cisternae as droplets of varying sizes (40 to 150 nm). Droplets have been observed also in the nuclear envelope. Since they occur therefore in all parts of the cytoplasmic membrane systems (Fig. 18-56B), they have been interpreted as markers of a physiologic continuity of the cell surface with all parts of the membranes of the apical cytoplasm.

After coursing through the membranous system, the droplets are discharged from the lateral surfaces of the absorptive cells at the nuclear level into the intercellular spaces, and so the basal part of the cell is bypassed. Lipid droplets, devoid of membranes, travel through the extracellular space toward the basal lamina, above which they accumulate in large clusters; they then erupt through this into the connective tissue spaces. From here they gain entrance to the lacteals by passing between endothelial cells. Although numerous lipid droplets can be seen entering the lacteals, only rarely do they occur in the blood capillaries. Physiologic experiments have indicated that triglycerides are selectively absorbed by the lymphatic vessels, whereas water-soluble, short-chain fatty acids enter the blood capillaries.

The observation that absorbed lipid droplets are closely invested by membranes in the apical cytoplasm strongly suggests that the droplets have entered the cell by pinocytosis and that the membranes are derived from the cell surface (Fig. 18-56A). It is known, however, that lipid is hydrolyzed in the intestinal lumen; thus it is possible that the products of hydrolysis have been absorbed by diffusion. In addition, it is known that triglyceride can be resynthesized by the microsomal fraction of these cells. Thus the droplets may reflect newly synthesized triglyceride which has accumulated within the endoplasmic reticulum. Although both pathways could explain the presence of lipid droplets within the cytoplasmic membrane system, it is likely that most of the lipid is absorbed by diffusion after initial hydrolysis (Fig. 18-56B). Compelling evidence is presented in studies which demonstrate that the initial phase of absorption is not temperature-dependent and thus most likely does not represent pinocytosis, which is an active process. In addition, observations following the exposure of the intestinal mucosa to lipid containing electron-opaque markers further suggest that pinocytosis is not a primary mechanism because the

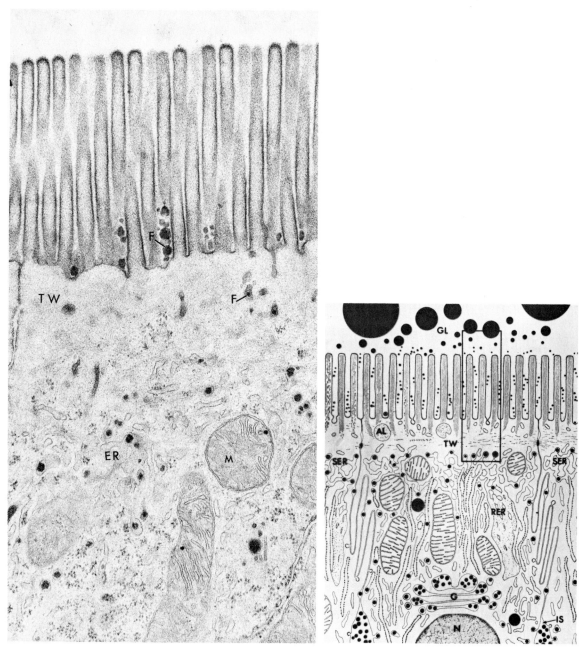

Figure 18-56   A. Electron micrograph of the apical part of an absorptive cell of the upper jejunum of a rat.   Linolenic acid containing 0.85 mg percent tristearin was instilled into the stomach.   One hour later, small droplets of fat (F) are found between the microvilli and within vesicles in the terminal web (TW).   Slender channels are invaginated from the plasma membrane at the bases of the intermicrovillus spaces.   Some droplets occur also within the tubules of the smooth endoplasmic reticulum (ER).   M, mitochondrion. ×28,000.   (Courtesy of S. Palay and J. P. Revel, 1964.)   B. Diagrammatic summary of the morphologic aspects of fat absorption by the absorptive cell of the small intestine.   (From Cardell et al.)

membrane-enclosed droplets are free of the accompanying markers.

The absorption of protein by the adult mammalian intestine is for the most part totally dependent upon initial hydrolysis prior to uptake by the absorptive cell. During postnatal development, proteins and other colloidal materials are taken into the absorptive cells of the distal small intestine without first being completely hydrolyzed. These accumulate in large supranuclear vacuoles resembling those seen in renal proximal tubule cells. As the gut matures, this structural manifestation disappears, along with most of the ability to absorb proteins and various colloidal materials.

Large intestine

The large intestine, or colon, begins at the ileocecal valve and consists of a *cecum* and *appendix;* the *ascending, transverse,* and *descending segments;* the *sigmoid colon;* and a terminal portion, the *rectum,* ending at the external orifice or *anus.* Its total length is roughly 150 cm in man.

COLON
The mucosa of the large intestine everywhere lacks villi; it has deep straight glands about two or three times as deep as those of the small intestine (about 0.5 mm). The lamina propria contains frequent solitary lymphatic nodules, often so large as to extend into the submucosa (Fig. 18-57). The submucosa contains the usual constituents plus large accumulations of fat cells.

The muscularis of the colon and cecum has a characteristic arrangement not found in the vermiform appendix or the more proximal portions of the alimentary tract. The longitudinal smooth muscle fibers of the outer layer gather into three equidistant longitudinal strands known as *taeniae* (G., bands). Between them, the longitudinal fibers form a thin, sometimes interrupted layer. Because of the tonus of the taeniae, the wall of the colon bulges outward as sacculations or *haustra* (L., buckets). Between these sacculations, the wall is thrown into crescentic *plicae semilunares* that project into the lumen. The ileocecal valve consists of two folds resembling such plicae. A peculiarity of the colon is that fascicles of longitudinal fibers from the taeniae frequently join the circular layer. This arrangement interrupts the continuity of the circular layer, and different intertaenial areas may contract independently.

The serosa is incomplete, since the ascending and descending limbs of the colon are retroperitoneal. It may contain lobules of fat that form pendulous projections (*appendices epiploicae*).

Epithelial cells The surface epithelium consists of a mixture of columnar absorptive cells, with striated borders, and mucous goblet cells. The crypts consist principally of tall mucous cells. In the human rectum, enterochromaffin cells occur at the bottom of the crypt. Epithelial proliferation occurs in the lower half to two-thirds of human rectal crypts to provide cells needed for the constant replacement. Replacement time in the human rectum has been estimated as 5 to 6 days.

The mucosa of the colon has two principal activities: (1) the absorption of water and of vitamins derived from bacteria and (2) the secretion of mucus, which serves as a protective lubricant. Some waste products and drugs are also excreted into the lumen through the epithelium.

CECUM AND VERMIFORM APPENDIX
The *cecum* is a blind pouch at the proximal end of the colon, and its terminal thin tip is known as the *vermiform appendix.* The structure of the cecum resembles that of the rest of the colon, and the vermiform appendix has a similar structure in miniature (Fig. 18-58), except that taeniae are absent. The glands are simple tubes, sometimes forked; the epithelium consists mainly of mucous cells. Lymphatic nodules are abundant and more or less confluent. The wealth of lymphatic vessels and lymphatic tissue is the most conspicuous histologic feature of the appendix (Fig. 18-59).

The lumen of the normal appendix in the adult, when empty, is thrown into folds separated by deep pockets. But this normal condition is found in scarcely 50 percent of individuals over 40 years of

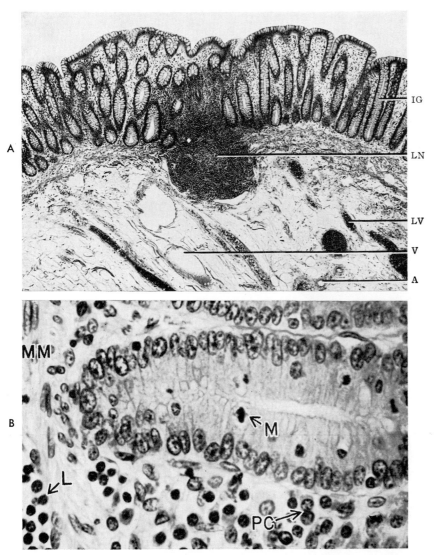

Figure 18-57   A. Longitudinal section of mucosa and submucosa of the human colon.   IG, intestinal gland; LN, lymphatic nodule, which has perforated through the muscularis mucosae into the submucosa; LV, lymphatic vessel filled with lymphocytes; V, vein; A, artery.   ×50.   B. Section through the base of a gland of the large intestine of a monkey.   M, mitotic figure in an epithelial cell; PC, plasma cells in the periglandular stroma; L, lymphatic vessel; MM, muscularis mucosae.   Bouin fixation.   ×600.

age because of a history of subclinical appendicitis.   Often the lumen is narrowed or even obliterated.   The epithelium and the underlying lymphatic tissue then disappear and are replaced by an axial mass of fibrous tissue.

RECTUM

The rectum is divided into two parts, an upper part that extends from the third sacral vertebra to the pelvic diaphragm, and a lower part, or anal canal, that continues down to the anus.   The lining of the

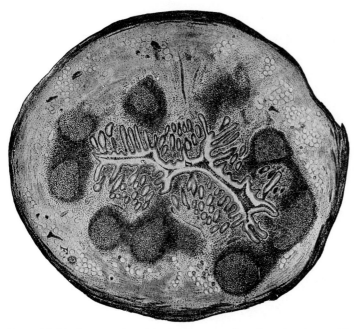

Figure 18-58   Cross section of the human appendix.   Note abundance of lymphatic nodules.   Only a part of the circular layer of the muscularis is included.   ×20.   (Sobotta.)

Figure 18-59   Lymphatic network in the human appendix as viewed from the surface.   Note enlargement of vessels over the nodules and valves in the larger vessels.   ×40.   (Teichmann.)

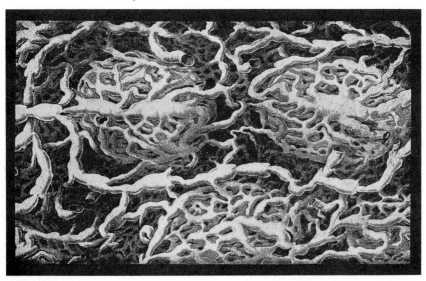

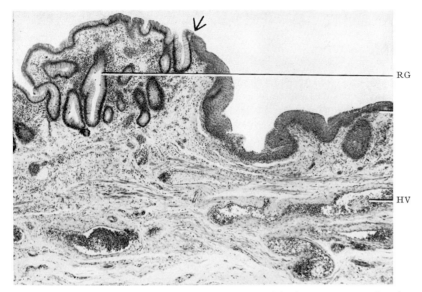

RG

HV

Figure 18-60   Longitudinal section through the junction of the human rectum and anal canal.   Arrow marks pectinate line.   RG, rectal gland; HV, hemorrhoidal vein in the submucosa.   ×35.

first part is thrown into several large, semilunar, circular folds, the *plicae transversales recti*. For most of its length the anal canal presents on its inner wall a number of longitudinal folds, the *anal columns*.

The mucous membrane of the first part of the rectum is similar to that of the colon, but its glands are somewhat longer (0.7 mm) and are composed almost completely of mucous cells. Solitary lymphatic nodules are present. A continuous layer of longitudinal muscle is present. The rectum has no mesentery, and the serosa is replaced by adventitial connective tissue.

The lower portion of the rectum, or anal canal, is 2 to 3 cm in length and roughly elliptical in cross section. It ends at the anus, where its lining becomes continuous with the external skin. In the anal canal, the epithelium changes abruptly from simple columnar to stratified cuboidal at the *pectinate line* (Fig. 18-60). The anal columns join one another somewhat below this line, creating pocketlike anal valves. Above each valve is a recess termed an *anal sinus*. At this level the muscularis

mucosae disappears. The uncornified epithelium of the canal changes into typical keratinized stratified squamous epithelium at the anus proper. In the lower part of the anal canal a few isolated sebaceous glands make their appearance.

The skin immediately around the anus forms the *zona cutanea*. Sweat glands are absent from the region immediately bordering the anus, but at a distance of 1.0 to 1.5 cm there is an elliptical zone, 1.5 cm wide, containing simple tubular glands, the *circumanal glands*. These are apocrine sweat glands, being the terminal representatives of the milk line (see Chap. 24). They secrete an oily fluid that is related, in lower mammals, to sexual activity.

The outer layers of the anal canal include a very vascular submucosa, which contains blood vessels, numerous nerves, and Pacinian corpuscles. The veins form the large hemorrhoid plexus (Fig. 18-60) and are especially susceptible to varicosities. The circular layer of the muscularis becomes thickened at its termination, forming the internal anal sphincter. Beyond this, striated muscle fibers surround the orifice, forming the external anal sphincter.

References

ORAL CAVITY

BEIDLER, L. N., and R. L. S. SMALLMAN: Renewal of Cells within Taste Buds, *J. Cell Biol.*, **27**:263 (1965).

HASHIMOTO, K., R. J. DIBELLA, and G. SHKLAR: Electron Microscopic Studies of the Normal Human Buccal Mucosa, *J. Invest. Derm.*, **47**:512 (1966).

LISTGARTEN, M. A.: Electron-microscopic Study of the Gingivo-dental Junction of Man, *Amer. J. Anat.*, **119**:147 (1966).

MATTERN, C. F. T., W. A. DANIEL, and R. I. HENKIN: The Ultrastructure of the Human Circumvallate Papilla. I. Cilia of the Papillary Crypt, *Anat. Rec.*, **167**:175 (1970).

MURRAY, R. G., A. MURRAY, and S. FUJIMOTO: Fine Structure of Gustatory Cells in Rabbit Taste Buds, *J. Ultrastruct. Res.*, **27**:444 (1969).

PROVENZA, D. V.: "Oral Histology," J. B. Lippincott Company, Philadelphia, 1964.

SCHROEDER, H. E.: Melanin Containing Organelles in Cells of the Human Gingiva. I. Epithelial Melanocytes, *J. Periodont. Res.*, **4**:1 (1969).

SCHROEDER, H. E., and M. A. LISTGARTEN: Fine Structure of the Developing Epithelial Attachment of Human Teeth, "Monographs in Developmental Biology," vol. 2, S. Karger AG, Basel, 1971.

SCHROEDER, H. E., and J. THEILADE: Electron Microscopy of Normal Human Gingival Epithelium, *J. Periodont. Res.*, **1**:95 (1966).

SCHUMACHER, S.: Die Mundhohle, Die Zunge, Der Schlundkopf, in W. von Möllendorff and W. Bargmann (eds.), "Handbuch der mikroskopischen Anatomie der Menschen," vol. 5, pt. 1, Springer-Verlag OHG, Berlin, 1927.

SKOUGAARD, M. R.: Cell Renewal, with Special Reference to the Gingival Epithelium, *Advances Oral Biol.*, **4**:261 (1970).

ZALEWSKI, A. A.: Combined Effects of Testosterone and Motor, Sensory, or Gustatory Nerve Reinnervation on the Regeneration of Taste Buds, *Exp. Neurol.*, **24**:285 (1969).

SALIVARY GLANDS

HAND, A. R.: Nerve-acinar Cell Relationships in the Rat Parotid Gland, *J. Cell Biol.*, **47**:540 (1970).

LEESON, C. R.: Structure of Salivary Glands, in C. F. Code and W. Heidel (eds.), "Handbook of Physiology," vol. 2, sec. 6, chap. 1, American Physiological Society, Washington, 1967.

LEPPI, T. J.: Gross Anatomical Relationships between Primate Submandibular and Sublingual Salivary Glands, *J. Dent. Res.*, **46**:359 (1967).

LEPPI, T. J., and S. S. SPICER: The Histochemistry of Mucins in Certain Primate Salivary Glands, *Amer. J. Anat.*, **118**:833 (1966).

MUNGER, B. L.: Histochemical Studies on Seromucous- and Mucous-secreting Cells of Human Salivary Glands, *Amer. J. Anat.*, **115**:411 (1964).

STRUM, J. M., and M. J. KARNOVSKY: Ultrastructural Localization of Peroxidase in Submaxillary Acinar Cells, *J. Ultrastruct. Res.*, **31**:323 (1970).

TAMARIN, A.: Myoepithelium of the Rat Submaxillary Gland, *J. Ultrastruct. Res.*, **16**:320 (1966).

TAMARIN, A., and L. M. SREEBNY: The Rat Submaxillary Salivary Gland. A Correlative Study by Light and Electron Microscopy, *J. Morph.*, **117**:295 (1965).

TANDLER, B.: Ultrastructure of the Human Submaxillary Gland. I. Architecture and Histological Relationships of the Secretory Cell, *Amer. J. Anat.,* **111**:287 (1962).

TANDLER, B., C. R. DENNING, I. D. MANDEL, and A. H. KITSCHER: Ultrastructure of Human Labial Salivary Glands. I. Acinar Secretory Cells, *J. Morph.,* **127**:383 (1969).

TANDLER, B., and L. L. ROSS: Observations of Nerve Terminals in Human Labial Salivary Glands, *J. Cell Biol.,* **42**:339 (1969).

TOMASI, T. B., JR., and J. BIENENSTOCK: Secretory Immunoglobulins, *Advances Immun.,* **9**:11 (1968).

ZIMMERMAN, K. W.: Die Speicheldrusen der Mundhohle und die Bauchspeichel-druse, in W. von Möllendorff and W. Bargmann (eds.), "Handbuch der mikroskopischen Anatomie der Menschen," vol. 5, pt. 1, Springer-Verlag OHG, Berlin, 1927.

ESOPHAGUS

PARAKKAL, P.: An Electron Microscopic Study of the Esophageal Epithelium in the Newborn and Adult Mouse, *Amer. J. Anat.,* **121**:175 (1967).

STOMACH

BENSLEY, R. R.: The Gastric Glands, in E. V. Cowdry (ed.), "Special Cytology," 2d ed., vol. 1, Paul B. Hoeber, Inc., New York, 1932.

FORSSMAN, W. G., L. ORCI, R. PICTET, A. E. RENOLD, and C. ROUILLER: The Endocrine Cells in the Epithelium of the Gastrointestinal Mucosa of the Rat. An Electron Microscope Study, *J. Cell Biol.,* **40**:692 (1969).

FORTE, T. M., and J. G. FORTE: Histochemical Staining and Characterization of Glycoproteins in Acid-secreting Cells of Frog Stomach, *J. Cell Biol.,* **47**:437 (1970).

GROSSMAN, M. I., and I. N. MARKS: Secretion of Pepsinogen by the Pyloric Glands of the Dog, with Some Observations on the Histology of the Gastric Mucosa, *Gastroenterology,* **38**:343 (1960).

ITO, S.: Anatomic Structure of the Gastric Mucosa, in C. F. Code and W. Heidel (eds.), "Handbook of Physiology," vol. 2, sec. 6, chap. 41, American Physiological Society, Washington, 1967.

LINDERSTROM-LANG, K.: Distribution of Enzymes in Tissue and Cells, *Harvey Lect.,* **34**: (1938).

MAC DONALD, W. C., J. S. TRIER, and N. B. EVERETT: Cell Proliferation and Migration in the Stomach, Duodenum, and Rectum of Man: Radioautographic Studies, *Gastroenterology,* **46**:405 (1964).

PLENK, H.: Der Magen, in W. von Möllendorff (ed.), "Handbuch der mikroskopischen Anatomie der Menschen," vol. 5, pt. 2, Springer-Verlag OHG, Berlin, 1932.

RUBIN, W., M. D. GERSHON, and L. L. ROSS: Electron Microscope Radioautographic Identification of Serotinin-synthesizing Cells in the Mouse Gastric Mucosa, *J. Cell Biol.,* **50**:399 (1971).

RUBIN, W., L. L. ROSS, M. H. SLEISENGER, and F. H. JEFFRIES: The Normal Human Gastric Epithelia. A Fine Structural Study, *Lab. Invest.,* **19**:598 (1968).

SEDAR, W. W.: Uptake of Peroxidase into the Smooth-surfaced Tubular System of the Gastric Acid-secreting Cell, *J. Cell Biol.,* **43**:179 (1969).

STEVENS, C. E., and C. P. LEBLOND: Renewal of the Mucous Cells in the Gastric Mucosa of the Rat, *Anat. Rec.,* **115**:231 (1953).

SMALL INTESTINE

BENNETT, G.: Migration of Glycoprotein from Golgi Apparatus to Cell Coat in the Columnar Cells of the Duodenal Epithelium, *J. Cell Biol.,* **45:**668 (1970).

BROWN, A. L.: Microvilli of the Human Jejunal Epithelial Cell, *J. Cell Biol.,* **12:**623.

CARDELL, R. R., S. BADENHAUSEN, and K. R. PORTER: Intestinal Absorption in the Rat. An Electron Microscopical Study, *J. Cell Biol.,* **34:**123 (1967).

CHENG, H., J. MERZEL, and C. P. LEBLOND: Renewal of Paneth Cells in the Small Intestine of the Mouse, *Amer. J. Anat.,* **126:**507 (1969).

CLARK, S. L., JR.: The Ingestion of Proteins and Colloidal Materials by Columnar Absorptive Cells of the Small Intestine in Suckling Rats and Mice, *J. Biophys. Biochem. Cytol.,* **5:**41 (1959).

CLEMENTI, F., and G. E. PALADE: Intestinal Capillaries. I. Permeability to Peroxidase and Ferritin, *J. Cell Biol.,* **41:**33 (1969).

FERREIRA, M. H., and C. P. LEBLOND: Argentaffin and Other "Endocrine" Cells of the Small Intestine in the Adult Mouse. II. Renewal, *Amer. J. Anat.* **131:**331 (1971).

FLOREY, H. W.: The Secretion and Function of Intestinal Mucus, *Gastroenterology,* **43:**326 (1962).

GAGE, S. H., and P. A. FISH: Fat Digestion, Absorption, and Assimilation in Man and Animals as Determined by the Dark-field Microscope, and a Fat-soluble Dye, *Amer. J. Anat.,* **34:**1 (1924).

ITO, SUSUMU: The Enteric Surface Coat on Cat Intestinal Microvilli, *J. Cell Biol.,* **27:**475 (1965).

LADMAN, A. J., H. A. PADYKULA, and E. W. STRAUSS: A Morphological Study of Fat Transport in the Normal Human Jejunum, *Amer. J. Anat.,* **112:**389 (1963).

LEBLOND, C. P., and B. MESSIER: Renewal of Chief Cells and Goblet Cells in the Small Intestine as Shown by Radioautography after Injection of Thymidine-H³ into Mice, *Anat. Rec.,* **132:**247 (1958).

MERZEL, J., and C. P. LEBLOND: Origin and Renewal of Goblet Cells in the Epithelium of the Mouse Small Intestine, *Amer. J. Anat.,* **124:**281 (1969).

MILLER, D., and R. K. CRANE: The Digestive Function of the Epithelium of the small Intestine. II. Localization of Disaccharide Hydrolysis in the Isolated Brush Border Portion of Intestinal Epithelial Cells, *Biochim. Biophys. Acta,* **52:**293 (1961).

MOOG, F.: The Functional Differentiation of the Small Intestine. VIII. Regional Differences in the Alkaline Phosphatases of the Small Intestine of the Mouse from Birth to One Year, *Develop. Biol.,* **3:**153 (1961).

NEUTRA, M., and C. P. LEBLOND: Synthesis of the Carbohydrate of Mucus in the Golgi Complex as Shown by Electron Microscope Radioautography of Goblet Cells from Rats Injected with Glucose-H³, *J. Cell Biol.,* **30:**119 (1966).

PADYKULA, H. A.: Recent Functional Interpretations of Intestinal Morphology, *Fed. Proc.,* **21:**873 (1962).

PADYKULA, H. A., E. W. STRAUSS, A. J. LADMAN, and F. H. GARDNER: A Morphologic and Histochemical Analysis of the Human Jejunal Epithelium in Nontropical Sprue, *Gastroenterology,* **40:**735 (1961).

PALAY, S. L., and L. J. KARLIN: An Electron Microscopic Study of the Intestinal Villus, I and II, *J. Biophys. Biochem. Cytol.,* **5:**363, 373 (1959).

PATZELT, V.: Der Darm, in W. von Möllendorff (ed.), "Handbuch der mikroskopischen Anatomie der Menschen,'' vol. 5, Springer-Verlag OHG, Berlin, 1936.

STRAUSS, E. W.: Morphological Aspects of Triglyceride Absorption, in C. F. Code and W. Heidel (eds.), ''Handbook of Physiology,'' vol. 3, sec. 6, chap. 71, American Physiological Society, Washington, 1968.

TRIER, J. S.: Morphology of the Epithelium of the Small Intestine, in C. F. Code and W. Heidel (eds.), ''Handbook of Physiology,'' vol. 3, sec. 6, chap. 63, American Physiological Society, Washington, 1968.

WILSON, T, H.: ''Intestinal Absorption,'' W. B. Saunders Company, Philadelphia, 1962.

WRIGHT, R. D., M. A. JENNINGS, H. W. FLOREY, and R. LIUM: The Influence of Nerves and Drugs on Secretion by the Small Intestine and an Investigation of the Enzymes in the Intestinal Juice, *Quart J. Exp. Physiol.*, **30**:73 (1940).

LARGE INTESTINE

FLOREY, H. W.: Electron Microscopic Observations on Goblet Cells of the Rat's Colon, *Quart. J. Exp. Physiol.*, **45**:329 (1960).

HOLLMAN, K. H.: Über den Feinbau des Rectumepithels, *Z. Zellforsch.*, **68**:502 (1965).

LINEBACK, P. E.: Studies on the Musculature of the Human Colon, with Special Reference to the Taeniae, *Amer. J. Anat.*, **36**:357 (1925).

LORENZONN, V., and J. S. TRIER: The Fine Structure of Human Rectal Mucosa. The Epithelial Lining at the Base of the Crypt, *Gastroenterology*, **55**:88 (1968).

MARTIN, B. F.: The Goblet Cell Pattern of the Large Intestine, *Anat. Rec.*, **140**:1 (1961).

chapter 19

The liver and gallbladder

ALBERT L. JONES
AND
ELINOR SPRING
MILLS

General morphology and function

The liver is the largest *gland* in the human body, constituting approximately one-twentieth of the body weight in the neonate and one-fiftieth in the adult. It lies in the right upper quadrant of the abdominal cavity, beneath the diaphragm and attached to it. It is made up of four incompletely separated *lobes*. A thin connective tissue *capsule* (Glisson's capsule), usually covered by reflected peritoneum, lines the external surface of the liver. A definite hilus, the *porta hepatis,* is present, where vessels enter and ducts leave the liver, and the surface capsule becomes continuous with the internal stroma. Right and left *hepatic bile ducts* emerging from the gland unite in the porta hepatis to form the *hepatic duct* proper. A short distance outside the liver, the hepatic duct joins the *cystic duct* or *ductus choledochus,* which enters the duodenum about 10 cm below the pyloric-duodenal junction.

The liver has a dual blood supply. The *portal vein,* carrying blood which has already passed through the capillary beds of the alimentary tract, spleen, and pancreas, brings approximately 75 percent of the afferent blood volume to the liver. This blood is rich in nutrients and other absorbed substances but is relatively poor in oxygen. The *hepatic artery,* a branch of the celiac trunk, carrying well-oxygenated blood, supplies the remaining blood to the liver. Blood from branches of these two vessels mixes in passing through the sinusoids of the liver lobules (see Figs. 19-1 and 19-2). Sinusoidal blood flows toward the center of each lobule and is collected by the *central vein.* After leaving the lobules, the central veins unite to form the larger *sublobular* or *intercalated* veins which finally join the large *hepatic veins.* Blood returns to the heart via the *inferior vena cava.*

The classic structural unit of the organ is the

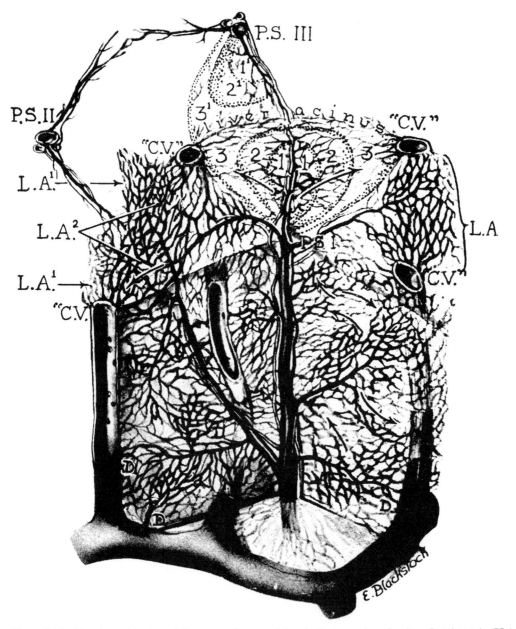

Figure 19-1 Vascular architecture of the human liver in relation to the parenchymal units. Portal canals (PS I, II, III), simple liver acini (LA, LA¹, LA²), central veins (CV), and circulatory zones of the simple liver acinus (1, 2, 3) are shown. The vertical vessel in the center of the drawing is a branch of the portal vein which on reaching the portal canal (PS I) ramifies into several terminals. Note the arcuate course of the terminal portal branches and the irregular arrangement of the simple acini. The parenchyma encompassed by PS I, II, and III corresponds to the peripheral boundary of a classic lobule. The liver acini, as the labels indicate, have terminal branches of the portal vein running through their morphologic axis and include segments of adjacent classic lobules. The sites where sinusoids open into the central vein are shown as holes in its wall. The large vessel at the base of the drawing is a sublobular vein, which runs along the base of the classic lobules and is formed from the central veins. (Drawing courtesy of A. M. Rappaport, Klin. Wschr., **38**:561, 1960.)

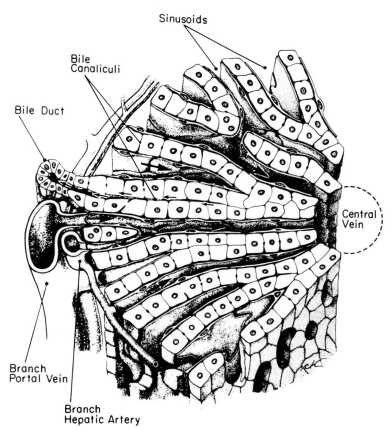

Sinusoids

Bile
Canaliculi

Bile Duct

Central
Vein

Branch
Portal Vein

Branch
Hepatic Artery

Figure 19-2   Direction of blood and bile flow within a segment of a liver lobule. The cell plates and sinusoids are radially disposed around the central vein (terminal hepatic venule). Blood, from terminals of the portal vein and hepatic artery within the portal canal, flows along the sinusoids (large arrows) and empties into the central vein. Bile flows (small arrows) in the opposite direction, toward the small bile duct in the portal canal. (Drawing courtesy of W. Bloom and D. W. Fawcett, "A Textbook of Histology," W. B. Saunders Company, Philadelphia, 1968. Drawing based on illustration from A. W. Ham, "Textbook of Histology," J. B. Lippincott Company, Philadelphia, 1965.)

hepatic lobule, a polyhedral prism of tissue approximately 2 mm long and 0.7 mm wide containing anastomosing plates of parenchymal cells and a labyrinthine system of blood sinusoids.   Branches of the afferent blood vessels and bile ducts run along the edges of the polyhedron, and the central vein runs throughout its center.   *Bile,* produced by the parenchymal cells, is secreted into minute *bile capillaries* or *canaliculi* between the glandular epithelial cells.   At the periphery of the lobule, bile flows into small *bile ductules,* or canals of Hering, and eventually into the larger *bile ducts.*   The liver is composed of approximately 1 million lobular units.

The liver is essential for life, and mammals survive subtotal hepatectomy mainly because the cells have extraordinary regenerative powers and the capacity to tolerate the increased metabolic demands.   The functional diversity and complexity of the liver are rivaled only by the central nervous system.   The liver functions both as an *exocrine* and an *endocrine gland.*   It secretes *bile,* which flows into the duodenum and contains, among other constituents, *bile salts* which emulsify dietary fats prior to digestion.   The liver takes up digested foodstuffs from the afferent blood and stores carbohydrate (glycogen), proteins, vitamins, and some lipids.   Stored substances not used by the hepatocyte can be released into the blood unbound (for example, glucose) or in association with a carrier (for example, triglyceride molecules complexed in a lipoprotein). The liver also synthesizes many substances in response to the body's demands: albumin and other plasma proteins, glucose, fatty acids for triglyceride synthesis, cholesterol, and phospholipids. The liver metabolizes both exogenous compounds such as drugs and insecticides and

endogenous compounds such as steroids and probably most other hormones. By virtue of its large vascular capacity, it serves as a major storehouse for blood. During embryogenesis and certain diseases of the adult, it is a site of hematopoiesis. Finally, its abundance of phagocytes makes the liver one of the principal filters for foreign particulate matter, especially for bacteria coming from the gut.

Histologic organization of the human liver

STROMA

Most of the liver's free surface, except for a small area within its diaphragmatic attachment, is covered by a single layer of flattened *peritoneal mesothelial cells*. Beneath the mesothelium lies a thin yet distinct *surface capsule* (Glisson's capsule) composed of regularly arranged collagen fibers, scattered fibroblasts, and a few small blood vessels. The capsule surrounds the four incompletely separated lobes and is thickest around the inferior vena cava and the hilus or porta hepatis. The capsule is reflected inwardly at the porta where its fibers merge with the denser connective tissue surrounding the vascular and biliary branches. Most of the fibrous hepatic stroma is derived from the connective tissue that passes into the liver through the porta. Within the interior of the organ, the connective tissue arborizes to such an extent that no segment of the parenchyma is more than a few millimeters away from one of its branches. Yet, it should be kept in mind that examination of liver sections following selective connective tissue staining procedures (for example, Mallory-Azan, silver impregnation, elastic fiber staining) and preparations of isolated hepatic stroma (that is, obtained by macerating away the parenchyma in water) reveals that, despite its size, under normal conditions, the large, bulky human liver contains relatively little connective tissue. Nevertheless, this connective tissue (1) provides an internal supporting framework for the hepatic parenchyma, (2) ensheaths most of the vessels and nerves, and (3) subdivides the parenchyma into *lobules*. The only connective tissue within the lobule is the *reticular network* between the sinusoidal endothelium and plates of paren-

chymal cells. The reticular fibers presumably support the liver parenchyma and also may keep the sinusoids open (see Fig. 19-3 for size and arrangement of reticular fibers). In addition, there is some evidence that when this reticular framework survives hepatic injury the parenchyma regenerates more rapidly and in a more orderly fashion (Rappaport, 1969). The failure to demonstrate fibroblasts in the sinusoidal areas with conventional light- and early electron-microscopic techniques fostered the widespread speculation that the reticular fibers in these regions are produced by cells other than fibroblasts. The endothelial cells lining the sinusoids were credited with fiber production, even though their ultrastructure revealed none of the usual features associated with the manufacture of extracellular proteins. However, recent electron-microscopic observations and autoradiographic studies have shown that normal livers do contain a few true fibroblasts within the sinusoidal lining. In addition, it has been suggested that a fat-containing perisinusoidal cell (that is, the so-called *Ito cell* or *lipocyte*) may be the progenitor of the perisinusoidal fibroblast, since fat cells in other tissues can be transformed into fibroblasts (Popper and Udenfriend).

At the periphery of the lobule, the reticular meshwork of the sinusoids becomes continuous with the *interlobular connective tissue,* which usually contains thick bundles of collagen, elastic fibers, and occasional fibroblasts. The term *Glisson's capsule* is sometimes applied to both the surface capsule and the internal connective tissue. However, because the interlobular tissue is not composed exclusively of fibrous tissue and in any

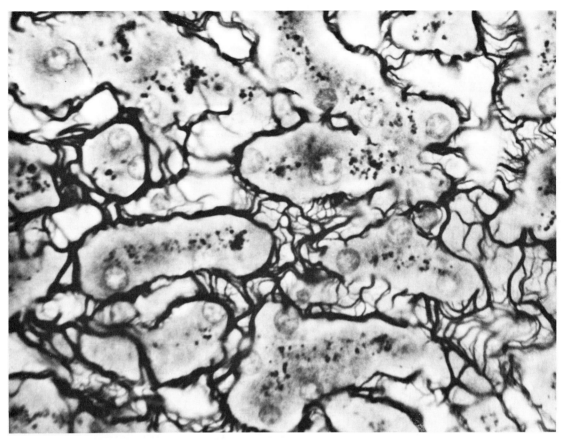

Figure 19-3 Photomicrograph of the human liver showing the close meshwork of reticular fibers in the perisinusoidal space between the parenchymal cells and the sinusoidal lining. A few littoral cell nuclei can be seen within the meshes of the reticulum. Silver, gold, hematoxylin, and Van Gieson's.

one site usually serves two or more contiguous lobules, the broader terms *portal canal, area, space, radicle,* and *tract* most commonly are used to designate the tissue in these regions. The fibrous stroma forms the bed of a portal canal. It ensheaths and carries the so-called *portal triad* (that is, branches of the hepatic artery, portal vein, and bile duct), lymphatic vessels, and nerves throughout the interior of the liver (see Fig. 19-4). The size of a portal canal depends upon its position in the branching connective tissue stroma. Large portal canals in the thicker branches of connective tissue may contain both large and small vessels derived from the portal vein and hepatic artery. The larger vessels carry blood to more distant sites, whereas the small vessels are usually terminal branches of the vein and artery carrying blood into the adjacent lobules. The smallest portal canals contain only terminal branches of the blood and biliary vessels. Sections through these regions usually reveal no more than four tubes (for example, venule from the portal vein, arteriole from the hepatic artery, lymphatic, and bile duct) embedded in a tiny isolated patch of loose connective tissue.

ALTERATIONS IN THE STROMA

Hepatic fibrosis or excess connective tissue is an early histologic sign of chronic liver disease; it is important to be able to recognize this phenomenon

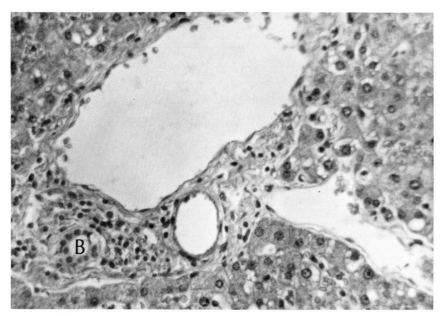

Figure 19-4   Photomicrograph of a portal canal from human liver.   Branches of the portal vein, hepatic artery, bile duct (B), and lymphatic vessel can be found within the connective tissue.   Note the large lumen in the portal vein and the cuboidal epithelium which lines the bile duct.   Mallory-Azan.   × 200.

in liver sections.   Fibrosis occurs primarily in three sites: (1) the portal canals, (2) around hepatocytes, and (3) around proliferating bile ductules that extend from the portal canals into the parenchyma. It is currently believed that parenchymal cell injury and / or degeneration is one of the primary stimuli for the formation of excess connective tissue.   The connective tissue elaborated under these conditions often forms new, irregular septa around nodules of regenerating parenchymal cells, preventing these cells from making appropriate connections with blood and biliary vessels, while the inelastic septa ultimately compress the nodules and restrict their growth.   As a result, blood and bile flow through the liver is impeded, cellular nutrition is impaired, and the organ often is unable to restore its normal architecture.   Factors responsible for stimulating fibroblasts, deposition, and catabolism of fibers are being investigated with the hope that the insidious fibrotic and cirrhotic changes associated with many liver diseases can be treated and controlled (see Popper and Udenfriend, 1970).

LOBULATION

The presence of small *histologic units* or *lobules* within the mammalian liver has been generally accepted since the pioneering observations of Wepfer (1664) and Malpighi (1666), but the validity and usefulness of the traditional definition of a hepatic lobule, based primarily upon the disposition of structural boundaries such as connective tissue septa and vessels within the liver lobes, have been questioned.   As a result, three primary schemata have been developed to describe the histologic and / or functional units of the liver.   The names *classic lobule, portal lobule,* and *liver acinus* have been assigned to the three interpretations.   Each concept was formulated under different circumstances, yet they are not mutually conflicting.   They represent different ways to interpret particular aspects of liver structure and function and thus facilitate our understanding of this organ (see Table 19-1).

The *classic lobule* was described above; it is a polyhedral prism of hepatic tissue about 1 mm by

2 mm whose boundaries are demarcated by connective tissue septa (portal canals) and/or the regular distribution of biliary and vascular vessels (portal triad). In cross section, the lobule is roughly hexagonal, but adjacent lobules are not perfectly aligned nor precisely the same size. In the angles of the hexagon are the portal areas containing connective tissue stroma and the portal triad or terminal branches of the hepatic artery, portal vein, and bile duct. The center of the lobule contains the *central vein* or *terminal hepatic venule* (the smallest subdivision of the hepatic veins) surrounded by a

Table 19-1   Important features of three concepts of liver lobulation

	Classic lobule	Portal lobule	Liver acinus
Cross-sectional appearance of three types of hepatic units. Classic lobules (hexagons) outlined in each diagram. Shaded regions show amount of tissue included in each unit and its relationship to classic lobules.	Central vein / Portal canals	Central vein / Portal canals	Central vein / Portal canals
Shape	Polygonal or hexagonal	Roughly triangular or wedge-shaped	Irregular; sometimes oval or diamond-shaped
Morphologic axis	Central vein	Portal area, especially interlobular bile duct	Terminal branches of portal triad lying along border of two adjacent classic lobules
Peripheral landmarks	Approximately six portal areas	Three (or more) central veins	Two (or more) central veins
Relationship to classic lobule	....	Encompasses those portions of all classic lobules which secrete bile into a common interlobular bile duct	Small sectors of two adjacent classic lobules
Direction of blood flow	From periphery (portal areas) to center (central vein)	From center (portal area) to periphery (central veins)	From center (portal area and edges of two adjacent classic lobules) to periphery
Direction of bile flow	From center toward periphery	From periphery to center	From periphery toward center
Advantages of concept	1 Emphasizes endocrine function of liver 2 Useful in understanding histologic changes associated with centrolobular necrosis (for example, CCl_4 poisoning)	1 Emphasizes exocrine function of liver (that is, bile secretion) 2 Makes histologic organization of a hepatic lobule comparable to those of most exocrine glands	1 Offers best explanation for gradient of metabolic activity or zonation within liver, that is, direct correlation between blood supply and metabolism 2 Helps to explain pattern of regeneration 3 Useful in understanding development of cirrhosis
Principal developers of concept	Wepfer; Malpighi; Mascagni; Kiernan; Müeller	Theile; Brissaud and Sabourin; Mall; Arey	Rappaport and coworkers; Novikoff and Essner

minute amount of connective tissue (see Fig. 19-5). One-cell-thick rows of *parenchymal* or *glandular epithelial cells* (hepatocytes) separated on either side by narrow vascular spaces, the *sinusoids,* radiate from the central vein to the portal areas at the periphery of the lobule. In histologic sections, the cell columns appear to be isolated branches or cords of parenchymal cells suspended in an underlying meshwork of blood sinusoids (see Fig. 19-6). Three-dimensional reconstructions of the lobule (Elias, 1949), however, show that the liver parenchyma has a more complicated arrangement than routine, two-dimensional, histologic sections indicate (Figs. 19-7 and 19-8). In short, these special preparations reveal that (1) the lobules are composed of a continuous system of communicating parenchymal *cell plates* or laminae and not single strands or columns of cells; (2) the parenchymal cells throughout an entire lobule are interconnected and subdivided by spaces or lacunae into anastomosing one-cell-thick plates; (3) the sinusoids run within the center, and the perisinusoidal *space of Disse* occupies the periphery of each lacuna; and (4) the lacunae form a continuous labyrinth within each lobule. In addition, stereograms of a liver lobule show that each lacuna opens directly into a *central space* containing the central vein. At the periphery of the lobule, however, the lacunae do not communicate freely with the portal areas. Instead, a *limiting plate* of hepatic cells, surrounding the circumference of the lobule, forms a nearly continuous wall between the interior of the lobule and the space occupied by the portal canals. Only tiny terminal branches of the hepatic artery, portal vein, and bile duct can penetrate the liver parenchyma via the occasional fenestrations in the limiting plate (see Figs. 19-2 and 19-8).

The *classic lobule* is best seen in those species (for example, pig, raccoon, camel, polar bear) in which relatively thick bands of interlobular connective tissue almost completely encapsulate each lobule (Fig. 19-9, see color insert). In man, lobulation is incomplete and poorly defined. The sparse perilobular connective tissue does not form a continuous boundary between contiguous lobules, and the parenchyma often appears to be coextensive between adjacent lobules. Nevertheless the approximate boundaries of a human classic lobule can be visualized by first locating a central vein and then following the successive, regularly placed portal triads which encircle the periphery of each lobule (Fig. 19-10, see color insert).

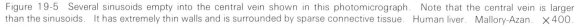

Figure 19-5   Several sinusoids empty into the central vein shown in this photomicrograph. Note that the central vein is larger than the sinusoids. It has extremely thin walls and is surrounded by sparse connective tissue. Human liver. Mallory-Azan. ×400.

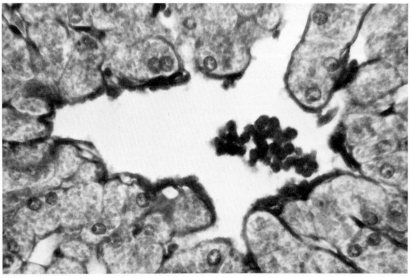

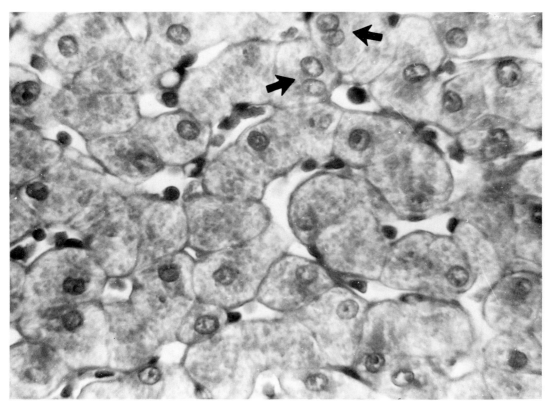

Figure 19-6 Liver parenchymal cells are shown at higher magnification in this photomicrograph. The cells are polyhedral, yet adjacent cells may vary in size and shape. The hepatic cells form branching and anastomosing single-cell-thick plates which are separated by the sinusoids (light areas). Arrows point to binuclear cells. Human liver. Mallory-Azan. ×600.

Blood flows from the portal canals (hepatic artery and portal vein) into the lobule, passes along the sinusoids, and is removed from the lobule by the central vein. Bile, however, flows in the opposite direction: from the parenchymal cells where it is formed to the interlobular bile ducts in the portal canals.

Although the classic lobule is regarded primarily as a structural unit, certain physiologic (for example, fat and glycogen deposition after a meal) and pathologic (for example, necrosis) changes often appear confined to specific areas within the lobule. Such changes may originate and spread through the territory of the classic lobule from either the peripheral (portal areas) or the central areas (central vein), producing an unusual circular gradient in which similar microscopic alterations appear in concentric bands or zones around the central vein (see Table 19-1). Because of this, certain histologists believe that the classic lobule can and should be regarded as both a structural and a functional unit of the liver.

The concept of the *portal lobule* began to emerge during the mid-nineteenth century as histologists discovered that, in most mammals, liver lobules are *not* well-defined anatomic units and that in many exocrine glands it is more convenient to consider a lobule as a *functional unit* rather than a segment of tissue enclosed by fissures or septa. As a result, in exocrine glands, the term *lobule* became synonymous with a group of secretory cells which release their product(s) into a common duct located in the center of the lobule. Subsequently, three lines of evidence suggested that the classic lobule was not

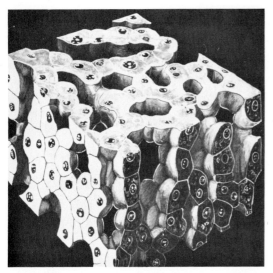

Figure 19-7   Stereogram of human liver showing that it contains a continuous mass of parenchymal cells. The parenchymal cells are arranged into plates, one cell in thickness, which anastomose with each other. The plates enclose spaces or lacunae containing the sinusoids. (Courtesy of H. Elias and J. C. Sherrick, "Morphology of the Liver," Academic Press, Inc., New York, 1969.)

the only logical unit to use in describing the liver parenchyma. Theile (1844) observed that when mammalian livers were crushed and washed in water the resulting specimen resembled a bunch of grapes: The lobules were clustered around branches of the portal vein. Brissaud and Sabourin (1844) reported that, in seal liver, lobules were formed by epithelial trabeculae radiating from portal canals rather than central veins. And Mall's (1906) studies of corrosion preparations, in which the portal, arterial, or biliary vessels had been injected in situ, demonstrated that arterial and portal vessels, bile ducts, lymphatics, nerves, and connective tissue all radiated from the portal areas. Eventually, these observations culminated in a new concept of hepatic lobulation called the *portal* or *functional lobule.*

The portal lobule is a roughly triangular or wedge-shaped prism of hepatic tissue. Its boundaries, however, are ill defined in most mammals except the seal. It encompasses those segments of three contiguous classic lobules which are drained by a common interlobular bile duct situated in a portal canal at their edge (see Table 19-1).

Figure 19-8   Summary of liver structure. (Courtesy of H. Elias and J. C. Sherrick, "Morphology of the Liver," Academic Press, Inc., New York, 1969.)

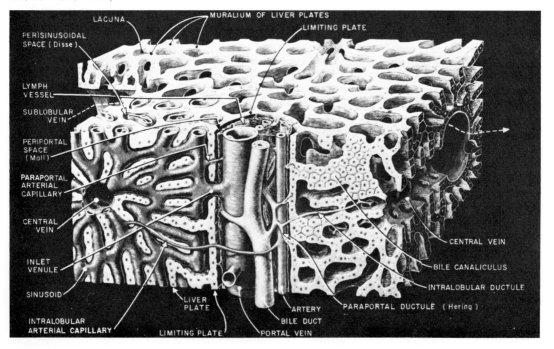

The morphologic axis of the portal lobule is the interlobular bile duct, and its peripheral limits are formed by three different "central" veins. According to this schema, bile flows from the periphery to the centrally located bile duct, and blood flows from the center of the lobule to the periphery. Hence, the pathways for bile drainage and blood flow are similar to most exocrine glands. Those who oppose the recognition and use of this concept often argue that it unduly emphasizes the liver's role as an exocrine gland, but since no valid judgment can be made about the relative importance of the exocrine and endocrine activities of the liver, both concepts deserve to be retained, each schema being useful, in its own way, to explain the myriad functions of the liver.

More recently, Rappaport and his colleagues (1969) have introduced the concept of the *liver acinus*. In certain respects this unit resembles the portal lobule, but it is much smaller and is usually described as the smallest functional unit within the liver. Observations of hepatic circulation in vivo and preparations of specially injected human liver casts revealed that the tissue around each central vein is derived from different sources, suggesting that this tissue is not one unit but a series of units or liver acini. The *simple liver acinus* is defined as a small, irregular mass of unencapsulated parenchymal tissue lying between two (or more) terminal hepatic venules ("central veins"). Its axis is a small radicle of the main portal canal containing a terminal portal venule, hepatic arteriole, bile ductule, lymph vessel, and nerves. In histologic sections, it includes only small segments of two adjacent classic lobules. The acini extend at right angles from the preterminal branches of the portal veins (at the edges of the classic lobules) to the central veins (see Figs. 19-1 and 19-11 and Table 19-2). The parenchyma is continuous between the classic lobules, and blood flows toward both central

Figure 19-11   Blood supply of the simple liver acinus. The oxygen tension and nutrient level of the blood in the sinusoids decrease from zone 1 through zone 3. Zones 1', 2', and 3' indicate corresponding volumes in a portion of an adjacent acinar unit. Circle A encloses the area commonly designated as periportal; B and C represent the areas more peripheral to the portal space (PS). THV, terminal hepatic venules. (From Fig. 1, A. M. Rappaport, Z. J. Borowy, W. M. Laugheed, and W. N. Lotto, Anat. Rec., **119**:11, 1954.)

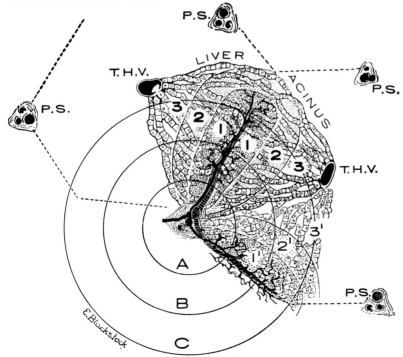

veins from the terminal branches of the portal veins. Although there is extensive communication among sinusoids, Rappaport et al. have found that the tissue within each acinus is supplied mainly by its parent vessels. Moreover, the cells within each acinus appear to be grouped into concentric zones around the axis of the acinus. Cells close to the axis and the terminal afferent vessels (for example, zone 1) are the first to receive blood and nutrients, the last to die, and the first to regenerate. Cells in more distant regions receive blood of poorer quality and also appear less resistant to damage. The concept of acinar circulatory zones has been extended by Rappaport to provide an explanation for the histologic appearance of many pathologic changes in the liver.

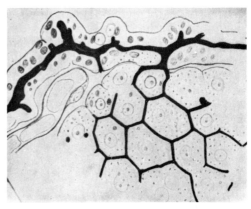

Figure 19-12 Drawing of a network of bile canaliculi in dog liver, showing the entrance of canaliculi into a terminal bile ductule at the edge of a lobule. Silver preparation. (Courtesy of H. Elias, Amer. J. Anat., **85**:379, 1949.)

PARENCHYMAL CELLS

The hepatic plates are composed of large, polyhedral parenchymal cells approximately 30 μm long and 20 μm wide (see Fig. 19-6). These cells make up approximately 80 percent of the cell population within the human liver (Gates et al., 1961). They are of different sizes: The smallest ones border perforations in the liver plate, and the largest ones are either polyploid or located in the corners where three cell plates meet. The six or more surfaces on each parenchymal cell are of three different types: (1) those adjacent to other parenchymal cells; (2) those bordering bile canaliculi; and (3) those touching the perisinusoidal space (Disse). At the light-microscopic level the plasmalemma appears fairly uniform and often indistinct, even though fine structural and histochemical studies reveal that the cell membrane undergoes characteristic modifications in each of these three sites. In optimal routine histologic preparations or following special procedures (for example, indigo blue staining, silver impregnation, or staining for adenosine triphosphatase), bile canaliculi are seen on surfaces between contiguous cells. These tiny channels follow an incomplete chicken-wire pattern along contiguous surfaces of parenchymal cells (see Fig. 19-12).

The nuclei are large, round, and usually centrally located. They contain one or more nucleoli and scattered clumps of chromatin. Generally the nuclei of parenchymal cells stain less intensely than the smaller nuclei of other cells in the liver. More-over, in the adult liver, parenchymal cell nuclei can be subdivided into several nuclear-size groups or classes (Doljanski, 1960). Polyploid nuclei, binucleated and multinucleated cells, are easily found. Adult mammalian livers contain 30 to 80 percent polyploid cells, and there appears to be good correlation between nuclear size and ploidy, that is, doubling of DNA content being accompanied by an approximate doubling of nuclear volume. The two nuclei of binuclear cells have roughly the same size and staining properties. Both nuclei divide simultaneously and are thought to arise from mononuclear cells through endomitosis. Binuclear cells can account for as much as 25 percent of the parenchymal cell population. The factors influencing the formation of polyploid and binuclear liver cells and the physiologic consequences of these phenomena are not understood. The work of Carriere (1969) and others suggests that aging and certain hormones regulate both the liver's mitotic index and the formation of the polyploid and binuclear cells. Mitotic activity, however, is rare in the intact normal adult liver (1 mitosis per 10,000 to 20,000 cells), and the minimum average life-span of a parenchymal cell is about 150 days. It is hoped that eventually new techniques will reveal more about the submicroscopic organization of these nuclei and their relation to ploidy, cell renewal, regeneration, and nuclear-cytoplasmic interactions.

The cytoplasm of the parenchymal cell is usually

granular; however, it can vary widely in appearance, often reflecting the functional and nutritional state of the cell. Usually large clumps of basophilic *ribonucleoprotein* and abundant mitochondria can be demonstrated throughout the cytoplasm. However, after a prolonged fast, the basophilic bodies decrease and the cytoplasm becomes predominantly eosinophilic. The Golgi complex ordinarily is located near a bile canaliculus, and usually there is more than one Golgi complex per cell. Stored materials such as glycogen and fat usually are not preserved in conventional histologic sections, but empty round vacuoles in the cytoplasm generally indicate the sites occupied by fat, and irregular empty spaces or flocculant, grainy cytoplasmic regions mark areas that were rich in glycogen.

It is generally assumed that all parenchymal cells can store or secrete any of the substances which are demonstrable histochemically (Fig. 19-13, see color insert). Disparities in the appearance and contents of the cytoplasm are thought to depend upon the position of the cell within the lobule and the time since the last meal. However, in our opinion, these problems have not been resolved and require additional work to determine how uniform liver cells are in metabolic capacity, nutritional requirements, and disease suceptibility (Table 19-2).

BLOOD VESSELS AND SINUSOIDS

The liver is highly vascularized, and its function is intimately related to the distribution and histology of its blood vessels. Blood is brought to the liver via the *portal vein* and *hepatic artery*. The livers of the dog, cat, and man receive a total blood flow of 100 to 130 ml per min per 100 gm tissue; of this, 70 to 75 percent is supplied by the portal vein and the remainder by the hepatic artery. Total hepatic blood flow is about one-quarter of the cardiac output. The hepatic arterial resistance is approximately 30 to 40 times greater than the portal resistance (Greenway and Stark, 1971).

The afferent blood vessels enter the organ at the *porta* and promptly form several large branches which initially course between the lobes ensheathed in the largest trabeculae of connective tissue and then follow the successive, graduated branchings of the stroma. The gross intrahepatic vascular anatomy has been studied by combined radiologic and injection-corrosion techniques. Specially in-jected plastic casts of adult human livers reveal that the liver can be divided into segments on the basis of its internal vasculature. Each branch of the afferent vessels entering the liver is essential for proper function since each one supplies blood to a specific area. Usually there are no anastomoses between the major branches and no accessory or additional portal veins or hepatic arteries which could provide the segments with an adequate blood supply should the major branches be impaired (Healey, 1970).

The incoming portal vein contains no valves, and its lumen is much larger than the lumen of the accompanying hepatic artery. It bifurcates into two trunks in the porta which, in turn, divide into large branches or *rami venae portae* which are usually *interlobar* vessels. In man, branches of the portal vein with a diameter of 400 μm or more are called *conducting veins*. They are visible to the unaided eye and include the rami venae portae, their largest branches, and subbranches. These vessels are *large* and *medium-sized branches* of the portal vein. The histologic organization of the large conducting veins is like that of other large veins, with the exception that the portal vein contains no valves. The smaller branches of the conducting veins often lack a longitudinal layer of smooth muscle and are usually *interlobular*.

The smallest branches of the portal vein are called *distributing veins*. In man, these vessels have a diameter of 280 μm or less and are essentially endothelial tubes surrounded by a thin layer of smooth muscle fibers. They are found in the smallest portal canals and form the axis of the simple liver acinus. At intervals, they produce short *inlet venules* which pass through the limiting plate at the periphery of the lobule. Inlet venules arise perpendicularly from the axial distributing vein (see Fig. 19-14). The extreme ends of the inlet venules (terminal twigs) lead directly into the sinusoids; these terminal segments lack a muscle coat. Inlet venules, containing contractile endothelial cells, show sphincter activity that regulates the portal blood flow into the sinusoids. However, it is important to bear in mind that the amount of portal blood entering the liver depends upon the flow in the arteries which supply the gut regions drained by the portal vein (for example, branches of the celiac axis, superior and inferior mesenteric arteries).

Table 19-2   Cytochemical and ultrastructural evidence of metabolic heterogeneity in liver parenchymal cells

Substance or organelle	Experimental conditions		Distribution		References
	Animal	Method	Cytoplasm	Lobule	
Glycogen deposits	Fed	LM:* PAS or Best's carmine EM:* Lead stain	Throughout; often in close association with SER	Appears first in periphery of classic lobule or zone 1 of liver acinus	Deane, 1944; Novikoff and Essner, 1960
	Fasted 24 hr	LM: PAS or Best's carmine EM: Lead stain	Low or absent	Disappears last from cells around central vein (zone 3)	Deane, 1944
Fat droplets	Fed	LM: Sudan stains; oil red O; osmium impregnation	Random, throughout	Appear transiently after meal in central cells (zone 3)	Deane, 1944
	Ethanol treated	LM: Sudan stains; oil red O; osmium impregnation	Increased number of droplets; random, throughout	Most numerous in central cells (zone 3)	Elias and Sherrick; 1969
	Starved	LM: Sudan stains; oil red O; osmium impregnation	Increased after 24 hr; random, throughout	Depot fat appears first as droplets in peripheral cells (zone 1)	Rappaport, 1969
	Choline deficient	LM: Sudan stains; oil red O; osmium impregnation	Increased; random, throughout	Accumulate first in central cells (zone 3)	Rappaport, 1969
Bile acids	Fed	LM: barium chloride precipitation and acid fuchsin	Random, throughout	Most concentrated in peripheral cells (zone 1)	Deane, 1944
Acid phosphatase	Fed	LM, EM: modified Gomori lead salt technique	In lysosomes, especially peribiliary dense bodies	Activity highest in peripheral cells (zone 1)	Novikoff and Essner, 1960
Lysosomes (all categories)	Fed	EM: quantitative stereology	Peribiliary	Most in central cells (zone 3)	Loud, 1968
Krebs' cycle enzymes	Fed	LM, EM: tetrazolium salt techniques	In mitochondria	Activity highest in peripheral cells (zone 1)	Novikoff and Essner, 1960
Mitochondria	Fed	EM: quantitative stereology	Random, throughout	Smaller and more numerous in central cells (zone 3), ~800 per cell	Loud, 1968
Pentose shunt enzymes	Fed	LM, EM: tetrazolium salt techniques	Random, throughout	Activity highest in central cells (zone 3)	Isselbacher and Jones, 1964; Wachstein, 1959

Table 19-2   Cytochemical and ultrastructural evidence of metabolic heterogeneity in liver parenchymal cells (*Cont.*)

Substance or organelle	Experimental conditions		Distribution		References
	Animal	Method	Cytoplasm	Lobule	
Albumin	Fed	Fluorescent antibody techniques	Variable	No evidence of zonation; pronounced variation among adjacent cells	Hamashima et al., 1964
Rough endoplasmic reticulum	Fed	EM: quantitative stereology	Random, throughout	No zonation; about 25,000 μm^2 membrane area per cell	Loud, 1968
Smooth endoplasmic reticulum	Fed	EM: quantitative stereology	Throughout; often in association with glycogen	Membrane area in square micrometers per cell: periphery: 15,700 midzonal: 16,900 central: 21,600	Loud, 1968
Peroxisomes	Fed	EM: quantitative stereology	Random, throughout	Most numerous in central cells (zone 3), ~200 per cell	Loud, 1968

* Abbreviations: LM, light microscope; EM, electron microscope.

The largest intrahepatic branches of the hepatic artery are thick-walled. As the arteries branch and form smaller vessels, the muscle coat is reduced. Terminal branches contain only endothelium surrounded by a thin adventitia. Most of the blood within the hepatic arteries is distributed to the stroma, extrahepatic bile ducts, and gallbladder, and so only a very small volume enters the sinusoids directly. Blood from terminal branches of the hepatic artery usually enters the peribiliary or periductal capillary plexus within the portal canals. Small bile ducts are surrounded by one subepithelial capillary plexus, whereas larger bile ducts have a subepithelial and a submucosal plexus. These capillaries, in turn, usually are drained by small branches of the portal vein. As a result, most arterial blood reaches the hepatic sinusoids via an indirect route (see Fig. 19-15 for additional details).

The sinusoids, forming the rich intralobular vascular network, anastomose and converge toward the central vein. They differ from conventional capillaries in several aspects: They are larger and more variable in caliber (9 to 12 μm wide), their cell boundaries do not blacken with silver nitrate, and many of the cells are phagocytic. The sinusoid wall contains two types of cells: typical, flattened endothelial cells and large, fixed macrophages or *Kupffer cells*. The endothelial cell contains a small, compact nucleus, many micropinocytotic vesicles, small mitochondria, and only short profiles of rough ER scattered throughout the cytoplasm. The stellate-shaped Kupffer cells occur at various points along the sinusoidal lining (see Figs. 19-16 and 19-17). These cells contain larger, oval nuclei, more mitochondria, and more rough ER than the endothelial cells. They are active phagocytes, and their cytoplasm usually contains phagocytic vacuoles with amorphous debris, engulfed red blood cells, and/or iron.

The perisinusoidal space of Disse, surrounding the sinusoid wall, lies between the sinusoids and the parenchymal cells. Electron micrographs show

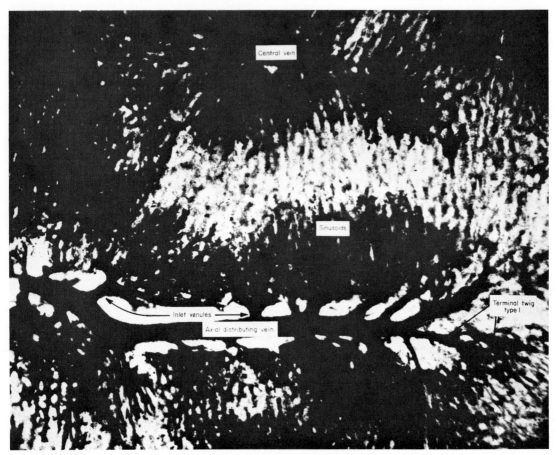

Figure 19-14   Thick section from a rabbit's liver, showing the terminal distribution and connections of the portal vein.   The preparation was made by injecting India ink into a mesenteric vein prior to sacrifice of the animal.   (Courtesy of H. Elias and J. C. Sherrick, "Morphology of the Liver," Academic Press, Inc., New York, 1969.)

that numerous parenchymal cell microvilli project into this space.   In addition, bundles of collagen can be seen in this region, but never in the abundance suggested by reticular fiber stains at the light-microscopic level.   Fat-laden lipocytes are found occasionally.   Their function is not understood, although they have been implicated in vitamin A metabolism and the production of fibroblasts.   On rare occasions, cells resembling the pericytes of the capillaries are observed.   Although hematopoietic cells are numerous in this region during fetal life, they are seldom seen in the adult except during chronic anemia.

The sinusoid lining in most mammals, except certain ruminants, appears discontinuous (Grubb and Jones, 1971; Wood, 1963).   Although some investigators (Wisse, 1970) believe that the discontinuities are artefacts, this opinion is not widespread at present.   The structure of the sinusoids is important for understanding how materials are exchanged between the blood and hepatic cells.   It is thought that in most mammals the sinusoid wall and the cells and fibers within the perisinusoidal space of Disse pose no significant morphologic barrier between the blood and the parenchymal cells.   This assumption is based on the following observations: (1) Gaps are often present between the attenuated processes of adjacent endothelial cells; (2) the fenestrae in the endothelial cells of most mammals contain no diaphragm; (3) the sinusoid endothelium of most mammals, except the ruminants, does not have a continuous basal lamina; and (4) the cells and reticular fibers in the perisinusoidal space do not form a continuous boundary. Hence it is pre- sumed that, in most mammals, fluid from the he- patic blood plasma passes through the discon- tinuities in the sinusoids and enters the space of Disse. Since the fluid bathes the microvilli project- ing into the space of Disse, it is suspected that this region may be a site for exchange of materials

Figure 19-15   Terminal branches of the hepatic artery in the rat. Arterioles (HA) and terminal arterioles (ha) give rise to cap- illaries (c) which surround bile ducts (BD). Capillaries arising from arterioles (PC) have well-developed sphincters. The periductal capillaries terminate by joining portal veins and/or sinusoids. A few capillaries join larger interlobular veins (PV), and some join terminal distributing veins (pv). Endothelial cell nuclei (EN) are usually located at or near the junctions of capillaries with other vessels. Sinusoids arising from capillaries are identical in structure to those arising from portal veins. At the periphery of the lobule all sinusoids resemble capillaries, having a complete basement membrane (BM) and unfenestrated endothelium. A short distance into the parenchyma they loose their basement membrane, become fenestrated, and are true sinusoids. There are numerous lymphatic vessels (L) and unmyelinated nerves (N, n) in the portal tissue. The nerves supply the smooth muscle of arterioles and precapillary sphincters. Occasionally small nerve fibers (n) are found in close relation to endothelial cells. (Cour- tesy of W. E. Burkel, Anat. Rec., **167**:333, 1970.)

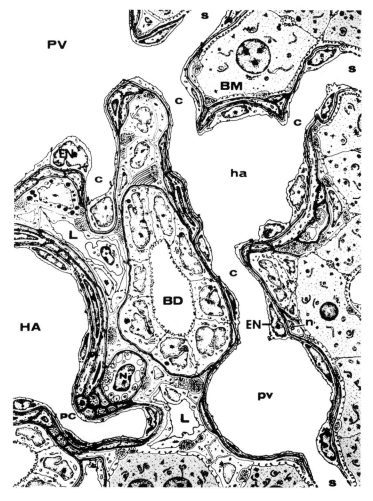

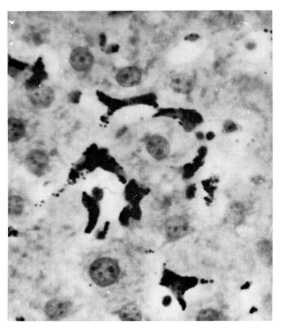

Figure 19-16 Kupffer cells within the sinusoid linings are phagocytic and belong to the reticuloendothelial system. They stand out as dark bodies in this photomicrograph because they have ingested carbon particles from the India ink which was injected intravenously before the animal was sacrificed. Rat liver. India ink vascular injection. Formol. H & E. ×700.

between the fluid and the parenchymal cells (see Figs. 19-17 and 19-18).

Blood leaves the lobule via the central vein or *terminal hepatic venule* which runs longitudinally through the middle of the lobule in the so-called *central space*. Central veins are lined by a simple endothelium covered by an external adventitia composed of a few spirally arranged connective tissue fibers. They are larger than sinusoids (45 μm in diameter), they travel alone, and their extremely thin walls contain numerous pores which communicate directly with the sinusoids. Several sinusoids can be seen opening into the central vein in Fig. 19-5. Note that there is no limiting plate of parenchymal cells as there is around the portal canal. At the periphery of the lobule, the central vein connects at right angles with a *sublobular* or *intercalated vein* (see Fig. 19-1). These vessels are larger than central veins. They are usually 90 to 200 μm in diameter, lined by endothelium, and

surrounded by a distinct inner circular and outer longitudinal layer of connective tissue fibers. Elastic fibers are numerous and arranged irregularly in nets throughout the walls. These veins course along the base of the lobules and enter the stromal trabeculae where they follow a solitary, isolated course, unaccompanied by other blood vessels or ducts. Sublobular veins ultimately form the *hepatic veins* (see Fig. 19-19).

The hepatic veins lack valves and have numerous anastomoses among their branches. The larger branches have a moderately well-developed tunica media and vasa vasorum. They usually travel alone and are surrounded by considerable amounts of connective tissue. Hepatic veins eventually join the *inferior vena cava.*

LYMPHATICS, TISSUE SPACES OF MALL, AND THE PERISINUSOIDAL SPACE OF DISSE

The liver's capsule and stroma contain numerous lymphatic vessels. Just beneath the capsule, *superficial lymphatic vessels* form loose plexuses which connect at intervals with the *deep lymphatic vessels* within the *portal canals* (see Fig. 19-20). Lymphatic capillary plexuses, coursing within the connective trabeculae, follow and surround branches of the portal vein, hepatic artery, and bile duct to their finest ramifications at the edge of the lobules. Because lymphatic capillaries have not been found between parenchymal cells, the origin and transport of liver lymph have been the subject of extensive investigation and controversy. The most widely accepted theory at present contends that the perisinusoidal space of Disse is the primary site for formation of liver lymph. The connections between the spaces of Disse and the lymphatic vessels in the terminal portal canals have not been demonstrated. This perplexing problem is complicated by the fact that the periphery of the lobule is surrounded by a limiting wall or plate of parenchymal cells. Elias and Sherrick (1969), however, suggest that in man, as fluid within the space of Disse reaches the edge of the lobules, it flows alongside the afferent blood vessels and leaves the lobules via the occasional fenestrations in the limiting plate. From there, the fluid enters the *periportal tissue space of Mall,* which lies between the portal connective tissue and the limiting plate (see

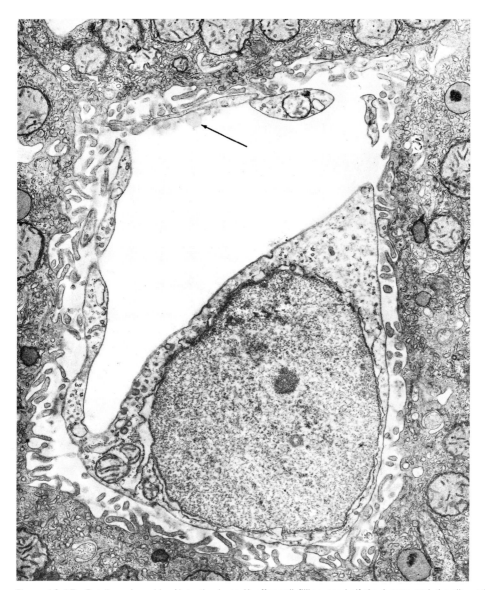

Figure 19-17   Rat liver sinusoid.   Note the large Kupffer cell filling one-half the lumen and the discontinuity of the sinusoidal lining.   A chylomicron is observed within the vascular space (arrow).   Approximately × 10,000.

Fig. 19-8).   Subsequently, the fluid diffuses from the space of Mall through the connective tissue and is collected by the lymphatic capillaries within the portal canal.   Lymph is then conveyed by progressively larger lymphatic vessels to the collecting vessels which leave the liver at the hilus.   On leaving the hilus, the lymph passes through the hepatic lymph nodes lying just below and above the diaphragm.

The large volume of lymph which leaves the liver contains more plasma proteins than lymph derived from other sources.   Although the bulk of liver lymph presumably is formed in the manner described above, a substantial portion of lymph may

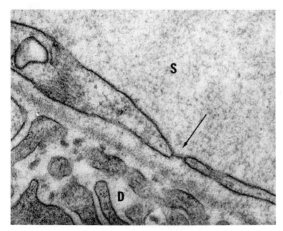

Figure 19-18   Endothelial lining of the sinusoid from sheep liver. Note the diaphragm covering one fenestra (arrow) and basal lamina. S, sinusoidal space; D, space of Disse. (From D. J. Grubb and A. L. Jones, Anat. Rec., **170**:75, 1971.)

originate directly from blood in the large branches of the hepatic and portal veins. These vessels are surrounded by small networks of lymphatics, and their vasa vasorum often contains lymph vessels.

NERVES

In man, nerves enter at the hilus. The fibers are mainly unmyelinated and from the autonomic nervous system. A few bundles of unmyelinated fibers and parasympathetic ganglion cells are found in the larger portal canals and capsule. Parasympathetic innervation of the liver is derived from preganglionic fibers in the dorsal efferent nucleus of the vagus. Sympathetic innervation is derived from preganglionic fibers (with cells of origin in T_7 to T_8 of the thoracic cord) which synapse in the celiac ganglion. Postganglionic sympathetic fibers from cells in the celiac ganglion are distributed to the hepatic arteries within the liver and the smooth muscle of the gallbladder. The arteries are thought to be innervated by sympathetic fibers only, whereas the bile ducts are innervated by sympathetic and parasympathetic fibers. Some fibers follow the vessels and ducts into the smallest portal canals, but it is questionable whether fibers penetrate the lobules and end on parenchymal cells. Thus, at present, the principal influence of the nervous system is thought to be exerted on the blood and biliary vessels.

Figure 19-19   A branch of the hepatic vein is shown surrounded by a considerable amount of connective tissue. These vessels usually travel alone. Human liver. Zenker formal in H & E.

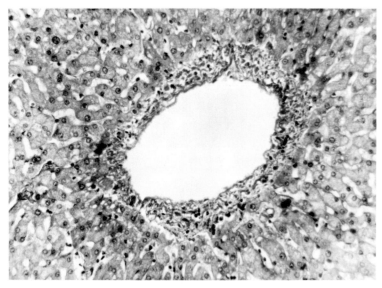

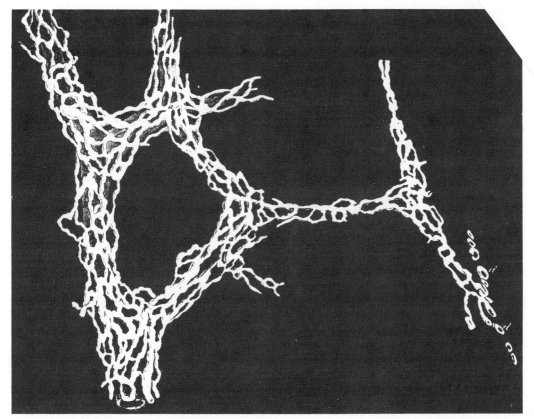

Figure 19-20   Network of lymphatic vessels. The vessels, shown in white, surround branches of the portal vein (to the left), connecting with superficial lymphatics in Glisson's capsule (to the right).   ×50.   (Teichmann.)

Ultrastructural and functional aspects of the parenchymal cells

ENDOPLASMIC RETICULUM AND GOLGI COMPLEX

Structure   Unlike most cells, both smooth and rough endoplasmic reticulum are well developed in hepatic parenchymal cells, although their relative quantities, precise position, and arrangement vary from cell to cell and may be significantly altered during different physiologic and experimental conditions.   In addition to the membrane-bound ribosomes of the rough ER, the liver cell contains many free ribosomes and polyribosomes which fluctuate

in response to various conditions (see Fig. 19-21).

The rough ER usually forms aggregates of parallel, flattened cisternae scattered randomly throughout the cytoplasm. They correspond to the *basophilic bodies* or *ergastoplasm* seen in specially stained histologic sections.   In the rat, the surface area of the rough and smooth membranes is equal in cells surrounding the central vein, but in the peripheral and midzonal cells, the rough ER has approximately 50 percent more surface area than the smooth (Loud, 1968).

The smooth ER is composed of a complex mesh-

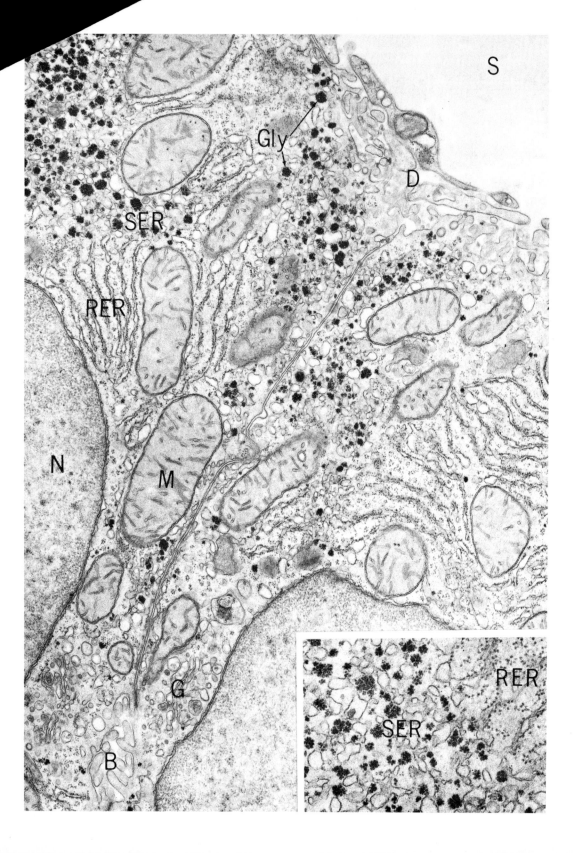

work of twisting, branching, and anastomosing tubules which frequently communicate with the rough ER and Golgi but never with the nuclear envelope. These tubules follow a highly tortuous course and often exhibit variations in caliber. Smooth ER in the liver often shows local specializations and almost invariably is associated with *glycogen*, although the functional significance of this relationship is unclear. In the rat, the surface area of the smooth ER is significantly higher in central (21,600 μm^2 per cell) and midzonal (16,900 μm^2 per cell) cells than in the peripheral cells (15,700 μm^2 per cell) (Loud, 1968).

Golgi profiles are numerous, and each parenchymal cell has been estimated to contain as many as 50 Golgi complexes (Claude, 1970), usually located near bile canaliculi. The fine structure of the Golgi complex is similar, but not identical, to those in other cell types. Each complex has three to five closely packed, parallel, smooth-surfaced cisternae and a variable number of vesicles. The bulbous ends of the cisternae and their associated large vesicles often are filled with electron-dense particles, 300 to 800 Å in diameter, which are thought to be the triglyceride-rich *very-low-density lipoproteins* (VLDL) which play an important role in the transport of lipids within the plasma (Jones et al., 1967; Hamilton et al., 1967; Mahley et al., 1969).

Function The liver microsomal fraction is known to participate in (1) the synthesis of albumin, fibrinogen, and other plasma proteins; (2) the synthesis of cholesterol for export and bile salt formation; (3) glucuronide conjugation of bilirubin, drugs, and steroids; (4) metabolism of drugs and steroids; (5) esterification of free fatty acids to triglycerides; and (6) the breakdown of glycogen.

All studies of protein synthesis for export (for example, albumin and other plasma proteins) show that protein synthesis is a function of the rough ER. The product is thought to leave the rough ER and migrate via the smooth ER to the Golgi complex and finally to the cell's vascular surface for release.

Cholesterol biosynthesis seems to be a function of the smooth ER. Evidence for this function came from the discovery that liver cells following phenobarbital administration were four times more active in cholesterol biosynthesis than control livers (Jones and Armstrong, 1965). (See Fig. 19-22.)

Many lipid-soluble drugs and steroids are metabolized and hydroxylated by the liver microsomal fraction. The microsomal *mixed-function oxidase system*, a chain of enzymes and cytochromes, such as NADPH cytochrome *c* reductase and cytochrome P_{450}, is thought to perform these functions. Although there is evidence that this functional chain occurs in both categories of ER, some investigators believe that the principal activity of the chain resides in the membranes of the smooth ER (Jones and Fawcett, 1966). Support for the latter view comes from the knowledge that some 200 lipid-soluble compounds with diverse chemical structure (for example, phenobarbital as against DDT) not only are metabolized by the microsomes but also promote a marked hypertrophy of the smooth ER and many of its enzymes and cytochromes. This type of response is considered adaptive since it enables the liver to more effectively metabolize the inducing substances. The value of such a response in the detoxification of drugs, certain carcinogens, and insecticides is obvious. In addition, progesterone and certain anabolic steroids also are inducers of liver smooth ER, its associated cytochrome P_{450}, and the mitochondrial enzyme Δ-aminolevulinic acid synthetase (ALA syn) (Jones and Emans, 1969) (see Fig. 19-23). Increased ALA syn activity results in increased heme production and stimulates the formation of cytochrome P_{450} (see Fig. 19-24). Interference with the terminal steps of heme synthesis produces an abnormal accumulation of porphyrin and the clinical condition of porphyria (Kaufman and Marver, 1970). As a result, it is currently assumed that sex steroids in some way regulate or influence the normal quantities of smooth ER and hence certain functional activities within the liver cells. The induction of liver ER and its subsequent effect on porphyrin and

Figure 19-21 Electron micrograph of two liver cells from the rat. S, sinusoid; D, space of Disse; Gly, glycogen; M, mitochondria; SER, smooth-surfaced reticulum; RER, rough-surfaced reticulum; B, bile canaliculi; G, Golgi apparatus; N, nucleus. Note the discontinuous endothelial lining, the association of glycogen with the SER (see insert), the flattened lamellar profiles of the RER, the microvilli within the space of Disse and bile canaliculus, and close relationships between the Golgi apparatus and bile canaliculi. ×27,000; insert ×45,000.

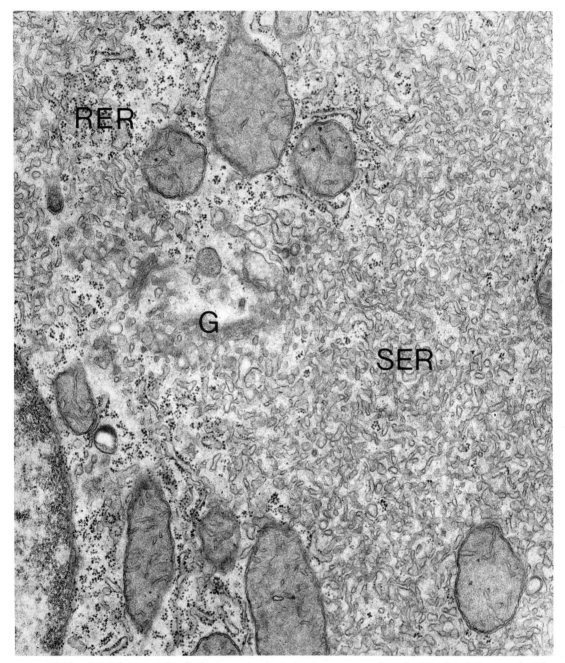

Figure 19-22 Liver cell from a phenobarbital-treated animal showing an extraordinary hypertrophy of the smooth-surfaced endoplasmic reticulum (SER). Because of its abundance, the smooth-membraned elements appear to crowd the profiles of rough-
surfaced endoplasmic reticulum (RER) into localized areas. The tangential section through the Golgi complex (G) shows several
areas of communication between this organelle and the SER. Approximately ×40,000. (From A. L. Jones and D. W. Fawcett,
J. Histochem. Cytochem., 14:215, 1966.)

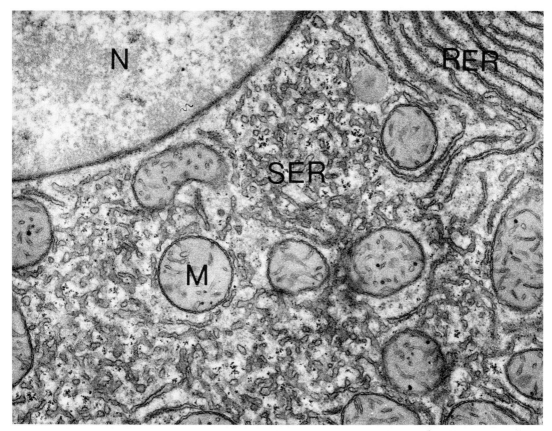

Figure 19-23   Certain synthetic and naturally occurring steroids produce a marked hypertrophy of the hepatic smooth-surfaced endoplasmic reticulum (SER).   Rough-surfaced endoplasmic reticulum (RER) can be observed partially wrapped around mitochondria during rapid membrane proliferation.   N, nucleus; M, mitochondria.   ×37,000.   (Courtesy of J. A. Hahn.)

drug metabolism should be considered by the physician when administering gonadal hormones for contraceptive purposes.

Deliberate controlled induction of microsomal enzymes, to increase glucuronyl transferase activity, has been found beneficial in certain cases of hyperbilirubinemia.   However, liver microsomal enzyme induction is *not* always beneficial.   First, membrane induction can alter the individual's response to therapeutic drugs; that is, the additional membranes may metabolize a drug at a new rate.   Hence, the dose-response relationships obtained for drugs administered to normal patients should *not* be assumed to apply to individuals with hypertrophied liver ER.   Second, hypertrophy of the ER often is accompanied by an increase in microsomal

hydroxylase activity, and some hydroxylated compounds are more dangerous than the parent compound.   One example is 3,4-benzpyrene, a relatively innocuous component of cigarette smoke, which on hydroxylation becomes a potent carcinogen.   Another example is carbon tetrachloride, long regarded as a powerful hepatotoxin.   Yet, it has been shown recently that the centrolobular necrosis associated with carbon tetrachloride poisoning is not caused by the parent compound, but rather by a free radical formed during its metabolism.

Fat metabolism is another important liver function associated with the ER.   In the parenchymal cell, free fatty acids not utilized for energy or membrane synthesis are reesterified into triglycerides.   A small amount of triglyceride is stored in cyto-

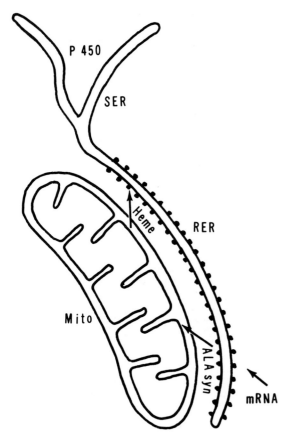

P 450

SER

Heme

RER

Mito

ALA syn

mRNA

Figure 19-24 The close association of the rough-surfaced reticulum with the mitochondria seen in electron micrographs is diagrammatically represented here. This relationship may be necessary for the production of smooth reticulum and cytochromes. Under the influence of messenger RNA (mRNA) the rough-surfaced endoplasmic reticulum (RER) synthesizes the enzyme Δ-aminolevulinic acid synthetase (ALA syn) which is transferred to the mitochondria. This results in an increased production of heme. Some heme is transferred back to the endoplasmic reticulum and utilized for the production of the microsomal heme protein P450. (From A. L. Jones and J. B. Emans in H. A. Salhanick, D. Kipnes, and R. L. Van de Wiele (eds.), "Metabolic Effects of Gonadal Hormones and Contraceptive Steroids," Plenum Press, New York, 1969.)

plasmic fat droplets and the remainder is released into the blood as VLDL (see Fig. 19-25). The VLDL particle is a lipid-protein complex. Its triglyceride, or fatty core, is encompassed by a surface apoprotein and a mixture of cholesterol and phospholipid. Presumably the particle is synthesized in the ER with the smooth ER forming the lipid and the rough

ER synthesizing the protein. The mechanism of complexing the two components is not understood.

Following synthesis, the lipoprotein is transferred through the smooth ER and is released from the cells. This may be accomplished in two ways: (1) smooth vesicles containing lipoproteins may bud off the smooth ER, migrate to the surface, and be released by exocytosis or (2) the lipoproteins within the smooth ER may be sequestered in Golgi vesicles, which in turn are released at the cell surface in a packet (see Figs. 19-25 and 19-26). This latter mode of transport is similar to that used by the pancreatic acinar cells for protein secretion. The recent intracellular localization of sugar nucleotide glycoprotein glycosyltransferases in Golgi-rich fractions from liver strongly suggests that the Golgi may be involved generally in glycoprotein production and in the addition of a carbohydrate component to the lipoprotein (see Fig. 19-27).

Membrane synthesis and turnover A number of important relationships between the subcellular structure and function of hepatic ER have been derived from the elegant studies of fetal and newborn rat livers by Dallner, Siekevitz, and Palade (1966). Three days prior to delivery, there is a marked increase in parenchymal cell glycogen. Although parenchymal cell rough ER is essentially fully developed, the activity of certain microsomal enzymes (for example, mixed-function oxidases and glucose-6-phosphatase) is nearly unmeasurable. Furthermore, there is little or no smooth ER in these cells. After birth, glycogen falls and smooth ER increases within the cells, while the activity of the above-mentioned enzymes begins to rise (although not all enzymes do so at the same rate) and the liver acquires the ability to metabolize certain drugs.

Following formation of ER within the hepatocyte, these membranes undergo constant renewal or turnover. The half-life of adult liver ER has been calculated to be 2 to $2\frac{1}{2}$ days (Schimke et al., 1968). Yet, it is becoming clear that not all components within these membranes turn over at the same rate. Moreover, recent studies of lipoprotein synthesis show that they can be synthesized and transported out of the liver cell within 5 min. Since each particle or packet of particles is surrounded by a portion of smooth ER and/or Golgi membrane,

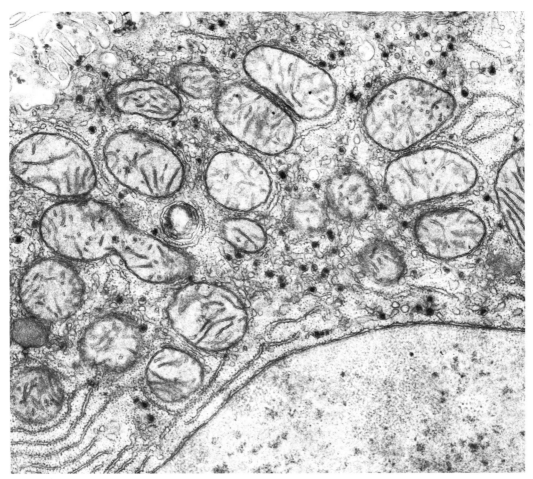

Figure 19-25 Portion of a rat liver cell engaged in the production and release of lipoproteins. The small 300- to 800-Å osmiophilic lipoprotein particles are enclosed within the cisternae of the smooth ER. Compare with diagram (Fig. 19-27). Many particles are near the vascular surface and within the space of Disse (upper left). Approximately ×25,000.

which accompanies the particle to the plasmalemma, it appears likely that membrane turnover might take minutes rather than days or hours, as previously thought.

LYSOSOMES

Structure Liver parenchymal cells contain many lysosomes (see Fig. 19-28). They can be found almost invariably within the cytoplasm bordering each bile canaliculus and Golgi complex. Lysosomes in these sites correspond to the so-called *peribiliary dense bodies* described by early histolo-

gists. These highly pleomorphic organelles vary in size, number, and position during different conditions. Since no two lysosomes look alike, their positive identification in electron micrographs requires that the intracellular particle be bounded by a single membrane and exhibit a positive staining reaction for acid phosphatase. Parenchymal cell lysosomes are usually 0.2 to 1 μm in diameter and contain variable amounts of material. Their contents may be homogeneous, heterogeneous, dense, or finely granular and may include myelin figures, pigment, intact or partially digested organelles, and/or inclusions.

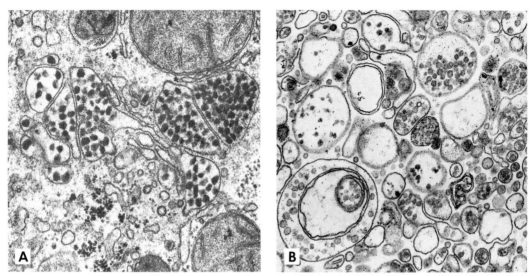

Figure 19-26   Electron micrographs of very-low-density lipoprotein particles within the Golgi complex of an intact liver cell (A) and within the membranes of the isolated Golgi-rich fraction (B) of rat liver. The lipoprotein particles can be further isolated from the Golgi membranes for analysis. Approximately ✕ 25,000. (Courtesy of R. L. Hamilton.)

Function   Lysosomes perform a number of digestive and lytic functions for the parenchymal cells. Under normal conditions, they catabolize certain unwanted exogenous substances, effete organelles, and inclusions. The latter two processes are especially important for maintenance and rejuvenation of the parenchymal cells since some products of digestion may be utilized by the cells for energy and repair; loss in liver mass and presence of increased numbers of lysosomes in livers of starved animals are associated with the mobilization and release of stored energy-producing substances needed to maintain the entire body. Hepatic lysosomes also appear to participate in the storage of iron. They normally contain ferritin-like substances and accumulate large quantities of these materials in iron storage diseases, for example, hemachromatosis and hemasiderosis. Nondigestible materials such as lipofuscin pigment accumulate in lysosomes or residual bodies of otherwise healthy liver cells and tend to increase in number as the individual ages.

There is now considerable evidence that lysosomes have an important role in the pathogenesis of many conditions. Hepatic lysosomes increase in viral hepatitis, cholestasis, and cell injury following anoxia, and the livers of children with Type 2 glycogenosis (Pompe's disease) lack the enzyme α-glucosidase and contain large glycogen deposits within their lysosomes (see Weissman, 1969, for review).

MICROBODIES (PEROXISOMES)

Structure   The microbody is a single membrane-bounded particle (approximately 0.2 to 1 μm in diameter) with a fine granular matrix. Each parenchymal cell has approximately 200 microbodies or one microbody per four mitochondria. Although some investigators have reported that microbodies are concentrated in regions rich in glycogen, others claim that they are randomly distributed throughout the cytoplasm. They vary greatly in size within the same cell; yet there appears to be no difference in enzymatic composition between small and large microbodies having the same structure. Hepatic microbodies in many mammals contain a crystalloid laminated core or nucleoid which distinguishes them from the denser peribiliary bodies, the lysosomes. The structure of the core varies greatly from species to species. In the hamster (Jones and Fawcett, 1966), it appears as a thin flexible sheet, whereas in the rat it is made up of tubules of two different sizes: small ones, approximately 45 Å in diameter, and large ones, 95 to 115 Å in diameter (see Fig. 19-29). The two types of tubules, in longitudinal section, produce the laminated appearance of the crystalloid. The core is thought to contain urate oxidase whereas catalase and D-amino acid oxidase presumably are present in the matrix. The livers of uricotelic animals, anthropoid primates, and man usually contain anucleoid microbodies deficient in urate oxidase. In some species the liver contains a mixture of nucleoid and anucleoid microbodies. This has been interpreted in

three ways: (1) that urate oxidase (the core material) is the last enzyme to be added to a new microbody; (2) that the two types may have slightly different functions; and (3) that there is an exchange of contents among microbodies.

Microbodies are thought to turn over quite rapidly under normal circumstances yet their origin and demise remain obscure. Numerous morphologic observations suggest that the liver microbodies are derived from the ER, but Legg and Wood (1970), on the basis of certain cytochemical data, suggest that they arise through fragmentation or budding from preexisting microbodies.

Figure 19-27 Diagrammatic representation of the possible steps in lipoprotein production and release. (Modified from A. L. Jones, N. B. Ruderman, and M. G. Herrera, J. Lipid Res., 8:429, 1967.)

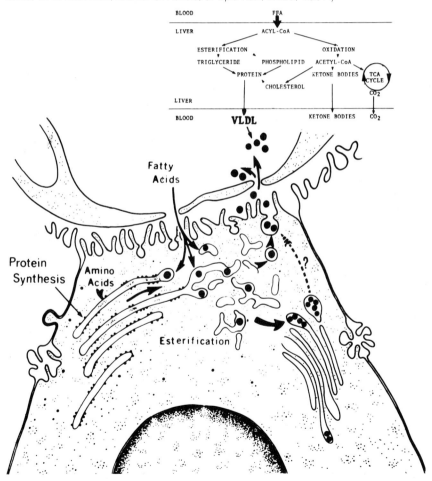

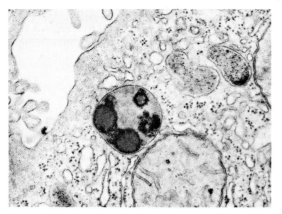

Figure 19-28   Three hepatic lysosomes near a bile canaliculus. Note the morphologic variation in their matrix and that they are bounded by a single membrane.   Approximately ×25,000.

The mitochondria appear to be randomly distributed throughout the cytoplasm.   However, there is good evidence that the number, size, shape, and enzymatic properties of liver mitochondria are related to the position of the cell within the lobule (Novikoff and Essner, 1960; Loud, 1968).

Mitochondria move about in the cytoplasm and undergo changes in structure and volume.   Such morphologic alterations are thought to reflect functional changes.   Swelling and contraction of isolated liver mitochondria occur in response to a number of endogenous substances such as hormones, calcium ions, phosphate ions, and fatty acids as well as changes in ion transport and os-

Figure 19-29   Microbodies.   In the rat, these single-membrane-bonded structures contain a crystalloid enmeshed in a homogenous matrix.   Both a cross section (a) and longitudinal section (b) of the crystalloid are observed in this micrograph. (See text.)   Approximately ×100,000.

Function   The physiologic significance of hepatic microbodies is not known although it is speculated that they may participate in any one or all of the following: disposal of hydrogen peroxide; metabolism of purines, lipids, and alcohols; oxidation of reduced NAD; and gluconeogenesis (see De Duve and Baudhuin, 1966, for review).   Human beings and certain mouse strains with little or no blood and liver catalase activity can survive satisfactorily; hence it appears that this constituent of the microbody is not essential for life.

Proliferation of hepatic microbodies occurs during embryologic development and early postnatal life, during recovery from partial hepatectomy, and following the administration of salicylates and ethyl-α-p-chlorophenoxyisobutyrate (CPIB or clofibrate).   The effects of the latter compound are particularly interesting because it is often used in the treatment of atherosclerosis (to lower serum triglycerides and cholesterol).   Presumably any one of these conditions could be used to explore the function and origin of liver microbodies.

MITOCHONDRIA

Parenchymal cells contain numerous well-developed mitochondria (approximately 800 per cell) (see Fig. 19-21).   In rat and human livers the mitochondria usually are *round* or *oblong* (for example, 0.5 to 1.5 μm in diameter, 1.5 to 4.5 μm in length). These organelles account for approximately 20 percent of the total nitrogen within each cell.

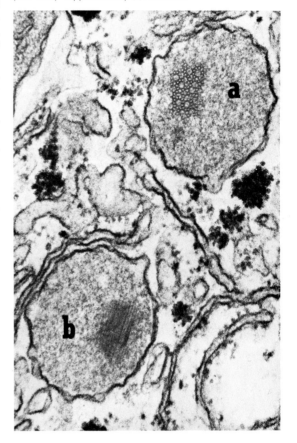

motic pressure. Although the precise meaning of these observations is not yet clear, it appears likely that both conformational and chemiosmotic changes are normally involved in energy transduction. The effects of swelling and contraction on the molecular organization and composition of the mitochondrial membranes are not yet complete; however, it appears that the flexibility of mitochondrial membranes depends, at least in part, upon the presence of unsaturated fatty acids (Packer, 1970).

Liver mitochondria are thought to be self-replicating bodies with a half-life of about 10.5 days. The presence of mitochondria within lysosomes has fostered the idea that the lysosomes destroy effete mitochondria. And the rapidity with which the mitochondria are thought to turn over, in comparison with the life-span of the cell, presumably accounts for the presence of a few atypical or abnormal mitochondria in otherwise healthy cells. The genesis of the liver mitochondrion, however, is still subject to conjecture. Budding or dividing mito-

chondria are not readily found in normal liver, but they are commonplace during recovery from simple riboflavin (Tandler et al., 1969) or dietary iron (Dallman and Goodman, 1971) deficiency. The giant mitochondria formed during the course of these diseases are restored to normal dimensions via division following the onset of replacement therapy. Fine-structural studies show that a transverse membranous partition or septum formed within the mitochondrion sequesters a small segment of the organelle from the main mitochondrial mass. Subsequently, this region is pinched off and the organelle returns to normal size. Although other theories have been put forth to account for the origin of liver mitochondria, the above theory is the most widely accepted at present.

Intramitochondrial inclusions have been described in hepatic mitochondria in a number of human diseases; however, their significance remains obscure.

The biliary space

BILE CANALICULI

The bile canaliculi are the smallest biliary spaces, ranging from 0.5 to 1.5 μm in diameter. They are usually centrally located between adjacent parenchymal cells (see Figs. 19-12 and 19-30). The bile canaliculi can be isolated from the remainder of the liver by maceration. Misinterpretation of this phenomenon resulted in the erroneous notion that the canaliculi were bounded by a separate cuticular wall. Electron-microscopic evidence has now clearly established that the limiting wall of the bile canaliculus is made up of local surface specializations on adjacent liver cells (Matter et al., 1969). Microvilli of the parenchymal cells protrude into the lumen of the canaliculi (see Fig. 19-21), and fine cytoplasmic filaments circumscribe the area beneath the canaliculi. They insert into desmosomes and extend into the core of the microvilli. The filament-rich pericanalicular ectoplasm of the liver and the terminal web area of the intestinal absorptive cell have similar staining reactions, indicating that they are composed, at least in part, of the same material (Biava, 1964). Histochemical prep-

arations, such as ATPase and alkaline phosphatase stains, have enabled us to clearly observe the biliary network with the light microscope. The finding of ATPase activity in this area suggests that bile secretion is an energy-requiring process.

The biliary space is separated from the other intercellular spaces by junctional complexes between the parenchymal cells. Immediately adjacent to the canalicular lumen is a tight junction (see Fig. 19-31). Lanthanum injected into the portal vein or retrograde up the common bile duct will not normally pass across this junction. Interestingly, when lanthanum is injected under increased pressure up the biliary tree, some particles pass across the tight junction (Matter et al., 1969). Because of this, it is speculated that certain components of bile, such as conjugated bilirubin, may gain access to the intercellular space by this route during times of chronic biliary obstruction. Another cellular attachment near the canaliculus is the nexus or gap junction. The membranes in this junction are parallel to one another with a 20-Å gap which normally will admit lanthanum. The function of the gaps is

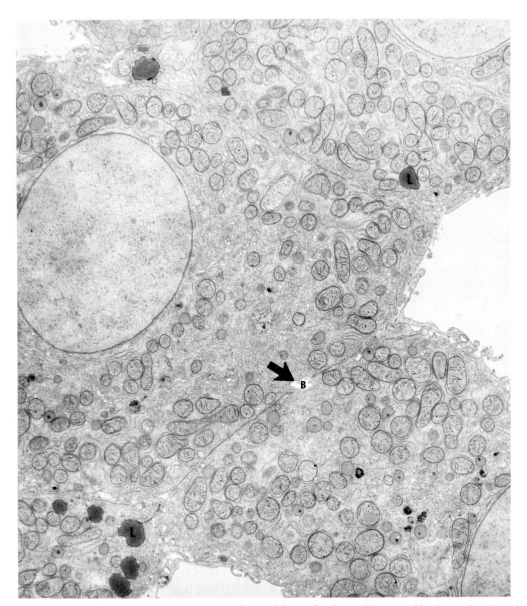

Figure 19-30 Low-power electron micrograph of several liver cells disposed between blood vascular channels or sinusoids. Note that the bile canaliculus (B) is centrally located between adjacent parenchymal cells. At this magnification one can appreciate the random distribution of the organelles. Golgi complexes, however, are almost always located between the nucleus and bile canaliculus. L, cytoplasmic lipid.

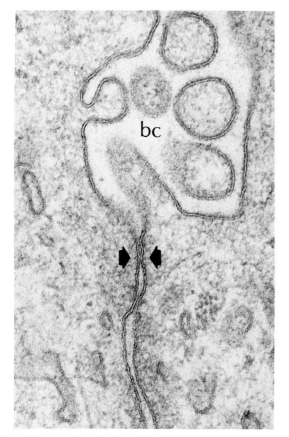

Figure 19-31 Tight junction adjacent to a bile canaliculus (bc) in rat liver. Note the focal merging of the two outer leaflets of the plasma membrane of the parenchymal cells (arrow). Approximately × 100,000. (Courtesy of D. Friend.)

by small vesicles to the Golgi cisternae where it is concentrated and later transferred into the bile canaliculus (Matter et al., 1969). It is possible that the secretory events leading from the Golgi to the canaliculi are so rapid that they are not observed by conventional techniques. Interestingly, retrograde injection of horseradish peroxidase into the biliary tree shows that this substance may return to the space of Disse through the liver cells in vacuoles which appear unassociated with the Golgi complex.

Other organelles, such as lysosomes and multi-vesicular bodies, are often found near the bile canaliculi, but like the Golgi complex, there is no direct evidence of their participation in bile formation or secretion.

When the flow of bile is impeded (cholestasis), certain architectural changes take place in the canaliculi. There is increased thickening of the ectoplasmic layers, and the canaliculi dilate with subsequent flattening and disorientation of the microvilli.

TERMINAL DUCTULES

Bile flows in the canaliculi to the periphery of the classic lobule and enters small terminal bile ductules or canals of Hering. These canals form short channels that convey bile from the canaliculi through the limiting plate and into the interlobular bile duct of the portal canals.

At first, one or two fusiform-shaped ductular cells share a canalicular lumen with a hepatocyte (see Fig. 19-32). Subsequently, they are lined by two to four cells which become cuboidal as the ductule nears the portal canal. The terminal ductules are smaller than the interlobular ducts, having diameters usually less than 15 μm. Many blunt microvilli project from their lumenal borders and junctional complexes. The nuclei are elongated and the mitochondria are smaller than those of neighboring hepatocytes. Endoplasmic reticulum is sparse, but the Golgi complex and pinocytotic vesicles are well developed, suggesting that the ductules are metabolically active. A basal lamina completely encompasses the ductules except at the point of contact between the hepatocytes and ductule cells.

The origin of the terminal ductule cell is a matter of debate. Some feel that it is derived from cells

still not clear but certain evidence indicates that they provide an electrical communication between cells. The nexus may be observed along any part of the plasmalemma between adjacent liver cells. Desmosomes, when included within the plane of section, appear near the canaliculi.

Curiously, only thin filaments are observed in the cytoplasm immediately adjacent to the canaliculus. Despite the fact that the Golgi complex is polarized toward the bile canaliculi, components of this complex are seldom observed passing through the ectoplasmic layer. However, intravascularly administered horseradish peroxidase is picked up at the vascular surface of liver cells and transported

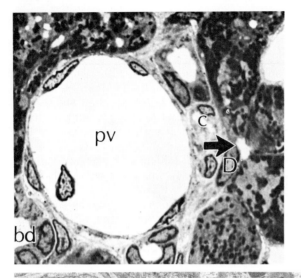

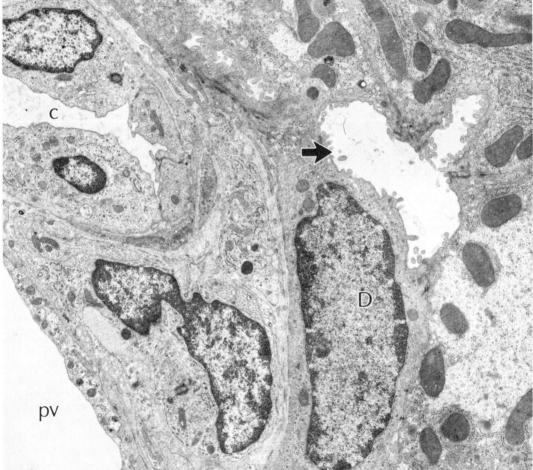

Figure 19-32 Adjacent to this portal canal a junction is seen between a terminal ductule cell and three hepatic parenchymal cells (arrow), by both light (upper figure; ×1100) and electron microscopy (lower figure; ×8000). Note the fusiform shape of the ductule cell and its basal lamina. pv, portal vein; c, capillaries; bd, bile duct; D, ductule cell. (Courtesy of R. L. Wood.)

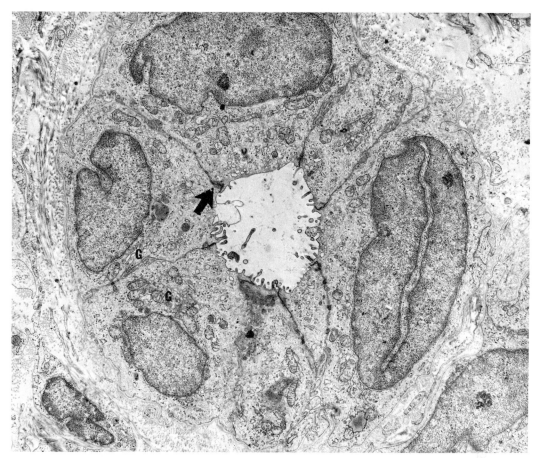

Figure 19-33   Small interlobular bile duct.   These ducts are encompassed by a thin basal lamina.   The cuboidal cells contain few organelles although pinocytotic vesicles are abundant and the Golgi complex (G), when included in the plane of section, is well developed.   Note the microvilli on their luminal surface and the apical zones of adhesion (arrow). Approximately ×12,000.

of the larger interlobular ducts, whereas others claim it is of parenchymal origin.   During chronic extrahepatic cholestasis, the ductule cells proliferate and almost completely replace the liver cells (Steiner et al., 1962).   Wilson believes they are primitive cells capable of differentiating into either parenchymal or bile epithelium.   Whatever their source or potentials, the epithelial cells of the terminal ductules are very unusual.

INTRAHEPATIC BILE DUCTS

Bile in the terminal ductules empties into *interlobular bile ducts* (30 to 40 μm in diameter) in the portal canals (see Fig. 19-4).   These ducts form a contin-

uous network of passageways whose size increases as they near the porta.   They are lined by a single layer of cuboidal or columnar epithelial cells which have microvilli on their lumenal surface (see Fig. 19-33).   The epithelium is surrounded by a basal lamina.   The basal nuclei are round and contain considerable chromatin often arranged like cartwheel spokes.   These cells, like those of the ductules, contain a prominent Golgi complex and vesicles considered to be pinocytotic.   Cholesterol crystals have been observed in the cytoplasm.   Occasionally, particles of mucus-secreting epithelium surrounded by a vascular plexus have been observed in the larger ducts.   The wall of the intrahepatic bile ducts is made up of dense fibrous tissue containing many elastic fibers. Smooth muscle fibers in the walls of the ducts near the hilus of the liver form the morphologic basis for the narrowing of the ducts in this location often seen in cholangiograms (Rappaport, 1969).

EXTRAHEPATIC BILE DUCTS

The extrahepatic ducts are enclosed by tall columnar cells. Their walls possess the same layers as the intestine, that is, mucosa, submucosa, muscularis, and adventitia. Tubular glands containing cells rich in mucopolysaccharides are occasionally noted at regular intervals in the submucosa. The wall of the extrahepatic ducts receives its blood supply from small branches of the hepatic and gastroduodenal arteries.

The *common hepatic duct* is approximately 3 cm long. It arises at the porta from the confluence of the right and left hepatic lobular ducts. It is joined by the *cystic duct* from the gallbladder to form the *common bile duct* (ductus choledochus) which is approximately 7 cm long and empties into the duodenum. Tubular glands containing PAS-positive cells are scattered along the length of the common duct. These glands are more extensive in a nongallbladder mammal such as the rat.

GALLBLADDER

Located on the undersurface of the right liver lobe and connected to the relatively rigid ducts of the biliary tree is a readily distensible bag: the gallbladder. In man, it is large enough to hold 30 to 50 ml of bile. The surface of the filled gallbladder is stretched evenly, but in the empty, contracted gallbladder it forms numerous elongated, decussating folds or rugae. The wall contains a surface epithelium, lamina propria, muscularis, and a serosa (see Fig. 19-34).

The mucosa contains an inner layer of simple columnar epithelium. The apex of each cell contains numerous microvilli (see Fig. 19-35), lateral junctional complexes, and associated tonofilaments. Desmosomes occur at frequent intervals

along the entire length of the lateral cell membranes. The Golgi is usually supranuclear and well developed. Rough ER and membrane-bounded granular inclusions are especially prominent in man. Mitochondria are numerous but relatively small.

The lamina propria is rich in blood vessels and connective tissue fibers. The muscularis consists of a number of layers of smooth muscle separated by a fairly extensive network of elastic fibers. The serosal coat is a broad connective tissue layer containing numerous collagen fibers and the blood vessels and lymphatics which supply the organ. Numerous nerves from the autonomic nervous system also can be noted on the serosal surface. Glands can be found occasionally in the lamina propria of the human gallbladder, especially near the neck. These glands contain goblet cells and a few cells which are identical to the argentaffin cells in the intestine. These so-called *mucous glands,* sparse in normal tissue, are moderately abundant in persons who have had chronic inflammation of the gallbladder. Yet it is difficult to tell whether a common pathologic factor promotes inflammation and stimulates the development of the glands or whether there is a secondary causal relationship between the development of cholecystitis and the presence of these glands.

Rokitansky-Aschoff crypts or *diverticula* are invaginations of the surface epithelium. Some of these crypts or sinuses extend through the entire width of the muscular layer. They favor bacterial retention and inflammation and are usually regarded as antecedents to pathologic changes.

Luschka's bile ducts are seen occasionally in some gallbladders. Serial sections reveal that these bile ducts, located along the hepatic surface of the gallbladder, open directly into the liver. The epithelium has a variable morphology but is generally similar to normal intrahepatic ducts. They are probably the consequence of some embryologic developmental disturbance.

The arterial supply of the gallbladder is via the *cystic artery* which usually rises from the right he-

Figure 19-34 Contracted gallbladder. Parts a (×3000) and c (×350) are scanning electron micrographs of the inner surface of guinea pig gallbladder. Part c shows the pronounced folding of the gallbladder mucosa. In a the bulging individual epithelial cells are covered with bristle-like microvilli. Compare with Fig. 19-35. Part b (×90) is a light micrograph of contracted human gallbladder. Note the diverticula (D) into the wall and the mucous gland (MG). The muscularis (M) is present but the serosa has been stripped off. Fixed in Zenker's fluid; H&E. (a and c from J. C. Mueller, A. L. Jones, and J. A. Long, Gastroenterology, vol. 62, 1972.)

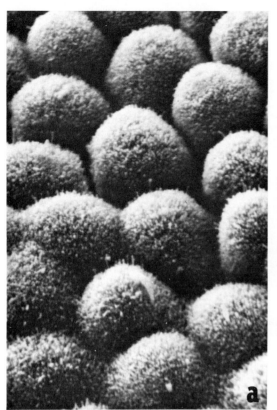

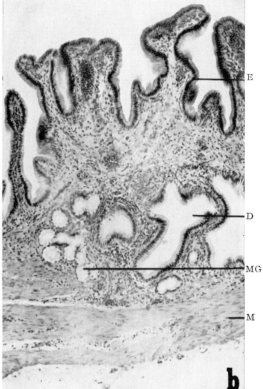

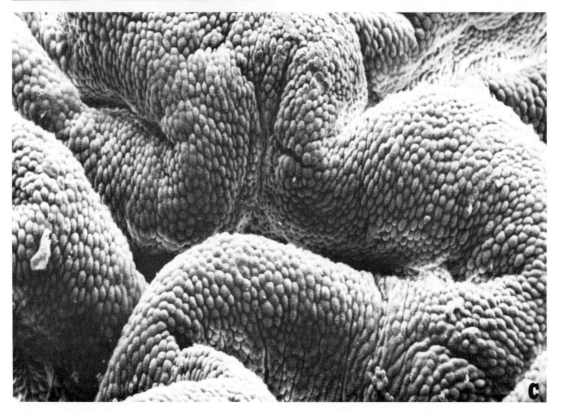

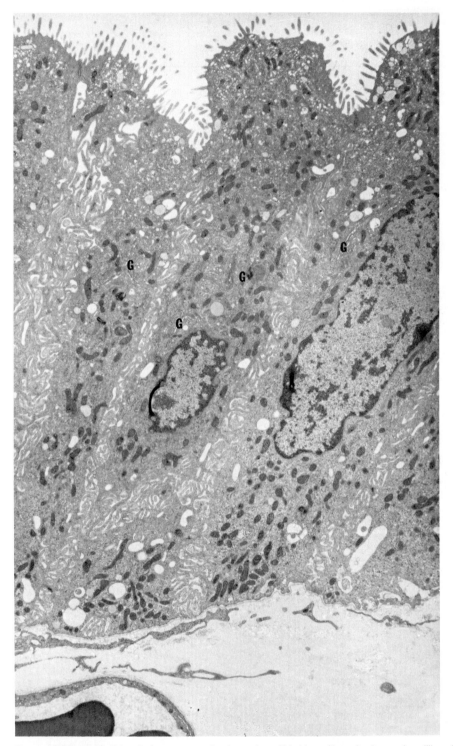

Figure 19-35 Epithelial cells from a normal guinea pig gallbladder. Note the long microvilli and the characteristic bulging of the apical region of the cell into the gallbladder lumen. The Golgi (G) apparatus is supranuclear, and the small mitochondria are distributed at random in the cytoplasm. Numerous pinocytotic vesicles and larger PAS-positive granules are in the apical cytoplasm. The lateral cell borders are markedly interdigitated, and a basal lamina encompasses the basal region of the cells. ×7000. (From J. C. Mueller, A. L. Jones, and J. A. Long, Gastroenterology, vol. 62, 1972.)

patic artery. At the gallbladder it divides into a superficial branch supplying the free or serosal surface and a deep branch which arborizes throughout the deeper, interior layers of the wall. These branches anastomose freely and may send twigs into the adjacent liver substance. Venous drainage from the gallbladder and cystic duct is via the *cystic vein* which ends in the right branch of the portal vein. Occasionally, some small venous branches may pass directly into the hepatic parenchyma and join the sinusoids. The lymph vessels of the gallbladder reportedly are intimately connected with lymph vessels of Glisson's capsule.

The neck of the gallbladder is continuous with the *cystic duct*. This duct retains all the layers of the wall of the gallbladder, is about 4 cm long, and joins the common hepatic duct. Its mucous membrane is thrown into a series of folds arranged in a spiral fashion around the tube (spiral valve) (see Fig. 19-36). Many nerve cells are found in the fibromuscular layer of the cystic duct.

CHOLEDOCHODUODENAL JUNCTION

The junction of the common bile duct, pancreatic duct, and the duodenum is an anatomic area of medical and physiologic importance. It regulates the flow of bile and pancreatic enzymes into the duodenum and governs the filling of the gallbladder. Occlusion of the choledochoduodenal junction by small gallstones or tumors results in cholestasis (and various sequelae).

In the human embryo, the ventral pancreatic and common bile duct arise from the hepatic diverticulum of the foregut. In the adult, the associated bile and pancreatic ducts pass obliquely through an opening in the circular musculature of the duodenum. The ducts empty their contents into a duodenal ampulla, the *ampulla of Vater*. The bile and pancreatic enzymes pass through the orifice in the ampulla into the lumen of the duodenum (see Fig. 19-36).

During passage through the intestinal wall, the associated bile and pancreatic ducts are invested by a common musculus proprius termed the *sphincter of Oddi*. The latter structure varies greatly among individuals but usually contains four subdivisions: (1) the *sphincter choledochus*, a strong annular sheath surrounding the common bile duct

prior to its junction with the pancreatic duct; (2) the *fasiculi longitudinales*, consisting of longitudinal muscle bundles which span the intervals between the two ducts from the margins of the fenestrae to the ampulla; (3) the *sphincter ampullae* or terminal musculature surrounding the ampulla of Vater; and (4) the *sphincter pancreaticus*, surrounding the intraduodenal segment of the pancreatic duct, prior to its junction with the ampulla.

Contraction of the sphincter choledochus prevents the flow of bile, whereas contraction of the fasiculi longitudinales shortens the ducts and facilitates the flow of bile into the duodenum. When both the pancreatic and common bile duct end in the ampulla, contraction of the sphincter ampullae may promote reflux of bile into the pancreatic duct, which, in turn, may result in pancreatitis.

Figure 19-36 The mucous membrane of the gallbladder and extrahepatic bile passages. The two sphincters are shown diagrammatically. (From "Grant's Method of Anatomy," The Williams & Wilkins Co., Baltimore, 1965.)

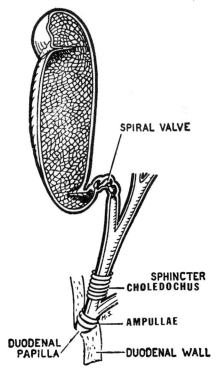

SPIRAL VALVE

SPHINCTER CHOLEDOCHUS

AMPULLAE

DUODENAL PAPILLA

DUODENAL WALL

BILE PRODUCTION AND TRANSPORT

Normally bile is continuously secreted from the hepatic parenchymal cells into the bile canaliculi. Fifteen milliliters of bile per kilogram of body weight is produced daily by adult human livers. Bile is secreted at a rate of approximately 0.6 ml per min in a 60-kg adult. The rate of synthesis and secretion depends largely on the blood flow to the liver. Bile is produced at a pressure of 200 to 300 mm H_2O. This pressure is regulated by the rate of secretion and viscosity of the bile, contractility of the gallbladder, and the resistance of the sphincter of Oddi.

The bile is an aqueous solution containing various organic and inorganic solutes. Bile salts, phospholipids, cholesterol, and bile pigments are the major organic solutes. Lecithin, the chief phospholipid, and cholesterol are insoluble in water but remain in solution even when the bile is concentrated by the gallbladder, presumably because they form mixed micelles with the bile salts. Indeed, Wheeler (1969) states that solubilization of cholesterol is possible only over a narrow range of concentrations of bile salts and lecithin. The protein concentration is very low in human bile, but electrolytes and glucose are found in practically the

Figure 19-37 Diagrammatic summary of some of the mechanisms involved in bile formation. The larger cells represent liver parenchymal cells and the smaller ones the bile duct system. [From H. O. Wheeler, in L. Schiff (ed.), "Diseases of the Liver," 3d ed., J. B. Lippincott, Philadelphia, 1969.]

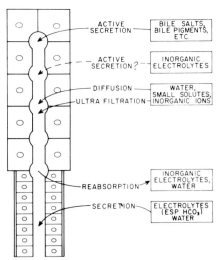

same concentration as they are in the blood. The latter two compounds probably enter the bile by simple diffusion, perhaps via the intercellular spaces of the parenchymal cells and then into the canaliculi. Other substances, such as bile salts, pigments, and sulfobromophthalein (BSP), a compound used in liver function tests to measure hepatic clearance, are approximately 100 times more concentrated in bile than in the blood, suggesting that they are actively secreted into the bile against the concentration gradient. Other compounds such as chloride and bicarbonate are less concentrated in the bile than in the plasma.

It has been suggested that there is some fluid reabsorption in the intrahepatic bile ducts (see Fig. 19-37). This is a well-established phenomenon in the gallbladder but direct studies are difficult in intrahepatic bile ducts. In the dog, the gastrointestinal hormone *secretin* appears to influence the secretory activity of the bile ducts; bile flow increases, the secretion becomes more watery, and it contains more sodium bicarbonate and less bile salts and pigments. Both secretin and cholecystokinin reportedly encourage the flow of bile into the intestinal lumen by inducing contraction of the gallbladder and relaxation of the sphincter of Oddi. Cholecystokinin is probably more potent in this regard than secretin. The parasympathetic vagus nerve is thought to contract the sphincter of Oddi between fatty meals.

The constituents in the bile that reach the intestine are not completely lost. Many are reabsorbed and transported by the portal blood to the liver for reexcretion (enterohepatic circulation). Most bile salts and the fatty acids from the phospholipid and cholesterol in the bile are reabsorbed.

In addition to providing a pool of bile for digestion of fat, the gallbladder also plays a role in concentrating the bile. Absorption in the normal gallbladder is confined largely to water and inorganic ions, especially sodium, calcium, chloride, and bicarbonate. In the dog, water is reabsorbed at a rate of 3 to 6 cm^3 an hour. This concentrates the bile 4 to 10 times (Cameron, 1970). In gallbladders known to be transporting fluid, Kaye et al. (1966) found that the intercellular spaces between the epithelial cells as well as the subepithelial spaces are distended. Studies of sodium localization showed high concentrations in the distended areas. ATPase activity was present along the lateral plasma membrane of the epithelial cells. Hence, it was concluded that solute from the bile is actively transported through the epithelial cell and across the lateral plasma membrane into the intercellular space.

The normal gallbladder secretes a small amount of mucus but the role of this process in the total economy of the organism is not understood.

The development of the liver and gallbladder

ORIGIN OF THE HEPATIC DIVERTICULUM

The liver primordium appears in human embryos (2.5 mm) during the middle of the third week of gestation. It begins as a thickening of the endodermal epithelium lining the cranioventral wall of the foregut near its junction with the yolk sac (that is, the anterior intestinal portal). The thickening rapidly develops into a ventral outgrowth which becomes hollow and lined by columnar epithelium. The cavity of the diverticulum is continuous with the region of the intestine destined to become the duodenum. As the diverticulum enlarges, it grows into the mesenchyme of the *septum transversum* and separates into (1) a cranial, hepatic portion which eventually forms the liver and intrahepatic bile ducts; (2) a smaller caudal, cystic portion which becomes the gallbladder, common bile duct, and cystic duct; and (3) a ventral portion which evolves into a segment of the head of the pancreas.

THE HEPATIC PARENCHYMA, SINUSOIDS, LIGAMENTS

As the hepatic diverticulum invades the septum transversum, the irregularly shaped endodermal cells migrate forward from the original invagination in the form of solid strands or cords. The cords grow between the two *vitelline veins* into the capillary network of the septum transversum that arises from these vessels. In so doing, the hepatic cords subdivide the capillaries in the plexus and become surrounded by them. This process ultimately leads to the development of the complicated adult pattern of the *parenchyma* and *sinusoids,* as the cell cords become hepatic plates and the capillaries become liver sinusoids. The hepatic plates at this stage are three to five cells thick and remain this way until several years after birth. Once the plates are formed, the liver cells become more regular in shape and are usually cuboidal. There are no binucleated cells until after birth and the cell volume increases as the cells undergo terminal differentiation. In the 10-mm, 6-week embryo, the liver is bilobed. Mesenchymal tissue from the septum transversum forms the *stroma, capsule,* and *mesothelium* of the liver. Reflections of peritoneum off the diaphragm onto the liver's surface will form the triangular and coronary ligaments, whereas the area of original contact with the septum transversum, which is not covered by peritoneum, forms the *bare area* of the liver.

HEMATOPOIESIS

By the tenth week, the liver constitutes approximately 10 percent of the body weight. Hematopoiesis within the liver commences at the 10-mm stage (6 weeks) and contributes much of this weight. For a short time the liver is the primary site for fetal blood formation. The hematopoietic cells are extravascular and in close contact with the parenchymal cells. The ratio of liver to body weight decreases during the last trimester when most hematopoietic sites within the liver disappear.

INTRAHEPATIC BILIARY TREE AND BILE CANALICULI

The first bile canaliculi appear as small vesicles between parenchymal cells of the sixth-week embryo, far in advance of bile secretion. During the sixth to ninth weeks, the remainder of the intrahepatic biliary tree begins to form and apparently is derived from limiting plate hepatocytes abutting the edges of the portal canals. It is thought that certain limiting plate hepatocytes, surrounding lumina or vesicles in the wall, are transformed into ductal epithelium as the mesenchyme penetrates the limiting plate. In later stages, connective tissue separates the transforming cells from the liver parenchyma. Bile production commences at 4 months of gestation. The bile flows into the gallbladder and then to the duodenum, producing the characteristic dark color of the meconium.

EXTRAHEPATIC BILIARY TRACT AND GALLBLADDER

Little is known about the early development of the extrahepatic biliary tract and gallbladder in man. However, as the originally hollow pars cystica elongates, its lumen is obliterated by the migration of cells into the original lumen. Hence, in the 6- to 7-mm embryo, the future gallbladder and common

Figure 19-38 Diagram showing development of liver veins. sv, sinus venosus; uv, umbilical veins; vv, vitelline veins; g, gut; dv, ductus venosus; a, caudal anastomosis of distal vitelline veins; d, diaphragm. [Courtesy of A. M. DuBois, The Embryonic Liver, in C. Rouiller (ed.), "The Liver" vol. 1, Academic Press, New York, 1963.]

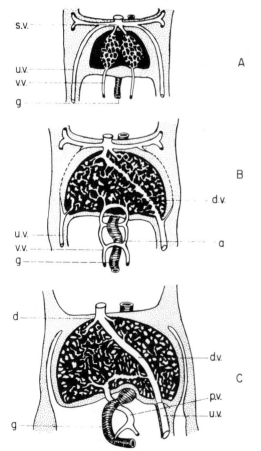

bile duct form a solid epithelial cord in the septum transversum just below the developing liver. Vacuolization of the solid cord produces a lumen in the common bile duct at 7.5 mm, the hepatic duct at 10 mm, the cystic duct at 16 mm, and the gallbladder at 18 mm. However, the gallbladder is not completely hollow until the third month. The mucosa, muscularis, and serosa of the gallbladder are established in the 29-mm embryo, but the mucosal folds are not formed until the very end of gestation.

Congenital atresia of the bile ducts can cause cholestasis and jaundice in the newborn. Untreated infants develop cirrhosis, liver failure, and portal hypertension and usually do not live longer than 2 years.

DEVELOPMENT OF THE HEPATIC VENOUS SYSTEM

The vasculature undergoes drastic changes during fetal life. In the 4.5-mm human embryo (5 weeks), the hepatic diverticulum and its associated capillaries (derived from the *vitelline veins*) lie between the right and left *umbilical veins* (Fig. 19-38A). During the 5-mm stage, the caudal segments of the vitelline veins begin to form three anastomoses. The anterior anastomosis is formed within the liver, whereas the middle and posterior form outside the liver, dorsal and ventral to the duodenum (Fig. 19-38B). As a result, two venous rings are formed. The right half of the upper ring and the left half of the bottom ring disappear by the 9-mm stage, and a new S-shaped vessel, composed of segments from the cross-connected vitelline veins, is formed. This vessel is the portal vein (Fig. 19-38C).

The efferent hepatic veins which drain the liver are derived from the vitelline veins proximal to the vitelline capillary plexus. In Fig. 19-38A, the vitelline veins are shown entering into the sinus venous, anterior to the liver. The stem of the right vitelline vein enlarges, and by the 9-mm stage it forms the termination of the inferior vena cava.

Except for very early stages, all maternal blood within the placenta flows through the umbilical veins. In the 5-mm embryo, the umbilical veins send ramifications into the liver (Fig. 19-38B). The right umbilical vein and proximal portions of the left umbilical vein disappear during the 6- to 7-mm stage. The remaining distal portion of the left umbilical vein supplies the liver with oxygenated blood from the maternal circulation (Fig. 19-38B).

The ductus venosus, which shunts blood directly from the left umbilical vein to the inferior vena cava, develops within the hepatic diverticulum during the 5- to 6-mm stage (Fig. 19-38B and C). The ductus venosus persists until birth, at which time it collapses and begins to atrophy. Eventually it forms a connective tissue remnant, the *ligamentus venosum*. Concomitantly, the left umbilical vein atrophies, forming the *ligamentum teres* which extends from the liver to the umbilicus.

References

AREY, L. B.: On the Presence of So-called Portal Lobules in the Seal's Liver, *Anat. Rec.*, **51**:315 (1932).

BEAMS, H. W., and R. L. KING: The Origin of Binucleate and Large Mononucleate Cells in the Liver of the White Rat, *Anat. Rec.*, **83**:281 (1942).

BIAVA, C. G.: Studies on Cholestasis: a Re-evaluation of the Fine Structure of Normal Human Bile Canaliculi, *Lab. Invest.*, **13**:840 (1964).

BOYDEN, E. A.: The Anatomy of the Choledochoduodenal Junction in Man, *Surg. Gynec. Obstet.*, **104**:641 (1957).

BRAUER, R. W.: Liver Circulation and Function, *Physiol. Rev.*, **43**:115 (1963).

BRUNI, C., and K. R. PORTER: The Fine Structure of the Parenchymal Cell of the Normal Rat Liver. I. General Observations, *Amer. J. Path.*, **46**:691 (1965).

BUCHER, N. L. R.: Experimental Aspects of Hepatic Regeneration, *New Eng. J. Med.*, **277**:686 (1967).

BURKEL, W. E.: The Fine Structure of the Terminal Branches of the Hepatic Arterial System of the Rat, *Anat. Rec.*, **167**:329 (1970).

BURSTONE, M. S.: New Histochemical Techniques for the Demonstration of Tissue Oxidase (Cytochrome Oxidase), *J. Histochem. Cytochem.*, **7**:112 (1959).

CAMERON, I. L.: Cell Renewal in the Organs and Tissues of the Nongrowing Adult Mouse, *Texas Rep. Biol. Med.*, **28**:3 (1970).

CAMERON, R., and P. C. HOU: "Biliary Cirrhosis," Charles C Thomas, Publisher, Springfield, Ill., 1962.

CARRIERE, R.: The Growth of the Liver Parenchymal Nuclei and Its Endocrine Regulation, *Int. Rev. Cytol.*, **25**:201 (1969).

CARRUTHERS, J. S., and J. W. STEINER: Fine Structure of Terminal Branches of the Biliary Tree. III. Parenchymal Cell Cohesion and "Intracellular Bile Canaliculi," *Arch. Path.*, **74**:117 (1962).

CHAPMAN, G. B., A. J. CHIARODO, R. J. COFFEY, and K. WIENEKE: The Fine Structure of Mucosal Epithelial Cells of a Pathological Human Gallbladder, *Anat. Rec.*, **154**:579 (1966).

CLAUDE, A.: Growth and Differentiation of Cytoplasmic Membranes in the Course of Lipoprotein Granule Synthesis in the Hepatic Cell. I. Elaboration of Elements of the Golgi Complex, *J. Cell Biol.*, **47**:745 (1970).

DALLMAN, P. R., and J. R. GOODMAN: The Effects of Iron Deficiency on the Hepatocyte: a Biochemical and Ultrastructural Study, *J. Cell Biol.*, **48**:79 (1971).

DALLNER, G., P. SIEKEVITZ, and G. E. PALADE: Biogenesis of Endoplasmic Reticulum Membranes. I. Structural and Chemical Differentiation in Developing Rat Hepatocyte, *J. Cell Biol.*, **30**:73 (1966).

DALLNER, G., P. SIEKEVITZ, and G. E. PALADE: Biogenesis of Endoplasmic Reticulum Membranes. II. Synthesis of Constitutive Microsomal Enzymes in Developing Rat Hepatocyte, *J. Cell Biol.*, **30**:97 (1966).

DE DUVE, C., and P. BAUDHUIN: Peroxisomes (Microbodies and Related Particles), *Physiol. Rev.*, **46**:323 (1966).

DEANE, H. W.: The Basophilic Bodies in Hepatic Cells, *Amer. J. Anat.*, **78**:227 (1946).

DEANE, H. W.: A Cytological Study of the Diurnal Cycle of the Liver of the Mouse in Relation to Storage and Secretion, *Anat. Rec.*, **88**:39 (1944).

DEANE, H. W.: The Cytology of the Mouse Liver in a Controlled Diurnal Cycle, *Anat. Rec.*, **84**:477 (1942).

DOLJANSKI, F.: The Growth of the Liver with Special Reference to Mammals, *Int. Rev. Cytol.*, **10**:217 (1960).

DU BOIS, A. M.: The Embryonic Liver, in C. Rouiller (ed.), "The Liver," vol. 1, p. 1, Academic Press, Inc., New York, 1963.

ELFVING, G.: Crypts and Ducts in the Gallbladder Wall, *Acta Path. Microbiol. Scand.*, **49** (Suppl. 135): 1960.

ELIAS, H.: A Re-examination of the Structure of the Mammalian Liver. I. Parenchymal Architecture; II. The Hepatic Lobule and Its Relation to the Vascular and Biliary Systems, *Amer. J. Anat.*, **84**:311, **85**:379 (1949).

ELIAS, H., and J. C. SHERRICK: "Morphology of the Liver," Academic Press, Inc., New York, 1969.

ESSNER, E., and A. B. NOVIKOFF: Localization of Acid Phosphatase Activity in Hepatic Lysosomes by Means of Electron Microscopy, *J. Biophys. Biochem. Cytol.*, **9**:773 (1961).

FAWCETT, D. W.: Observations on the Cytology and Electron Microscopy of Hepatic Cells, *J. Nat. Cancer Inst.*, **15**:1475 (1955).

FULLER, R. W., and E. R. DILLER: Diurnal Variation of Liver Glycogen and Plasma Free Fatty Acids in Rats Fed ad Libitum or Single Daily Meal, *Metabolism*, **19**:226 (1970).

GATES, G. A., K. S. HENLEY, H. M. POLLARD, E. SCHMIDT, and F. W. SCHMIDT: The Cell Population of Human Liver, *J. Lab. Clin. Med.*, **57**:182 (1961).

GREENWAY, C. V., and R. D. STARK: Hepatic Vascular Bed, *Physiol. Rev.*, **51**:23 (1971).

GRUBB, D. J., and A. L. JONES: Ultrastructure of Hepatic Sinusoids in Sheep, *Anat. Rec.*, **170**:75 (1971).

HAMASHIMA, Y., J. G. HARTER, and A. H. COONS: The Localization of Albumin and Fibrinogen in Human Liver Cells, *J. Cell Biol.*, **20**:271 (1964).

HAMILTON, R. L., D. M. REGEN, M. E. GRAY, and V. S. LE QUIRE: Lipid Transport in Liver. I. Electron Microscopic Identification of Very Low Density Lipoproteins in Perfused Rat Liver, *Lab. Invest.*, **16**:305 (1967).

HAYWARD, A. F.: The Structure of Gallbladder Epithelium, *Int. Rev. Gen. Exp. Zool.*, **3**:205 (1968).

HEALEY, J. E.: Vascular Anatomy of the Liver, *Ann. NY Acad. Sci.*, **170**:8 (1970).

HERING, E.: The Liver, in S. Stricker (ed.), "Manual of Human and Comparative Histology," vol. 2, The New Sydenham Society, London, 1872.

JONES, A. L., and D. T. ARMSTRONG: Increased Cholesterol Biosynthesis Following Phenobarbital Induced Hypertrophy of Endoplasmic Reticulum in Liver, *Proc. Soc. Exp. Biol. Med.*, **119**:1136 (1965).

JONES, A. L., and J. B. EMANS: The Effects of Progesterone Administration on Hepatic Endoplasmic Reticulum: an Electron Microscopic and Biochemical Study, in H. A., Salhanick, D. Kipnes, and R. L. Van deWiele (eds.), "Metabolic Effects of Gonadal Hormones and Contraceptive Steroids," Plenum Press, New York, 1969.

JONES, A. L., and D. W. FAWCETT: Hypertrophy of the Agranular Endoplasmic Reticulum in Hamster Liver Induced by Phenobarbital (with a Review of the Functions of This Organelle in Liver), *J. Histochem. Cytochem.*, **14**:215 (1966).

JONES, A. L., N. B. RUDERMAN, and M. GUILLERMO HERRERA: Electron Microscopic and Biochemical Study of Lipoprotein Synthesis in the Isolated Perfused Rat Liver, *J. Lipid Res.*, **8**:429 (1967).

KADENBACH, B.: Synthesis of Mitochondrial Proteins: Demonstration of a Transfer of Proteins from Microsomes into Mitochondria, *Biophys. Biochim. Acta*, **134**:430 (1966).

KAUFMAN, L., and H. S. MARVER: Biochemical Defects in Two Types of Human Hepatic Porphyria, *New Eng. J. Med.*, **283**:954 (1970).

KAYE, G. I., H. O. WHEELER, R. T. WHITLOCK, and N. LANE: Fluid Transport in the Rabbit Gallbladder. A Combined Physiological and Electron Microscopic Study, *J. Cell Biol.*, **30**:237 (1966).

LEBLOND, C. P., and B. E. WALKER: Renewal of Cell Populations, *Physiol. Rev.*, **36**:255 (1956).

LEGG, P. G., and R. L. WOOD: New Observations on Microbodies. A Cytochemical Study on CPIB-treated Rat Liver, *J. Cell Biol.*, **45**:118 (1970).

LOUD, A. V.: A Quantitative Sterological Description of the Ultrastructure of Normal Rat Liver Parenchymal Cells, *J. Cell Biol.*, **37**:27 (1968).

MAHLEY, R. W., R. L. HAMILTON, and V. S. LE QUIRE: Characterization of Lipoprotein Particles Isolated from the Golgi Apparatus of Rat Liver, *J. Lipid Res.*, **10**:433 (1969).

MALL, F. P.: A Study of the Structural Unit of the Liver, *Amer. J. Anat.*, **5**:227 (1906).

MATTER, ALEX, L. ORCI, and C. ROUILLER: A Study on the Permeability Barriers between Disse's Space and the Bile Canaliculus, *J. Ultrastruct. Res.*, **11** (Suppl): (1969).

MUELLER, J. C., A. L. JONES, and J. A. LONG: Topographical and subcellular anatomy of the guinea pig gallbladder. Gastroenterology. vol. **62**, 1972.

MYRON, D. R., and J. L. CONNELLY: The Morphology of the Swelling Process in Rat Liver Mitochondria, *J. Cell Biol.*, **48**:291 (1971).

NOVIKOFF, A. B.: Cell Heterogeneity within the Hepatic Lobule of the Rat, *J. Histochem. Cytochem.*, **7**:240 (1959).

NOVIKOFF, A., and E. ESSNER: The Liver Cell: Some New Approaches to Its Study, *Amer. J. Med.*, **29**:102 (1960).

NOVIKOFF, A. B., D. H. HAUSMAN, and E. PODBER: The Localization of Adenosine Triphosphate in Liver: *In Situ* Staining and Cell Fractionation Studies, *J. Histochem. Cytochem.*, **6**:61 (1958).

PACKER, L.: Relation of Structure to Energy Coupling in Rat Liver Mitochondria, *Fed. Proc.*, **29**:1533 (1970).

PETERS, T., J. T. DANZI, and C. A. ASHLEY: Effect of the Rate of Albumin Synthesis on the Proportion of Hepatocytes Containing Demonstrable Serum Albumin, *Fed. Proc.*, **27**:775 (1968).

PETERS, T., B. FLEISCHER, and S. FLEISCHER: The Biosynthesis of Rat Serum Albumin. IV. Apparent Passage of Albumin through the Golgi Apparatus during Secretion, *J. Biol. Chem.*, **246**:240 (1971).

POPPER, H., and S. UDENFRIEND: Hepatic Fibrosis. Correlation of Biochemical and Morphologic Investigations. *Amer. J. Med.*, **49**:707 (1970).

RAPPAPORT, A. M.: Anatomic Considerations, in Leon Schiff (ed.), "Diseases of the Liver," 3d ed., pp. 1–49, J. B. Lippincott Company, Philadelphia, 1969.

RIGATUSO, J. L., P. G. LEGG, and R. L. WOOD: Microbody Formation in Regenerating Rat Liver, *J. Histochem. Cytochem.*, **18**:893 (1970).

SABOURIN, C.: Recherches sur l'anatomie normale et pathologique de la glande biliaire de l'homme, Alcan, Paris, 1888.

SASSE, D.: Chemorphology der Glykogensynthese und des Glykogengehalts während der Histogenese der Leber, *Histochemie,* **20**:159 (1969).

SCHACHTER, H., I. JABBAL, R. L. HUDGIN, and I. PINTERIC: Intracellular Localization of Liver Sugar Nucleotide Glycoprotein Glycosyltransferases in a Golgi-rich Fraction, *J. Biol. Chem.,* **245**:1090 (1970).

SCHIMKE, R. T., R. GANSCHOW, D. DOYLE, and I. M. ARIAS: Regulation of Protein Turnover in Mammalian Tissues., *Fed. Proc.,* **27**:1223 (1968).

SCHREIBER, G., R. LESCH, V. WEINSSEN, and J. ZÄHRINGER: The Distribution of Albumin Synthesis Throughout the Liver Lobule, *J. Cell Biol.,* **47**:285 (1970).

STEINER, J. W., and J. S. CARRUTHERS: Studies on the Fine Structure of the Terminal Branches of the Biliary Tree. I. The Morphology of Normal Bile Canaliculi, Bile Pre-ductules (Ducts of Hering) and Bile Ductules, *Amer. J. Path.,* **38**:639 (1961).

STEINER, J. W., and J. S. CARRUTHERS: Studies on the Fine Structure of the Terminal Branches of the Biliary Tree. II. Observations of Pathologically Altered Bile Canaliculi, *Amer. J. Path.,* **39**:41 (1961).

STEINER, J. W., J. S. CARRUTHERS, and S. R. KALIFAT: The Ductular Cell Reaction of Rat Liver in Extrahepatic Cholestasis. I. Proliferated Biliary Epithelial Cells, *Exp. Molec. Path.,* **1**:162 (1962).

TANDLER, B., R. A. ERLANDSON, A. L. SMITH, and E. L. WYNDER: Riboflavin and Mouse Hepatic Cell Structure and Function. II. Division of Mitochondria during Recovery from Simple Deficiency, *J. Cell Biol.,* **41**:477 (1969).

WEISSMAN, G.: Lysosomes, *New Eng. J. Med.,* **273**:1084 (1965).

WHEELER, H. O.: Secretion of Bile, in Leon Schiff (ed.), "Diseases of the Liver," 3d ed., pp. 84–102, J. B. Lippincott Company, Philadelphia, 1969.

WILSON, J. W., and E. H. LEDUC: Movements of Macrophages Studied with the Use of Thorotrast, *J. Nat. Cancer Inst.,* **10**:1348 (1950).

WISSE, E.: An Electron Microscopic Study of the Fenestrated Endothelial Lining of Rat Liver Sinusoids, *J. Ultrastruct. Res.,* **31**:125 (1970).

WOOD, R. L.: Evidence of Species Differences in the Ultrastructure of the Hepatic Sinusoid, *Z. Zellforsch.,* **58**:679 (1963).

chapter 20   The pancreas   SUSUMU ITO

The human pancreas is a large retroperitoneal gland, often more than 20 cm long, lying on the posterior wall of the abdominal cavity behind the stomach. The *head* of the pancreas lies in the curve of the C-shaped duodenum and is joined by a slightly constricted region, or *neck,* to the *body,* or main part of the gland. The thin-tailed portion extends across the abdominal cavity to the spleen. The fresh pancreas is almost white, with a slight pink tinge owing to its vascularity. Unlike other abdominal organs, the pancreas lacks a well-defined capsule. Instead, the outer limit on its ventral aspect is a thin layer of connective tissue and peritoneal mesothelium. The gland is subdivided by delicate connective tissue septa into lobules of a size just visible with the naked eye. Blood and lymphatic vessels, nerves, and excretory ducts run in these septa.

The pancreas is both an exocrine and endocrine gland, and these functions are carried out by distinctly different groups of cells. Digestive enzymes are formed by acinar cells and are delivered by a duct system to the duodenum. Pancreatic hormones regulating carbohydrate metabolism are produced by the cells in the *islets of Langerhans,* which are clusters of endocrine cells embedded within the lobules of acinar tissue. The islets have no duct system; their products, like those of other endocrine glands, are released directly into the circulatory system. ·

The exocrine pancreas

HISTOLOGY OF THE EXOCRINE PANCREAS

The cells responsible for the enzyme-rich pancreatic secretions are the pancreatic *acinar cells,* serous-type cells which form the compound tubuloacinar or tubuloalveolar glands. Clusters of *acini* and their duct systems are separated by areolar connective tissue, which is continuous with that outlining the pancreatic *lobules* (Fig. 20-1). The acinus is composed of a single layer of pyramidal cells with their narrow apical ends bordering the lumen and their broad bases resting on a thin basement membrane and reticular connective tissue. The terminal portions of the pancreatic duct system extend into the acini so that the flattened duct cells are interposed between some of the acinar cells and the lumen.

Figure 20-1 Photomicrograph of human pancreas. Two islets of Langerhans and a number of small intralobular ducts are present in the acinar tissue. An interlobular duct is shown at the lower right. ×160.

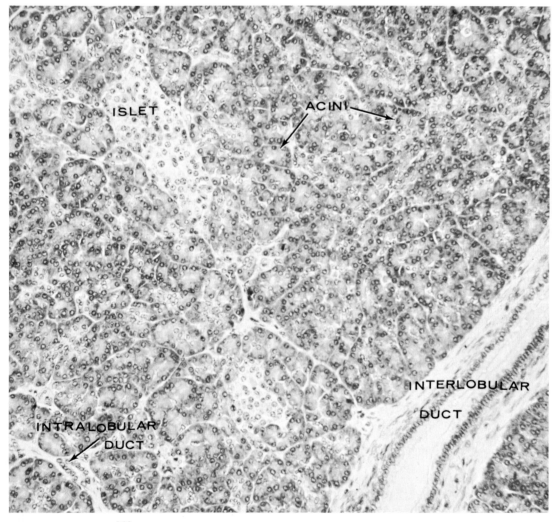

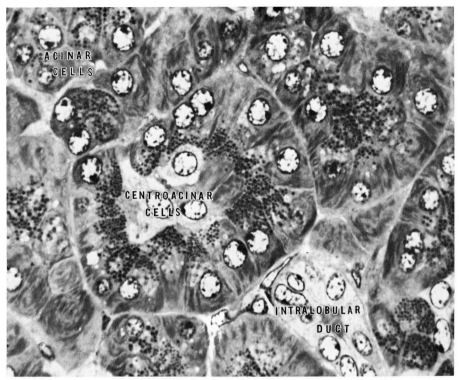

Figure 20-2 Photomicrograph of human pancreas showing several acini and an intralobular duct. Note the preservation of fine cytologic detail in the acinar cells. The apical zymogen granules, the lightly stained supranuclear Golgi complex, and the striated appearance of the basal ergastoplasm are evident. Centroacinar and intralobular duct cells are lightly stained. Formalin fixation, postosmicated, and Epon embedded. Toluidine blue stain. ×1,120.

These duct cells within the acinus are known as the *centroacinar cells* (Fig. 20-2).

In the pancreas of the fasting individual, the apical portion of the acinar cells is laden with many refractile secretory granules, the *zymogen granules*. These possess acidophilic staining properties in routine histologic sections. The intensely basophilic basal portion of the cell appears lamellar or filamentous in favorable light-microscopic preparations (Fig. 20-2). Long before the biochemical nature of this basophilic material was known, it was named *ergastoplasm*. Its strong affinity for basic dyes is now known to be due to a high concentration of ribonucleoprotein. Interspersed with the ergastoplasm are moderate numbers of filamentous mitochondria. A well-developed Golgi complex located in the supranuclear region may be stained by special silver- or osmium tetroxide–impregnation techniques. The precise location of the Golgi complex in the cell varies with the abundance of zymogen granules, being nearer the apex of the cell when few granules are present and supranuclear or lateral to the nucleus during phases in which the apical cytoplasm is filled with stored granules. The basally placed nuclei of the acinar cells are spherical and contain prominent nucleoli. Occasional cells are binucleate.

BLOOD VESSELS, NERVES, AND LYMPHATICS

The arterial blood supply to the pancreas is from the celiac and superior mesenteric arteries, which send branches into the gland along the ducts and in the connective tissue septa. Veins generally accompany the arteries and drain to the portal or the splenic vein. The nerve supply arises from the celiac plexus; bundles of nerve fibers accompany the blood vessels, finally terminating as fine branches on the acini. Myelinated nerves from the vagus are also found in the interlobular connective tissue. Occasional Pacinian corpuscles may be found within the pancreas. The distribution of the lymphatic system within the organ remains to be elucidated.

FINE STRUCTURE OF THE PANCREATIC ACINAR CELL

The fine structure of the pancreatic acinar cells is generally similar to that of other serozymogenic cells, such as serous cells of the salivary glands and the pepsinogenic cells of the gastric glands. Their common characteristics are the presence of an extraordinary abundance of rough endoplasmic reticulum (ER) and the accumulation of zymogen granules.

The predominant organelle in the basal cytoplasm of the pancreatic acinar cell is the rough ER, a membrane system of meandering tubules and flattened cisternae which have numerous ribosomes attached to the cytoplasmic surface (Figs. 20-3 and 20-4). Free ribosomes are also found in abundance in the cytoplasmic matrix. Mitochondria with typical transversely oriented cristae and varying numbers of dense intramitochondrial granules are sequestered between elements of the granular reticulum and along the lateral plasma membrane. Chromatin in the nucleus is generally dispersed, but there is a peripheral accumulation of chromatin adjacent to the nuclear envelope except at the nuclear pores. The outer, ribosome-studded membrane of the nuclear envelope is occasionally continuous with the endoplasmic reticulum. One or two prominent nucleoli are often located adjacent to the nuclear envelope. There are two distinctive zones in the nucleolus. One region, formed of granules resembling the cytoplasmic ribosomes, is arranged into coarse strands that form the nucleolonema; a second finely granular component, which is localized in the interstices, resembles chromatin in its structural appearance.

The extensive Golgi complex is formed of smooth-surfaced membranes arranged in lamellar arrays of flat cisternae with many associated small vesicles and larger vacuoles. Some of the Golgi vacuoles contain flocculent material of intermediate density; others have a dense substance similar to the zymogen granules. These are condensing vacuoles in transitional stages of zymogen granule formation. Direct continuity of the ER and the smooth-surfaced membranes of the Golgi complex are rarely, if ever, observed. However, continuities of the ER with smooth-surfaced vacuolar dilations associated with the Golgi complex have been reported. The relative infrequency of these connections suggests that they may be transitory. In addition to the components of the Golgi complex, one or two centrioles may be found in the cell center, but centrioles are more frequently observed in the apical cytoplasm just beneath the luminal plasma membrane.

Zymogen granules are generally concentrated in the apical cytoplasm just beneath the plasma membrane. The granules are variable in size, the largest measuring up to 1.5 μm in diameter. They are preserved as membrane-limited spherical granules whose density appears to vary with preservation technique. No ordered internal structure has been observed. The interstices between the granules are packed with ribosomes and ER membranes. When few or no granules are present, the rough ER and free ribosomes are distributed throughout the cell.

The luminal end of the cell has a few stubby microvilli coated with a thin layer of fine, radiating, filamentous material. The plasma membranes of adjacent cells are fused into well-developed zonulae occludentes. The relatively straight lateral cell membranes are separated from one another by a narrow space of uniform width, joined by occasional desmosomes. A thin amorphous basement membrane, or lamina, with its associated collagen fibers, underlies the smooth-contoured base of the cell. The acinar cell cytoplasm also contains some dense, membrane-limited lysosome-like bodies, as well as a few multivesicular bodies.

THE DUCTS

Although the smallest ducts are not conspicuous in the usual histologic preparations, an extensive duct system permeates the organ. The apical borders of the acinar cells form the lumina of the acini. Unlike the salivary glands, in which the acini are found at the ends of the intercalated ducts, the pancreatic acinar cells tend to extend into the ducts, so some duct cells are apparently included

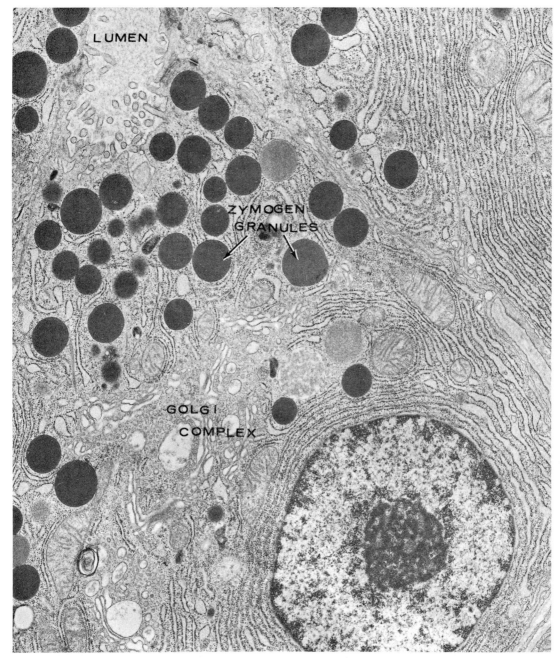

Figure 20-3 Electron micrograph of a human pancreatic acinar cell. The abundant granular endoplasmic reticulum and the store of dense zymogen granules are distinguishing features of this cell. In the supranuclear cytoplasm there is a prominent Golgi complex with zymogen granules in various formative stages. A profile of a zymogen granules whose contents have been discharged into the lumen is present at the apical border. A nucleus with a prominent nucleolus is present near the base of the cell. ×11,500. (All electron micrographs of the human exocrine pancreas were prepared from tissue blocks courtesy of A. Like.)

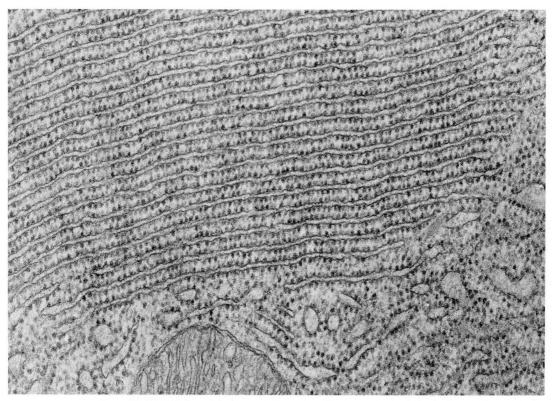

Figure 20-4 Electron micrograph of a small part of a pancreatic acinar cell from the bat. Part of a mitochondrion and a lamella, as well as tubular array of ribosome-studded endoplasmic reticulum, are illustrated. ×65,000.

in the lumen of the acinus and are therefore known as the *centroacinar cells.*

The fine structure of the centroacinar cells and the cells of the small ducts are similar (Figs. 20-5 and 20-6). Both have a sparse covering of microvilli on the free border, and the lateral cell membrane is fairly straight in the centroacinar cells. However, there is considerable interdigitation of intralobular duct cells. The cytoplasm appears empty, in contrast to the acinar cells. The duct cells have a few small mitochondria, a little Golgi complex, and only small amounts of endoplasmic reticulum.

Secretory ducts such as those in salivary glands are not found in the pancreas. The intralobular or intercalated ducts of the pancreas serve as tributaries to the larger *interlobular ducts* located in the connective tissue septa (Fig. 20-1). These interlobular ducts are formed by columnar cells, which appear similar to those of the smaller ducts but are intermingled with occasional goblet cells like those in the intestine. Argentaffin cells are also found in the simple columnar epithelium of the larger pancreatic ducts. The interlobular ducts join the main pancreatic duct, the duct of Wirsung, which traverses the entire length of the organ. Near the duodenum it runs along the ductus choledochus and either joins it or independently enters the ampula of Vater. An accessory duct, the duct of Santorini, located cranial to the main pancreatic duct, is also present. These large ducts are enveloped in a layer of dense connective tissue containing some elastic fibers. Arteries, veins, and lymphatic vessels as well as sympathetic ganglion cells and nerves, which are mostly unmyelinated, are found in the connective tissue surrounding the ducts.

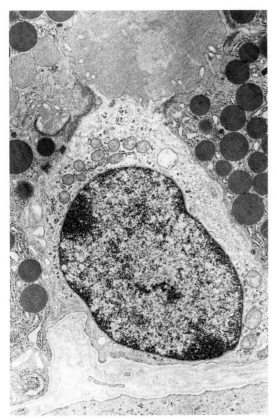

Figure 20-5 A low-power electron micrograph of a human centroacinar cell bordering the luman of a pancreatic acinus. Note the low density of the centroacinar cell cytoplasm and the paucity of cytoplasmic organelles. A basal lamina underlies the duct and acinar cell. The interconnected zymogen granules of low density near the upper left corner are granules which may be discharging their contents into the lumen. × 10,000.

SECRETORY ACTIVITY

The pancreas normally releases its secretions into the intestine when chyme from the stomach enters the duodenum. Secretion may be stimulated experimentally by activation of the vagus nerve, by administration of drugs such as pilocarpine, or by injections of the intestinal hormones secretin or pancreozymin. The pancreatic secretions are highly alkaline, and their enzymes are activated when neutralized by the acidic gastric chyme.

The secretory mechanism of the pancreatic acinar cells studied by direct observations combined with the study of tissue sections prepared by special techniques led investigators to postulate that zymogen granules were formed in the basal ergastoplasm, condensed in the Golgi zone, and stored in the apical cytoplasm. More recently, studies using radioactive amino acids and light and electron-microscopic autoradiography, correlated with biochemical studies of cell fractions, have fully substantiated the early morphologic observations and interpretations.

On the basis of extensive morphologic and biochemical studies of various functional changes of the guinea pig pancreatic acinar cells, Palade and Siekevitz (1958) have postulated that the zymogen is synthesized by the ribosomes on the endoplasmic reticulum. The newly formed enzymes are then transferred to the lumen of the cisternae and, in the guinea pig pancreas, become visible as dense intracisternal granules. Although the mechanism for the transport of material is not clear, the zymogen is apparently transferred to the Golgi complex by an intermediary reticulum.

In the Golgi complex the zymogen is further concentrated in *condensing vacuoles* to the fully formed zymogen granules, which are enclosed in a smooth-surfaced membrane and stored in the apical cytoplasm. The morphologic process of zymogen secretion from the acinar cell is accomplished by the coalescence of the membrane limiting the zymogen granule with the apical plasma membrane. This results in the release of zymogen directly into the lumen.

Caro and Palade (1964) used a radioactively labeled amino acid, [3H]leucine and were able to localize specific sites of synthesis, concentration, and storage of zymogen by making autoradiographs of thin tissue sections and examining them in the electron microscope. It is interesting to note that all these studies using newly developed techniques substantiate the hypothesis made in 1875 by R. Heidenhain, who studied the cytology of the pancreatic acinar cells in various physiologic states.

The time period required for the synthesis of zymogen is quite short. Palade, Siekevitz, and Caro (1962) found that less than 45 min was necessary for a labeled amino acid to be secreted as a component of pancreatic juice. Using light-microscopic autoradiographs of incorporated [3H]leucine, Warshawsky, Leblond, and Droz (1963) showed that the mean life-span of a zymogen

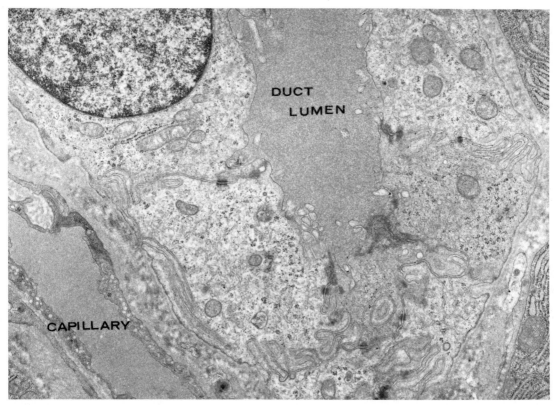

Figure 20-6   Electron micrograph of a small intralobular duct.   The cytoplasm of the duct cells is of low density and contains small mitochondrion and free ribosomes as well as granular and smooth-surfaced endoplasmic reticulum.   Occasional cilia, as shown in the lumen, are present in the ducts.   A small capillary with fenestrated endothelial cells is present in the adjacent connective tissue.   ×13,000.

granule in the rat pancreas is about 47.7 min. The synthesis of zymogen begins in the ergastoplasm within 2 to 5 min and the product is found 15 min later in the Golgi complex.   The enzymes are then stored or secreted from the apical cytoplasm.   Studies by Jamieson and Palade (1971) have shown that discharge of zymogen granules does not require continuous protein synthesis but depends on respiratory energy.   The localization of the pancreatic enzymes chymotrypsin and carboxypeptidase in the zymogen granules was demonstrated histochemically by fluorescein-labeled antibody techniques.

The human pancreas secretes about 2 liters of fluid per day.   At least nine enzymes as well as water, bicarbonate, and salts are found in pancreatic juice.   The presence of the proteolytic enzymes trypsinogen, chymotrypsinogen, and carboxypeptidase has been demonstrated in isolated zymogen granule fractions.   Pancreatic amylase, an enzyme that breaks down carbohydrate, has been found in both zymogen and soluble fractions.   Also present in pancreatic juice are fat-splitting enzymes, lipase and lecithinase, and the nucleic acid–hydrolyzing enzymes, ribonuclease and deoxyribonuclease.

Experimental stimulation of pancreatic secretion by the intestinal hormone secretin elicits a bicarbonate-rich, watery secretion with little enzyme, which apparently comes from the intralobular and interlobular duct cells rather than the acinar cells. Further evidence for this secretory activity lies in the histochemical demonstration of carbonic anhydrase in the duct cells.   Injections of a second hormone, pancreozymin, extracted from the duodenal mucosa, produce a flow of enzyme-rich pancreatic secretion originating from the acinar cells. The mechanism of the action of secretin and pancreozymin on the pancreas is not clear, but these hormones clearly play a major role in the control of enzyme secretion.

Even before the use of hormonal stimulation of pancreatic secretion, physiologists had found that both stimulation of the vagus nerve and administration of pilocarpine produce an enzyme-rich secretion similar to that obtained with pancreozymin.

The endocrine pancreas

The endocrine cells of the pancreas are found in scattered groups throughout the organ and are commonly designated as the *islets of Langerhans,* or simply as the pancreatic islets or islands. These occur as clusters of a few to hundreds of cells embedded in the acinar tissue (Figs. 20-1 and 20-7. and Fig. 20-8, see color insert). Occasional single islet cells may be found among the exocrine secretory cells of the pancreatic acini. The distribution of islets is variable, but in man they are more numerous in the tail of the organ. It has been estimated that approximately 1 million islets are present in a human pancreas.

The islet is highly vascular, with numerous capillaries that probably touch every endocrine cell. In contrast, the acinar tissue is rather poorly supplied with capillaries. This pronounced difference allows for the demonstration of the islets of Langerhans by perfusion with dyes.

In routine histologic preparations, the islet cells show no strikingly individual characteristics. They appear as islands of lightly stained cells (Fig. 20-7) surrounded by a thin layer of reticular fibers. The cells are smaller than those in the surrounding exocrine tissue, so the nuclei appear more closely packed. Appropriate fixation and staining techniques reveal the presence of several cell types. The two most common are the larger, flamed-shaped *alpha,* or *A,* cells which compose about 20 percent and the smaller *beta,* or *B,* cells which compose about 75 percent of the islet cells. The A cells are sometimes absent in the smaller islets and when present tend to be located peripherally.

Both cell types contain characteristic secretory granules whose relative solubility originally distinguished A cells from B cells. The secretory granules of the A cells are preserved by alcohol or Formalin-containing fixatives, whereas the B cell

granules are soluble in alcohol. If both types of granules are preserved by an appropriate fixative such as Zenker-Formol or Bouin's, differences in the staining affinities of the granules can be seen. With

Figure 20-7 Photomicrograph of an islet of Langerhans and the surrounding acini in human pancreas. The different islet cell types cannot be distinguished in routine preparations. Hematoxylin and phloxine. ×380.

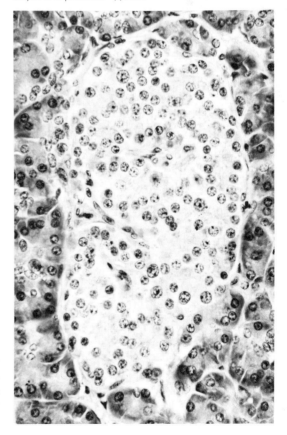

the Gomori aldehyde fuchsin method (Fig. 20-8, see color insert) the A cells contain deep-purple-staining granules and the B cell granules are red.

A third cell type encountered less frequently (about 5 percent) contains small granules with still different staining properties. These cells were first found in human pancreatic islets and designated *delta,* or D cells. They are most numerous in primates but have been described in many other species. A staining characteristic of some of the D cell granules is their capacity to reduce silver nitrate to give the argentaffin reaction. In addition to these cells, a fourth type of agranular, clear cell, the *C* cell, has been observed in the guinea pig pancreas. The nature and significance of these infrequent cell types is unclear. Various possibilities, such as variations in the secretory cycle or degenerative stages of the A or B cells, have been suggested to explain the C and D cells.

Fine structure of the islet cells

Osmium tetroxide fixation preserves the A and B cell secretory granules as dense, membrane-limited structures. The A cell granules are opaque and spherical. After aldehyde fixation an outer mantle of less-dense material fills the space between the dense core and the sac (Fig. 20-10). The structure of the A cell granules appears to be a relatively consistent characteristic among all mammals. The cytoplasm of the A cell contains a well-developed Golgi complex, a moderate amount of rough ER, and free ribosomes. A few small filamentous mitochondria are encountered in the cytoplasmic matrix, which has an overall low density when contrasted with the acinar cells (Fig. 20-7). The nucleus of the A cell tends to be deeply indented or lobulated.

The B cells contain variable numbers of granules (Fig. 20-9), which have distinct morphologic characteristics in different species. In some mammals (rat, mouse, rabbit, guinea pig) the B cell contains granules that are generally similar in size but less opaque than those of the A cells. Furthermore, a large clear space is present between the B cell secretory granule and its limiting membrane. In other species (man, dog, cat, bat), the secretory granules are dense, crystalloid structures in a pale homogenous matrix, enclosed within a loosely fitting limiting membrane (Fig. 20-9). The B cell has a Golgi complex which is more prominent than that of the A cell and contains more rough ER and free ribosomes. The concentration of the reticulum, however, is lower than in the acinar cell. The granules in the B cell tend to be located between the round or ovoid nucleus and the plasma membrane bordering the capillary.

The D cell has not been extensively studied in many species, but it has been described in some as containing numerous membrane-enclosed granules of moderately low density (Fig. 20-11). Islet cells containing no characteristic granules, the C cells, have few organelles and the cytoplasmic matrix is of very low density. Some investigators regard the C and D cells as functional variants of either the A or B cells rather than as separate cell types.

A thin basement membrane or lamina and varying amounts of connective tissue may delineate the islet cells from the acinar cells and extend into the island. However, in many areas the plasma membranes of islet cells are closely apposed to the acinar cell membranes with no intervening basement lamina. Desmosomes are only rarely encountered joining islet cells. However, the cell membranes have folds that are interdigitated with adjacent cells or project into the intercellular space. Distinct basement laminae are always found bordering the base of the capillary endothelium and the adjacent islet cell. The endothelial cells of pancreatic capillaries in both acinar and islet tissues are the fenestrated type. Circular fenestrations are found in attenuated areas of the endothelial cell; they measure some 50 to 100 nm across and appear to have a thin diaphragm extending across the pore.

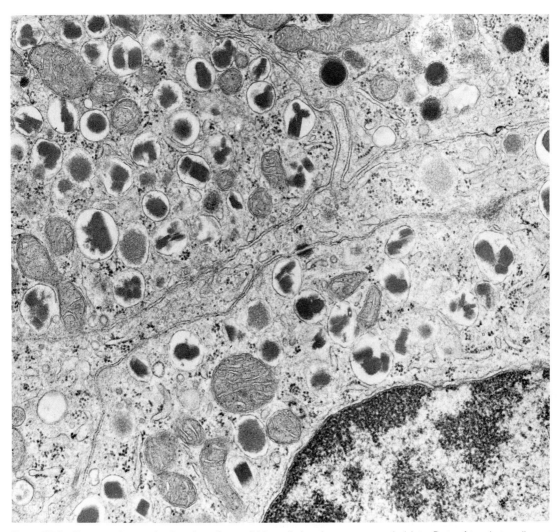

Figure 20-9 Electron micrograph of portion of several islet cells in a human pancreatic islet. Parts of two beta cells containing numerous distinctive crystalline granules in a pale matrix and enclosed by a loose-fitting sac occupy much of this illustration. For comparison a fragment of an A cell is included at the upper right. Desmosomes are relatively infrequent between islet cells, but one is shown near the center of the figure. ×30,000. (Courtesy of A. Like.)

SECRETORY ACTIVITY

Histophysiologic studies on the islets of Langerhans have provided a growing understanding of this endocrine tissue. It is now clear that the islets produce the hormone *insulin,* which stimulates the deposition of glycogen in liver and skeletal muscle and also regulates glucose metabolism. Insulin is important for the proper function of the enzyme hexokinase, which brings about phosphorylation of glucose during both the metabolic degradation of glucose and its incorporation into glycogen. When insulin is present in insufficient amounts or is inactive, glucose is not utilized properly. This causes a rise of the blood glucose level and the excretion

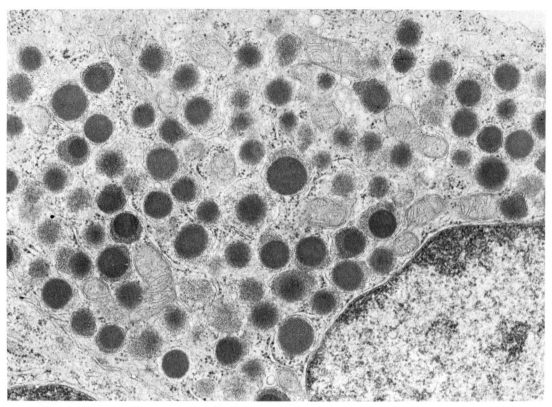

Figure 20-10 Electron micrograph of a portion of an A cell. The dense granules of the human alpha cells are embedded in a material of lower density, the mantal, and enclosed by a smooth membrane. Mitochondrion and granular endoplasmic reticulum are also present. ×31,000. (Courtesy of A. Like.)

of abundant and sweet urine, which is characteristic of diabetes mellitus.

The discovery that the pancreas was involved in carbohydrate metabolism was the result of physiologic studies by Minkowski in the 1880s on pancreatectomized dogs. His assistant noted that flies were attracted to the urine, which was found to contain sugar. The hormonal nature of the islet cell secretions was clearly established by studies in which pancreatic ducts were ligated and in other experiments in which pancreatic tissue was implanted subcutaneously in animals that had been pancreatectomized. In neither of these experimental conditions did glycosuria occur, indicating that a necessary regulating factor was being secreted into the bloodstream by pancreatic cells.

The proof of the origin of pancreatic insulin was

established when insulin was isolated from the whole pancreas. Early attempts to extract pancreatic hormones were unsuccessful because of the proteolytic action of the acinar cell enzymes. However, ligating the pancreatic ducts caused degeneration of the acinar cells but no change in the islets. An extract of such organs was found by Banting et al. (1922) to contain a protein capable of alleviating diabetes mellitus. It was subsequently found that this hormone, insulin, was not inactivated by acid or alcohol, although the exocrine digestive enzymes were destroyed. By using these methods, the direct isolation of insulin from pancreatic tissue was possible.

Insulin is synthesized in the pancreatic islet by the B cell. Histologic examination of the remaining pancreas of animals made diabetic by removing a major part of the pancreas reveals a sequence of changes including degranulation of the cell, followed by hydropic degeneration which may accompany glycogen accumulation. Finally, there is complete degeneration of the B cells. These cytologic alterations are interpreted as the result of pathologic hyperactivity of these cells. Similar changes in the B cells are obtained in animals whose blood glucose concentrations have been experimentally elevated or who have been given excessive amounts of growth hormone.

Further study of islet function has been made possible by the drug *alloxan,* which produces a marked and permanent diabetes mellitus in experimental animals. After an initial increase in B granules, there is a degranulation of the B cells, followed by cell fragmentation. Although alloxan is specific for pancreatic B cells, it also damages other tissues; however, doses of alloxan sufficient to produce diabetes allow the other cells to recover.

The prolonged administration of insulin results in a lowered blood glucose concentration, and the appearance of the B cells suggests that they are in a state of reduced secretory activity. There is an uncommon disease in man, hyperinsulinism, which is due to a tumor of islet tissue in which B cells predominate and produce an excess of insulin with consequently reduced blood glucose levels.

The direct localization of insulin in the B cells has been accomplished with fluorescent antibody techniques and by the direct isolation and assay of these cells for insulin. Lacy and Williamson (1962)

Figure 20-11 Electron micrograph of a portion of a fetal human delta cell and part of an adjacent alpha cell. The granules of the cell type are of lower density, homogeneous composition, and enclosed by a tight fitting membrane. ×25,000. (Courtesy of A. Like.)

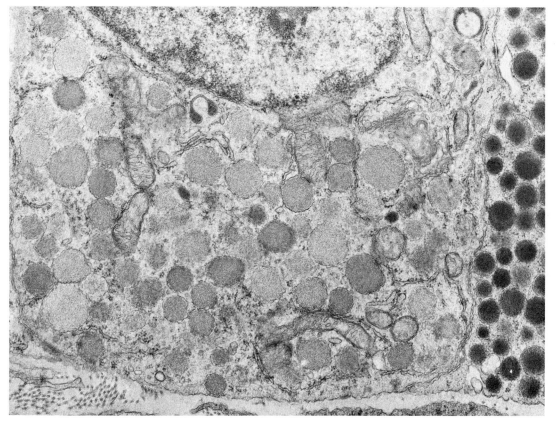

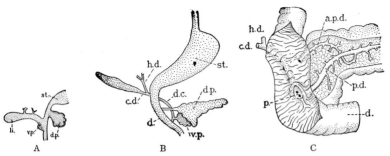

Figure 20-12   A and B. Diagram of the pancreas of human embryos, 10 and 15 mm.   C. Dissection of duodenum and pancreas of adult human. a.p.d., accessory pancreatic duct; c.d. cyst duct; d., duodenum; d.c., ductus choledochus; d.p. dorsal pancreas; h.d., hepatic duct; li., liver; p., duodenal papilla; p.d., pancreatic duct; st., stomach; v.p., ventral pancreas.

have calculated that each B cell of the rabbit contains 1.7 μU of insulin.

Evidence for the precise endocrine function of the A cell is less clear than for the B cell. However, there is good indication that the A cells are the source of *glucagon,* a hormone which affects sugar metabolism by accelerating liver glycogenesis and raising blood glucose. The localization of glucagon in the islet is suggested by the greater amount that can be isolated from the tail than from the head of the pancreas. Furthermore, the uncinate process of the dog pancreas is apparently devoid of A cells and no glucagon has been extracted from this region. Evidence for the origin of glucagon from the A cells is suggested by the undiminished amounts of glucagon extractable from the pancreases of alloxan diabetic rats and by immunofluorescent antibody studies which indicate that glucagon is localized in A cells.

Little is known of the contents of the C and D cells of the islets or of their physiologic roles.

Development of the pancreas

The pancreas arises in the human embryo during the fourth week of gestation as two separate outpocketings of the intestinal tube near the level of the common bile duct. These primordia, the dorsal and ventral pancreases, later meet and fuse (Fig. 20-12A and B). The dorsal portion enlarges much more rapidly and becomes the tail, body, and part of the head of the adult pancreas, and the ventral pancreas contributes to the remaining portion of the head. The duct of the ventral pancreas becomes the main outlet, which empties directly into the duodenum or into the common bile duct. The duct of the dorsal pancreas becomes the accessory pancreatic duct, which lies slightly cranial to the main duct and is smaller (Fig. 20-12C).

During development, the pancreas forms a ramifying system of tubules composed of a single layer of undifferentiated cells. These differentiate into *duct cells, acinar cells,* and *islet cells.* The duct cells retain some regenerative capacity in the adult organ. In addition to the differentiated duct cells in the adult pancreas, there are small tubular arrays of undifferentiated cells from which new acinar and islet cells will arise. Differentiated acinar tissues and islet cells are first found in the fetal pancreas during the third or fourth month of gestation.

References

BANTING, F. G., C. H. BEST, J. B. COLLIP, W. R. CAMPBELL, and A. A. FLETCHER: Pancreatic Extracts in the Treatment of Diabetes Mellitus, *Canad. Med. Ass. J.*, **12**:141 (1922).

BAUM, J. B., B. E. SIMMONS, R. H. UNGER, and L. L. MADISON: Localization of Glucagon in the Alpha Cells in the Pancreatic Islet by Immunofluorescent Techniques, *Diabetes*, **11**:371 (1962).

BECKER, V.: Histochemistry of the Exocrine Pancreas, in A. V. S. de Reuck and M. P. Cameron (eds.), "The Exocrine Pancreas," Ciba Foundation Symposium, Little, Brown, Boston, 1962.

BENCOSME, S. A., R. A. ALLEN, and H. LATTA: Functioning Pancreatic Islet Cell Tumors Studied Electron Microscopically, *Amer. J. Path.*, **42**:1 (1963).

BENSLEY, R. R.: Studies on the Pancreas of the Guinea Pig, *Amer. J. Anat.*, **12**:297 (1911).

CARAMIA, F.: Electron Microscopic Description of a Third Cell Type in the Islets of the Rat Pancreas, *Amer. J. Anat.*, **112**:53 (1963).

CARO, L. G., and G. E. PALADE: Protein Synthesis, Storage, and Discharge in the Pancreatic Exocrine Cell. An Autoradiographic Study, *J. Cell Biol.*, **20**:473 (1964).

COVELL, W. P.: A Microscopic Study of Pancreatic Secretion in the Living Animal, *Anat. Rec.*, **40**:213 (1928).

DE DUVE, C.: Glucagon: The Hyperglycaemic Glycogenolytic Factor of the Pancreas, *Lancet*, **2**:99 (1953).

DIXIT, P. K., I. P. LOWE, C. B. HEGGESTAD, and A. LAZAROW: Insulin Content of Microdissected Fetal Islets Obtained from Diabetic and Normal Rats, *Diabetes*, **13**:71 (1964).

EKHOLM, R., T. ZELANDER, and Y. EDLUNG: The Ultrastructural Organization of the Rat Exocrine Pancreas. I. Acinar cells, *J. Ultrastruct. Res.*, **7**:61 (1962).

GOMORI, G.: Observations with Differential Stains on Human Islets of Langerhans, *Amer. J. Path.*, **17**:395 (1941).

HERMAN, L., T. SATO, and P. J. FITZGERALD: The Pancreas, in S. M. KURTZ (ed.), "Electron Microscopic Anatomy," Academic Press, New York, 1964.

ICHIKAWA, A.: Fine Structural Changes in Response to Hormonal Stimulation of the Perfused Canine Pancreas, *J. Cell Biol.*, **24**:369 (1965).

JAMIESON, J. D., and G. E. PALADE: Condensing Vacuole Conversion and Zymogen Granule Discharge in Pancreatic Exocrine Cells: Metabolic Studies, *J. Cell Biol.*, **48**:503 (1971).

LACY, P. E.: The Pancreatic Beta Cell: Structure and Function, *New Eng. J. Med.*, **276**:187 (1967).

LACY, P. E., and J. R. WILLIAMSON: Quantitative Histochemistry of the Islets of Langerhans. II. Insulin Content of Dissected Beta Cells, *Diabetes*, **11**:101 (1962).

LAZAROW, A.: Cell Types of the Islets of Langerhans and the Hormones They Produce, *Diabetes*, **6**:222 (1957).

LAZARUS, S. S., and B. W. VOLK: Histochemical and Electron Microscopic Studies of a Functioning Insulinoma, *Lab. Invest.*, **11**:1279 (1962).

LIKE, A. A.: The Ultrastructure of the Secretory Cells of the Islets of Langerhans in Man, *Lab. Invest.*, **16**:937 (1967).

LIKE, A. A., and W. L. CHICK: Studies in the Diabetic Mutant Mouse. II. Electron Microscopy of Pancreatic Islets, *Diabetologia*, **6**:216 (1970).

MARSHALL, J. M.: Distributions of Chymotrypsinogen, Procarboxypeptidase, Desoxyribonuclease, and Ribonuclease in Bovine Pancreas, *Exp. Cell Res.*, **6**:240 (1954).

MUNGER, B. L., F. CARAMIA, and P. E. LACY: The Ultrastructural Basis for the Identification of Cell Types in the Pancreatic Islets. II. Rabbit, Dog and Opossum, *Z. Zellforsch.*, **67:**776 (1965).

OPIE, E. L.: Cytology of the Pancreas, in E. V. Cowdry (ed.), "Special Cytology," 2d ed., vol. 1, Hoeber-Harper, New York, 1932.

PALADE, G. E.: Functional Changes in the Structure of Cell Components, in T. Hayashi (ed.), "Subcellular Particles," Ronald Press, New York, 1959.

PALADE, G. E., P. SIEKEVITZ, and L. G. CARO: Structure, Chemistry and Function of the Pancreatic Exocrine Cell, in A. V. S. de Reuck and M. P. Cameron (eds.), "The Exocrine Pancreas," Ciba Foundation Symposium, Little, Brown, Boston, 1962.

RENOLD, A. E.: Insulin Biosynthesis and Secretion—A Still Unsettled Topic. *New Eng. J. Med.*, **282:**173 (1970).

SIEKEVITZ, P., and G. E. PALADE: A Cytochemical Study on the Pancreas of the Guinea Pig. I. Isolation and Enzymatic Activities of Cell Fractions, *J. Biophys. Biochem. Cytol.*, **4:**203 (1958).

SIEKEVITZ, P., and G. E. PALADE: A Cytochemical Study on the Pancreas of the Guinea Pig. II. Functional Variations in the Enzymatic Activity of Microsomes, *J. Biophys. Biochem. Cytol.*, **4:**309 (1958).

SJÖSTRAND, F. S.: The Fine Structure of the Exocrine Pancreas Cells, in A. V. S. de Reuck and M. P. Cameron (eds.), "The Exocrine Pancreas," Ciba Foundation Symposium, Little, Brown, Boston, 1962.

THOMAS, T. B.: Cellular Components of the Mammalian Islets of Langerhans, *Amer. J. Anat.*, **62:**31 (1937).

WARSHAWSKY, H., C. P. LEBLOND, and B. DROZ: Synthesis and Migration of Proteins in the Cells of the Exocrine Pancreas as Revealed by Specific Activity Determination from Radioautographs, *J. Cell Biol.*, **16:**1 (1963).

ZIMMERMANN, K. W.: Die Speicheldrüsen der Mundhöhle und die Bauchspeicheldrüse, in W. von Möllendorff (ed.), "Handbuch mikroskop. Anat. Menschen," vol. 5, pt. 1, Springer Verlag, Berlin, 1927.

chapter 21   The respiratory system

SERGEI P. SOROKIN

The respiratory system consists of the lungs and a number of associated structures whose primary functions are to provide the living organism with oxygen from the air and to remove excess carbon dioxide from the bloodstream. The system is composed of three functional parts: a conducting portion, a respiratory region, and a ventilating mechanism. The *conducting portion* of the system includes the nasal cavity and associated sinuses, the nasopharynx, the larynx, the trachea, and the branching bronchial passages of the lungs. Collectively they warm, moisten, and filter the inspired air before it reaches the expansive *respiratory region* of the lungs, located distal to the bronchial tubes. There the cellular barrier between inspired air and bloodstream is sufficiently thin to promote rapid exchange of gases. An efficient musculoelastic mechanism moves air over the respiratory surface and forms a third functional part of the system. The components of this *ventilating mechanism* include the thoracic cage and its intercostal muscles, the muscular diaphragm, and the elastic connective tissue of the lungs. During inspiration, contraction of the muscles raises the ribs and lowers the floor of the thoracic cavity to increase its volume and to expand the lungs. During expiration, the muscles relax; elastic recoil of the expanded pulmonary tissue causes the thorax to contract. In forced expiration the natural recoil is abetted by contraction of the abdominal and external intercostal muscles, which decrease the volume of the thoracic cavity and lungs beyond their normal resting levels.

Nasal cavity and sinuses

The surfaces of the nasal cavity are covered by two types of lining: a *respiratory mucosa* that warms and moistens the air, and an *olfactory mucosa* that houses the receptors of smell. As the first segment of the conducting portion of the respiratory tract, the cavity is most fully developed in warm-blooded animals, where it is well separated from the oral cavity by the hard palate. The olfactory mucosa occupies a large proportion of the nasal lining of keen-scented animals such as carnivores and rooting ungulates; it is greatly restricted in primates and other forms that have a poor sense of smell. The respiratory mucosa is well developed in both the keen- and the feebly scented. In the former, the mucosa is both more highly folded and more extensive in area; moistening the air enhances olfaction.

Figure 21-1 Section through the nasal septum of a monkey, showing hyaline cartilage on the left and the richly glandular nasal mucosa on the right. Masson's trichrome stain. ×50.

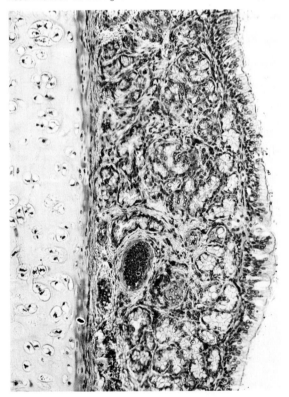

RESPIRATORY MUCOSA

The nasal cavity is divided into symmetric halves by the nasal septum (Fig. 21-1), which contains hyaline cartilage. Stratified squamous epithelium of the facial skin continues through the nostrils into the *vestibule*, beneath the projecting cartilaginous portion of the nose. There large hairs and associated sebaceous glands form the first defense against the entry of particulate matter. Posteriorly the hair and glands become sparse, and the epithelium thins as it approaches the paired openings to the principal nasal chambers, located within the skull. These are smooth-sided along the septum but are convoluted laterally by turbinate projections from the underlying ethmoid and inferior turbinated bones, and each forms a narrow, ribbon-like passage for air. Their surfaces total some 160 cm^2 in man and are coated with a mucous film. These anatomic arrangements help to promote turbulence in air flow; this assures the mucous film effective contact with the air stream. The epithelium beneath is pseudostratified, ciliated, and columnar. Goblet cells are abundantly but unevenly distributed within it, since they concentrate in sheltered regions. More exposed portions of the epithelium, such as that over the turbinates, may have small areas of transition to a stratified squamous lining. In fine structure, this epithelium resembles the epithelium of the trachea and bronchi described later.

Numerous branched, tubuloalveolar glands extend into the underlying connective tissue as invaginations of the epithelium. They resemble minor salivary glands, having short ducts and acini both lined by secretory cells. These vary widely in type within a mucous to serous range, and the cellular makeup of a typical gland varies with the species. In general, mucous cells occur nearer the openings of the glands along the ducts and acini, whereas serous cells occur more peripherally in the acini or in demilunes beyond them. The larger ducts occasionally contain a distinct columnar epithelium that separates the secretory cells from the surface lining of the nasal cavity, but the columnar cells lack basal striations and give no indication of participation in the secretory process.

Beneath the epithelium, the connective tissue is of fairly uniform composition until it blends into the periosteal and perichondrial layers of the nasal skeleton. Epithelium and glands are enveloped in a richly collagenous connective tissue. Mononuclear leukocytes may infiltrate the tissue freely or may occur as nodular aggregations.

Vascular supply The vascular supply to the nose is rich and has several unusual features. Although some differences in distributional pattern exist among mammals, the respiratory and olfactory mucosae usually have separate arterial supplies: the sphenopalatine and the ethmoidal arteries, respectively. Both vessels and their branches anastomose rather freely throughout their subdivisions. The main vessels to the respiratory mucosa lie next to the periosteum in a latticework pattern that becomes a close-meshed net as they run either obliquely or horizontally forward across the nasal septum and lateral walls. In contrast, arteries to the olfactory region spread out in a radial array. The main respiratory arteries send out superficial arcading branches; from them, other vessels run perpendicularly toward the surface, where they divide into arterioles that supply a network of capillaries just beneath the epithelium, and into others for the glands and the submucosal tissues. Arteriovenous anastomoses are common, particularly where the vasculature is richest, as in the path of the inspiratory stream and in the swell bodies described below (Fig. 21-2). These communicating vessels are tortuous; in their thick walls the medial smooth muscle has an epithelioid appearance, and the intima lacks an internal elastic membrane. As befits a secretory mucosa, the subepithelial and periglandular capillaries are fenestrated whereas the deeper ones are not. The veins are rather more conspicuous than the arteries, particularly where they lie over the arteries, as they do in man, dogs, cats, and rabbits. There they exist as a superficial, fine-meshed plexus of small vessels and a deeper, coarser latticework of thick-walled tubes. These drain into larger veins at the anterior and posterior ends of the nasal cavity. In addition, a well-developed lymphatic system is present.

Over the middle and inferior turbinates the superficial venous plexus consists of cavernous, thin-walled vessels that lack muscular septa but otherwise resemble erectile tissue (Chap. 26). This is the region of the *swell bodies*. In man and in other animals, blood flow is so regulated there that hourly periods of swelling occur alternately on the two sides of the nasal cavity, causing a reduction in air flow on the affected side and an upward deflection of the air stream on inspiration. Most of the respired air passes through the neighboring passage, giving the mucosa on the occluded side time to recover from dessication and haply assisting the narial muscles in directing air to the olfactory region. This physiologic cycle is regulated autonomically. Engorgement results from constriction of the deeper veins and dilatation of the arterioles that feed the plexus through capillaries. Adrenergic fibers from the superior cervical ganglion not only form rich networks over the arteries and arterioles, as in other vascular beds, but over the veins as well, particularly in the swell bodies. They exert a tonic, vasoconstrictive action. Cholinergic nerves from the pterygopalatine ganglion promote vasodilatation and secretion by the glands. In the olfactory region, on the other hand, blood flow is not clearly affected by either sympatho- or parasympathomimetic agents.

Histophysiology From the rear of the nasal cavity forward, the numerous circulatory loops each receive fresh arterial blood; but blood flow in the

Figure 21-2 Arterial supply to the nasal mucosa. (After J. D. K. Dawes and M. M. L. Prichard, J. Anat., **87**:311, 1953.)

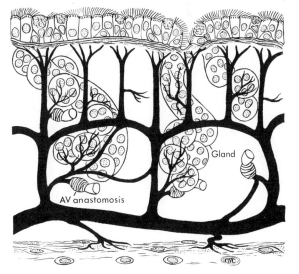

Gland

AV anastomosis

superficial vessels of each loop generally counters the flow of inspired air, and the whole forms a compound countercurrent system.   Viewed from the surface, the small vessels are set in rows as in a heat exchanger.   These are ranked most closely under surfaces most exposed to the inspiratory system, where glands are particularly abundant as well.   In an engineer's terms, the nose is said to function like a scrubbing tower supplied with fresh fluid at successive levels.   Despite a fractional-second contact time with the nasal mucosa, the inspired air is more efficiently cleared of ozone, sulfur dioxide, and other water-soluble polutant gases—far better than by the oropharynx.   These gases are dissolved in the mucous carpet overlying the epithelium and are partially absorbed and partially carried off to the pharynx by ciliary action.

OLFACTORY MUCOSA

The olfactory mucosa of man is limited to an area that covers some 500 mm^2 of the roof of the nasal cavity and upper portions of the nasal septum. Compared with the respiratory mucosa, its pseudo-stratified columnar lining is taller, and the glands

beneath are of a serous rather than mixed type (Fig. 21-3).   The mucosa produces an ample fluid secretion in which odored substances are dissolved before being detected by cells of the epithelium. Three cell types predominate: *olfactory cells, sustentacular cells,* and *basal cells.*   Olfactory cells are bipolar neurons.   The others combine characteristics of epithelial and Schwann cells.   The tall sustentacular cell is differentiated along secretory lines, whereas the short basal cell is undifferentiated and remains able to divide and to transform into either of the mature types.   Special methods, such as silver impregnation or staining with methylene blue, are needed in order to distinguish the cells clearly by light microscopy.   In routine sections identification is aided by a tendency for the round nuclei of olfactory cells to occur at a level between those of the basal cells and the ovoid nuclei of the supporting cells.

Individual olfactory cells within the epithelium respond differently to various odors; nonetheless these receptors all look alike.   They are widest about the nucleus and from there taper into two processes, an apically directed *dendrite* and a centrally directed *axon.*   Unlike many neurons, the cell

Figure 21-3   Vertical section through the olfactory region of an adult human being.   ×400.

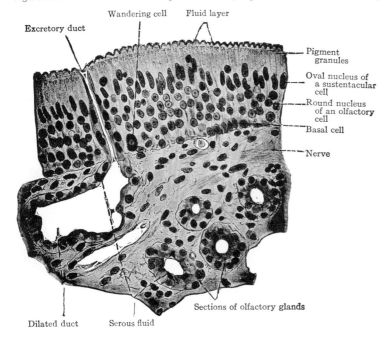

Wandering cell   Fluid layer

Excretory duct

Pigment granules

Oval nucleus of a sustentacular cell

Round nucleus of an olfactory cell

Basal cell

Nerve

Sections of olfactory glands

Dilated duct   Serous fluid

body contains little ergastoplasm, but a supranuclear Golgi apparatus and other organelles are present in moderation. The dendrite, approximately 1 μm in thickness, is crowded with microtubules that run along its length in parallel courses. Its apical end extends above the surface of the epithelium as a bulbous *olfactory knob,* which contains basal bodies, mitochondria, and profiles of agranular reticulum and bears a tuft of cilia. Among different vertebrates the shape of this knob and the number of cilia present are highly variable characteristics of this cell. Frequently the knob measures about 4 μm high by 1.5 μm thick, and the cilia number 6 to 12 (Fig. 21-4). These have the dimensions and "9 + 2" axial structure of typical cilia for a few micrometers, then abruptly narrow to half the usual diameter for the remainder of their length. Ciliary tubules within the distal segment change in configuration from doublets to singlets and gradually diminish in number. The shafts may be as long as 80 μm in cats, and the distal segment may be four or five times longer than the proximal segment in frogs. These measurements differ in other species. Olfactory cilia rarely exhibit motility. Their distal segments are too thoroughly enmeshed with other cilia and microvilli in the surface fluid to beat effectively. More certainly, they greatly increase receptor cell exposure to odorate substances.

Below the nucleus the olfactory cell becomes drawn into a threadlike axon. As its diameter approximates 0.2 μm, the process is just visible in the light microscope. It extends below the basal lamina to join axons from adjacent cells in forming small fascicles, which become invested by Schwann cells. The fascicles penetrate the cribriform plate of the ethmoid bone and become grouped into *fila olfactoria.* These lead into the ipsilateral member of the paired *olfactory bulbs,* where the axons synapse.

Among cells of the olfactory epithelium the sustentacular cells are the most numerous and most conspicuous. They differ in histochemical attributes from olfactory cells but share some of them, such as a capacity for reducing TPN (NADP), with basal cells and those of the glands beneath. These cells are rich in organelles, notably a supranuclear Golgi apparatus and a tightly compacted agranular reticulum. Together with numerous lipid-rich granules, the reticulum may fill the apical cytoplasm.

Apart from lysosomes, other membrane-bounded granules are present. They give the cells a secretory complexion even if the granules differ in appearance from one species to another. Along the apical surface microvilli are prominent. Laterally the cells form the usual variety of junctional contacts with adjacent olfactory and sustentacular cells, but so-called *gap junctions* have not been observed. As a rule, these cells are spaced so as to separate adjacent olfactory cells. Moreover, they ensheath the dendritic and axonal processes of those neurons in mesaxons and in this respect resemble gliocytes. Metabolic exchanges evidently occur along the sustentacular-olfactory interfaces. Accordingly the supportive function of these cells can be understood broadly. Toward the base of the epithelium, olfactory axons become ensheathed in processes from basal cells, only these are finger-like rather than sheet-like and the wrapping is discontinuous (Fig. 21-4).

Beneath the olfactory epithelium the connective tissue contains the branched tubuloalveolar glands of Bowman and myelinated fibers of the trigeminal nerve, in addition to unmyelinated olfactory axons, Schwann cells, and the usual elements of connective tissue. Cuboidal cells of Bowman's glands contain secretory granules and discharge a serous fluid onto the olfactory surface by way of excretory ducts, which are lined by flattened cells (Fig. 21-3). The glands secrete continuously and provide fresh solvent for odored substances. The fibers of the trigeminal nerve terminate in slender processes that extend into the epithelium. Some of them synapse with nonciliated brush cells sparsely distributed there (Fig. 21-4) and elsewhere in the nasal and pulmonary linings. In the nose these cells possibly play a minor role in olfaction, for some trigeminal input reaches the olfactory bulbs. They may also provide sensory input for the sneeze reflex. Blood vessels to the olfactory region supply a rich subepithelial capillary plexus and a deeper one of veins. Lymphatics run among the veins, and the tissue blends into the subjacent perichondrium and periosteum.

Histophysiology   It has proved more difficult for man to form concepts about olfaction than to conceptualize the processes of seeing and hearing. For one thing, he has no experience of olfaction to compare with his working knowledge of the other modalities gained from centuries spent in building optical devices, musical instruments, and the like. Accordingly, olfactory structure-function relationships remain crudely understood. Notwithstanding, the olfactory cell is recognized as the primary receptor for smell, because only this cell type degenerates after sectioning of the olfactory nerves. Moreover, it resembles known sensory cells of the eye and ear in such details as the presence of some type of cilia at the apex, in the microtubular arrays between the apex and main body of the cell, and in the sheathing of its proc-

Figure 21-4 Olfactory epithelium, showing three-dimensional and ultrastructural aspects.

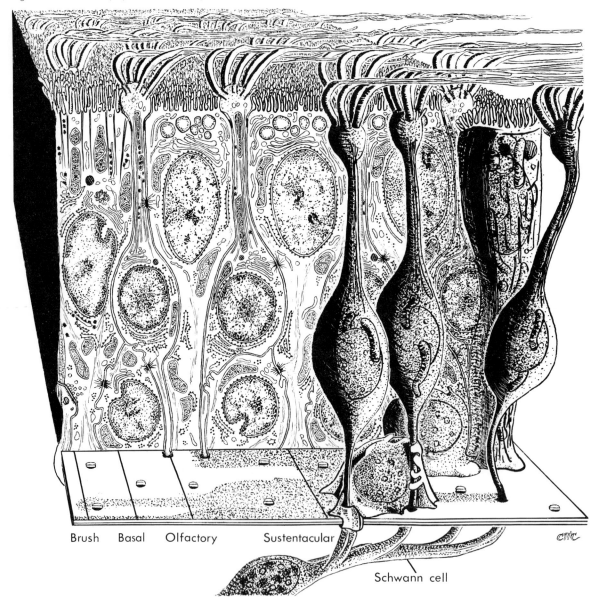

Brush   Basal   Olfactory   Sustentacular

Schwann cell

esses by other elements of the epithelium. If an odored substance is added to the surface fluid, this is reflected by a change in electrical potential recorded along the nerve. The change in potential probably is a summation of several activating and inhibitory discharges, including a negative potential representing the olfactory cell's initial response to stimulation and a positive potential associated with secretion by neighboring cells. Stimulation of the olfactory cell apparently results from depolarization of the plasma membrane covering distal portions of the cilia, for in extending through an often thick surface coating, these processes make first contact with the stimulating substance. In exceptional instances olfactory cells are not provided with cilia, but then the surface coating is thin and depolarization occurs on the microvilli.

It is not known precisely how the olfactory cells become stimulated, nor how collectively they are able to discriminate among a vast range of odors. Most vertebrate receptors seem to respond to a fairly wide range of substances. Insects possess an additional class of highly specific receptors for pheromones, which trigger stereotyped behavioral responses, but, although such responses are recognized as well in mammals, the receptors for them have not been identified in the olfactory epithelium. Clinical data provide evidence for less than 100 specific anosmias in man; this is but one reason to believe that his olfactory cells respond to a limited number of "primary odors," with a range being perceived by differential action. Experimental evidence furthermore suggests that human olfactory discrimination often correlates with the shape of the stimulant molecules; this has led to a stereochemical theory of olfaction and a search for specific receptor proteins along the cell surface. Such a theory can account for the remarkable phenomenon of olfactory adaptation, whereby odors first noticed on entering a room are soon forgotten; but it must be conceded that the primary odors for man may not be the same as those for another animal. Moreover, the theory must become reconciled to certain cases where stereochemically related compounds provoke dissimilar responses.

If the foregoing is uncertain, it is even less clear how olfactory neurons interact electrically with adjacent cells in the absence of gap junctions or other interfacial specializations considered prerequisite to electrical coupling. Nonetheless, signals are received from the epithelium and become partially integrated with other input in the cell bodies of the neurons before being transmitted along the axon. Axons from adjacent cells at first run in parallel but become intermixed as they enter the outermost layer of the olfactory bulb, so that the projection of the epithelium onto the bulb is not precisely topographic as it is in projections of the retina or cochlea on nuclei of the brain. The olfactory axons branch and synapse with dendrites of second-order neurons, termed *mitral* or *tufted* cells, within spherical tangles of neuropil, termed *olfactory glomeruli*. Signals from about 1,000 olfactory cells converge on each second-order cell. In mammals each second-order cell sends its one main dendrite to a single glomerulus so that a given glomerular system represents a specific group of olfactory cells and can be so projected centrally. In the bulb, numerous subsidiary circuits connect neurons of the mitral series with smaller granule cells, as evidenced by the presence of dendrodendritic, dendroaxonal, and somatodendritic synapses between them. These circuits provide a basis for amplifying or inhibiting incoming signals and are abetted by feedback to the granule cells from higher centers. Recordings made from olfactory bulbs of human subjects seem to show that at this level odor quality is coded as patterns of frequency components, whereas odor detection is dependent on adequate signal strength and its characterization on still greater amplitude. From the bulbs, incoming signals are passed to third-order neurons in the olfactory cortex and nearby subcortical regions at the base of the forebrain. These higher centers and the olfactory bulbs interact directly or indirectly with more caudal parts of the brain, including the thalamus and hypothalamus. Olfactory sensations are represented bilaterally, owing to the presence of interbulbar fibers and cross connections at higher levels.

VOMERONASAL ORGANS

The vomeronasal (Jacobson's) organs are paired tubular structures located in the floor of the nasal cavity along each side of the septum. Their cavities are lined in part by an *accessory olfactory epithelium* and open by ducts either to the nasal or oral cavities. They are well developed in many mammals but in primates exist only during embryonic life. The accessory epithelium and the glands beneath resemble their counterparts in the olfactory mucosa, but accessory olfactory cells often lack cilia and their axons lead to small *accessory olfactory bulbs,* located one to a side. These are like olfactory bulbs of amphibians, which are simple in structure and do not possess segregated glomerular systems, as do the mammalian bulbs. The function of these organs is unknown; it is likely they are more involved than the olfactory mucosa with behavioral responses related to specific odors.

PARANASAL SINUSES

The paranasal sinuses are blind pockets that reach the nasal cavity through narrow openings. Their linings are continuous with the nasal mucosa and are similar in type, although less highly developed. Much of the epithelium is simple, ciliated, and columnar; the glands are smaller; and the connective tissue is reduced in amount. The sinuses contribute to the humidification of the nasal cavity. In keen-scented carnivores, portions of the sphenoidal and frontal sinuses may be occupied by ethmoturbinal bodies and serve as extensions of the olfactory area.

Nasopharynx

The pseudostratified ciliated columnar lining and glands of the nasal mucosa continue into the upper or nasal portion of the pharynx. With some interruption by stratified epithelium as the oropharynx and larynx are crossed, a similar covering is found in the remaining major conducting portions of the respiratory tract. In the pharynx, however, the mucosa becomes thinner and generally rests directly upon skeletal muscle, being separated from it by a broad elastic layer. Below the *fornix,* or roof of the pharynx, a zone of stratified columnar epithelium may extend for short distances as the lining undergoes transition to the noncornified, stratified squamous epithelium typical of the oral cavity and oropharynx. Ventrally, stratified squamous epithelium covers most of the nasal surface of the soft palate; laterally the ciliated epithelium extends

downward around the openings of the eustachian tubes, which are similarly lined. The midline *pharyngeal tonsil* is located on the dorsal wall of the nasopharynx. Patches of stratified squamous epithelium are common on its surface, but pseudostratified columnar cells predominate. Ordinarily small, the tonsil may become quite large in childhood and, together with lymphoid tissue near the auditory orifices, constitute the *adenoids.* Stratified squamous epithelium is continued below the oropharynx into the laryngeal pharynx, where the respiratory tract becomes separated from the alimentary tract at the entrance to the larynx. During swallowing movements, food is excluded from the nasopharynx by the contraction of the pharyngopalatine muscles and the retraction of the uvula between them.

Larynx

The larynx is a hollow, bilaterally symmetric structure framed by cartilages, bound together by ligaments and muscles, and located between the pharynx and the trachea. It acts primarily as a valve to prevent swallowed food from entering the lower respiratory tract, but it is a tone-producing instrument as well, and in man it has important additional functions in the production of speech. The anatomic valve itself is termed the *glottis* and

consists of a pair of lateral mucosal folds, the *vocal folds,* located partway inside the larynx. The size of the glottal aperture changes with circumstance. Partly open during quiet breathing, it widens to permit deep inspiration but closes prior to swallowing and before intrathoracic or intraabdominal pressures are raised. During phonation the aperture fluctuates rapidly between slightly open and fully closed positions.

GENERAL STRUCTURE

The larynx (Fig. 21-5) is based on a ring-shaped *cricoid* cartilage which rests upon the trachea. Above, the ventral and lateral walls of the larynx are framed largely by a shield-like *thyroid* cartilage, which articulates with the side of the cricoid by means of two *inferior cornua* and with the hyoid bone by means of two *superior cornua*. A pair of pyramidal, *arytenoid* cartilages arise from the dorso-cranial surface of the cricoid cartilage and delimit the dorsal wall. The summit of each is capped by a small *corniculate* cartilage. A midline *epiglottis* extends cranially from within the thyroid to define the ventral border of the laryngeal entrance, becomes attached to the hyoid bone, and thereafter ends as a clublike protuberance in the pharynx. These framing cartilages are linked to each other by means of striated *intrinsic muscles,* whose ori-

gins and insertions are confined to laryngeal structures. They are also interconnected by means of dense connective tissue, notably a sheet-like cricothyroid membrane and several thyrohyoid ligaments. The latter, together with the *extrinsic muscles,* help to attach the larynx to adjacent structures. In effect, the larynx is suspended from the hyoid bone and to some extent can slide up and down within a sleeve of connective tissue in accommodating itself to functional needs.

Within the larynx the mucosa is thrown into three pairs of lateral folds. The first pair stretches between the tips of the arytenoid cartilages and the epiglottis at the laryngeal entrance, frequently being stiffened by small *cuneiform* cartilages embedded within. These are the *aryepiglottic folds.* The *ventricular folds,* or false vocal folds, are next, and the true *vocal folds* are last. Both of these may contain slight cartilaginous support, especially near their dorsal points of attachment, respectively, to the ventricular and vocal processes of the arytenoids. Both insert on the thyroid cartilage ventrally. Above the vocal folds the laryngeal space (*vestibule*) is roughly triangular in cross section, and between vocal and ventricular folds the side walls recess to form the *laryngeal ventricles.* Below the vocal folds the lumen (*atrium*) gradually becomes cylindrical.

The glottis The glottal aperture is bordered by a pair of *vocal ligaments,* one to each side within the vocal folds, and from them it receives its configuration. The ligaments are bands of elastic connective tissue that extend from the arytenoid cartilage of each side to insert partly on a midline point on the thyroid cartilage (Fig. 21-7) and partly on portions of the cricothyroid membrane adjacent. The vocal folds also contain striated muscle fibers of the thyroarytenoid group, which lie lateral to the ligaments on each side and insert into the thyroid and arytenoid cartilages. Being suspended between these two cartilages, both of which articulate with the cricoid, each vocal fold is affected whenever the cartilages are moved. Since the intrinsic muscles interconnect the laryngeal cartilages, by their actions they serve to regulate the glottis. By the same token, they move the ventricular folds as well, though to a lesser extent. The principal actions to affect the glottal aperture are those that rock the arytenoids on the cricoid and those that rock and

Figure 21-5   Diagram of the human larynx showing the dorsal aspect on the left and a cutaway view of ventricular and vocal folds on the right.   Approximately × 1.5.

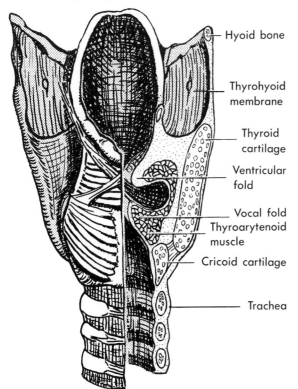

Hyoid bone

Thyrohyoid membrane

Thyroid cartilage

Ventricular fold

Vocal fold
Thyroarytenoid muscle

Cricoid cartilage

Trachea

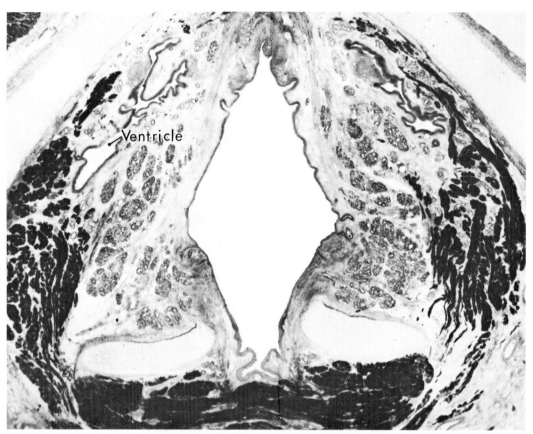

Figure 21-6 Cross section of the human larynx at the level of the ventricular folds. Muscles (arytenoideus and ventricularis portion of thyroarytenoideus) and glands are revealed by their reaction for succinic dehydrogenase. The ventricular appendixes extend between the folds and the thyroid cartilage (top of picture). ×10.

glide the thyroid on the cricoid. When the arytenoids are rotated outward (action of the posterior cricoarytenoid muscles) the glottis opens. Conversely, when they are rotated inward (lateral cricoarytenoids and interarytenoids), or when they are approximated in a gliding motion (arytenoid), it closes. When the thyroid is tilted forward (cricothyroids) or the cricoid is pulled backward (lateral cricothyroids and extrinsic cricopharyngeus) the vocal folds stretch, and when the thyroid is tilted backward (thyroarytenoids) they relax. Such muscular actions are related primarily to the valvular function of the glottis, for not all are essential to phonation. In phases of deglutition the larynx is moved principally by the extrinsic muscles. The

intrinsic muscles nevertheless contribute to this process by drawing the arytenoid cartilages forward against the epiglottis to help close off the larynx (thyroarytenoids, aryepiglottics, and arytenoid).

HISTOLOGY

Epithelium and glands The mucosa of the larynx is continuous with that of the pharynx and the trachea and exhibits features of both. Stratified squamous epithelium from above extends partway into the larynx, over the aryepiglottic folds laterally and somewhat further ventrally, where it covers the entire lingual side of the epiglottis and the upper half of its laryngeal aspect. It is also present at other points of wear, such as over the vocal folds and the arytenoid cartilages.   Elsewhere this gives way to a pseudostratified, ciliated, columnar lining after passage through a transitional zone of stratified columnar epithelium.   The pseudostratified epithelium and its associated glands resemble those of the trachea and bronchi and function similarly in conditioning the inspired air and in adding to the protective coating of mucus spread over the epithelial surface.   Much of this is swept up to the larynx from the lower respiratory tract and in turn is driven into the pharynx by local ciliary action.

Figure 21-7   Cross section of the human larynx at the level of the true vocal folds.   The vocal ligaments are elevated above part of the laryngeal ventricles on each side.   ×8.

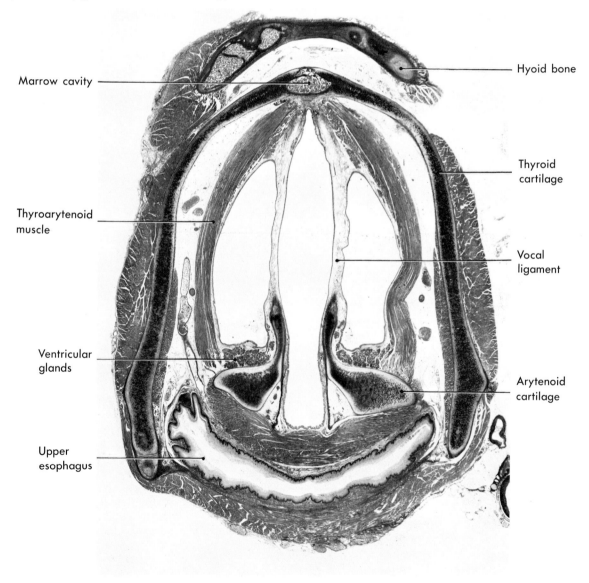

The laryngeal glands are small, branching, tubulo-alveolar invaginations of the epithelium. They occur in groups and generally remain confined to the lamina propria. Exceptionally they may penetrate parts of the framing cartilages. Most frequently, as in man, these deep excursions occur only in relation to the epiglottis and give that cartilage a uniquely pockmarked appearance. The glands are especially abundant along the rim of the aryepiglottic fold; these are *arytenoid glands*. Many occur as well in the ventricular folds (Fig. 21-6) and in the dorsal wall of the laryngeal ventricles. They are absent from the vocal ligaments and only gradually reappear toward the base of the vocal folds, whence they increase and eventually encircle the laryngeal space at the level of the cricoid cartilage. Most of the glands produce a mucous secretion that stains less brilliantly with PAS and differs in other ways from the mucus of goblet cells. Accordingly, they can be considered *seromucous* glands, keeping in mind the limitations of the term.

Figure 21-8   Part of a seromucous acinus in the epiglottis of the little brown bat, showing an intraepithelial nerve ending with synaptic vesicles.   ×12,000.

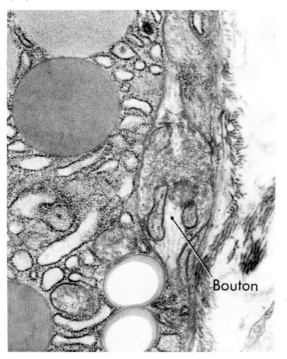

Bouton

Like their counterparts in the nose and in conducting airways of the lungs, the laryngeal glands are regulated by unmyelinated nerves. These frequently penetrate the basal laminae of acini and ramify among the secretory cells as thread-like processes each bearing one or more swellings charged with predominantly clear (cholinergic) synaptic vesicles (Fig. 21-8). In addition to glands, a few taste buds occur at the base of the epiglottis.

Connective tissue   Within the larynx the usual elements of connective tissue are combined in a great variety of textures. Beneath the epithelium this tissue is a rather loose lamina propria, but this becomes denser around solid structures and so is not everywhere distinct from the encircling submucosa. All cell types are represented, as are all the fibers, but elastic fibers are unusually abundant. These are heaviest in the glottis where they are bundled in parallel arrays to make up the vocal ligaments, which may be regarded as thickenings of the submucous cricothyroid membrane. The fibers of this membrane diminish in size and number in caudal parts of the vocal folds, and the lamina propria above it becomes particularly loose so that it offers little resistance to edematous swelling. Consequently, during laryngeal infections it sometimes threatens the airway with obstruction. Small lymphoid nodules and migratory leukocytes frequently occur in this tissue, as might be expected from its proximity to the outside environment. Such nodules rarely are found near the glottis but become prominent below in the atrial part of the larynx. In capillaries supplying the epithelium and glands, fenestrated plaques appear in the endothelium at points where the vessels closely approach the basal laminae. The capillaries drain into venous plexuses situated more deeply. The lymphatic system is similarly arranged with a superficial network leading to a deeper plexus of larger vessels.

Cartilage   The laryngeal cartilages not only furnish examples of all the main histologic types of cartilage but illustrate some of the variations to be found within each type. Early in life all are hyaline cartilages. Later on, most of the cuneiforms and corniculates, part of the epiglottis, and the apices and vocal processes of the arytenoids become converted to elastic cartilage, and smaller portions of the epiglottis and the arytenoids become fibrocartilage. In sum, the larger structural cartilages remain hyaline, whereas the smaller ones become elastic. The fiber-containing cartilages of the larynx differ from each other most conspicuously in the patterns made by their fibrous networks. These follow lines of stress and may be curved and interlacing in the epiglottis but are straight and parallel where the vocal ligaments join the arytenoids. Certain differences are seen as well among the hyaline cartilages. For example, the capsular matrix often is more basophilic in the thyroid cartilage than in the others. However, any of the hyaline cartilages may ossify with age, and a marrow cavity may form inside the bone (Fig. 21-7). Among these variant cartilages the epiglottis stands out, for, although its cells unquestionably are chondrocytes, its matrix is sparse, variously admixed with other connective tissue cells and fibers, and closely intruded on by adjacent tissues. In some species it resembles *chondroid tissue* of lower vertebrates more than typical mammalian cartilage.

Muscle and nerves All the laryngeal muscle is cross-striated muscle, an unusual tissue to find in tubular viscera of vertebrates but present there as well as in adjacent portions of the esophagus. Functionally this muscle enables the larynx to carry out its specialized tasks. Phylogenetically it reflects the development of this region from the visceral skeletal system derived from splanchnic mesoblast and formed into cartilages and muscles of the mandibular, hyoid, and branchial arches. At first intended to expand and contract the pharynx for purposes of feeding and respiration, the muscles were later put to new uses as the branchial arches became transformed into the skeleton of the larynx. The intrinsic muscles seem to be composed of fiber types in the intermediate to red range, judging from criteria discussed in the chapter on muscle. The fibers are small and strongly reactive for the mitochondrial enzyme succinic dehydrogenase. Furthermore, electron micrographs of these muscles show that the mitochondria frequently occur in subsarcolemmal and interfibrillar chains. In bats, cricothyroid fibers additionally possess a highly developed sarcoplasmic reticulum. Such visible features might well help these muscles to achieve short refractory periods and rapid contrac-

tility, but alone they are an inadequate basis for predicting muscular performance. More certainly, physiologic characteristics of skeletal muscles are greatly influenced by their innervation.

The larynx is extensively represented in both sensory and motor cortex, and the muscles are under fine control. This is projected through the pyramidal system to motor neurons in the *nucleus ambiguus,* and signals reach the larynx through branches of the vagus nerve. One of these, the superior laryngeal nerve, innervates the cricothyroid muscle through its external branch. Other intrinsic muscles are controlled by the recurrent laryngeal nerve. Afferent impulses from the larynx initiate the cough reflex, mediate a general chemical sense, and influence reflex activity in swallowing. Sensory and secretomotor impulses are carried predominantly by the internal branch of the superior laryngeal nerve. It represents most of the region above the glottis and the subglottal region as well, through communication with the recurrent nerve. Sensory input travels this path to cell bodies in the *nodose ganglion.* Sensation from part of the area of the epiglottis is carried to the *petrous ganglion* of the glossopharyngeal nerve, whose domain is in the vicinity of the nasopharynx. Sympathetic innervation to the larynx is much as described in the section on the trachea. Owing to the small size of laryngeal motor units as well as to the widespread autonomic and sensory innervation of the region, laryngeal tissues are richly supplied with nerves. These are arranged in superficial and deep plexuses.

ROLE OF THE LARYNX IN PHONATION
Speaking and singing are characteristic human activities controlled by large segments of the human brain and effected principally by means of the larynx, other parts of the respiratory system, and structures in the mouth. In these activities, the mouth is relatively more important to speech and the larynx to singing. In both cases the glottis is the usual source of *voiced sound,* which is produced by the passage of air driven by elevated subglottic pressure through the closed vocal folds. These part intermittently to emit puffs of air, and this alternately compressed and rarefied air is delivered to the airways above, which act as resonating cavities. Voiced sound has a fundamental fre-

quency determined by the mass of the vocal ligaments, their length, and their tension. This acoustic system has been likened to that of a reed organ pipe, where air is passed from a wind chest through the reed and into the organ pipe. In man, however, the driving pressure, the pitch of the reed (glottis), and the size of the resonant cavity all are variable and not fixed. In singing, the larynx is called on to produce fundamental tones of greatly varied pitch, whereas for speech only a limited range is called for, centering around 125 cycles per second for men and around 225 for women. Moreover, certain sounds of speech, such as the f in fast, are not voiced but produced with an open glottis, whereas others, such as the h in hat, are produced by gradual closure, or aspiration. The resonant cavities are of importance because, depending upon their size and shape, they reinforce the fundamental tone and tones of higher pitch derived from the overtone series, beginning with a frequency of about 400 cycles per second. The laryngeal vestibule and the nasopharynx form a resonant cavity in the neck that automatically tunes itself to the frequency sung, because as the pitch is raised the larynx slides upward and shortens the cavity. The nasal cavity and sinuses are tuned to certain frequencies only, as their dimensions are fixed. The oral cavity is formed into a very finely tunable resonator regulated by movements of the tongue, the jaws, the soft palate, and the lips. It can be seen that speech sounds are generated principally in the mouth and not in the larynx; for spoken sounds can be whispered, and this is done with a partially open glottis. Roughly speaking, vowel sounds are steady-state sounds and consonants are transient ones, exceptions being the nasal sounds m and n, the rolled r, and the sustained s. Each vowel sound is characterized by a set of fixed pitches to which the oral resonator is tuned. This sound is excited by a laryngeal tone of equal or lower pitch. It is precisely when words are sung to high tones that the different requirements of singing and speech become clear; for if the laryngeal tone is higher than the ones needed to excite a certain vowel sound, the vowel cannot be pronounced correctly.

Glottic structure related to phonation It is believed that during phonation the edges of the closed glottis are driven apart by subglottic pressure but are drawn together again by a Bernoulli force and by *elastic recoil* of the vocal folds. This is the summation of the tension in stretched elastic fibers of the vocal ligaments and the tension exerted between antagonistic pairs of intrinsic muscles, principally the cricothyroids acting against the thyroarytenoids. Certain other muscles are involved as well, such as those acting to hold the folds together. The loudness of sound emitted from the larynx increases as the vocal folds are approximated, and when the glottis is closed, further increases result largely from increases in subglottic pressure. It has been argued that the *vocalis* muscle, the part of the thyroarytenoid group that lies adjacent to the vocal ligament, influences both character and volume of laryngeal sound by helping to open the vocal folds during phonation. This argument is based upon claims that some of the vocalis fibers insert on the vocal ligaments instead of on the cartilages. Such claims have been disputed convincingly in the case of man, although it is true some vocalis fibers insert into the cricothyroid membrane below the glottis. The argument remains a vital one in relation to the larynx of certain bats who use bursts of intense laryngeal ultrasound for purposes of echolocation.

On the whole, laryngeal muscles act more to alter the pitch and mode of vibration of the vocal folds than to initiate phonation or to amplify its intensity. Characteristically, these results can be achieved in more than one way. For example, the pitch of the laryngeal sound can be changed either by altering the tension, the length, or the mass of the vocal ligaments, or by causing only part of their length to vibrate. Similarly, by thinning out the edges of the glottal aperture the mode of vibration can be changed and the falsetto tone then results. All these changes require complex muscle action. In trained singers they seem to involve the intrinsic muscles more and extrinsic muscles less than they do in the case of vocal amateurs.

Human ventricular folds, pervaded by glands, are not well suited to phonation. They close over the closed glottis prior to coughing. Old-time singers made use of this action to initiate their vocal attack in a maneuver known as *coup de glotte*. In echolocating bats, however, these folds may be as thin and flexible as the true vocal folds.

Trachea

The trachea or windpipe is a hollow tube originating at the base of the larynx and ending below at the *carina,* where it bifurcates to form the main airway, or *primary bronchus,* of each lung. Like the other conducting portions of the respiratory system, the trachea conditions the air as it passes to the lungs and provides protection from dust and airborne infection. It runs close to the ventral surface of the neck largely unstrengthened by neighboring tissues. Consequently, it would collapse during forceful inspiration, or on inspiration against a closed glottis, were it not reinforced by a skeleton of cartilage embedded in its wall. This represents a part of the visceral skeleton of vertebrates, homologous to the fifth branchial arch of fish, and, like the laryngeal cartilages, adapted to new uses by terrestrial forms. To some extent, tracheal structures seem to reflect divergent *branchial* and *pulmonary* influences exerted on them during development. Although retaining a midline position and in large measure the bilateral symmetry associated with it, the trachea acquires a more radial plan of organization than that possessed by the larynx, and the tissues become arranged in concentric layers of mucosa, submucosa, an incomplete muscularis, and adventitia. This radial plan becomes fully developed in the bronchi and serves as the organizational basis for succeeding intrapulmonary airways.

HISTOLOGY

Epithelium and glands The tracheal mucosa closely resembles that of the nose and nasopharynx and is virtually identical with that in the lower part of the larynx and in the pulmonary bronchi. It is secretory, harboring many exocrine glands and being lined by a pseudostratified columnar epithelium in which *ciliated* and *mucous* cells predominate. This epithelium is taller in large mammals than in small ones. It may vary in appearance even among individuals of the same species, since it is sensitive to irritation and responds by increasing in height while its mucous cells and the glands beneath undergo hypertrophy. With more intense or prolonged irritation, portions of the epithelium may assume a stratified squamous form through a process of change termed *squamous metaplasia* by pathologists. This change arguably is within the epithelium's normal expressive range, since islands of stratified squamous cells normally occur in exposed parts of the pseudostratified lining of the upper airway and remain stable for a lifetime. In addition to ciliated and mucous cells, *basal* (short) cells stand out because their nuclei form a row close to the basement lamina to give the epithelium its apparently stratified appearance. These cells do not extend to the free surface and evidently serve as a reserve population for the epithelium. Other types of cells have minority representation but often escape notice completely because their distinguishing features are poorly resolved by light microscopy.

As seen by electron microscopy, at least six different cell types make up this laryngobronchial epithelium. Ultrastructural characteristics of these cells are illustrated in Fig. 21-9. The epithelium exhibits moderately high levels of activity for mitochondrial enzymes associated with oxidative phosphorylation and for lysosomal enzymes. Much of this activity is attributable to the ciliated and mucous cells. In ciliated cells the mitochondria tend to concentrate just below the apical cytoplasm which contains the ciliary basal bodies. The basal bodies are ranged in a single layer and number about 300 per cell. Each is a centriole that has produced a cilium, and these extend from the basal bodies through the surface microvillous layer and into the lumen of the airway. At the base of these cells one sometimes sees one or two centrioles unassociated with cilia. The supranuclear region is occupied by the Golgi apparatus and various lysosomal elements, including a few large residual bodies. Ciliated cells have only moderate numbers of ribosomes, either free or attached to membranes of the endoplasmic reticulum, so that the appreciable cytoplasmic basophilia of this epithelium is ascribable in larger measure to the mucous cells. These resemble goblet cells of the small intestine and exhibit characteristics of protein-secreting cells: an extensive, cisternal ergastoplasm housed in the lower part of the cell, a supranuclear Golgi apparatus, and an apical cytoplasm charged with membrane-bounded but ofttimes coalescing mu-

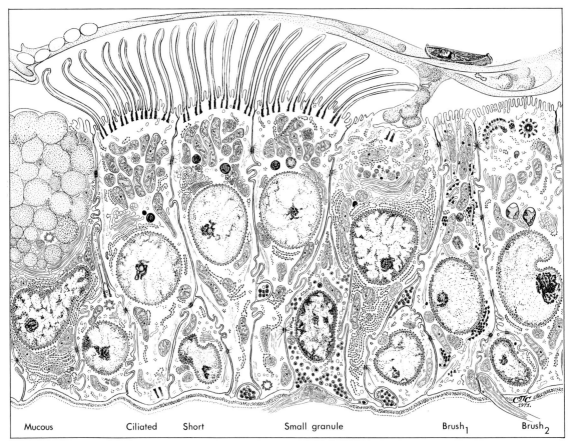

Figure 21-9   Diagram showing ultrastructural characteristics of cells in the laryngobronchial epithelium.

Mucous	Ciliated	Short	Small granule	Brush₁	Brush₂

cous droplets.   In these cells the centrioles usually are seen amidst the secretory material in the apical cytoplasm.   When secretion occurs, the droplets are shed along with some of the cytoplasmic threads separating them.   Thereafter the centrioles seem to become active in reconstituting the apical plasmalemma.   A cell that has just released its secretion no longer is identifiable by light microscopy as a mucous cell and becomes another nonciliated cell in the epithelium.   Collectively these are called *brush* cells, a term that recognizes their microvillous border as one of few distinctive features.   Among this heterogeneous group a small number have been shown to possess epitheliodendritic (afferent) synapses with nerve processes that reach the cells from the underlying connective

tissue (Fig. 21-9, brush₁).   Consequently, these brush cells have been considered sensory receptors.   They have numerous glycogen granules as well as a preponderance of agranular reticulum in their cytoplasm.   In other brush cells, precursors of the basal bodies or intermediates in some other differentiative process may occur in the cytoplasm (Fig. 21-9, brush₂), indicating that these cells are immature and have recently replaced cells that have been cast off from the epithelium.   Basal (short) cells often contain strands of a keratinoid material in the cytoplasm but otherwise appear even less differentiated than the immature brush cells.

Small-granule cells occupy a basal position in the epithelium along with the short cells.   These unusual cells possess many small (1000 to 3000 Å) dense cored granules that resemble the neurosecretory granules of adrenal medullary cells (Chap. 31), which are rich in catecholamines. They extend slender processes containing these granules among the epithelial cells and along the basement lamina. Small-granule cells occur either singly or in small clusters; they are closely associated with nerve processes, many bearing synaptic vesicles, that are directed toward the epithelium. Similar cells are widely although sparsely distributed elsewhere in the epithelium and glands of conducting airways in the respiratory system. Judging from morphologic evidence, it appears that these cells participate as effectors in the integration of secretory processes. The conducting airways also contain intraepithelial nerves. These are typical nervous processes containing parallel microtubular arrays along much of their length. They ramify throughout the lower part of the epithelium in potential spaces between the lateral surfaces of the cells. These spaces open up somewhat when the cells become distended with fluid; more frequently they are obliterated, and adjacent cell membranes appear tightly interlocked. The cells are joined to each other on the sides by desmosomes and near the apical surface by junctional complexes.

Tracheal glands share essential features and a certain variability as to cell type with the glands of the larynx and pulmonary bronchi. In man they are mixed mucous glands with serous crescents, and they occur in far greater numbers than in the otherwise similar tracheas of the great apes. Around the tracheal lumen the glands generally extend into the submucosa. They are more highly developed dorsally where they may penetrate the muscularis to enter the adventitia. A more detailed discussion of the cell types in these glands will be found in the section on bronchi.

Connective tissue   The connective tissue compartments of the trachea are not as well defined as they are in the walls of the alimentary tract (Chap. 18). This is especially true of small mammals where the total thickness of the tracheal wall is meager. In man one distinguishes a lamina propria, a submucosa, and an adventitia. The lamina propria of the mucosa is a loose tissue containing interwoven collagenous and elastic fibers, many small vascular channels, and the usual fixed and wandering cells of connective tissue. The elastic fibers are joined into a continuous network in which the heavier fibers run in a predominantly longitudinal direction but are interconnected by slender fibrils. Peripherally these fibers become condensed into an *elastic membrane* that demarcates the lamina propria from the submucosa (Fig. 21-16), which contains the distributing vessels and larger lymphatics of the tracheal wall. The submucosa has relatively fewer elastic fibers and more collagen than the propria; these fibers run in bundles among the glands and serve to bind the elastic network of the propria to the enveloping cartilaginous skeleton. The submucosa ends by blending into the perichondrium of the cartilages.

Cartilage   The tracheal cartilages are irregular, crescentic rings embedded in a fibrous connective tissue that forms a tube about the submucosa. There are 16 to 20 cartilages in man. These are evenly spaced within the fibrous membrane, which normally is not fully stretched and so permits some tracheal movement. They sometimes branch, and adjacent cartilages sometimes fuse with one another, but all are incomplete dorsally where the trachea contacts the esophagus. These gaps are bridged by fibrous tissue and bands of smooth muscle joining the ends of the cartilages. Near the tracheal bifurcation a few longitudinal muscle fibers run outside the transverse bands to link a number of the cartilages with the dorsal portion of the carinal ridge. This area receives additional support from the last cartilage, which extends under the bifurcation as well as around the sides of the trachea. In animals subject to unusually high transtracheal pressures, the tracheal skeleton may be modified in different ways. In seals the tracheal rings are supplemented by smaller cartilages embedded in the fibrous membrane, and the whole structure is stiffened; in bats the cartilages overlap each other like roofing tiles and provide additional buttressing at little cost in flexibility. Topographically, the tracheal skeleton occupies the innermost portion of the adventitia, but over the dorsum the muscularis takes up the corresponding part of the wall. Developmentally, the cartilage layer is distinct from the rest of the adventitia; the cartilages appear as independent chondrifications within a continuous, crescentic, cartilage-forming rudiment, which persists in adult life as the fibrous membrane. Histologically, the cartilages are hyaline but become fibrous with age. The perichondrium is virtually inseparable from the fibrous membrane and is thicker on the outer than on the inner surface of the rings. External to this region the adventitia becomes an areolar tissue rich in fat cells. It carries nerves and blood vessels to the trachea, receives its lymphatic drainage, and blends into tissues of the neck and of the mediastinum.

NERVES, BLOOD VESSELS, AND LYMPHATICS

The nervous, vascular, and lymphatic supplies to the trachea are independent of those to the lungs, although they resemble their counterparts in the walls of the larger pulmonary airways and function in concert with them. The trachea receives visceral afferent fibers and sympathetic and parasympathetic efferents. In its innervation it differs from the pharynx or larynx principally in lacking a branchial motor component. The courses of individual fibers are all but impossible to trace because the sensory and autonomic nerves all contribute to plexuses formed about the viscera and while crossing them frequently exchange fibers. Rostral to the trachea such a plexus occurs in the lateral and dorsal walls of the pharynx, and caudally another (*pulmonary plexus*) occurs around the tracheal bifurcation. Some of the fibers in these networks end in the trachea. *Visceral afferent* fibers leave the trachea and adjacent structures through branches of the vagus nerve and travel to the nodose ganglion, or else they separate in the pharyngeal plexus and pass through the sympathetic trunk to reach cell bodies in the dorsal root ganglia of cervical and upper thoracic nerves. Cell bodies of preganglionic *sympathetic* efferents occur at upper thoracic levels of the spinal cord. Postganglionic fibers are said to originate from the three cervical ganglia and from the upper thoracic portion of the sympathetic trunk. Preganglionic *parasympathetic* fibers originate in the dorsal motor nucleus of the vagus and synapse with second-order neurons located in small tracheal ganglia embedded in the adventitia and submucosa. Fibers of all the foregoing types reach the tracheal wall chiefly from the left side through the left recurrent nerve, but some reach it from the right through the vagus and its right recurrent branch.

Tracheal tissues receive systemic blood through branches of the inferior thyroid arteries. These ramify in the submucosa and near the carina anastomose with bronchial arteries, which supply the bronchi walls. Venous blood drains through the thyroid venous plexus and returns to the systemic circuit via the middle and inferior thyroid veins. Tracheal lymphatics lead out laterally to a few paratracheal nodes located beside the recurrent nerves, and to nodes of the superior deep cervical chain.

The lungs

EXTERNAL FORM

The primary bronchi of the right and left lungs arise in the mediastinum from the bifurcation of the trachea. They follow a short extrapulmonary course and together with the main pulmonary vessels and nerves enter the hilum of their respective lungs. These occupy the thoracic cavity which is smaller on the left than on the right owing to the position of the heart. Consequently, the right lung is always larger than the left and almost always is subdivided into a greater number of *lobes*. The lobes are separated from each other to varying degrees among different animal species but are confluent medially in the vicinity of the main bronchus. In man there are three on the right and two on the left, but in many mammals the right lung has a fourth, infracardiac lobe extending between the heart and the diaphragm. Where the heart strongly inclines to the left, as in the insectivores, the left lung has but one lobe. Just as the lungs can be subdivided into lobes, the lobes can be subdivided into smaller units, termed *bronchopulmonary segments, subsegments*, and *lobules;* these are demarcated to varying degrees by fissures on the lobar surfaces. For all its varied appearance, the outward form of the lung imperfectly reflects its underlying structure, for a sheet of visceral pleura covers the surfaces. In providing an airtight capsule the pleura effectively conceals the system of airways, together with associated respiratory tissue and vascular supplies, that form the structural basis of the organ.

INTERNAL STRUCTURE

The lungs of birds and mammals are structurally the most complex of vertebrate lungs. Each is marvellously adapted to supply the large amounts of oxygen that these animals use; avian and mammalian lungs nevertheless differ basically from each other in the organization of conducting and respiratory regions. This chapter is concerned only with mammalian lungs, which share a single structural plan among all their prototherian, metatherian, and eutherian representatives. Wide variations on this plan nevertheless occur in some mammalian groups, especially among the marine mammals.

Each lung is organized fundamentally about its system of airways, metaphorically termed the *bronchial tree*. In this system the primary bronchus is a trunk that divides into a number of branches. These subdivide into smaller branches, and so on until tiny, thin-walled spaces are reached, where respiratory exchange takes place. In such an arrangement a given branch of the bronchial tree will ventilate a definite part of the respiratory surface. As a system of air conduits, the bronchial tree is best visualized in casts prepared by filling all but the last few generations of branches with latex or plastic casting materials, for then the branching pattern can be studied to advantage (Fig. 21-10). If the entire bronchial tree is cast, it takes on the form of the intact lung and appears solid.

The three-dimensional structure of the lungs is fully achieved by superimposing additional branching systems on the basic bronchial tree. The most important of these is the pulmonary vascular circuit consisting of the pulmonary arteries, capillaries, and veins (Figs. 21-41 and 21-42, see color insert). The arteries spread over the dorsolateral surfaces of the bronchial tree and follow its divisions precisely until in the respiratory region the vessels divide into capillaries. The bronchial arteries, pulmonary lymphatics, and nerves all follow the bronchial tree as closely as the pulmonary artery does; they also ramify along the pulmonary vessels and extend into the pleura. Pulmonary veins form at the boundaries

between regions ventilated by adjacent bronchi and run within interfacial connective tissue to the main pulmonary veins, which are suspended from the ventral surfaces of the bronchi. A common adventitia of connective tissue invests the bronchial tree and associated blood vessels. It continues outward along the veins where it blends in with the surrounding septal tissue. At the surface this tissue becomes confluent with the connective tissue of the visceral pleura. The branching systems in the lungs thereby become bound together and linked through septa to capsular tissue at the surface. The larger of these septa run out to the lobar fissures and hence are *interlobar septa*. Others follow planes of separation between the segments of a lobe and are *intersegmental septa;* still others less regularly subdivide smaller parts of the lung.

Bronchopulmonary segments   Clinical interest in the branching pattern of human lungs usually extends to the level of bronchopulmonary segments. These are supplied by branches of the lobar bronchi or by branches that immediately follow them; consequently segmental bronchi are third- or fourth-order branches. There are three segments in the right upper lobe, two in the middle, and five in the lower lobe. On the left there are five altogether in both divisions of the upper lobe and five in the lower lobe. From the preceding it can be seen that the segments carry their own arterial supply, which branches with the bronchi, and that they are bounded by connective tissue septa. At this level the bronchial tree rarely exhibits an unusual branching pattern. When anomalies occur, they do so at predictable sites, and the segmental artery is displaced along with the bronchus. This makes it feasible for surgeons to perform successful partial resections of the lungs in cases of serious pulmonary disease.

Branching of the airways   The most typical mammalian lungs are adapted to fit comfortably within long, narrow, and deep thoracic cavities such as many quadrupeds possess. In these the primary bronchi run caudally from the hilum toward the dorsomedial inferior angle of each lung. Secondary bronchi arise predominantly as outward directed lateral branches of the primary bronchi. They also form a dorsal and a less complete ventral series and

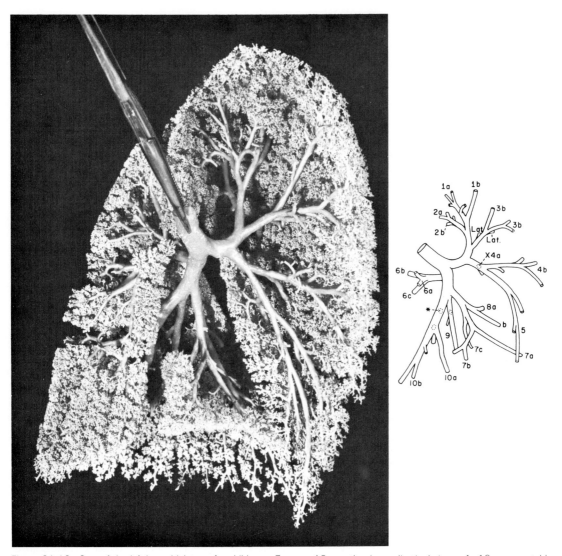

Figure 21-10 Cast of the left bronchial tree of a child, age 7 years, 10 months, in mediastinal view.   1–10, segmental bronchi; ×4a, displaced subsegmental branch; *, subsuperior bronchus of lower lobe.   ×0.8. (Courtesy of E. A. Boyden and D. H. Tompsett.)

rarely an internal lateral one as well. The primary bronchus thereby serves as an axis for each lung. The secondary branches are largest cranially and smallest caudally. They are given off fairly regularly, the lateral branches in alternation with the dorsoventral sets. In man the lungs are squeezed into a short, broad, and shallow thorax; accordingly, the pattern of bronchial branching is atypical. In-

formed opinion holds that the primary bronchi of man are not true axial structures but that they give rise to three secondary bronchi in the right lung and two in the left. These become the lobar bronchi, and each develops its own pattern of branching.

Like the trachea, many of the subsidiary bronchi branch by unequal dichotomy, whereby the smaller of two diverging bronchi veers more from the path of its parent than the other. From this viewpoint, the bronchial tree consists of a sequence of unequal branchings that vary in number, depending on whether counts are made in long or in short segments. In man as many as 25 generations can be counted in the longest segmental bronchi, making the maximum number of divisions 27 or 28 starting from the primary bronchus. Nevertheless, because of the variation in size of bronchi belonging to the same branching order, and because of the variability in the number of generations between the trachea and the respiratory zone, the bronchial tree is not adequately described in this manner but yields more useful information when approached in other ways. These are discussed below.

The caliber of the airways and the angles of branching have been measured in bronchial trees of human and canine lungs. These data enable one to estimate patterns of air flow and the effectiveness of ventilation in various parts of the lung more accurately than is possible when calculations are based on abstract models. In these species the distance from the carina to the respiratory surface (the *bronchial path length*) varies considerably in different parts of the lung. This inequality represents an accommodation of the bronchial tree to available space and is smaller in man than in the long-chested dog, where the paths range from 2 mm to 12 cm, beginning with the base of the lobar bronchus. Other things being equal, bronchi of equal caliber have about the same number of terminal airways, and these lead to an approximately equal area of respiratory surface. Nevertheless, where the bronchial path is longer, its airways are of larger caliber than where the path is shorter; a lowered airway resistance is compensation for the long path. The main defect in this arrangement is that the respiratory surface at the end of these long pathways is exposed to a disproportionately large volume of residual air in the bronchial tree (the *anatomical dead space*), and under certain circumstances this may lead to unequal ventilation of ambient air in different regions of the lung.

As the bronchi bifurcate, the total cross-sectional area of the airway increases by a factor of about 1.3 in each of the first five generations and then by somewhat more. If the total cross-sectional area is measured at successive distances from the

carina, it is seen to reach a peak and then to decline. At first the increments due to branching predominate over the decrements due to termination of the smaller bronchial paths. Subsequently the terminations predominate. The effect of these anatomic arrangements is to make the conducting portions of the lungs as small as possible. In living specimens the airway is flexible and changes its configuration with each breathing cycle. It has been likened to a gradually expanding funnel on inspiration but to a more cylindrical vessel on expiration, owing to changes in the diameters of distal bronchi (Fig. 21-11).

Along the distal half of a bronchial pathway the airways divide at regular intervals, often forking obtusely and always decreasing in caliber after branching. Further along, a fairly abrupt transition leads to a region where branching is frequent and the branches are short and slender. In man these patterns can be seen in bronchograms made after instilling radiopaque material in the bronchial tree. The coarser branching occurs at 0.5- to 1-cm intervals along an axial path of several centimeters; the finer branching occurs at intervals of 2 to 3 mm and extends about 1 cm farther (Fig. 21-12). The fine-meshed pattern is found in the distal part of all bronchial pathways whether they end deep in the lungs or near the pleural surface. By means of correlated histologic study it has been established that the final branches of this network are terminal conducting airways. The respiratory portion of the lung begins immediately afterward, the region ventilated by one terminal radiating from the outlet for a distance of 2 to 5 mm.

The larger airways of the lungs are called *bronchi* and the smaller ones are called *bronchioles*. These are essentially anatomic terms but a fairly characteristic histologic appearance is associated with each. In man the bronchi comprise some 9 to 12 generations, beginning with the primary bronchus and ending with airways having a caliber of approximately 1 mm. The bronchioles begin as branches of the smallest bronchi and in man continue for up to 12 generations before ending as terminal bronchioles. A range is given because the number of bronchial and bronchiolar divisions vary, depending on the segment counted. Histologically, bronchi cannot be distinguished from bronchioles on the basis of a single characteristic. For

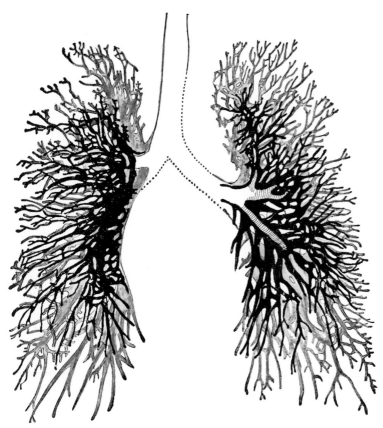

Figure 21-11   Bronchial tree.   Tracings made from x-ray shadows.   Gray, inspiration; black expiration.   (Courtesy of C. C. Macklin.)

Figure 21-12   Centimeter and millimeter branching patterns in the peripheral airway.   The end branches are terminal bronchioles.   About natural size.   (After L. Reid and G. Simon, Thorax, **13**:103, 1958.)

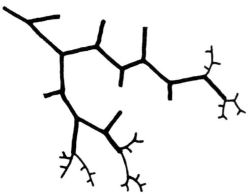

example, it is often stated that bronchi contain cartilage in their walls whereas bronchioles do not. With such definitions one soon runs into terminologic difficulty: In the howling monkey and in many microchiropteran bats there is virtually no intrapulmonary cartilage (Fig. 21-13).   On the other hand, in whales the cartilage extends to well beyond the conducting airways.   In man it is continued for varying distances along the part of the bronchial tree having the centimeter-branching pattern; the millimeter-branching airways are safely termed bronchioles.

Bronchi   For a short distance beyond their origin, extrapulmonary bronchi retain the structural organization of the trachea and a similar histologic appearance in the mucosa, submucosa, muscularis,

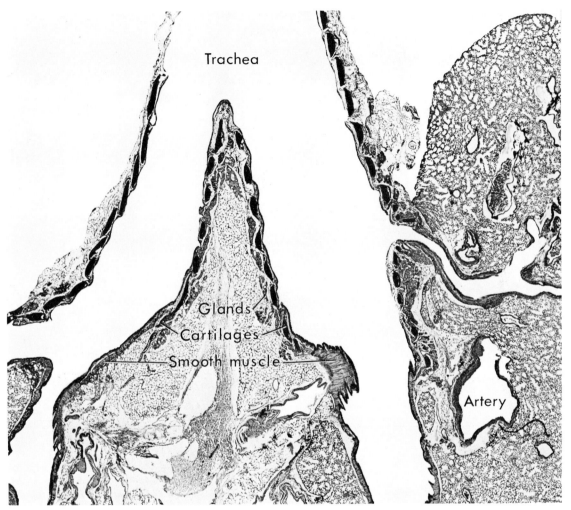

Figure 21-13   Section of a bat's lung near the hilum showing the trachea and primary bronchi and part of the right lung.   Glands are coextensive with the cartilage of the bronchial wall and in this species occur largely in the adventitia.   Iron hematoxylin. ×30.

and adventitia.   Gradually two major changes become manifest: (1) the cartilaginous rings become less regular and (2) the muscularis develops into a complete ring of smooth muscle located between the submucosa and the cartilage.   At first the bronchial cartilages only become shorter and narrower than those of the trachea, but not far beyond the hilum they become highly irregular in shape. Viewed in cross sections of the bronchi, the cartilages often seem isolated (Fig. 21-14), but viewed in three dimensions they remain part of a comprehensive skeletal framework.   At bronchial bifurcations they often are saddle-shaped.   Further along the airway they become reduced to solitary fragments.   As in the trachea, the cartilages are hyaline, although parts of them are infiltrated with elastic fibers, especially in the smaller bronchi.   The muscularis becomes a more prominent layer as the cartilages decline.   It is made up of numerous fascicles of some 20 to 30 cells each (Figs. 21-13

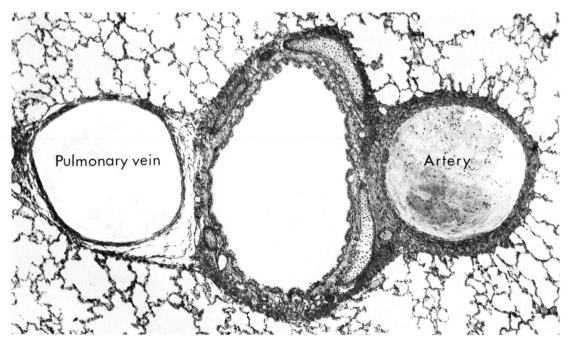

Figure 21-14   Cross section of a bronchus in a kitten.   Mallory azan stain.   ×85.

Figure 21-15   Adenosine triphosphatase activity in the lung of a beaver.   The bronchial smooth muscle is strongly reactive (black).   Gomori method, pH 9.4.   ×350.

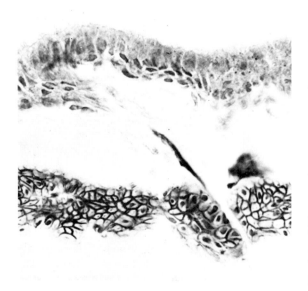

and 21-15).   These fascicles can be identified as separate entities, but in the bronchi they are closely packed into a continuous layer, and they all follow fairly similar circular or spiral courses about the airway.   Some muscle fibers in the outer part of the muscularis are attached to the fibrous membrane that envelopes the cartilages.   This membrane also serves as an attachment for numerous fine elastic and collagenous fibers that cross the muscularis to join heavier fibrous networks in the connective tissue beneath the epithelium.

As the bronchial generations are traced, the airway gradually undergoes a change from a histologic appearance typical of bronchi (Fig. 21-14) toward one typical of bronchioles.   With continued branching, the bronchial wall decreases in thickness, but all layers of the wall are not decreased proportionately.   The disproportion alone accounts for most of the change in appearance.   As the bronchi become smaller, the pseudostratified epithelium becomes lower.   Connective tissue compartments internal to the muscularis become reduced in width. In small bronchi the lamina propria becomes so thin that the fibers of its elastic membrane lie immediately beneath the epithelium. The submucosa remains appreciably thick where it houses the acini of the bronchial glands. It contains branches of the bronchial arteries, which supply nutrient capillary beds for the airway. Near the hilum it contains the bronchial veins as well.

If the cells and collagenous fibers of an inflated lung are digested away, a skeleton of elastic tissue remains, perfect in its preservation of the outlines of the bronchial tree, the pulmonary alveoli, and the blood vessels (Figs. 21-16 and 21-17). In the airways the elastic skeleton comprises mainly the longitudinally oriented proprial fibers and elastic fibers in the fibrocartilaginous membrane of the inner adven-

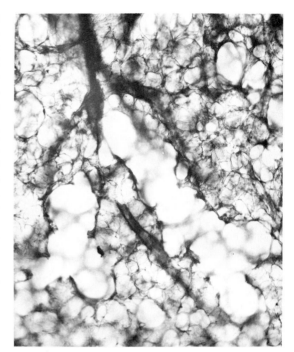

Figure 21-17 Thick section of a rat lung prepared to show the elastic fiber skeleton. Resorcin-fuchsin stain. ×80.

Figure 21-16 Cross section of a child's bronchus stained for elastic fibers. These are formed into an elastic membrane between the epithelium and muscularis, into a circular pattern in the muscularis, and into a longitudinal adventitial network. The cartilage is partly elastic. ×150.

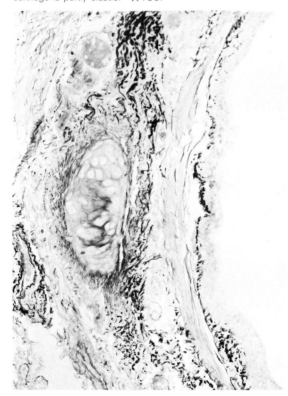

titia. Submucosal fibers serve to suspend the mucosa from the outer layers of the airway and to support the blood vessels and glands within the submucosa. Consequently, these fibers take a more radial course overall than the proprial fibers. In the muscularis the fibers run in various, often circular directions. Reticular fibers are distributed with the elastic fibers. They lie just beneath the epithelial basement lamina and form a delicate tracery around individual stromal cells. The coarser collagenous fibers are everywhere present in the connective tissues but are densest in the common investments of the major pulmonary septa, vessels, and bronchi.

Bronchial glands The bronchial glands closely resemble the numerous small glands located in the upper air passages. They are coextensive with the cartilaginous skeleton. Accordingly, along certain bronchial paths in man they come as close as 2 to 3 cm from the pleura but approach less closely in other paths. In bats they scarcely extend beyond the hilum (Fig. 21-13). Surface mucous cells and these glands together produce the secretions that coat the surfaces of the airways. The relative contributions of the two sources differ according to the species studied; this difference is compounded in the presence of chronic disease. As glands disappear from the airway, the surface mucous cells often increase in number. They are carried further into the bronchial tree than the glands and end in the bronchioles. The glands are supplied by bronchial vascular beds furnished with fenestrated capillaries (Fig. 21-18). As described in the section on the larynx, glandular acini are penetrated by both sensory and secretomotor nerve endings. In contrast, the overlying pseudostratified epithelium has sensory but few motor endings. This difference may be the explanation why the glands readily secrete after stimulation of parasympathetic nerves, whereas the surface cells respond more clearly to local irritation.

The major constituents of the glands are both mucous and serous epithelial cells, the myoepithelium, and at times some unspecialized, cuboidal

Figure 21-18 Endothelial fenestrations in a glandular capillary in the bronchial wall of an opossum. ×12,000.

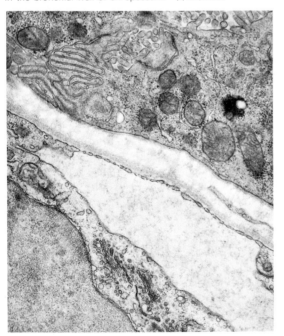

lining cells in the larger ducts. Minor constituents include small-granule cells similar to those in the surface epithelium and a number of unusual cell types that are inconspicuous in paraffin sections and, lacking mucoid droplets, are usually classified as serous cells. There is evidence that the human bronchial tree secretes several types of mucins; nevertheless it is not certain whether the secretions are produced by one or by several different cell types. In the glands four acid glycoproteins are found—two sialomucins and two sulfomucins—and they are distributed differentially among the mucous cells. These cells resemble the surface mucous cells in fine-structural characteristics and in possessing secretory droplets that tend to coalesce. Since the surface cells of the larger airways produce sulfomucin and those more peripheral produce sialomucin, it would seem that all these products are made by cells similar in appearance. Nonetheless, in some species the bronchial glands possess still other mucoid cells. These have small secretory droplets like those in surface mucous cells of the gastric glands (Chap. 18). Even less is known about the serous cells than the mucous cells, but among unusual cells grouped in this category, human glands have an acidophilic *oncocyte* and opossums have a *hydrotic* cell that seems capable of performing osmotic work. Stellate *myoepithelial* cells are found in the acini and partway up the ducts. They rest on the epithelial side of the basement lamina and encircle the secretory cells with their processes. They possess ultrastructural features of smooth muscle and by their contraction help to expel the contents from secreting glands (Fig. 21-19).

Bronchioles At some point along any given bronchial path the airway, having lost its bronchial characteristics, gradually acquires new ones; the airway is then called a bronchiole (Fig. 21-20). It retains the radial organization of preceding passages but no longer is lined by a laryngobronchial type of epithelium, nor has cartilage, glands, or a continuous muscularis. New features are (1) a columnar epithelium in which a unique type of secretory cell displaces the mucous cell; (2) a proportional increase, compared with large bronchi, in the thickness of the muscularis; and (3) a separation of smooth muscle fascicles by connective tissue (Fig. 21-21). This

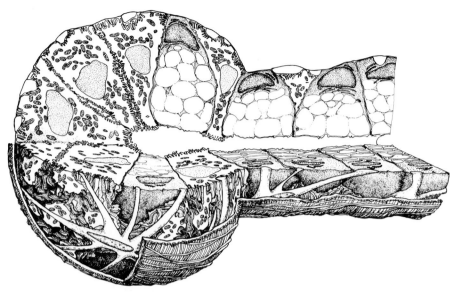

Figure 21-19 Diagram showing a three-dimensional view of the acinus and duct of a bronchial gland. (Drawing by G. Pederson-Krag in S. Sorokin, Amer. J. Anat., **117**:311, 1965.)

Figure 21-20 Bronchiole and small pulmonary artery in a kitten's lung. Mallory azan stain. ×125.

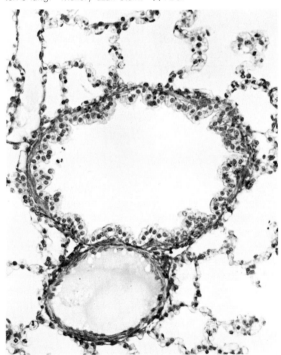

effectively unites all connective tissue compartments of the bronchiolar wall into one investing mass.

Two major cell types, more of them ciliated than nonciliated, line the bronchioles (Fig. 21-22). The ciliated cells are similar to those in the bronchi except that they are shorter. The nonciliated *bronchiolar* cells (Clara cells) give the epithelium its special character. These are tall, dome-shaped cells that protrude into the bronchiolar lumen to the tips of the cilia. Accordingly, in sections of bronchioles the epithelium has a scalloped contour. With a basal ergastoplasm and apical, membrane-bounded droplets, bronchiolar cells can be classified among serous cells; but they contrast with them for possessing an unusual abundance of agranular reticulum in the supranuclear and apical cytoplasm (Fig. 21-23). This predominates over the Golgi lamellae, the lysosomal particulates, the apical centrioles, and other normal features of the region. In rodents, rabbits, and in man, bronchiolar cell mitochondria are unusually large, globose bodies with a voluminous matrix and few cristae (Fig. 21-23). In other species they are more conventional in appearance. Where the mitochondria are unusual, the secretory droplets seem to have

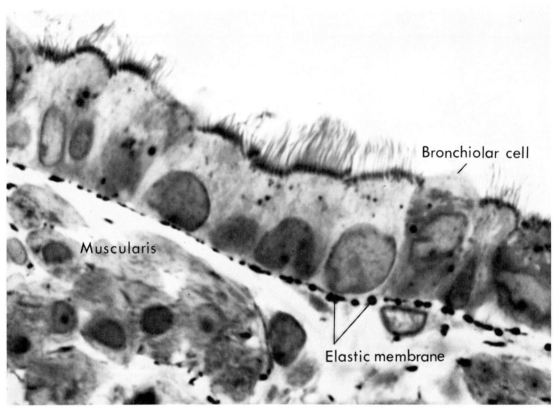

Figure 21-21   Longitudinal section of bronchiolar epithelium of a rat, showing ciliated and bronchiolar cells.   Beneath the epithelium, bundles of smooth muscle are separated by connective tissue.   Toluidine blue.   ×1,440.

a high lipid content; otherwise they resemble the zymogen granules of many cells.   The granules are released from the apical cytoplasm, but little else is known about the function of these cells, except that in some species glycogen synthesis takes place along the agranular membranes.   Among minor components of the bronchiolar epithelium, small-granule cells frequently cluster in the lower part of the epithelium, and the presumably sensory brush cell has also been reported present.

As in many water-permeable epithelia, cytoplasmic leaflets extend from the lateral surfaces of both ciliated and nonciliated cells to intermingle with those from adjacent cells (Fig. 21-22).   Moreover, capillary loops close to the basement lamina have discrete, fenestrated areas facing the epithelium.   These features occur elsewhere along the

conducting airways and in the body.   They are a part of a mechanism to provide regulated water transport across the epithelium.

Reconstructions of the bronchiolar wall have shown the smooth muscle to be formed into a geodesic network.   The separate fascicles of muscle branch and anastomose so that some fibers run circularly and others obliquely.   Through this arrangement the force of contraction is exerted perpendicular to the wall.   Owing to the comparative strength of the muscularis in the bronchioles, contractions are felt there more strongly than in the bronchi.   Like muscles of the alimentary tract, those of the airway are activated by parasympathetic fibers and are known to undergo peristaltic movements.   They participate in the cough reflex and increase bronchial tone in cold weather.   They also relax during inspiration and contract at the end of expiration, thereby helping bronchial fiber systems to return distended airways to resting dimensions.

THE RESPIRATORY ZONE

Respiratory bronchioles and subdivisions   Each terminal bronchiole divides into two daughter branches called *respiratory bronchioles*. These resemble the terminal bronchiole in all but one respect: here and there the walls are interrupted by saccular outpocketings called *alveoli*, where respiratory gas exchange takes place (Figs. 21-25 to 21-27). At once possessing a respiratory surface and a bronchiolar structure, respiratory bronchioles are aptly named. Subsequently the number of al-

veoli increase with each branching of the airway, and after about five divisions from the terminal bronchiole, the pathway ends in grape-like clusters of alveoli. As these branches are traversed, the fraction of the wall taken up by alveoli increases, until the wall becomes little more than a series of openings into the alveoli. At that point the branches still retain the appearance of a conduit and are called *alveolar ducts*. Futher on, the tubular sense is lost, and the remaining spaces are called, successively, *atria, alveolar sacs,* and *alveoli* (Fig. 21-29). The respiratory surface aerated by one terminal bronchiole is partitioned among the alveoli located all along the succeeding branches.

In adult man there normally are three orders of respiratory bronchioles, and where they are not

Figure 21-22   Electron micrograph of bronchiolar epithelium of a bat, showing bronchiolar (upper left) and ciliated cells and the lateral interdigitations between cells.   ×7,000.

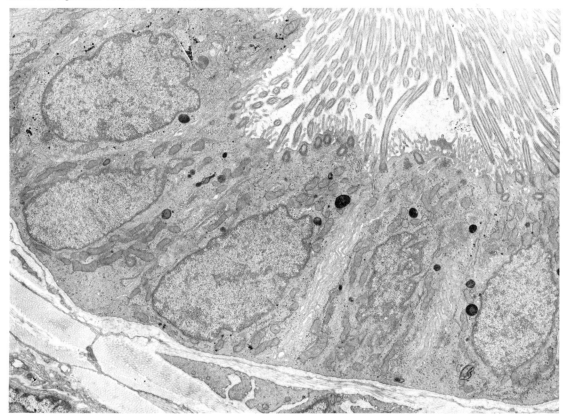

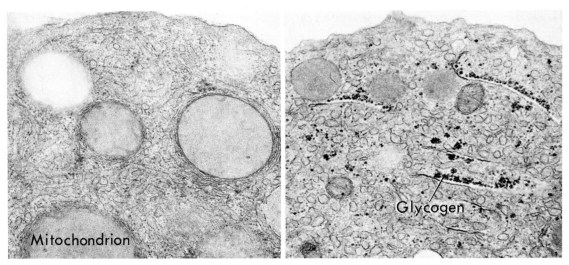

Figure 21-23   Detail of apical cytoplasm in bronchiolar cells of a mouse (left) and a bat (right).   ×30,000.

interrupted by alveoli, the walls are lined by a low columnar epithelium containing ciliated and bronchiolar cells.   At the alveolar rim these cells become continuous with the thin alveolar lining.   Beneath the epithelium the muscularis remains prominent within an investment of connective tissue that contains vascular beds and pulmonary nerves (Fig. 21-24) and is carried into the alveolar walls. The respiratory bronchioles are followed by about two generations of *alveolar ducts*.   Along their highly alveolated walls the ducts exhibit bronchiolar characteristics only in the few places where a group of columnar epithelial cells cover underlying bands of muscle and connective tissue.   The muscle forms a terminal sphincter at the outlet of the last alveolar duct and almost always ends there (Fig. 21-28).   Evidently because the bronchiolar and alveolar epithelia are closely related biologically, alveolar epithelial cells sometimes are admixed in the lining of the ducts.   The alveolar ducts open into *atria*, which are vestibules communicating with the multilocular *alveolar sacs*.   Occasionally one but usually two or more sacs arise from each atrium.   These are irregular cavities surrounded by pulmonary *alveoli,* which are the individual locules of the sacs.   The alveoli are the smallest subdivisions of the respiratory tree.   Within a given lung they are of fairly uniform size, but their dimensions are proportioned to the metabolic rate of the ani-

mal, being smallest (30 μm) in shrews and bats and largest (1,100 μm) in the large and sluggish Sirenia.   In man, a total of some 300 million alveoli is divided between the lungs, and individual alveoli measure about 200 μm in diameter.   Beyond the alveolar ducts the elastic fibers abandon their predominantly longitudinal course along the airway and form a complex network of fibers which come together to encircle the successive openings of atria, alveolar sacs, and alveoli.

Functional respiratory units   Those interested in pulmonary function have long sought to define functional subdivisions within the respiratory surface, aiming for an ideal unit that is at the same time modular and well defined anatomically.   Such is the nonuniformity of the lungs that the ideal is unattainable, for it is one thing to find structurally similar units in this region, and it is another to find them uniform in size and shape.   Moreover, the *average* size of these units is scaled up or down, depending on the animal possessing them.   Among a wide range of mammals the size of such units is roughly commensurate with lung volume, which is proportional to body weight, and with respiratory surface area, which varies linearly and directly with basal oxygen consumption.   The best anatomic unit is the *acinus,* which is simply the terminal bronchiole and all its branches.   In man it has dimen-

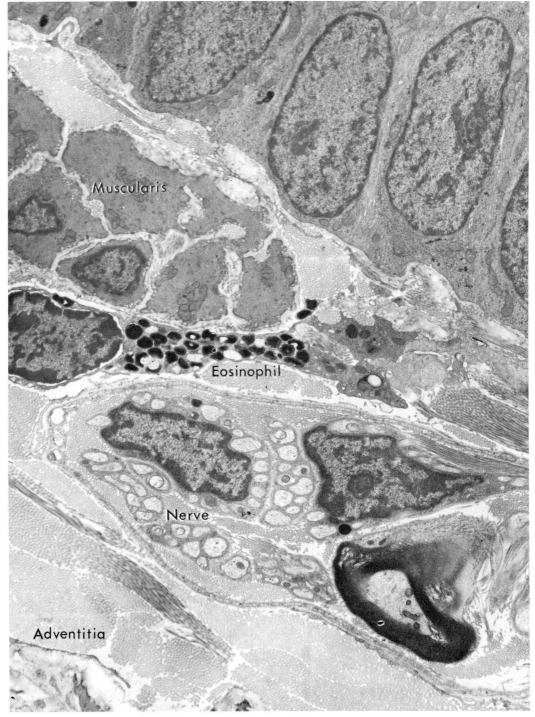

Figure 21-24 Electron micrograph showing connective tissue within the bronchiolar wall. A nerve passes from outside the muscularis into the submucosal space. ×8,000.

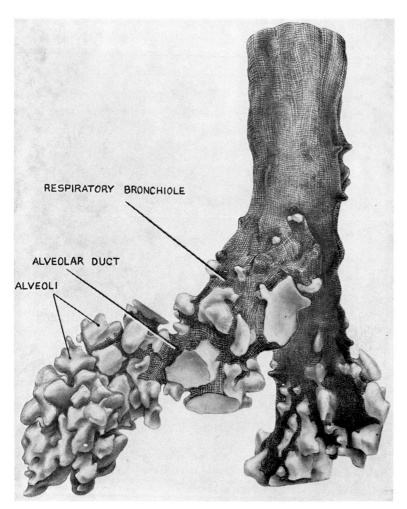

RESPIRATORY BRONCHIOLE

ALVEOLAR DUCT

ALVEOLI

Figure 21-25   Cast model of a respiratory bronchiole with its subdivisions.   Several alveolar ducts have been represented as removed.   The cross-hatching represents the approximate extent of the muscular coat along the bronchial tree.   (From J. L. Bremer, Carnegie Institute Contrib. Embryol., 1935.)

sions of millimeter size and is divided by its first-order respiratory bronchioles into two hemiacini. These differ in size and shape from each other and from those of other acini, the free variations on a simple pattern arising from a competition among branches for available space.   A larger peripheral unit is the (secondary) *lobule,* supposedly formed by connective tissue septa passing into the lung from the pleura.   Unfortunately, such septa are well defined only near the pleura and not deep within the lungs, and they do not demarcate equal volumes of lung.   Consequently, this lobule has been redefined for the human lung in terms of the branching pattern in the peripheral airway (Fig. 21-12).   It consists of a cluster of three to five acini whose terminal bronchioles arise close by one another at the end of a given centimeter-branching bronchial path.   Such a unit measures 1 to 2 cm^2 in volume and is of a convenient size for use in radiologic studies on patients.

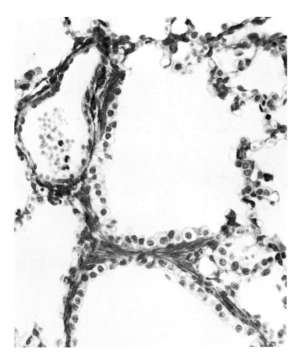

Figure 21-26 Respiratory bronchiole of a kitten. Note the low columnar epithelium on the left and the alveoli on the right. Mallory azan stain. ×125.

Alveolar organization The alveolar wall is specialized toward promoting diffusion between external and internal environments. As at any exposed surface, an epithelium covers a vascularized connective tissue space, but in the alveolar wall the epithelial and connective tissue layers are both very thin, and the blood vessels form the richest capillary network in the body (Fig. 21-30). In details of organization these walls are similar in most mammalian lungs. Between adjacent alveoli a framework of elastic and collagenous fibers supports a meshwork of anastomosing pulmonary capillaries. The vessels are woven through the framework much as vines are woven through a trellis. In marine mammals, alveolar capillaries run in two beds, one on each of two adjacent alveolar surfaces, being separated from each other by a central connective tissue septum rich in cells and fibers, and from the alveolar air by a layer of epithelium. Through reduction in the connective tissue and through forma-

tion of extensive anastomoses, these capillary beds are rationalized by most other mammals into one system that serves adjacent alveoli. The connective tissue septum, having become thin and pliant, no longer occupies a distinctly central position but fills the interstices between the capillaries (Figs. 21-29 and 21-31). When alveoli abut against the pleura, the septa, or large blood vessels instead of against each other, the alveolar connective tissue blends in with the tissue of the adjacent structure. At such points only do alveoli contact lymphatic capillaries, for these vessels do not penetrate interalveolar septa except when the septa are rather thick, as in whales.

The alveolar epithelium is inhomogeneous, con-

Figure 21-27 Respiratory bronchiole of a bat reacted for acid phosphatase. Ciliated cells and alveolar macrophages (2) are strongly reactive; great alveolar cells (1) and bronchiolar cells (3), less so. Burstone's method. ×200.

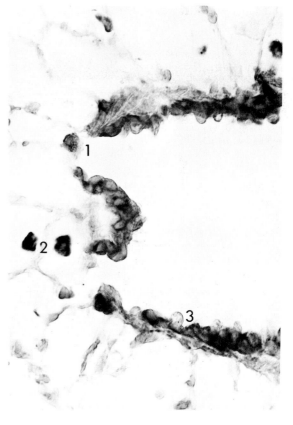

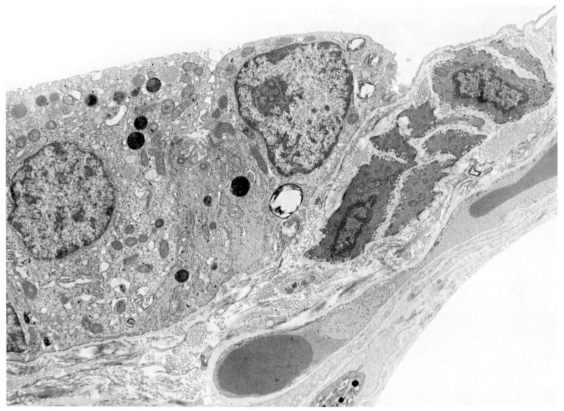

Figure 21-28 Transition from the alveolar duct to the atrial space. Bronchiolar cells, a great alveolar cell, and a squamous alveolar cell are in continuity. The terminal muscle sphincter lies beneath. ×5,000.

sisting principally of attenuated *squamous alveolar* cells and pleomorphic *great alveolar* cells. The connective tissue beneath the epithelium makes up about a third of the thickness of the total air-blood barrier, which in rats averages about 1.5 μm with a range from 0.1 to several micrometers. Where the alveolar diffusion barrier is thinnest, the capillary loops press against the epithelium so that connective tissue is excluded and epithelium and endothelium are separated by only a submicroscopic basement lamina (Fig. 21-36). Compared with a single 1-μm micrococcus, this membrane does not present a formidable obstacle to invasion by microorganisms. Nonetheless, to judge by the absence of chronic inflammatory cells from the region, alveolar surfaces normally are not threatened by invasion. Credit for this falls on the *alveolar macro-*

phages, which move along surfaces coated by epithelial secretions and effectively police the alveoli. Capillaries within alveolar walls all belong to the pulmonary vascular circuit and do not have endothelial fenestrations. Nevertheless, when the vascular compartment of the animal is overloaded and the filtration pressure rises, the pulmonary capillaries then leak fluid and small proteins through clefts between endothelial cells. Excessive leakage into the alveoli is prevented by the alveolar epithelium, which possesses tight junctions and remains relatively impermeable until damaged.

Between the capillaries one or more small, slit-like *alveolar pores* can be seen in thick sections that have been fixed and dried in an expanded state (Fig. 21-32). These pores connect adjacent alveoli and are fully open in expanded lungs. They are then about 10 to 15 μm in diameter and are encircled by a few elastic and reticular fibers. These pores are the best known among several kinds of accessory communications between adjacent air spaces. Others exist at the levels of respiratory bronchioles and alveolar ducts, where short circuits can occur between the airway and alveoli of the same or of adjacent acini. Still others come into being as a result of aberrant branching within the acini, and they interconnect airways of adjacent bronchial paths either directly or indirectly. The latter provide relatively major intercommunications, perhaps through passages as large as 0.2 mm in diameter. These accessory channels normally may serve as a fine control in equalizing interacinar pressures, but the extent to which they are present varies greatly with the species. In canine lungs these paths are plainly evident; in man they are apparent; but in pigs they are difficult to demonstrate. Where a terminal bronchiole is obstructed, the alveoli connected to it can be ventilated through these collateral channels. They may also serve as routes for the spread of pneumonia or neoplasm.

Alveolar cells There are three major types of cells in alveolar walls: endothelial cells of capillaries,

Figure 21-29 Diagram of the respiratory subdivisions in the lung, showing a respiratory bronchiole, alveolar ducts, and subdivisions. Smooth muscle (dark cells) ends in the alveolar ducts. The atria (circled) are spaces bounded by the termination of the alveolar duct, on one end, and the openings of the alveolar sacs, on the other. In addition, major features of the alveolar walls are presented.

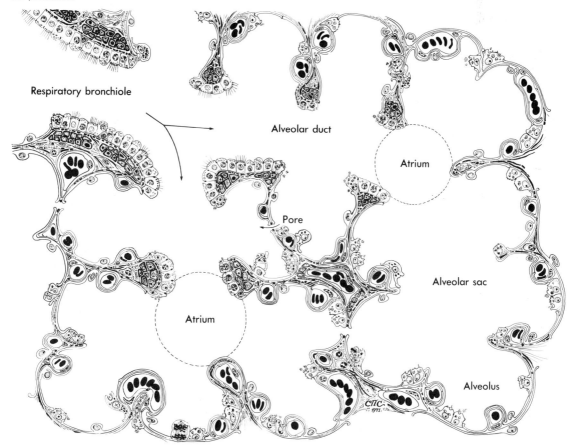

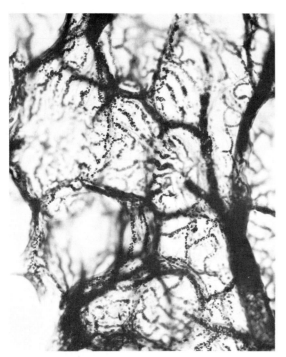

Figure 21-30 Thick section of adult human lung, showing the distribution of small blood vessels within the alveolar walls. ×125.

lamina as a thin sheet and joins other epithelial cells making up the continuous alveolar lining. In many mammals the attenuated portions of the cytoplasm are so thin as to be below the resolving limit of the optical microscope (0.2 μm); in bats the layer may approach 250 Å, a thickness of little more than apical and basal plasmalemmae combined. For this reason a controversy raged for years whether or not a complete alveolar epithelium existed, but the question was resolved by electron microscopy. Squamous alveolar cells have inconspicuous metabolic activity as revealed histochemically, and much of it must be directed toward maintaining surfaces so extensively exposed to alveolar air. These cells are rather deficient in ergastoplasm and other cytoplasmic organelles, but those present are distributed fairly evenly among perinuclear and peripheral regions. Pinocytotic vesicles occur in small numbers at both basal and apical surfaces, and from the latter short microvilli here and there extend into the alveolar space. Squamous cells are capable of using pinocytotic action to take up small amounts of protein from the alveoli; exceptionally they store protein aggregates within the cytoplasm. Their main role is that of providing an intact surface of minimum thickness readily permeable to gases. The plasmalemmae of cells are the main barriers to diffusion in any multilayered biologic membrane, but they are freely permeable to gases, which dissolve in lipids.

Great alveolar cells (granular pneumonocytes, type II cells, large alveolar cells, alveolar cells) carry out other epithelial functions. These pleomorphic cells often have a roughly cuboidal shape. They rest on the epithelial basement lamina, sometimes occupying niches between capillary loops and sometimes standing upright in twos and threes along the alveolar surface (Fig. 21-29). However they are mixed in the epithelium, they are joined to their neighbors by the same type of continuous tight junctions that binds all the epithelial cells together (Fig. 21-37). Great alveolar cells are identifiable in paraffin sections of lung because their nuclei are vesicular and relatively large and their cytoplasm appears vacuolated. At the light-microscopic level they stand out better in 1-μm plastic sections, and then the vacuoles are seen to be characteristic inclusions known as *multilamellar bodies* or *cytosomes* (Fig. 21-33).

squamous alveolar epithelial cells, and great alveolar cells. The capillaries resemble muscular capillaries and have been described above. By light microscopy they are difficult to distinguish from squamous alveolar cells because both cells are thin and elongate and their nuclei are small. An alveolar brush cell of unknown function is a minor constituent of the epithelium. The connective tissue normally contains only occasional fibrocytes, plasma cells, wandering leukocytes, and, rarely, a solitary smooth muscle fiber. Following severe challenge by acute or chronic infection, however, the connective tissue space enlarges and receives a variety of inflammatory cells from the bloodstream.

Squamous alveolar epithelial cells (membranous pneumonocytes, type I cells, small alveolar cells, pulmonary epithelial cells) appear widely separated from each other because, beyond the perinuclear region, the cytoplasm is abruptly attenuated (Fig. 21-35). Thereafter it extends over the basement

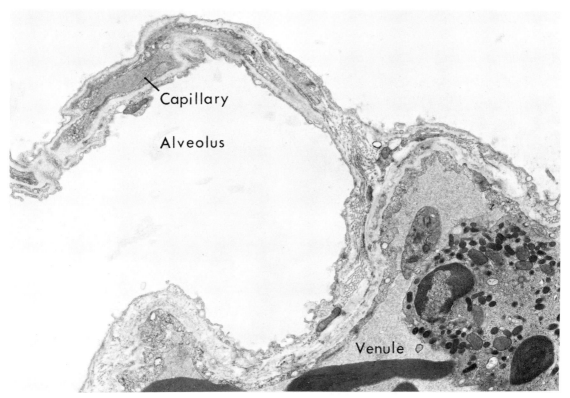

Figure 21-31   Interalveolar wall in the lungs, showing the central connective tissue space in continuity with a pulmonary venule. ×7,000.

Figure 21-32   Thick section of human lung prepared to demonstrate pores between adjacent alveoli. The pores are seen as light spots, the alveolar nuclei as dark spots on the walls. ×250.

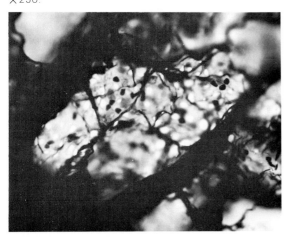

Great alveolar cells have considerable metabolic capacity (Fig. 21-34) at a level equaled in alveolar regions only by alveolar macrophages. Within the cytoplasm this capacity is reflected by the presence of well-developed mitochondria, but a secretory function is indicated even more strongly by the presence of a loosely ordered granular endoplasmic reticulum, an extensive and widely dispersed Golgi apparatus, numerous multivesicular bodies, and the multilamellar bodies (Fig. 21-37). The latter range in size up to 1 μm and occur among forms transitional in appearance between multivesicular bodies and the cytosomes (Fig. 21-38). Multilamellar bodies give histochemical reactions for phospholipids, mucopolysaccharides, and proteins, including reaction for several lysosomal hydrolases which are also found in the Golgi lamellae and in the multivesicular bodies. The cytosomes have been shown by autoradiographic studies to incorporate

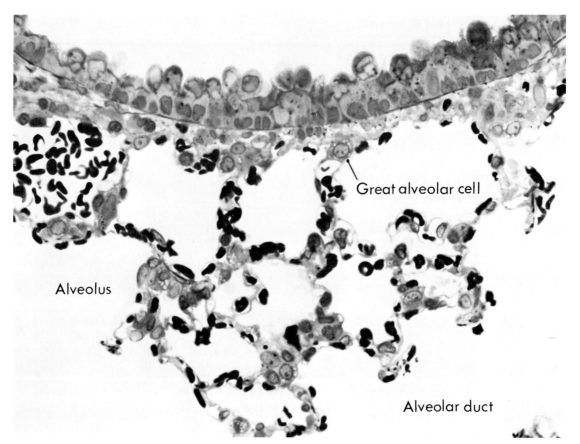

Figure 21-33 Light micrograph of a rat's lung showing bronchiolar epithelium (above) and respiratory tissue (below). Toluidine blue. ×400.

tritium-labeled choline, galactose, and leucine after these precursors first traverse the cell's synthetic centers. The cytosomes therefore are synthetic products of great alveolar cells and are associated with a lysosomal system that is biased to favor secretion. Synthesis and release occur continuously, the bodies being extruded singly from the apical microvillous border of the cell. The secretory material spreads over the alveolar surfaces and provides an extracellular coating with unusual surface activity. This is described below.

The alveolar surface coating consists of lipid and aqueous phases and contains a detergent substance, termed *surfactant,* whose active principles are substances related to the phospholipid dipalmitoyl lecithin. This material is interspersed with

water molecules at the alveolar surface, thereby reducing their mutual cohesiveness and consequently reducing the surface tension at the air-fluid interface. In the presence of surfactant, the work of breathing is reduced because the alveolar surface tension that tends to collapse alveoli is reduced, and this requires a lessened inspiratory force to oppose it. Surfactant stabilizes the alveoli as well. Since the pressure to overcome surface tension is greater in smaller than in larger alveoli, the larger of two interconnected alveoli would expand at the expense of the smaller. Nonetheless, as alveolar diameters fall, surface concentration of surfactant increases, thereby reducing surface tension. Respiratory distress syndrome is characterized by alveolar instability and often is due to surfactant deficiency.

Although the presence of a surface-active alveolar coating is not doubted, it has been difficult to present good images of the material in electron micrographs, and the most successful ones to date have been made in lungs fixed by intravascular rather than intratracheal perfusion of tissue fixative. In the former technique the extracellular lining is preserved as a superficial layer of phospholipids over a basal aqueous layer containing proteins and mucopolysaccharides. The upper layer consists of several lamellae each about 100 to 400 Å thick and resembles the crystalline phase of a polar lipid-water system. The basal layer is of variable thickness, and the substances dissolved there may possess properties more broadly related to defense postures than to surface activity.

Alveolar macrophages   Alveolar macrophages (alveolar phagocytes, dust cells) are preeminent among cells defending the respiratory region from contamination by microorganisms and inhaled particulate matter. They have long been distinguished by their vigorous phagocytic activity, which is in strong contrast to the virtual absence of such activity by other alveolar cells. They are most unusual, however, because they regularly scavenge the *surface* of the epithelium. In general, macrophages rarely migrate over epithelial surfaces and almost never do so in the absence of significant inflammation in the connective tissue beneath. The metabolic capacity of these cells is considerable and diverse. This is well documented because alveolar macrophages can be washed out from the lungs

Figure 21-34   Frozen section of alveolar walls in a bat's lung reacted for diphosphopyridine nucleotide reductase. Great alveolar cells and the phagocytes are the most reactive cells present; they compare in reactivity with the epithelial cells of the airways. ×600.

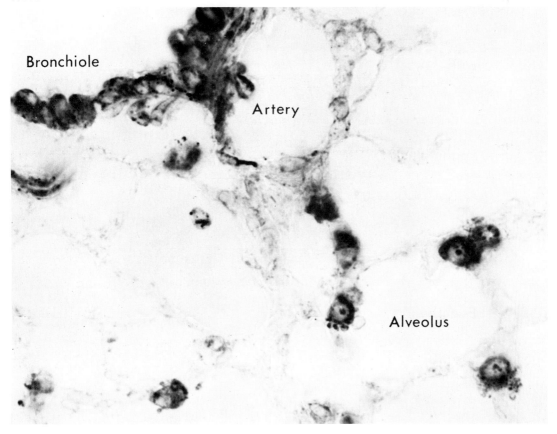

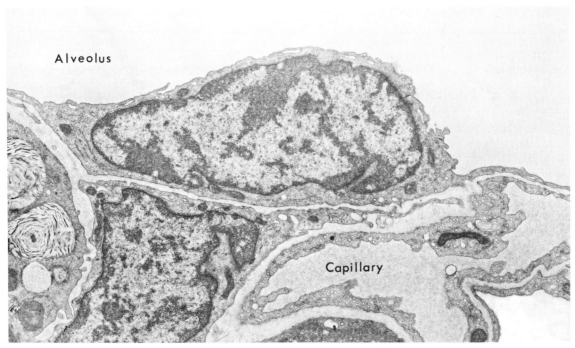

Figure 21-35   Squamous alveolar epithelial and neighboring cells in the alveolar wall.   (Courtesy of E. Schneeberger.)

Figure 21-36   Electron micrograph of the alveolar membrane of a rat.   The barrier between alveolar air and blood consists of a thin alveolar epithelium, a basement lamina, and the capillary endothelium.   Within the endothelial cell a network of fine-caliber agranular reticulum occupies the space between two mitochondria (mi).   Pinocytotic vesicles (pv) are seen in both epithelium and endothelium. $\times$15,000.

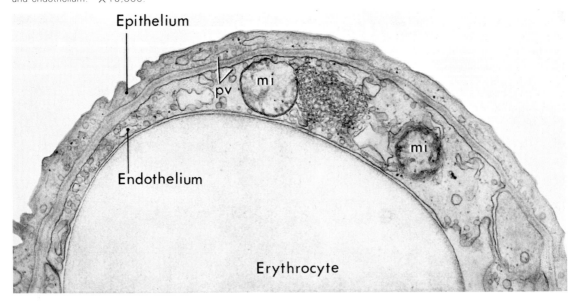

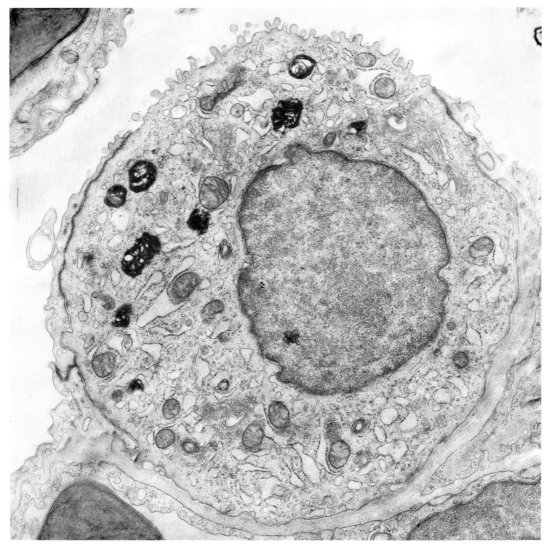

Figure 21-37   Great alveolar cell in the lungs of an opossum.   (From S. Sorokin, J. Histochem. Cytochem., **14**:884, 1966.)

through irrigation of the airway, and the resulting cell suspensions contain them in a high state of purity.   In addition to possessing a very well-developed lysosomal system organized along the usual lines of an intracellular digestive system (Fig. 21-27), these macrophages possess a reserve synthetic capacity that enables them to act in other than the most acute situations.

In most respects, alveolar macrophages resemble macrophages from other parts of the body. Pseudopodia extend from a peripheral ectoplasm free of organelles and inclusions.   A less fibrillar endoplasm within houses a euchromatic nucleus, the cytoplasmic organelles, and a great variety of dense bodies representing ingested matter enclosed within phagosomes (Fig. 21-40).   If the cell had been migrating when fixed, the nucleus might be displaced toward the rear, the advancing end would

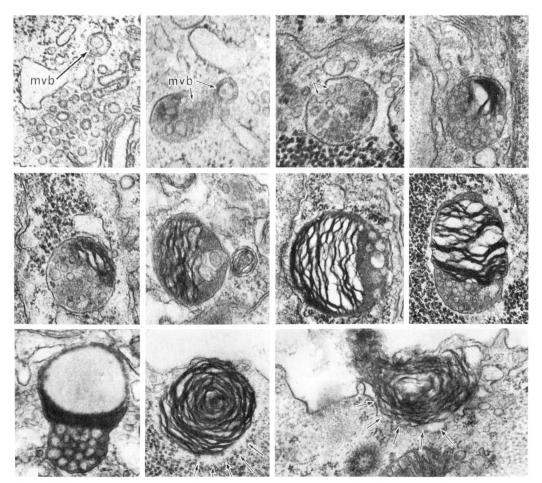

Figure 21-38   Sequence showing the development of cytosomes from small multivesicular bodies (mvb) through larger forms and on to secretion from the great alveolar cell.   (From S. Sorokin, J. Histochem. Cytochem., **14**:884, 1966.)

be broad, and the trailing end would taper into a firm tail to provide purchase for the cell (Fig. 21-39).   On the other hand, if the macrophage were examined in cell suspensions, it would be rounded and would reveal less.   In migrating phagocytes, coated vesicles (acanthosomes) occur at points along the advancing edges.   Within the cytoplasm the Golgi apparatus is well developed and surrounds a distinct, fibrillar centrosome, in which the centrioles reside.   From them microtubules radiate into the cytoplasm and organize the surrounding organelles about the centrosome.   The endoplasmic reticulum varies in extent with different

phases of cellular activity, but the agranular reticulum usually predominates over the granular.   Small rod-like mitochondria and free polysomes fill the available space.   Since the polysomes usually are unassociated with membranes, it can be assumed that most of the proteins synthesized are retained and not secreted by the cell.   Pinocytotic and coated vesicles, a few multivesicular bodies, transitional lamellae between the agranular reticulum and the Golgi apparatus, typical lysosomes, and phagosomes of a great variety of sizes and shapes take up much of the space and give the cytoplasm its pronounced lysosomal character.   The lysosomes

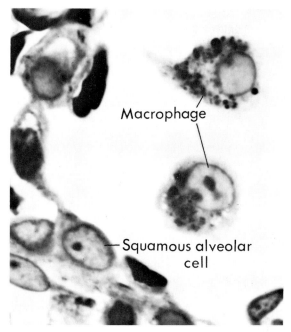

Figure 21-39   Macrophages in the alveolar space of a rat's lung.   Toluidine blue.   ×1,000.

sometimes have unusual configurations; these give alveolar macrophages of some animals a species-specific appearance.   For example, in rabbits the phagosomes contain dense circular inclusions, whereas in cats they contain lamellated material often in a radial configuration.   In man and among several rodents, however, typical lysosomes are admixed with larger phagosomes containing only assorted alveolar debris (Fig. 21-40).

Notwithstanding the alveolar macrophage functions by ingesting particulate matter and digesting it, many fundamental facts about the cell and its life cycle remain unknown.   The origin of the cell, the dynamics of its entrance and exit from the lungs, and the duration of its residence in alveolar walls and on the surface are imperfectly understood.   Alveolar macrophages are able to divide, but many consider them a population in transit, capable of a few divisions at best.   Various sources for these cells have been proposed, chiefly (1) hematopoietic tissues outside the lungs, (2) hematopoietic or connective tissues within the lungs, and (3) the alveolar epithelium, in particular the great alveolar cells.   Recent experimental work has pro-

Figure 21-40   Electron micrographs of alveolar macrophages obtained by bronchial lavage from human lungs.   Left, control; right, from a cigarette smoker.   ×6,000.   (Courtesy of A. J. Ladman.)

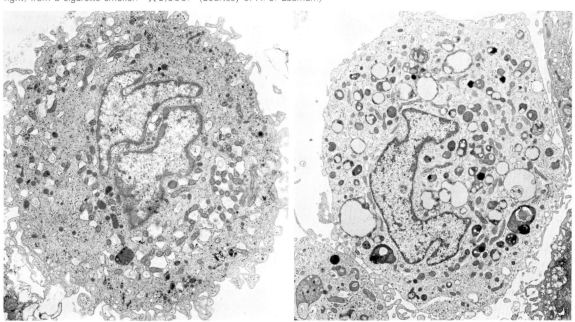

vided unequivocal evidence that at least some of the pulmonary macrophages are derived from hematopoietic cells. Under conditions where identifiable bone marrow cells are seeded into donor animals exposed to high doses of total body irradiation, it has been shown that all pulmonary macrophages originate from donor cells. Nevertheless, actively dividing populations of pulmonary cells would be compromised by the irradiation and consequently any intrapulmonary source of the macrophages would decline. Among hypothetical intrapulmonary sources, the great alveolar cell remains a plausible one; for the cell is highly plastic and along with the pulmonary endothelial cell it behaves like a stem cell, dividing into one daughter cell that remains in place and into another that leaves the area. Whether or not alveolar macrophages share a common origin with other macrophages of the body, they differ in enzyme content and levels of reactivity from blood-borne peritoneal macrophages of the same species. In particular, they differ from both peritoneal macrophages and heterophils in relying on oxidative phosphorylation to supply energy consumed during phagocytosis. Dust-laden macrophages leave the alveolar surfaces by migrating to the bronchial passages, where they are carried out to the pharynx and swallowed. A smaller number may enter the tissues where after death their contents are carried out along lymphatic channels.

PULMONARY CIRCULATION

The main blood supply to the lungs is furnished by the *pulmonary arteries*. These carry high volumes of blood at low pressures ($\frac{25}{5}$ mm Hg) from the right side of the heart to pulmonary capillaries in the alveolar walls. These are drained by *pulmonary veins*, which carry oxygenated blood to the left side of the heart. *Bronchial arteries* are small branches of the descending aorta that carry blood at systemic pressure ($\frac{120}{80}$ mm Hg) to the walls of most of the airway. *Bronchial veins* are present only near the hilum and form only accessory drainage from the bronchial wall toward the azygous veins. Consequently, blood from the two arterial systems drains into the pulmonary veins, and the three vascular systems form one integrated circuit. As described in the section on the internal structure of the lungs, the arteries branch with the bronchial tree, hence

alternate with the veins, which run in the septa between adjacent bronchi (Figs. 21-41 and 21-42, see color insert).

From the *pulmonary arterial* system branches are sent to airway tissues beginning at the level of the respiratory bronchioles. Distal to the alveolar duct the artery branches, and from the level of the atrium twigs are given off to the atria and a branch is sent to each alveolar sac. This divides into two, and the newly formed branches join the pulmonary capillary network (Fig. 21-30). Venules (Fig. 21-31) drain the distal ends of the sacs. *Pulmonary veins* have four origins: from capillaries of the pleura, alveolar ducts, and alveoli, and from the peribronchial venous plexus. The veins draining the airway frequently occur at points where bronchi or bronchioles divide and are called *bronchopulmonary veins*. They form the main channels for drainage of the bronchial arteries and are not anastomoses as that term is usually defined. *Bronchial arteries* run in the adventitia of the airways up to the respiratory bronchioles. Along their course they send branches through the muscularis. These divide into capillaries in the lamina propria. Deep to the capillaries venous plexuses are formed on both sides of the muscularis. The outer one contains the larger vessels that connect to the bronchopulmonary veins. Arterial branches also provide vasa vasorum for the pulmonary arteries and extend along interlobular septa to supply capillaries of the visceral pleura.

Several types of vascular anastomoses are found in the lungs. True anastomoses between bronchial and pulmonary arteries (Fig. 21-41, green, see color insert) are found in the peribronchial tissue near small peripheral bronchi and in the pleura. These vessels are small and have well-developed muscular walls. From them bronchial arteriovenous shunts (Fig. 21-41, green stripes, see color insert) branch off to the pulmonary veins, reaching them by way of the bronchopulmonary veins or by small peripheral pulmonary branches. These then are secondary anastomoses. There are also shortcuts to be found between parallel branches of bronchial arteries, and bronchial veins intercommunicate through the bronchial plexus. In healthy lungs the blood flow through these shunts is of small magnitude, and it passes from the bronchial to the pulmonary circuit.

Histologically the pulmonary arteries and veins resemble each other more closely than do corresponding vessels in other parts of the body; nevertheless, they preserve characteristics of arteries and veins. The arteries have relatively more muscle than the veins and to their smallest divisions possess internal elastic membranes (Fig. 21-43). The veins lack these but may contain less highly organized layers of elastic fibers at the same or at deeper levels (Fig. 21-44). Small mammals also possess cardiac muscle in the pulmonary veins, occurring either with smooth muscle or alone. Bronchial vessels generally resemble other systemic vessels of comparable size, but among small vessels

Figure 21-43 Section of rat lung stained for elastic fibers. A bronchus is cut in cross section above and a branch of the pulmonary artery lies below. A bronchial vessel (bron) is separated from the pulmonary artery by a lymphatic vessel (lym). Resorcin-fuchsin, lithium carmine, orange G. ×350.

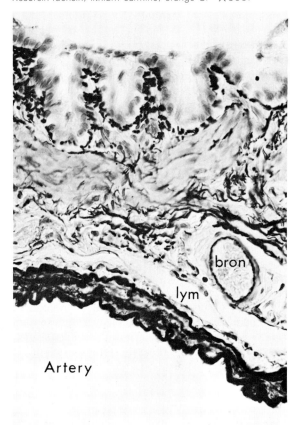

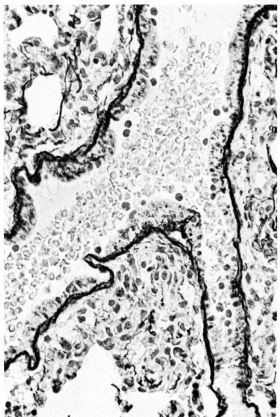

Figure 21-44 Longitudinal section of a branching pulmonary vein of a rat. The internal elastic membrane is absent. Resorcin-fuchsin, lithium carmine, orange G. ×350.

in both bronchial and pulmonary circuits of the lung, several specializations are found whose significance is yet to be learned.

Sympathetic discharge produces little effect on the pulmonary circulation. Mechanical factors, as well as the composition of the inspired gas, influence it more clearly. Vasoconstriction and increased flow result from hypoxia. Once constricted, the vessels may be relaxed by parasympathomimetic action.

No chemoreceptors have been found in the lung, but a glomus associated with the pulmonary trunk has been described. Histologically, it resembles the carotid body. It contains nests of epithelioid cells bound in connective tissue and richly supplied with blood from the pulmonary artery. Vagal and orthosympathetic fibers from the deep cardiac plexus provide innervation, but attempts to investigate glomar function have not given positive results.

LYMPHATICS

The lymphatics of the lung are abundant and form a closed system. A superficial set lies in the visceral pleura; a deep one accompanies the bronchi and pulmonary vessels (Fig. 21-41, see color insert). The sets interconnect at the hilum, where both enter the tracheobronchial lymph nodes. They also communicate near the origins of the pulmonary veins in the pleura and in the interlobar septa, which arise from the pleura.

The lymphatic vessels may be compared to thin-walled veins. The walls of the larger vessels have three layers; the smaller have no media (Fig. 21-43). They exhibit abrupt changes in diameter and near the hilum frequently have valves. Lymphatic capillaries attending pulmonary arterioles and venules extend to the alveoli; other such capillaries found in pulmonary septa and bronchi may reach adjacent alveoli as well.

Figure 21-45 Injected specimen showing well-developed superficial lymphatic channels on the visceral pleura. [From J. Lauweryns, in S. C. Sommers (ed.), "Pathology Annual," vol. 6, p. 365, Appleton-Century-Crofts, New York, 1971.]

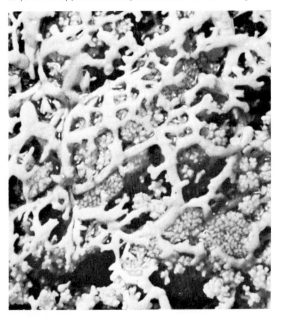

Within the lung, lymph flows centripetally along lymphatics of the bronchial tree and the pulmonary arteries. At the bifurcations of bronchi, the fluid passes through lymphatic tissue. Pleural lymph reaches the hilar lymphatics either through the well-developed superficial channels (Fig. 21-45) or by way of the deep lymphatics (Fig. 21-46). Inspiratory movements promote drainage of the system.

NERVES

Fibers from both homolateral and contralateral vagus nerves and from the sympathetic chain contribute to the posterior and smaller anterior pulmonary plexuses located at the hilum. From there fibers are sent to the bronchial tree, the blood vessels, and the visceral pleura. Along the bronchi an adventitial plexus contains ganglion cells and the larger nerve bundles. A second plexus lies superficial to the cartilages and consists largely of postganglionic parasympathetic efferents. Both plexuses come together in the smaller bronchioles and extend to the alveolar ducts. Fibers destined for bronchial or bronchiolar smooth muscle enter the muscularis from its outer aspect. Those destined for the epithelium and glands pass between the muscular bundles into the submucosa (Fig. 21-24) where they run for short distances before turning into the innervated structures.

Stimulation of the vagus produces contraction of the bronchial muscle and discharge of the glands. Sympathetic discharge, or administration of sympathomimetic agents, inhibits the vagus and dilates the bronchi. The periarterial plexus extends to the capillaries. The visceral pleura is innervated directly from the hilum, as well as by nerves that accompany the bronchial arteries through the pulmonary septa. Sensory endings occur in the pulmonary epithelium or just beneath it, as in the atria. They also occur in the smooth muscle and connective tissue septa. They are connected to large medullated fibers that run to the nodose ganglia of the vagus nerves. The intraepithelial endings have been described in the sections on epithelium and glands.

PLEURA

The *visceral pleura* is closely applied to each lung. It is covered by a simple mesothelium whose cells

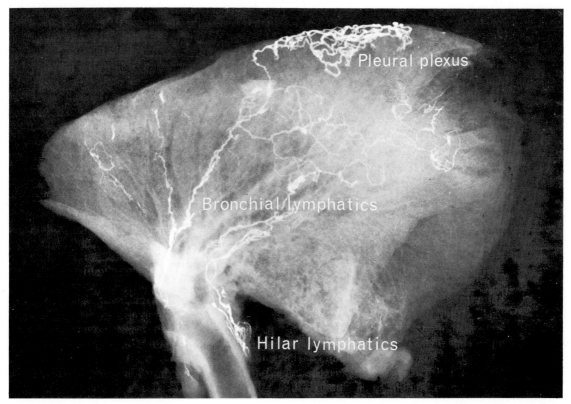

Figure 21-46 Injected specimen of adult human lung, showing the intercommunication between superficial and deep pulmonary lymphatics. [From J. Lauweryns, in S. C. Sommers (ed.), "Pathology Annual," vol. 6, p. 365, Appleton-Century-Crofts, New York, 1971.]

are notable for the complexity of their junctions and the luxuriance of their brush border. They rest on a thin layer of dense fibrous tissue. Beneath lies the relatively thick connective tissue, rich in elastic fibers, that continues into the interlobar and interlobular septa of the lung. The dense pleural sheet

effectively prevents leakage of air into the thoracic cavity. The *parietal pleura,* a thicker and less elastic membrane, contains fat cells. The vascular supply to the visceral pleura is derived from both pulmonary and systemic circuits; the parietal supply is entirely systemic.

Development of the lungs

The airways of the lung develop from a midline endodermal bud, the *laryngotracheal groove,* located on the floor of the pharynx between the sixth arches. This bud branches to form the two primary bronchi and their arboreous subdivisions. The larynx develops from adjacent pharyngeal structures.

The future connective tissue adjacent to the pulmonary epithelium is derived from a relatively cellular mesenchyma, originally located next to the laryngotracheal groove. It accompanies the invading endodermal buds. These advancing tissues migrate amid a relatively acellular mesenchyma,

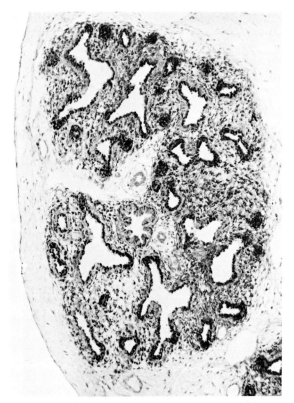

Figure 21-47   Section of a lobule from a 3.5-month fetal human lung, demonstrating glycogen (black). A central bronchiole is surrounded by tissue containing budding bronchial branches. These have cuboidal epithelium. Connective tissue surrounds the lobule; the parietal pleura is at the left. PAS method. ×125.

which gives rise to the blood vessels, interlobar septa, pulmonary pleura, and cartilage. The growing tips, or *terminal buds,* of the expanding bronchial tree appear to be centers of much of the morphogenetic activity of the lungs, for they early reveal histochemical specialization and exhibit concentrated mitotic activity. These phenomena account in some degree for the successive branching of the developing bronchial tree; however, differences between the configurations of right and left lungs become apparent early.

Fetal lungs have a glandlike structure. Their terminal portions are lined by a cuboidal epithelium (Fig. 21-47). Capillaries lengthen into loops that stretch overlying cells, and the epithelium begins to attenuate before the first breaths are drawn. Prenatal inspiratory movements and possibly contractions of smooth muscle in the bronchial tree help to shape the alveoli. At birth, lungs of various species differ greatly in histologic and histochemical maturity. It is not the presence of a thin alveolar epithelium so much as the development of an adequate pulmonary vasculature that is critical to the survival of premature infants. On this basis the extreme limit of viability has been placed at 4.5 months, but the chances of survival increase dramatically when alveoli appear.

Within a few hours after birth the lungs fill with air. At that time proprioceptive and other chemically mediated mechanisms produce a decrease in pulmonary vascular resistance and increase in blood flow. These effects are enhanced by the opening of new circulatory routes on expansion of the lungs. Some time later the *ductus arteriosus* closes, and the definitive pulmonary circuit comes into being.

In man few nonrespiratory branches are added to the bronchial tree after birth; in dogs their number may decrease. This is because alveolar formation is essentially a centripetal process superimposed on the centrifugal process that resulted in the laying down of the bronchial tree. The neonatal human lung contains shallow alveoli within a peripheral zone made up of clusters of thin-walled saccules. These alveoli enlarge in the immediate postnatal period as the terminal region is remodeled. This is followed by the onset of retrograde alveolarization. As development proceeds, respiratory bronchioles become transformed into alveolar ducts, and bronchioles become respiratory bronchioles. The number of alveoli continue to increase until early adolescence, but the shorter bronchial pathways complete their development before then. The formation of accessory respiratory pathways at acinar and bronchiolar levels evidently is a byproduct of this postnatal reorganization.

References

ALLISON, A. C.: The Morphology of the Olfactory System in the Vertebrates, *Biol. Rev.*, **28**:195 (1953).

BARNETT, C. H.: A Note on the Dimensions of the Bronchial Tree, *Thorax,* **12**:175 (1957).

BOYDEN, E. A.: Development of the Human Lung, in V. C. Kelley (ed.), "Brennemann's Practice of Pediatrics," vol. 4, chap. 64, Harper & Row, New York, 1971.

BOYDEN, E. A.: The Structure of the Pulmonary Acinus in a Child of $6\frac{2}{3}$ Years, *Anat. Rec.*, **169**:282 (1971).

BOYDEN, E. A., and D. H. TOMPSETT: The Postnatal Growth of the Lung in the Dog, *Acta Anat.*, **47**:185 (1961).

BRAIN, J.: The Uptake of Inhaled Gases by the Nose, *Ann. Otol.*, **79**:529 (1970).

CAUNA, N., and K. H. HINDERER: Fine Structure of Blood Vessels of the Human Nasal Respiratory Mucosa, *Ann. Otol.*, **78**:865 (1969).

CHEVALIER, G., and A. J. COLLET: In vivo Incorporation of Choline-^{3}H, Leucine-^{3}H and Galactose-^{3}H in Alveolar Type II Pneumocytes in Relation to Surfactant Synthesis. A Quantitative Radioautographic Study in Mouse by Electron Microscopy, *Anat. Rec.*, vol. **174,** 1972.

COURNAND, A.: Pulmonary Circulation, Its Control in Man, with Some Remarks on Methodology, *Science,* **125**:1231 (1957).

DANNENBERG, A. M., JR., M. S. BURSTONE, P. C. WALTER, and J. W. KINSLEY: A Histochemical Study of Phagocytic and Enzymatic Functions of Rabbit Mononuclear and Polymorphonuclear Exudate Cells and Alveolar Macrophages, *J. Cell Biol.*, **17**:465 (1963).

DAWES, J. D. K., and M. M. L. PRICHARD: Studies of the Vascular Arrangements of the Nose, *J. Anat.*, **87**:311 (1953).

FISCHER, H., H. BÖRSIG, and E. EDEN: Studien über den Bau des Bindegewebsgerüstes der Trachea bei verschiedenen Säugetieren, *Gegenbaur Morph. Jahrb.*, **102**:227 (1962).

FLOREY, H., H. M. CARLETON, and A. Q. WELLS: Mucus Secretion in the Trachea, *Brit. J. Exp. Path.*, **13**:269 (1932).

GODLESKI, J. J., and J. D. BRAIN: The Origin of Alveolar Macrophages in Mouse Radiation Chimeras, *J. Exptl. Med.*, **136**:630 (1972).

GOODRICH, E. S.: "Studies on the Structure and Development of Vertebrates," Dover Publications, Inc., New York, 1958.

HAM, A. W., and K. W. BALDWIN: A Histological Study of the Development of the Lung, with Particular Reference to the Nature of Alveoli, *Anat. Rec.*, **81**:363 (1941).

HAYEK, H. VON: Cellular Structure and Mucus Activity in the Bronchial Tree and Alveoli, in A. V. S. de Reuck and M. O'Connor (eds.), "Pulmonary Structure and Function," Ciba Foundation Symposium, Little, Brown and Company, Boston, 1962.

HEISS, R.: Der Atmungsapparat, in W. von Möllendorff (ed.), "Handbüch der Mikroskopischen Anatomie des Menschen," Springer-Verlag OHG, Berlin. 1936.

HONJIN, R.: Experimental Degeneration of the Vagus, and Its Relation to the Nerve Supply of Lung of the Mouse, with Special Reference to the Crossing Innervation of the Lung by the Vagi, *J. Comp. Neurol.*, **106**:1 (1956).

HONJIN, R.: On the Nerve Supply of the Lung of the Mouse, with Special Reference to the Structure of the Peripheral Vegetative Nervous System, *J. Comp. Neurol.*, **105**:587 (1956).

KRAHL, V. E.: The Glomus Pulmonale: Its Location and Microscopic Anatomy, in A. V. S. de Reuck and M. O'Connor (eds.), "Pulmonary Structure and Function," Ciba Foundation Symposium, Little, Brown and Company, Boston, 1962.

LAUWERYNS, J.: The Blood and Lymphatic Microcirculation of the Lung, in S. C. Sommers (ed.), "Pathology Annual," vol. 6, p. 365, Appleton-Century-Crofts, New York, 1971.

LAUWERYNS, J.: L'angioarchitecture du Poumon, *Arch. Biol., (Liege),* **75**(Suppl.):771 (1964).

LELONG, M., and R. LAUMONIER: Histological and Histochemical Evolution of the Foetal Lung, in J. F. Delafresnaye and T. E. Oppé (eds.), "Anoxia of the New-born Infant, a Symposium," Charles C Thomas, Publisher, Springfield, Ill., 1954.

MACKLEM, P. T.: Airway Obstruction and Collateral Ventilation, *Physiol. Rev.,* **51**:368 (1971).

MACKLIN, C. C.: The Pulmonary Alveolar Mucoid Film and the Pneumonocytes, *Lancet,* **266**:1099 (1954).

MACKLIN, C. C.: Pulmonic Alveolar Vents, *J. Anat.,* **69**:188 (1935).

MACKLIN, C. C.: The Musculature of the Bronchi and Lungs, *Physiol. Rev.,* **9**:1 (1929).

MILLER, W. S.: "The Lung," 2d ed., Charles C Thomas, Publisher, Springfield, Ill., 1947.

NEGUS, V.: "The Comparative Anatomy and Physiology of the Nose and Paranasal Sinuses," E. Livingstone and S. Livingstone, Edinburgh, 1958.

OREN, R., A. E. FARNHAM, K. SAITO, E. MILOFSKY, and M. L. KARNOVSKY: Metabolic Patterns in Three Types of Phagocytizing Cells, *J. Cell Biol.,* **17**:487 (1963).

PATTLE, R. E.: Properties, Function and Origin of the Alveolar Lining Layer, *Proc. Roy. Soc. (London), Ser. B,* **148**:217 (1958).

PFAFFMANN, C. (ed.): Olfaction and Taste, "Proceedings of the Third International Symposium," Rockefeller University Press, New York, 1969.

PROCTOR, D. F.: Physiology of the Upper Airway, in W. O. Fenn and H. Rahn, (eds.), "Handbook of Physiology," sec. 3, Respiration, vol. 1, p. 309, Waverly Press, Baltimore, 1965.

REID, L.: The Secondary Lobule in the Adult Human Lung with Special Reference to Its Appearance in Bronchograms, *Thorax,* **13**:110 (1958).

REID, L., and G. SIMON: The Peripheral Pattern in the Normal Bronchogram and Its Relation to Peripheral Pulmonary Anatomy, *Thorax,* **13**:103 (1958).

ROSS, R. B.: Influence of Bronchial Tree Structure on Ventilation in the Dog's Lung as Inferred from Measurements of a Plastic Cast, *J. Appl. Physiol.,* **10**:1 (1957).

SCHAEFFER, J. P.: The Mucous Membrane of the Nasal Cavity and the Paranasal Sinuses, in E. V. Cowdry (ed.), "Special Cytology," vol. 1, Paul B. Hoeber, Inc., New York, 1932.

SCHNEEBERGER, E., and M. J. KARNOVSKY: The Influence of Intravascular Fluid Volume on the Permeability of Newborn and Adult Mouse Lungs to Ultrastructural Protein Tracers, *J. Cell Biol.,* **49**:319 (1971).

SOROKIN, S.: The Cells of the Lungs, in P. Nettesheim, M. G. Hanna, Jr., and J. W. Deatherage, Jr. (eds.), "Morphology of Experimental Respiratory Carcinogenesis," CONF 700501, p. 3, U.S. Atomic Energy Commission, Oak Ridge, Tenn., 1970.

SOROKIN, S.: A Morphologic and Cytochemical Study on the Great Alveolar Cell, *J. Histochem. Cytochem.,* **14**:884 (1966).

SOROKIN, S., H. A. PADYKULA, and E. HERMAN: Comparative Histochemical Patterns in Developing Mammalian Lungs, *Develop. Biol.*, **1**:125 (1959).

TENNEY, S. M., and J. E. REMMERS: Comparative Quantitative Morphology of the Mammalian Lung: Diffusing Area, *Nature* **197**:54 (1963).

TOBIN, C. E.: Human Pulmonic Lymphatics, *Anat. Rec.*, **127**:611 (1957).

TOBIN, C. E.: Lymphatics of the Pulmonary Alveoli, *Anat. Rec.*, **120**:625 (1954).

WEIBEL, E.: Die Blutgefässanastomosen in der menschlichen Lunge, *Z. Zellforsch.*, **50**:653 (1959).

WEIBEL, E. R., and J. GIL: Electron Microscopic Demonstration of an Extracellular Duplex Lining Layer of Alveoli, *Respiration Physiol.*, **4**:42 (1968).

WOLSTENHOLME, G. E. W., and J. KNIGHT (eds.): ''Taste and Smell in Vertebrates,'' J. & A. Churchill, London, 1970.

chapter 22 The urinary system

RUTH ELLEN BULGER

There are those who say that the human kidney was created to keep the blood pure, or more precisely, to keep our internal environment in an ideal balanced state. I would deny this. I grant that the human kidney is a marvelous organ, but I cannot grant that it was purposefully designed to excrete urine, or even to regulate the composition of the blood, or to subserve the physiological welfare of *Homo sapiens* in any sense. Rather I contend that the human kidney manufactures the kind of urine that it does, and it maintains the blood in the composition which that fluid has, because this kidney has a certain functional architecture: and it owes that architecture not to design or foresight or any plan, but to the fact that the earth is an unstable sphere with a fragile crust, to the geologic revolutions that for 600 million years have raised and lowered continents and seas, to the predacious enemies, and heat and cold, and storms and droughts, the unending succession of vicissitudes that have driven the mutant vertebrates from sea into fresh water, into desiccated swamps, out upon the dry land, from one habitation to another, perpetually in search of the free and independent life, perpetually failing for one reason or another to find it.[1]

[1] Homer W. Smith, "Studies in the Physiology of the Kidney," p. 66, University of Kansas, University Extension Division, Lawrence, Kans., 1939.

Introduction

COMPONENTS OF THE URINARY SYSTEM

The normal human urinary system consists of two kidneys, two ureters, a bladder, and a urethra. The kidneys elaborate a fluid product called urine; the ureters, two fibromuscular tubes, conduct the urine to a single urinary bladder where the fluid accumulates for periodic evacuation via the single urethra which connects the bladder to the exterior.

KIDNEY FUNCTION

The kidneys make significant and sometimes vital contributions to several important functions:

1. The excretion of waste products of metabolism

2. The elimination of foreign substances and their breakdown products

3. The maintenance of the extracellular fluid volume

4. The regulation of the amount and type of various salts to be retained or excreted by the body

5. The regulation of total body water

6. The control of acid-base balance

The kidneys carry out these various functions because of their architecture: gross, histologic, cytologic, and chemical. This particular architecture results from the modeling and remodeling which occurred during the long evolutionary process in which animals were subjected to varying environmental conditions. Three separate kidneys have developed during evolution: the pronephros, the mesonephros, and the metanephros. This evolutionary experience is repeated in each human embryo with the serial development of three separate kidneys and the subsequent degeneration of the first two during early embryonic life. In each of these kidneys there are filtering devices capable of developing a fluid which the adjacent tubules then modify. The filter has become more efficient and the tubule more complex during evolution.

Three separate physiologic processes are involved in the formation of urine by the adult metanephric kidney: (1) filtration, (2) secretion, and (3) reabsorption. The first step in the formation of urine is a *filtration* process in which an ultrafiltrate of plasma is created. The filtering membrane retains most large proteins within the blood, but a small amount of albumin (MW approximately 70,000) passes into the filtrate. As it passes down the tubule, the filtrate is altered by *secretion,* in which additional substances are moved by the lining cells of the tubule from the surrounding renal interstitium into the filtrate within the tubular lumen, and *reabsorption,* whereby substances are moved from the intratubular filtrate across the tubular cells back into the renal interstitium. The fluid that emerges at the end of the tubule is the net result of these three processes and is called *urine.*

Urine production in the mammalian kidney is a grossly inefficient process. In man, every 24 hr 180 liters of fluid are filtered by the renal corpuscles into the tubular lumen of the kidney, but normally only 1 or 2 liters of urine are produced. The remainder of the filtered fluid is reabsorbed across the tubular epithelium to reenter the blood vascular system. This process requires a large expenditure of energy.

The kidney

The kidneys of man are paired, bean-shaped organs which lie in the retroperitoneal space on the posterior aspect of the abdominal cavity. The lateral border on each kidney is convex, and the medial border is concave. Normally one kidney is found on either side of the vertebral column, with their upper margins near the upper region of the twelfth thoracic vertebra. The upper poles lie closer to the vertebral column than the lower poles, and so the long axis of the kidney is parallel with the psoas muscles. The kidney is surrounded by a fibrous capsule and situated within a mass of fatty tissue.

The medial concave border is penetrated by a vertical slit called the *renal hilus.* Branches of the renal artery, vein, lymphatics, and nerves, as well as an expanded part of the ureter (called the *pelvis*), pass through the hilus to the renal parenchyma. The renal hilus communicates with a flattened cavity within the kidney called the *renal sinus*. Within the sinus, the expanded pelvis of the ureter branches into three or four major calyxes which in turn branch to form seven to fourteen minor calyxes. Loose connective tissue and fat tissue found within the sinus provide a region through which the vessels and nerves pass.

When the kidney is bisected into dorsal and ventral portions (Fig. 22-1), it can be seen to be divided into a cortex and a medulla. The cortex consists of a broad outer zone of dark red substance and projections which extend toward the renal sinus (called the *renal columns* because of their columnar profile in a section of kidney). The medulla is composed of a variable number of conical structures of lighter, striated appearance called *medullary pyramids*. They are situated with their bases adjacent to the outer zone of cortex, and their apices pro-

ject into the renal sinus. The apex of each medullary pyramid is capped by a funnel-shaped minor calyx. Urine produced by the kidney exits at the medullary apex and is funneled by a minor calyx into the remainder of the extrarenal collecting system.

The kidney is divided into units called *lobes*. One lobe consists of a conical medullary pyramid and the cortical substance which surrounds it like the cap of an acorn. The kidneys of some animals, such as rodents, consist of only one lobe (unilobar). However, multilobar human kidneys contain from six to eighteen lobes. During human fetal life, the lobes develop separately and are demarcated by deep clefts between them (Fig. 22-2). In postnatal life, however, these clefts are generally obliterated and the organ appears to have a smooth surface, although the lobes still exist within the kidney.

At intervals along the base of each medullary

Figure 22-1 Gross anatomic appearance of a human kidney, at three-fifths its natural size. The tissue has been bisected to reveal elements of the internal structure. (From H. Braus, ''Anatomie des Menschen,'' Springer-Verlag OHG, Berlin, 1924.)

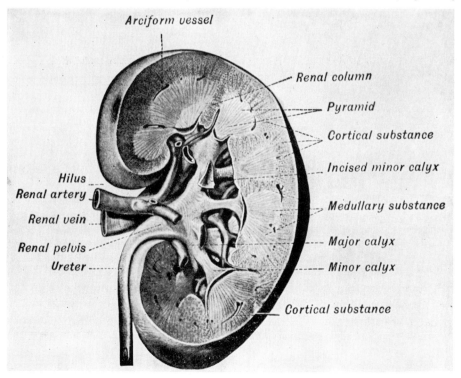

Arciform vessel

Renal column

Pyramid

Cortical substance

Incised minor calyx

Hilus

Renal artery

Medullary substance

Renal vein

Renal pelvis

Major calyx

Ureter

Minor calyx

Cortical substance

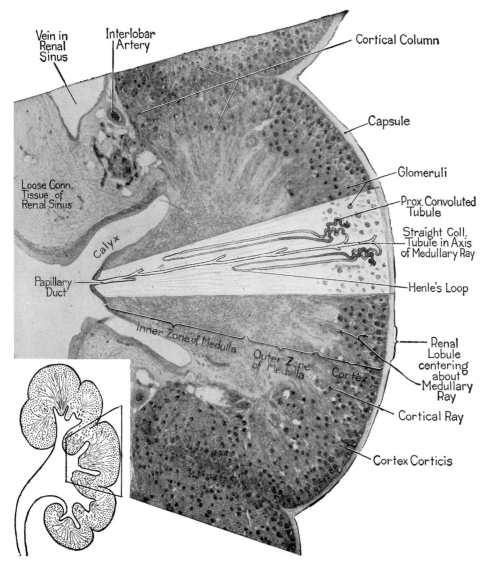

Figure 22-2 Photomicrograph showing one lobe of a metanephric kidney from a 6-month-old human fetus. The inset outlines the part of the kidney which appears in the photograph. The schematic diagram in the center of the lobe shows the position and arrangement of the renal tubules around a straight collecting tubule. ×18. (From B. M. Patten, "Human Embryology," 3d ed., McGraw-Hill Book Company, New York, 1968.)

pyramid, striated elements called *medullary rays* penetrate into the cortex. Although they resemble the medullary substance because of their striated appearance, the medullary rays are considered part of the cortex. Each medullary ray forms the center of a small cone of renal parenchyma called a *lobule*.

An additional zonation can be seen in the gross structure of the medulla, which is divided into an *outer zone* adjacent to the cortex and an *inner zone* including the medullary tip (which is called the *papilla*). The outer zone, in turn, consists of an outer and inner stripe. The zones seen grossly are a reflection of the differing morphologies of the regions of the renal secretory units and of their orientation within the kidney (Fig. 22-3).

FUNCTIONAL ANATOMY OF THE URINIFEROUS TUBULE

The functional unit of the kidney is the uriniferous tubule. Each kidney in man contains approximately one million of these units. The uriniferous tubule is composed of a long convoluted portion called the *nephron* and a system of *intrarenal collecting ducts*. Each of these segments was derived from a different embryologic primordium. The nephron developed from the metanephrogenic blastema (tissue from the caudal region of the urogenital ridge),

whereas the collecting ducts were derived from the ureteric bud (a diverticulum of the mesonephric duct). In spite of this dual derivation, a gradual transition is seen in the structure and function at the junction of these two regions, and so the term *nephron* has recently been used synonymously with uriniferous tubule by some investigators. In this chapter, however, the term nephron will not include the intrarenal collecting ducts.

Nephron   The nephron is composed of several regions of diversified morphology, but all of them are characterized by cells that have an elaborate shape with numerous lateral interdigitating processes. The blind end of the nephron is indented

Figure 22-3   Schematic diagram of a cortical and a juxtamedullary nephron, showing the relationship of segments of the nephron to the zones of the kidney which can be seen grossly.

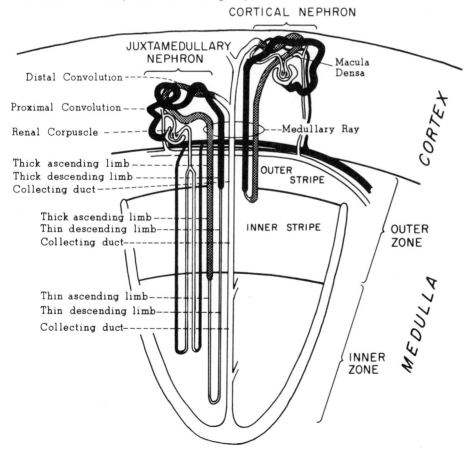

by a network of capillaries and supporting cells to form a filtering body called the *renal corpuscle*. In addition, the nephron consists of the following: (1) a neck, (2) a proximal convoluted tubule, (3) a straight region of the proximal tubule, (4) a thin limb, (5) a straight region of the distal tubule, (6) a macula densa region of the distal tubule, and (7) a distal convoluted tubule.

Nephrons are situated within the kidney in a characteristic position (Fig. 22-2) with the renal corpuscles and proximal convoluted tubules situated within the cortex. The straight portion of the proximal tubule, the thin limb segment, and the straight portion of the distal tubule form a looping

structure called the *loop of Henle,* which enters into the medullary pyramid by way of a medullary ray, forms a hairpin loop within the medulla, and returns to the cortex via the same medullary ray. As the straight portion of each distal tubule enters the cortex, it passes adjacent to its originating renal corpuscle, forming the macula densa of the distal tubule, and then continues as the distal convoluted segment.

Although all nephrons have these regions, two separate types of nephrons have been described. Presumably there is a continuum between these two types. The *cortical* nephrons are characterized by a renal corpuscle located in the peripheral region

Figure 22-4   Sections of kidney cortex cut perpendicular to the capsule in A and parallel to the capsule in B to show the medullary rays and the convoluted tubules which lie between them. × 80.

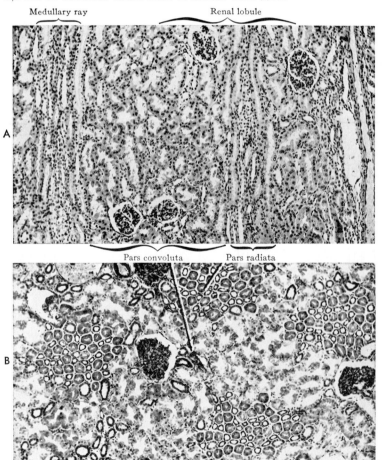

Medullary ray   Renal lobule

A

Pars convoluta   Pars radiata

B

of the cortex and by a short loop of Henle which may lack a thin limb segment. The *juxtamedullary* nephrons are characterized by a larger renal corpuscle located in the cortex adjacent to the medulla, a longer convoluted tubule, and a long loop of Henle with a lengthy thin limb segment. Even though the nephrons differ in length, each region of all nephrons tends to occupy a certain position in the kidney as a whole, causing the gross zonation described earlier (Fig. 22-3). For example, the thin limbs are seen in the inner stripe of the outer zone of the medulla and in the inner zone of the medulla whereas the proximal and distal convoluted tubules are located only in the cortex.

The nephrons empty into a complex system of collecting ducts. In human kidneys, the cortical nephrons tend to empty singly into a terminal collecting duct whereas several juxtamedullary nephrons empty into an arched collecting duct which courses peripherally in the cortex and then enters the medullary ray. These cortical collecting ducts merge while traversing the medullary ray and medullary pyramid and empty as several large collecting ducts at the apex of the medullary pyramid.

Renal corpuscle The nephron begins with a renal corpuscle which is located in the cortex and is roughly oval in shape (Fig. 22-4). Estimates of their diameter in man range from 150 to 250 μm. Each renal corpuscle consists of tufts of anastomosing capillaries and their supporting cells, which have developed within a double-walled capsule formed by half of the S-shaped bend in one end of the developing renal tubule. A renal corpuscle therefore has some resemblance to a balloon (the capsule) with a fist (the capillaries) punched into it. The outer wall of the capsule is called the *parietal* layer; the inner wall is the *visceral* (*glomerular*) layer. The space between the two walls of the capsule is called *Bowman's space*. The epithelium of this visceral wall covers the anastomosing capillaries much like a glove covers each finger of a hand. Between the epithelium and the capillaries is an extracellular layer, the glomerular *basement membrane* (*basal lamina*).

At one region of the renal corpuscle, called the *urinary pole*, the parietal layer of capsular epithelium is continuous with the epithelium of the neck of the tubule (Fig. 22-5). Bowman's space is

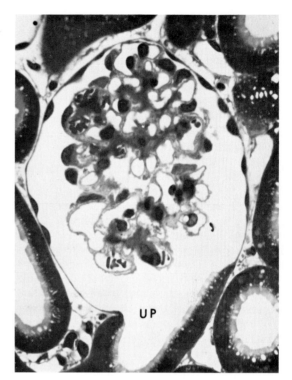

UP

Figure 22-5 Renal corpuscle of an epoxy resin section from a rat kidney, showing the urinary pole (UP). Toluidine blue. ×520.

therefore continuous with the lumen of the remaining nephron, so that fluid formed by filtration within the renal corpuscle enters the lumen of the proximal convoluted tubule. Another region of the renal corpuscle located roughly opposite the urinary pole is called the *vascular pole* (Fig. 22-6). It is marked by the point of entrance of the afferent arteriole and the exit of the efferent arteriole. The afferent arteriole enters the renal corpuscle and divides into four or more primary branches. Each of these branches becomes a network of anastomosing capillaries which forms a lobule. The lobule has a stalk or supporting region called the *mesangial region*. The capillaries within a lobule reunite to form the efferent arteriole which exits from the vascular pole. Since the efferent arteriole again breaks up to form a second capillary network, such an arrangement constitutes a portal system—an arterial portal system, in contrast to the venous portal system in the liver. The second capillary network surrounds the tubules and is therefore called the *peritubular capillary network*. Some authors describe a differing morphology at the vascular pole of juxtamedullary nephrons (Ljungqvist, 1964). In their descriptions, the afferent arteriole is continuous with the efferent arteriole, and the capillaries to the renal corpuscle exit from the side of this arteriolar shunt. Because of the anatomy of the arterioles in the juxtamedullary region, if the renal corpuscle dies, an aglomerular vessel can form. These vessels have been called the *vasa rectae verae*.

The renal corpuscle therefore consists of the following parts: (1) the parietal epithelium of the capsule, (2) the visceral epithelium of the capsule, (3) the glomerular basement membrane (basal lamina), (4) the endothelium of the glomerulus, and (5) the intraglomerular mesangial region (Figs. 22-5 to 22-7). These will be considered in order.

THE PARIETAL EPITHELIUM OF BOWMAN'S CAPSULE
The parietal epithelium consists of a layer of simple squamous cells which bulge into Bowman's space in the region of their nuclei. They are polygonal in outline and rest on a thick basement membrane

Figure 22-6 Renal corpuscle of an epoxy resin section from a rat kidney, showing the afferent and efferent vessels (arrows) at the vascular pole. ×320.

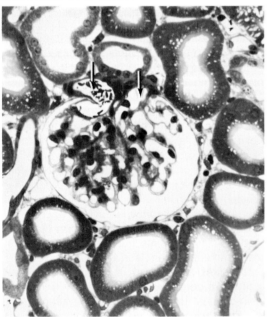

which in some cases appears to be multilayered. At the vascular pole, the parietal epithelium is reflected to form the visceral layer.

THE VISCERAL EPITHELIUM OF BOWMAN'S CAPSULE
The visceral epithelium closely embraces the entire network of glomerular capillaries and consists of cells which have a complex shape. The cells, which are frequently called *podocytes*, do not rest on the basement membrane for long regions but tend to sit somewhat removed in Bowman's space. The cells have long primary processes called trabeculae. The trabeculae in turn branch to form secondary and tertiary processes. All three of these kinds of processes again branch to form thin, club-shaped terminal processes called *pedicels* (little feet) which interdigitate in a complicated manner with similar processes from adjacent cells. This is well demonstrated in a scanning electron micrograph taken by Arakawa (1970) (Fig. 22-8). The pedicels form a layer along the glomerular basement membrane. This elaborate interdigitation results in an extensive pattern of narrow slits between the pedicels. In electron micrographs, these slits seem to be bridged by a thin layer of material of unknown composition called the *filtration-slit membrane*, which is thinner than a cell membrane and appears to be similar to the diaphragms seen across the pores of fenestrated capillaries and across nuclear pores. The podocytes have nuclei which are large and irregular in shape and tend to be indented on one side in the region of the Golgi apparatus. They contain abundant protein secretory equipment, numerous fine filaments, and microtubules.

GLOMERULAR BASEMENT MEMBRANE (BASAL LAMINA)
In adult human beings, the basement membrane is thick, with a mean diameter of approximately 320 to 340 nm (Jorgensen, 1966). It is thinner in very young children and in most experimental animals. The basement membrane stains with periodic acid–Schiff (PAS) reagent. It appears to contain a collagen-like protein and a mucopolysaccharide rich in sialic acid. It is composed of three layers: an electron-dense central layer, the lamina densa, and a less dense layer on either side, the lamina rara externa (adjacent to the glomerular podocytes) and a lamina rara interna (adjacent to the capillary endothelium). In the stalk region of each capillary loop, the basement membrane does not surround

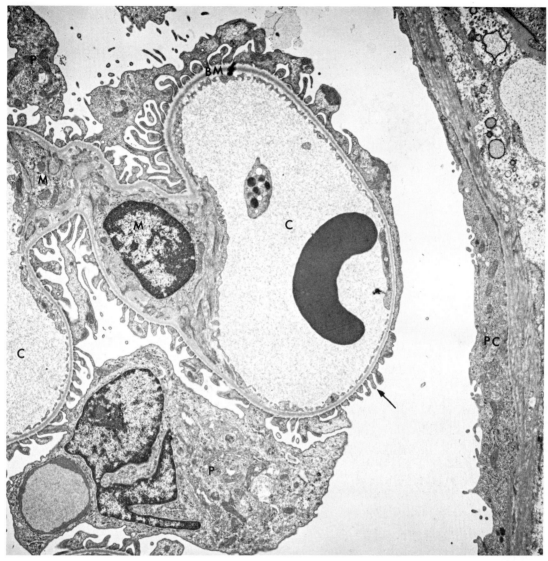

Figure 22-7   Electron micrograph from a renal corpuscle, showing capillaries (C), glomerular podocytes (P), with their small processes called pedicels (arrow), mesangial cells (M), and the glomerular basement membrane (BM). A portion of a parietal cell (PC) can be seen at the right.   ×6,100.

the entire endothelium but instead appears to be reflected with the glomerular epithelial cells from which it is presumably largely derived (Fig. 22-7).

ENDOTHELIUM   The endothelium consists of a simple squamous layer of fenestrated cells.   The cells are extremely thin, except at the stalk region of the capillary where their nuclei bulge into the lumen.   In this region the cells can have complex processes extending into the capillary lumen.   The fenestrae of this particular endothelium differ from those found in the more typical fenestrated endothelium of the peritubular capillaries and of other regions of the body in that the pores appear to be more irregular in shape and larger in size (approxi-

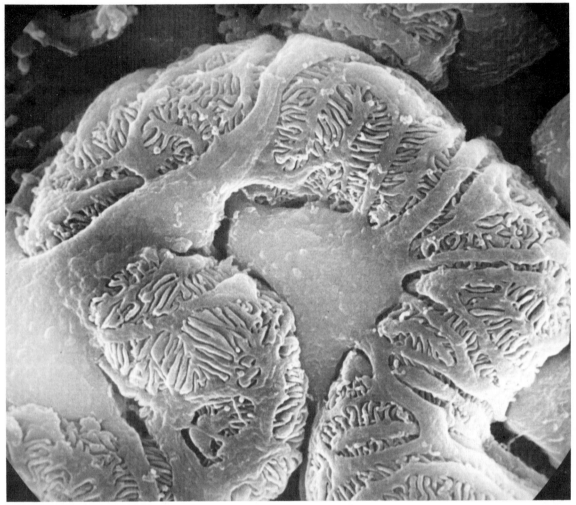

Figure 22-8 Scanning electron micrograph of a capillary loop from a normal rat kidney glomerulus, showing the processes of podocytes interdigitating along the surface of the capillary wall. ×4,500. (Fig. 4, M. Arakawa, Lab. Invest., **23**:489, 1971.)

mately 50 to 100 nm in diameter). Although pores in fenestrated endothelium are generally bridged by a thin diaphragm, only a few of the fenestrae of the glomerulus are bridged by diaphragms. Both of these modifications (large-sized pores and few diaphragms) would increase the permeability of this endothelium.

INTRAGLOMERULAR MESANGIAL REGION The mesangial or stalk region of the capillary tuft consists of a population of cells and the matrix material in which they are embedded. The cells appear similar

to pericytes seen adjacent to vessels elsewhere in the body. Each cell contains a small, densely staining nucleus, fine filaments especially abundant along the cell membranes, and dense cytoplasmic plaques located along the cell membrane. The cells have long processes, some of which can penetrate the mesangial matrix underlying the capillary endothelium to come into contact with the endothelial cell. In some cases, these processes appear to project through the endothelium into the lumen of the capillary. The function of these mesangial cell projections is at present unknown. Mesangial cells are of particular importance because they have a propensity to divide in certain kidney diseases. The mesangial matrix appears to be an amorphous substance with less electron density than the lamina densa of the basement membrane. It appears to be continuous with the lamina rara interna. The function of the mesangial region is at present unresolved but it might provide support for the capillaries or have a contractile or a phagocytic function. The intraglomerular mesangial region is continuous with the extraglomerular mesangial region (part of the juxtaglomerular apparatus) and in certain experimental circumstances can be seen to contain granulated cells like those of the extraglomerular mesangium.

FUNCTION OF THE RENAL CORPUSCLE Because of its morphology, the renal corpuscle behaves as a filtering device which allows the passage of water and ions but retains large objects such as cells and even large protein molecules. Since a small amount of albumin penetrates the filter, it appears to be near the effective pore size of the filtration barrier. The barrier is complex and, as can be seen in Fig. 22-9, consists of three morphologic structures: (1) the fenestrated endothelium, (2) the glomerular basement membrane, and (3) the slits between pedicels which are bridged by the filtration-slit membrane. Each of these barriers restricts structures of a particular size. Tracer molecules of various sizes have been used to determine the limits of the permeability of each of the barriers. The capillary endothelial pores limit the passage of red blood cells and other formed elements of the blood but allow the passage of a molecule such as ferritin (MW 450,000) (Farquhar et al., 1961). The basement membrane serves to restrict the passage of ferritin and to be a relative barrier to the passage of catalase (MW 240,000) (Venkatachalam et al., 1970). Molecules of myelo-

Figure 22-9 Electron micrograph of the filtration barrier from a rat renal corpuscle, showing a red blood cell (RBC) within a capillary lumen, an endothelial cell (E) with fenestrations, a basement membrane (BM), and a layer of interdigitating pedicels (Pe). ×71,700.

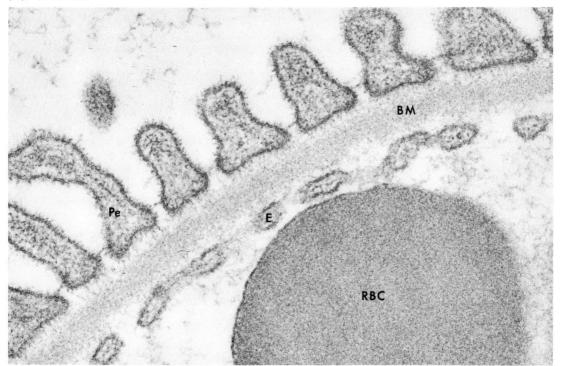

peroxidase (MW 170,000) appear to penetrate the basement membrane but to be retained by the filtration-slit membrane (Graham and Karnovsky, 1966). Horseradish peroxidase (MW 40,000) penetrates the filtration-slit membrane (Graham and Karnovsky, 1966).

Several morphologic features favor the production of a large volume of glomerular filtrate. The kidney has a large renal blood flow (approximately 20 to 25 percent of the cardiac output) and, because of the vascular arrangement of the kidney, almost all the blood must pass through a renal corpuscle. In addition, a contractile efferent arteriole helps to maintain a high filtration pressure along the entire glomerular capillary bed. Also, as has been mentioned earlier, the endothelial pores are larger and the majority appear to lack a diaphragm. The complex shape of the podocytes increases the area of the intercellular channels through which the filtrate can pass to gain access to Bowman's space, and these are limited only by a thin diaphragm.

The pressure relationships of the renal corpuscle also favor filtration. The hydrostatic pressure in the glomerular capillaries is nearly 90 mm Hg, whereas the opposing hydrostatic pressure of Bowman's space is only 15 mm Hg. The oncotic pressure within the capillaries is approximately 30 mm Hg, but almost no oncotic pressure is present within Bowman's space. The resulting glomerular filtration pressure is therefore equal to (90 − 15) − (30 − 0) or 45 mm Hg. This high pressure results in an average of 180 liters of glomerular filtrate being formed each 24 hr in a normal human adult.

Neck segment The transition region which connects the renal corpuscle with the proximal tubule is called the *neck segment*. It is not well developed in mammalian kidneys. The neck shows variation in structure and even in its presence in differing species. In rat kidneys, no neck segments are seen (Fig. 22-5), whereas in mouse kidneys, cells like those lining the proximal convoluted tubule have been observed to line the wall of Bowman's capsule. In man, however, certain nephrons have a short neck segment lined with simple squamous epithelium like the lining of the parietal wall of Bowman's capsule (Fig. 22-33). In cystinosis (a relatively rare inherited metabolic disease), these

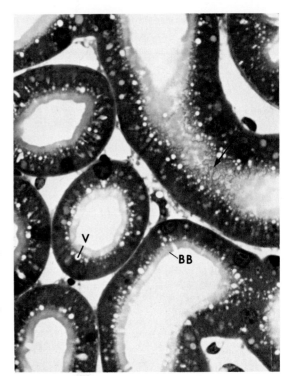

Figure 22-10 Profiles of proximal convoluted tubules in the cortex of a rat kidney embedded in epoxy resin. Note the brush border (BB) lining the lumen and the vacuoles (V) of the apical endocytotic apparatus. In the upper right-hand corner of the picture, the section cuts parallel to the surface of the cell in such a way that one can see the elaborate apical interdigitations of these cells (arrow). ×570.

flattened epithelial cells extend for a greater length and constitute the Swan neck deformity (Darmady and Stranack, 1957).

Proximal tubule The proximal tubule is composed of segments differing somewhat in their morphology, histochemical reactions, and vulnerability to various toxins. Two of these are most frequently distinguished: a *proximal convoluted portion,* which comprises the longest tubule in the cortex and hence the one most frequently seen in random section, and a *straight portion (pars recta)* of the proximal tubule, which enters an adjacent medullary ray and turns toward the renal sinus to form the first part of the loop of Henle which penetrates into the medulla.

The lumen of the functioning proximal tubule is wide open in life because of the blood pressure. Anything that interrupts the blood supply to the organ will make the proximal tubular lumens collapse. To preserve the morphology of the living animal, an adequate filtration pressure must be maintained during fixation. This can be done by dripping the fixative on the kidney surface, by rapid freezing procedures, by microperfusion of single tubules, or by intravascular perfusion of fixative solutions.

PROXIMAL CONVOLUTED TUBULE   The proximal convoluted tubule is the longest and largest segment of the mammalian nephron, averaging approximately 14 mm in length and 30 to 60 μm in diameter. It is lined by a single layer of cells that have an elaborate shape, a well-developed microvillus (or brush) border along the lumen, an active endocytotic apparatus, and an abundant acidophilic cytoplasm (Figs. 22-10 to 22-12).

The cells exhibit an extensive system of lateral processes which interdigitate with corresponding

Figure 22-11   Electron micrograph of portions of three proximal convoluted tubules, showing the microvillus brush border (BB), the abundant endocytotic apparatus (EA), and the numerous elongated mitochondria (M) oriented perpendicular to the tubular basement membrane.   ×3,100.

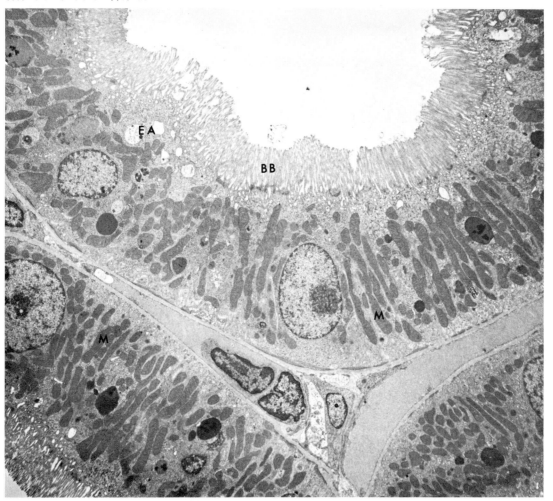

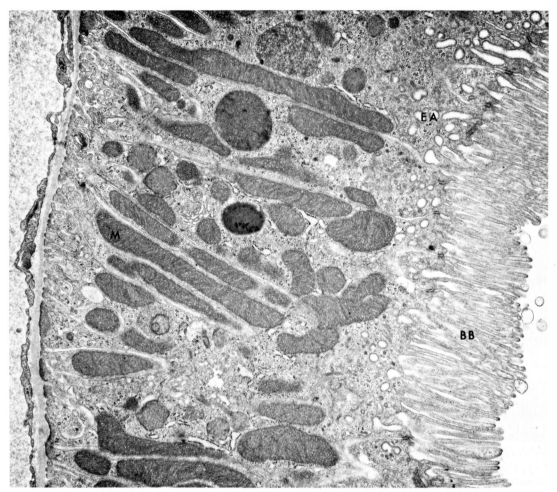

Figure 22-12   Electron micrograph of a proximal convoluted tubule, showing details of the microvillus brush border (BB), the endocytotic apparatus (EA), the numerous mitochondria (M) seen in the basal part of the cell, and the compartments formed by the lateral interdigitating processes from adjacent cells.   ×9,600.

lateral processes from adjacent cells. Large ridges extend the full height of the cell. More extensive but smaller interdigitating processes are also present in the apical region, and an especially prominent and elaborate system of primary and secondary interdigitations exist in the basal half of the cell (Fig. 22-13). These lateral interdigitating processes greatly increase the area of lateral cell membrane and form an extensive labyrinth of lateral intercellular spaces. The lateral processes are generally wide enough to contain one layer of large mito-

chondria which are oriented with their long axes from cell apex to cell base; this orientation causes the pattern of basal striations seen in the basal cytoplasm of well-fixed kidneys.

One of the major functions of the proximal tubule is to reduce the volume of glomerular filtrate by approximately 80 percent of its original volume. This is accomplished by the active transport of sodium ions out of the proximal convoluted tubular cells into the lateral intercellular spaces by a Mg^+-dependent Na^+-K^+ activated ATPase pump presum-

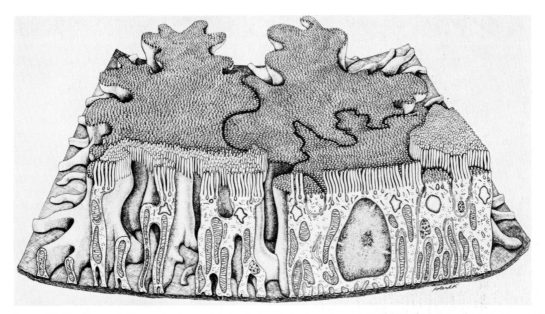

Figure 22-13 Diagram of a proximal convoluted tubular cell to show the elaborate interdigitations that occur between adjacent cells. Some interdigitating processes extend the full height of the cells, whereas smaller elaborate interdigitations occur in the basal and apical regions. (From Fig. 5, R. Bulger, Amer. J. Anat., **116**:237, 1965.)

ably located within the lateral cell membrane. The abundant mitochondria located next to the lateral cell membranes provide the ATP for this transport. Because of the electric charge of the sodium ions pumped into the lateral space, chloride ions follow passively, and this accumulation of ions causes an osmotic movement of water into this labyrinthine system. The increased hydrostatic pressure thus created in the lateral spaces in turn forces fluid out through the porous basement membrane into the renal interstitium.

The brush border lining the luminal surface of the cells consists of long, closely packed, microvilli which are covered by the apical cell membrane (Fig. 22-14). An extracellular mucopolysaccharide coats these microvilli (Fig. 22-15). The microvilli of the proximal tubule appear to reabsorb amino acids and sugars in a manner similar to those of the intestinal striated border. Isolated segments obtained from rabbit renal cortex that are rich in brush border membrane contain a high concentration of two disaccharides and several ATPases (Berger and Sacktor, 1970). Similar preparations have also been shown to bind L-proline. This has

Figure 22-14 Electron micrograph from a portion of a proximal convoluted tubular cell, showing the finger-like microvilli that make up the brush border region. The processes are surrounded by a layer of apical cell membrane. ×18,300.

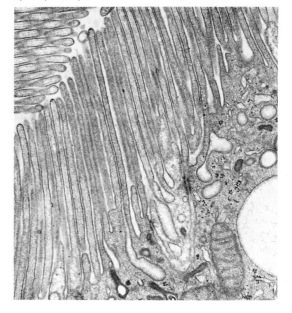

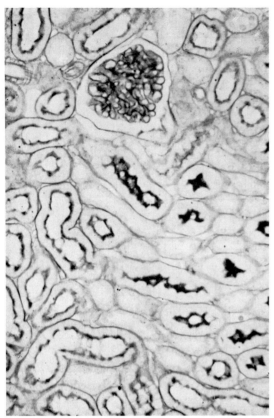

Figure 22-15   PAS reaction in mouse kidney.   A positive reaction is seen in the brush border of the proximal tubules and in the basement membranes of the tubules and of the renal corpuscle.   ×300.   (Courtesy of H. W. Deane.)

been interpreted as evidence for the probable site of the initial step in the transtubular transport of the amino acid (Hillman and Rosenberg, 1970).

Although the glomerular filtrate contains only a low concentration of protein, the volume of filtrate is so large that several grams of protein are filtered each day (Fig. 22-16).   The proximal tubule reabsorbs this filtered protein.   The cell therefore contains a prominent endocytotic apparatus which includes the following components: (1) Tubular invaginations of the apical cell membrane are located between the bases of the microvilli and extend down into the apical cytoplasm.   The protein appears to be bound to the layer of fuzz (glycocalyx) radiating from the cell membrane (Fig. 22-17).   (2)

A series of small vesicles are thought to bud from the bases of the tubular invaginations and presumably to ferry the trapped protein molecules to the next component of the endocytotic apparatus.   (3) Large apical vacuoles form by the fusion of the small vesicles (Fig. 22-18).   (4) Condensing vacuoles condense the proteins.   When tracer proteins such as horseradish peroxidase are injected into the vessels of a mammal, they are seen first within the lumen of the tubular invagination, second in the vesicles, third in the apical vacuoles, fourth within the condensing vacuoles, and finally within lysosomes.   Studies using horseradish peroxidase as a

Figure 22-16   Electron micrograph from a renal corpuscle of an animal that had received horseradish peroxidase prior to fixation. The dense reaction product can be seen in the capillary lumen (C) within the pores (P) of the endothelium and within the basement membrane (BM).   The material is filtered into Bowman's space (BS).   ×30,000.

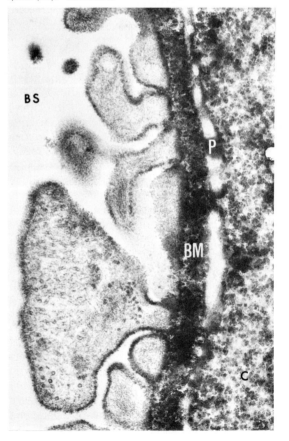

molecular tracer and the histochemical reaction for acid phosphatase as a lysosomal tracer when done simultaneously (Straus, 1964) have shown that within 60 min both the acid hydrolases and the absorbed protein can be seen within the same bodies. This presumably occurs by the fusion of primary or secondary lysosomes with elements of the endocytotic apparatus (Fig. 22-19). In general, proteins sequestered within lysosomes appear to be destined for breakdown into amino acids with their subsequent reuse by the animal. In the kidney, undigested residues within lysosomes can be released from the cell by fusion of the lysosomal membrane with the cell membrane at the luminal surface.

Figure 22-17 Electron micrograph of the apical region of a proximal convoluted tubular cell which was in the process of taking up horseradish peroxidase. The reaction product can be seen within the apical invaginations (arrow) formed by the apical plasma membrane and in apical vacuoles (AV). ×17,100.

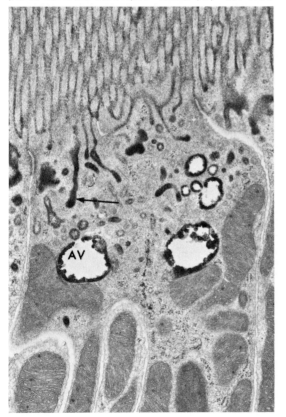

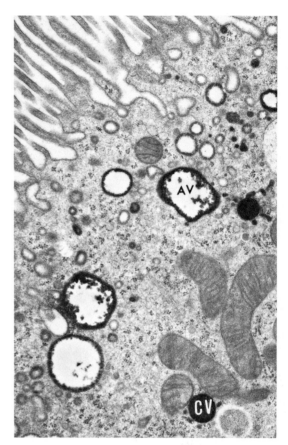

Figure 22-18 Electron micrograph of the apical region of a proximal tubular cell which was in the process of taking up horseradish peroxidase. The reactive product can be seen in apical vacuoles (AV) and in condensing vacuoles (CV) within the apical cytoplasm. ×13,700.

The proximal tubular cells contain a large, round, centrally located nucleus with a prominent nucleolus. The Golgi apparatus lies in a supranuclear position and appears to consist of a large number of vesicles and membrane cisterns. Proximal tubular cells also contain microbodies (Fig. 22-20), with a dense matrix substance, often with a core-like nucleoid, and in some species plate-like structures (marginal plates) along the surface. The bodies are frequently surrounded by the smooth endoplasmic reticulum (ER). Microbodies have been called peroxisomes (De Duve and Baudhuin, 1966) because they contain enzymes concerned with cellular metabolism of hydrogen peroxide. In addition, they

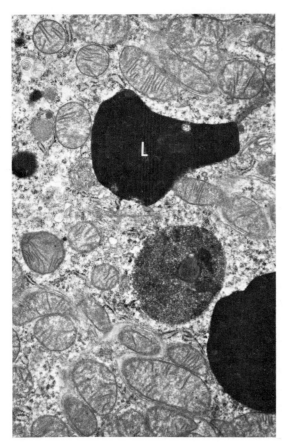

Figure 22-19 Electron micrograph of the basal region of a proximal convoluted tubular cell that had taken up horseradish peroxidase 3 days prior to fixation. The reaction product can be seen within lysosomes (L) in the basal cytoplasm. ×11,500.

may function in gluconeogenesis since it is well known that proximal tubular cells utilize fatty acids as an energy source. The proximal tubular cells are bound together by an extremely short tight junction and an intermediate junction. Desmosomes are only infrequently seen.

In addition to the functions already discussed, the proximal tubule reabsorbs bicarbonate by the secretion of hydrogen ions into the tubular lumen. This leads to the formation of carbonic acid which breaks down into carbon dioxide and water. A number of exogenous organic acids (such as penicillin) and organic bases are actively secreted into the tubular fluid by the proximal tubule. The struc-

ture which accomplishes these functions has not been identified.

STRAIGHT PART OF THE PROXIMAL TUBULE   The straight part of the proximal tubule begins in the medullary ray and penetrates into the medulla for varying lengths, depending upon whether the nephron is of the cortical or juxtamedullary type.   The straight part ends near the lower border of the outer stripe of the outer zone of the medulla where it abruptly changes into the cells of the thin limb of Henle's loop (Fig. 22-3).

The cells in the straight part of the proximal tubule are similar to those of the convoluted seg-

Figure 22-20 Electron micrograph showing microbodies (Mb) from a proximal convoluted tubular cell of a primate (Galago). The microbody is characterized by a single membrane surrounding it, a dense homogeneous matrix, dense bodies within the matrix, called nucleoids (N), and, in certain species, plate-like structures along the edge of the body, called marginal plates (MP). ×50,400.

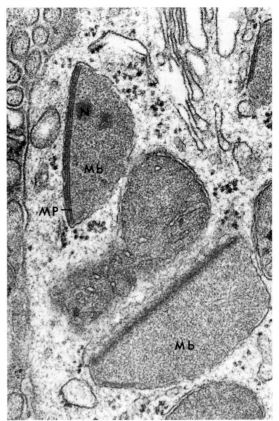

ment, but they appear to be lower in height and have a less elaborate shape (Fig. 22-21). The mitochondria, although still abundant, are smaller and more randomly distributed throughout the cell. The brush border is frequently well developed and PAS-positive. The cells contain fewer lysosomes and a less well-developed endocytotic apparatus. However, microbodies are more prominent in this region of the tubule.

Thin limb of the loop of Henle   The thin limb segment can be short or absent in cortical nephrons and occurs largely on the descending limb, or it can be long, reaching far into the inner medulla in juxta-

medullary nephrons, with both descending and ascending thin limb segments. In human nephrons, approximately 14 percent of the nephrons have long loops of Henle, whereas the remainder are cortical nephrons. The tubule is approximately 20 to 40 μm in diameter. The thin limb segment is lined by a thin squamous epithelium whose wall is approximately 1 to 2 μm in height (Fig. 22-22). Although the epithelium is therefore thicker than the endothelium, it is somewhat difficult to distinguish from endothelium in paraffin sections. In the region of the nucleus, the cell bulges into the lumen. Although there are species differences, the cells of the thin limb are also elaborate in shape with lateral

Figure 22-21 Electron micrograph of the straight part of the proximal tubule from a normal human kidney. The cells are of less elaborate shape, and the mitochondria are more circular in profile. The brush border (BB) and lysosomes (L) can be seen. ×16,000.

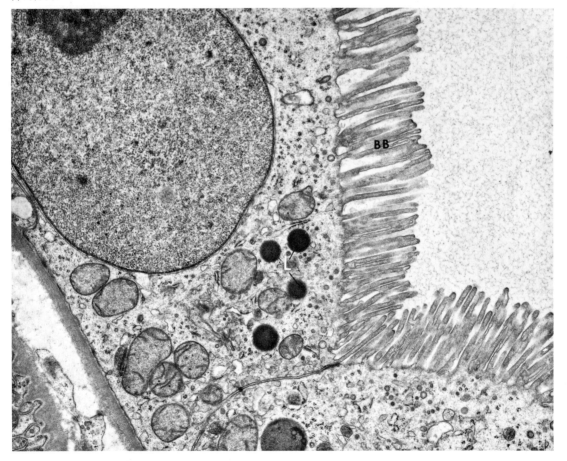

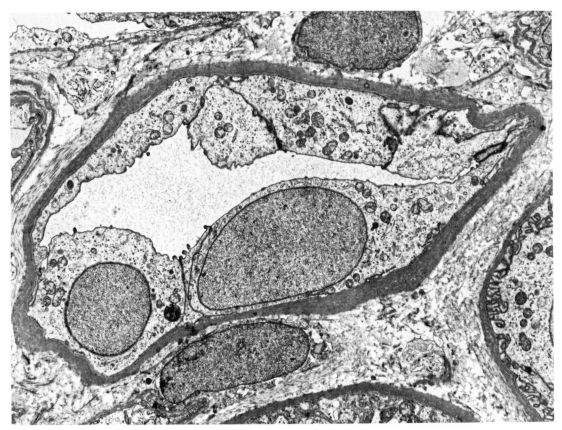

Figure 22-22   Electron micrograph of the thin limb segment from a normal human kidney.   The number of processes seen indicates that the cells are elaborate in shape; however, man has a much simpler cell shape in this region than most experimental animals.   ×9,600.

interdigitating processes which generally are the full thickness of the epithelium.   The early thin limb cells contain many lateral extensions, have abundant microvilli, and a few small round mitochondria.   The shape of the cells of the thin limb become less complex throughout its course so that in the last part of the thin ascending limb, fewer interdigitating processes are seen and fewer microvilli are present.   Although the morphology of thin descending and ascending limbs is similar except for these changes in cell shape, the two limbs are believed to have different functions.

It was noted early that birds and mammals were the only two species whose nephrons had loops of Henle and were the only animals that could produce hypertonic urine.   It was also noted that the fluid in the cortex was isosmotic with plasma, whereas there was an increasing osmotic concentration of the medulla as one approached the papillary tip.   It was therefore postulated that the loop of Henle plays an important role in concentrating urine by serving as a countercurrent multiplier system.

The loop of Henle is believed to function in the following manner.   The thin (and thick) ascending limb actively pumps sodium ions from the tubular fluid into the extracellular space.   In this region, the permeability to water appears to be low, so with the exit of the sodium ions the luminal fluid becomes hypotonic and the sodium ions are trapped in the medullary interstitium.   This hypothesis will be further discussed in the section Function of the Distal Nephron.   A passive role has been postulated for the thin descending limb.   Some physiologists believe that the thin descending limb is highly permeable to water but not to solutes, whereas others believe it is permeable to both.

Distal tubule   The distal tubule is composed of three regions: the straight part of the distal tubule (pars recta), the macula densa, and the distal convoluted tubule.

STRAIGHT PART OF THE DISTAL TUBULE   The straight part of the distal tubule begins near the border of the inner and outer medulla in a transition from the thin ascending limbs.   In some species such as rat, this transition appears to be fairly abrupt, and in others such as man, it is gradual.   The straight part of the distal tubule forms the third component of the loop of Henle and completes the looping structure by returning through the medulla and the medullary ray to the renal corpuscle from which the tubule arose.   The cells of the ascending thick limb are extremely irregular in shape with most of their interdigitations extending from the lumen to the basal region of the cell (Fig. 22-23).   Although this straight part resembles the convoluted part of the

Figure 22-23   Electron micrograph of the ascending thick part of the distal tublue from a normal human kidney.   The cells are highly interdigitated, and the lateral processes contain large mitochondria.   ×12,800.

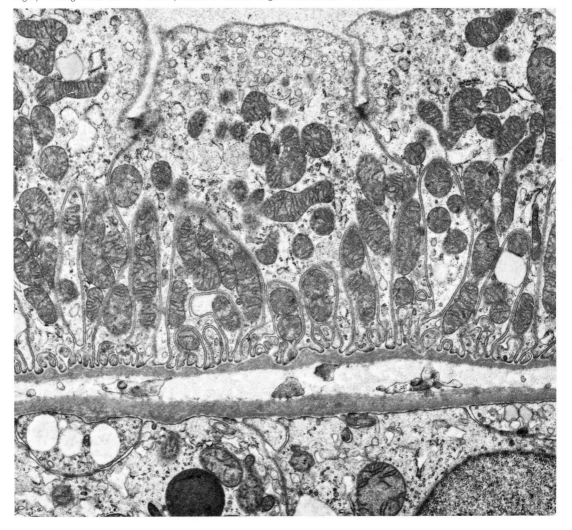

distal tubule, the cells are shorter and therefore their nuclei bulge into the lumen. A few microvilli are seen along the cell surface. The lateral interdigitating processes contain numerous mitochondria which appear to be involved with the lateral cell membrane in the active transport of sodium ions from the tubular luminal fluid which occurs in this region. The permeability of the tubule to water is low in this region and therefore water does not become osmotically equilibrated and the luminal contents remain hypotonic to blood.

MACULA DENSA   As the distal tubule returns to the renal corpuscle of its origin, it runs adjacent to the efferent arteriole, the extraglomerular mesangium, and the afferent arteriole. In this region, the cells in the wall of the distal tubule are narrow and their nuclei are close together. In stained sections the nuclear accumulation causes a dense region, hence the name *macula densa* (Fig. 22-26). This association of the distal tubule with the two arterioles and the extraglomerular mesangium is called the *juxtaglomerular apparatus* and will be discussed under that heading later in the chapter.

DISTAL CONVOLUTED TUBULE   The distal convoluted tubule is shorter (approximately 5 mm) than the proximal tubule and hence fewer profiles are seen in a random section of the cortex. The diameter of this tubule is somewhat variable, being approximately 20 to 50 μm. The cells appear to be shorter, and more nuclei are seen in a cross-sectional profile than in the proximal tubule (Figs. 22-24 and 22-25), because, in part anyway, many cells are binucleate. Because the cells are short, distal tubules frequently have a larger luminal diameter than proximal tubules. The cells do not have a brush border but a few luminal microvilli are seen. The endocytotic apparatus is not well developed; however, a few vacuoles and lysosomes can be seen within the cells. The cytoplasm appears somewhat less acidophilic than in the proximal tubule. In the basal region of the cytoplasm, lateral processes interdigitate with those from adjacent cells, forming an extensive lateral intercellular labyrinthine space like that seen in the proximal tubule (Fig. 22-26). The processes contain large mitochondria and form a pattern of basal striations similar to that seen in the proximal tubule. The active transport of sodium ions from the tubular filtrate can continue in this segment of the nephron. The nuclei appear to lie in the apical cytoplasm near the lumen. A continuous basement membrane surrounds the tubule.

A gradual morphologic change is seen between the last region of the distal tubule and the collecting duct. The interdigitating processes of the distal tubular cells become less extensive. Intercalated (dark) cells similar to those described in the collecting duct appear in the latter region of the distal tubule.

Intrarenal collecting ducts   The collecting ducts can be divided into three regions: the initial segment found in the cortex (Figs. 22-27 to 22-29), the medullary segment found in the upper medulla, and the large papillary ducts in the apex of the papilla (Fig. 22-30). This division is somewhat arbitrary because there is a gradual transition in the form of the collecting ducts from their beginning to their end.

Figure 22-24   Light micrograph of two distal convoluted tubules from a rat kidney embedded in epoxy resin. The cells contain large mitochondria but lack a brush border.   × 1,000.

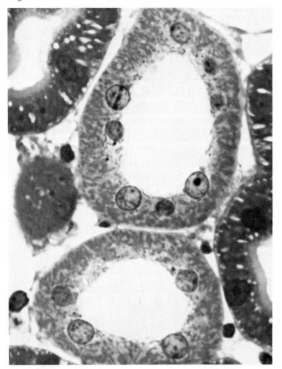

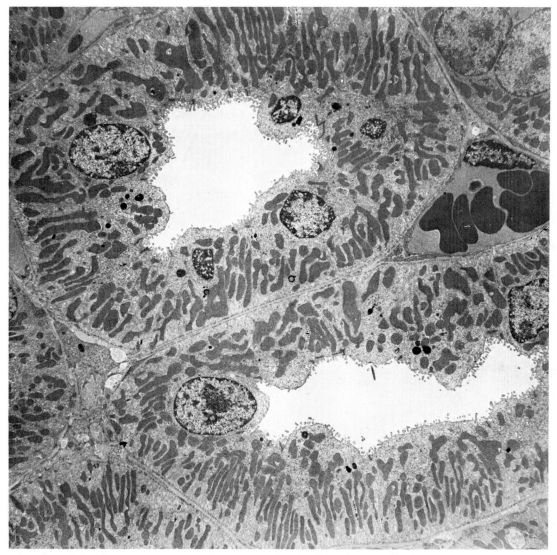

Figure 22-25   Electron micrograph of two distal convoluted tubular profiles, showing the large number of mitochondria contained in these cells and the few small microvilli which line the lumen but do not form a brush border.   The nuclei lie in an apical position.   ×2,800.

Initial segment   The initial segment includes the connecting portion from the distal convoluted tubule to the collecting tubules, which in cortical nephrons empties directly into a terminal collecting duct, and an arched portion formed by the confluence of several connecting pieces from juxtamedullary nephrons.   The arched portion begins deep in the cortex and ascends and then turns to descend into a medullary ray.   The number of nephrons which empty into arched collecting ducts prior to entrance into a terminal collecting duct versus those entering singly varies with the species.   In humans both types occur.

Two types of epithelial cells line the collecting

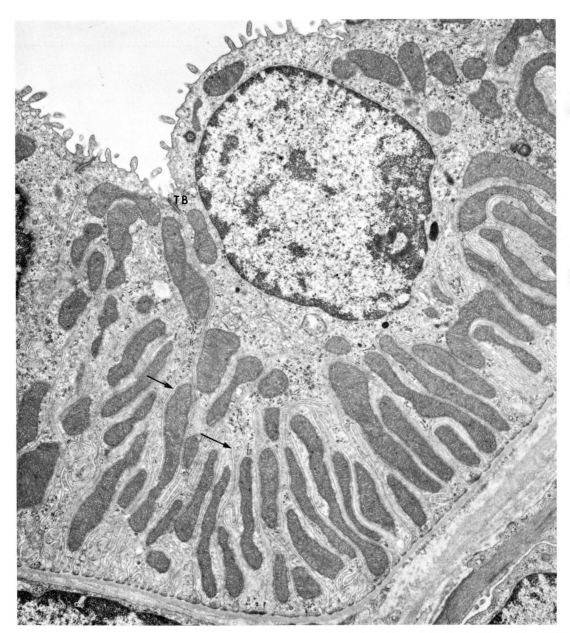

Figure 22-26 Electron micrograph of a distal convoluted tubule, showing the lateral intercellular labyrinth (arrows) formed by the interdigitation of lateral processes in the basal region of the distal tubular cells. The large elongate mitochondria occupy these processes. The cell nucleus occupies an apical position. The cell surfaces are joined apical-laterally by prominent terminal bars (TB), and the apical cell membrane has only small microvilli. ×10,300.

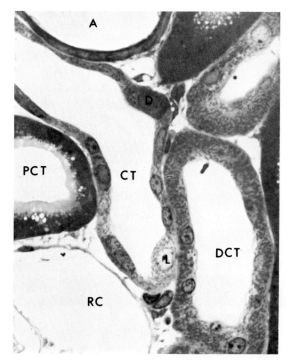

Figure 22-27   Light micrograph of a cortical collecting tubule (CT) from a rat kidney embedded in epoxy resin. Light (L) and dark (D) cells lining this tubule can be identified. Profiles of proximal (PCT) and distal (DCT) convoluted tubules, an arteriole (A), and a renal corpuscle (RC) can be seen. ×670.

tubule (Figs. 22-28 and 22-29). The principal (light) cells are low cuboidal cells with well-defined cell margins; round, centrally placed nuclei; a fairly pale staining cytoplasm; and multiple, small, randomly oriented mitochondria. In electron micrographs, these cells are seen to have a few small microvilli and a basal cell region which contains some small, short, interdigitating processes as well as some tortuous infoldings of the basal cell membrane.

Interspersed between the principal cells are intercalated (dark) cells, which have a more intensely staining cytoplasm and contain more mitochondria which are located all around the nucleus. These cells have more microvilli on their luminal surfaces, and their apical cytoplasm contains a large number of vesicles. Dark cells are seen throughout the cortex and in some of the medulla but do not exist in the papillary region. The dark cells are seen to vary in number with varying states of acid-base balance and may play a role in urine acidification (reviewed by Myers et al., 1966).

Medullary collecting ducts   The medullary collecting ducts are similar in structure to the cortical ones although the cells gradually increase in height.

Papillary ducts   The convergence of the collecting tubules within the kidney leads to the formation of several large straight collecting tubules called papillary ducts (or ducts of Bellini) (Fig. 22-30). These large collecting ducts have a diameter of 200 to 300 μm. They empty their contents into the minor calyxes through small holes on the surface of the papillary apex. This surface is called the *area cribrosa* (Fig. 22-31).

Function of the distal nephron   Since a gradual transition occurs in the function of the distal tubule and collecting duct, the two regions are often referred to as the distal nephron and discussed together.

CONCENTRATION AND DILUTION OF URINE (Fig. 22-32)   The mammalian kidney can rid the body of water by producing a copious volume of dilute urine or conserve water by producing a small amount of concentrated urine. It manages this because it contains a countercurrent multiplier (the loop of Henle) and two countercurrent exchangers [the looping medullary vessels (vasa recta) and the large collecting ducts passing through the medullary interstitium].

The ascending limb of the loop of Henle pumps sodium ions into the medullary interstitium from the tubular lumen. The water permeability of this region is low, and so osmotic equilibration does not occur. Because of the shape of Henle's loop, many of the sodium ions are trapped within the medulla. This produces an increasingly hypertonic environment as the papilla of the medulla is approached. In man the osmolarity of the interstitium may reach 1,200 milliosmoles per liter at the papillary tip. The collecting ducts again course through the medulla to empty at its apex. If they are permeable to water, the hypertonic environment of the medulla becomes a driving force to remove water from the tubular lumen by osmosis. The water permeability of the collecting ducts is controlled by

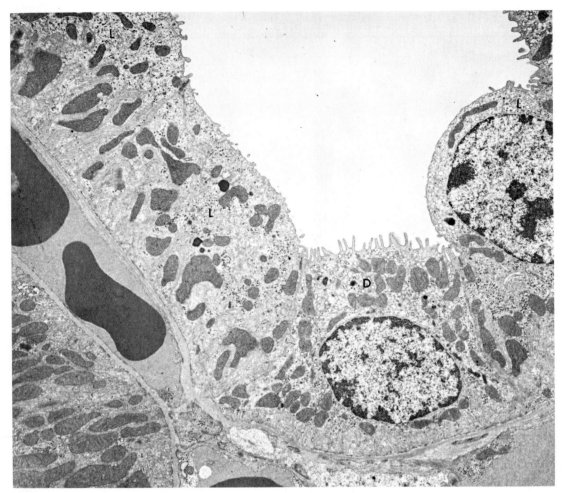

Figure 22-28   Electron micrograph of a cortical collecting tubule from a rat kidney, showing light cells (L) and a dark cell (D) The dark cell is characterized by numerous mitochondria and an elaborate pattern of the apical cell membrane forming folds and microvilli.   Abundant apical vesicles are also seen in the dark cell.   ×5,600.

an antidiuretic hormone (ADH).   When blood levels of this hormone are high, the permeability of the collecting duct to water is increased and therefore water leaves the tubular fluid in the collecting duct by osmosis, producing a concentrated urine.   The fluid entering the distal tubule is always hypotonic, and sodium ions can continue to be pumped out of the distal tubular lumen.   Therefore, when the titer of circulating ADH is low and the collecting duct permeability to water is decreased, a dilute urine will be produced.

ACIDIFICATION OF URINE   Although about half of the bicarbonate ion is reabsorbed in the proximal tubule, the distal nephron still plays an important role in acid-base balance.   It is the site of continued reabsorption of bicarbonate with resulting secretion of hydrogen ions, it is the site of secretion of hydrogen ion into the tubular lumen for buffering with anions of weak acids and of the acidification of the urine, and it is the site of conversion of ammonia to ammonium ions (although the ammonia might be produced elsewhere in the kidney).

SODIUM-ION–POTASSIUM-ION EXCHANGE   The distal nephron is also the site at which the hormone aldosterone stimulates sodium-ion reabsorption and potassium-ion secretion.

THE JUXTAGLOMERULAR APPARATUS

At the vascular pole of the renal corpuscle, a specialized portion of the distal tubule, the macula densa, comes into an intimate relationship with the afferent and efferent arterioles as well as with a pad of cells called the *extraglomerular mesangium* (Barajas, 1970; Barajas and Latta, 1967).   Unmyelinated nerve endings are associated with these structures.   These four entities (the afferent arteriole, the efferent arteriole, the macula densa, and the extraglomerular mesangium) constitute the jux-

taglomerular apparatus (Figs. 22-33 and 22-34).

Modified smooth muscle cells in the wall of the afferent (and sometimes the efferent) arteriole in this region produce granules which can be identified by their staining properties and have been shown to contain the hormone renin (pronounced as in renal).   These modified smooth muscle cells are called *juxtaglomerular cells*.   Although the modified cells still contain intracellular filaments and dense bodies like other smooth muscle cells, they have more rough ER, a large Golgi apparatus, and a number of membrane-bounded secretory granules in various states of production, condensation, and storage (Fig. 22-35).

The *macula densa* comprises the cells lining the wall of the distal tubule between the ascending

Figure 22-29   Electron micrograph of light cells from a human collecting tubule.   These cells have a somewhat less elaborate contour to their cell membranes than do those of the rat.   ×7,700.

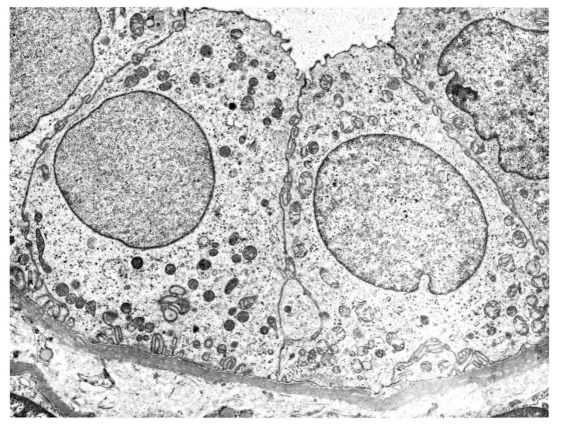

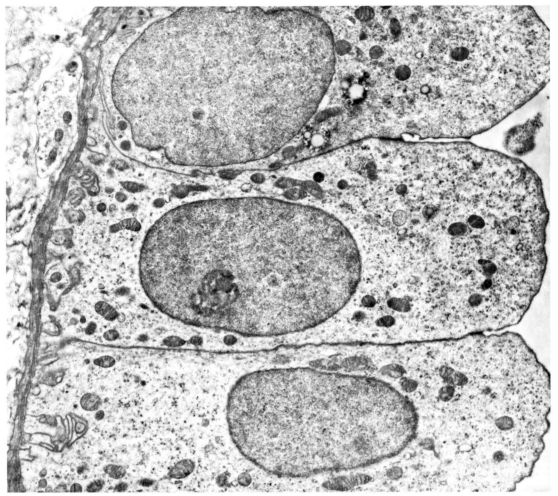

Figure 22-30 Electron micrograph of a medullary collecting tubule from a normal human kidney. Medullary collecting cells are taller than cortical ones but still contain some basal membranous infoldings and oval mitochondrial profiles. ×30,700.

straight portion and the distal convoluted portion. The macula densa appears as a dense spot because the cells of this region are narrower than in adjacent portions of the tubule, and so the nuclei are closer together. In addition, the interdigitations generally seen in the basal cytoplasm of distal tubular cells are oriented parallel to the basement membrane instead of perpendicular to it. Some of these processes extend close to the juxtaglomerular cells and to the cells of the extraglomerular mesangium. The macula densa cells have mitochondria which ap-

pear shorter and more randomly oriented. The cells appear to be polarized toward the basal surface, and the Golgi apparatus is found lateral or basal to the nucleus. Because of its unique location, this region could be a sensing device of some parameter in the distal tubular fluid content and could affect the granulated cells in the arteriolar wall. The cells of the *extraglomerular mesangium* (sometimes called *Polkissen, Lacis cells,* or *polar cushion*) form a cushion of cells between the walls of the afferent and efferent arterioles. These cells

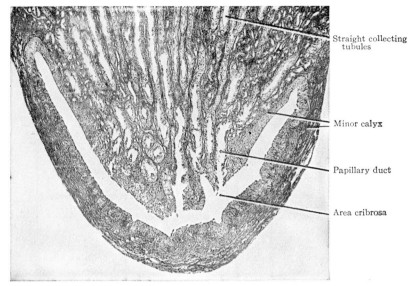

Straight collecting
tubules

Minor calyx

Papillary duct

Area cribrosa

Figure 22-31   Longitudinal section of the kidney papilla of a rhesus monkey, showing the area cribrosa and the wall of the minor calyx.   ×40.

resemble the intraglomerular mesangial cells with which they are contiguous.   Although some of the cells contain granules, the majority are filled with fine intracytoplasmic filaments, dense attachment bodies at the cell membrane, and the usual organelles.

In response to a decrease in the extracellular fluid volume in an animal, the juxtaglomerular apparatus releases the enzyme renin which acts on a plasma α-2-globulin, called *angiotensinogen,* and releases an inactive decapeptide known as angiotensin I.   A converting enzyme, presumably located in the lung, converts angiotensin I to the octapeptide angiotensin II, which is the trophic hormone for the zona glomerulosa of the adrenal cortex and causes the release of aldosterone.   Aldosterone then stimulates the distal nephron to reabsorb sodium ions in exchange for hydrogen or potassium ions.   Since sodium is the major extracellular ion, its renal retention leads to an increase in the extracellular fluid volume of the animal.   Angiotensin II is also a potent vasoconstrictor.

RENAL INTERSTITIUM

The cortical interstitium is small in normal animals.   However, in a variety of disease processes the interstitium increases in volume and becomes fibrotic.   Around the vessels, the interstitium is abundant (Swann and Norman, 1970).   Two main cell types are seen within the cortical interstitium. The most frequently seen is the fibroblast.   The second is a cell in the mononuclear series which, under certain circumstances, can be seen to contain a large number of phagocytic vacuoles and lysosomes.   Fine collagen bundles traverse the cortical interstitium.   Under normal circumstances, the interstitium also contains a fluid reabsorbate which is in transit from the lumen of the tubules to the capillaries.

In contrast, the interstitium of the medulla is much more abundant; it contains a population of elongate interstitial cells whose long axes lie perpendicular to the long axes of the tubules in that region (Fig. 22-36).   The cells are characterized by long, branching processes which come close to vessels and tubules and in some circumstances

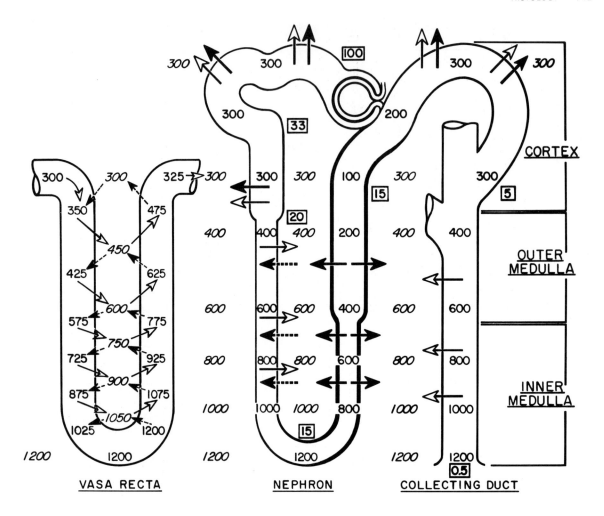

VASA RECTA

NEPHRON

COLLECTING DUCT

CORTEX

OUTER MEDULLA

INNER MEDULLA

➡ Na Active Transport

⇢ Na Passive Diffusion

⇨ H₂O Passive Diffusion

☐% Glomerular Filtrate Remaining at Each Level of Tubule

Figure 22-32 Summary of water and ion exchanges in the nephron during production of hypertonic urine, and of countercurrent exchange across the vasa recta to preserve the osmolar gradient. Numbers represent concentration of urine, blood, and interstitium in milliosmoles per liter. (Redrawn and modified from R. F. Pitts, "Physiology of the Kidney and Body Fluids," Year Book Medical Publishers, Inc., Chicago, 1963; courtesy of W. Roth.)

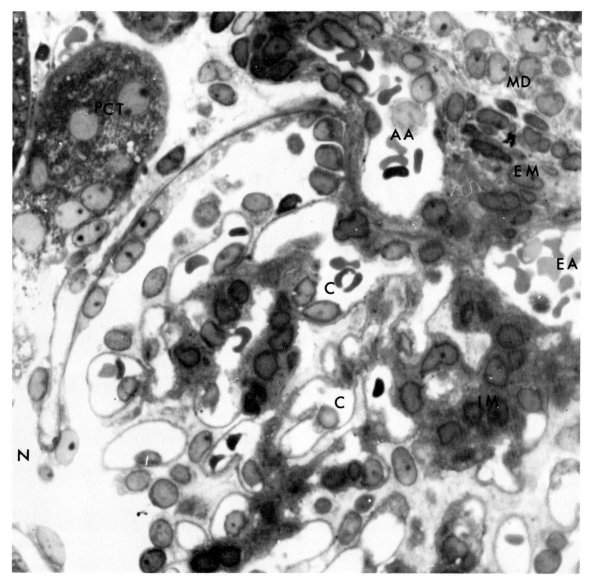

Figure 22-33 Light micrograph of a juxtaglomerular apparatus from a human renal corpuscle showing the macula densa (MD), the afferent arteriole (AA), the efferent arteriole (EA), the extraglomerular mesangium (EM), the intraglomerular mesangium (IM), the capillary loops (C), a neck region (N), and a proximal convoluted tubule (PCT). ×760.

appear to encircle them. The most unique feature of these cells is that they contain a variable number of lipid droplets within their cytoplasm. In addition, the cytoplasm contains fine intercellular filaments, rough ER, numerous lysosomes, and other organelles. The cells appear to be partially surrounded by a layer of material which resembles basement membrane (external lamina) and also extends into the intercellular space around the cells, forming a network. Small bundles of collagen, flocculent material, and fine filaments (approximately 13 nm in diameter with an electron-lucent core) are seen

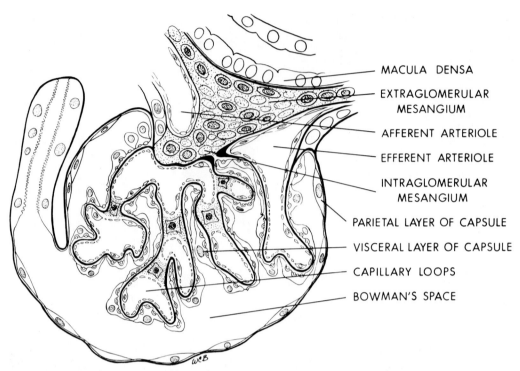

MACULA DENSA

EXTRAGLOMERULAR
MESANGIUM

AFFERENT ARTERIOLE

EFFERENT ARTERIOLE

INTRAGLOMERULAR
MESANGIUM

PARIETAL LAYER OF CAPSULE

VISCERAL LAYER OF CAPSULE

CAPILLARY LOOPS

BOWMAN'S SPACE

Figure 22-34 Diagram of the juxtaglomerular apparatus redrawn and simplified from Fig. 22-33 to show the four elements of the juxtaglomerular apparatus as well as the position of the capillaries, mesangial cells, and epithelial cells of the renal corpuscle.

within the intercellular matrix.   Several functions have been proposed for these unique interstitial cells including (1) that they elaborate the interstitial matrix; (2) that they are contractile and presumably by contraction play a role in the concentration of urine; (3) that they are phagocytic; and (4) that they produce the vasodepressor substances that have been isolated from the renal interstitium in certain animals, which are most likely prostaglandins E_2 and A_2 (Westura et al., 1970; McGiff et al., 1970; Muehrcke et al., 1970).

BLOOD VESSELS

Arteries The *renal arteries* generally arise from the lateral region of the abdominal aorta at the level of the first and second lumbar vertebrae.   Each artery runs downward and laterally and then usually divides into an *anterior* and *posterior division* before

it reaches the renal hilus.   The anterior division runs in front of the renal pelvis; the posterior division enters the renal sinus behind the renal pelvis. Although there appears to be variation in the next branching, five *segmental* branches are generally described.   The anterior division branches into the upper, middle, and lower segmental arteries, and the posterior division becomes a posterior segmental artery.   The fifth, or apical, segment can arise from either the anterior or posterior division or from branches of both divisions.   While in the renal sinus, the segmental arteries branch to form interlobar arteries which enter the renal columns adjacent to the renal pyramids.   At the base of the renal pyramid, the *interlobar* artery branches into many *arcuate arteries* that run across the base of the medullary pyramid near the cortico-medullary junction (Figs. 22-37 and 22-38).   The arcuate arteries give off branches called *interlobular* arteries

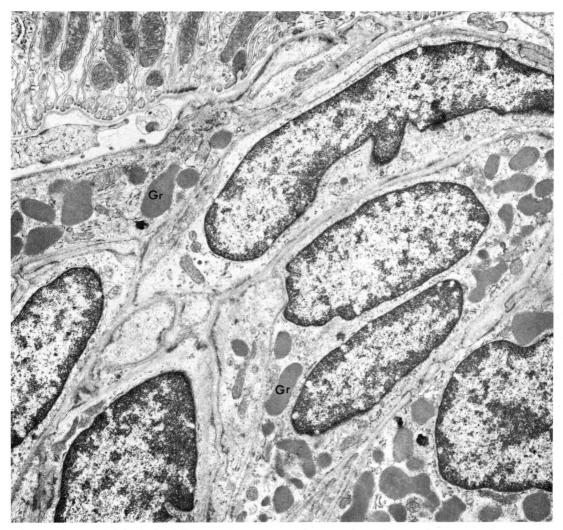

Figure 22-35 Electron micrograph showing juxtaglomerular cells from a rat kidney. The juxtaglomerular granules (Gr) can be seen within the cytoplasm of the modified smooth muscle cells. ×9,300.

which course peripherally in the cortex midway between medullary rays (hence between renal lobules).   As the interlobular arteries ascend, they give off *afferent arterioles* which can serve one or more renal corpuscles.   The afferent arteriole enters the renal corpuscle and forms several lobules of capillary networks.   Anastomosis occurs between the capillaries in any lobule, but not between capillaries of adjacent lobules.   The capillaries then converge to form the efferent arteriole which exits from the renal corpuscle at the vascular pole.

Postglomerular capillary circulation   The efferent arterioles leave the renal corpuscle and divide into a second capillary network (Fig. 22-38).   The morphology of these capillaries differs, depending on whether the renal corpuscle is of the cortical or juxtamedullary type.   The efferent arterioles from

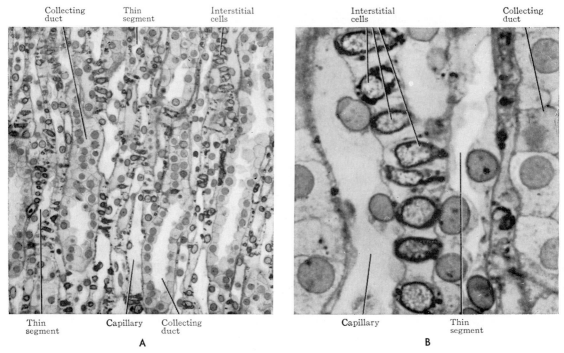

Figure 22-36 Light micrograph of sections taken of the renal pyramid from a rat kidney, showing the horizontal, ladder-like array of interstitial cells located in this region. Epoxy resin section, toluidine blue. A, ×275; B, ×1,100.

cortical nephrons are short and divide to form a tortuous *peritubular capillary network* supplying the associated convoluted tubules. It appears that the blood in this capillary network flows rapidly in the direction opposite to that of the fluid in the tubular lumen (Steinhausen et al., 1970).

The majority of efferent arterioles from juxta-medullary nephrons divide to form several parallel unbranched vessels called the *arteriolae rectae spuriae* (Fig. 22-39). These vessels descend into the medullary pyramid, where they make a hairpin turn and ascend again in the region adjacent to the descending limb forming a vascular countercurrent exchanger (Fig. 22-40). The descending limbs are called *arteriolae rectae,* and the ascending limbs are called *venae rectae.* The walls of the arteriolar vessels in the outer medulla have a thicker endothelium (2 to 4 μm) than the walls of the ascending venous vessels. The venous vessels are lined by fenestrated capillaries. The vessels form capillary

plexuses at various levels throughout the medullary pyramid. Blood flow through the medulla is much smaller in volume and slower in flow rate than that in the cortex, and so the inner medulla has a lower oxygen supply and derives most of its energy from glycolysis.

Veins The venous supply in the kidney is quite irregular, and anastomoses occur between its vessels. Near the renal capsule, small venules drain in a star-like pattern, forming the stellate veins which, in turn, form the interlobular veins which course adjacent to the interlobular arteries and receive numerous tributaries from the cortical peritubular capillary network. The interlobular veins empty into the arcuate veins which extend across at the level of the cortico-medullary junction. The arcuate veins also receive blood from the venous branches of the vasae rectae. Interlobar veins are formed by the confluence of arcuate veins; these

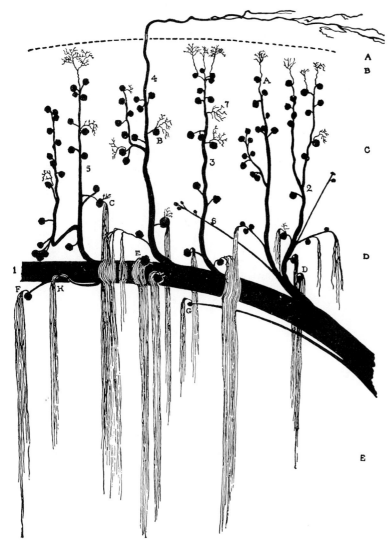

Figure 22-37 Diagram to represent the finer arterial distribution of the kidney. A. Capsule. B. Subcapsular zone. C. Cortex. D. Juxtamedullary zone. E. Medulla. The arcuate artery (1) gives off numerous interlobular arteries. The long, straight arteriolae rectae can be seen passing down into the medulla.

course adjacent to the medullary pyramid in company with the corresponding artery. The confluence of these vessels forms the renal vein. On the right side of the body, the renal vein is short, but on the left side of the body it is longer and receives blood from the gonadal, suprarenal, and inferior phrenic veins.

Lymphatics Lymphatic vessels have been identified accompanying the larger renal vessels and appear to be more prominent around the arteries than around the veins. They have been identified along the interlobular, arcuate, interlobar, segmental, and renal arteries and veins (Fig. 22-41) (Kriz and Dieterich, 1970). In the region of the renal sinus, they

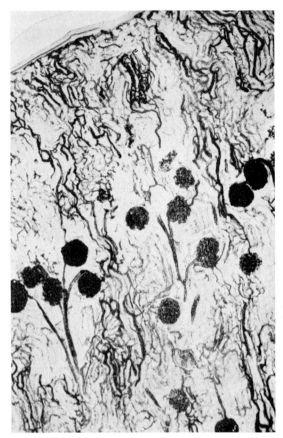

Figure 22-38   Arteries of the dog kidney were infused with a gelatin solution and therefore have visualized the interlobular arteries, the afferent arterioles, the glomerulus, the efferent arterioles, and the peritubular capillary anastomoses around the tubules.   ×46.

converge into several large trunks which exit via the renal hilus.   The lymph is then drained into nodes along the inferior vena cava and aorta.   The lymphatics that accompany the interlobular vessels anastomose with a rich supply of lymphatics in the renal capsule and perirenal tissue.   Lymph vessels have not been well demonstrated within the cortical parenchyma.   In addition, Rawson (1949), studying tumor penetration via renal lymphatics, identified lymph capillaries beginning at the tip of the medullary pyramid and extending peripherally to empty into lymphatic vessels at the base of the medullary pyramid.

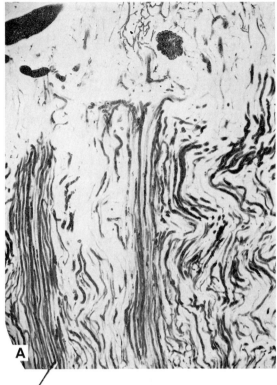

Arteriolae
rectae spuriae

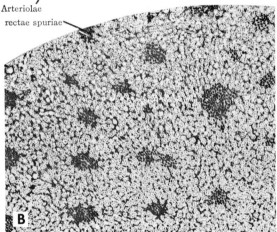

Figure 22-39   Arteriolae rectae spuriae of a dog.   Arteries were infused with colored gelatin.   A. Radial section through the base of a renal pyramid, showing origin of tassels of arterioles at the junction of cortex and medulla.   ×45.   B. Transverse section of pyramid showing islands of arteriolae rectae spuriae.   ×42. (Courtesy of D. Fawcett.)

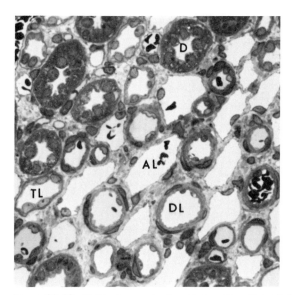

Figure 22-40   Light micrograph of a cross section through a bundle of vasa recta (center) from the outer medulla of a human kidney. Note the patterned array with thick-walled descending limbs of the vasa recta (DL) being surrounded by thin-walled ascending limbs of the vasa recta (AL). The straight part of the distal tubule (D) and some thin limb sections (TL) can also be identified.   ×420.

INNERVATION

Many autonomic nerve fibers which form the renal plexus accompany the renal artery and its branches to the kidney. The majority of these fibers are from the sympathetic division of the autonomic nervous system. The fibers are derived from cell bodies located mainly in the celiac and aortic ganglia. The sympathetic fibers innervate renal blood vessels to cause vasoconstriction. In addition, some authors believe that parasympathetic fibers of the autonomic nervous system derived from the vagus nerve also enter the kidney. Sensory fibers have been described as well. When these sensory fibers are cut, renal pain is blocked. Although numerous light microscopists describe nerve endings along the wall of the renal tubules and within the renal corpuscle, electron microscopists have not recognized them and have identified nerve endings only along the renal vessels, in the juxtaglomerular apparatus, and in the renal interstitium. Nerves have not been identified penetrating the basement membrane of any tubule or within the renal corpuscle. Since the nerve fibers to the kidney are cut during renal transplantation, it is obvious that the kidney can function adequately without an extrinsic nerve supply.

Extrarenal collecting system

EXCRETORY PASSAGES

Urine is conveyed from the kidney to the bladder where it is stored. When the bladder becomes appropriately distended, the micturition reflex causes emptying of the bladder, and the urine leaves via the urethra. Urine is excreted through the minor calyxes (Fig. 22-42), the major calyxes, the renal pelvis, the ureter (Fig. 22-43), the bladder, and the urethra. The walls of all but the latter are similar in their basic structure, being composed of an inner mucosal layer, a middle muscularis layer, and an external adventitial coat of connective tissue which binds the structure to the surrounding connective tissue. The upper portion of the bladder extends into the pelvic cavity and therefore is covered by parietal peritoneum and hence has a serosa. The thickness of the three layers of the wall increases from the minor calyxes to the bladder.

Mucosa   While the urine is being conveyed and stored within the extrarenal collecting system, only small changes occur in its composition. A specialized lining layer called *transitional epithelium* along the lumen of the excretory passages and the bladder is responsible for this low permeability (Fig. 22-44). This intact epithelium seems to be a barrier to the rapid diffusion of salt and water. In addition, transitional epithelium gives a distensibility to the lining layer. The epithelium generally is said to be two to three cells thick in the minor calyxes, four to five cells thick in the ureter, and six or more cells thick in the empty bladder. The superficial cells of the transitional epithelium appear large and rounded and sometimes contain large polyploid nuclei in their superficial layer. When the epithelium is stretched, such as in the filling bladder, it becomes much thinner and the surface cells are

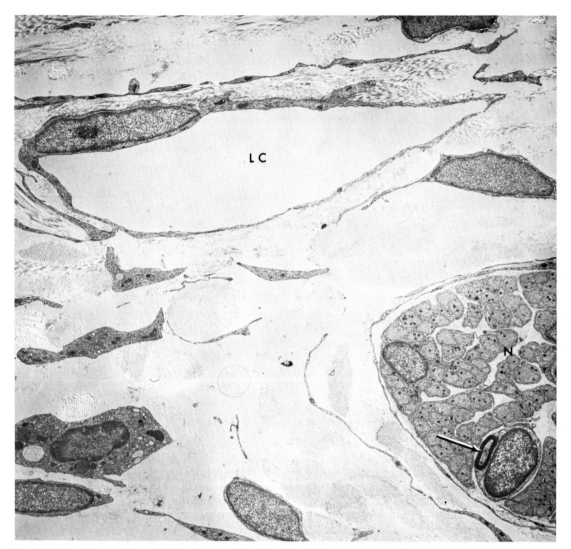

Figure 22-41   Electron micrograph showing a renal lymph capillary (LC) accompanying a large vessel within the renal parenchyma. A nerve (N) can be seen in the upper right-hand corner which consists almost entirely of unmyelinated fibers.   However, one myelinated axon can be identified (arrow).   ×3,300.

stretched into a squamous layer. The distensibility of the transitional epithelium results not only from a change in shape of the cells from rounded to flat but also from certain other anatomic features. The surface of the luminal cells is characterized by an irregular contour with small V-shaped indentations which penetrate into the cell (Figs. 22-45 and 22-46). The apical cytoplasm contains stacks of fusiform vesicles which are limited by a membrane of the same thickness as the apical plasma membrane (12 nm). It appears that the fusiform vesicles are formed from the surface membrane when the bladder is relaxing. This is demonstrated by placing a marker such as ferritin in the lumen of

folding allows for considerable increase in luminal diameter.

Muscularis The muscular layer of the excretory passages usually consists of two layers of smooth muscle. Although the precise orientation of the muscle is complex, the inner layer appears to be oriented predominantly in a longitudinal fashion whereas the outer layer is oriented predominantly in a circular fashion. In addition, the layers of smooth muscle differ from those of the gastrointestinal tract in that they are penetrated by connective tissue in such a manner that bundles of smooth muscle are seen.

The muscle layers are thinnest in the minor calyxes but two layers of muscle are present (Fig. 22-42). The inner layer is attached to the base of the medulla and contains longitudinal fibers. The outer layer follows a more circumferential path with anterior and posterior loops which cross on the anterior and posterior sides of the calyx (Van den

Figure 22-43 Light micrograph showing the wall of a dog ureter lined by transitional epithelium (TE), lamina propria (LP), muscularis (M), and a layer of adventitia (A) containing vessels. ×120.

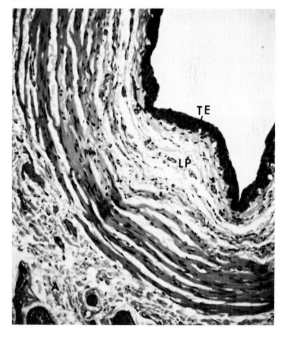

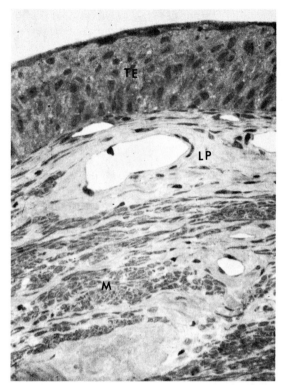

Figure 22-42 Light micrograph showing the wall of a minor calyx. The calyx is lined by transitional epithelium (TE), a lamina propria (LP), and muscularis (M).

the bladder and observing its uptake into the fusiform vesicles (Porter and Bonneville, 1968). In addition, the epithelial cells beneath the surface appear to have numerous lateral interdigitations and projections which disappear during distension. Only a few small desmosomes are seen between the cells of the transitional epithelium. Capillaries lie close beneath the basement membrane of the epithelium (Fig. 22-47).

Lamina propria The lamina propria is composed of a fairly dense layer of collagenous connective tissue which becomes somewhat looser in the lower region near the muscularis. There is no submucosa in the wall. When the excretory passages are empty, the mucosa is folded. When the organ is distended, the mucosa can be stretched flat; this

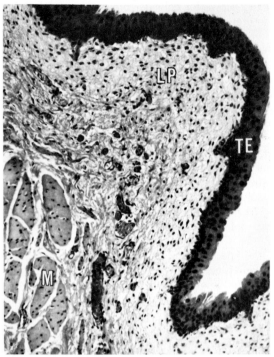

Figure 22-44   Light micrograph of part of the wall of a dog bladder, showing the transitional epithelium (TE), the lamina propria (LP), and part of the muscularis (M).   ×500.

Bulcke et al., 1970).   This layer extends higher up and forms a ring around the base of the medullary pyramid.   The calyxes act as funnels whose walls contract in waves that move the fluid from the medullary pyramid into the renal pelvis.

The walls of the renal pelvis and the upper two-thirds of the ureter contain the same two layers of smooth muscle which continue to be found in bundles; however, they are thicker than in the walls of the calyxes.   In the lower third of the ureter, an additional outer longitudinal layer of smooth muscle is found.   Periodic peristaltic waves proceed down the ureter, forcing urine into the bladder.   No definite pacemaker initiating these waves has been found.

The ureters pierce the bladder wall obliquely, and the inner longitudinal layer of smooth muscle inserts into the lamina propria of the bladder.   Because of the oblique course of the ureters through the wall of the bladder, their walls are pressed together as

the bladder distends.   The likelihood of urine refluxing into the ureters is therefore decreased.

BLADDER

The bladder is a reservoir for urine and varies in size and shape as it is filled (Fig. 22-44).   Three layers of smooth muscle with complex orientation have been described in the thick wall of the bladder.   The middle layer is the most prominent.   Because of the tortuosity of the muscle, it is difficult to delineate clearly these various layers in a random histologic section.   In the region of the trigone, an internal sphincter is formed by the orientation of smooth muscle around the opening of the urethra.

Blood vessels   Blood vessels penetrate the walls of the excretory passages and enter the muscularis where they supply it with an abundant capillary network.   A plexus is then formed within the lamina propria of the mucosa, and branches form a rich plexus of capillaries which are located just beneath the epithelium (Fig. 22-47).   In the deeper layers of the walls of the pelvis and ureters, abundant lymph vessels are seen accompanying these blood vessels.

Nerves   The bladder is supplied by both sympathetic and parasympathetic divisions of the autonomic nervous system.   The sympathetic fibers traverse the inferior hypogastric plexus and form a plexus in the adventitia of the bladder wall, the *plexus vesicalis.*   These sympathetic fibers appear to play little role in micturition.   The preganglionic fibers of the parasympathetic division which supply the bladder arise from the spinal cord in the second, third, and fourth sacral levels.   The fibers traverse to the bladder via the pelvic nerve and the inferior hypogastric plexus where they intermingle with the sympathetic fibers and synapse with ganglion cells located within the adventitia and muscularis of the bladder wall.   These fibers are important for micturition.   Afferent sensory fibers from the bladder traverse the pelvic and hypogastric nerves.

URETHRA

The urethra is a fibromuscular tube through which urine passes from the urinary bladder to the exterior.   In the male, the urethra is long (approximately 20 cm) and also serves for the passage of seminal

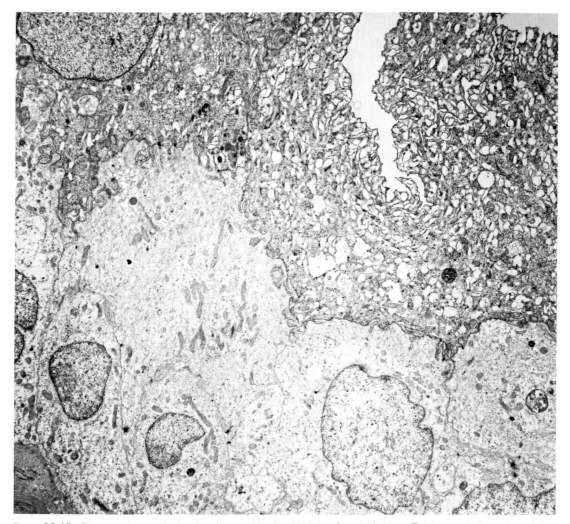

Figure 22-45 Electron micrograph showing the transitional epithelium of a rat bladder. The large cells lining the apical surface are characterized by an irregular contour to their apical plasma membrane and by numerous fusiform vesicles within their cytoplasm. ×31,500. (Courtesy of F. Remington.)

fluid during ejaculation. In the female, it is short (approximately 3 to 5 cm). Since the male and female urethra differ in structure, they will be considered separately.

Male urethra The male urethra can be divided into three segments. It begins at the neck of the bladder and extends through the prostate gland (prostatic portion), through the pelvic and urogenital diaphragm (membranous portion), and finally

through the root and body of the penis to the tip of the glans penis (spongy part, or anterior part).

The *prostatic portion* of the urethra is approximately 3 to 4 cm in length. It extends through the prostate gland where multiple small prostatic ducts enter. On the posterior wall of the prostatic urethra, a conical elevation called the *veru montanum* (or *colliculus seminalis*) is located. A blind invagination called the *prostatic utricle* extends into the substance of the prostate at the summit of this

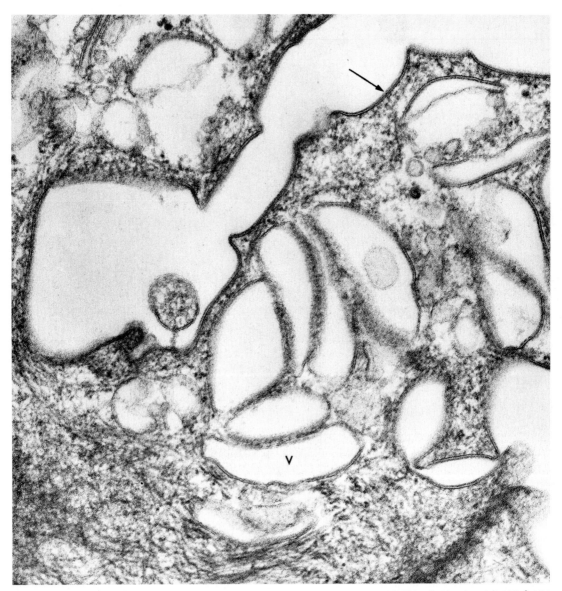

Figure 22-46 Electron micrograph of the surface cell membrane of a transitional epithelial cell, showing the 120-Å-thick apical plasma membrane (arrow) and similar membranes surrounding fusiform vesicles (V) in the cytoplasm. ×6,600.

region. The prostatic utricle is thought to represent a vestige of the fused caudal ends of the Mullerian or paramesonephric duct, which in the female form the uterus and most of the vagina. The ejaculatory ducts enter the urethra on each side of the opening of the prostatic utricle. The urethra in this region is lined by transitional epithelium. The lamina propria is highly vascular. Two coats of smooth muscle bundles surround the mucosa in which the inner has bundles oriented longitudinally and the outer bundles are circular in orientation. The circular muscular bundles are a continuation of the thickened circular region at the bladder outlet, called the *internal sphincter* of the bladder.

The *membranous portion* of the male urethra runs from the apex of the prostate to the bulb of the corpus cavernosus penis, traversing the urogenital and pelvic diaphragms. It is therefore surrounded by striated muscle fibers which form the *external sphincter* of the bladder. The epithelium in this region is stratified or pseudostratified columnar.

The *spongy portion* (anterior) is approximately 15 cm long and extends through the bulb, body, and glans of the penis encased by the corpus cavernosum urethrae (spongiosum). The lumen of the urethra is dilated within the region of the bulb (intrabulbar fossa) and in the glans (novicular fossa). The epithelium lining most of the urethra in this region is pseudostratified columnar (Fig. 22-48), with patches of stratified squamous epithelium. In the novicular fossa the epithelium becomes strati-

Figure 22-47 Electron micrograph of the base of the transitional epithelium, showing a capillary (C) separated from the epithelium only by the basement membranes (BM). ×6,900. (Courtesy of F. Remington.)

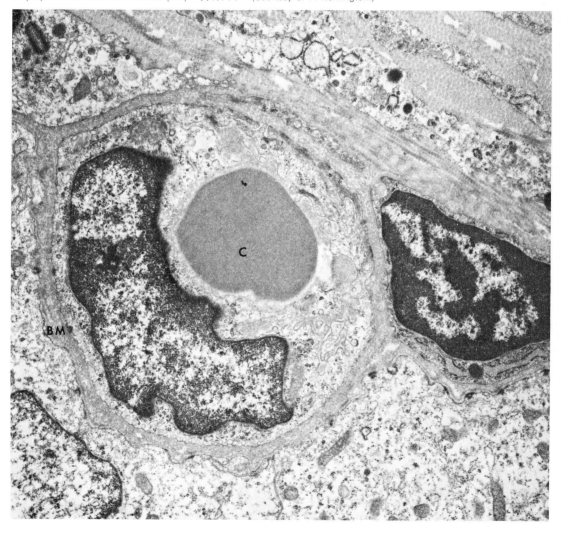

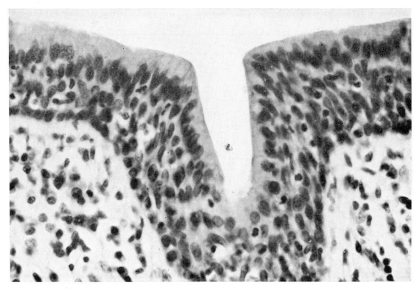

Figure 22-48   Psudostratified epithelium lining the cavernous portion of the human male urethra.   ×450.

Figure 22-49   Transverse section of the human female urethra.   Picric acid–sublimate fixation.   ×10.   (Von Ebner.)

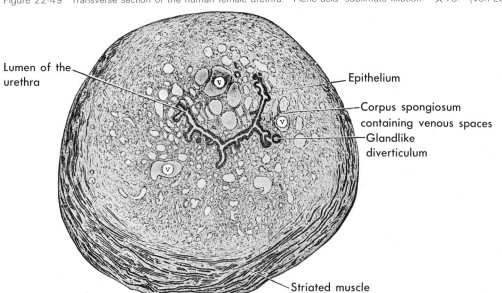

Lumen of the urethra

Epithelium

Corpus spongiosum
containing venous spaces

Glandlike
diverticulum

Striated muscle

fied squamous. The ducts of the bulbourethral glands enter the spongy segment of the urethra. Mucus-secreting glands (glands of Littre) also empty into the urethra throughout its length. However, they are most frequently found within this spongy portion.

Female urethra   The female urethra is relatively short, approximately 3 to 5 cm long. The lumen is crescentic in outline, and most of it is lined with stratified squamous epithelium (Fig. 22-49). Pseudostratified columnar epithelium may also be found. Within the epithelium some nests of mucus glands may be found. The lamina propria consists of a wide zone of vascular connective tissue which contains many thin-walled veins. The muscularis of the female urethra is similar to that in the bladder neck. An inner longitudinal layer of smooth muscle bundles is surrounded by a thicker layer of smooth muscle with circular orientation. The outer circular fibers are continuous with those in the internal sphincter of the urethra. The outer circular layer is reinforced with striated muscle fibers of the constrictor muscle of the urethra.

References

ARAKAWA, MASAAKI: A Scanning Electron Microscopy of the Glomerulus of Normal and Nephrotic Rats, *Lab. Invest.*, **23**:489–496 (1970).

BARAJAS, LUCIANO: The Ultrastructure of the Juxtaglomerular Apparatus as Disclosed by Three-dimensional Reconstructions from Serial Sections, *J. Ultrastruct. Res.*, **33**:116–147, (1970).

BARAJAS, LUCIANO, and HARRISON LATTA: Structure of the Juxtaglomerular Apparatus, *Circ. Res.*, **20, 21** (Suppl. II):15–28 (1967).

BERGER, SOSAMMA J., and BERTRAM SACKTOR: Isolation and Biochemical Characterization of Brush Borders from Rabbit Kidney, *J. Cell Biol.*, **47**:637–645 (1970).

BULGER, RUTH ELLEN: The Shape of Rat Kidney Tubular Cells, *Amer. J. Anat.*, **116**:237–255 (1965).

BULGER, RUTH ELLEN, and BENJAMIN F. TRUMP: Fine Structure of the Rat Renal Papilla, *Amer. J. Anat.*, **118**:685–722 (1966).

CLARK, S. L., JR.: Cellular Differentiation in the Kidneys of Newborn Mice Studied with the Electron Microscope, *J. Biophys. Biochem. Cytol.*, **3**:349–362 (1957).

DARMADY, E. M., and F. STRANACK: Microdissections of the Nephron in Disease, *Brit. Med. Bull.*, **13**:21 (1957).

DE DUVE, CHRISTIAN, and PIERRE BAUDHUIN: Peroxisome (Microbodies and Related Particles), *Physiol. Rev.*, **46**:323–357 (1966).

DU BOIS, A. M.: The Embryonic Kidney, in Charles Rouiller and Alex F. Muller (eds.), "The Kidney," vol. 1, pp. 1–59, Academic Press, Inc., New York, 1969.

FARQUHAR, M. G., S. L. WISSIG, and G. E. PALADE: Glomerular Permeability. I. Ferritin Transfer across the Normal Glomerular Capillary Wall, *J. Exp. Med.*, **113**:47 (1961).

GOTTSCHALK, C. W., and M. MYLLE: Micropuncture Study of the Mammalian Urinary Concentrating Mechanism: Evidence for the Countercurrent Hypotheses, *Amer. J. Physiol.*, **196**:927 (1959).

GRAHAM, R. C., and MORRIS J. KARNOVSKY: Glomerular Permeability. Ultrastructural Cytochemical Studies Using Peroxidases as Protein Tracers, *J. Exp. Med.*, **124**:1123–1134 (1966).

HARPER, J. T., HOLDE PUCHTLER, SUSAN N. MELOAN, and MARY S. TERRY: Light-microscopic Demonstration of Myoid Fibrils in Renal Epithelial, Mesangial and Interstitial Cells, *J. Microscopy,* **91**:71–85 (1970).

HICKS, R. M., and B. KETTERER: Isolation of the Plasma Membrane of the Luminal Surface of Rat Bladder Epithelium, and the Occurrence of a Hexagonal Lattice of Subunits Both in Negatively Stained Whole Mounts and in Sectioned Membranes, *J. Cell Biol.,* **45**:542–553 (1970).

HILLMAN, RICHARD E., and LEON E. ROSENBERG: Amino Acid Transport by Isolated Mammalian Renal Tubules. III. Binding of L-proline by Proximal Tubule Membranes, *Biochim. Biophys. Acta,* **211**:318–326 (1970).

HOLLINSHEAD, W. HENRY: Renovascular Anatomy, *Postgrad. Med.,* **40**:241–246 (1966).

JORGENSEN, FINN: "The Ultrastructure of the Normal Human Glomerulus," Munksgaard, Copenhagen, 1966.

KRIZ, W., and H. J. DIETERICH: The Lymphatic System of the Kidney in Some Mammals. Light and Electron Microscopic Investigations, *Z. Anat. Entwicklungsgesch,* **131**:111–147 (1970).

LJUNGQVIST, A.: Structure of the Arteriole-Glomerular Units in Different Zones of the Kidney, *Nephron,* **1**:329–337 (1964).

MC GIFF, JOHN C., KEITH CROWSHAW, NORBERTO A. TERRAGNO, and ANDREW J. LONIGRO: IV. Renal Interstitial Cells: Prostaglandins and Hypertension. Release of a Prostaglandin-like Substance into Renal Venous Blood in Response to Angiotensin II, *Circ. Res.,* **26**:I-121–I-130 (1970).

MÖLLENDORFF, W. VON: Der Exkretionsapparat, "Handbüch der mikroskopischen Anatomie des Menschen," vol. 7. pt. 1, Springer-Verlag OHG, Berlin, 1930.

MUEHRCKE, ROBERT C., ANIL K. MANDAL, and FREDERICK I. VOLINI: IV. Renal Interstitial Cells: Prostaglandins and Hypertension. A Pathophysiological Review of the Renal Medullary Interstitial Cells and Their Relationship to Hypertension, *Circ. Res.,* **26**, **27**:I-109–I-119 (1970).

MYERS, CHARLES E., RUTH ELLEN BULGER, C. CRAIG TISHER, and BENJAMIN F. TRUMP: Human Renal Ultrastructure. IV. Collecting Duct of Healthy Individuals, *Lab. Invest.,* **15**:1921–1950 (1966).

OSVALDO, LYDIA, and HARRISON LATTA: The Thin Limbs of the Loop of Henle, *J. Ultrastruct. Res.,* **15**:144–168 (1966).

PITTS, R. F.: "Physiology of the Kidney and Body Fluids," Year Book Medical Publishers, Inc., Chicago, 1963.

PORTER, KEITH R., and MARY A. BONNEVILLE: "Fine Structure of Cells and Tissues," Lea & Febiger, Philadelphia, 1968.

RAWSON, A. J.: Distribution of the Lymphatics of the Human Kidney as Shown in a Case of Carcinomatous Permeation, *Arch. Path.,* **47**:283 (1949).

RHODIN, J.: Anatomy of Kidney Tubules, *Int. Rev. Cytol.,* **7**:485–534 (1958).

RICHET, G., J. HAGEGE, and M. GABE: Correlation between Bicarbonate Transfer and Morphology of Tubular Cells Distal to Henle's Loop in the Rat, *Nephron,* **7**:413–429 (1970).

ROUILLER, CHARLES: General Anatomy and Histology of the Kidney, in Charles Rouiller and Alex F. Muller (eds.), "The Kidney," vol. 1, pp. 61–156, Academic Press, Inc., New York, 1969.

SMITH, H. W.: "The Kidney, Structure and Function in Health and Disease," Oxford University Press, New York, 1951.

SMITH, HOMER W.: "Studies in the Physiology of the Kidney," University of Kansas, University Extension Division, Lawrence, Kans., 1939.

SPERBER, I.: Studies on the Mammalian Kidney, *Zool. Bidrag. Uppsala,* **22**:249–431, 1944.

STEINHAUSEN, MICHAEL, GEORG-M. EISENBACH, and RAINER GALASKE: A Counter-current System of the Surface of the Renal Cortex of Rats, *Pfluegers Arch. Europ. J. Physiol.,* **318:**244–258 (1970).

STRAUS, WERNER: Cytochemical Observations on the Relationship between Lysosomes and Phagosomes in Kidney and Liver by Combined Staining for Acid Phosphatase and Intravenously Injected Horseradish Peroxidase, *J. Cell Biol.,* **20:**497–507 (1964).

SWANN, H. G., and RICHARD J. NORMAN: The Periarterial Spaces of the Kidney, *Texas Rep. Biol. Med.,* **28:**317–335 (1970).

TISHER, C. C., R. E. BULGER, and B. F. TRUMP: Human Renal Ultrastructure. III. The Distal Tubule in Healthy Individuals, *Lab. Invest.,* **18:**655–668 (1968).

TISHER, C. C., R. E. BULGER, and B. F. TRUMP: Human Renal Ultrastructure. I. Proximal Tubule of Healthy Individuals, *Lab. Invest.,* **15:**1357–1394 (1966).

TRUETA, J., A. E. BARCLAY, P. DANIEL, K. J. FRANKLIN, and M. M. L. PRICHARD: "Studies of the Renal Circulation," Blackwell Scientific Publications, LTD., Oxford, 1947.

VAN DEN BULCKE, C., E. N. KEEN, and H. FINE: Observations on Smooth Muscle Disposition in the Urinary Tract, *J. Urol.,* **103:**783–789 (1970).

VENKATACHALAM, M. A., R. S. COTRAN, and M. J. KARNOVSKY: An Ultrastructural Study of Glomerular Permeability in Aminonucleoside Nephrosis Using Catalase as a Tracer Protein, *J. Exp. Med.,* **132:**1168–1182 (1970).

VENKATACHALAM, M. A., M. J. KARNOVSKY, H. D. FAHIMI, and R. S. COTRAN: An Ultrastructural Study of Glomerular Permeability Using Catalase and Peroxidase as Tracer Proteins, *J. Exp. Med.,* **132:**1153–1167 (1970).

WESTURA, EDWIN E., HARTMUT KANNEGIESSER, JAMES D. O'TOOLE, and JAMES B. LEE: IV. Renal Interstitial Cells: Prostaglandins and Hypertension. Antihypertensive Effects of Prostaglandin A_1 in Essential Hypertension, *Circ. Res.,* **26, 27:**I-131–I-140 (1970).

ZIMMERMANN, K. W.: Zur Morphologie der Epithelzellen der Saugetierniere, *Arch. Mikrobiol. Anat.,* **78:**199–231 (1911).

chapter 23   The female reproductive system

RICHARD J. BLANDAU

The female reproductive system (Fig. 23-1) is composed of an internal group of organs situated within the pelvis and consisting of the *ovaries,* the *oviducts* (also called *uterine* or *fallopian tubes*), the *uterus,* and the *vagina.* The external genitalia comprise the *mons pubis,* the *labia minora,* the *labia majora,* and the *clitoris.* The mammary glands, though not genital organs, are an important appendage to the reproductive system (see Chap. 24). The ovaries are paired organs situated on either side of the uterus, each 2 to 5 cm long, 1.5 to 3 cm wide, and 0.8 to 1.5 cm thick. The size of the ovaries varies greatly from week to week during each menstrual cycle or during pregnancy; this is related to the number and stage of development of the growing follicles and corpora lutea. To study the ovaries of any animal intelligently, it is important to know at which stage of the reproductive cycle they were removed.

The ovary is attached to the broad ligament by a double fold of peritoneum, the *mesovarium* (Figs. 23-1 and 23-2). The mesovarium is attached to the ovary only along one margin, the *hilum.* The *suspensory ligament* of the ovary (Fig. 23-1) is a fold of peritoneum which is directed upward over the iliac vessels and contains the ovarian vessels. The mesovarium and the suspensory ligaments often contain significant amounts of smooth muscle fibers whose rhythmic contractions, particularly at the time of ovulation, move the ovaries closer to the fimbriae of the oviducts.

SEXUAL MATURATION (PUBERTY)

The female sexual organs normally remain in an infantile state during approximately the first 10 years of life. In the succeeding 2 to 4 years there occurs a gradual enlargement of the reproductive organs, accompanied by growth of the breasts, changes in the contours of the body, and the appearance of axillary and pubic hair. This period of sexual development culminates in the appearance of the first menses (*menarche*) at an average age of 13.5 years. In a recent study of 30,000 menstrual cycles in women between 15 and 39 years of age, the average cycle length was 29 days with a standard deviation of 7.46 days. Mature reproductive life, characterized by recurring menstrual cycles, lasts until about the forty-fifth to the fiftieth year of life. The human female then enters a period known as the *menopause* (also referred to as the *climacteric* or "change of life") during which reproductive cycles become irregular, lengthen, and eventually cease. Thereafter, in the *postmenopause* period, the reproductive organs are atrophic and functionless.

The internal organs

THE OVARIES

The ovaries are remarkable organs which store from the time of birth all the eggs the human female will ever have. They also secrete cyclically hormones that are essential for the postnatal growth and development of the secondary sex organs and the mammary glands.

Each ovary is covered by a continuous mesothelium composed of a single layer of cuboidal epithelium. Because of the tenuous attachment of this layer of cells to the underlying stroma, it is often brushed off in making the histologic preparation. Each ovary consists of an outer cortex and a central medulla (Fig. 23-2). The demarcation between these two areas is often indistinct (Fig. 23-3). Embedded within the loose connective tissue of the medulla are nerves, lymph vessels, and many large blood vessels. The arteries are often coiled and

Figure 23-1 Reproduction organs of the female human being.

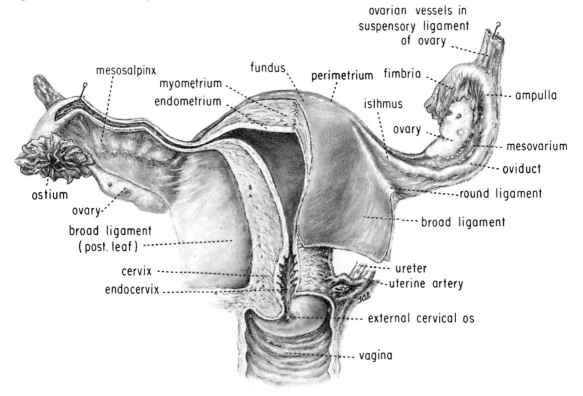

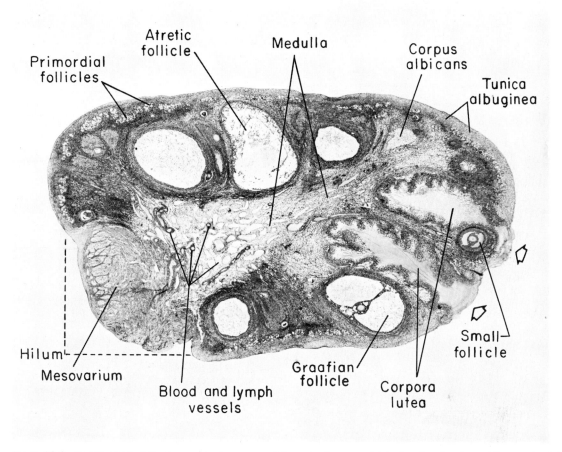

Figure 23-2   Unretouched photomicrograph of an ovary of the cat.   Arrows point to the site of rupture of two ovarian follicles 1 hr before the ovary was removed and fixed.   ×12.

tortuous as they pass toward the cortical zone. This arrangement allows them to adapt readily during the phases of rapid ovarian enlargement, ovulation, and corpus luteum formation.   The medulla may also contain remnants of a closed ductular system, the *rete ovarii*.   These are small and irregularly arranged ducts, lined by a single layer of low cuboidal epithelium.   Embryologically, they are homologous to the *rete testes* in the male gonads. They have no function in the female but on occasion they may become cystic.

The stroma of the cortex is composed of closely packed spindle-shaped cells (Fig. 23-3) arranged in irregular whorls except near the periphery where they form a dense, fibrous, collagenous connective tissue layer, the *tunica albuginea* (Figs. 23-2 and 23-3).   Elastic fibers are few or absent.   A few smooth muscle cells have been described as scattered in the cortical stroma in the ovaries of rats and monkeys.

At the time of birth, in the human female 300,000 to 400,000 oocytes are embedded in the stroma of the cortex of both ovaries.   Of these, only 420 to 480 may ovulate during the entire reproductive life of the individual and only about 5 percent of these will be fertilized.   During each

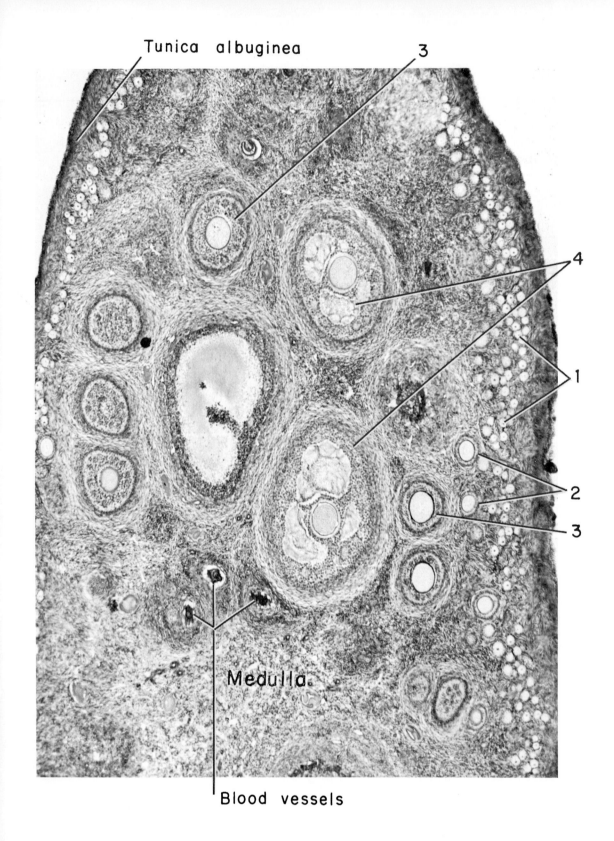

Tunica albuginea

3

4

1

2

3

Medulla.

Blood vessels

menstrual cycle, 15 to 20 follicles may grow to a considerable size (Fig. 23-3), but all of these except the one that will ovulate will degenerate. The majority of the remaining oocytes are destined to degenerate and disappear from the cortex by the process of *atresia,* which begins during the fetal period, is accentuated postnatally, and continues throughout the reproductive life span. More will be said concerning the various types of atresia later in this chapter.

Primordial or unilaminar follicles The cortex of the ovary, particularly in the young female, contains large numbers of individual *primordial* or *unilaminar* follicles (Fig. 23-3) consisting of a large, round oocyte surrounded by a single layer of flattened and elongated *follicular* or *granulosa* cells. A primordial follicle (Fig. 23-4) is composed of an oocyte and the follicular cells surrounding it, resting on a basement membrane. Because the oocyte is a cell of such large size (25 to 30 μm), its circumference may be surrounded by several flattened *follicular cells* in section. The plasma membranes of the oocyte and the follicular cells at this stage are relatively smooth, closely apposed to one another, and at certain places connected by desmosomes. The oocyte (Fig. 23-4) has a large vesicular nucleus with finely dispersed chromatin and one or more large nucleoli. The nuclear envelope bears well-developed pores. A well-developed Golgi apparatus with short tubular profiles may be located near the nucleus. The round mitochondria have typical cristae. The endoplasmic reticulum (ER) is represented by numerous small vesicles. The cytologic characteristics of the oocytes easily distinguish them from the follicular cells or any of the other cells in the cortical stroma (Fig. 23-3).

Growth of follicles As the oocyte begins to grow, the flattened follicular cells become cuboidal (Fig. 23-3) and proliferate rapidly to form a stratified epithelium. These follicles are now *multilaminar.* The multilaminar epithelium rests on a distinct *basement membrane (membrana limitans externa)*

(Fig. 23-5) which stains brilliantly with the PAS method. The basement membrane is exceptionally homogeneous and relatively highly polymerized, and it separates the *stratum granulosum* from the *theca interna* (Fig. 23-6). As the egg grows, a clear, refractile, highly polymerized membrane, the *zona pellucida (mucoid oolemma)* (Fig. 23-7), is interposed between the oocyte and the immediately adjacent follicular cells. The origin of the zona pellucida is uncertain; some believe it is formed from secretions of the follicular cells that immediately surround the egg, whereas other investigators suggest that peripheral Golgi bodies in the oocyte itself have some function in its formation.

As the zona pellucida appears, the plasma membrane of the oocyte forms numerous microvilli (Fig. 23-7) that extend into the zonal membrane. At the same time, irregularly arranged and sinuous cytoplasmic projections from the follicular cells (Fig. 23-7) penetrate the zona and make contact with the plasma membrane of the egg. Some follicle cell processes may penetrate deeply into the ooplasm of the oocyte. Thus, despite the presence of a rather thick zona pellucida (5 μm in the mature ovum), the egg and follicular cells maintain plasma membrane contact throughout the period of growth and until about the time of ovulation.

The theca cone As the follicle begins to grow and becomes multilaminar, it tends to sink deeper into the cortical stroma, while the surrounding stromal cells become arranged into a circumferential sheath to form the *theca folliculi* (Fig. 23-5). The growing follicle is then directed toward the ovarian surface by the formation of a wedge-shaped *thecal cone* (Fig. 23-8) whose details are not seen unless the follicle is sectioned in the proper plane. The directional movement of the thecal cone toward the surface moves the numerous oocytes stored in the cortex (Fig. 23-8) laterally so that they are not unduly compressed by the rapidly growing and expanding follicles. The stromal cells constituting the theca folliculi differentiate into an inner glandular and vascularized layer, the *theca interna* (Fig.

Figure 23-3 Photomicrograph of a rabbit ovary showing (1) numerous primordial follicles with a single layer of flattened follicular cells, (2) unilaminar follicles with a single layer of cuboidal epithelium, (3) multilaminar follicles without antra, and (4) vesicular follicles with follicular antra. Note the increase in size of the egg as the follicle grows, and the presence of the zona pellucida in 2, 3, and 4. $\times$100.

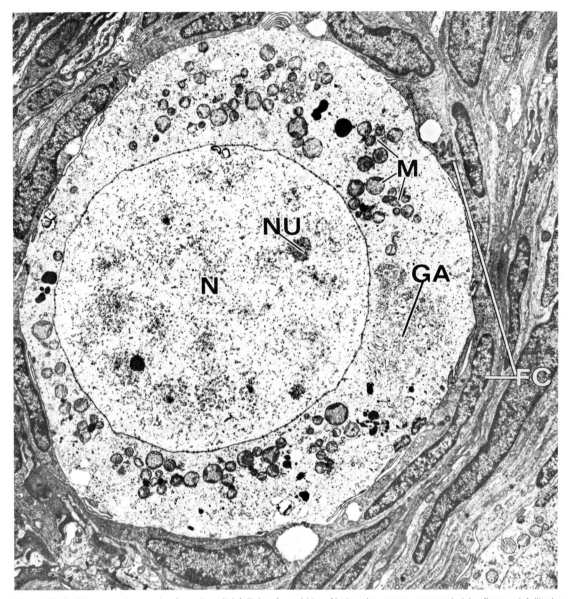

Figure 23-4   Electron micrograph of a primordial follicle of a rabbit.   Notice the oocyte surrounded by flattened follicular epithelium (FC) and the absence of zona pellucida.   The cytoplasm of the oocyte contains some characteristic round mitochondria (M), a few strands of endoplasmic reticulum, and numerous free ribosomes.   N, nucleus; NU, nucleolus; GA, Golgi apparatus. ×4,500.   (Courtesy of F. J. Silverblatt.)

23-6), and an outer layer of connective tissue cells, the *theca externa*.   The boundary between the two thecal layers is indistinct, as is that between the theca externa and the surrounding stroma.   The theca interna is composed of fibroblast-like cells which multiply to form a number of concentric layers of cells.   In later stages of follicular growth these cells enlarge and differentiate into steroid-secreting cells. They appear either ovoid or spindle-shaped and have rounded nuclei. Lipid droplets are abundant and may be visualized, particularly if stained with fat stains. When the follicle ovulates, the thecal gland cells persist for only a short time before undergoing degeneration, and they soon disappear completely. Numerous small blood vessels penetrate the theca externa to supply the complex vascular plexus of the theca interna (see Fig. 23-14B). Blood vessels do not enter the layers of follicular epithelium until after ovulation.

Development of the vesicular follicle When the follicular cells have proliferated into 6 to 12 layers,

there appear among them small lakes of follicular fluid which stain positively with the PAS reaction and are called the *Call-Exner bodies* (Fig. 23-9). They are thought to represent the precursors of follicular fluid. In some animals, such as the rabbit, the Call-Exner bodies are numerous and much more obvious than in the ovarian follicles of women. The accumulations of follicular fluid enlarge and coalesce to form a fluid-filled cavity, the *follicular antrum* (Figs. 23-9 and 23-10). The *liquor folliculi* is a clear, viscid fluid rich in hyaluronic acid. In sectioned material it often has a granular appearance and stains a pale pink with the PAS method. An ovarian follicle with a completely formed antrum

Figure 23-5 A multilaminar, growing follicle with a distinct basement membrane separating the follicular epithelium from the theca folliculi of a rabbit. ×350.

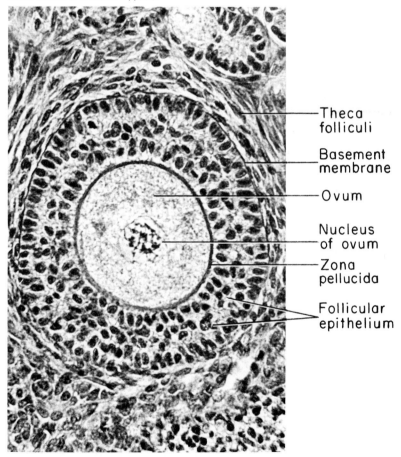

Theca
folliculi

Basement
membrane

Ovum

Nucleus
of ovum

Zona
pellucida

Follicular
epithelium

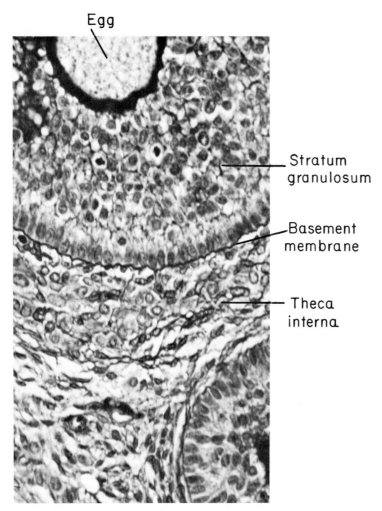

Egg

Stratum granulosum

Basement membrane

Theca interna

Figure 23-6   Section from a multilaminar follicle of a rabbit, showing the thickness of the basement membrane and the transformation of the theca interna into steroid-secreting cells.   ×850.

is described as a *secondary* or *vesicular* follicle. By the time antrum formation begins, the oocyte has attained its full size (125 to.150 μm in human beings) and is encompassed by a fully developed zona pellucida.   The follicle continues to enlarge until it reaches a diameter of 8 to 10 mm or more (Figs. 23-11A and B).

The earliest phase of follicular growth which precedes antrum formation is not under hormonal control, whereas all the growth subsequent to and including liquor folliculi formation is dependent entirely upon the action of gonadotrophic hormones secreted by the adenohypophysis.   The follicle has no endocrine function prior to the formation of an

Figure 23-7   Electron micrograph of a peripheral sector of a mouse oocyte, its zona pellucida, and the associated follicular cells. Notice the numerous microvilli from the oocyte and the sinuous processes from the follicle cells penetrating the zona pellucida. ZP, zona pellucida; MV, microvillus; GC, Golgi complex; L, lipid; FCP, follicle cell processes; N, nucleus.   ×7,800.   (Courtesy of D. L. Odor.)

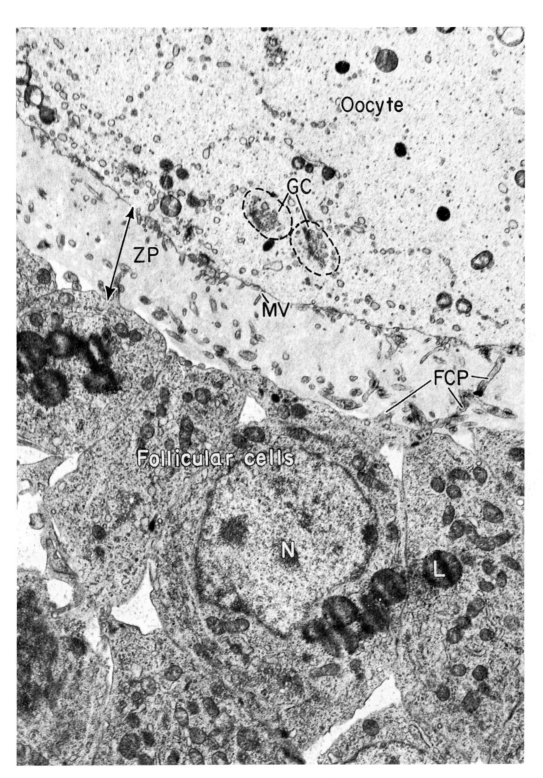

Oocytes   Theca
cone

Mesothelium
(Germinal
epithelium)

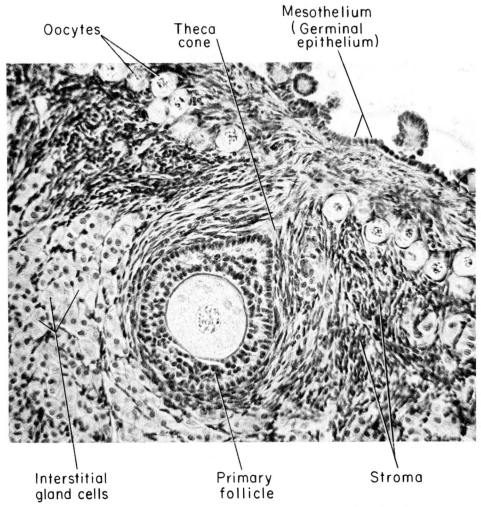

Interstitial
gland cells

Primary
follicle

Stroma

Figure 23-8 The appearance of the theca cone in a growing follicle. Note how the primary oocytes are moved aside as the follicle expands toward the surface. ×300.

antrum, whereas after this event it becomes an endocrine body that secretes estrogens and, just before and after ovulation, both estrogens and progestins. In most vesicular follicles the egg, surrounded by several layers of follicular cells, assumes an eccentric position, giving an appearance of a small hillock protruding into the antrum (Fig. 23-11A). The follicular cells encompassing the egg constitute the *cumulus oophorus*. The zona pellucida is surrounded by a single continuous layer of follicular cells, the *corona radiata* (Fig. 23-11B),

which are anchored to the zona by cytoplasmic processes that penetrate the zona (Fig. 23-7).

The preovulatory follicle The discharge of a mature ovum at ovulation results from a series of complex cytologic and growth changes within the egg itself and in the follicular and thecal cells surrounding it. Why only certain of the primordial follicles begin to grow and develop during any particular reproductive cycle is still a mystery.

In the human female, follicles require 12 to

14 days to reach maturity and attain the preovulatory stage. As the follicles reach their maximum size, they may occupy the full thickness of the ovarian cortex and bulge above the surface of the ovary (Fig. 23-11A).

Maturation division of the ovum Before an egg can be fertilized, it is essential that its *diploid* number of chromosomes (46) be reduced to the *haploid* number (23). This process begins before the egg is discharged from the follicle and involves the for-

mation of the *first polar body* (Fig. 23-12), which results in the very unequal cytoplasmic division. In order to understand fully the various steps in this complex process, the reader is urged to review the process of meiosis.

In the human female all the oocytes complete the earliest stages of meiosis during the fetal period, and so postnatally the chromosomes are in the *dictyotene* or "resting" stage of meiosis. They will remain in this stage throughout the reproductive life or until the oocyte begins the period of preovulatory

Figure 23-9   A multilaminar, vesicular follicle of a rabbit in which the Call-Exner vacuoles are prominent. Fusion of these results in an enlarged antrum filled with follicular fluid.   ×120.

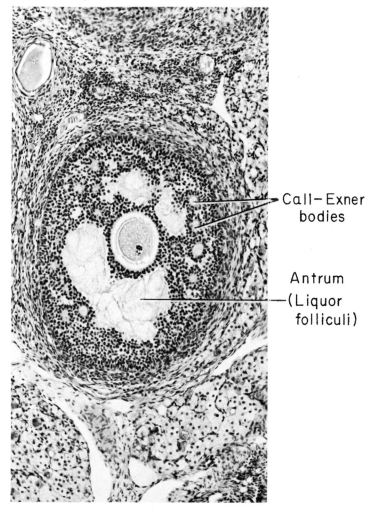

Call—Exner bodies

Antrum (Liquor folliculi)

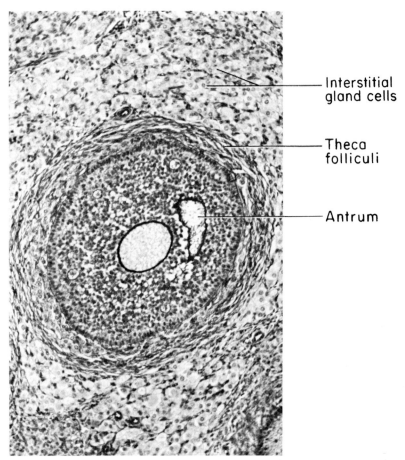

Interstitial gland cells

Theca folliculi

Antrum

Figure 23-10 The early formation of an antrum, the concentric arrangement of the cells of the stroma to form the theca folliculi, and the arrangement and appearance of the interstitial gland cells of a rabbit ovary. ×100.

growth, at which time the process of meiosis is resumed. In the formation of the first polar body, the *vesicular nucleus* or *germinal vesicle* moves to a position just beneath the *oolemma*, the plasma membrane of the egg (Fig. 23-12B); the chromatids, still attached at their chiasmata, condense and become visible at the microscopic level. The nuclear membrane disappears, and a spindle with fine spindle fibers is formed and assumes a position paratangential to the surface. The chromosomes are grouped on the metaphase plate of the spin-

dle. The spindle then rotates 90° to the egg surface. A small bleb of clear cytoplasm is extruded from the egg and half of the chromosomes are discharged into it (Fig. 23-12C). The first polar body is quickly pinched off and comes to lie free within the perivitelline space (Fig. 23-12D). A second spindle forms immediately and the chromosomes remaining in the egg become arranged on the metaphase plate. This is the condition of the egg at the time of ovulation (Fig. 23-12E and F), and it has required approximately 8 to 10 hr

Figure 23-11 Photomicrograph of preovulatory follicles of (A) rat and (B) rabbit. Notice the separation of the cumulus oophorus from the stratum granulosum. Notice also the secretion of the secondary follicular fluid, expecially in B.

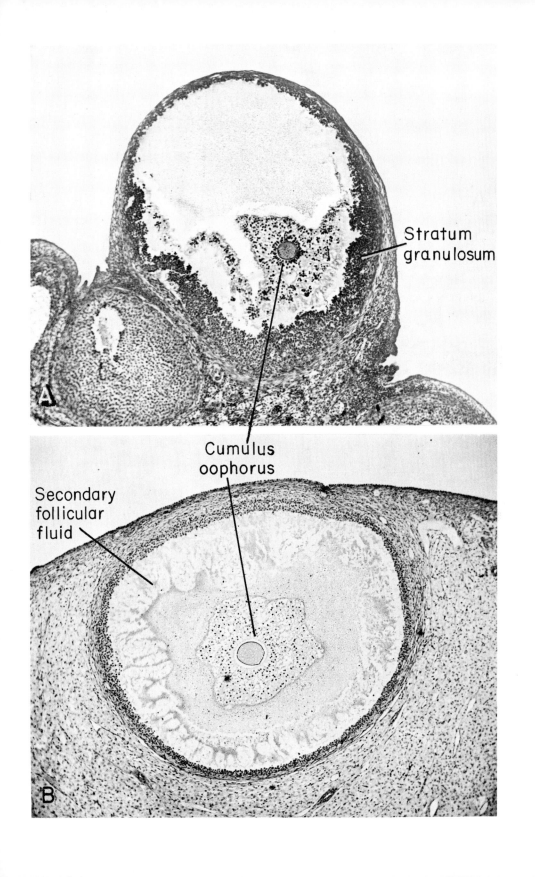

Stratum granulosum

Cumulus oophorus

Secondary follicular fluid

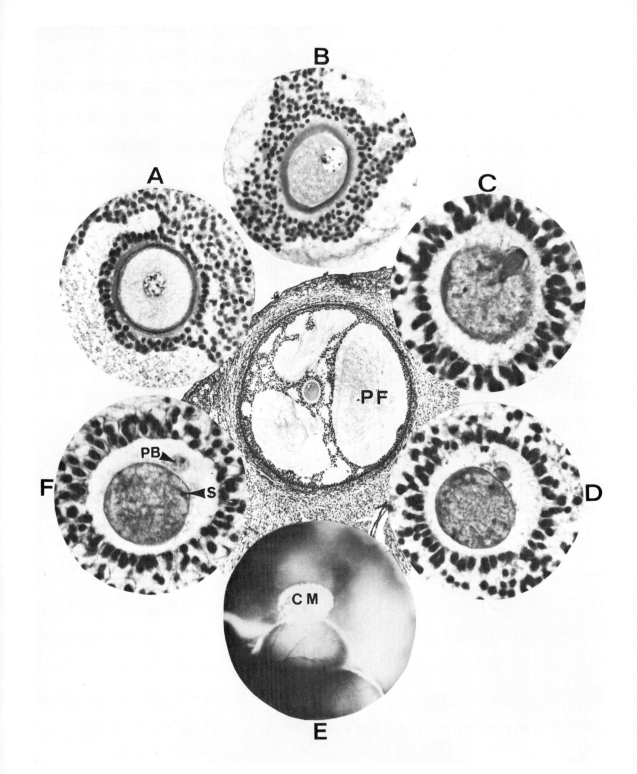

to attain this condition. The formation of the *second polar body* in the second meiotic division must await the transport of the ovulated egg into the ampulla of the oviduct and its penetration by a spermatozoon.

The size of the preovulatory follicle increases significantly during the 12 to 15 hr prior to rupture, the period of *preovulatory swelling.* It involves (1) a rapid growth of the follicle itself, (2) the secretion of a thinner *secondary follicular fluid* (Fig. 23-11B) at an increased rate, and (3) late in this phase an increased inward folding of the stratum granulosum and theca (Fig. 23-11A; see also Fig. 23-15A). Changes occur also in the cumulus oophorus preparatory to freeing the ovum from the stratum granulosum. The intercellular cement anchoring the cumulus cells to one another depolymerizes so that they separate from one another (Fig. 23-11A and B). This separation appears to be related to the action of the luteinizing hormone secreted by the adenohypophysis.

In some animals the cumulus mass, with its enclosed egg, floats free within the antrum (Fig. 23-11B); in others, the strands of cumulus remain attached to the follicle wall until ovulation.

Ovulation The sequence of events leading to the rupture of the follicle and expulsion of the egg is still a mystery. The appearance of a bulging follicle above the surface of the ovary may give the impression that increasing intrafollicular pressure leads to its rupture. However, careful measurements of intrafollicular pressure just before ovulation reveals that there is no significant increase in pressure even at the moment of rupture. Approximately 30 min before a follicle ruptures, the stratum granulosum, the theca folliculi, and tunica albuginea become thinned out progressively (Fig. 23-13) in a restricted area on the surface of the follicle. This bulging area is called the *stigma* or *macula pellucida.* It has been suggested that collagenase may depolymerize the collagen fibers in the region of the stigma, weak-

ening the follicular wall. This is an attractive theory, but conclusive evidence is not yet available.

Just before ovulation, a nipple-like cone bulges above the surface of the follicle. Its membranous covering appears similar to the basement membrane which separates the follicular cells from the theca. Within a few minutes, this membrane ruptures (Fig. 23-13D), expelling the ovum enclosed in the cumulus oophorus. This event is called *ovulation* (Figs. 23-13E and 23-14A see color insert), and the ovulated egg can now be termed the *gamete.* Ovulation has been observed many times in various living anesthetized laboratory animals and recorded cinematographically. In rats and rabbits a rather slow extrusion of the follicular contents was observed. The time between rupture of the stigma and discharge of the ovum averaged 72 sec when the egg was preceded by some of the thin follicular fluid and 126 sec when the cumulus oophorus was extruded first. In many mammals, including primates, the viscous follicular fluid is not completely expressed from the antrum during ovulation. It may remain adherent to the site of the stigma (Fig. 23-14A see color insert) until it is swept from the ovarian surface by the cilia lining the fimbriated end of the oviduct.

Formation of the corpus luteum The ovulated follicle is transformed rapidly into a new, highly vascularized, glandular structure, the *corpus luteum* or *luteal gland.* It is called the *corpus luteum of ovulation* if pregnancy does not follow. If pregnancy ensues, it is called the *corpus luteum of pregnancy.* In pregnancy, the corpus luteum grows much larger and lasts longer.

Even before ovulation the wall of the follicle tends to become folded or plicated (Fig. 23-15A). The plicae are retained (Fig. 23-15B) as the follicle is transformed into a corpus luteum and are a characteristic feature of the fully formed luteal body. The transformation of the ovulatory follicle into a corpus luteum involves, first of all, the depolymer-

---

Figure 23-12 Stages in the formation of the first polar body in a preovulatory follicle (PF) of the rat. A. The centrally located vesicular nucleus at the beginning of the preovulatory growth phase. B. The movement of the nucleus to the periphery of the egg. C. Formation of the first polar body. D. Abstriction of the polar body vesicle and the compacted chromosomes remaining within the egg. E. An ovulated follicle from a 16-mm motion picture. CM, cumulus mass. F. Section of this cumulus mass, showing the first polar body (PB) and the second maturation spindle (S), with the remaining chromosomes on the metaphase plate.

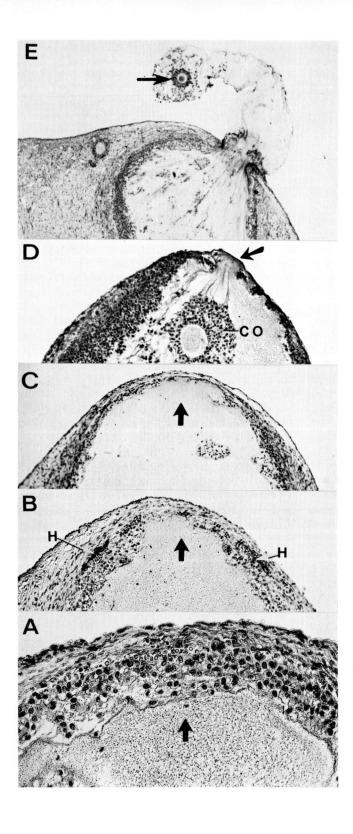

ization of the basement membrane that originally separated the granulosa cell layers from the theca. This allows the connective tissue cells and blood vessels to invade the stratum granulosum (Fig. 23-16). The granulosa cells of the ovulatory follicle that will become the luteal cells of the corpus luteum begin to undergo cytomorphosis even before ovulation. The large preovulatory follicle secretes both estrogen and progesterone. Mitoses are seldom seen in the glandular parenchyma cells of the developing corpus luteum but are noted in the rapidly developing endothelium of the blood vessels which invade it.

The *luteal cells* enlarge and become polyhedral in shape and filled with lipid droplets (Fig. 23-17A). In ordinary histologic preparations the cytoplasm of the luteal cells contains numerous empty vacuoles whose lipid contents are dissolved out by the organic solvents used in processing the tissues. Several types of luteal cells have been described but it is not known whether these are transition stages in the differentiation of a single cell type or represent distinct cell species. An interesting feature of the developing corpus luteum is the rapid invasion of the stratum granulosum with connective tissue elements and sprouts of capillary endothelium. The connective tissue forms a delicate reticulum supporting the luteal cells. A complex rete network of capillaries forms throughout the gland. With time, larger blood vessels are formed (see Fig. 23-14B see color insert). The formation of the vascular network in the developing corpus luteum is remarkably similar to that seen during the development of the vascular supply in any embryonic organ.

In electron micrographs of the corpus luteum, the luteal cells have mitochondria with tubular cristae and an abundant smooth ER so characteristic of steroid-secreting cells. The fully formed corpus luteum secretes both estrogens and progestins. If the egg is not fertilized, the corpus luteum lasts for about 14 days. With its demise (Fig.

23-17B), the rate of secretion of estrogens and progestins drops, and it begins to undergo involution. The luteal cells become filled with complex lipids and degenerate. With time, a hyaline intercellular material accumulates, and the former corpus luteum assumes the appearance of an irregular white, hyaline scar, the *corpus albicans* (Fig. 23-18). The corpus albicans may persist for many months before it gradually disappears. If, on the other hand, the egg is fertilized and implants into the endometrium of the uterus, the corpus luteum persists. It enlarges to 2 to 3 cm to become the *corpus luteum of pregnancy*. During pregnancy, the corpus luteum remains functional for several months and then gradually declines up to full term. Involution is accelerated after delivery, leading to the formation of a corpus albicans. A corpus albicans formed from a corpus luteum of pregnancy may last for years.

Atresia of follicles As mentioned earlier, atresia, or degeneration of eggs and follicles, at all stages of follicular development is a prominent feature in the life of the ovaries. Large numbers of oocytes degenerate and disappear during the fetal and early postnatal periods. It has been proposed that a primary cause of atresia during these early periods is the disruption or loss of the follicular cells encompassing each oocyte. This suggests that, if the life of the oocyte is to be maintained, the follicular cells must be in continuous and intimate contact with the plasma membrane of the egg. Among the groups of follicles that grow to a large size in each menstrual cycle, only one, as a rule, attains full maturity and ovulates. All the remaining large vesicular follicles and many of the smaller ones undergo atresia.

Atresia of a vesicular follicle may occur in many different ways (Fig. 23-19A, B, and C) but always with the usual signs of cell degeneration, such as pycnosis and chromatolysis of the nuclei and shrinkage and dissolution of the cytoplasm. The

Figure 23-13 Stages in the formation of the stigma or macula pellucida in an ovulating follicle. A. Several hours before ovulation the stratum granulosum is still quite thick, as are the theca and tunica albuginea. B. One-half hour before ovulation hemostasis (H) appears in the region of the stigma. There is a significant thinning out of the follicular cells and stroma. C. A few minutes before rupture the follicular cells have almost disappeared, as has the stromal tissue in the region of the stigma. D. The stigmal cap lifts away and the free cumulus oophorus (CO) streams toward the opening. E. Ovulation is completed but the viscous antral fluid still adheres to the site of rupture.

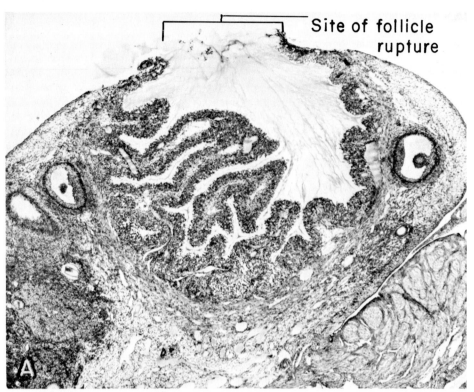

Site of follicle
rupture

A

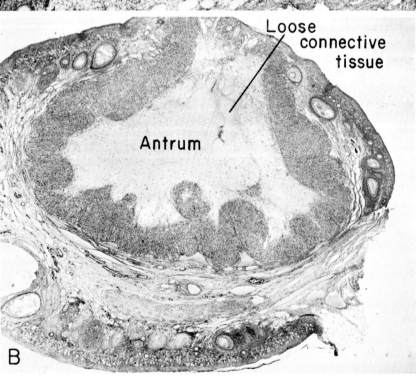

Loose
connective
tissue

Antrum

B

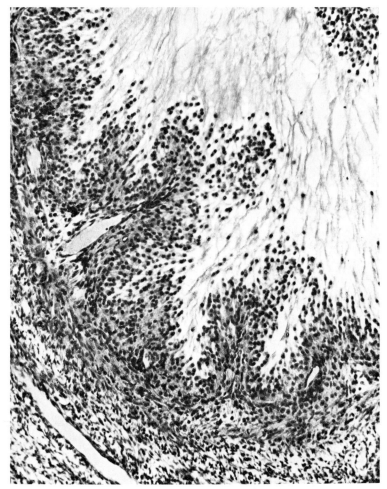

Figure 23-16 Section of the wall of a corpus luteum of a monkey one day after ovulation. Connective tissue and blood vessels are invading the stratum granulosum. ×100.

ooplasm cytolyzes, often leaving only the remnant of the zona pellucida (Fig. 23-19C) to mark the location of the ovum. Macrophage invasion of atretic follicles is a constant feature. The zona pellucida, composed of complex mucopolysaccharides, is more resistant, but eventually it, too, is broken down and engulfed by macrophages.

Occasionally, the basement membrane separating the follicular cells from the theca interna increases in thickness, assumes a corrugated hyaline-like appearance, and is called the *glassy membrane*. In some atretic follicles the cells of the theca interna enlarge, become epithelioid (Fig. 23-19B), and may be arrayed in a radial or cord-like fashion. These cords of cells may be separated from one another by delicate connective tissue

Figure 23-15 Photomicrograph of two stages in the development of the corpus luteum of the cat. A. The recent site of rupture as well as the remarkable foldings of the stratum granulosum. B. Several days later the luteal cells appear glandular and the antrum is being invaded by a loose connective tissue.

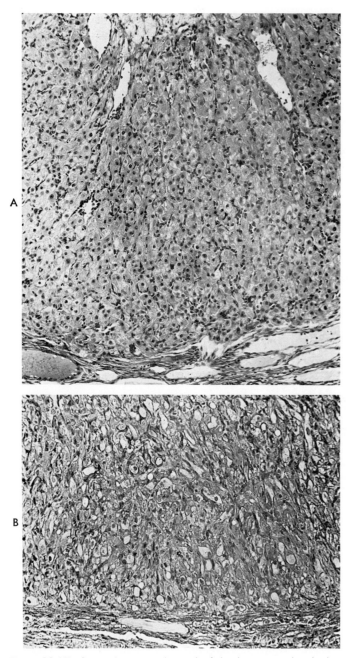

Figure 23-17 Corpus luteum at the peak of development and early degeneration in the monkey. A. Corpus luteum 8 or 9 days after ovulation. Cavity at top of picture. B. Corpus luteum first day of menstrual flow. Cells shrunken, extensive lipid vacuolation, nuclei pycnotic. ×95. (Courtesy of G. E. Corner.)

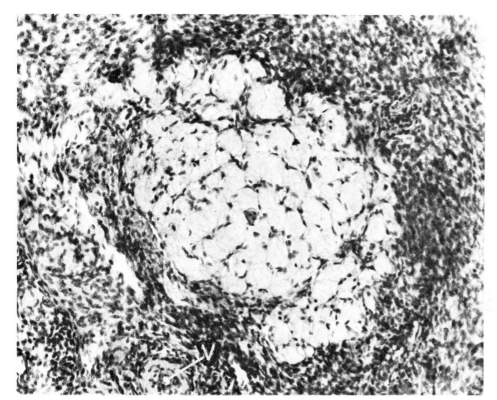

Figure 23-18   Corpus albicans in human ovary.

fibers and a capillary network. The cells are often filled with lipid droplets, giving them an appearance of an old corpus luteum.

The interstitial gland   The origin, development, and endocrine function of the *interstitial gland* or *interstitial cells* of the ovary have been the subject of much confusion and controversy. In many mammals, such as the rabbit (Figs. 23-8 and 23-10) and women (Fig. 23-20), clusters or cords of large, epithelioid cells with cytology and vascularity typical of endocrine glands are dispersed in the cortical stroma. These are referred to collectively as the *interstitial gland* or *interstitial cells*. Cytologically, they resemble luteal cells to a remarkable degree.

The interstitial gland is present periodically in the ovary of the human female from before birth until well after the menopause. The interstitial cells are thought to originate from the cells of the theca

interna of degenerating large secondary follicles or degenerating vesicular follicles of all sizes. The theca interna of the very large preovulatory follicles that are not destined to ovulate have already differentiated into functional thecal gland cells and therefore cannot be transformed into interstitial glandular tissue.

Differentiation of interstitial gland tissue is cyclic and is probably related to the rhythmic atresia of the various crops of vesicular follicles during the menstrual cycle or pregnancy. The role of the interstitial gland cells in normal ovarian physiology is yet to be completely defined. Studies on steroidogenesis in the ovarian stroma in women shows that it principally synthesizes estrogens. In rabbits, on the other hand, interstitial cells are stimulated directly by gonadotrophins to synthesize and secrete 20α-OH-progesterone. Many believe that the interstitial gland plays a significant role in providing estrogens for the growth and development of the

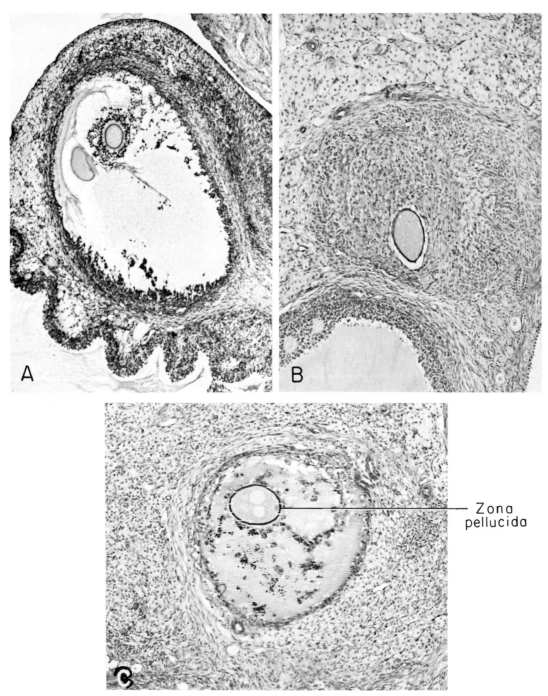

Figure 23-19   Follicular atresia.   A. Cat.   B. Rabbit.   C. Monkey.   A. Large follicle cells of stratum granulosum and egg degenerating.   B. Antrum filled with glandular-appearing cells, egg degenerated but zona pellucida still intact.   C. Theca interna contributing to interstitial gland tissue; follicular cells cytolyzed and zona pellucida remains.

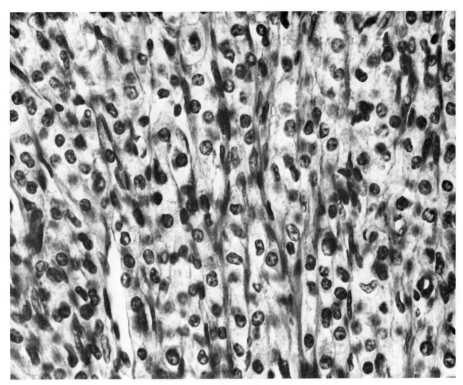

Figure 23-20 Mature interstitial gland tissue at 8 1/2 months of gestation in a woman. Notice the arrangement of the glandular cells and the nuclei of the capillary endothelium between the rows of cells. ×840. (Courtesy of H. W. Mossman.)

secondary sex organs during the prepubertal period.

Other groups of epithelioid cells may be found in the region of the hilum of the ovary and are called *hilus cells*. These cells are usually associated with vascular spaces and unmyelinated nerve fibers. They appear glandular, contain lipids, cholesterol esters, and lipochrome pigments and are identified best during pregnancy and at the onset of the menopause. Tumors or hyperplasia of the hilus cells usually leads to masculinization. Although the evidence is tenuous, it is suggested that these cells secrete steroids related to androgens.

Vessels, nerves, lymphatics The ovaries have a rich blood supply from several sources (Fig. 23-14B). The principal arteries are the ovarian arteries which arise from the aorta below the level of the renal vessels. They travel a relatively long course through the infundibulopelvic ligaments to reach the ovaries. The ovarian arteries anastomose with the uterine arteries which are branches of the hypogastrics.

The veins accompany the arteries and often form a complex plexus of vessels in the hilum. Of principal interest is the cyclic change and continuous reorganization of the vascular pattern of the ovaries as crops of follicles and corpora lutea grow, perform their function, and degenerate. Thus, with each cycle, an extensive blood and lymphatic system develops to support the growth and cytodifferentiation of various cells.

The ovary has a lymphatic system (Fig. 23-21) whose ubiquity and complexity are seldom appreciated. Large numbers of lymphatic vessels are organized around the developing follicles and corpora lutea. The extrinsic lymphatic drainage follows a course to the aortic, preaortic, and para-aortic lymph nodes in the pelvis.

In developing follicles, the lymphatics are arranged in a basket-like network within the theca

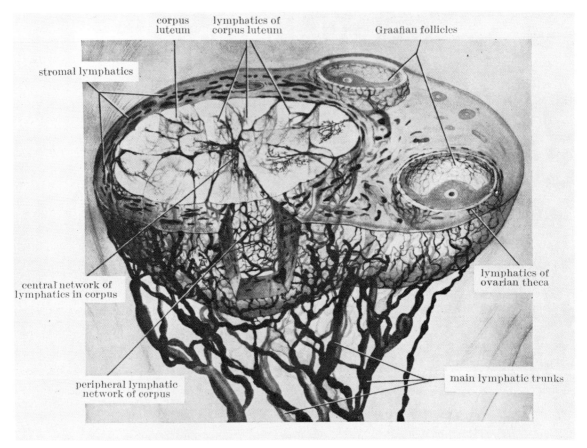

corpus luteum

lymphatics of corpus luteum

Graafian follicles

stromal lymphatics

central network of lymphatics in corpus

lymphatics of ovarian theca

peripheral lymphatic network of corpus

main lymphatic trunks

Figure 23-21 Diagram showing the arrangement of lymphatics within and around a corpus luteum, Graafian follicles, and stroma in the ovary of the ewe.   (Courtesy of B. Morris.)

folliculi but, like the blood vessels, do not penetrate into the stratum granulosum.   The corpora lutea, however, are heavily infiltrated by lymphatic vessels (Fig. 23-21).   The lymphatic capillaries often have open intercellular junctions (Fig. 23-22) so that materials from the interstitial pores can readily enter the vessels.   It has been shown in the ewe, for example, that coincident with the formation of the corpus luteum lymph flow from the ovary increases significantly.   It has been suggested that there may be an association between the synthesis and secretion of steroid hormones by the corpus luteum and an increase in capillary permeability.

Nerves The nerves of the ovaries are derivatives of the ovarian plexus and uterine nerves.   All vessels and nerves enter the ovary through the hilum.

Most of the nerves are nonmyelinated and sympathetic and supply the muscular coats of aterioles. Some nonmyelinated fibers form plexuses around multilaminar follicles.   Whether nerves are associated also with the generalized smooth muscle cells in the ovary is unknown.   A few sensory nerve endings have been described in the ovarian stroma.

THE OVIDUCTS
The oviducts extend bilaterally from the uterus to the region of the ovary (Fig. 23-1).   They provide the necessary environment for fertilization and segmentation of the egg until it attains the morula stage of development.   The fertilized egg remains within the oviduct for a total of 3 days before it enters the uterus.

The oviducts in the sexually mature human female are 10 to 12 cm in length. They are suspended by a rather loose mesentery, the *mesosalpinx* (Fig. 23-23A and B), a derivative of the broad ligament. Each oviduct may be divided into several linear segments distinguishable by gross examination and by study of transverse sections taken at different levels throughout the tube. These are the *interstitial* segment which pierces the uterine wall, the *isthmus* (Fig. 23-1) which comprises approximately two-thirds of the oviduct, and the

somewhat more dilated *ampulla* (Fig. 23-1) which extends from the isthmus to the funnel-shaped orifice, the *infundibulum*. The free margin of the infundibulum is extensively folded and fluted, giving it a fimbriated or tentacle-like appearance (Figs. 23-1 and 23-23A). In many mammals the fimbriated end of the infundibulum embraces the ovary at the time of ovulation, almost completely enclosing it and forming the *ovarian bursa*. Such an intimate relationship of the fimbriae to the ovary has not

Figure 23-22   Low-power electron micrograph of a blood capillary and two adjacent lymphatics in the ovarian stroma of a rat. Notice the open junctions (J) (lines) in the endothelium of both lymphatics.   ×8,000.   (Courtesy of B. Morris.)

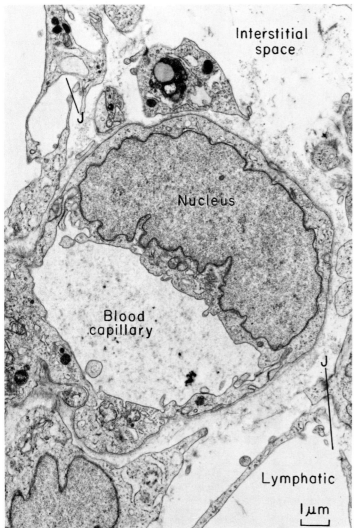

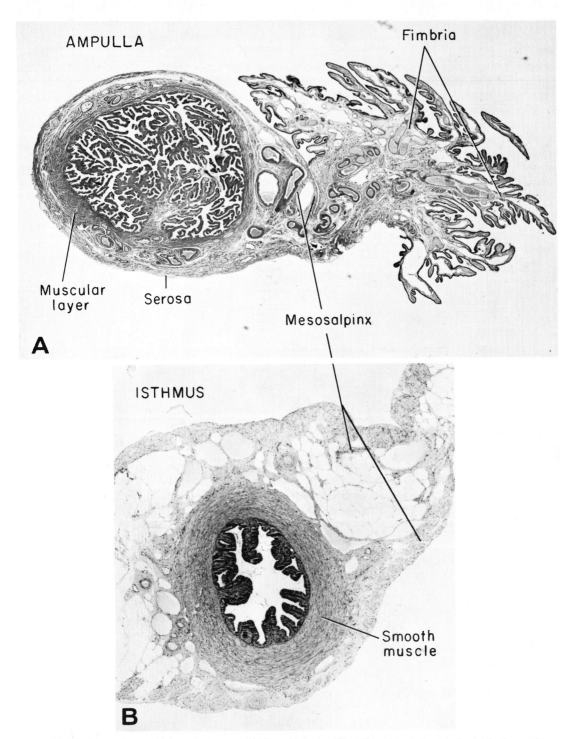

AMPULLA

Fimbria

Muscular
layer

Serosa

Mesosalpinx

A

ISTHMUS

Smooth
muscle

B

Figure 23-23   Photomicrograph through the ampulla (A) and isthmus (B) of the oviduct of a rabbit.   In A, the section was cut to include some of the fimbria.

been observed in the human female. The wall of the oviduct consists of a complex mucous membrane, a muscular layer, and, peripherally, a serosa.

The mucosa Throughout the length of the oviduct, the mucous membrane extends into the lumen in a linear system of complex folds which are elaborately branched, especially in the ampulla (Fig. 23-23A) where in a cross section they appear as a complex labyrinth of spaces. In the isthmus the folds are much less complex and are primarily simple, longitudinal ridges (Fig. 23-23B). The mucosal folds throughout the oviduct are quite thin and are composed of a surface epithelium of columnar cells resting on a lamina of connective tissue (Fig. 23-24). Many of the cells are ciliated and are interspersed among nonciliated cells that appear to be glandular (Fig. 23-24). The ciliated cells of the oviduct are most numerous on the fimbrial surface of the infundibulum, somewhat less so in the ampulla, and fewer still in the isthmus and interstitial segments. The cilia of the oviduct exhibit the basal body complexes and fibrillar arrangements typical of cilia elsewhere (Fig. 23-25).

The epithelium of the oviduct of the human female shows cyclic hypertrophy and atrophy during each menstrual cycle. The ciliated cells may vary in height from 30 μm at about the time of ovulation to 15 μm or less during the late luteal phase or shortly before the onset of menstruation. After the menopause, the epithelium is of the low cuboidal type and there are fewer ciliated cells.

The development of cilia in the oviduct is in some manner dependent on the presence of the ovary. In women born without ovaries no ciliated cells develop and the mucosal folds are little more than broad ridges. In addition, it has been shown recently that removal of the ovaries from a sexually mature rhesus monkey causes a dramatic atrophy of the oviduct epithelium with complete loss of cilia from the epithelial cells. If the castrate animal is injected with estrogens, the ciliated epithelium is completely restored. Experiments such as these demonstrate dramatically the processes involved in

Figure 23-24 Photomicrograph showing the ciliated and glandular cells of the surface epithelium of the ampulla of the oviduct of the monkey. (Courtesy of R. Brenner.)

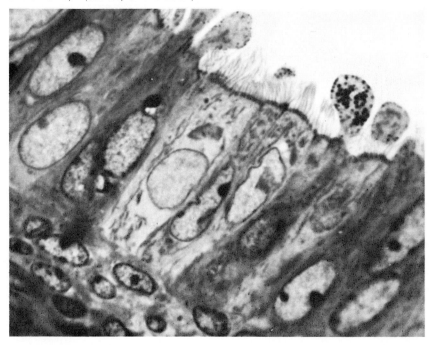

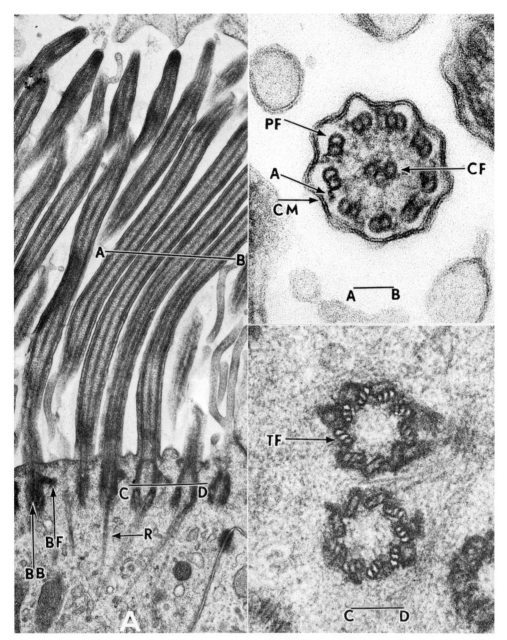

Figure 23-25   A. Typical cilium and basal body complex.   Each basal body (BB) has a basal foot (BF) and proximal rootlets (R).   ×30,000.   The line A–B through the cilia represents the transverse section seen on the upper right.   The line C–D through the basal body represents the transverse section seen on the lower right.   A–B. Cross section of a typical cilium. There are nine peripheral double fibrils (PF) and two single central fibrils (CF).   A short projection or "arm" (A) is present on each peripheral doublet.   The cilium is bounded by a ciliary membrane (CM).   ×160,000.   C–D. Cross sections of typical basal bodies.   In each basal body there are nine peripheral triplet fibrils (TF) embedded in a dense material.   The core of the basal body is much less dense and lacks central fibrils.   ×130,000.   (Courtesy of R. Brenner.)

ciliogenesis and dependence of ciliated cells of the reproductive tract upon hormones for their full development and function.

The cilia of the fimbria all beat toward the ostium of the oviduct and play an important role in sweeping the ovulated eggs from the surface of the ovary and into the ampulla of the oviduct. Even though the mucosa of the ampulla is relatively well ciliated and all the cilia beat in the direction of the isthmus, it appears that egg transport through the ampulla is caused primarily by peristaltic muscular contractions. The role of ciliary beat in the ampulla is at present unknown.

After ovulation, the egg, embedded in the cumulus oophorus (Fig. 23-14A see color insert), is transported from the site of ovulation to the lower end of the ampulla in approximately 10 min. The ampulla is normally the site of sperm penetration and fertilization. Fifteen to eighteen hours after fertilization the egg has been freed of all its cumulus cells; it then moves into the isthmus where its transport is slowed, requiring approximately 2 days to reach the uterus.

It is usually assumed that all the cilia in the oviducts of mammals beat toward the uterus. It has been found recently, at least in the rabbit, that the ciliated cells on the surfaces of some of the longitudinal ridges in the isthmus of the oviduct beat in the direction of the ovary whereas others on adjacent ridges beat in the direction of the uterus. Whether currents set up by this alternate ciliary movement play any role in the passage of spermatozoa to the ampulla is unknown. It should be pointed out that the rate of passage of spermatozoa through the oviducts to the site of fertilization (the ampulla) is much too fast to be accounted for by their own motility. Although evidence is not complete, it appears that both muscular and ciliary activity are primarily responsible for the rapid movement of spermatozoa through the oviducts.

The mucous membrane of the oviduct rests directly upon the tunica muscularis with no intervening submucosa. The lamina propria of the mucous membrane is thin, consisting of a delicate, loose connective tissue extending into the folds and containing a few scattered muscle cells.

Muscularis The muscularis of the oviduct consists, in general, of an inner circular or spiral layer and an external layer of rather poorly defined longitudinal fibers (Fig. 23-23A and B). There are no distinct boundaries between the two. A third, inner layer of longitudinal muscles has been described in the proximal isthmus in the oviducts of the human female. There is an obvious increase in the thickness of the circular muscle layers as the isthmus approaches the uterus. The peritoneal coat of the oviduct is covered by a thin serosa.

UTERUS

The uterus is a hollow, pear-shaped organ with a thick muscular wall. It receives the oviducts and opens into the vagina through the cervical canal (Fig. 23-1). It lies in the pelvic cavity interposed between the bladder and rectum. Its size varies among nonpregnant women but average dimensions are length, 6.3 cm; breadth, 4.5 cm; and thickness, 2.5 cm. The expanded rostral portion is referred to as the *body* or *corpus uteri*, and the caudal portion, a part of which protrudes into the upper vagina, is the *cervix*. The cervical canal passes from the uterine cavity through the cervix and opens into the vagina. The opening visible from the vaginal vault is called the *external os* (Fig. 23-1). The term *fundus* refers to the dome-shaped upper portion of the body of the uterus from which the oviducts extend. The body of the uterus is flattened anteroposteriorly, and the lumen appears as a transverse slit. The cavity of the uterus is confluent with the lumina of the oviducts.

The wall of the uterus is composed of an internal layer, the *endometrium* (mucosa); a middle layer, the *myometrium* (muscularis); and an external layer, the *perimetrium* (serosa) (Fig. 23-1). It should be noted that the posterocaudal third of the uterus does not have a serosa, since this portion of the uterus lies below the peritoneal reflection. The connective tissue of the broad ligament at the lateral edges of the uterus is termed the *parametrium*.

Endometrium Beginning at puberty and continuing until the menopause, the uterine mucosa undergoes cyclic changes in structure and secretory activity. The terminal event in each cycle is a partial destruction and sloughing of a portion of the endometrium, accompanied by some extravasation of blood, an event termed *menstruation*. The endometrium is a complex mucous membrane (Fig.

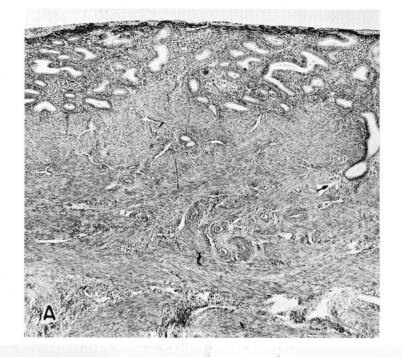

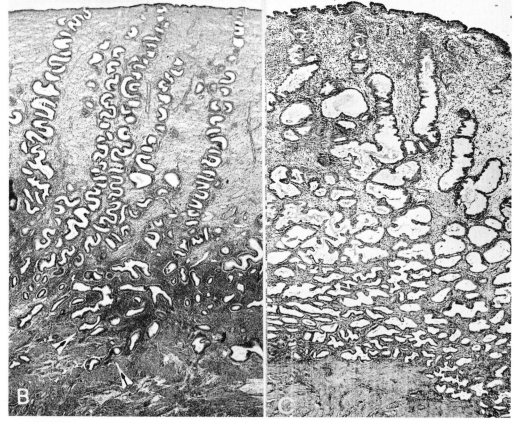

23-26). Its height varies from 1 to 7 mm, depending on the phase of the menstrual cycle. It consists of a simple columnar epithelium and a wide lamina propria, the *endometrial stroma*. It is firmly attached to the myometrium without any intervening submucosa. The stroma contains many simple tubular *uterine glands* (Fig. 23-26B) which open onto the surface of the mucosa, extend deep into the endometrial stroma, and end blindly near the muscularis. Occasionally, they are branched in the area adjacent to the myometrium. The epithelium lining the glands and that covering the surface appear identical. Occasionally, patches of ciliated cells may be seen either within the glands or on the surface epithelium facing the lumen. There is a basement membrane beneath the epithelium of both the glands and surface epithelium. The stroma in which the uterine glands are embedded resembles mesenchyme tissue (Fig. 23-26C); the cells are loosely arranged and stellate in appearance and often have oval nuclei.

The endometrium is usually divided into two layers or zones (Fig. 23-27), differing in their morphology and function: a *lamina basalis* or *basal layer* and a *lamina functionalis* or *functional layer*.

The basal layer is applied directly to the myometrium and occasionally may extend into small pockets in the muscularis (Fig. 23-26A and B at arrows). Dr. Carl Hartman once removed all the endometrial tissue from the uterus of a menstruating rhesus monkey by scrubbing it away with cotton swabs. At the end of the next menstrual cycle, he was surprised to find a completely regenerated endometrium. This was a dramatic demonstration of the regenerative capacity of the endometrium even from the bits of tissue tucked into the small pockets of the myometrium.

There is considerable variation in the thickness of the basal layer of endometrium. Its stroma is much more cellular and fibrous than that of the functional zone. The basal layer undergoes few obvious microscopic changes during a menstrual cycle and serves principally as a source of tissue for the cyclic regeneration of the functional layer. The functional layer rises from the basal layer toward the lumen of the uterus and is the site of the principal cyclic changes in the endometrium which prepare a bed for the fertilized ovum. The endometrial tissue, and particularly the functional zone, undergoes a constantly changing histologic picture which is related directly to the secretion of the various hormones by the ovary.

The epithelial cells during the early proliferative phase are tall columnar cells (Fig. 23-28) with numerous long, narrow microvilli extending from their surfaces. Their nuclei may be elongated or quite irregular in shape, their mitochondria are relatively small, and their Golgi complexes assume a supranuclear position. Many cells show cytoplasmic inclusions and granules of varying size and shape. At this stage in the cycle, glycogen is not discernible by electron microscopy. Dramatic changes in the cytology of cells (Fig. 23-29) are seen during the midsecretory phase, at the time the corpus luteum is secreting actively. The mitochondria are larger and are surrounded by narrow tubules of rough ER. Large aggregates of glycogen, as well as numerous polyribosomes, are present. During the later secretory phase, the apical portions of the cells are filled with glycogen. The apical cell membrane becomes distended and ruptures, releasing glycogen and other cytoplasmic components into the lumen. During the premenstrual or degenerative phase (Fig. 23-30), the mitochondria are significantly smaller and lysosomes increase in number. Myelin figures or lipid droplets have formed within the remaining glycogen deposits.

A very elaborate and unique vascular system is developed in anticipation of an implanting embryo, and this should be explored in some detail. The uterine artery gives off 6 to 10 *arcuate arteries* (Fig. 23-27) which extend between the outer and middle third of the myometrium and have *radial branches* inward to supply the endometrium. There may be 20 or more radial branches (sometimes called *submucous vessels*) from each arcuate artery. The *spiral arteries* (Fig. 23-27) are particularly characteristic of the endometrium. They pass through the basalis and extend into the functional zone. The proximal part of the vessel is an unchanging seg-

Figure 23-26 Photomicrograph of human endometrium during the menstrual cycle and pregnancy. A. Shedding of the stratum functionalis has been completed, and its regeneration has just begun. B. Early secretory endometrium. C. Gestational endometrium, fourteenth day of pregnancy. Notice the arrows pointing out stratum basalis tissue in crypts of myometrium.

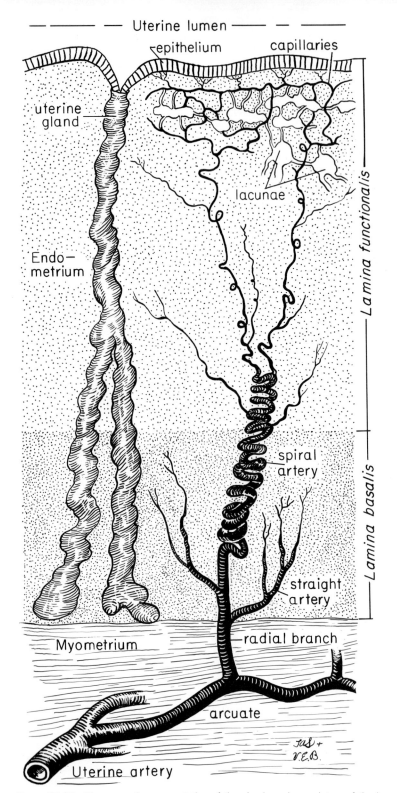

Figure 23-27 Diagrammatic representation of the glands and vasculature of the human endometrium.

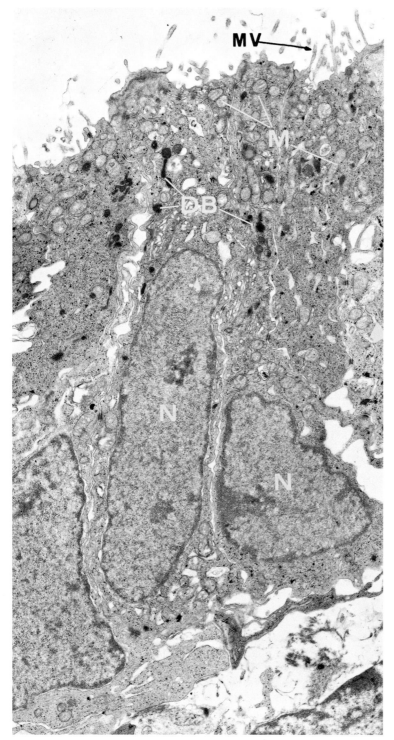

Figure 23-28 Electron micrograph of human epithelial cells during the early proliferative phase. N, nucleus; M, mitochondria; DB, dense bodies; MV, microvilli. ×10,500. (Courtesy of E. R. Friedrich.)

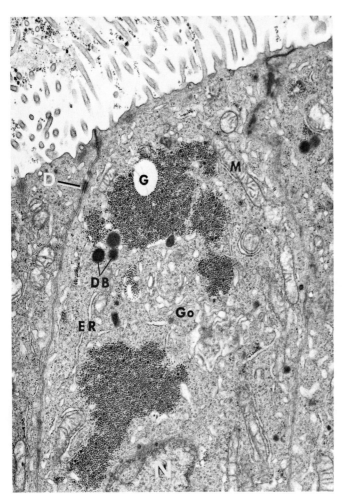

Figure 23-29   Electron micrograph of the apical cell portion of the midsecretory phase of human endometrium.   Notice the large glycogen deposits (G), the slightly dilated Golgi structure (Go), and a few remaining dense bodies (DB).   D, desmosome; ER, endoplasmic reticulum; M, mitochondria.   ×11,400.   (Courtesy of E. R. Friedrich.)

ment whereas the distal end is subject to repeated degeneration and regeneration with each menstrual cycle.   The typical development of the spiral arteries is dependent on a certain ratio of estrogens and progestins.   Branches of the spiral vessels serve the tissues of the basalis as independent arteries or arterioles.   These *straight arteries* (Fig. 23-27) are not subject to the actions of hormones.

As the spiral vessels traverse the functionalis they divide into several terminal arterioles which frequently anastomose with one another.   These,

in turn, connect with a complex rete network of capillary units and *lacunae* (Fig. 23-27).   The lacunae are very thin, dilated units which vary greatly in size.   These structures are ordinarily not classified as part of the venous system but rather are terminal *ectatic capillaries* or *connecting lacunae* and are defined as part of the arterial vasculature. The venules and veins also form an irregular network with sinusoidal enlargements called *collecting lacunae* which appear largest during the late secretory phase of the cycle.   The endometrial veins flow into

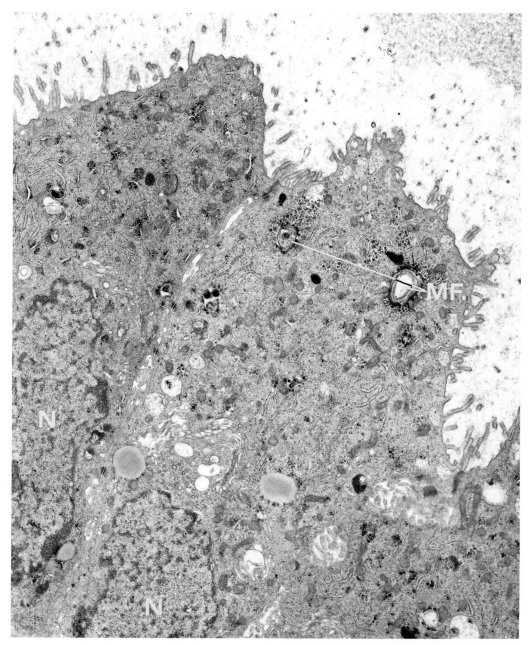

Figure 23-30 Premenstrual phase of human endometrium. Apical cell portions with small mitochondria and lysosomes; myelin figures (MF) forming within the glycogen deposits. ×11,400. (Courtesy of E. R. Friedrich.)

a venous plexus concentrated at the basalis-myometrial border.

Cyclic changes in the endometrium

During a menstrual cycle, the endometrium passes through three successive phases which correspond to the functional activity of the ovary: The *proliferative* (or *follicular*) *phase* is concurrent with the growth of the follicles and estrogen secretion, the *secretory* (or *luteal*) *phase* coincides with the functional life of the corpus luteum, and the *menstrual phase* lasts through the period of menstrual bleeding.

Proliferative phase   During the proliferative phase, the endometrium increases in thickness from about 1 to 2 or 3 mm. The endometrial glands become longer and more numerous. Many mitoses may be seen throughout the epithelium and the stroma. The epithelial cells, particularly in the glands, become taller and accumulate a considerable store of glycogen basal to the nucleus. No doubt other presecretory substances accumulate as well. The luminal surface of the epithelium is even and the cell membranes distinct and unbroken. The glands are either straight-walled or slightly wavy. They secrete a thin mucoid. The stroma during this time is rich in mucoid substance.

In the proliferative phase, the coiled arteries lengthen with the regrowth of the endometrium and extend through more than half its thickness. They are lightly coiled.

Secretory phase   Remarkable modifications of the endometrium ensue within a day or two after ovulation has occurred. The glands become irregularly coiled and the glandular epithelium begins to secrete. The lumen of each gland becomes filled with a mucoid fluid rich in nutrients, particularly glycogen. The glycogen moves from a subnuclear position to the apical surface and, as described earlier, is discharged from the cells. The glands enlarge and often become sacculated, especially in the deeper third of the mucosa. The endometrium gradually becomes more edematous and may increase in thickness to 5 or 6 mm. This increase is due primarily to swelling of the tissues rather than to proliferation of cells. The mesenchymatous cells of the stroma share in this edematous condition. During the luteal phase, the coiled arteries lengthen and become more spiral. Near the end of the cycle, rather characteristic decidual changes are often seen in the stromal cells.

Menstrual phase   Reduction in hormonal activity of the corpus luteum 4 to 5 days prior to the appearance of menstruation has a profound effect on the endometrium. Changes in the hemodynamics of blood flow in the functionalis is of primary significance in understanding the process of menstruation. The endometrium becomes ischemic and stops secreting. The functionalis shrinks, owing to loss of ground substance and water. The stromal cells become closely packed and densely stained. The lumina of the glands are reduced or obliterated in the general collapse of the endometrium. There is an intermittent constriction of the spiral vessels, resulting in reduced arterial and venous blood flow and stasis in the capillaries. Approximately 2 days after the endometrium begins its decline, the epithelium becomes disrupted and blood, uterine fluid, and desquamated bits of the mucosa are sloughed from the functionalis and discharged via the vagina. This period of bloody vaginal discharge, lasting roughly 5 days, is termed the *menses*. The menstrual process begins with extravasation of blood from capillaries or from arterioles into the stroma. This blood forms small hematomas that coalesce and rupture onto the mucosal surface. Fragments of mucosa detach, leaving exposed stroma and naked vessels. The disintegrating functionalis becomes tattered and soaked with blood. Desquamation of tissue continues until the stratum functionalis is discarded.

Menstrual blood is both arterial and venous. Clotting is inhibited, and hemostasis is dependent upon vasoconstriction. Arterial bleeding is intermittent and brief, coincident with the period of relaxation of the coiled arteries, whereas bleeding from veins is a light but protracted seepage. The coiled arteries are shed piecemeal and more slowly than the neighboring stroma and glands, and so they often protrude from the denuded surface of the menstruating endometrium. As the coiled portion is breaking up, contraction bands that occur beneath the coiled portion mark the extent of the arterial shedding. Small tufts of clotted blood fill the lumina at the tips of the coiled vessels. The straight arteries serving the stratum basalis do not become constricted during menstruation; hence, the stratum basalis remains well supplied with blood during the sloughing of the functionalis.

The functionalis is usually lost entirely, leaving only the basalis with the exposed blind ends of the glands. Elsewhere the mucosal surface is denuded and raw. With the cessation of hemorrhage and the concomitant initiation of the development of a new set of ovarian follicles, remnants of healthy uterine epithelium, particularly from the mouths of the glands, proliferate rapidly and provide the denuded areas with an epithelial covering.

The gravid cycle After ovulation, it takes about 3 days for the fertilized ovum to reach the uterus. The zygote undergoes rapid embryonic growth and by the fifth day develops into a *blastocyst*. By the early part of the second week of the luteal phase, it becomes embedded in the uterine mucosa (*implantation, nidation*). At this time, the peripheral cellular elements of the blastocyst (the *chorion*) begin secreting a hormone known as *human chorionic gonadotrophin* (HCG) which helps sustain the life and function of the corpus luteum beyond the usual limits of a menstrual cycle. The growth of the endometrium is not interrupted; there is no menstrual flow, and this circumstance is commonly denoted as the *first missed period*. A secretory or progestational endometrium becomes a *gestational endometrium* (Fig. 23-26C) simply by the fact of pregnancy. It undergoes further progestational development during the early weeks of pregnancy.

The cervix The mucosa lining of the cervix, the *endocervix*, is continuous with that of the body of the uterus (Fig. 23-1) but differs sharply in both its epithelium and underlying stroma. The cervix uteri (Fig. 23-31) encloses the cervical canal which is approximately 3 cm long and slightly distended in the middle portion. The mucous membrane, 3 to 5 mm thick, forms very complex, deep furrows or compound clefts called the *plicae palmatae* (Fig. 23-32). These folds run in longitudinal, transverse, and oblique directions and form a very irregular arrangement which may penetrate the entire thickness of the mucosa. This arrangement of folds is often misinterpreted as being a system of branching tubular glands of the compound racemose variety. The basic pattern, then, of the epithelium of the

cervical canal is a complex system of clefts with accessory folds and tunnel-like projections. The lining epithelium of the plicae palmatae consists of a single layer of tall, mucus-secreting cells. Some of the epithelial cells are ciliated, with the cilia beating toward the vagina. The height of the cells and the position of their nuclei vary with the time of the cycle and their secretory activity. During the proliferative and secretory phases, the epithelial cells synthesize mucus and other substances and package them in membrane-bounded vacuoles (Fig. 23-33). The cells laden with these materials stain poorly, and their nuclei are pushed to the base of the cells (Fig. 23-34). During active secretion, the nuclei rise to the center of the cells (Fig. 23-35) as the secreted mucus distends the lumina of the glands. Occasionally, some of the plicae become occluded and dilate with secretions. Such cysts are called *Nabothian follicles* (Fig. 23-31). The cervical canal is usually filled with mucus. The biochemical and biophysical characteristics of the mucus vary with the time in the cycle.

The mucosa of the cervix does not take part in the menstrual changes, and so it is not sloughed. After the menopause, the mucosa shrinks, the glandular epithelium becomes gradually flattened, and the secretory activity is arrested.

Myometrium The musculature of the uterus forms a thick tunic that is composed of three muscle layers somewhat blended because of complex interconnecting bundles and interspersed by considerable connective tissue. Well-defined muscle layers are not easily discernible over the body of the uterus. In general, the cells in the central portion of the muscularis are more circularly disposed, whereas those to either side tend to be directed obliquely or longitudinally. The middle region of the muscularis contains many large blood and lymphatic vessels (*stratum vasculare*). Over the cervix, the muscularis is layered in a relatively defined manner; there are an inner and outer longitudinal and a middle circular layer. Elastic fibers, though few and peripherally located in the uterus, are abundant in the outer wall of the cervix.

In the nonpregnant uterus the muscle cells are about 0.25 mm in length. During pregnancy, they increase in number and in size and may reach a length of 5 mm by the end of gestation, with a

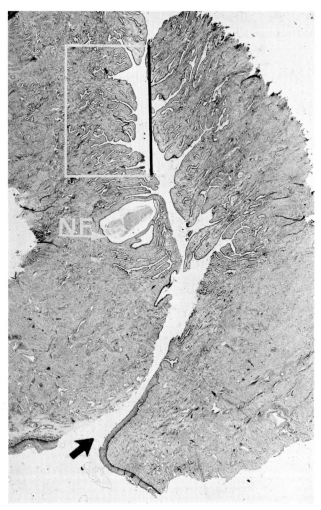

Figure 23-31   Longitudinal section of a human cervix uteri (proliferative phase of menstrual cycle).   Arrow indicates lumen; NF, Nabothian follicle.   Figure 23-32 is an enlargement of the rectangular box.   H&E stain.   ×9.   (Courtesy of E. R. Friedrich.)

commensurate increase in cell thickness. New smooth muscle cells are added by differentiation from embryonic connective tissue cells and probably by division of preexisting smooth muscle cells. Since many of these remain after childbirth, the uterus does not revert to its virginal size. Other changes accompanying the distension of the pregnant uterus are increase in elastic tissue peripheral to the myometrium, striking growth of the blood vessels, and a thinning out of the muscle layers.

Perimetrium   The pelvic peritoneum surrounding the uterine tubes and most of the uterus constitute

their serosa. It extends from the sides of the uterus, forming the broad ligaments through which blood and lymph vessels and nerves reach the uterus on each side. The larger vessels are exceptionally tortuous.

Embedded in the perimetrium are the sympathetic ganglia and plexuses. The sympathetic supply to the uterus is derived from the hypogastric plexus, and the parasympathetic supply is by the way of rami from the second, third, and often the fourth sacral nerves. Large nerve trunks enter the uterus at the cervix and extend to all parts of the body and fundus. The musculature and blood vessels are abundantly supplied, and some fibers ramify in the endometrium, forming a network around the glands. Nothing is known about the significance of these fibers or what happens to them during the cyclic sloughing and regeneration of the superficial layer of the endometrium. No ganglia cells have been found within the wall of the uterus.

VAGINA

The vagina is a thick-walled fibromuscular tube that forms the lowermost segment of the reproductive tract and connects the uterus with the outside of the body. The wall consists of a *mucosa,* a *muscularis,* and a heavy covering of connective tissue. The lumen of the vagina is flattened anteroposte-

Figure 23-32   Enlargement of marked area in Fig. 23-31. Notice the arrangement and complex pattern of the plicae palmatae. ×40. (Courtesy of E. R. Friedrich.)

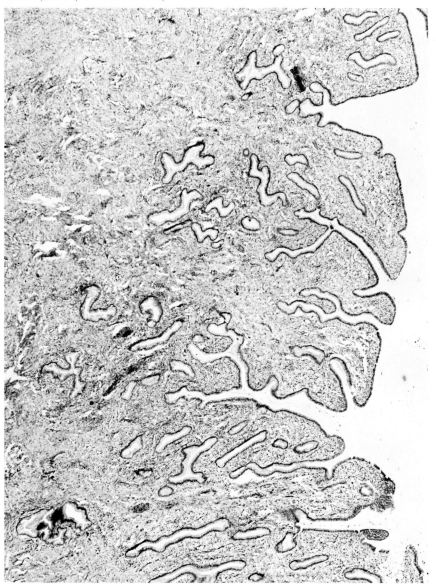

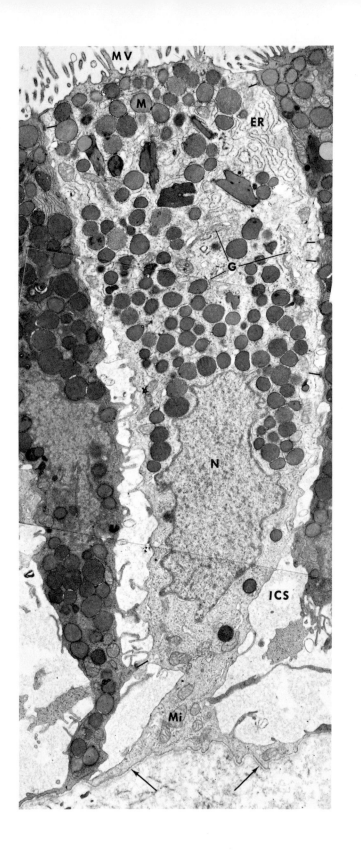

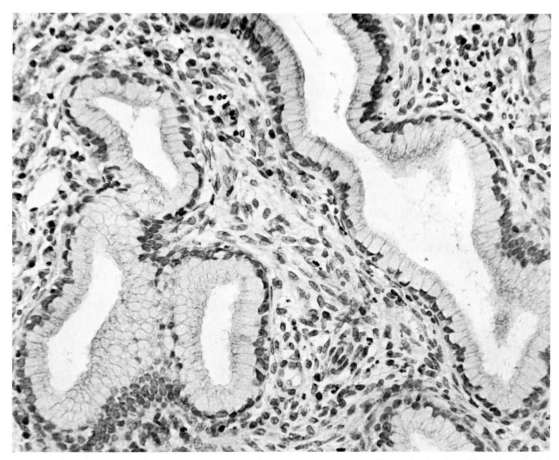

Figure 23-34 Epithelium of human cervical glands. Cells laden with mucus. Notice the basal position of the nuclei. H&E stain. ×350. (Courtesy of E. R. Friedrich.)

riorly. The mucosa is thrown into numerous transverse folds or *rugae* (Fig. 23-1).

The mucous membrane consists of a stratified squamous epithelium many cell layers thick, resting on a papillated lamina propria (Fig. 23-36). Cells in the outer layers are greatly flattened and may contain keratohyaline granules, but they are not strictly cornified. At midcycle they all contain an abundance of glycogen. Some of the superficial layer of the vaginal epithelium may be shed at or near the time of menstruation (Fig. 23-37) and is referred to, in parallel with the uterine mucosa, as the *functionalis*.

The vagina is lubricated by mucus which originates from the cervix. There are no glands in the mucosa of the human vagina.

In the lamina propria subjacent to the vaginal epithelium, there is a wide band of rather dense fibrous connective tissue that is succeeded peripherally by a layer of loose connective tissue in which are many blood vessels. Beyond this lies the muscle coat. Elastic fibers are plentiful beneath the

Figure 23-33 Electron micrograph of endocervical epithelial cells. ⟶, basement membrane; N, nucleus; G, Golgi complexes; ER, granular endoplasmic reticulum; M, mucous granules; MV, microvilli; ⎯, desmosomes; ICS, intercellular pores. ×9,400. (Courtesy of E. R. Friedrich.)

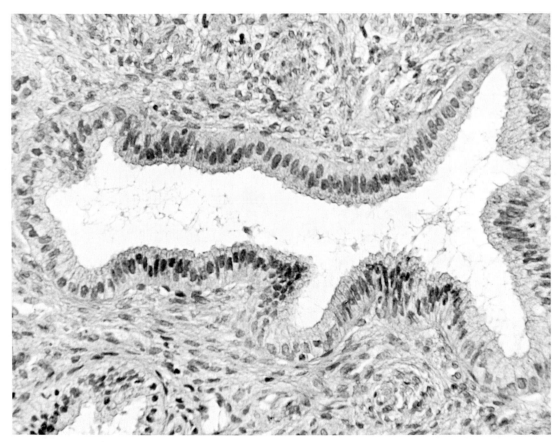

Figure 23-35 Epithelium of human cervical glands in active secretion. Notice the change in the position of the nuclei and the secretory materials within the lumen. H&E stain. ×350. (Courtesy of E. R. Friedrich.)

epithelium and present sparingly elsewhere in the fibromuscular wall. Diffuse lymphoid tissue and solitary nodules (Fig. 23-36) are present occasionally in the mucous membrane. From these arise the lymphocytes which, along with granulocytes, invade the epithelium in large numbers in each menstrual cycle. The great accentuation in numbers, particularly of granulocytes before, during, and after menstruation, is apparent also in the vaginal smears.

The muscularis of the vagina is composed of an inner and an outer layer. In the outer portion there are bundles of longitudinal smooth muscle cells that are continuous with corresponding cells in the myometrium. Where the two muscle layers meet, the inner circular cells are interwoven with the outer longitudinal ones. Striated muscle cells form a sphincter around the introitus of the vagina.

The vagina has an external coat composed of a firm inner layer well supplied with elastic fibers and an outer layer of loosely arranged connective tissue which blends with that of surrounding organs.

Blood and lymphatic vessels are abundant in the wall of the vagina. The veins in the rugae are particularly numerous and large, and during sexual excitement they stimulate erectile tissue. The vaginal wall receives myelinated and unmyelinated nerve fibers. The latter form a ganglionated plexus in the external fibrous coat and supply the muscularis and blood vessels. The myelinated fibers terminate in special sensory organs in the mucosa.

The surface cells of the vaginal epithelium undergo continuous desquamation and constitute the bulk of the cells seen in a vaginal smear. In sub-human primates and many lower forms, the free cells in the vagina vary in number, type, and form in a regular and predictable manner, correlating with events in the reproductive cycle. In women

Figure 23-36 Photomicrograph of an oblique section through the vaginal wall of a monkey recovered a few hours after ovulation. Notice the lymph nodule (LN) in the submucosa. C is a cross section of a connective tissue core. Imagine the deep papilla at X cut in cross section.

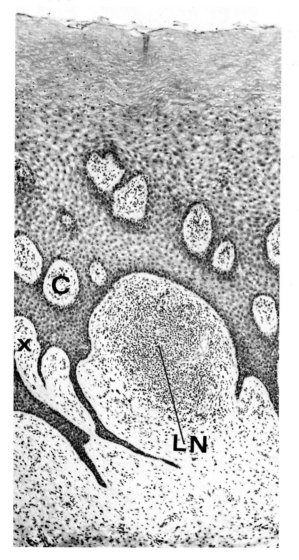

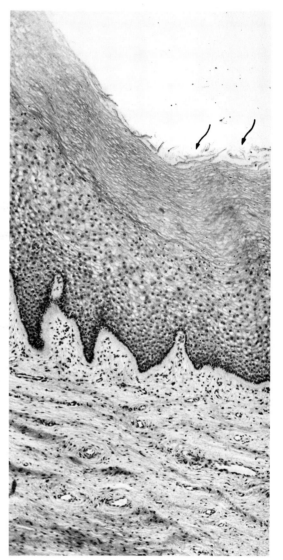

Figure 23-37 Photomicrograph of the vaginal mucosa in the fornix near the cervix in a monkey. Notice that the papillae are not as extensive. There is some peeling of the superficial layers (arrows) of stratified squamous epithelium. H&E stain. ×300.

the vaginal epithelium varies little with the cycle, and smears are mainly useful in determining whether the vaginal mucosa is atrophic or under effective estrogen stimulation.

The glycogen stores in the superficial cells of the vaginal epithelium are fermented to lactic acid by certain acid-forming bacteria which thus influence the pH of the vaginal fluid. The glycogen accumulation correlates with the amount of estrogen stimulation, being greatest at the time of ovulation. With diminished estrogen titer, as after ovulation, there is less glycogen formed and less broken down and so the pH of the vaginal fluid shifts toward alkalinity; this favors the development of infectious organisms such as staphylococci, *Escherichia coli*, trichomonas, and *Monilia albicans*. The ability of estrogen to reduce the vaginal pH and increase the thickness of the epithelial wall accounts for its effectiveness in the treatment of various vaginal infections that are especially common in children and postmenopausal women.

External sex organs (external genitalia)

These comprise the *labia majora* and *minora, clitoris,* and *vestibular glands*. The labia majora are homologous with the scrotum of the male. They are composed of skin and a thin layer of smooth muscle. In adulthood, the outer surface is covered with coarse pubic (genital) hair, with numerous sebaceous and sweat glands. The labia minora are devoid of hair, are covered by a stratified squamous epithelium, and enclose a highly papillated vascular core of loose connective tissue. Sebaceous glands, not connected with hair follicles, occur on both sides. Enhanced pigmentation is due to melanin granules in the deep strata of the epithelium.

The *clitoris* is an erectile body and is the homologue of the corpora cavernosa of the penis. It is mainly composed of two small cavernous bodies and a poorly developed *glans clitoridis*. The clitoris is covered with a thin layer of stratified squamous epithelium overlying a vascular stroma with high papillae and containing many such specialized sensory nerve terminations as Meissner's corpuscles, Pacinian corpuscles, and Krause's end bulbs.

The *vestibule* is the space at the vaginal portal flanked by the labia. The epithelium differs from that of the vagina in possessing glands. The *lesser vestibular glands* secrete mucus and are situated mainly about the clitoris and urethral outlet. There is in addition a pair of *large vestibular glands* (*glands of Bartholin*), which are located in the lateral walls of the vestibule. They correspond to the bulbourethral glands of men and are similar in structure; they are the tubuloacinar type and are lined with columnar cells that produce a whitish, mucoid, lubricating fluid.

The *hymen* consists of fine-fibered vascular connective tissue covered on both sides with a mucous membrane similar to that of the vagina.

References

BAKER, T. G., and L. L. FRANCHI: The Fine Structure of Oogonia and Oocytes in Human Ovaries, *J. Cell Sci.*, **2**:213 (1967).

BARTELMEZ, G. W.: Histological Studies on the Menstruating Mucous Membrane of the Human Uterus, *Carnegie Inst. Contrib. Embryol.*, **24**:141 (1933).

BASSETT, D. L.: The Changes in the Vascular Pattern of the Ovary of the Albino Rat during the Estrous Cycle, *Amer. J. Anat.*, **73**:251 (1943).

BLACK, E.: Quantitative Morphological Investigations of Follicular System in Women, *Acta Endocr.*, **8**:33 (1951).

BLANDAU, R. J.: Biology of Eggs and Implantation, in W. C. Young (ed.), "Sex and Internal Secretions," 3d ed., vol. 2, chap. 14, p. 797, The Williams & Wilkins Company, Baltimore, 1961.

BLANDAU, R. J.: Ovulation in the Living Albino Rat, *Fertil. Steril.*, **6**:391 (1955).

BRENNER, R. M.: Renewal of Oviduct Cilia during the Menstrual Cycle of the Rhesus Monkey, *Fertil. Steril.,* **20:**599 (1969).

CORNER, G. W.: The Histological Dating of the Corpus Luteum of Menstruation, *Amer. J. Anat.,* **98:**377 (1956).

CRISP, T. M., D. A. DESSOUKY, and F. R. DENYS: The Fine Structure of the Human Corpus Luteum of Early Pregnancy and during the Progestational Phase of the Menstrual Cycle, *Amer. J. Anat.,* **127:**37 (1970).

DANFORTH, D. N.: The Fibrous Nature of the Human Cervix and Its Relation to the Isthmic Segment in Gravid and Nongravid Uteri, *Amer. J. Obstet. Gynec.,* **53:**541 (1947).

FLUHMANN, C. F.: The Glandular Structure of the Cervix Uteri, *Surg. Gynec. Obstet.* **106:**715 (1958).

HAFEZ, E. S. E., and R. J. BLANDAU: The Mammalian Oviduct, "Comparative Biology and Methodology," The University of Chicago Press, Chicago, 1969.

HERTIG, A. T.: The Primary Human Oocyte: Some Observations on the Fine Structure of Balbiani's Vitelline Body and the Origin of the Annulate Lamellae, *Amer. J. Anat.,* **122:**107 (1968).

HERTIG, A. T., and E. C. ADAMS: Studies on the Human Oocyte and Its Follicle. I. Ultrastructural and Histochemical Observations on the Primordial Follicle Stage, *J. Cell Biol.,* **34:**647 (1967).

JACOBSON, H. N., and O. NIEVES: Intrinsic Nerve Fibers of the Primate Endometrium, *Exp. Neurol.,* **4:**180 (1961).

MARKEE, J. E.: The Morphological and Endocrine Basis for Menstrual Bleeding, *Progr. Gynec.,* **2:**63 (1950).

MARKEE, J. E.: Menstruation in Intraocular Endometrial Transplants in the Rhesus Monkey, *Carnegie Inst. Contrib. Embryol.,* **28:**220 (1940).

MORRIS, B., and M. B. SASS: The Formation of Lymph in the Ovary, *Proc. Roy. Soc. (London), Ser. B,* **164:**577 (1966).

MOSSMAN, H. W., M. J. KOERING, and D. FERRY, JR.: Cyclic Changes of Interstitial Gland Tissue of the Human Ovary, *Amer. J. Anat.,* **115:**235 (1964).

ODOR, D. L.: The Temporal Relationship of the First Maturation Division of Rat Ova to the Onset of Heat, *Amer. J. Anat.,* **97:**461 (1955).

PAPANICOLAOU, G. N.: The Sexual Cycle in the Human Female as Revealed by Vaginal Smears, *Amer. J. Anat.,* **52:**519 (1933).

PRIBOR, H. C.: Innervation of the Uterus, *Anat. Rec.,* **109:**339 (1951).

RYAN, K. J., Z. PETERS, and J. KAISER: Steroid Formation by Isolated and Recombined Ovarian Granulosa and Thecal Cells, *J. Clin. Endocr. Metab.,* **28:**355 (1968).

RYAN, K. J., and R. V. SHORT: Formation of Estradiol by Granulosa and Theca Cells of the Equine Ovarian Follicle, *Endocrinology,* **76:**108 (1965).

SCHMIDT-MATTHIESEN, H.: "The Normal Human Endometrium," McGraw-Hill Book Company, New York, 1963.

STRASSMAN, E. O.: The Theca Cone and Its Tropism toward the Ovarian Surface, a Typical Feature of Growing Human and Mammalian Follicles, *Amer. J. Obstet. Gynec.,* **41:**363 (1941).

VICKERY, B. H., and J. P. BENNETT: The Cervix and Its Secretions in Mammals, *Physiol. Rev.,* **48:**135 (1968).

WITSCHI. E.: Migration of the Germ Cells of Human Embryos from the Yolk Sac to the Primitive Gonadal Folds, *Carnegie Inst. Contrib. Embryol.,* **32:**67 (1948).

chapter 24   The mammary gland

WILLIAM U. GARDNER

Man normally has two mammary glands, one over each pectoral region. There may also be accessory *nipples* (a condition called *hyperthelia*), accessory *areolae* (pigmented areas around nipples), and accessory mammary glands (a condition called *hypermastia*), the supernumerary structures being located most frequently along the embryonic *mammary* (*milk*) *line* that extends from the medial-axillary area to the groin.

Localized ectodermal thickenings at one or more intervals on each embryonic mammary line mark the location of future mammary glands and nipples. The number and location of the thickenings and hence of the future mammary glands are characteristic of the species and, within the species, of the sex and genotype. Breasts and nipples at sites remote from the usual mammary line have been described.

The localized thickenings of the embryonic ectoderm appear first in 8-mm human embryos (approximately 30 days). About 12 days later (25-mm embryo), epithelial cords extend from the localized thickenings into the underlying mesenchyma. From 15 to 25 cords ultimately develop in the human female. Eventually the cords acquire lumina and become the primary ducts of the several future lobes of the mammary gland. Only primary and secondary ducts develop during embryonic and fetal stages (Fig. 24-1). The breast at birth is a rudimentary, multiple, branched tubular gland. Only during the onset of sexual maturity in the female does the complexity of the branched tubular gland increase with the appearance of tertiary, quaternary, and more minute branching (Fig. 24-2). During recurring menstrual cycles and especially during pregnancy, the breast becomes a multiple, compound tubuloalveolar structure as the terminal alveoli form. After lactation ceases, the glands regress, the small terminal alveoli are resorbed, and the gland reverts essentially to a compound tubular structure.

The breast undergoes changes during the life

cycle of the individual; it also undergoes striking changes during the reproductive cycle—pregnancy and lactation—and less extensive changes during the menstrual cycles. The mammary glands of the human male usually remain rudimentary although sometimes, especially at puberty, some transient proliferation may occur (*gynecomastia*).

Nipple

The nipples develop by different fundamental processes in different animals. In the mouse a circular epithelial cleft, which later canalizes, separates the nipple from the adjacent skin. In some species, especially animals such as the cow and sheep, the mesenchyma proliferates to form the teat. In man, a special stroma containing numerous bundles of smooth muscle develops which, with a minimum of connective tissue proliferation, forms a nipple with erectile capacity. In man nipples are not evident at birth as elevated structures and usually only become evident with the approach of sexual maturity. Nipples do not form in males of some species, such as the rat and mouse, although rudimentary mammary ducts may persist. The formation of nipples in female embryos of some species can be prevented by injection of male hormone (testosterone) into the pregnant mother at critical stages of embryonic mammary development. The nipple and the glandular mammary tissues are separate entities developmentally and functionally.

Nipples grow when estrogenic hormones are injected or are present in the female. The direct application of small amounts of estrogenic hormone to one nipple stimulates its growth without influencing the other. Unlike the mammary secretory epithelium, the nipple is directly responsive to estrogens.

The nipple is covered by a stratified squamous epithelium that is continuous with the openings of the major excretory ducts of the gland and peripherally with the relatively hairless and pigmented areola. In pigmented individuals, the nipple and areola are more heavily pigmented than the adjacent skin after sexual maturity is attained. The accumulation of melanin in the deeper layers of the epidermis increases, particularly during pregnancy and when estrogenic hormones are given. The pinkish color of the nipple of immature or blond individuals is due to the long dermal papillae and proximity of blood vessels to the surface.

The dermis of the nipple and areola has relatively long papillae and contains little or no adipose tissue. An interlacing network of somewhat circularly arranged smooth muscle fibers is located in the dermis (Fig. 24-3). In the nipple area muscle fibers from the circular network project radially and are continuous with elastic fibers that terminate in the dermal papillae, hence the wrinkled and pitted appearance of the skin. Three types of glands occur in the dermis of the nipple and areolar sebaceous glands, some of which open into the mammary ducts; apocrine glands in the more distal areola; and accessory mammary glands in the tubercules of Montgomery at the periphery of the areola.

Figure 24-1 A. Drawing of a section through a rudimentary mammary gland of a 200-mm fetus, showing portions of five different epithelial cords extending from the central bud into the adjacent connective tissues. ×50. B. Reconstruction of the breast of a 6-month-old fetus, showing approximately 15 epithelial cores extending from the primitive nipple. Some cords show small branches. ×6.5. (From B. M. Patten, "Human Embryology," 2d ed., McGraw-Hill Book Company, New York, 1952.)

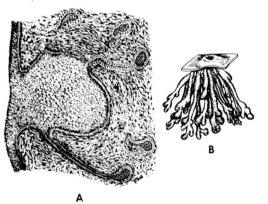

A   B

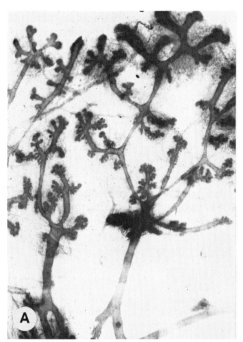

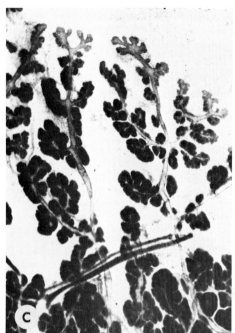

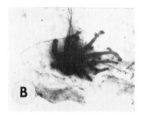

Figure 24-2   A. Photograph of an area of the mammary gland of a 2-year-old male macaque monkey that had several injections of estrogen during 9 weeks.   The terminal ducts (upper part) are large, intensely stained, with numerous mitotic figures.   The ducts nearer the nipple terminate in numerous small branches that will form intralobular ducts.   B. Photograph of the mammary gland of a 2-year-old male monkey, showing primary ducts.   ×2.   C. Area of the mammary gland of a male macaque monkey, showing a development of smaller ducts peripherally and of lobules of alveoli centrally (lower part of photograph).   This monkey had received estrogen for 22 weeks.   All preparations were stained with Mayer's hemalum and dissected to remove overlying stroma.

Innervation of nipple and mammary gland

In general, the dermal innervation of the breast resembles that of other skin areas.   The dermal papillae of the nipple and areola contain a number of free-fiber nerve endings (Fig. 24-4).   Meissner-like nerve endings are also found in the dermal papillae of the areola.   In the underlying dermis are multibranched free-fiber nerve endings and looped endings.   The skin around the areola contains neural plexuses around hair follicles and, in the superficial area, expanded nerve endings (Merkel's disks).   Krause-like end bulbs and Ruffini-like nerve endings are found in the deeper layers of the der-

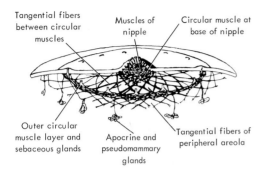

Figure 24-3   Schema of the arrangement of smooth muscles in the areola and nipple in the nonerected condition. The position of the more superficial sweat glands, deeper apocrine glands, and pseudomammary glands (glands of Montgomery) are shown in relation to the muscles. (From A. Dabelow, "Handbüch mikroskopischen. Anatomic des. Menschen," vol. 3, pt. 3, Springer-Verlag OHG, Berlin, 1957.)

mis. Pacinian corpuscles have been found in the deeper layers of the dermis and in deeper parts of the gland.

The larger sphincteric ducts of the nipple are surrounded by unmyelinated nerve fibers that supply the muscle fibers. Unmyelinated nerve fibers follow the blood vessels in the interlobular stroma of the breast. They supply the smooth muscles of the larger ducts and the blood vessels. Tactile acuity of the breast area is slight; few nerves arise in the superficial dermis but afferents arising in the deeper dermis provoke, through reflex connections, a contraction of the areolar and nipple musculature and a release of a galactagogue, presumably oxytocin, from the posterior lobe of the pituitary. The motor innervation of the vascular, muscular, and accessory glandular tissue of the breast is largely, if not

Figure 24-4   Diagrammatic presentation of the different types and distribution of nerve endings in the dermis of the nipple, areola, adjacent skin, and mammary parenchyma as revealed by staining with methylene blue. Branched free-fiber endings are most numerous in the nipple (1). Small free fibers also end in the dermal papillae of the nipple and areola (1'). The ducts are supplied by nonmyelinated fibers (2). Meissner-like endings are found in the dermal papillae of the areola (3), and small looped-fiber endings (4) are located throughout the dermis. Krause-like (7) and Ruffini-like bulbs are found in the deeper layers of the dermis. Hair follicles (5) have the usual distribution of nerves. Merkel's discs (8) were only in the hairy areas. Some investigators have observed Pacinian bodies in the deeper stroma of the breast. (From M. R. Miller and M. Kasahara, Anat. Rec., **135**:155, 1959.)

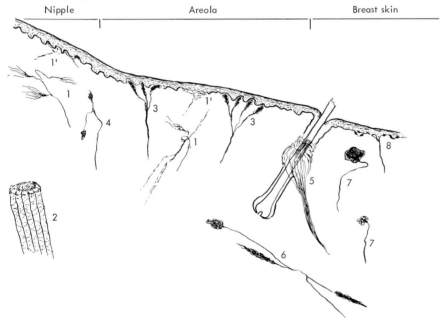

entirely, through sympathetic postganglionic fibers. Acetylcholinesterase-containing fibers supply the muscles of the sphincters of the primary ducts in the nipple. Adrenergic agents cause vascular constriction and some dilatation of the larger mammary ducts. The myoepithelial cells of the alveoli and smaller ducts are not innervated but contract upon exposure to oxytocin, which is released by the posterior pituitary gland.

Mammary parenchyma

The mammary gland in its functional state is a compound tubuloalveolar gland. The larger ducts open at the nipple where a stratified squamous epithelium is continuous with the two-layered columnar epithelium of the primary duct. The larger ducts are lined by an inner tall columnar layer and an outer cuboidal layer of epithelial cells. The smaller ducts have a single layer of columnar epithelial cells and the smallest ducts as well as the alveoli have irregularly dispersed deep *myoepithelial cells* (*basket cells*) near the basement membrane. The height of the cells of the ducts and alveoli depends upon the functional state of the gland and their relative distension (Fig. 24-5, see color insert). A distinct basement membrane surrounds all the epithelial components. The basement membrane in turn is surrounded by a loose stroma, especially about the smallest intralobular ducts and alveoli. The intralobular stroma contrasts sharply with the interlobular stroma; it contains larger and more compactly arranged collagenous fibers and relatively fewer elastic fibers. The stroma of the breast develops at the same time as the parenchyma of the gland. The initial growth about the ducts is made into a loose vascular-fatty subcutaneous tela. The "fatty lobules" or "fat organ" into which the ducts project, and in which the lobules develop, contribute both the looser intralobular stroma and the more compact interlobular stroma. In some species the mammary epithelium will grow only in a fatty stroma.

The lactating mammary gland produces milk which contains unique proteins, casein, lactoglobulin, and lactalbumin; a unique sugar, lactose; and a high concentration of fat. The fats, sugars, and proteins are all produced by the same cells. The fats first appear in the secretory cells as small droplets at about the level of the nucleus; these droplets enlarge as they become more apically located (Fig. 24-6). The fat droplets are always surrounded by smooth membranes and even retain the membrane as they are pinched off from the apex of the cell. Incidentally, fat is found in the epithelial cells of the smaller ducts and alveoli of nonlactating breasts. The proteins first appear in the Golgi area, and are located in smooth membrane vacuoles that may be derived from the Golgi membranes. Aggregates of electron-dense materials accumulate in these vacuoles. The vacuoles move to the free surface of the cell; their membranes become continuous with the surface membrane and thus extrude their contents (reversed pinocytosis). Where lactose and milk salts are elaborated and how they are extruded are unknown. Milk secretion is not an apocrine type of secretion, as was once thought.

Studies of fine structure (Fig. 24-5) have also revealed microvilli on the luminal surface of the secretory cells and terminal bars or desmosomes. The cellular membranes are only slightly interdigitated and in close approximation with the basement membrane except where myoepithelial cells intervene. The cytoplasm contains rather large mitochondria (five or more for each central section) that differ slightly in size with changes of secretory activity, endoplasmic reticulum less compactly arranged than in hepatic cells and much increased during lactation, an apical Golgi body that is more conspicuous during lactation, and lysosomes (dense bodies). The latter may contain a cathepsin, an acid phosphatase, and, in some species, ferritin as well. Mitochondrial fractions of breast tissue show seven- to nine-fold increases in some enzymes, such as succinic dehydrogenase and cytochromic oxidase, when the gland is secreting.

The myoepithelial cells of the lactating breast show an affinity for silver stains and contain enough

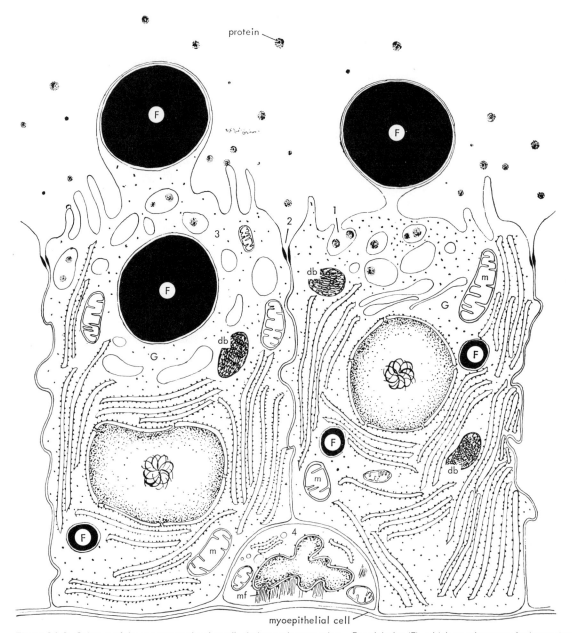

Figure 24-6 Schema of the mammary alveolar cells during active secretion. Fat globules (F), which may be several micrometers in diameter, first appear as small, membrane-surrounded structures in the cytoplasm at about the level of the nucleus. Details of their origin are unknown. They are pinched off the apical surface, carrying investing membranes with them. Electron-dense protein aggregates first appear in smooth-membrane vesicles in the Golgi region (G) and move in their vacuoles to the apical surface, where they are extruded (1). Some smooth-membrane vacuoles contain no granules (3), and some contain several aggregates. The myoepithelial cells with irregular nuclei (4) are located on the basement membrane and contain myofibrils (mf). Dense bodies or lysosomes (db) occur frequently in all cells and contain acid phosphatase and possibly a cathepsin. Desmosomes (2) are present. Mitochondria (m) are present at random. (Adapted from W. Bargmann and A. Knoop, Z. Zellforsch., 49:344, 1959; K.-H. Hollmann, J. Ultrastruct. Res., 2:423, 1959; and H. Miyawaki and Y. Nishizuka, Gann, 53:107, 1962.)

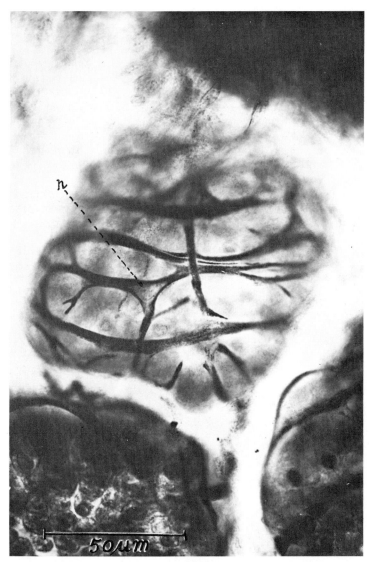

Figure 24-7 Branching myoepithelial cell of a small contracted alveolus of a lactating goat, stained by silver impregnation. The nucleus of one myoepithelial cell is shown by n. (From K. C. Richardson, Proc. Roy. Soc. (London), Ser. B, **136**:30, 1949.)

alkaline phosphatase to outline their structures when the tissues are exposed to suitable procedures (Fig. 24-7). Each cell has an irregular nucleus, a branching or stellate shape, and always is located adjacent to the basement membrane. Myofibrils have been observed, and actual contraction has been seen when the cells have been exposed to oxytocin.

Breast during the menstrual cycles

The areola begins to enlarge with the approach of sexual maturity and thereafter a sex difference in size exists. Variations in size and pigmentation of the areola are genetically determined and independent of body size.

During and after puberty, the extent of the branching mammary ducts increases by terminal growth, and probably cyclically during the menstrual cycles; at least, cyclic changes occur in the breasts of adult women. The amount of fat in adjacent stroma begins to increase cyclically at puberty. It is not related to the extent of epithelial growth or body size. Some lobules of alveolar tissue probably form in the breasts of older nulliparous women. The growth is centrifugal: lobules composed of alveoli first appear near the nipple and later develop peripherally (Fig. 24-2). During the recurring menstrual cycles, the ducts grow to the extent determined by inherent factors that limit the extent of breast parenchyma. The amount of lobular growth may vary from individual to individual, but very few alveoli are present in comparison with the gland during late pregnancy.

During the latter part of the menstrual cycles of adult women, the alveoli and smaller ducts increase in size (Fig. 24-8). They regress during the men-

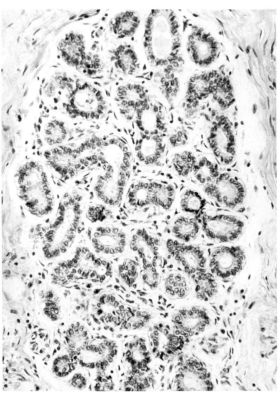

Figure 24-8 Part of a mammary lobule at the beginning of the menstrual period. The alveoli are slightly distended, contain secretion, and are lined by cuboidal or columnar cells. The stroma is vascular, and the small bundles of collagenous fibers are separated by matrix. (From F. W. Foote and F. W. Stewart, Ann. Surg., **121**:6, 1945.)

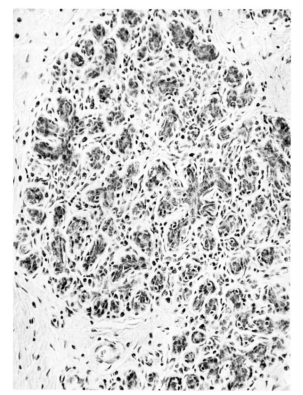

Figure 24-9 Part of a mammary lobule on the eighth day after the onset of menstruation. The epithelial cells are now arranged in strands or groups without lumina, and their cytoplasmic mass has been greatly reduced. The stroma is less vascular; it contains relatively more collagen and less nonfibrous matrix. (From F. W. Foote and F. W. Stewart, Ann. Surg., **121**:6, 1945.)

strual and early postmenstrual period (Fig. 24-9). The changes in the breast during the menstrual cycle may be only a general trend, as inconstancies exist from one individual to another; repeated samples from the same individual have not been studied.

Cyclic changes in volume of the breasts also are associated with edema and hyperemia of the mammary glands. When cyclic swelling of the breast occurs, it is usually greatest during the premenstrual period.

Regression and involution of the mammary gland

Lactation can continue for long periods if milk is removed regularly; women may nurse their offspring for several years. Milk production usually declines or stops during late pregnancy; it also stops if the milk is not removed. When milk removal stops, the glands become distended and the epithelial lining of the alveoli and ducts assumes a columnar or even a squamous state. The capillaries are compressed. After a few days the amount of intraductal secretion decreases and the distended alveoli and ducts become smaller. The secretion is withdrawn without significant assistance from macrophages. The secretions are apparently changed to soluble substances and carried away in tissue fluid and blood with very little foreign-body reaction. The epithelial cells themselves acquire pycnotic nuclei, lose their intracellular and finally their cellular membranes, and seem to autolyze in the alveolar space. Whole alveoli—in some animals almost all the alveoli—are resorbed. It seems that those processes leading to the growth of the parenchyma and stroma are reversed during involution. During sexually active life, the amount of postparturitional or postlactational involution is not so extensive as after the menopause or after ovariectomy. The regressed glands have the capacity to become functional mammary glands upon proper stimulation. A low level of function can be retained for a long period.

The life cycle of the mammary epithelial cell is not known but the incidence of mitosis is low and hence replacement is slow. The progressive decrease in milk production after the peak of lactation is probably due to cell loss through involution without subsequent replacement.

Endocrine control of mammary growth and function

The mammary glands are recent phylogenetic adaptations for the nourishment of postnatal young. The endocrine environment necessary for their growth is particularly complicated. Although mammary growth can be induced in some gonadectomized animals by injection of estrogens such as estradiol, this is not true for all species. Complete mammary glands will develop in estrogen-treated monkeys, only mammary ducts in most rodents, and no mammary growth at all in dogs given estrogens. In some species the injection of progesterone with estrogen provokes additional or complete mammary growth. Hypophysectomized animals, unless pregnant, will show little mammary response when estrogens are given, or even estrogens and progesterone. Some hormone from the pituitary gland, probably either prolactin or the growth hormone (somatotropin), is necessary for complete mammary glands in rodents given estradiol and progesterone. Optimal mammary growth in vitro requires, in addition, adrenal cortical hormones and especially insulin, and these hormones abet mammary growth in vivo. The possibility exists that both mammary parenchymal and stromal components must be properly influenced by hormones for mammary growth. Because lactation involves the conversion of relatively large amounts of food energy into milk, milk production can be influenced indirectly by modifications of digestion and assimilation at other than mammary levels.

Reference has already been made to the reflex stimulation of the release of oxytocin and its effect upon the myoepithelial cells. The posterior lobe of the pituitary and the anterior pituitary are thus involved in the secretion of milk. As noted elsewhere

(Chap. 27), the production or release of hormones from the pituitary gland is probably under hypothalamic control.

Species differences exist in mammary responses to hormones. Few critical studies have been done upon mammary growth in man. The pituitary gland is certainly essential for lactation, however, and indirect evidence indicates that it may be essential for mammary growth.

References

AGATE, F. J.: The Growth and Secretory Activity of the Mammary Glands of the Pregnant Rhesus Monkey (*Macaca mulatta*) Following Hypophysectomy, *Amer. J. Anat.*, **90**:257 (1952).

BARGMANN, W., and A. KNOOP: Über Die Morphologie der Milchsekretion: Licht- und Elekromen-mikroskopische Studien an der Milchdrüse der Ratte, *Z. Zellforsch., skop. Anat.*, **49**:344 (1959).

BÄSSLER, R.: Beiträge zur Morphologie der Kindlichen Brustdrüse, *Frankfurt. Z. Path.*, **69**:37 (1958).

COWIE, A. T., and S. J. FOLLEY: The Mammary Gland and Lactation, in W. C. Young (ed.), "Sex and Internal Secretions," 3d ed., chap. 10, The Williams & Wilkins Company, Baltimore, 1961.

DABELOW, A.: Die Milchdrüse, in W. von Möllendorff (ed.), "Handbuch mikroskopischen Anatomie des Menschen," vol. 3, pt. 3, Springer-Verlag OHG, Berlin, 1957.

DAWSON, E. K.: A Histological Study of the Normal Mamma in Relation to Tumor Growth. I. Early Development to Maturity, *Edinburgh Med. J.*, **41**:653 (1934).

DEMPSEY, E. W., H. BUNTING, and G. B. WISLOCKI: Observations on the Chemical Cytology of the Mammary Gland, *Amer. J. Anat.*, **81**:309 (1947).

FAULKIN, L. J., and K. B. DE OME: Regulation of Growth and Spacing of Gland Elements in the Mammary Pad of the C$_3$H Mouse, *J. Nat. Cancer Inst.*, **24**:953 (1960).

FOOTE, F. W., and F. W. STEWART: Comparative Studies of Cancerous versus Non-cancerous Breasts. I. Basic Morphologic Characteristics, *Ann. Surg.*, **121**:6 (1945).

GARDNER, W. U., and G. VAN WAGENEN: Experimental Development of the Mammary Gland in the Monkey, *Endocrinology*, **22**:164 (1938).

GIACOMETTI, L., and W. MONTAGNA: The Nipple and Areola of the Human Female Breast, *Anat. Rec.*, **144**:191 (1962).

HOLLMANN, K.-H.: L'ultrastructure de la glande mammaire normale de la souris en lactation, *J. Ultrastruct. Res.*, **2**:423 (1959).

HOLMES, R. L.: Alkaline Phosphatase in the Rabbit Mammary Gland, *Nature (London)*, **178**:311 (1956).

HOWE, A., K. C. RICHARDSON, and M. S. C. BIRBECH: Quantitative Observations on Mitochondria from Sections of Guinea Pig Mammary Gland, *Exp. Cell Res.*, **10**:194 (1956).

INGLEBY, H.: Normal and Pathological Proliferation of the Breast with Special Reference to Cystic Disease, *Arch. Path.*, **33**:573 (1942).

LASFARGUES, E. Y.: Cultivation and Behavior *in vito* of the Normal Mammary Epithelium of the Adult Mouse. II. Observations on the Secretory Activity, *Exp. Cell Res.,* **13:**553 (1957).

LINZELL, J. L.: The Silver Staining of Myoepithelial Cells, Particularly in the Mammary Gland, and Their Relation to the Ejection of Milk, *J. Anat.,* **86:**49 (1952).

LYONS, W. R.: The Direct Mammotropic Action of Lactogenic Hormones, *Proc. Soc. Exp. Biol. Med.,* **51:**308 (1942).

MC CANN, S. M., R. MACK, and C. GALE: Possible Role of Oxytocin in Stimulating the Release of Prolactin, *Endocrinology,* **64:**870 (1959).

MILLER, M. R., and M. KASAHARA: The Cutaneous Innervation of the Human Female Breast, *Anat. Rec.,* **135:**153 (1959).

MIYAWAKI, H., and Y. NISHIZUKA: Electron Microscopic Study of Precancerous Lesions in the Mammary Glands of Mice: Constant Association of Virus-like Particles with Hyperplastic Nodules, *Gann,* **53:**107 (1962).

MONTAGNA, W., and G. H. BOURNE: Some Histochemical Observations on the Resting Human Mammary Glands, *Acta Anat.,* **31:**231 (1957).

OZZELLO, L., and F. D. SPEER: The Mucopolysaccharides in the Normal and Diseased Breast, Their Distribution and Significance, *Amer. J. Path.,* **34:**993 (1958).

RAWLINSON, H. E.: The Iron Content of the Resting Mammary Glands of Normal and Tumor-bearing C_3H Mice, *Acta Un. Int. Cancr.* **12:**711 (1956).

RAWLINSON, H. E., and G. B. PIERCE: Visible Intraepithelial Iron in the Mammary Glands of Various Species, *Science,* **117:**33 (1953).

RAYNAUD, A., and J. RAYNAUD: Fréquence des malformations mammaires chez le foetus femelles de souris provenant de mères ayant recu une injection de dipropionate d'estradiol, au cours de le gestation, *C. R. Soc. Biol.,* **149:**1233 (1955).

RICHARDSON, K. C.: Contractile Tissue in the Mammary Gland, with Special Reference to Myoepithelium in the Goat, *Proc. Roy. Soc. (London), Ser. B,* **136:**30 (1949).

SOEMARWOTO, I. N., and H. A. BERN: The Effect of Hormones on the Vascular Pattern of the Mouse Mammary Gland, *Amer. J. Anat.,* **103:**403 (1958).

SPEERT, H.: The Normal and Experimental Development of the Mammary Gland of the Rhesus Monkey, with Some Pathological Correlations, *Carnegie Inst. Contrib. Embryol.,* **32:**9 (1948).

WAUGH, D., and E. VAN DER HOEVEN: Fine Structure of the Human Adult Female Breast, *Lab. Invest.,* **11:**220 (1962).

WELLINGS, S. R., and K. B. DE OME: Milk Protein Droplet Formation in the Golgi Apparatus of the C_3H/Crgl Mouse Mammary Epithelial Cells, *J. Biophys. Biochem. Cytol.,* **9:**479 (1961).

chapter 25 The human placenta

HELEN A. PADYKULA

The placenta is a transient organ characteristic of mammals that mediates physiologic exchange between the mother and the developing embryo-fetus. It is important at the outset to understand that the placenta has both fetal and maternal parts and is, therefore, composed of cells of two different genotypes. This is a biologic situation with important immunologic implications since the placental-fetal complex may be viewed as a homograft of foreign tissue. The following general definition, derived from Mossman's (1937) monograph, is a useful one to remember. The placenta consists of "an intimate apposition or fusion of the fetal membranes with the uterine mucosa for the purpose of carrying out physiological exchange." Thus, to understand what a placenta is in morphologic terms, it is essential to know the structure of the extraembryonic membranes and also of the progestational uterine endometrium.

The functions of this maternal-fetal complex are manifold. The placenta must serve temporarily as a fetal lung, kidney, intestine, and probably as a

fetal liver as well; furthermore, it is a complex endocrine organ. Oxygen and nutrients are transferred across the placenta from the maternal blood to the fetal blood; carbon dioxide and various metabolic waste products are transported in the reverse direction. The placental association places the fetal bloodstream in close proximity to the maternal bloodstream, but normally these two bloodstreams do not mix. They are separated by tissue layers called the *placental barrier*.

The placenta varies considerably in its morphology among the orders of mammals. This diversity makes it quite unique when compared with organs, such as the lung, kidney, or liver, which are relatively similar among different mammals. Placental diversity has phylogenetic significance which is most likely related to the evolutionary modifications that occurred in the vertebrate extraembryonic membranes as they were modified for intrauterine development. In this chapter the discussion is limited to the human placenta. However, it should be emphasized that thorough understanding of the placenta of primates is derived only through a knowledge of comparative placentation (Mossman, 1937; Amoroso, 1952) and, going even farther back phylogenetically, through a knowledge of the development of birds and reptiles. The reader is advised to review the structure and function of the extraembryonic membranes of the chick and pig as well as the histophysiology of the primate uterus (see standard texts of embryology and Chap. 23). The most complete collection of human placental specimens ever gathered together may be studied in a recent excellent monograph by Boyd and Hamilton (1970) which is a rich source of information on placental morphology.

Viviparous animals, when compared with ovipa-rous forms, have relatively small ova that contain little stored nutrient. The human ovum, as it is shed from the Graafian follicle, is 100 to 150 μm in diameter and is surrounded by a thick glyco-protein coat, the *zona pellucida* (Fig. 25-1) and a variable number of corona radiata cells. Fertiliza-tion occurs in the ampulla of the fallopian tube. As the newly formed zygote passes through the fallopian tube, it undergoes holoblastic cleavage (Fig. 25-2) and forms a solid mass of cells called the *morula*. Between 84 and 96 hr after ovulation the morula enters the uterus; fluid begins to accu-mulate among the cells, a central cavity appears, and the *free blastocyst* is formed (Fig. 25-3). The blastocyst exists free in the uterine secretions for

Figure 25-1   A living human secondary oocyte cultured in pyruvate Krebs-Ringer medium. Under in vitro conditions, human oocytes obtained from ovarian follicles proceed with meiosis, form the first polar body (PB), and mature to the metaphase II stage. The cumulus cells have been removed; the zona pellucida (ZP) is present. Scale marker, 20 μm. (From J. F. Kennedy and R. P. Donahue, Science, **164**:1292, 1969.)

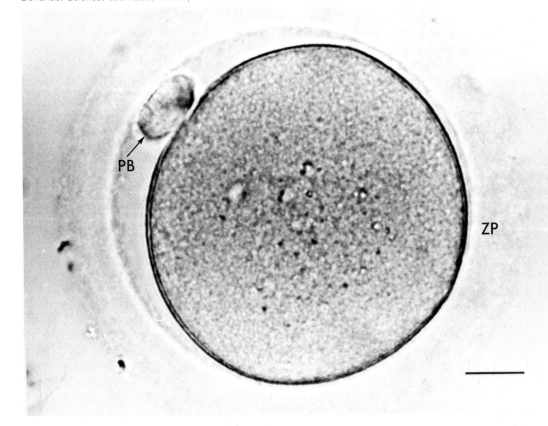

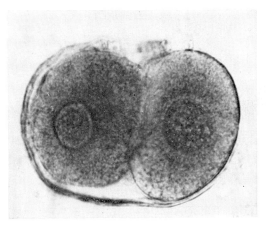

Figure 25-2 Two-cell stage of the human zygote, probably 1½ to 2½ days old, obtained from the fallopian tube. The zona pellucida still surrounds the blastomeres. ×400. (Courtesy of A. T. Hertig and J. Rock.)

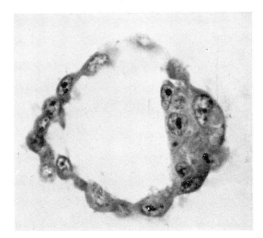

Figure 25-3 Normal human free blastocyst approximately 4½ days old obtained from the uterine cavity. Observe the layer of primitive trophoblastic cells surrounding the blastocyst cavity, and the inner cell mass located at one pole. The zona pellucida has almost completely disappeared. ×600. (Courtesy of A. T. Hertig and J. Rock.)

approximately 3 days, since the youngest attached human blastocyst is estimated to be 7½ days of age (Fig. 25-5).

The human blastocyst, like those of most mammals, is nearly spherical (Fig. 25-3). The precursor of the parenchyma of the placenta, the *trophoblast* ("nutritive layer"), makes a precocious appearance as a thin layer of extraembryonic cells that surround a fluid-filled cavity and a mass of embryo-forming cells (the inner cell mass) attached at one pole of the inner surface of the trophoblast. The trophoblast is the outer component of the *chorion,* the outermost extraembryonic membrane. Before implantation the zona pellucida is shed, and the blastocyst begins to implant in the highly glandular progestational uterus at approximately day 21–22 of the menstrual cycle. Currently the biology of the mammalian blastocyst is an area of intensive investigation which is considered to be related to the development of effective fertility control. For a compilation of recent studies the reader is referred to Blandau (1971).

Implantation

The human blastocyst usually implants on the upper posterior wall of the body of the uterus near the midsagittal plane. As the trophoblastic cells come into contact with the uterine epithelium, they begin to proliferate and soon form an attachment to the uterine wall (Fig. 25-4). As we trace placental differentiation, it will become evident that the trophoblast forms the parenchyma of the fetal placenta and that it constitutes the major element of the placental barrier.

The blastocyst of the rhesus monkey begins to implant on the ninth day after fertilization (Fig. 25-4). The trophoblastic cells proliferate rapidly in a coronal area at the embryonic pole of the blastocyst, and several points of attachment to the uterine epithelium are established. In the few subprimate mammals that have been studied, the trophoblast forms desmosomes and apical junctional complexes with the uterine epithelium. This intimate ultrastructural association suggests that the uterine epithelium does not recognize the genetic "foreignness" of the trophoblast.

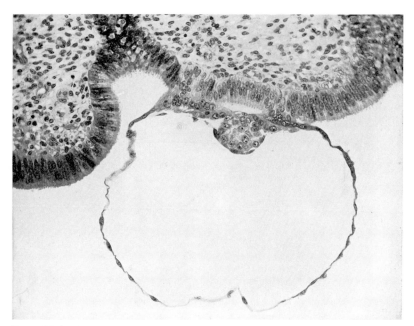

Figure 25-4 Eight-to-nine-day blastocyst of a rhesus monkey becoming attached to the endometrium. Syncytial trophoblast is conspicuous at the embryonic pole and is penetrating the uterine epithelium. The embryo-forming cells (the future germ disc) form a discrete mass which is separated from the cavity of the blastocyst by primitive endoderm. ×200. (Courtesy of C. H. Heuser and G. L. Streeter.)

Figure 25-5 Seven-day human implantation site in the edematous 22-day secretory endometrium. The trophoblast, which is here in direct contact with the uterine stroma, has proliferated to form a thick solid plate of syncytiotrophoblast and cytotrophoblast. The embryo-forming cells constitute a bilaminar germ disc which lies just below the thick plate of trophoblast. The blastocyst cavity is collapsed here. ×300. (Courtesy of A. T. Hertig and J. Rock.)

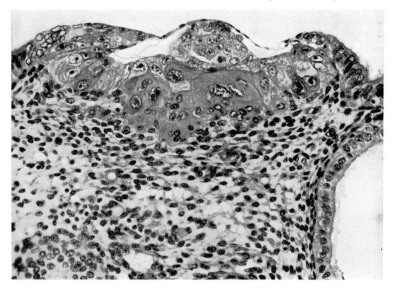

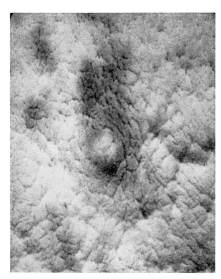

Figure 25-6   Surface view of the human endometrium and implantation site on the eleventh day of development. Sections through this specimen are shown in Figs. 25-7 and 25-8. ×8. (Courtesy of A. T. Hertig and J. Rock.)

tening, translucent area, a little less than 1 mm in diameter, surrounded by a bright red area which reflects a modification of blood vessels in the adjacent stroma. Microscopic examination of sections of this 11-day implant reveals that rapid growth and differentiation of the trophoblast have occurred around the entire circumference (Fig. 25-8). At this time two types of trophoblast are clearly evident: an inner layer of primitive cytotrophoblast composed of individual cells and a broad outer layer of primitive syncytial trophoblast. The syncytium now possesses spaces called *lacunae* that contain maternal blood. The lacunae communicate with each other and with maternal sinusoids and veins;

Figure 25-7   Section through an 11-day human implantation site in the 25-day secretory endometrium. The invading blastocyst has achieved an interstitial position, being located immediately below the endometrial surface. The whole expanse of the endometrium is evident with its dilated, coiled glands heavy with secretion. See Fig. 25-8 for enlargement of the implantation site. ×20. (Courtesy of A. T. Hertig and J. Rock.)

The youngest known attached human blastocyst (approximately $7\frac{1}{2}$ days) is shown in Fig. 25-5.[1] The local surface epithelium has disappeared, and the trophoblast is in contact with the connective tissue. The trophoblast, which is in the form of a thick plate, has differentiated into the *syncytiotrophoblast*, a multinucleated cytoplasmic mass or syncytium which arises by the fusion of separate cells of the *cytotrophoblast*. Intact superficial maternal capillaries course through the primitive syncytial trophoblast of this early implant.

The human embryonic complex undergoes *interstitial implantation*; it sinks into the endometrial connective tissue and becomes enclosed by it. By the eleventh day the interstitial position is achieved and the uterine epithelium covers over the site (Figs. 25-6 to 25-8). A view of the endometrial surface at the implantation site of a normal 11-day human embryo is shown in Fig. 25-6. The embryonic complex resides in a slightly raised, glis-

[1] Our knowledge of early human development is derived primarily from the important studies of A. T. Hertig and J. Rock. For a comprehensive bibliography of their work, see the paper by Hertig, Rock, and Adams published in 1956.

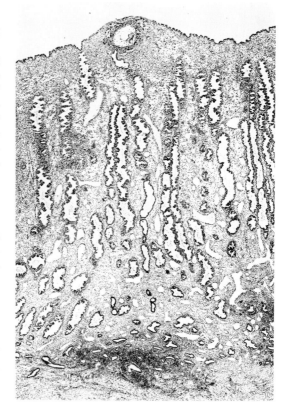

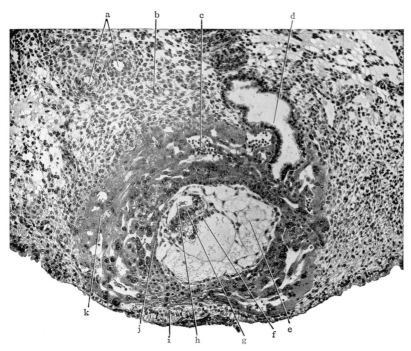

Figure 25-8 Section through an 11-day human implantation site in the 25-day secretory endometrium. Within the syncytial trophoblast (k) is an intercommunicating network of lacunar spaces which contain some maternal blood (c). The bilaminar embryonic germ disc is apparent in the center of the implant, with the amniotic cavity above and the yolk sac cavity below. Above the embryo and to the right is an enlarged secretory endometrial gland (d), whereas above and to the left the edematous stroma contains a coiled artery (a, b). e, exocoelom; f, endoderm forming part of the yolk sac; g, ectodermal embryonic shield; h, amniotic cavity enclosed by amnion which is delaminating in situ; i, repairing endometrial epithelium; j, cytotrophoblast. ×100. (Courtesy of A. T. Hertig and J. Rock.)

these vascular connections allow the initiation of the maternal circulation. The appearance of the placental hormone, *human chorionic gonadotrophin* (HCG), in the maternal circulation at this time provides evidence that a functional maternal vascular connection has been established. This early endocrine activity by the trophoblast provides a convenient basis for early recognition of pregnancy in human beings.

At this early stage of development, two extraembryonic membranes, not involved in the formation of the human placenta, are also being differentiated (Fig. 25-8). The *amnion* is a dome-like membrane that encloses a fluid-filled cavity over the embryonic plate. At this time the embryonic disc is bilaminar and consists of a thick plate of ectoderm and a thin ventral layer of endoderm. The *yolk sac* is attached to the ventral surface of the embryonic disc; its cavity is lined dorsally by the primitive endoderm and elsewhere by a layer of flattened cells. The confluent spaces in the loose extraembryonic mesenchyme surrounding the yolk sac represent the exocoelom. Although the yolk sac is involved in placentation in subprimate mammals, it never establishes contact with the chorion in man (Fig. 25-12), and its function is unknown.

Establishment of the placental villi and circulation

The third week of pregnancy (days 14 to 21) is a period of intense trophoblastic growth and differentiation, a time when the significant placental relationships are established. By the fifteenth day the maternal circulation through the syncytial trophoblast becomes fully functional, as lacunae become large and confluent and connect with endometrial arteries as well as with the veins. Cords of trophoblast, called *primary chorionic villi,* begin to extend outward from the surface of the chorion, owing to rapid proliferation of the cytotrophoblast which provides a fundamental cellular mechanism for expansion of the fetal placenta. After the fifteenth day, mesenchyme appears in the proximal attached portions of the cords and extends progressively toward their growing distal ends (Fig. 25-9). As mesenchyme forms in the cores of the villi, they are gradually converted from primary chorionic villi into *secondary villi.* Each secondary villus contains a core of mesenchyme surrounded by a continuous sheath of cytotrophoblast which is covered, in turn, by a mantle of syncytial trophoblast. The maternal blood flows through large intercommunicating spaces that have arisen from the confluence of the lacunae of the primitive syncytium, which are now referred to collectively as the *intervillous space* (Fig. 25-10). The surface of the syncytiotrophoblast is bathed directly by circulating maternal blood at this early time in gestation.

The distal tips of the secondary villi are now solid columns (*cytotrophoblastic cell columns*) which unite peripherally to form the *trophoblastic shell* (Figs. 25-10 and 25-11), which encloses the entire implant and is the outermost frontier of embryonic

Figure 25-9 Section through a 16-day human implantation site. Observe the embryonic shield with the amniotic cavity (i) above it and the yolk sac cavity (c) below it. The dark chorion encloses the large exocoelom (j) and is connected to the embryo by the mesodermal body stalk (b). Secondary villi containing cores of mesoderm and angioblasts are differentiating (d). Peripheral to these is a lamina composed largely of cytotrophoblast, constituting cell columns (f) and the developing trophoblastic shell (e). Surrounding the latter is the decidua. Below, separating the implant from the uterine cavity, is a broad zone of decidua capsularis (g). a, decidua basalis; k, intervillous space; h, dilated maternal venous sinus. ×30. (Courtesy of A. T. Hertig and J. Rock.)

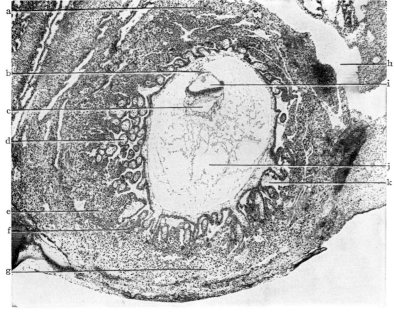

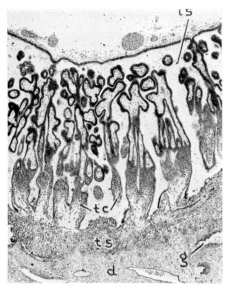

Figure 25-10 Section through the placenta of a rhesus monkey on the twenty-ninth day of gestation. Secondary chorionic villi are visible; each villus consists of a core of mesoderm surrounded by a darkly stained mantle of cytotrophoblast and syncytium which borders the intervillous space (is) through which maternal blood circulates. The tips of the villi extend downward as columns of cellular trophoblast (primary villi). The distal ends of these trophoblastic cell columns (tc) unite on the periphery of the growing placenta to form the trophoblastic shell (ts). The latter merges indistinctly with the underlying decidually transformed endometrium (d). g, uterine gland. Iron-hematoxylin stain. × 5.

tissue. It is composed principally of cellular trophoblast but also contains irregular strands of peripheral syncytial trophoblast, some of which penetrate quite deeply into the endometrium and make contact with the uterine blood vessels. The arrangement of the cytotrophoblast in the columns and shell provides a mechanism for lengthening the villi and for circumferential expansion of the fetal placenta. In addition, the cytotrophoblast proliferates in localized areas on some villi, creating the *cytotrophoblastic cell islands* which become conspicuous later in pregnancy (Fig. 25-23).

Embryonic blood vessels appear in the cores of the villi and form the *tertiary* placental villi. Also the primordium of the umbilical cord makes its appearance through the formation of the *body stalk* (Fig. 25-11) which is the homologue of the allantoic stalk in other groups of mammals. This mesodermal primordium connects the caudal part of the

embryonic shield with the chorion to form a *chorio-allantoic placenta*. By subsequent differentiation and elongation, the body stalk forms the *umbilical cord* which contains *umbilical vessels*. Thus the newly formed blood vessels of the placental villi become connected through the umbilical vessels with the embryonic heart; toward the end of the third week, fetal blood begins to circulate in the capillaries of the villi. The placental villi are now supplied by both maternal and fetal blood, and physiologic exchange is thereby greatly enhanced.

The allantoic stalk of most mammals contains an endodermal diverticulum of the hindgut which, in association with the allantoic mesoderm, forms the allantoic sac. In man and the monkey the endodermal diverticulum of the hindgut remains rudimentary and microscopic (Fig. 25-11).

Figure 25-11 Section through the 18- to 19-day human placental site. The curved germ disc has differentiated to the stage of Hensen's node and the primitive groove. The yolk sac (ys) contains blood islands. The body stalk (bs), which is partly penetrated by an endodermal diverticulum. connects with the chorionic mesoderm. Secondary placental villi (v) are evident; their distal ends are solid masses of cytotrophoblast that fuse peripherally to form the trophoblastic shell (ts). × 15. (Courtesy of A. T. Hertig and J. Rock.)

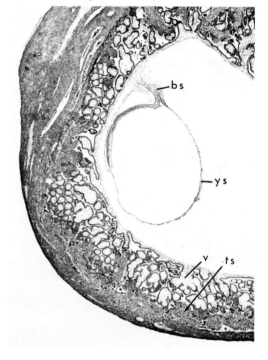

Placental (chorionic) villi

The structural and functional unit of the human fetal placenta is the *villus*. It brings the fetal blood-stream close to the maternal blood for physiologic exchanges. It constitutes the placental barrier that regulates the transport of substances between the bloodstreams. At the same time the villous structure creates a tremendous trophoblastic surface that facilitates transport. As the villi differentiate, they become longer and highly branched, and they are described by some investigators as resembling trees rooted in the chorionic plate, with branches extending into the intervillous space (Figs. 25-12 and 25-22A, see color insert). At term, approximately 11 square meters of surface area have been

Figure 25-12 Normal human gestation sac at 40 days, carefully separated and removed from the uterus. The chorion laeve has been removed to reveal the relationships of the embryo and extraembryonic membranes. The embryo is most immediately enclosed by the amnion. The chorionic membrane encloses the exocoelom into which the small yolk sac extends. The placental villi project outward from the chorionic plate; at this early stage, the villi are diffusely distributed over the entire chorionic surface. ×3.5. (Carnegie Institution of Washington.)

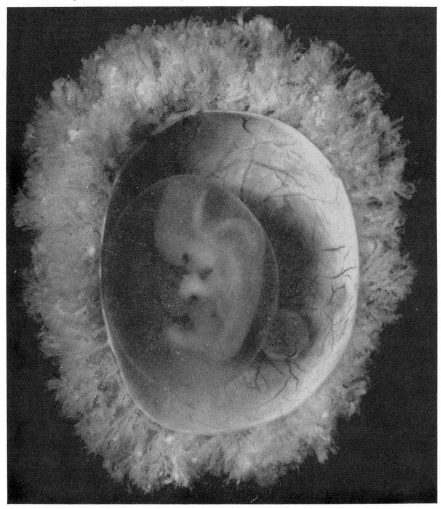

differentiated on the placental villi; this calculation does not include the further amplification created by microvilli on the free trophoblastic surface.

The morphology of the villi has been difficult to interpret at the microscopic level, since only pieces of the branches are seen in sections (Fig. 25-29). It is clear, however, that the main or *stem villi* are attached to the chorionic plate (Fig. 25-22). During pregnancy each stem villus subdivides longitudinally at its distal end to create villi of a second or third order. These, in turn, form still smaller branches, some of which terminate in the trophoblastic shell (basal plate) and are called *anchoring villi*. The *terminal* (or free) villi extend freely into the intervillous space and contain sinusoidal capillaries. Each stem villus and its branches has a separate fetal blood supply; this unit has been designated a *fetal cotyledon*. Differing interpretations of the form of the fetal cotyledon occur in the literature; some investigators describe a tree-like configuration (Fig. 25-22A, see color insert) whereas others think that the branches of the stem villus form a barrel-like configuration that encloses a central cavity (Fig. 25-22B, see color insert). The number of fetal cotyledons appears to decrease from approximately 320 in early gestation to 60 at term (Boyd and Hamilton, 1970). However, concomitantly the total surface area for transport is expanded by an increase in the number of terminal villi coupled with a decrease in their diameter.

In the early placenta the villi occur all over the surface of the chorion (Fig. 25-12). Basally, in association with the thick well-vascularized endometrium, the villi branch elaborately and grow in length. They constitute the *chorion frondosum* and eventually give rise collectively to the gross discoidal form of the definitive placenta. The endometrial connective tissue in this region is called the *decidua basalis*. Over the outer chorionic wall, which bulges toward the uterine cavity, the villi are much shorter and here, by the third month of gestation, the villi and the associated *decidua capsularis* dwindle, leaving the *chorion laeve*. As the fetus enlarges and its membranes expand, the chorion laeve eventually fuses with the *decidua vera* of the

Figure 25-13   Cross section of a young human placental villus, showing an axial mesodermal core surrounded by the two-layered trophoblastic epithelium composed of an inner cellular layer of Langhans' cells (cytotrophoblast) and an outer layer of syncytium (syncytial trophoblast). Vacuoles of various sizes occur in the syncytium.   ×550. (Courtesy of W. J. Hamilton and R. J. Gladstone.)

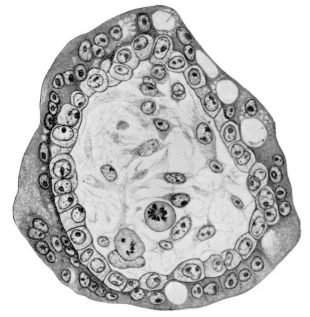

opposite uterine wall, thereby obliterating the uterine cavity. Consult a textbook of mammalian embryology for illustration of these relationships.

The villus of the early placenta has a loose mesenchymal core that is covered by two layers of trophoblast (Figs. 25-13; 25-14, color insert; 25-15; and 25-16, color insert). The inner or cytotrophoblastic layer is composed of large *Langhans' cells* that have large nuclei and a slightly basophilic cytoplasm. Overlying the Langhans' cells is a more basophilic layer of relatively thick syncytiotrophoblast. Mitoses occur in the Langhans' layer but not in the syncytium; in vivo isotopic labeling of dividing nuclei with [³H] thymidine has

established that in the rhesus monkey the Langhans' cytotrophoblast produces the syncytium (Fig. 25-15). The Langhans' cells decrease in number after the fifth month of pregnancy; at term, relatively few remain. Thus, the Langhans' layer is a germinal bed of cells that multiply, transform, and then fuse with the syncytium to cause its expansion. These germinal cells store a considerable amount of glycogen during the first 4 to 6 weeks of gestation; thereafter the glycogen store diminishes.

The undifferentiated state of the Langhans' cells is evident also in their ultrastructure (Fig. 25-18). Free ribosomes are common in the cytoplasm

Figure 25-15 Radioautographs showing the incorporation of tritiated thymidine into the placental villi of the rhesus monkey. A. One hour after an intravenous injection of [³H] thymidine, only the nuclei of the cytotrophoblastic (C) or Langhans' cells are labeled. B. However, 48 hr after such an injection, a high percentage of syncytiotrophoblastic (S) nuclei carry the label. ×600. (Courtesy of A. R. Midgley and G. B. Pierce.)

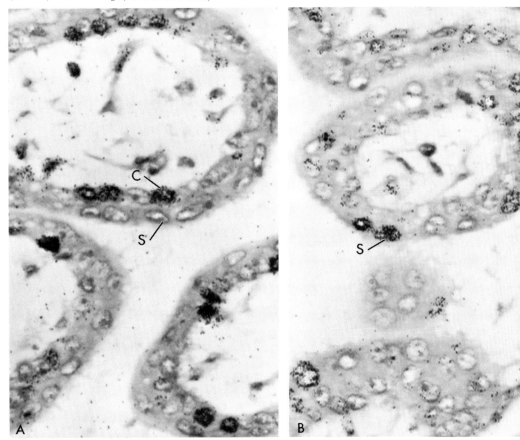

insert; 25-15; 25;16, color insert; 25-17; and 25-18). By its position and prevalence, it must be the chief regulator of transport and, in addition, it is most likely the site of synthesis of both the steroid and protein placental hormones (see below). The syncytiotrophoblast is a continuous layer of multinucleated cytoplasm that forms a complete covering over the multitudinous villi. A significant structural-functional point is the apparent absence of intercellular space in this absorptive surface. All substances entering or leaving the fetal blood must therefore pass through the syncytial cytoplasm. This layer, which is thick early in gestation, becomes progressively thinner as gestation advances (Fig. 25-19). As the Langhans' layer becomes discontinuous, the syncytium comes increasingly in contact with the basal lamina.

The free surface of the syncytium interacts directly with the maternal blood and is modified into a profusion of highly pleomorphic microvilli (Fig. 25-18). In addition, the syncytial surface is extended by larger projections in the form of ridges that are studded with microvilli. The elaborate and irregular form of the surface projections suggests tremendous mobility of the superficial cytoplasm. Some are pseudopods and contain cytoplasmic organelles; others consist of club-like microvilli. Like the conspicuous microvillous borders of the small intestine and proximal tubule of the kidney, this placental border is rich in alkaline phosphatase activity. Between the microvilli are small, bristle-coated pits or caveolae which may be involved in macromolecular uptake. Relatively large tabs of syncytium, such as that illustrated in Fig. 25-16 (see color insert), often project into the intervillous space. In normal pregnancy, such nucleated syncytial sprouts are liberated into the intervillous space and enter the maternal venous system. They get as far as the maternal pulmonary capillaries but apparently do not enter the systemic arterial system. Later in pregnancy even whole villi are released into the maternal circulation (Ramsey, 1971). The significance of this remarkable phenomenon is unkown.

A conspicuous feature of the nuclei of the syncytiotrophoblast is their tendency to clump close together (Fig. 25-24). They are usually located in the basal cytoplasm and are larger in younger

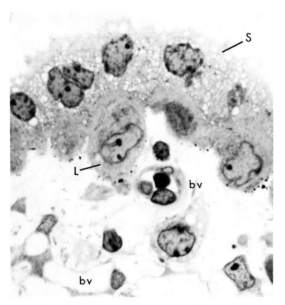

Figure 25-17   Human placental villus at 10 weeks. The cytoplasm of the syncytiotrophoblast (S) appears vacuolated. The nuclei of the syncytium have a heavier chromatin pattern than those of Langhans' cells (L). Fetal blood vessels (bv) are generally not closely apposed to the trophoblast. Plastic section, 2 μm, toluidine blue.   ×600.

whereas rough endoplasmic reticulum (ER) is relatively sparse; the Golgi complex seems to be the best-developed portion of the cytoplasmic membrane system. The mitochondria are larger than those of the syncytium. The Langhans' cells are associated with each other and with the syncytium by desmosomes and tight junctions; their basal surfaces rest on a basal lamina. Transitional cells with ultrastructural characteristics occur intermediate between those of Langhans' cells and syncytium, and evidence of cell fusion between these transitional cells and the syncytium has been obtained. Remnants of fusion are represented in the syncytial cytoplasm by fragments of cell membranes, desmosomes, and even intercellular spaces. Thus, the multinucleate condition of the syncytiotrophoblast originates in the same manner as that of skeletal muscle fibers, that is, by the fusion of initially separate cells.

The placental syncytium is a remarkable structural differentiation (Figs. 25-13; 25-14, color

stages than later in gestation. Vacuolation of the cytoplasm is common during the first 3 months (Fig. 25-17), but the ultrastructural basis of this has not been adequately defined. The superficial cytoplasm, especially in the early syncytium, is distinctly acidophilic; the ultrastructure of this region shows a concentration of smooth-surfaced vesicles of various sizes and relatively few endoplasmic reticulum elements. In contrast, the basal and perinuclear cytoplasm is intensely basophilic (Fig. 25-16, see color insert), reflecting a high concentration of both free ribosomes and rough ER, whose cisternae are often dilated (Fig. 25-18) and contain a moderately dense material. This elaborate system of rough-surfaced membranes suggests that this trophoblastic layer is invloved in the synthesis of proteins for

Figure 25-18   Electron micrograph of the human placenta at 4 months' gestation. The two trophoblastic layers are evident; the syncytiotrophoblast (S) is attached to the subjacent germinal cytotrophoblast or Langhans' cells (L) by desmosomes (D). The Langhans' cells lie on the basal lamina (arrow). A thin layer of connective tissue intervenes between the trophoblastic complex and the underlying blood vessel (BV). The free surface of the syncytium is modified into an irregular microvillous border. The superficial cytoplasm of the syncytium contains vesicles and irregularly shaped vacuoles. Rough endoplasmic reticulum is abundant in the syncytium but relatively sparse in the Langhans' cells. The undifferentiated cytoplasm of the Langhans' cells contains many free ribosomes. G, Golgi complex. ×15,000. (Courtesy of A. C. Enders.)

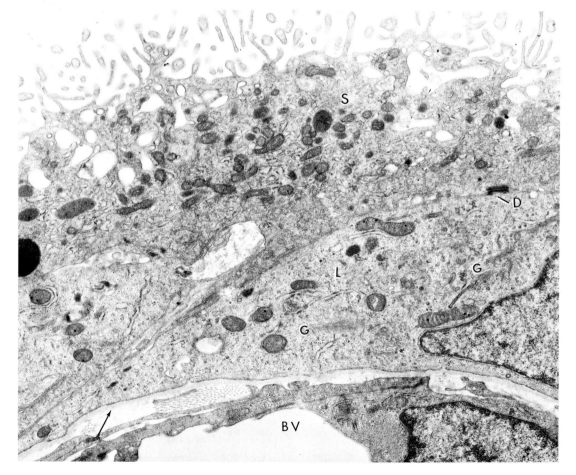

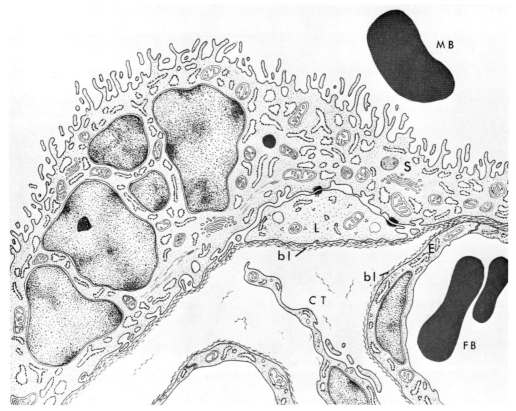

Figure 25-19 Diagram of the human placental barrier near term. The maternal blood (MB) is separated from the fetal blood (FB) by the syncytiotrophoblasts (S), occasional Langhans' cells (L), basal lamina of the trophoblast (bl), fetal connective tissue (CT), basal lamina (bl) of the fetal capillary, and the fetal endothelium (E). (Courtesy of A. C. Enders, 1965.)

export, perhaps serum proteins and the two placental protein hormones, HCG and human chorionic somatomammotropin (HCS) (see below). Smooth ER is inconspicuous or absent.

Another significant ultrastructural feature of the syncytium is the presence of large cytoplasmic granules surrounded by smooth membranes. Smaller granules with similar appearance are associated with the Golgi apparatus. It is not known whether these granules represent secreted or absorbed material. Golgi complexes are distributed at intervals in the syncytium. Slender filamentous mitochondria occur throughout the cytoplasm. Glycogen is stored in the syncytiotrophoblast only during the first month and disappears by the end of the second month.

A significant cytochemical feature of the syncytium is the presence of numerous birefringent, sudanophilic droplets throughout gestation. These lipid droplets have cytochemical properties similar to those of steroid-producing cells of the gonads and adrenal cortex. These cytochemical comparisons have long suggested that the syncytium may be responsible for the secretion of the placental steroids, estrogen and progesterone. This suggestion has been given more substance by the localization within the villous trophoblast of Δ^5-3β-hydroxysteroid dehydrogenase, an enzymatic complex involved in the biosynthesis of steroid hormones.

The stroma of the villi is initially a loose mesenchyme which becomes more densely collagenous with advancing gestation. Two types of cells occur

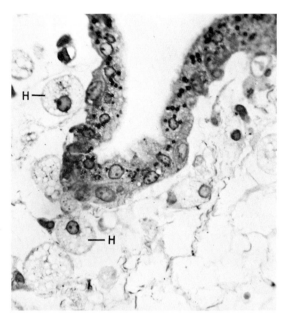

Figure 25-20 Human placental villus at 10 weeks. The two-layered trophoblast rests on a rather loose mesenchymal stroma. Within the loose meshwork of reticular fibers and mesenchymal or fibroblastic cells lie the highly vacuolated Hofbauer cells (H). See Fig. 25-21. Plastic section, 2μm, toluidine blue. ×450.

in this fetal connective tissue, fibroblasts and a unique cell type called the *Hofbauer cell*. The fibroblasts possess the usual ultrastructural features of this cell type elsewhere, where they are known to be the elaborators of collagen and ground substance. The Hofbauer cells are large, elliptical, and vacuolated; they are most numerous in the early placenta (Fig. 25-20). Ultrastructural and cytochemical evidence suggests that they are similar to macrophages (Fig. 25-21). It is interesting that they are located in a separate extracellular compartment that is free of collagen fibrils and is delimited from the rest of the stroma by the processes of fibroblasts. The specific function of the Hofbauer cells remains speculative.

Branches of the umbilical arteries and vein course through the stroma of the stem villi and their branches (Figs. 25-22, see color insert, and 25-23). The terminal (free) villi possess an anastomosing network of nonfenestrated capillaries that are sinusoidal in their proportions; they may exceed 50 μm in diameter (Fig. 25-24). These wide vessels allow an unusually small decrease in the blood pressure from the umbilical artery to the umbilical vein.

Junction of maternal and fetal tissues

The region of confrontation between fetal and maternal tissues is interesting from an immunologic point of view, since cells of two different genotypes are in intimate association. It is the region of placental attachment, and nothing is known about the cohesive forces which bind the trophoblast to the decidua here. At birth this region of attachment will become the region of separation as the *deciduate placenta* is shed.

In the early placenta the outermost fetal tissue, the trophoblastic shell, is formed by the fusion of solid columns of cytotrophoblast at the distal tips of the secondary villi. The trophoblastic shell comes into close association with the *decidua*, which is the designation for the endometrium of the pregnant uterus. The cells of the two genotypes intermingle here, and it is difficult to distinguish between them in a routine preparation. From the time of implantation a peculiar extracellular material

called *fibrinoid* accumulates around the fetal cytotrophoblasts (Figs. 25-25 to 25-27); the term fibrinoid describes a group of substances related to fibrin. In later development this junctional zone of intermingling maternal and fetal cells is referred to as the *basal plate*. During the second half of pregnancy, the basal plate thins out, and the maternal and fetal cells become mixed in a complex manner.

The cellular relationships of the basal plate are incompletely described and remain a challenge to specialists in the subject. It is useful to remember, however, that the decidual cells are derivatives of the uterine connective tissue and, as such, are surrounded by collagen fibrils. The fetal cells tend to be surrounded by fibrinoid. Also the cytotrophoblastic cells are epithelial derivatives and are held together by desmosomes (Fig. 25-27). It is significant that these peripheral cytotrophoblastic cells differ considerably in their ultrastructure and cyto-

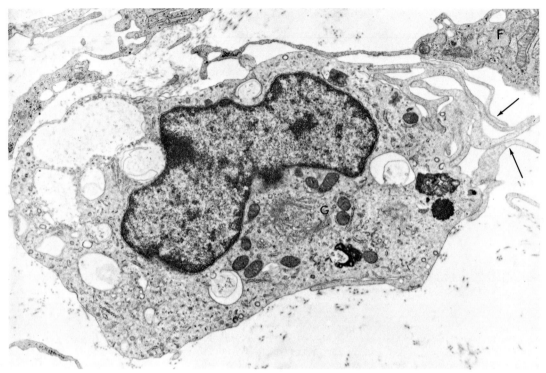

Figure 25-21   Electron micrograph of a Hofbauer cell in the human placenta at 3 months gestation.   The Hofbauer cells have ultrastructural features resembling those of tissue macrophages.   The cell surface appears highly mobile, with broad cytoplasmic extensions (arrows) suitable for engulfing materials.   Vacuoles of varying size and content are conspicuous, along with some dense bodies.   G, Golgi complex; F, fibroblast.   ×9,000.   (Courtesy of A. C. Enders.)

chemistry from the Langhans' cytotrophoblast on the villi.   Their cytoplasm is strongly basophilic (Fig. 25-25) and contains a well-developed rough ER (Fig. 25-27), whereas the Langhans' cell cytoplasm is faintly basophilic and has little rough ER (Fig. 25-18).   The peripheral cytotrophoblastic cells later in gestation contain fine glycoprotein granules.   To some investigators, these cells bear some resemblance to the gonadotrophin-secreting basophils of the anterior pituitary and thus might be the producers of chorionic gonadotrophin.   Investigators attempting to localize the site of secretion of HCG by immunohistochemical procedures have usually used only samples of the villous portion of the placenta.   Most of these studies identify the syncytium as the probable synthesizer of both HCG and HCS.   Further work must still be done to establish with certainty the sites of synthesis of the pro-

tein hormones.   Since the cytotrophoblast of the basal plate, cell columns, and cell islands has the cytologic features of cells that synthesize protein for export, they should be studied further.

The separated uterine surface of the delivered placenta shows elevated convex subdivisions of *maternal cotyledons* (lobes) that are demarcated by grooves.   The position of the maternal cotyledons corresponds roughly to that of the fetal cotyledons.   *Placenta septa* occupy the intercotyledonary grooves of the basal plate into the intervillous space.   Investigators disagree whether these septa are maternal or fetal in origin or whether they have a dual origin.   Attempts to distinguish maternal from fetal cells by identifying Barr bodies or female sex chromatin, when a male fetus occurs, have not resolved this controversy.

The nature of the immunologic relationship of the

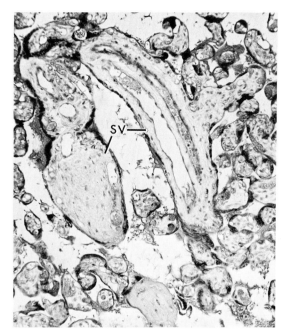

Figure 25-23 Branches of the stem villi in the human placenta at term. In the branches of the stem villus (SV) at the right, a fetal artery and vein course through its core. In addition, a branch point is evident in this stem villus. Eosin-methylene blue. ×100.

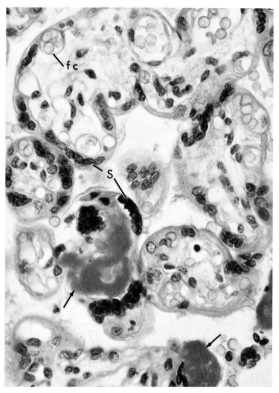

Figure 25-24 Human placental villi at term. Fetal sinusoidal capillaries (fc) are now closely apposed to the syncytiotrophoblast (S). The stroma is denser than in early gestation. Hyalinization of the villi is evident (arrows). In certain areas the nuclei of the syncytium are crowded together and form dense clusters. Eosin-methylene blue. ×450.

trophoblast with the uterine epithelium and with the decidua is of considerable theoretical and practical importance. Also, once maternal circulation is established, the maternal blood cells in the intervillous space are washed against the fetal syncytium. Early embryonic tissue is antigenic, the mother is immunologically competent, and yet gestation proceeds to term without a typical local immune response by the mother. Considerable effort is being directed toward the possibility that ex-

tracellular coats, such as the cell coat (glycocalyx) of the epithelia, or extracellular deposits, such as fibrinoid, may constitute an immunologic barrier. In addition, the nature of the antigenicity of the trophoblast remains to be defined.

Placental circulation

The gross anatomy of the placenta reflects strongly the vascular arrangement. A pattern of blood flow through the *definitive discoidal placenta* was illustrated by Ramsey and Harris in 1966 (Fig. 25-22A, see the color insert). More recently, a somewhat modified interpretation of blood flow

has been presented by Freese. The two umbilical arteries are continuous with the fetal internal iliac arteries and carry blood that is rich in carbon dioxide from the fetus to the placenta. In the chorionic plate they divide into numerous placental arteries that spread fanwise; from these radial

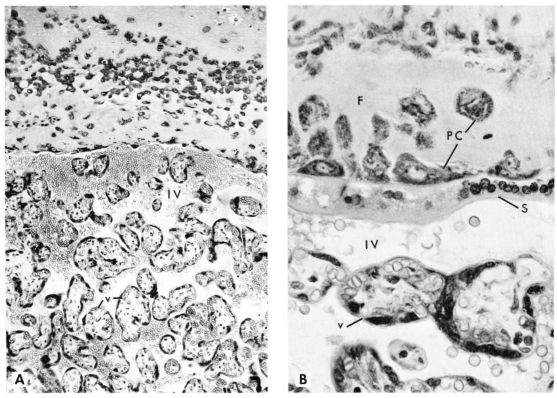

Figure 25-25   Human placenta at term, showing the composition of the basal plate at two different magnifications.   The upper part of each photomicrograph shows the basal plate whereas the lower part contains placental villi (v) and the intervillous space (IV).   In the basal plate, the peripheral cytotrophoblastic cells (PC) possess conspicuous cytoplasmic basophilia, a major cytochemical feature of this cell type.   Note also that these epithelial cells are embedded in fibrinoid (F).   Maternal blood is evident in the intervillous space, and the fetal blood vessels are packed with erythrocytes.   Note in B that syncytium (S) clothes the fetal aspect of the basal plate.   Eosin-methylene blue.   A, ×100; B, ×450.

trunks, vertical branches are given off which ramify into the stem villi and their numerous branches. The branching form of the villus is followed by the blood vessels.   The fetal arteries branch and rebranch to break up finally into the *sinusoidal capillary bed* of the smallest villi (Fig. 25-24).   Throughout gestation, newly formed capillaries invade the syncytial buds on the growing tips of the villi and thus the volume of the capillary bed increases steadily during pregnancy.   Each stem villus (that is, fetal cotyledon) with its ramifications is autonomous.   The number of fetal cotyledons decreases from approximately 320 in early gestation to 60 at term.   To keep pace with the growing fetus, fetal cotyledons increase in weight and length, instead of spreading the area of placental attachment.

The circulation of maternal blood commences during the second week; the fetal circulation is established by the end of the third week.   The vascularity becomes increasingly rich on both maternal and fetal sides.   Early in pregnancy, the fetal capillaries lie in a central position in the villus but, as pregnancy advances, these thin-walled, anastomosing, endothelial tubes with their large lumina come to lie just beneath the surface of the trophoblast.   The venous blood is returned from the multitude of terminal villi through a system of veins which accompany the arteries.   These lead eventually to the single *umbilical vein* that carries oxygenated blood back to the fetus where it connects with the ductus venosus. The fetal circulation through the placenta is maintained by a pressure head; it has been demonstrated in the fetal lamb that at term the pressure gradient between the umbilical arteries and umbilical vein is approximately 65 mm Hg. The placental capillary pressure is much above that of other capillary beds and also exceeds the pressure in the maternal intervillous space. The umbilical arteries, as well as the sinusoidal capillaries in the villous stem, have large lumina, and this keeps the pressure high.

Maternal blood enters the intervillous space through open-ended uteroplacental arteries (endometrial spiral arteries) that penetrate the basal plate. At the point of entry the arteries have terminal dilations. These are the remarkably modified coiled arteries of the nonpregnant endometrium which have been rebuilt from invading cytotrophoblasts. The tunica media is largely replaced by trophoblast. It is interesting that the trophoblast does not, however, invade the uteroplacental veins. There is generally one arterial entry opening usually at the center of a fetal cotyledon (Fig. 25-22B, see color insert). Recent observations indicate a correspondence between the fetal and maternal cotyledons. This unifying concept defines the cotyledon as the maternal and fetal circulating units, and the location of the spiral artery determines the position of the cotyledons.

The maternal blood from the uteroplacental artery spurts into the intervillous space of a fetal cotyledon in "fountain-like jets" (Fig. 25-22, see color insert). It has been assumed that the force of this jet stream sweeps aside the free terminal villi, especially near the point of arterial entry (Fig. 25-22A, see color insert). According to another interpretation, the jet stream is directed into a central, villous-free cavity of the fetal cotyledon (see Freese). Since the maternal arterial blood pressure is greater than the pressure in the intervillous space, the arterial stream is driven toward the chorionic plate; then as the pressure of the stream decreases, lateral dispersion occurs. Lateral dispersion has been visualized in living pregnant rhesus monkeys by x-ray cinematographic means. The blood then falls back in a fountain-like

spray to bathe the extensive surface of the syncytiotrophoblast, and exchanges between the two bloodstreams occur. Blood may also circulate from one cotyledon to another through perforations in the septa. Finally it drops back into venous openings that are distributed along the basal plate. The venous pressure is lower than that of the intervillous space; thus differences in the blood pressure of the arteries, intervillous space, and veins control the maternal circulation in the placenta. The maternal

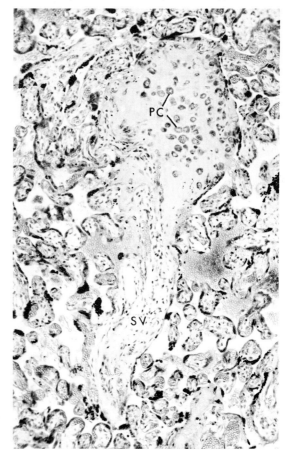

Figure 25-26 Human placenta at term, showing a portion of a stem villus (SV) with an associated cell island of peripheral cytotrophoblast (PC). The large stem villus occupies the center of the photomicrograph and is surrounded by numerous sections through the finely branched villous tree. The peripheral trophoblastic cells stain darkly because of their high cytoplasmic content of ribonucleoprotein. Eosin-methylene blue. ×100.

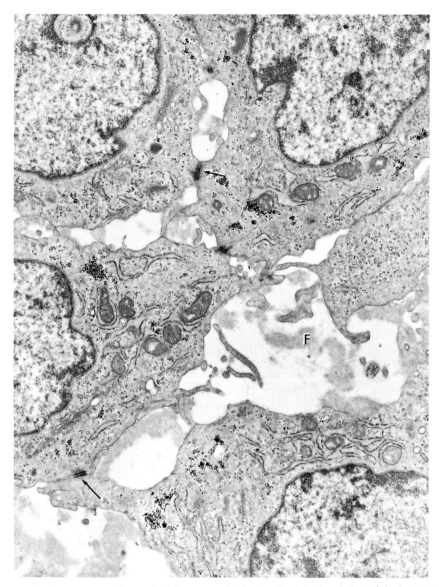

Figure 25-27 Electron micrograph of the cytotrophoblastic cells of the basal plate of the human placenta at 3 months gestation. The peripheral cytotrophoblastic cells are joined together at intervals by desmosomes (arrows); also large intercellular spaces contain a relatively amorphous dense material called fibrinoid (F). Conspicuous components of the cytoplasm are rough endoplasmic reticulum, mitochondria, Golgi complex, and glycogen particles. ×15,000. (Courtesy of A. C. Enders.)

and fetal bloodstreams move in more or less opposite directions, but investigators tend to agree that countercurrent flow does not occur, at least in the primate placenta. For discussion of the possible arrangements of flow in the two bloodstreams, see Dawes (1968).

Comparative placentation

The human placenta may be described as *hemochorial, villous, discoidal,* and *deciduate.* To understand the meaning of this classification it is necessary to appreciate comparative placentation, a topic beyond the scope of this chapter. Detailed information on comparative placentation can be found in the works of Grosser (1927), Mossman (1937), Amoroso (1952), and Wislocki and Padykula (1961). Briefly, however, the yolk sac and allantois fuse with the chorion in different mammals to form various placental relationships. In human beings, only a chorioallantoic placenta is formed. The chorioallantoic placentas of mammals can be classified according to gross form or on the basis of the histologic structure of the placental barrier. The gross form is related to the distribution of villi (or lamellae) over the surface of the chorion. The early human placenta starts out with the villi quite uniformly distributed over the outer surface of the chorion; this gross arrangement is described as a *diffuse placenta* (Fig. 25-12). It differentiates into a definitive form that is *discoidal* in shape, that is, the villi are arranged in the form of a disc (Fig. 25-22, see color insert). Other gross forms are cotyledonary (ruminants) or zonary (carnivores).

The histologic classification introduced by Grosser is based on the microscopic structure of the placental barrier. Grosser's classification is derived from the number of maternal tissue layers that intervene between the maternal and fetal circulations (Fig. 25-28) and thus has functional implications. When the chorion is apposed to an

Figure 25-28 Chorioallantoic barriers of sow, sheep, cat, and man near full term. This reinterpretation of Grosser's classification indicates that the differences in the widths of the various types of placental barriers may not be so great as generally believed. The fetal capillaries (fc) and maternal capillaries (mc) are heavily outlined, in the human placenta, the maternal capillaries have been eroded, and the maternal blood circulates through the intervillous space. In the epitheliochorial placenta of the sow and in the syndesmochorial placenta of the sheep, the fetal capillaries penetrate deeply into the trophoblast, and the maternal capillaries push into the overlying tissue. These morphologic modifications decrease significantly the distance between the two bloodstreams. Furthermore, the placental barriers of the sheep and cat are practically identical with respect to the number of layers separating the two bloodstreams. (Prepared by G. B. Wislocki in consultation with E. C. Amoroso.)

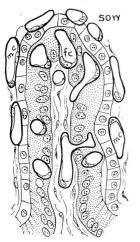
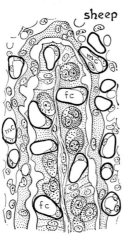
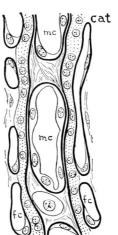
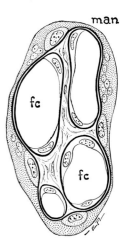

intact (epithelial) endometrium, this relationship is described as *epitheliochorial* (for example, pig, horse). In the *syndesmochorial* placenta (ruminants), the uterine epithelium is destroyed, leaving the connective tissue stroma exposed to the trophoblast. In the *endotheliochorial* placenta (for example, carnivores) most of the connective tissue surrounding the maternal capillaries is destroyed, thus placing the trophoblast in close association with the maternal endothelium. In the *hemochorial* placenta (for example, bats, higher primates, some insectivores, and rodents), the maternal blood comes into direct contact with the chorionic villi or lamellae through the loss of the maternal capillary endothelium. In this type of placenta the endometrium becomes transformed into decidua and is partially destroyed. At birth there may be considerable bleeding (man and monkey) as the *deciduate* placenta is shed. Although Grosser's scheme is generally useful and valid, recent ultrastructural observations have indicated that it is an oversimplification from the morphologic point of view (see Fig. 25-28) and thus most likely from a functional point of view as well.

The human placental barrier

Early in implantation the hemochorial nature of the human placental barrier is established, as maternal blood circulates through the lacunae lined by syncytium (Fig. 25-8). As the villi form and expand, the thickness of the barrier decreases progressively as the Langhans' cells disappear, the syncytium flattens into a thin layer, and the sinusoidal capillaries assume a position closer to the basement membrane. Thus the barrier is composed entirely of fetal tissue. The branches of the villous tree become progressively smaller and more numerous (Fig. 25-29). Concomitant with this progressive structural change, there may be alterations in permeability to many substances.

The placental barrier at term varies in its thickness; it can be as thin as 2 μm but some areas are as thick as 60 μm. Evidence is gathering that regional differences may exist along the barrier. A substance passing from the maternal blood to the fetal blood first encounters the free surface of the syncytium, which is highly modified to form a multitude of pleomorphic microvilli and other surface projections. Small molecules presumably are transferred through the plasma membrane of the elaborate evaginations to enter the syncytium. Uptake of macromolecular substances may occur through pinocytosis, since invaginations of the plasma membrane are frequent and are in close association with small vesicles. The pathway of absorption through the syncytium is unknown. Although membrane-limited droplets have been reported in the syncytium, it is not known whether they represent absorption or secretion, since the abundant endoplasmic reticulum of the syncytium may be involved in both activities. The ultrastructure of the syncytium is quite similar to that of thyroid follicular cells, which are also involved in the two-way traffic of secretory and absorptive functions.

The basal surface of the syncytial trophoblast borders on either Langhans' cells or on the epithelial basal lamina directly; the latter relationship becomes more common as gestation proceeds (Fig. 25-19). At term the basal cytoplasm is modified to form narrow infoldings as well as foot-like processes. Associated with these invaginations there are often relatively large irregular gaps between the syncytium and the epithelial basement lamina. This structural amplification of the basal surface may be related to transport from the fetal toward the maternal blood. The epithelial basal lamina rests on a thin layer of connective tissue, and occasionally the processes of fibroblasts may intervene between the epithelium and the capillary. The endothelial cells rest on their own basal lamina, with their junctions closely apposed. Pinocytotic vesicles occur on both surfaces of the cells. In some regions the connective tissue layer may be obliterated and the two basal laminae become closely apposed or fused.

Thus, at the ultrastructural level, the three-layered hemochorial placental barrier becomes further subdivided into at least five ultrastructural layers: syncytium, trophoblastic basal lamina,

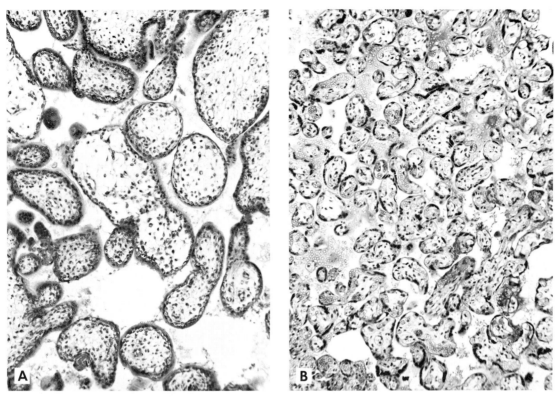

Figure 25-29   Human placental villi at 10 weeks (A) and at term (B).   Both photomicrographs were taken at the same magnification.   Note that as gestation proceeds the branches of the villous tree become progressively finer and more numerous.   Also, the placental barrier becomes thinner and fetal capillaries come in close apposition to the trophoblastic cover.   H&E.   ×100.

connective tissue layer, endothelial basal lamina, and endothelium.   Since it is known that there is considerable regulation of the substances trans-ferred between the two bloodstreams, the mechanism of regulation must be distributed among these ultrastructural layers.

Functions of the placenta

The transport activities of the placenta are complex since the numerous materials required for the synthesis of fetal tissues must be transferred and the waste products of fetal metabolism removed.   In general, small molecules cross more readily than larger ones.   The building blocks for proteins, phospholipids, and polysaccharides are transferred from the maternal blood to support the synthesis of large molecules in the fetus.   An exception to this is the transfer of antibodies across the human placenta; the transmission of passive immunity is a prenatal event in man and depends on the capacity to transport intact protein molecules.   Although it is generally believed that gases and water pass by means of simple diffusion, this concept is currently being questioned.   There is abundant evidence for the existence of active transport mechanisms in the placenta, since glucose, certain other sugars, and amino acids are clearly transported by energy-requiring processes.   The regulatory effect of such a process is illustrated in the example of the diabetic mother. Her high blood glucose results in some increase in fetal blood sugar, but the fetal level is always considerably less than the maternal level. Of the various components of the placental barrier, the one that is most likely concerned with the mechanism of regulation is the syncytium.

The placenta is a multipotential endocrine gland that can perform some of the functions of the anterior pituitary and ovary. In some species, including man, the ovaries can be removed quite early in pregnancy without affecting its course; the placental steroids maintain an appropriate gestational environment. Two protein hormones are produced that mimic certain functions of the adult pituitary, human chorionic gonadotrophin (HCG) and human chorionic somatomammotropin (HCS). The latter hormone is also referred to as a human placental lactogen (HPL). HCG is a glycoprotein hormone with inherent FSH and LH activities; however, its function in normal pregnancy is unknown. HCS is a single polypeptide chain that is remarkably similar to human growth hormone (HGH) in molecular weight and in the number and sequence of amino acids. Both HGH and HCS have growth-promoting, lactogenic, as well as metabolic effects, and this led to the suggestion that HCS is the growth hormone of pregnancy. The placenta has all the enzymatic machinery needed to synthesize progesterone from acetate or cholesterol but lacks two enzymes needed for estrogen synthesis; however, these are present in the fetal adrenal and possibly the fetal liver. Thus, estrogen is synthesized by the integrated endocrine activity of the *feto-placental unit*. The concept of the feto-placental unit was introduced in 1962 by Diczfalusy who defines it as follows: ''. . . the fetus and placenta form a functional unit to carry out biosynthetic reactions together, which the placenta *per se* or the fetus *per se* are incapable of completing.''

Immunocytochemical procedures have shown that HCG and HCS are localized almost exclusively in the syncytiotrophoblast of the placenta. Thus there is a strong possibility that the syncytium is the site of synthesis of both of these protein hormones, although available evidence indicates that the peripheral cytotrophoblast should still be considered as a possible site of origin. The recent demonstration of the presence of HCG in the rough endoplasmic reticulum of the syncytium provides evidence that it is synthesized there (Dreskin et al, 1970). Most investigators believe that the syncytiotrophoblast may also be the site of synthesis of progesterone and estrogen. The occurrence in the syncytium of the special lipid droplets that are characteristic of steroid-synthesizing cells of the gonads and adrenals and also of Δ^5-3β-hydroxysteroid dehydrogenase supports this possibility. A troublesome ultrastructural point, however, is the paucity or absence of smooth ER in the syncytium; this organelle is characteristically abundant in other steroid-synthesizing cells, such as those of the gonads and adrenal. Thus cytochemical evidence suggests that the syncytiotrophoblast may be capable of synthesizing not only protein but steroid hormones as well, and this unique possibility deserves further exploration.

The trophoblast resembles the hepatic parenchyma in its wide range of both anabolic and catabolic activities. For example, it has been shown that placental tissue can synthesize fatty acids and steroids from acetate or pyruvic acid. It performs conversions of substrate; for example, androgens are converted to estrogens and glucose to fructose. It is not surprising that the placenta exhibits great biochemical complexity, since it performs the multiple functions usually associated with the lungs, kidneys, endocrine glands, liver, and intestinal mucosa of the adult organism.

Biologists have looked to the placenta as a major factor in the forces which initiate birth. It has been suggested that the placenta undergoes age changes as gestation proceeds. The principal morphologic age changes in the human placenta are the accumulation of fibrin and fibrinoid and the hyalinization of the syncytium (Figs. 25-24 and 25-25) (see review by Wislocki, 1956). However, it is not at all certain that these changes limit placental function. There is some evidence of waning physiologic activity near term, but on the whole it has been difficult to pinpoint the functional changes as being related to senescence. As fetal organs differentiate and acquire their characteristic functions, it is possible that the placenta may relinquish some of its activities. However, interrelations between placental differentiation and fetal differentiation remain for the most part undefined. The concept of the fetoplacental unit, which rests entirely, so far, on evidence related to steroid metabolism, is an important step in this direction. The "life-span" of the human placenta is normally less than 266 days. Thus the placenta provides an interesting model for studying differentiation, since kaleidoscopic changes in morphology, function, and chemical composition occur in a relatively short time.

Umbilical cord

The human umbilical cord is a translucent, glistening, white "rope" of tissue that is fetal in origin. It extends from the umbilicus to the placenta and reaches a length of 35 to 50 cm at term. It consists of two *umbilical arteries* and one *umbilical vein* embedded in an abundant mucous connective tissue (Fig. 25-30, see color insert). It is covered by an epithelium which is initially single-layered and becomes stratified late in gestation. In transverse sections, the arteries usually appear constricted, whereas the vein is generally open. The umbilical cord and its peculiar blood vessels usually exhibit torsion; there is an average of 11 spiral turns, but the number is proportional to the length of the cord. From the umbilicus to the placenta, the caliber of the blood vessels increases, but the vein normally remains larger than the arteries.

Mucous connective tissue is highly characteristic of the umbilical cord. In this specialized stroma, the ground substance is unusually abundant. This slippery, gelatinous material, rich in mucopolysaccharide, is also called *Wharton's jelly.* It fills the relatively large intercellular spaces that are located among the interlacing bundles of collagenous fibers. The intense metachromasia of Wharton's jelly suggests the presence of acid mucopolysaccharide (Fig. 25-30, see color insert). Collagen fibers are plentiful, but elastic and reticular fibers are rare or absent except in the umbilical vessels. The cells of this connective tissue are a primitive form of fibroblast, larger and more stellate than the fibroblasts of adult areolar tissue. In routine preparations, the outlines of these cells are difficult to recognize, and only their nuclei are evident. Like many other embryonic cells, they have a rich store of glycogen. Capillaries, lymphatic vessels, and nerves are absent from the human umbilical cord.

The *umbilical arteries* are peculiar in their structure. Their relatively thick muscular walls are heavily impregnated with metachromatic ground substance. Unlike muscular arteries elsewhere, they do not have an elastica interna. Instead, their walls contain a diffuse network of elastic fibers which is especially dense beneath the intima. The arteries have a thick muscular coat but there is lack of agreement about the arrangement and number of layers of smooth muscle fibers. There is no elastica externa, and the tunica adventitia is replaced by mucous connective tissue.

The wall of the *umbilical vein* is quite muscular, being composed of intermingled longitudinal, oblique, and circular smooth muscle fibers. Its elastic component is less conspicuous than that of the umbilical arteries; elastic fibers are limited to an elastica interna which is a primary feature used to distinguish the vein from the arteries. The smooth muscle cells of both umbilical arteries and vein are rich in glycogen. These fetal vessels are devoid of innervation and vasa vasorum.

The human umbilical cord is a derivative of the body stalk (Fig. 25-11), which is considered to be the homologue of the allantoic mesoderm. The endodermal component of the allantois extends the entire length of the cord as a slender epithelial tube. At birth, however, it is represented by only a strand of epithelial cells in the vicinity of the umbilicus. In addition, the stalk of the yolk sac, surrounded by an extension of the body cavity, occurs in the umbilical cord in early development. This stalk contains the endodermal vitelline duct and the vitelline vessels enclosed in a slender strand of mesoderm. The loop of intestine from which the yolk stalk originates may also extend into the cord; ordinarily it is retracted into the abdomen by the time of birth, but if not, umbilical hernia results. Usually the stalk of the yolk sac and its vitelline vessels, together with the coelom of the cord, have been obliterated some time before birth, so that no traces of them remain in the cord.

References

AHERNE, W., and M. S. DUNNILL: Morphometry of the Human Placenta, *Brit. Med. Bull.*, **22**:5 (1966).

AMOROSO, E. C.: Placentation, in A. S. Parkes (ed.), "Marshall's Physiology of Reproduction," vol. 2, chap. 15, Longmans, Green & Co., Inc., London, 1952.

BLANDAU, R. J. (ed.): "The Biology of the Blastocyst," The University of Chicago Press, Chicago, 1971.

BLANDAU, R. J.: Biology of Eggs and Implantation, in W. C. Young (ed.), "Sex and Internal Secretions," 3d ed., vol. 2, chap. 14, The Williams & Wilkins Company, Baltimore, 1961.

BOYD, J. D., and W. J. HAMILTON: "The Human Placenta," W. Heffer & Sons, Ltd., Cambridge, England, 1970.

CRAWFORD, J. M.: Vascular Anatomy of the Human Placenta, *Amer. J. Obstet. Gynec.*, **84**:1543 (1962).

DAWES, G. S.: "Foetal and Neonatal Physiology," Year Book Medical Publishers, Inc., Chicago, 1968.

DICZFALUSY, E.: Steroid Metabolism in the Foetal-Placental Unit, in A. Pecile and C. Finzi (eds.), "The Foeto-Placental Unit," Excerpta Medica Foundation, Amsterdam, 1969.

DRESKIN, R. B., S. S. SPICER, and W. B. GREENE: Ultrastructural Localization of Chronic Gonadotropin in Human Term Placenta, *J. Histochem. Cytochem.*, **18**:862 (1970).

ENDERS, A. C.: Fine Structure of Anchoring Villi of the Human Placenta, *Amer. J. Anat.*, **122**:419 (1968).

ENDERS, A. C.: Formation of the Syncytium from Cytotrophoblast in the Human Placenta, *Obstet. Gynec.*, **25**:378 (1965).

ENDERS, A. C., and B. F. KING: The Cytology of Hofbauer Cells, *Anat. Rec.*, **167**:231 (1970).

ENDERS, A. C., and S. J. SCHLAFKE: Cytological Aspects of Trophoblast-Uterine Interaction in Early Implantation, *Amer. J. Anat.*, **125**:1 (1969).

FREESE, U. E.: The Uteroplacental Vascular Relationship in the Human, *Amer. J. Obstet. Gynec.*, **101**:8 (1968).

GROSSER, O.: "Früenentwicklung, Eihautbildung und Plazentation des Menschen und der Saügetiere, Bergmann, Munich, 1927.

HAGERMAN, D. D., and C. A. VILLEE: Transport Functions of the Placenta, *Physiol. Rev.*, **40**:313 (1960).

HARRIS, J. W. S., and E. M. RAMSEY: The Morphology of Human Uteroplacental Vasculature, *Contrib. Embryology*, **38**:45 (1966).

HERTIG, A. T., J. ROCK, and E. C. ADAMS: A Description of 34 Human Ova within the First 17 Days of Development, *Amer. J. Anat.*, **98**:435 (1956).

LOBEL, B. L., H. W. DEANE, and S. L. ROMNEY: Enzymic Histochemistry of the Villous Portion of the Human Placenta from Six Weeks of Gestation to Term, *Amer. J. Obstet. Gynec.*, **83**:295 (1962).

MARTIN, C. B., JR., and E. M. RAMSEY: Gross Anatomy of the Placenta of Rhesus Monkeys, *Obstet. Gynec.*, **36**:167 (1970).

MIDGLEY, A. R., JR., G. B. PIERCE, JR., G. A. DENEAU, and J. R. G. GOSLING: Morphogenesis of Syncytiotrophoblast in Vivo: an Autoradiographic Demonstration, *Science*, **141**:349 (1963).

MOSSMAN, H. W.: Comparative Morphogenesis of the Foetal Membranes and Accessory Uterine Structures, *Carnegie Inst. Contrib. Embryol.*, **26**:129 (1937).

RAMSEY, E. M.: Placental Vasculature and Circulation, in R. O. Greep (ed.), "Handbook of Physiology," vol. 00, sec. 00, chap. 00, American Physiological Society, Washington, D.C., 1972.

REYNOLDS, S. R. M.: Formation of Fetal Cotyledons in the Hemochorial Placenta. A Theoretical Consideration of the Functional Implications of Such an Arrangement, *Amer. J. Obstet. Gynec.,* **94:**425 (1966).

THIEDE, H. A., and J. W. CHOATE: Chorionic Gonadotropin Localization in the Human Placenta by Immunofluorescent Staining. II. Demonstration of HCG in the Trophoblast and Amnion Epithelium of Immature and Mature Placentas, *Obstet. Gynec.,* **22:**433 (1963).

VILLEE, D. B.: Development of Endocrine Function in the Human Placenta and Fetus, *New Eng. J. Med.,* **281:**473 (1969).

WILKIN, P.: Morphogenese, in J. Snoeck (ed.), "Le Placenta humain—Aspects morphologiques et fonctionnels," pp. 23–70, Masson, et al, Paris, 1958.

WISLOCKI, G. B.: Morphological Aspects of Ageing in the Placenta, *Ciba Found. Colloq. Ageing,* **2:**105 (1956).

WISLOCKI, G. B., and H. S. BENNETT: Histology and Cytology of the Human and Monkey Placenta, with Special Reference to the Trophoblast, *Amer. J. Anat.,* **73:**335 (1943).

WISLOCKI, G. B., and H. A. PADYKULA: Histochemistry and Electron Microscopy of the Placenta, in W. C. Young (ed.), "Sex and Internal Secretions," 3d ed., vol. 2, chap. 15, The Williams & Wilkins Company, Baltimore, 1961.

WYNN, R. M.: Morphology of the Placenta, in N. S. Assali (ed.), "Biology of Gestation," vol. 1, pp. 94–184, Academic Press, Inc., New York, 1968.

chapter 26   The male reproductive system

AARON J. LADMAN

The male reproductive system consists of primary sex organs, the two *testes,* and a set of accessory sexual structures. The testes form the male sex cells, *spermatozoa,* and also secrete a hormone, *testosterone,* which is responsible for the growth and function of the accessory male sex organs and for the development of other attributes of masculinity, such as beard, deep voice, and strong musculature. The accessory sexual organs comprise the excretory ducts in which spermatozoa are matured and prepared for discharge, an associated group of glands that contribute fluid secretions to the semen, and the *penis*. The general arrangement of the structures of the male reproductive system is shown schematically in Fig. 26-1.

Testis

The testis is an ovoid body lying in the scrotum. It communicates with the urethra by means of an excurrent duct system. The testis is covered by a tough, compact, fibrous coat, the *tunica albuginea* (Fig. 26-2), composed of collagenous connective tissue with an admixture of elastic fibers. There is a thin layer of squamous cells on the outer surface of this coat, which is the mesothelial lining of the scrotal sac reflected over the testis. The inner surface of the tunica albuginea is less dense and contains numerous blood vessels, the *tunica vasculosa*. At the posterocephalic margin of the testis, the tunic thickens to form the *mediastinum testis*. Ducts, blood vessels, and nerves enter or leave the testis through the mediastinum.

From the mediastinum delicate connective tissue septula, carrying small vessels, radiate into the testis, dividing it into about 250 lobules (Fig. 26-2).

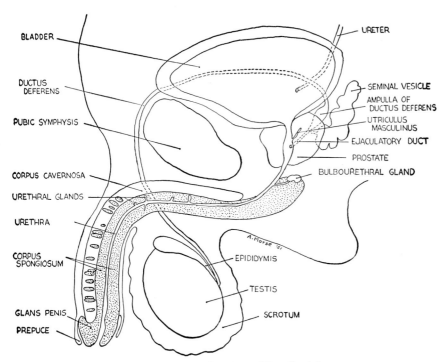

Figure 26-1   Male reproductive organs, median view.   (After Eberth.)

VASCULAR AND NERVOUS CONNECTIONS TO THE TESTIS

It is a distinctive feature of mammals that the testicular artery becomes highly convoluted as it approaches the testis and is surrounded by the venous *pampiniform plexus,* a thermoregulatory device for preheating or precooling the blood.   Some branches of the testicular artery enter the testis through the mediastinum, whereas others pass over the periphery of the testis in the tunica vasculosa. Arterioles enter the septula both from the mediastinum and from the periphery.   Branches leave the septula and form capillary plexuses around the convoluted tubules.   Veins accompany the arteries.   Lymphatic vessels are numerous in the tunica albuginea and extend along the tubules.   The testes have both a vasomotor and a sensory innervation. Nerves from the spermatic plexus form a net in the deeper part of the tunica albuginea and from there reach the walls of the tubules and the Leydig cells.

SEMINIFEROUS TUBULE

Each testicular lobule contains one to three greatly convoluted, sperm-producing *seminiferous tubules.*   These are mostly arches (Fig. 26-3) which connect at each end with a space in the mediastinum, the *rete testis* (Fig. 26-2)—a portion of the excurrent duct system.   Anastomoses and branching of the tubules are common in man.   Rarely, a tubule may terminate blindly at one end.   The seminiferous tubules derive from and preserve the fundamental pattern of the sex cords of the embryonic testis.   Uncoiled, the seminiferous tubules measure up to 80 cm in length and are only 150 to 250 μm in width.   In man the combined length of the seminiferous tubules in one testis is approximately 255 meters.   They are ensheathed by a heavy basement membrane composed of lamellae of collagenous fibers and an interlamellar space of varying size occupied by one or more layers of flattened cells (Fig. 26-4).   These cells contain many extremely fine cytoplasmic filaments which are believed to be contractile. In histologic sections of testis, the conspicuous structural elements are the convoluted tubules (Fig. 26-5), which will have been cut in many different planes. The lumina of the tubules are usually filled with free sperm or the tails of sperm that are still attached to supporting cells of Sertoli in the wall of the tubule. The intertubular spaces are filled with loose connective tissue with some elastic fibers and the cells of Leydig (see below).

SEMINIFEROUS EPITHELIUM

The seminiferous tubules are lined by a highly specialized stratified epithelium, termed the *seminiferous* or *germinal epithelium*. The cells touching the basement membrane are of two types, *spermatogonia* and Sertoli cells. The seminiferous epithelium proliferates from the spermatogonia and is composed of a succession of different generations of cells arranged in ill-defined, concentric layers (Figs. 26-5 and 26-6). These include, from the periphery to the lumen of the tubule, *spermato-*

Figure 26-2   Transverse section of the testis of an adult man.   ×4.   (Von Möllendorff.)

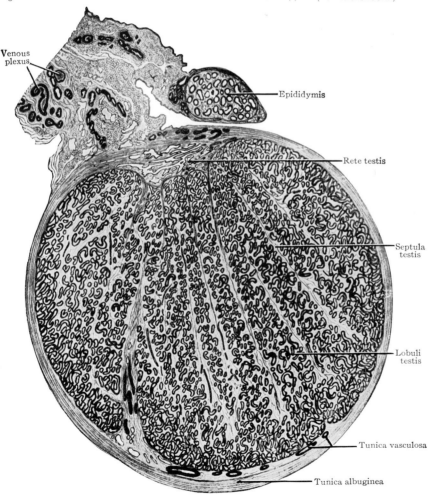

Venous plexus

Epididymis

Rete testis

Septula testis

Lobuli testis

Tunica vasculosa

Tunica albuginea

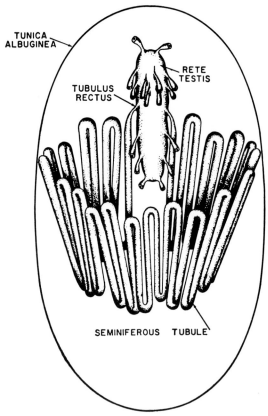

TUNICA
ALBUGINEA

TUBULUS
RECTUS

RETE
TESTIS

SEMINIFEROUS   TUBULE

Figure 26-3 Diagrammatic representation of the arched nature and the connections of a seminiferous tubule with the rete testis in an adult rat. (From Figure 13, Y. Clermont and C. Huckins, Amer. J. Anat., **108**:87, 1961.)

gonia, spermatocytes (primary and secondary, but the latter are not always found because they divide soon after formation), spermatids, and spermatozoa. In transverse sections of the tubules in most mammals, the cells of any given generation are all at a uniform stage of cell division or differentiation and are disposed around the entire circumference of the tubule. In man, however, cells at an identical stage in spermatogenesis may occupy only part of the circumference of the tubule (Fig. 26-22).

Spermatogonia Spermatogonia are 12 μm in diameter and constitute a high proportion of the cells bordering on the limiting membrane of the seminiferous tubule. Being a primitive type of cell, they

have no specialized features and few distinguishing characteristics. The nuclei are round or slightly ovoid, approximately 6 to 7 μm in diameter, with granular chromatin and one or more large vacuolar spaces rich in glycogen (Figs. 26-6 and 26-7). Nucleoli are usually attached to the nuclear membrane. The cytoplasm stains lightly, has a faint, granular texture, and may possess a crystal of Lubarsch approximately 1.0 × 7.0 μm. This inclusion is composed of closely packed parallel arrays of dense filaments interspersed with dense granules (Sohval et al., 1971) (Fig. 26-8). All spermatogonia have the diploid number of chromosomes and divide only by mitosis.

The mechanism whereby spermatogonia differentiate and yet continue to renew their source has recently been clarified. From a given mitosis both daughter spermatogonia are destined either to differentiate or to remain as part of the stock of primitive spermatogonia termed the stem cells. In man and most other species studied, these two categories of spermatogonia, often designated as type A (stem cells) and type B (derivative cells), can be recognized by special staining. Two subcategories of type A spermatogonia based on nuclear staining have been described in man. These are termed pale (Ap) and dark (Ad) (Fig. 26-7). In rodents, further subdivisions of the stages of spermatogonial differentiation have been described (Huckins and Oakberg, 1971). Type A spermatogonia undergo mitosis to perpetuate themselves as well as to differentiate into type B cells (Fig. 26-7). Type B cells can divide by mitosis several times before they differentiate into spermatocytes. A single stem cell may divide into as many as 16 primary spermatocytes (Huckins and Oakberg, 1971). Since cytoplasmic bridges are present in spermatogonia (Fig. 26-9) and persist until the formation of spermatozoa (Fig. 26-10), a cytoplasmic syncytium encompassing 64 or more spermatozoa may have a common stem cell progenitor. What initiates stem cell differentiation remains an intriguing problem for research.

Primary spermatocytes As a result of the last mitotic division of type B spermatogonia, primary spermatocytes form and immediately go into an interphase or resting stage. They are easily distinguished by their large size (18 μm) and prominent nuclei with evenly distributed fine chromatin granules (Figs. 26-5 and 26-6). They are located immediately central to the spermatogonia and seldom touch the limiting membrane. They divide only once; this is a meiotic division which reduces the number of chromosomes to the haploid condition. The lengthy prophase of this meiotic division, preceded by a duplication of the DNA, involves extensive rearrangements of the chromatin threads. The nuclei progress through the leptotene, zygotene, pachytene, and diplotene steps to diakinesis (see *meiosis,* (Chap. 1).

Secondary spermatocytes These cells have a diameter of 12 μm and arise from primary spermatocytes after the first meiotic division. Following a brief interphase stage, they proceed through the second meiotic division to yield haploid spermatids. The nucleus of a resting secondary spermatocyte is approximately 7 μm and can be distinguished from a primary spermatocyte and early spermatid on the basis of size, round shape, central position, and deeply staining chromatin, and a few large chromophilic globules (Figs. 26-5 to 26-7). Because secondary spermatocytes differentiate

Figure 26-4   Section of a human seminiferous tubule, showing the myoid nature of the cytoplasmic filaments within the surrounding connective tissue cells. Approximately ×20,000. (Courtesy of M. H. Ross.)

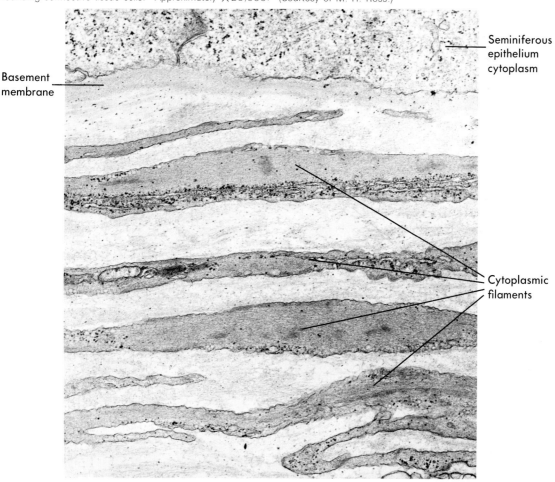

Basement membrane

Seminiferous epithelium cytoplasm

Cytoplasmic filaments

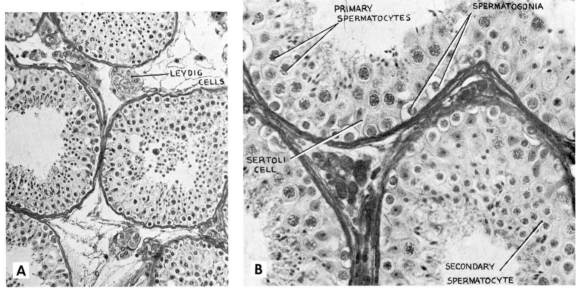

Figure 26-5 Sections of normal human testes. A. Testis of a man aged 26. ×160. B. Testis of a man aged 34. Sperm count 120 million per ml. All stages of spermatogenesis are shown. ×360. (Courtesy of W. O. Nelson.)

quickly, they are only rarely seen in sectioned material.

Spermatids Spermatids are about 8 μm in diameter. They border on the lumen and, in all except the earliest forms, their nuclei are located eccentrically (Fig. 26-6). The nucleus undergoes an elongation and an apparent reduction in size during the transformation of spermatids into spermatozoa (see later). Intercellular bridges (Fig. 26-10) linking many spermatids provide evidence that cytokinesis of differentiating spermatid precursors has been incomplete. The appearance of spermatids grouped in clusters of 8 or 16 adds further support to this view (Huckins and Oakberg, 1971).

Spermiogenesis The term *spermiogensis* refers specifically to the morphologic transformation of

spermatids into spermatozoa (Fig. 26-11). The major features of this process involve elaboration of a nuclear cap from the Golgi apparatus, condensation of the nucleus, formation of a motile flagellum, and extensive shedding of cytoplasm.

These changes begin by eccentric displacement of the nucleus and the appearance of a localized grouping of Golgi membranes, often into a concentric configuration. The Golgi apparatus elaborates an acrosomal system composed of a single membrane-enclosed vesicle, the *acrosomal vesicle,* containing a single large granule, the *acrosome* (Fig. 26-12). The vesicle and granule continue to enlarge through further vacuolar contributions from the surrounding Golgi substance. The acrosomal system becomes applied to the nucleus, and the position of the acrosome establishes the anterior pole of the spermatid. The cytoplasm shifts cau-

Figure 26-6 The six ''cellular associations'' in the human seminiferous epithelium. Each of these combinations of cells corresponds to a stage of the cycle of the seminiferous epithelium. Ser, Sertoli cell; Ad and Ap, dark and pale type A spermatogonia; B, type B spermatogonia; R, resting primary spermatocyte; L, leptotene spermatocyte; Z, zygotene spermatocyte; P, pachytene spermatocyte; Di, diplotene spermatocyte; Sptc-Im, primary spermatocyte in division; Sptc-II, secondary spermatocyte in interphase; Sa, Sb₁, Sb₂, Sc, Sd₁, Sd₂, spermatids at various steps of spermatogenesis. (Courtesy of C. G. Heller and Y. Clermont.)

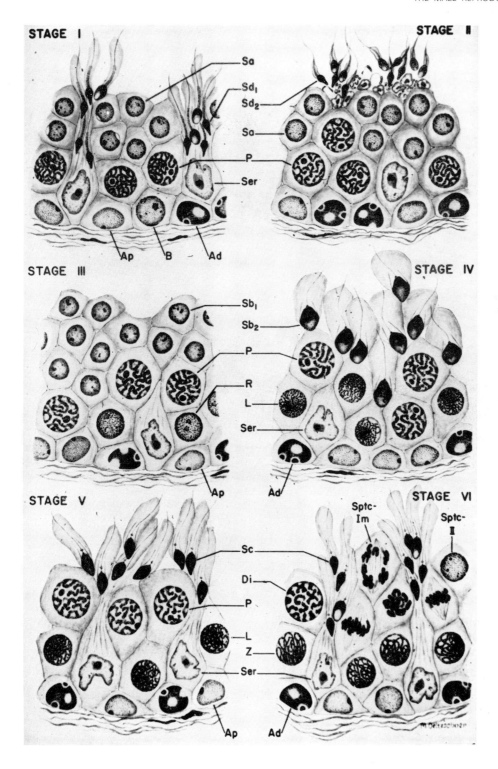

STAGE I

STAGE II

Sa
Sd₁
Sd₂
Sa
P
Ser
Ap   B   Ad

STAGE III

STAGE IV

Sb₁
Sb₂
P
R
L
Ser
Ap
Ad

STAGE V

STAGE VI

Sptc-Im
Sptc-II
Sc
Di
P
L
Z
Ser
Ap   Ad

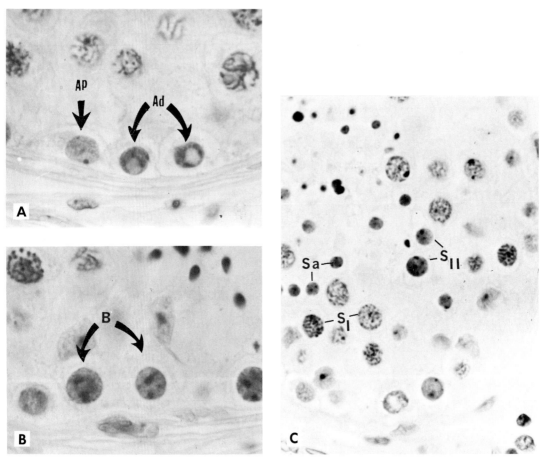

Figure 26-7 Sections of human seminiferous epithelium, illustrating various cell types. A. Two types of spermatogonia, the Ap (with pale nucleus) and the Ad (with dark nucleus containing a clear vacuole). ×1,200. B. Type B spermatogonia is larger than type A, and more than one nucleolus may be present. ×1,200. C. Two classes of spermatocytes, the primary spermatocytes, S_I, in various stages of the first meiotic division, secondary spermatocytes, S_{II}, positioned closer to the lumen and of smaller size, and the spermatids, Sa, of still smaller nuclear and overall cell size. ×800. (Courtesy of M. J. Rowley et al.)

dally, carrying with it the acrosomal vesicle, which collapses over the anterior two-thirds of the nucleus to form a double-layered *head cap* (Figs. 26-13 and 26-14). In most mammals studied, the acrosome remains as a dense structure at the anterior pole of the nucleus, and in different species it exhibits extreme variation in size and shape. In man it flattens out and loses its identity as a discrete structure before spermiogenesis is complete.

Information concerning the development of the acrosomal system has been greatly aided by the fact that the acrosome and head cap are prominently stained by the PAS reaction. Clermont and Leblond (1955) subdivided spermiogenesis into a series of steps based on this staining. Six such steps are found in man (Fig. 26-6).

While the acrosome and head cap are being elaborated, two cylindrical centrioles situated at right angles to each other move from a position near the nucleus to the periphery of the cell opposite the forming acrosome. Formation of the axial filaments of the tail is initiated by the distal centriole. The centrioles move back to the nucleus along the long axis of the cell without interrupting the formation of the filamentous core of the tail. The proximal centriole, a rosette of nine sets of three tubules each (Figs. 26-15 and 26-16), attaches itself to the caudal pole of the nucleus while the distal centriole continues to elaborate the flagellum. As the cytoplasm shifts caudad, mitochondria gather end to end and arrange themselves spirally about the proximal portion of the tail filament, forming the *mitochondrial sheath* of the middle piece (Figs. 26-16 and 26-17).

As spermiogenesis proceeds, the nuclei begin to elongate, the Feulgen-positive granules (DNA) become uniform in size and evenly dispersed, except for some clear spaces. These "vacuoles" disappear, and in the final stages the nuclei assume a homogeneous appearance and stain deeply. The extra cytoplasm of this late spermatid is later shed and appears in the lumen of the tubes as anucleate masses, termed *residual bodies* (Fig. 26-11). The RNA of the residual bodies condenses so that they stain with uniform intensity.

Spermatozoa The human *spermatozoon* has a head and a tail and is approximately 60 μm long. Segments of the tail, in order of their proximity to the head, are designated the *middle piece, principal piece,* and *end piece* (Figs. 26-15 to 26-17). The middle piece, a segment about 5 to 7 μm long and a little over 1 μm thick, contains, in addition to the proximal portion of the tail filament, the mitochondrial sheath (Figs. 26-16 and 26-17) and next to the nucleus a "neck" region comprising two elongate centrioles at right angles to each other. The principal piece forms the main portion of the flagel-

Figure 26-8 Crystal of Lubarsch (arrow) in a type A spermatogonium. The spermatogonium rests on a double basement lamina (BL) and is surrounded by Sertoli cell cytoplasm containing lipid droplets (Lip). ×7,100. (From A. Sohval et al., J. Ultrastruct. Res., **34**:83–102, 1971.)

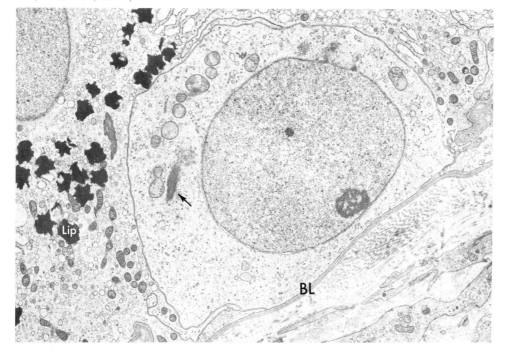

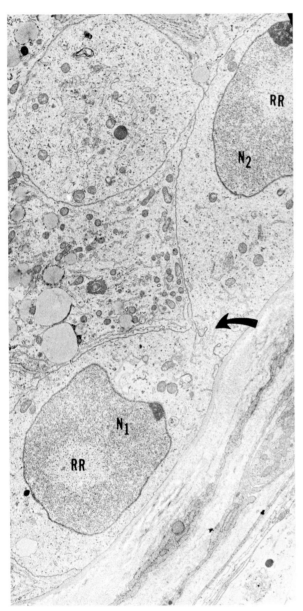

Figure 26-9   Normal human testis.   Two Ad (dark) spermatogonia (N_1 and N_2) connected by an intercellular bridge (arrow).   RR are areas of rarefaction which correspond to the vacuole seen by light microscopy.   ×6,100.   (Courtesy of M. J. Rowley and C. G. Heller.)

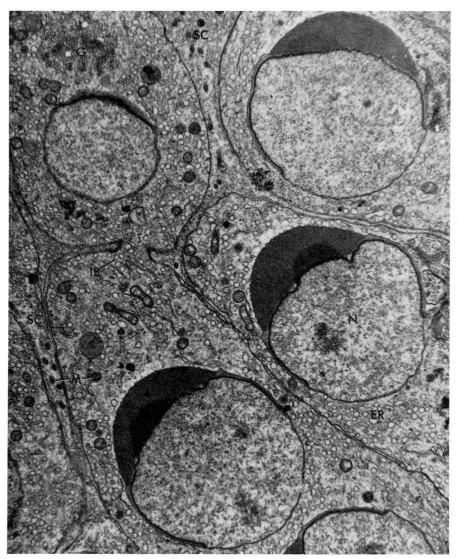

Figure 26-10   Electron micrograph of seminiferous epithelium of a guinea pig, showing early spermatids linked syncytially by an intercellular bridge (IB).   Note also portions of Sertoli cells (SC), acrosome, Golgi complex (G), and endoplasmic reticulum (ER). The mitochondria (M) in the Sertoli cells are smaller and more dense than those of the germinal cells.   ×8,000.   (Courtesy of D. W. Fawcett and S. Ito.)

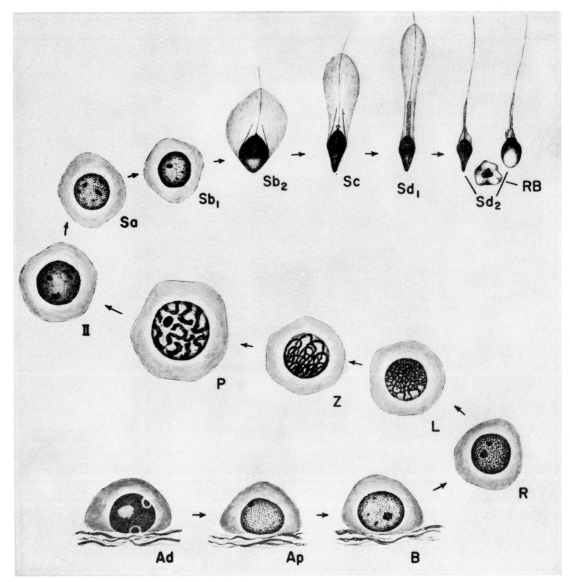

Figure 26-11 Drawing showing the evolution of spermatozoa in man. Labels same as in Figure 26-6. RB, residual body. (Courtesy of C. G. Heller and Y. Clermont.)

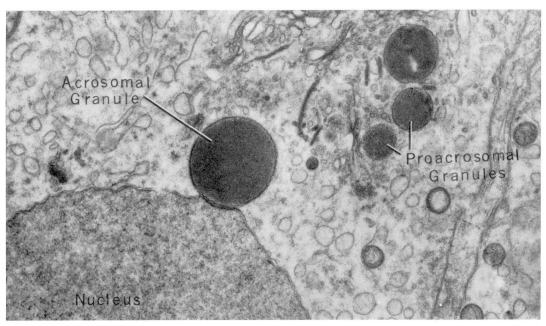

Figure 26-12 Electron micrograph showing an early stage in the formation of the acrosomal system of a guinea pig. Proacrosome in the Golgi substance. The membrane-bounded acrosomal granule has already taken up a position on, and established the anterior pole of, the nucleus. ×16,000. (Courtesy of D. W. Fawcett and R. D. Hollenberg.)

Figure 26-13 Spermatid showing the acrosomal vesicle and enclosed denser granules in a guinea pig. ×16,000. (Courtesy of D. W. Fawcett and R. D. Hollenberg.)

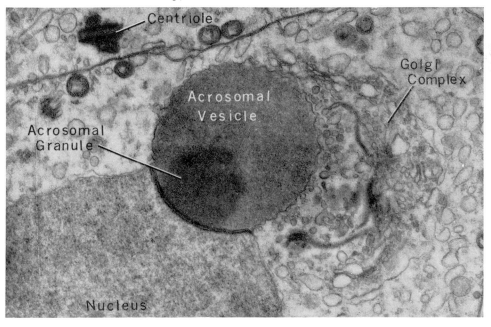

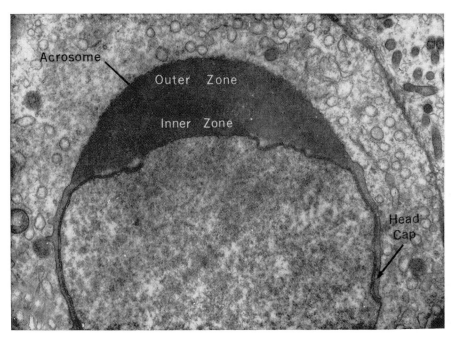

Figure 26-14   Acrosome spreading over the anterior pole of the spermatid nucleus to form the head cap in a guinea pig.   The Golgi complex has moved from this region, and enlargement of the acrosome has ceased.   (Courtesy of D. W. Fawcett and R. D. Hollenberg.)

lum and is about 45 μm in length.   The filamentous core is enclosed in a sheath composed of *circumferential fibers* (Fig. 26-17).   These are semicircular in shape and end on opposite sides of the principal piece in two *longitudinal columns,* which are thickenings of the sheath that extend the length of the principal piece.   The circumferential fibers branch and anastomose.   The end piece is simply the terminal segment (5 μm) of the flagellum, in which the central filamentous complex is bare (Figs. 26-15 and 26-17).

Transverse sections of the sperm tail show that it is organized in basically the same "9 + 2" pattern as that of motile cilia or flagella throughout the animal kingdom.   The axial filament consists of 20 microtubules arranged in nine peripheral pairs and one central pair (Fig. 26-17).   In the middle piece and proximal portion of the principal piece there is an additional and more peripheral set of nine coarse fibers, which are usually of uneven size.   Although these additional fibers are presumed

to aid motility, our knowledge concerning their nature or function is still incomplete.

Sertoli cells   The Sertoli cells are columnar cells which extend through the seminiferous epithelium and touch on the basement membrane.   In mature testes the Sertoli cells are much fewer in number than germinal cells and are spaced quite regularly along the tubules (Figs. 26-5, 26-6, and 26-18).   The principal distinguishing histologic features of the Sertoli cells concern the nucleus, which has a polymorphous shape, a folded nuclear membrane, and a prominent, large nucleolus that stains unevenly (Figs. 26-18B and 26-19).   The nucleolus has an eosinophilic central core and an irregular basophilic rim.   The cytoplasm contains many fibrils, filamentous mitochondria, lipid droplets, granules staining with iron hematoxylin, glycogen, and, in man only, a slender crystalloid of Charcot-Böttcher (Fig. 26-19).   The Sertoli cells do not normally undergo mitosis.

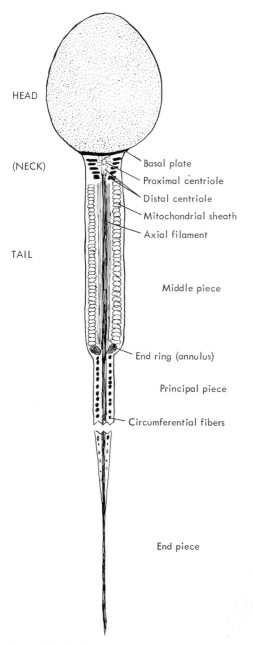

HEAD

(NECK) — Basal plate
— Proximal centriole
— Distal centriole
— Mitochondrial sheath
— Axial filament

TAIL

Middle piece

— End ring (annulus)

Principal piece

— Circumferential fibers

End piece

Figure 26-15 Diagram of a mature human spermatozoon.

Spermatids appear to embed themselves in Sertoli cell cytoplasm in great numbers (Figs. 26-6 and 26-20). It is thought that the Sertoli cells provide food for them; this view is based on the variation in quantity and distribution of glycogen and lipid in Sertoli cells during spermatogenic activity, indicating that sperm may consume these substances. Any condition which interferes with spermatogenesis results in a marked accumulation of lipid in Sertoli cells. Some cases of infertility may be related to Sertoli cell dysfunction and the resultant failure of spermatozoa to mature normally. The electron microscope has shown that spermatids are separated from Sertoli cell cytoplasm by a continuous space between adjacent plasma membranes (Fig. 26-20). Recent studies have revealed that the Sertoli cell forms part of the blood-testis barrier which keeps certain macromolecules from gaining access to the lumen of the seminiferous tubule and to those spermatogenic elements whose processes have an intimate contact with the lumen (Fig. 26-20).

The Sertoli cells are very resistant to noxious agents and the aging process. In experimental animals, such conditions as cryptorchidism and toxic debilitation may result in a near-total loss of germinal epithelium with virtually no effect on Sertoli cells (Fig. 26-18). Hypophysectomy results in a reduction of the seminiferous epithelium to one or two layers of cells, nearly all of which are Sertoli cells. The nuclei of Sertoli cells undergo marked changes at puberty, suggesting that they are subject to androgen control.

SPERMATOGENESIS

The term *spermatogenesis* refers to the process whereby spermatozoa evolve from spermatogonia.

The cycle of the seminiferous epithelium Examination of the seminiferous epithelium in rodents reveals the repeated occurrence of combinations of cells in certain steps in the formation of the different generations of germ cells. For instance, spermatids at a given step in spermiogenesis occur only in combination with spermatogonia and primary and secondary spermatocytes at a particular step in development. These groupings of cell types, termed *cellular associations*, are of fixed composi-

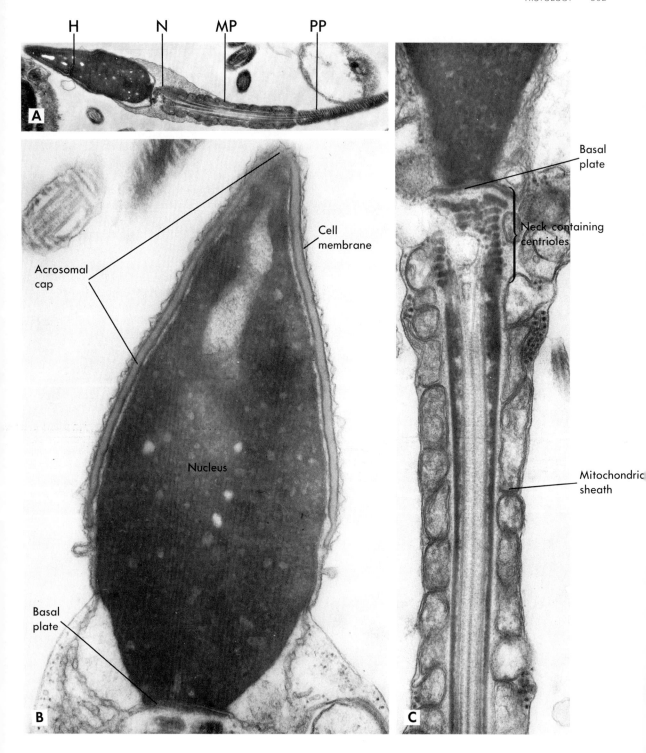

H   N   MP   PP

A

Acrosomal cap

Cell membrane

Nucleus

Basal plate

B

Basal plate

Neck containing centrioles

Mitochondrial sheath

C

Middle piece   Principal piece   End piece

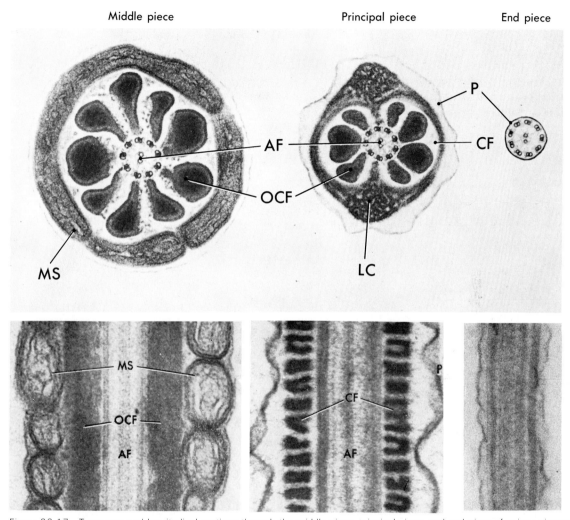

Figure 26-17   Transverse and longitudinal sections through the middle piece, principal piece, and end piece of guinea pig spermatozoa.   The internal core of the middle piece consists of a central pair of fibers, the axial filament (AF), surrounded by nine
peripheral pairs of fibers and nine outer coarse fibers (OCF).   MS, mitochondrial sheath.   In the principal piece, the circumferential fibers (CF) of the sheath are continuous with the opposed longitudinal columns (LC).   P, plasmalemma.   All similar magnifications.   (Courtesy of D. W. Fawcett.)

Figure 26-16   Ejaculated human sperm.   A. H, head; N, neck; MP, middle piece; and PP, principal piece are seen.   ×7,500.
B. Details of the head include the plasma membrane, acrosomal cap, nucleus, and basal plate.   ×37,500.   C. Elements of the
neck and middle piece regions are clearly shown.   ×36,500 (Courtesy of Dr. L. Zamboni.)

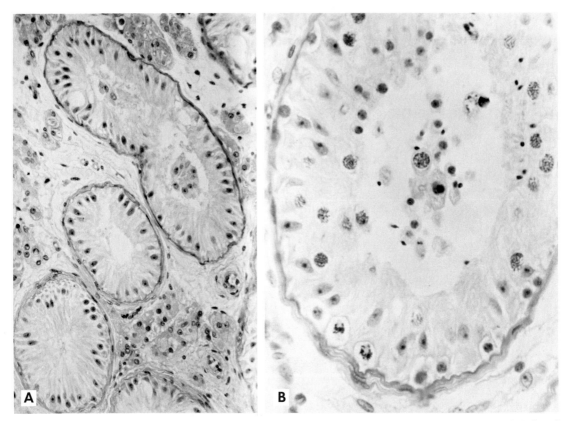

Figure 26-18 Biopsy samples of human testis. A. 42 weeks following 600-rads testicular x-ray radiation. Only Sertoli cells line the seminiferous tubules. ×160. B. Recovery beginning 2 years after 100-rads testicular x-ray irradiation. Various stages in the spermatogenic cycle can now be identified. ×400. (Courtesy of M. J. Rowley and C. G. Heller.)

tion, and they appear in a fixed sequence. Thus each recognized cell grouping represents a stage in a cyclic process, and the series of successive stages occurring between two appearances of the same cellular association is defined as the *cycle of the seminiferous epithelium*. The number of such stages in a cycle is constant for any given species; the rat has 14, the guinea pig 12, and man 6 (Fig. 26-6); the stages are designated by Roman numerals. If it were possible to examine in the living state the cut end of a seminiferous tubule of the rat, all 14 stages would occur in succession and the series (cycle) would repeat itself time after time. Although each cycle involves the differentiation of a new crop of spermatogonia and the liberation of a new crop of spermatozoa, the span of spermatogenesis involves several cycles, usually four to five.

The stages are of unequal duration, some lasting only a few hours whereas others take days, but the duration of any given stage and of the complete cycle is constant for a given species.

The wave of the seminiferous epithelium In most mammals examined, except man, a given cellular association occupies a length or segment of the seminiferous tubules. Each such segment corresponds to a stage of the cycle of the seminiferous epithelium and is numbered accordingly. The segments are disposed along the tubule in consecutive

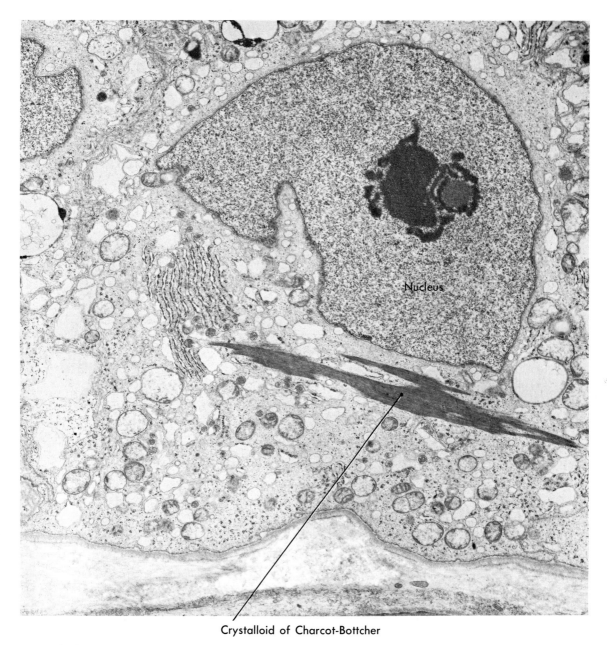

Crystalloid of Charcot-Bottcher

Nucleus

Figure 26-19   Human Sertoli cell showing a slender cytoplasmic crystalloid of Charcot-Böttcher.   ×10,000.   (Courtesy of M. J. Rowley.)

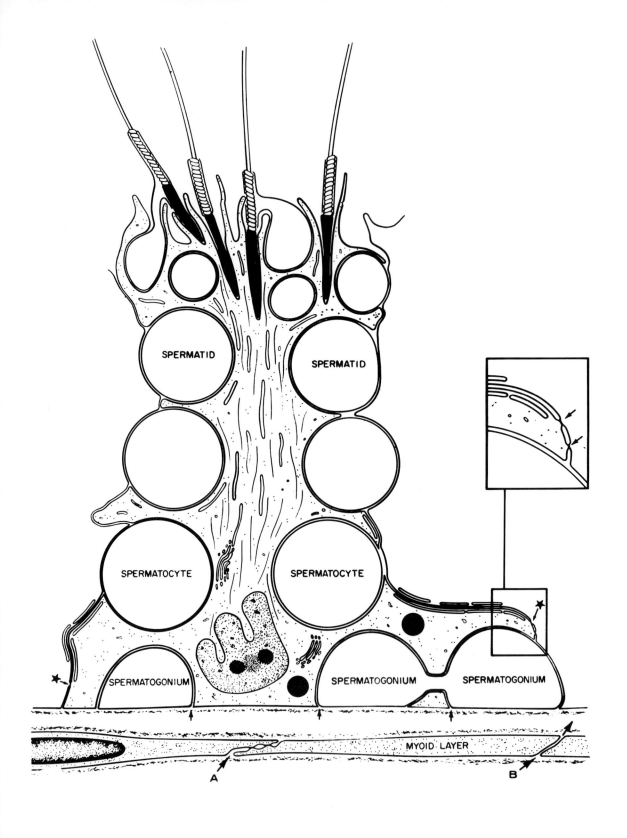

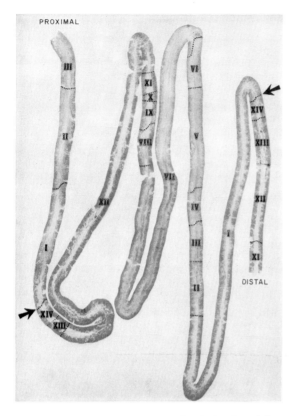

PROXIMAL

DISTAL

Figure 26-21 Longitudinal section of an isolated seminiferous tubule of rat testis, showing a wave of the seminiferous epithelium. Fourteen segments representing the 14 stages of the cycle of the seminiferous epithelium are arranged in continuous numerical and distally descending order to form a so-called wave. The limits of the wave are indicated by arrows. Note the difference in lengths of the several segments and the variability in length of segments of a given type (compare segments I, II, and XII). (From Fig. 7, B. Perey, Y. Clermont, and C. P. Leblond, Amer. J. Anat., **108**:55, 1961.)

order to form what is termed, somewhat inaccurately, a *wave of the seminiferous epithelium* (Fig. 26-21). Each wave consists of the complete series of segments representing the recognized cellular associations for that species. The segments are disposed distally along the seminiferous tubule in descending order and form a continuous succession of waves. Rats, for example, show an average of 12 waves per tubule. The descending order of the sequence of segments applies to both limbs of the tubular arches, reading distally from the rete testis (see below). The continuous successions of waves in each limb meet distally near the midpoint of the arch. At this point, designated the *site of reversal,* the order of the sequence of segments reverses. The reversal is due to the shift in the direction of progression from distal to proximal along the tubule. At points where the seminiferous tubules branch, the continuity of the descending order is not broken.

In distinguishing between waves and cycles of the seminiferous epithelium, it is important to bear in mind that the cycle refers to changes taking place over a period of time at a given point along the seminiferous tubule, whereas the wave refers to the distribution of different cellular associations along the tubule at any given time.

The average length of each tubular segment correlates roughly with the *relative* duration of the corresponding cellular association or stage of the cycle. In rats, the several segments in a wave vary in average lengths from 0.4 to 3.2 mm, and the stages they represent vary from 6 to 62.8 hr. However, according to Perey, Clermont, and Leblond (1961), there is no strict proportionality between segmental length and duration of the

Figure 26-20 Diagram depicting the localization of the blood-testis barrier and the compartmentalization of the germinal epithelium by tight junctions between adjacent Sertoli cells. Note the germ cells and their relationship to a columnar Sertoli cell. The primary barrier to substances penetrating from the interstitium is the myoid layer. The majority of cell junctions in this layer are closed by a tight apposition of membranes as indicated at A. Over a small fraction of the tubule surface, the myoid junctions exhibit a 200-Å-wide interspace and are therefore open as depicted at B. Material gaining access to the base of the epithelium by passing through open junctions in the myoid layer is free to enter the intercellular gap between the spermatogonia and the Sertoli cells. Deeper penetration is prevented by occluding junctions (stars) on the Sertoli-Sertoli boundaries. These tight junctions constitute a second and more effective component of the blood-testis barrier. In effect, the Sertoli cells and their tight junctions delimit a *basal* compartment in the germinal epithelium, containing the spermatogonia and early preleptotene spermatocytes, and an *adluminal* compartment, containing the spermatocytes and spermatids. Substances traversing open junctions in the myoid cell layer have direct access to cells in the basal compartment, but to reach the cells in the adluminal compartment, substances must pass through the Sertoli cells. (From M. Dym and D. W. Fawcett, Biol. Reprod. **3**:308–326, 1971.)

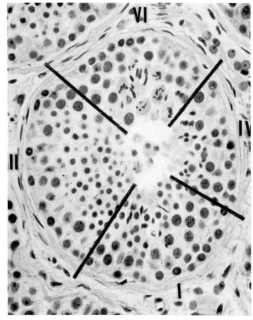

stages of the cycle. For example, in rats, segment VI has a length equal to about 2 percent of the wave, whereas the duration of stage VI is 9.2 percent of the cycle. The lengths of segments and of waves vary considerably but the duration of stages and of cycles is constant.

In man the segments are not sharply demarcated and form a mosaic in which each segment involves only a portion of the circumference of the tubule (Figs. 26-22 and 26-23). Man, therefore, does not exhibit a wave of the seminiferous epithelium. However, it is believed that the fundamental pattern of the cycle of the seminiferous epithelium is as characteristic of man as of other mammalian species.

Duration of spermatogenesis By studying the fate of radio-labeled germ cells in man, Heller and Clermont have determined that the cycle lasts 16 days ($\pm$1 day) (Fig. 26-24) and that the process of spermatogenesis extends over approximately four cycles (Fig. 26-25) for a duration of close to 64 days. Since hormone treatment has failed to alter the time period of either the cycle of the seminiferous epithelium or of spermatogenesis as a whole, these processes may be regarded as biologic constants.

Figure 26-22 Photomicrograph showing in a single cross section of a seminiferous tubule of man four different and well-demarcated stages of the cycle of the seminiferous epithelium. ×40. (From Fig. 16, Y. Clermont, Amer. J. Anat., **112**:50, 1963.)

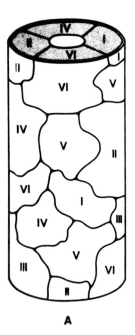

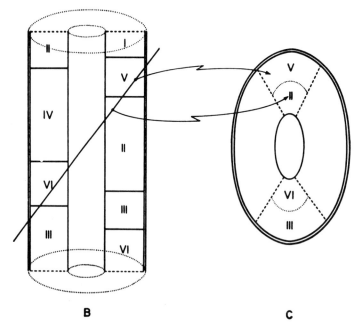

A   B   C

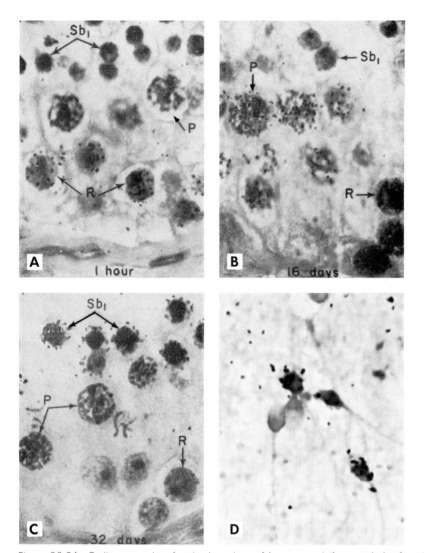

Figure 26-24   Radioautographs of stained sections of human seminiferous tubules from biopsies collected at 1 hr (A) and at 16 days (B) and 32 days (C) after a single injection of [³H] thymidine.   R, resting spermatocyte; P, pachytene spermatocyte; Sb_1 is a step in spermiogenesis.   At 1 hr (A), the labeled material is in the resting primary spermatocytes; at 16 days (B) it is in the pachytene primary spermatocytes; at 32 days, it is in early spermatids.   Labeled sperm (D) appear in the ejaculate 58 days after thymidine administration.   A, B, and C are at ×1,000 (courtesy of C. G. Heller and Y. Clermont); D is at ×1,350 (courtesy of M. J. Rowley, F. Teshima, and C. G. Heller).

Figure 26-23   Diagrammatic representation of a portion of a seminiferous tubule of man in (A) whole mount, (B) longitudinal section, and (C) oblique section, showing the random and mosaic-type distribution of areas occupied by six different cellular associations (that is, stages I to VI).   In oblique sections, dual or incomplete cell associations may appear in any given area along the wall of the tubule.   (Courtesy of C. G. Heller and Y. Clermont.)

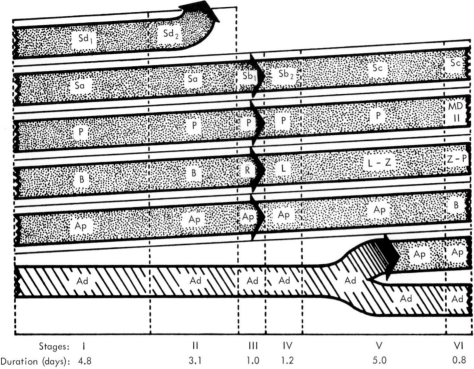

Figure 26-25   Diagrammatic representation of the assessed duration of spermatogenesis in man.   The composition of the six cellular associations or stages of the cycle is shown by letters.   The stippled bands represent the number of cycles which occur in spermatogenesis.   The bottom and top arrows represent the start and end of spermatogenesis; the other arrows show the direction of cellular development.   The width of the stages is proportional to their duration.   Spermatogenesis extends over 4 cycles for a total of approximately 64 days.   Ad, spermatogonia with dark nucleus.   Ap, spermatogonia with light nucleus.   B, type B spermatogonia; R, resting primary spermatocyte; L, leptotene spermatocyte; Z, zygotene spermatocyte; P, pachytene spermatocyte; MD, maturation division; II, secondary spermatocyte; Sa, Sb, Sc, Sd, Sd_2, spermatids at various steps of spermatogenesis.   (Courtesy of C. G. Heller and Y. Clermont.)

INTERSTITIAL CELLS
(CELLS OF LEYDIG)

Clumps of rounded or fusiform cells, the *interstitial cells* of the testis or *cells of Leydig,* are found in the angular spaces between the seminiferous tubules.   The rounded cells are thought to be mature secretory forms, and the more slender variety probably represent a transitional stage in the differentiation of interstitial cells from primitive spindle-shaped cells in the lamina propria of the seminiferous tubules.   The definitive interstitial cells constitute a diffuse endocrine gland and are almost the entire source of the androgenic hormone secreted by the male gonad.   There are marked species differences in the abundance of interstitial cells.

Mature human interstitial cells (Fig. 26-26) aggregate in clusters or are thinly scattered along blood vessels.   They have a large, round, and somewhat wrinkled nucleus and a centrosome.   The cytoplasm is strongly acidophilic, has a fine granular texture, and contains lipid droplets, mitochondria, Golgi apparatus, pigment granules, refractile globules, and protein *crystals of Reinke* (Fig. 26-26).   These are all better visualized by electron microscopy (Fig. 26-27), which also reveals an additional cytoplasmic constituent, a rich elaboration of small, smooth-surfaced vesicles and anastomosing, tubular membranes of smooth ER (Fig. 26-28).   Such dispositions of smooth ER seem to be characteristic of steroid hormone-secreting cells.   Ribosomes are sparse and are seen only in the cytoplasmic matrix. The mitochondria are notable by their inconstancy in size and shape, and they usually have cristae exhibiting tubular structure rather than the more common lamellar arrangement. Lipid droplets are comparatively scarce, usually spherical in outline, and of homogeneous density. Lipochrome pigment granules are abundant, especially in older men, and are seen as heterogeneous conglomerations of dense granules. Present also are other granules, with and without enclosing membranes and of uncertain nature. Protein crystals of Reinke are the most conspicuous and curious cytoplasmic constituents of these cells (Fig. 26-27). They are of inconstant occurrence among

individuals and among the cells of a given individual. The crystals show wide variance in size and form but are often rectilinear and may be 20 μm long and 3 μm thick. The angles may be sharp or rounded. The crystals are composed of macromolecules about 150 Å in diameter, which, being evenly spaced at about 190 Å, present a highly ordered pattern of internal structure. In addition, aggregates of hollow cylinders are sometimes seen, whose structure suggests a relationship with the crystals. By histochemical techniques, the interstitial cells show the presence of cholesterol, ascorbic acid, lipases, esterase, leucyl-aminopeptidase, succinic dehydrogenase, cytochrome oxidase, and 3-β-ol dehydrogenase.

The Leydig cells, though numerous at birth owing to the stimulation of the fetal testis by chorionic gonadotrophin, largely revert to fibroblast-like cells during the first year. They reappear in increasing numbers just prior to pubescence. In fully developed testes, the interstitial cells rarely undergo mitosis.

ENDOCRINE FUNCTIONS OF THE TESTIS

In addition to producing sperm cells, the testis secretes into the bloodstream an androgenic steroid hormone, *testosterone,* which is essential for puberal development and structural and functional maintenance of the male accessory reproductive organs. The interstitial cells are responsible for secretion of the testicular androgenic hormone.

The characteristic structure and endocrine function of the interstitial cells are sustained and controlled by the hypophyseal gonadotrophic hormone LH (*luteinizing hormone*), also known as ICSH or *interstitial cell-stimulating hormone.* In the absence of LH, the interstitial cells undergo severe atrophy and cease functioning. The completely atrophic Leydig cell is spindle-shaped, the amount of cytoplasm is greatly reduced, and the nucleus is extremely pycnotic. The lipid droplets also disappear. The maintenance of the structure and the spermatogenic function of the seminiferous tubules is, on the other hand, dependent upon the action of the *follicle-stimulating hormone* (FSH) (see Chap. 27).

The functions of the germinal epithelium (gamete production) and of the Leydig cells (testosterone

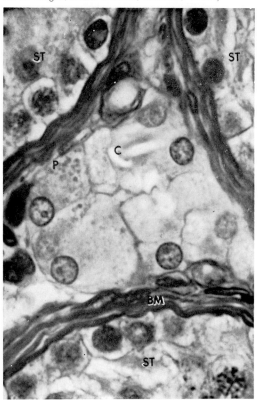

Figure 26-26 Interstitial cells in the human testis. Granular pigment (P) and negative images of crystals of Reinke (C) can be seen in the cytoplasm. Seminiferous tubule (ST); basement membrane (BM). ×1,500. (From Fig. 1, D. W. Fawcett and M. H. Burgos, Amer. J. Anat., **107:**257, 1960.)

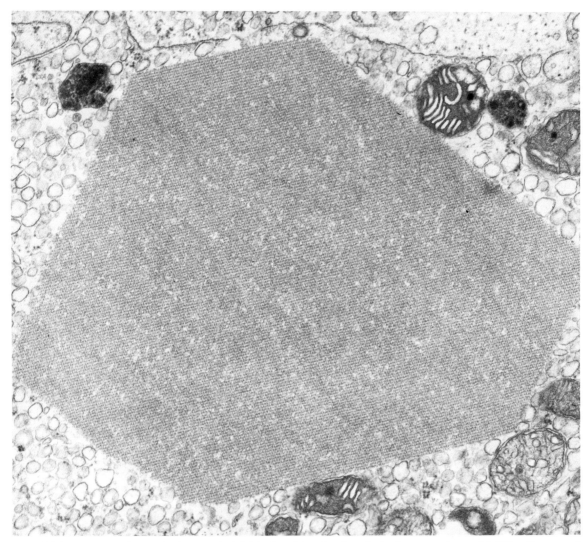

Figure 26-27   Electron micrograph of a crystal of Reinke found in a Leydig cell of a human testis.   ×16,400.   (Courtesy of M. J. Rowley.)

production) can be selectively altered by a variety of drugs.   Both activities can be depressed by estrogen whereas diamines suppress spermatogenesis without disturbing Leydig cell function.   Administration of human chorionic gonadotrophin and high dosages of clomiphene increase hormone release and completely turn off spermatogenic activity.

IONIZING RADIATION

Graded doses of ionizing radiation administered directly to human testes (Fig. 26-18) evoke correspondingly graded biologic responses consisting of reduction in sperm count, denuding of the germinal epithelium, and prolongation of the time for cellular recovery.   In general, the lower the dosage, the less dramatic is the cell loss, and the more rapid the recovery.

RELATION OF THE SCROTUM TO THE TEMPERATURE REQUIREMENTS OF THE TESTES

The germinal cells in the seminiferous tubules are peculiarly susceptible to injury by temperatures above that of the scrotum, which in man is 1.5 to 2.5°C lower than that of the abdominal cavity. When the testes of mature male animals (rats, guinea pigs) are retracted into the abdomen and rendered cryptorchid by surgical means, the seminiferous epithelium degenerates. The Sertoli cells are not reduced in number, nor does this procedure cause any early impairment of the androgenic function of the Leydig cells, as shown by the fact that

Figure 26-28 Electron micrograph of interstitial cells of an opossum, showing free ribosomes and a smooth-surfaced, tubular endoplasmic reticulum. The mitochondria are of uneven size, and their internal membranes are sparse and of a tubular nature. ×15,000. (Courtesy of D. W. Fawcett.)

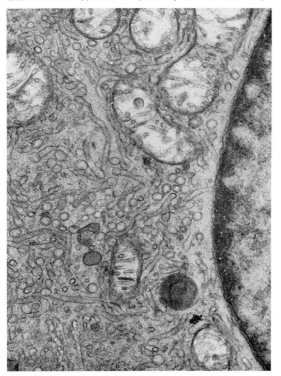

the accessory sexual organs are maintained at normal adult size for at least 6 to 8 months, after which they may gradually become smaller. This evidence of a delayed decline in the secretory activity of the interstitial cells is reflected also by a waning sex drive; the reason for this failure is not clear. In addition to the possibility of tubular injury at body temperature, fevers are well known to induce temporary infertility. If the condition of nondescent of the testes in adolescent patients is allowed to persist too long, both the spermatogenic and the masculinizing functions of the testes may be irreparably damaged.

EXCURRENT DUCT

The course taken by spermatozoa in passing from the seminiferous tubule to the outside of the body, sketched for an initial survey of all the structures concerned (Figs. 26-1 and 26-29), is as follows: The seminiferous tubules open into a labyrinth of flattened spaces, the *rete testis*. From the rete, several ducts, the *ductuli efferentes*, pass directly outside the testes to communicate with a common duct, the *ductus epididymidis*. The latter takes an irregularly convoluted course through the epididymis (see below) and, just before leaving it, becomes the *ductus deferens*, which extends to the *urethra*. Next to the urethra is a constricted portion of the ductus deferens called the *ejaculatory duct*.

Tubuli recti and rete testis The convoluted seminiferous tubules within a given testis lobule are mainly in the form of loops, each end of which joins the *rete testis* (Fig. 26-29). Terminally the tubules taper down, straighten out, and join the rete at acute angles. The tapering portion is lined primarily by Sertoli cells. The straight segments are termed the *tubuli recti*, or *straight tubules*. They are lined with cuboidal epithelial cells and are confluent with the rete testis (Fig. 26-2), a labyrinth of spaces in the mediastinum. The rete has a low cuboidal epithelium, some cells of which are provided with a central flagellum. There are no smooth muscle cells surrounding the tubuli recti or the rete, only a limiting membrane.

Ductuli efferentes In man, 10 to 15 ductules, the ductuli efferentes (Fig. 26-29), emerge from the

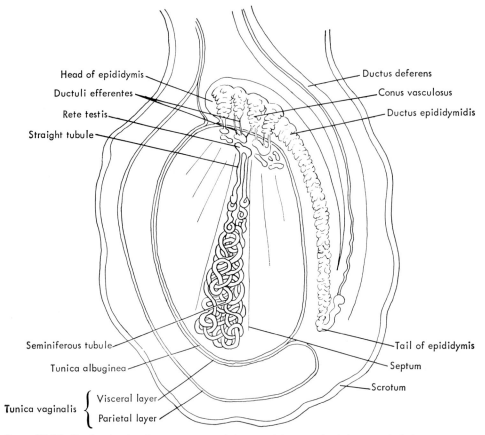

Head of epididymis
Ductuli efferentes
Rete testis
Straight tubule

Ductus deferens
Conus vasculosus
Ductus epididymidis

Seminiferous tubule
Tunica albuginea

Tunica vaginalis { Visceral layer
Parietal layer

Tail of epididymis
Septum
Scrotum

Figure 26-29 Testis, showing the arrangement of ducts and the scrotal relations, vertical view.

mediastinum and connect the rete with the ductus epididymidis. Each ductus efferens is coiled into a cone-shaped mass in the head of the epididymis. Centripetal folds in the epithelium give the inner surface of these ducts a festooned appearance (Fig. 26-30). The epithelium is pseudostratified and characteristically consists of alternating patches of columnar and cuboidal cells, the latter forming evenly spaced pockets on the luminal surface. The epithelial cells, both tall and short, contain fat, pigment, and other granules, and produce a secretion which may cling bleb-like to the cell surface. Both types of cells are ciliated in man; however, in the opossum, ciliated cells intermingle with nonciliated cells which have microvilli on their luminal

surfaces (Fig. 26-31) that are believed to play a role in the absorption of fluids from the luminal contents. The cilia beat in the direction of the epididymis and aid the passage of sperm.

In addition to the cells bordering on the lumen, there are occasional cells submerged in the epithelium and resting on the thin basement lamina (Fig. 26-32). Termed *basal cells,* these are fairly widely distributed along the reproductive tract.

The epithelium rests on a basement lamina that is surrounded by a layer of circular smooth muscle fibers several cells thick. It is significant that from the testis to the urethra the sperm duct has a muscular coat. Once spermatozoa have been carried to the ductuli efferentes by the flow of luminal fluid, their further transport is assured by muscular action. The muscle layer thickens toward the ductus epididymidis. Among the muscle cells there are elastic fibers which, like those of the ductus epididymidis and ductus deferens, first appear at puberty.

Ductus epididymidis   The ductus epididymidis in man is a highly tortuous tube 4 to 5 meters in length. The coils of this duct, together with the entwining connective tissue and surrounding tunic, form the *epididymis* (Fig. 26-29). The duct is lined with pseudostratified epithelium consisting of tall columnar cells and rounded basal cells (Fig. 26-32). The surface cells contain secretory granules and, sometimes, pigment. On their luminal

surfaces are long extensions or ''king-sized'' microvilli; earlier these were named *stereocilia* (Fig. 3-22), yet they are nonmotile and do not have basal bodies. The epithelium possesses a variable amount of cytoplasmic basophilia, fine lipid granules, and other nonlipid hyaline granules.

The epididymal duct has a basement membrane and a thin lamina propria encircled by smooth muscle (Fig. 26-32) with the fibers oriented circularly. The muscle layer is very thin over most of the length of the tube, but it thickens and longitudinal fibers appear near the ductus deferens. Outside the muscle layer, loose connective tissue is molded about the duct and constitutes the interstitium of the epididymis.

Blood vessels and nerves are found in the fibrous stroma. The nerves form, in addition to perivascular nets, a thick *plexus myospermaticus* provided with autonomic ganglia. The plexus is found in the muscle layer, which it supplies, sending fibers also into the mucosa. In the ductus deferens and seminal vesicles, this plexus is said to be more highly developed than in the epididymis.

Ductus deferens   The ductus deferens (Fig. 26-1) is a paired, thick-walled tube which is continuous with the ductus epididymidis and extends to the *prostatic urethra*. Near the prostate the lumen widens and appears as a spindle-shaped enlargement, the *ampulla*. At the distal end of the ampulla the duct is joined by the seminal vesicles. From this point it continues to the urethra as the *ejaculatory duct*. The wall of the ductus deferens is composed of three well-defined layers: the *mucosa, muscularis,* and *adventitia* (Fig. 26-33).

The mucosa protrudes into the lumen in several low longitudinal folds. The epithelium is similar in structure to, but not so tall as, that in the ductus epididymidis. Many of the columnar cells have nonmotile stereocilia which are matted together, forming cones (Fig. 26-34). The cilia tend to disappear toward the ampulla. A delicate basement lamina is present. The lamina propria is made dense by a heavy infiltration of elastic fibers. The ductus is surrounded by a smooth muscle coat 1 to 1.5 mm thick. The fibers of the inner and outer layers are arranged longitudinally and those of the middle layer, circularly. The adventitia is com-

Figure 26-30   Section of ductus efferens from a 15-year-old boy.   ×225.

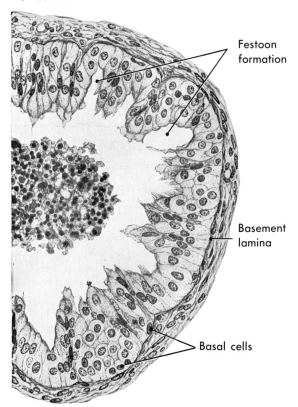

Festoon formation

Basement lamina

Basal cells

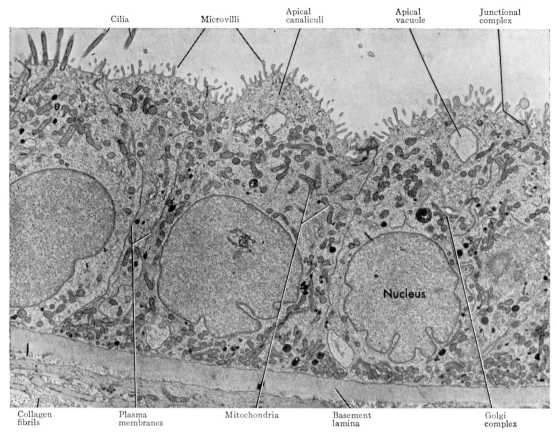

Cilia   Microvilli   Apical canaliculi   Apical vacuole   Junctional complex

Nucleus

Collagen fibrils   Plasma membranes   Mitochondria   Basement lamina   Golgi complex

Figure 26-31 Section through the beginning of a ductus efferens of the opossum. The simple columnar epithelium is composed of ciliated and nonciliated cells having basally positioned nuclei, numerous mitochondria, and other cell organelles. The luminal surfaces of the nonciliated cells possess microvilli; in the apical cytoplasm of these cells are many canaliculi, small vesicles, and larger vacuoles. Junctional complexes can be identified at the distal apposition of the lateral plasma membranes. Basally, tongues of cytoplasm of contiguous cells interdigitate extensively. The epithelium rests upon a thickened basement lamina. ×10,000.

posed of a fibrous covering of the muscle layer and loose connective tissue which blends with that of contiguous structures.

Ampulla The longitudinal folds in the mucosa of the ductus deferens extend into the ampulla, where they increase in height and become branched. The ampulla has a wide lumen (Fig. 26-35), and its muscular coating is thinner, with less distinct layers, than elsewhere in the ductus deferens. The longitudinal layers separate into long strands which terminate toward the ejaculatory ducts.

Ductus ejaculatorius The proximal portion of each ductus deferens extending from the ampulla to the urethra is reduced in width and is known as the *ductus ejaculatorius*, or *ejaculatory duct* (Fig. 26-35). These ducts penetrate the prostate gland and open into the urethra on a thickened portion of the urethral mucosa known as the *colliculus seminalis* or the *verumontanum* (Fig. 26-36). The mucous membrane, cast into numerous thin folds, forms glandular diverticula similar to, but less elaborate than, those in the ampulla. The epithelium (Fig. 26-37) is pseudostratified or simple columnar,

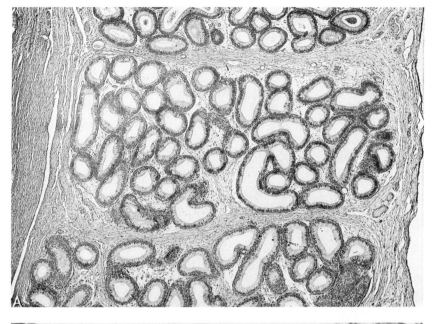

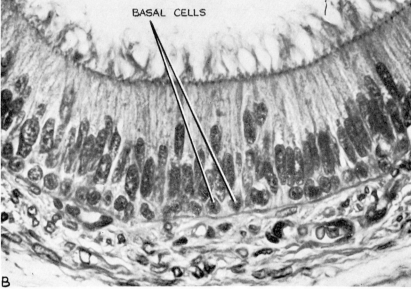

BASAL CELLS

Figure 26-32   Epididymis, human.   A. Vertical section through the body of epididymis.   ×27.   B. Section of wall of the ductus epididymidis.   Note stereocilia, terminal bars, basal cells, and muscular and adventitial tunics.   ×500.

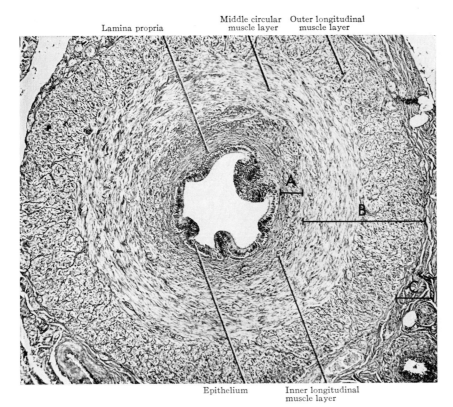

Lamina propria   Middle circular   Outer longitudinal
       muscle layer   muscle layer

Epithelium   Inner longitudinal
                muscle layer

Figure 26-33 Photomicrograph of a transverse section of the human ductus deferens. A, Mucosa; B, muscularis; C, adventitia. ×50.

Figure 26-34 Epithelium lining of the human ductus deferens. Approximately ×600.

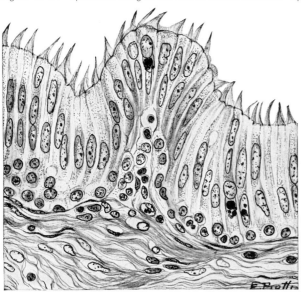

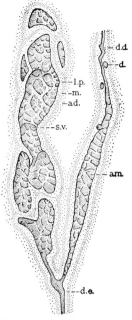

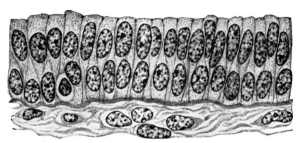

Figure 26-37   Pseudostratified columnar epithelium from the ejaculatory duct of a 34-year-old man.   ×800.   (Stieve.)

Figure 26-35   Ductus deferens and seminal vesicle.   Natural size and relations.   ad, adventitia; am, ampulla; d, diverticulum; dd, ductus deferens; de, ejaculatory duct; m, muscularis; sv, seminal vesicle; lp., lamina propria.   (Eberth.)

Figure 26-36   Transverse section through the human verumontanum.   ×16.   (Stieve.)

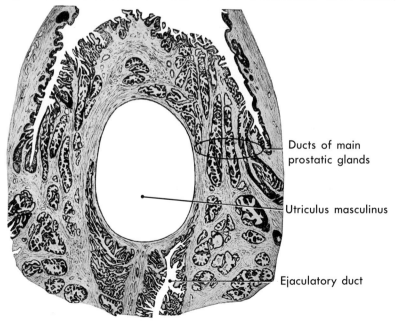

Ducts of main prostatic glands

Utriculus masculinus

Ejaculatory duct

becoming transitional near the urethral orifice. The ejaculatory ducts have a muscular coating, except that the wall of the intraprostatic portion is composed of the fibromuscular stroma of the prostate.

For a description of the male urethra, see Chap. 22.

Associated glands and organs

GLANDS ASSOCIATED WITH EXCURRENT DUCT

Seminal vesicles The seminal vesicles arise as outgrowths from the ductus deferens distal to the ampulla (Fig. 26-35). They develop into elongated hollow organs, whose walls are pocked with small, sac-like evaginations. Each saccule is honeycombed by thin folds of mucosa (Fig. 26-38) which extend deep into the lumen. These branch into secondary and tertiary folds which join to form numerous irregular spaces, all of which communicate with the larger central lumen. These are not true glands; the arrangement merely increases the secretory surface area. The folds are covered with a pseudostratified epithelium consisting of tall, columnar, nonciliated cells that reach the surface, and basal cells identical with those seen elsewhere in the excurrent duct. The secretory cells have a single ovoid nucleus and contain colorless vacuoles, a lipochrome pigment, and some Sudan-staining lipid.

Additional detail has been observed in the secretory cells of the seminal vesicle by using the electron microscope. The cytoplasm contains few mitochondria and is packed with rough ER, some channels of which appear to communicate with the prominent supranuclear Golgi complex that exhibits large secretory vacuoles containing dense secretory granules.

The abundant secretion formed in the seminal vesicles is a viscid material with a yellowish tinge. The height of the cells and their secretory activity are dependent upon the action of testosterone. After castration, the seminal vesicles shrink, cease forming seminal fluid, and the epithelium is reduced to low cuboidal.

The seminal vesicle has a basement membrane, a tunica propria that contains elastic fibers and extends over the entire vesicle, a smooth muscle coat consisting of inner circular and outer longitudinal fibers, and an adventitial layer.

Prostate The prostate, like the seminal vesicles, is a major secretory contributor to the seminal plasma. The prostate (Fig. 26-39) surrounds the urethra near the neck of the bladder and consists of three groups of glands arranged somewhat con-

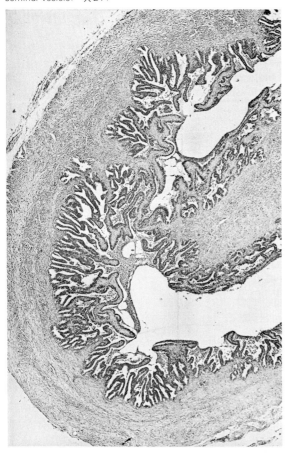

Figure 26-38 Longitudinal section of a diverticulum of a human seminal vesicle. ×27.

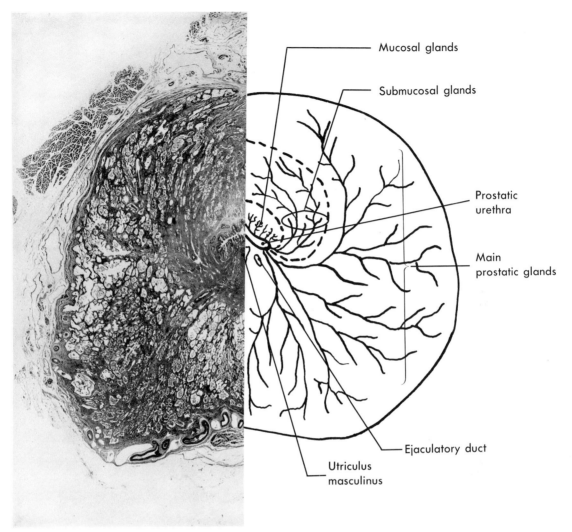

Figure 26-39   Normal human prostate in transverse section at left.   4× (From L. M. Franks, Ann. Roy. Coll. Surg. Eng., **14**:92, 1954.)   Diagram of the glandular composition added at right.

centrically around the urethra.   The smallest are the periurethral mucosal glands.   Immediately peripheral to them are the submucosal glands (Fig. 26-39).   The main prostatic gland is the largest and is grouped into four or five lobes consisting of 30 to 50 tubuloalveolar branched glands.   The ducts of the mucosal glands open at various points into the urethra, whereas those of the submucosal and main glands open onto the posterolateral urethral sinus near the verumontanum (Fig. 26-36).

In each lobe the glands are embedded in a markedly fibromuscular stroma which aids in the ejaculatory discharge of the prostatic fluid.

The glandular epithelium in the prostate is normally simple cuboidal (Fig. 26-40) to columnar. In some of the alveolar recesses there may be small darkly staining basal cells with supranuclear secretory granules; the secretion consists of similar granules and larger vesicular structures which may represent the detached portions of the cells (apocrine

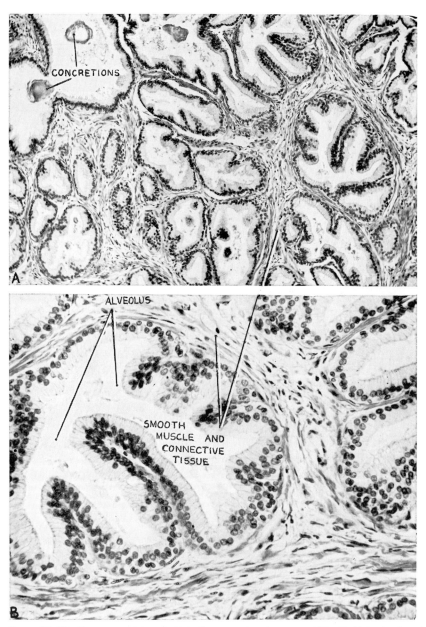

CONCRETIONS

A

ALVEOLUS

SMOOTH
MUSCLE AND
CONNECTIVE
TISSUE

B

Figure 26-40   Human prostate. A. Note fibromuscular stroma.   ×90.   B. Note simple columnar epithelium, few basal cells, secretion in lumen.   ×275.

secretion) as well as desquamated cells. Near the outlet of the ducts, the epithelium changes to the transitional type characteristic of the bladder and prostatic urethra. Histochemically, the prostatic epithelium is remarkable for the abundance of acid phosphatase that occurs throughout the cytoplasm. As seen by electron microscopy (Fig. 26-41), the prostatic epithelial cells possess luminal microvilli and an abundance of rough ER, except in the region of the Golgi structure. Apically the ER membranes are moderately distended. Castration changes are marked by collapse of these distended membranes, the increased number of liposomes, and a loss of basophilia and acid phosphatase. These and other cellular changes are reversed by the administration of testosterone.

In the prostatic alveoli, of older persons especially, there are concretions of various forms, 0.2 to 2 mm in diameter (Fig. 26-40); in sections they may exhibit concentric layers (Fig. 26-42) and show double refraction with polarized light. Their reactions to treatment with iodine solutions indicate their starchy nature. They are probably deposited around fragments of cells. The larger concretions sometimes obstruct the prostatic ducts and cause distension of the gland. Octahedral crystals also occur in the prostatic secretion.

The prostate is surrounded by a fibroelastic capsule with some smooth muscle fibers on its inner aspect. These muscle fibers connect with others that penetrate between the prostatic lobules. In many rodents one pair of the lobes of the prostate is differentiated to supply a secretion which coagulates the seminal fluid in the vagina, forming a vaginal plug.

The *utriculus prostaticus* (*uterus masculinus*) is a small pouch on the dorsal wall of the urethra which opens on the verumontanum between the orifices of the two ejaculatory ducts (Figs. 26-36 and 26-39).

BULBOURETHRAL GLANDS

The two *bulbourethral glands,* or *Cowper's glands,* are pea-sized structures situated one on each side of the urethral bulb and connected with the urethra by fairly long ducts. These are compound tubulo-alveolar glands; the end pieces may be rounded sacs or simple tubes. The epithelium is one-cell-layered (Fig. 26-43). The cells in different acini vary greatly in height and appearance. In the resting state, they are columnar with granular cytoplasm and have a clear, spherical nucleus. At the peak of secretion, the acini are almost filled; the tall clear cells have their nuclei flattened against the basal lamina. The cells appear to be filled with mucus, although acidophilic spindle-shaped bodies are also present. In acini distended by secretion the cells may be markedly flattened. Basket cells may also be found. The glands are divided into small lobules by septa composed of connective tissue and striated muscle. The excretory ducts are lined with columnar epithelium, except near the urethral outlet where it becomes pseudostratified columnar. The coating of the ducts is made of fibrous tissue and a thin layer of smooth muscle. The secretion product is a glairy, mucus-like substance. It is poured into the urethra under erotic stimulation and probably acts as a lubricant.

SPERMATIC CORD

In the *spermatic cord* are numerous arteries, veins, lymphatics, and nerves, and the rudiment of the processus vaginalis. The numerous veins constitute the pampiniform plexus. Their walls are usually provided with a very thick musculature including both circular and longitudinal fibers. The outer wall of the cord is made up of striated muscle fibers of the tube-like cremaster muscle.

PENIS

The penis is an elongate organ consisting principally of the urethra and three parallel cavernous bodies. The paired *corpora cavernosa penis* are placed dorsally, and beneath them in the midline is the single *corpus cavernosum urethrae* (*spongiosum*) that originates as an expanded portion, the *bulbus urethrae,* and terminates as the *glans penis,* a structure at the end of the penis having the appearance of a blunted cone. The urethra lies in the center of the spongiosum. A dense fibroelastic connective tissue layer, the *tunica albuginea,* binds the three cavernous bodies together (Fig. 26-44) and also provides an attachment for the skin over the shaft of the penis. The deeper fibers of this tunic are organized as an albuginea around each cavernous body. Those surrounding the corpora

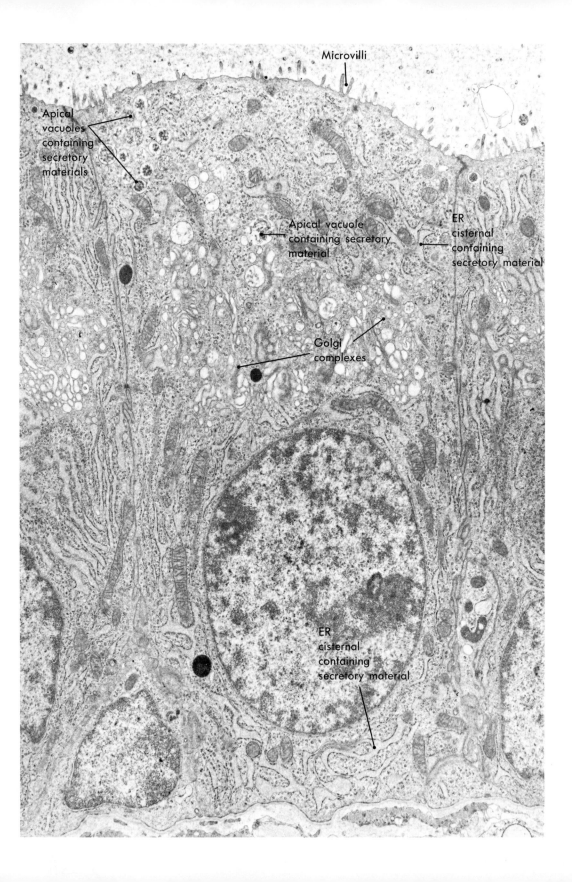

Microvilli

Apical
vacuoles
containing
secretory
materials

Apical vacuole
containing secretory
material

ER
cisternal
containing
secretory material

Golgi
complexes

ER
cisternal
containing
secretory material

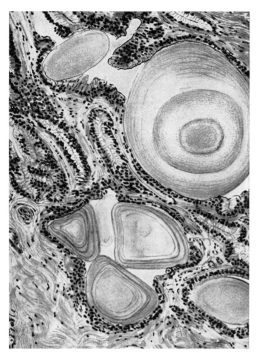

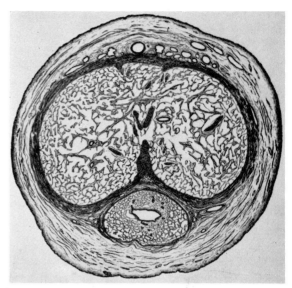

Figure 26-44   Cross section of the penis of a 23-year-old man. The septum between corpora cavernosa penis is incomplete. Section is from distal one-third of the organ. (Stieve.) ×2.5.

Figure 26-42   Section of the human prostate, showing concretions. ×90.

Figure 26-43   Section through part of a lobule of the bulbourethral gland. (Stieve.) ×90.

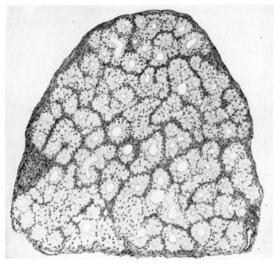

cavernosa penis fuse in the midline to form a septum in the penis which becomes incomplete distally (Fig. 26-44). The albuginea enclosing the spongiosum contains circularly arranged smooth muscle fibers and is thinner and more elastic than that of the paired cavernous bodies.

The cavernous bodies are composed of true erectile tissue that increase in size by filling with blood and change from a flaccid to a rigid state, thereby producing an erection of the penis. These bodies are honeycombed by a complex network of venous spaces (Fig. 26-45) separated by trabeculae. The trabeculae are lined with typical vascular endothelium and have connective tissue and smooth muscle in the wall. Blood enters these spaces from two sources: Capillaries in the walls of the trabeculae drain into the spaces, but the more important supply for the purpose of erection is the terminal branches of arteries which course through the walls of the trabeculae and empty directly into the spaces. These are the *helicine arteries,* so called because in the flaccid penis they

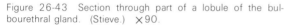

Figure 26-41   Columnar cells of the epithelium of ventral prostate of a 28-day-old rat. These cells possess enlarged Golgi complexes, dilated cisternae of rough endoplasmic reticulum, and vacuoles containing dense secretory material. ×12,000. (Courtesy of C. J. Flickinger.)

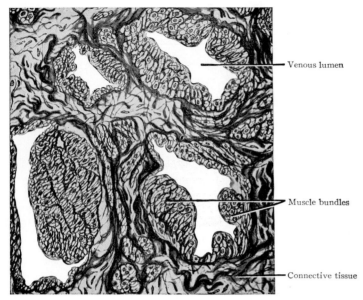

Venous lumen

Muscle bundles

Connective tissue

Figure 26-45   Section showing venous spaces in corpus cavernosum urethrae.   ×200.   (Von Möllendorff.)

are coiled and twisted. They have heavy muscular walls, with subendothelial thickenings of the longitudinal muscle fibers that partly occlude the lumen. The veins draining the cavernous bodies have such thick walls that they resemble arteries; they contain abundant columns of inner longitudinal muscle fibers that make the lumen crescentic or star-shaped. The erectile tissue of the glans penis consists only of convolutions of large veins (Fig. 26-46), and it does not reach the same state of rigidity as the shaft of the erect penis.

Recent studies of the vascular events associated with the process of erection and detumescence of the penis have clarified our understanding of these important processes. The presence of arteriovenous (AV) anastomoses which occur between the deep artery of the penis and the peripheral venous return has been reaffirmed (Fig. 26-47). Hemodynamic experimental work in human beings has shown that blood flow into the cavernous spaces of 20 to 50 ml per min will produce erection without the necessity of postulating a venous closing mechanism. Since parasympathetic activity on the AV complex is required to increase blood flow to the cavernous spaces, it is suggested that concomitant sympathetic activity produces contraction

of arterioles supplying the rest of the penis. This combined autonomic interplay assures a rigid intromittent organ through which sperm can be discharged into the vaginal vault. Relaxation of such autonomic activity after sexual excitement reduces blood flow to the cavernous spaces and shunts most of the blood to the peripheral venous vessels, thereby returning the penis to its flaccid condition (see legend of Fig. 26-47).

The skin of the penis is thin, elastic, fat-free, and somewhat more deeply pigmented than that covering the body. Coarse pubic hairs are present at the root of the organ; elsewhere over its shaft there are only lanugo hairs. At the forward end of the penis, the skin is attached to the *corona of the glans* and forms a circular fold, the *prepuce* (foreskin) that overlies the glans. The inner surface of the prepuce differs from the skin elsewhere on the penis by having a thinner epidermis and being free of sebaceous and sweat glands (the skin of the glans is glabrous). Over the body of the penis there is a subcutaneous layer of smooth muscle fibers which is continuous with the *tunica dartos* of the scrotum. On the *corona glandis* sebaceous glands occur in the absence of hair follicles.

The penis is abundantly supplied with spinal,

sympathetic, and parasympathetic nerve fibers. The sensory fibers of the medullated spinal nerves (*dorsal nerves of the penis*) terminate in many types of sensory ending; as tactile corpuscles in the papillae of the dermis, as end bulbs of Krause and Pacinian corpuscles in the superficial connective tissue, and as genital corpuscles found in or near the cavernous bodies. Free sensory endings also occur. The sympathetic and parasympathetic nerves are a continuation of the prostatic plexus and supply the numerous smooth muscles of the trabeculae and the cavernous blood vessels. The glans is peculiar in that it has no receptors for light touch, warmth, or cold; however, end bulbs are present.

SEMEN

This secretion consists of spermatozoa suspended in a complex fluid derived from the accessory sex glands which empty into the excurrent duct system. The ejaculate is about 3 ml in volume and contains approximately 200 to 300 million spermatozoa. In man, three main glandular systems contribute successively to the ejaculate. The first portion comes from the prostate gland and is a thin, milky emulsion that is slightly alkaline. In addition the bulk of the acid phosphatases are solely derived from the prostate. The second portion comprises

the secretions from the testes, ductus epididymidis, and ductus deferentes and therefore contains the highest concentration of spermatozoa. The third portion possesses the highest concentration of fructose, a substance specific for the seminal vesicles and a prime energy source for motile sperm. Prostaglandins, a family of biologically active lipids found in high concentrations in human seminal fluid, are derived from the seminal vesicles and presumably the testis. Their biologic properties as regulators of smooth muscle activity exert a considerable influence upon the implantation process. Much research is currently in progress concerning the abortifacient potential of the prostaglandins.

The average transit time of human spermatozoa from the Sertoli cell through the ductular system to their appearance in the ejaculate is 12 days (range 1 to 21 days).

The fertilizing power of sperm increases as they move distally along the ductus epididymidis, and it has been assumed that this maturing process is aided by substances contributed to the luminal contents by the epithelium. Ligation experiments and dye injections indicate, quite to the contrary, that the main function of the ductus epididymidis is absorptive and not secretory. Ligation of the excurrent duct system near the testis produces extreme edema of that organ, whereas ligation at

Figure 26-46 Section through the glans penis of an adult man. Anastomosing veins with circular and longitudinal smooth muscle cells in their coats. Sensory nerve corpuscle to the left. ×275.

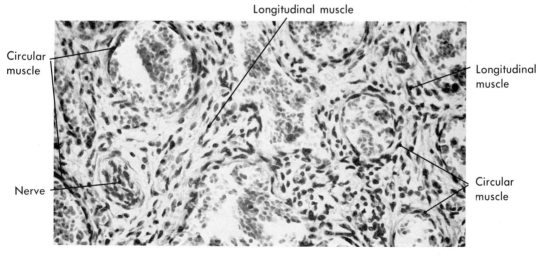

Longitudinal muscle

Circular muscle

Longitudinal muscle

Nerve

Circular muscle

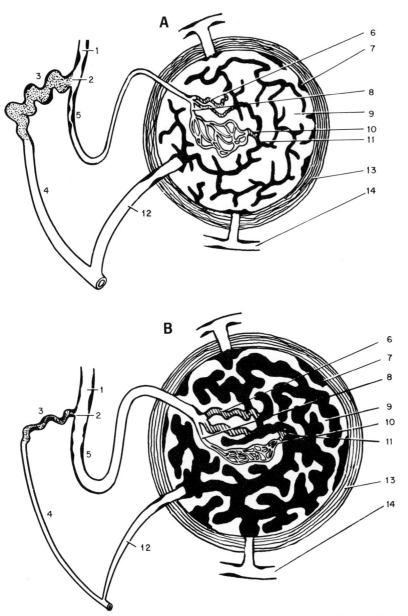

Figure 26-47 Vascular relationships of the human penis. A. In the flaccid state, blood flows toward the corpora cavernosa in the deep artery of the penis (1). This vessel possesses intimal cushions which tend to regulate blood flow. Almost all the blood passes directly into (2) an arteriovenous anastomosis (3) which is usually dilated in this state and connects with efferent veins (4). Minimal amounts of blood pass to the corpora cavernosa. At a point inside the corpora, this artery (5) divides into two branches, the helicine artery (6) that empties almost immediately into the blood spaces of the erectile tissue (7, 11), and the nutritive artery (8) of the trabeculae (9) which, after breaking up into a capillary network, re-forms into a small vein (10) and empties into the cavernous space (11). Cavernous spaces are drained by veins which have internal cushions (12, 14). These pierce the tunica albuginea (13) and constitute the efferent venous return. B. During erection, blood flow in the deep artery of the penis (1) increases. The opening (2) of the arteriovenous anastomosis (3) is reduced by active vasoconstriction resulting in a slightly dilated artery (5) passing through the tunica albuginea (13) into the cavernous body. The helicine arteries (6) dilate, the cavernous spaces (7) fill with blood while the nutritive vessel (8) and its venous junction (10) with the cavernous space (11) become compressed. Blood flow leaving the cavernous body (12, 14) is not reduced despite the internal structure of these emergent veins. (Adapted and modified from G. Conti, Acta Anat., 5:217–262, 1952.)

more distal points, especially beyond the proximal third of the epididymis, produces little or no edema. Thus fluids contributed to the lumen of the seminiferous tubule are reabsorbed by the ductuli efferentes and the proximal portion of the ductus epidiymidis. Sperm are stored in great abundance in the tail of the epididymis where an ionic medium keeps them immotile and conserves their energy store; this medium is probably produced as a special function of the epithelium in this area. Indeed, in the epididymis of some rodents and large mammals, four to eight distinct regions have been recognized. The appearance and cytochemistry of the epithelium, as well as its capacity to take up dyes or reabsorb luminal fluids, differ markedly in these regions.

References

BRANDES, D.: The Fine Structure and Histochemistry of Prostatic Glands in Relation to Sex Hormones, *Int. Rev. Cytol.*, **20**:207 (1966).

BURGOS, M. H., R. VITALE-CALPE, and A. AOKI: Fine Structure of the Testis and Its Functional Significance, in A. D. Johnson, W. R. Gomes, and N. L. Vandenmark (eds.), "The Testis," vol. 1, chap. 9, pp. 551–649, Academic Press, Inc., New York, 1970.

CARPENTER, M. P., and B. WISEMAN: Prostaglandins of Rat Testis, *Fed Proc.*, **29**:248 (Abstract) (1970).

CHANG, K. S., F. K. HSU, S. T. CHAN, and Y. B. CHAN: Scrotal Asymmetry and Handedness, *J. Anat.*, **94**:534–548 (1960).

CHRISTENSEN, A. K., and D. W. FAWCETT: The Fine Structure of Interstitial Cells of the Mouse Testis, *Amer. J. Anat.*, **118**:551 (1966).

CHRISTENSEN, A. K., and D. W. FAWCETT: The Normal Fine Structure of Opossum Testicular Interstitial Cells, *J. Biophys. Biochem. Cytol.*, **9**:653 (1961).

CLERMONT, Y.: The Cycle of the Seminiferous Epithelium in Man, *Amer. J. Anat.*, **112**:35 (1963).

CLERMONT, Y., and C. P. LEBLOND: Spermiogenesis of Man, Monkey, Ram and Other Mammals as Shown by the "Periodic Acid-Schiff" Technique, *Amer. J. Anat.*, **96**:229 (1955).

CONTI, G.: L'érection du pénis humain et ses bases morphologico-vascularies, *Acta Anat.*, **5**:217–262 (1952).

DE KRETSER, D. M., K. J. CATT, and C. A. PAULSEN: Studies on the *in vitro* Testicular Binding of Iodinated Luteinizing Hormone in Rats, *Endocrinology*, **88**:332–337 (1971).

DORR, L. D., and M. J. BRODY: Hemodynamic Mechanisms of Erection in the Canine Penis, *Amer. J. Physiol.*, **213**:1526–1531 (1967).

DYM, M., and D. W. FAWCETT: The Blood-Testis Barrier in the Rat and the Physiological Compartmentation of the Seminiferous Epithelium, *Biol. Reprod.*, **3**:308–326 (1970).

ELIASSON, R.: Prostaglandin—Properties, Actions and Significance, *Biochem. Pharmacol.*, **12**:405–412 (1963).

FAWCETT, D. W.: A Comparative View of Sperm Ultrastructure, *Biol. Reprod.*, **2** (Suppl.): 90–127 (1970).

FAWCETT, D. W., and M. H. BURGOS: Studies on the Fine Structure of the Mammalian Testis. II. The Human Interstitial Tissue, *Amer. J. Anat.*, **107**:245 (1960).

FAWCETT, D. W., and R. D. HOLLENBERG: Changes in the Acrosome of Guinea Pig Spermatozoa during Passage through the Epididymis, *Z. Zellforsch.*, **60**:276 (1963).

FLICKINGER, C. J.: Ultrastructural Observations on the Postnatal Development of the Rat Prostate, *Z. Zellforsch.*, **113:**157–173 (1971).

HAMILTON, D. W.: Steroid Function in the Mammalian Epididymis, *J. Reprod. Fertil.* (Suppl.), **13:**89–97 (1971).

HELLER, C. G., M. F. LALLI, and M. J. ROWLEY: Factors Affecting the Testicular Function in Man, "Pharmacology of Reproduction," vol. 2, Pergamon Press, New York, 1966.

HELLER, C. G., P. WOOTTON, M. J. ROWLEY, M. F. LALLI, and D. R. BRUSCA: Action of Radiation upon Human Spermatogenesis, *Proc. 6th* Pan-Amer. Congr. *Endocr., Excerpta Med.*, 1965.

HUCKINS, C.: The Spermatogonial Stem Cell Population in Adult Rats. I. Their Morphology, Proliferation and Maturation, *Anat. Rec.*, **169:**533–557 (1971).

HUCKINS, C., and E. F. OAKBERG: Cytoplasmic Connections between Spermatogonia Seen in Whole Mounted Seminiferous Tubules from Normal and Irradiated Mouse Testes, *Anat. Rec.*, **169:**344 (1971).

KARIM, S. M. M., and G. M. FILSKIE: Therapeutic Abortion using Prostaglandin F$_2$ Alpha, *Lancet*, **1:**157–159 (1970).

KORMANO, M., and H. SUORANTA: Microvascular Organization of the Adult Human Testis, *Anat. Rec.*, **170:**31–39 (1971).

LADMAN, A. J.: The Fine Structure of the Ductuli Efferentes of the Opossum, *Anat. Rec.*, **157:**559 (1967).

LADMAN, A. J., and W. C. YOUNG: An Electron Microscopic Study of the Ductuli Efferentes and Rete Testis of the Guinea Pig, *J. Biophys. Biochem. Cytol.*, **4:**219 (1958).

MASON, K. E., and S. L. SHAVER: Some Functions of the Caput Epididymis, *Ann. NY Acad. Sci.*, **55:**585 (1952).

NEWMAN, H. F., J. D. NORTHRUP, and J. DEVLIN: Mechanism of Human Penile Erection, *Invest. Urol.*, **1:**350–353 (1964).

NICANDER, L.: Studies on the Regional Histology and Cytochemistry of the Ductus Epididymidis in Stallions, Rams and Bulls, *Acta Morph. Neerl. Scand.*, **1:**337 (1958).

OAKBERG, E. F.: Spermatogonial Stem-cell Renewal in the Mouse, *Anat. Rec.*, **169:**515–532 (1971).

PEREY, B., Y. CLERMONT, and C. P. LEBLOND: The Wave of the Seminiferous Epithelium in the Rat, *Amer. J. Anat.*, **108:**47 (1961).

ROWLEY, M. J., J. D. BERLIN, and C. G. HELLER: The Ultrastructure of Four Types of Human Spermatogonia, *Z. Zellforsch.*, **112:**139–157 (1971).

ROWLEY, M. J., F. TESHIMA, and C. G. HELLER: Duration of Transit of Spermatozoa through the Human Male Ductular System, *Fertil. Steril.*, **21:**390 (1970).

SOHVAL, A. R., Y. SUZUKI, J. L. GABRILOVE, and J. CHURG: Ultrastructure of Crystalloids in Spermatogonia and Sertoli Cells of Normal Human Testis, *J. Ultrastruct. Res.*, **34:**83–102 (1971).

SPEROFF, L., and P. W. RAMWELL: Prostaglandins in Reproductive Physiology, *Amer. J. Obstet. Gynec.*, **107:**1111–1130 (1970).

STIEVE, H.: Männliche Genitalorgane, in W. von Möllendorff (ed.), "Handbüch mikroskopischen Anatomie des Menschen," vol. 7, pt. 2, Springer-Verlag OHG, Berlin, 1930.

ZAMBONI, L., and M. STEFANINI: The Fine Structure of the Neck of Mammalian Spermatozoa, *Anat. Rec.*, **169:**155–172 (1971).

ZAMBONI, L., R. ZEMJANIS, and M. STEFANINI: The Fine Structure of Monkey and Human Spermatozoa, *Anat. Rec.*, **169:**129–154 (1971).

chapter 27 The hypophysis (pituitary gland)

NICHOLAS S. HALMI

Introductory remarks on endocrine tissues

The *endocrine glands* are also known as *ductless glands* or *glands of internal secretion*. Their parenchymal cells manufacture specific products, termed *hormones,* which they usually secrete into the bloodstream. Hormones act as chemical regulators of the functions of specific tissues elsewhere in the body or of the somatic cells generally. The specific structure affected is spoken of as the *target organ* of the hormone concerned. The endocrine glands constitute one of the great coordinating mechanisms of the body, the other being the nervous system. The two systems are intimately linked in their functions. The focus of neuroendocrine integration is the adenohypophysis, which regulates a number of target glands (thyroid, adrenal cortex, gonads) and is in turn controlled by ''release'' and ''inhibitory'' factors produced in hypothalamic neurons and conveyed to the adenohypophysis through its blood vessels. Both the nervous and the endocrine system participate in the maintenance of

a steady physiologic state and are therefore described as having a *homeostatic* or *homeokinetic* role.

The glands which are universally recognized as endocrine glands are the hypophysis, thyroid, parathyroids, adrenals (each consisting of medulla and cortex), gonads, and islets of the pancreas. The placenta, when present, also elaborates hormones. Some other organs (intestine, kidney) have endocrine functions in addition to their dominant activity. The number of hormones produced by the endocrine glands ranges from one (testis) to nine (hypophysis).

Endocrine glands have no ducts, and their cells secrete into vascular channels. Most endocrine glands are primarily comprised of parenchyma and blood vessels, with little stroma. The parenchymal cells are usually polyhedral epithelial cells, arranged with at least one surface abutting upon the wall of a blood or lymph vessel. Their cytoplasm generally

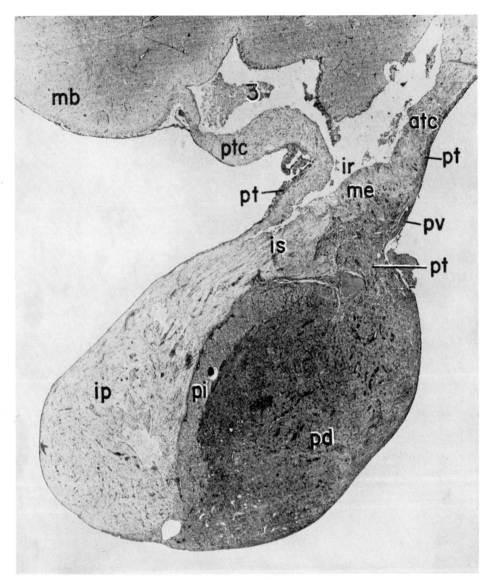

Figure 27-1   Midsagittal section through a rabbit hypophysis that is in connection with the hypothalamus.   This shows the pars distalis (pd), the pars intermedia (pi), the infundibular process (ip), the infundibular stem (is), the pars tuberalis (pt), a portal vessel (pv), the median eminence (me), anterior and posterior portions of the tuber cinereum (atc and ptc), the third ventricle (3) with its infundibular recess (ir), and the mammillary body (mb).   Azan.

contains either clear vacuoles filled with lipid material or granules that are denser than the cytoplasm and have specific affinities for certain dyes.   The presence of these cytoplasmic inclusions is not, however, a necessary condition for the elaboration of hormones.   Cells which produce steroid hormones (for example, those of the adrenal cortex) contain lipid droplets; those whose products are peptide or protein hormones (like the cells of the anterior pituitary lobe) have secretion granules in their cytoplasm. The abundance of these droplets or granules correlates better with the amounts of hormones stored than with their secretion rate.

The endocrine glands have an exceptionally rich blood supply; the thyroid and adrenals are among the most vascular tissues in the body. This is a reflection of their intense metabolic activity and of the fact that the bloodstream both supplies the materials from which hormones are synthesized and carries away the released hormones.

Hypophysis (pituitary gland)

GROSS STRUCTURE AND SUBDIVISIONS

The hypophysis lies at the base of the brain, to which it is linked by a stalk, the *infundibular stalk*. In man the stalk is long and slants forward from the brain to the hypophysis. The hypophysis is flattened on the superior surface and is distinctly elongated in the transverse plane. Average measurements of the gland are 1.3 cm (transverse) by 1 cm (sagittal) by 0.5 cm (vertical). It weighs less than 1 gm in adults, being somewhat heavier in females than in males. The hypophysis undergoes some enlargement during pregnancy and may weigh up to 1.5 gm in multiparae. The hypophysis in man, as in most mammals, rests in a depression in the sphenoid bone, the *sella turcica*. The dura mater of the brain extends across this bony depression as a diaphragm, the *diaphragma sellae,* and is reflected over the surface of the hypophysis to form a fibrous connective tissue capsule. There is a hole in the diaphragm through which the pituitary stalk extends. In the sellar fossa the capsule of the hypophysis lies against the periosteum lining the sella.

By gross inspection, the hypophysis is seen to consist of two lobes. The anterior lobe is pinkish and composed of soft, friable glandular tissue; the posterior lobe is white, more fibrous, and firmer in consistency. On microscopic examination, other structural components of the hypophysis are revealed (Fig. 27-1). A small portion, connected with and extending upward from the anterior lobe, surrounds the pituitary stalk in collar-like fashion, forming the *pars tuberalis*. Between the two major parts of the hypophysis lies a thin cellular partition which is termed the *intermediate lobe,* or *pars intermedia*. The hypophysis is attached to the brain by means of the infundibulum, consisting of an elongated *infundibular stem* and the so-called *median eminence,* which contains the *infundibular recess* of the third ventricle. The infundibular stem thickens beneath the diaphragma sellae and continues as the button-shaped *pars nervosa,* or *infundibular process*. The stem attaches to the brain at the median eminence. The pars nervosa, stem, and median eminence constitute the neurohypophysis (see Fig. 27-1). In man, the median eminence is poorly developed. The pars nervosa and the pars intermedia are intimately fused. This gland is structurally so complex that the terms *anterior lobe* and *posterior lobe,* though well established in the literature of endocrinology and eminently useful because they indicate the two most important functional parts of the hypophysis, do not encompass the entire gland. A much-used classification of the structural components of the whole hypophysis is given in Table 27-1. The infundibular stem and the pars tuberalis which surrounds it constitute the *hypophyseal stalk*.

HISTOGENESIS OF THE HYPOPHYSIS

The adenohypophysis and the neurohypophysis have different embryologic origins. The former arises as an invagination (Rathke's pouch) of the lining of the future oral cavity, whereas the nervous component develops as a downgrowth (infundibulum) from the floor of the diencephalon (Fig. 27-2A). The two anlagen are closely situated and soon establish

Table 27-1   Divisions of the hypophysis

Major division	Subdivisions
Adenohypophysis	Pars tuberalis
	Pars intermedia—intermediate lobe
	Pars distalis—anterior lobe
Neurohypophysis	Pars nervosa or infundibular process— posterior lobe
	Infundibulum
	Infundibular stem
	Median eminence (of tuber cinereum)

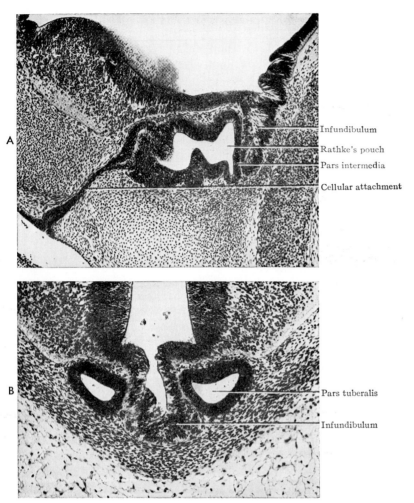

Infundibulum

Rathke's pouch

Pars intermedia

Cellular attachment

Pars tuberalis

Infundibulum

Figure 27-2 Development of the human hypophysis. A. A 17-mm embryo. Midsagittal section through the bulbous end of Rathke's pouch and the adjacent infundibulum. The cellular strand marks the point of origin of the epithelial component of the hypophysis. B. Median section through the hypophysis of a midterm fetus. (Courtesy of B. Romeis.)

contact. The stem of tissue connecting the nervous lobe to the brain is retained in the adult as the core of the pituitary stalk. The attachment of Rathke's pouch to the roof of the oral cavity is lost early in embryonic life, but rudiments are sometimes found as a cellular strand in the sphenoid bone and as a nest of glandular tissue, known as the *pharyngeal pituitary,* at the site of origin in the nasopharynx. The pharyngeal pituitary may produce functional pituitary tumors. At least one hormone

(growth hormone) has been identified in its cells.

Figure 27-2B illustrates well what happens as the development of Rathke's pouch proceeds. It aligns itself early against the rostral surface of the infundibulum and develops into three separate glandular portions: (1) the rostral wall of the pouch, which thickens very markedly to form the pars distalis; (2) the caudal wall, which becomes a very thin layer of cells that fuses with the neural outgrowth and is known as the pars intermedia; and (3) the bilateral thickenings of the wall on the dorsolateral aspects of Rathke's pouch, which form two horn-like extensions that pass around the infundibular stem, one on each side, forming a collar of tissue, the pars tuberalis.

BLOOD SUPPLY OF THE HYPOPHYSIS

The hypophysis derives its blood supply from two sets of arteries: a pair of inferior hypophyseal arteries that arise from the internal carotids and supply the pars nervosa, and several superior hypophyseal arteries emanating from the internal carotids and from the posterior communicating ar-

Figure 27-3 Diagram of the hypophyseal blood supply. The following structures are labeled: optic chiasm (o ch), supraoptic nucleus (sn), periventricular nucleus (pn), third ventricle (3d v), tuberal nuclei (tn), tuber cinereum (tc), median eminence (me), pars tuberalis (pt), tuberal plexus (tp), capillary loops from tuberal plexus (cl), internal carotid (ic), superior hypophyseal arteries (sha), infundibular stem (is), portal vessels (pv), pars distalis capillaries (pdc), pars intermedia (pi), pars nervosa capillaries (pnc), inferior hypophyseal artery (iha), hypophyseal veins (hv), and cavernous sinus (cs). (Drawing by G. Buckley.)

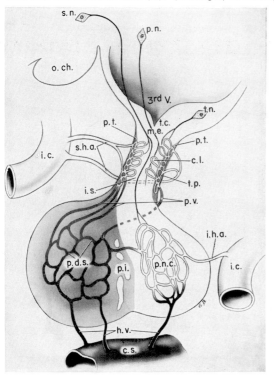

tery of the circle of Willis. The superior arteries feed a capillary plexus in the pars tuberalis which gives off capillary loops that penetrate the median eminence and infundibular stem. This plexus is drained by portal vessels that pass down the pars tuberalis and supply the capillaries in the pars distalis. A set of short inferior hypophyseal arteries feeds the outer layer of the pars distalis in man. The portal vessels are so called because, like the portal vein of the liver, they are interposed between two sets of capillaries, one in the pars tuberalis and infundibular stem, and another in the pars distalis. Anastomoses between the capillaries of the pars nervosa and those of the anterior lobe exist but are not abundant. The venous drainage of both the pars distalis and the pars nervosa is by way of hypophyseal veins that empty into the cavernous sinus (Fig. 27-3).

The hypophyseal "portal circulation" is a remarkably constant feature throughout the vertebrate groups. Although the hypothalamic and hypophyseal blood supplies are separate except for a few capillary anastomoses, the portal vessels are believed to provide the morphologic basis for the regulation of the anterior lobe by the hypothalamus; hypothalamic nerve fibers end around the capillary loops in the infundibular stem, and substances that have traveled along them (neurohormones, hypophysiotropic factors) can be released there into the bloodstream; the blood, thus enriched, is carried to the pars distalis by the portal vessels, and the neurohormones can then influence the cells of this part of the adenohypophysis. The hypophyseal portal circulation provides the vascular part of what is called the *neurovascular link* between the hypothalamus and the pituitary.

NERVE SUPPLY OF THE HYPOPHYSIS

Nerve fibers originating from hypothalamic cells are an integral part of the neurohypophysis and are discussed in that context. Nerve fibers of the infundibular stalk do not appear to extend into the pars distalis, but in some mammals nerve fibers leave the pars nervosa to terminate about cells of the pars intermedia. Although some postganglionic sympathetic and possibly also parasympathetic nerve fibers can be found in the adenohypophysis, there is no evidence that their function is anything other than vasomotor.

Adenohypophysis

In spite of its small size, the adenohypophysis elaborates seven hormones: growth hormone (somatotropin, STH), prolactin, thyrotropin (TSH), the gonadotropins (LH and FSH), adrenocorticotropin (ACTH), and melanocyte-stimulating hormone (MSH).

MICROSCOPIC STRUCTURE

Pars tuberalis The pars tuberalis forms a collar of cells 25 to 60 μm thick around the neural stalk. It is thickest anterior to the stalk and frequently incomplete on the posterior aspect. The cells are arranged in short cords or globular clusters and occasionally as small follicles. Nests of squamous cells are often found in or around the pars tuberalis. They were believed to give rise to tumors (craniopharyngiomas), but such groups of squa-

mous cells are seldom seen in children, whereas craniopharyngiomas are most commonly discovered during the second decade of life.

Pars intermedia In most species this portion of the adenohypophysis is quite distinct. In some mammals (for example, the whale) and in birds, it is lacking. In such animals a dural septum separates the pars distalis from the pars nervosa. In man the pars intermedia is rudimentary. Its cells often surround colloid-filled cysts and merge imperceptibly with those of the pars distalis. Sometimes a remnant of Rathke's cleft persists; in such cases the pars intermedia cells are those posterior to the lumen. They are either chromophobes or basophils. The cells lining follicles may be ciliated. A unique feature of the human gland is the invasion of the pars nervosa by basophilic (specifically β_1)

Figure 27-4 Portions of the human pars nervosa. A. Basophilic cells of the intermediate lobe (top) invading the pars nervosa. Masson's trichrome. B. Tubular glands (t) surrounded by lymphocytes in the pars nervosa. Note a blood vessel (v) and a large intermediate lobe cyst (ic). Gomori's trichrome.

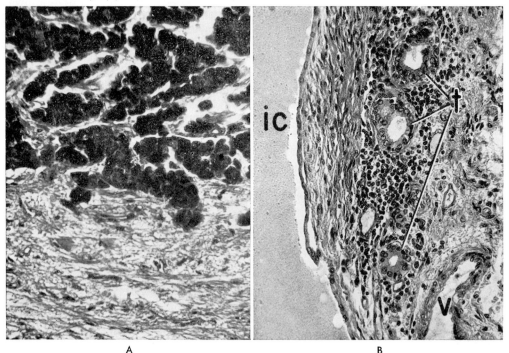

A

B

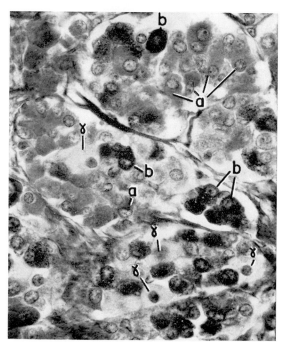

Figure 27-5 Portion of a human pars distalis. Note reticular fibers dividing cell nests; see also acidophils (a), basophils (b), and γ cells (γ). PAS-hematoxylin-orange G.

cells of the pars intermedia (Fig. 27-4A). Such displaced cells may be quite numerous or altogether absent. Tubular (salivary type) glands surrounded by loose lymphoid tissue (Fig. 27-4B) can sometimes be seen in the pars nervosa next to the pars intermedia.

Pars distalis The pars distalis forms about 75 percent of the hypophysis. The cells in the pars distalis are arranged mainly in cords between which are large-bore capillaries. Some cells appear to be in clusters, others in twisted cords, and still others form small, well-defined follicles whose lumina may contain colloid. There is very little connective tissue in any part of the hypophysis, and in the pars distalis only a light meshwork of reticular fibers is present. These are entwined around the basement membranes of the cells and the capillaries (Fig. 27-5).

The classic nomenclature distinguishes three main types of cells in the pars distalis: *acidophils, basophils,* and *chromophobes.* These were said to

constitute about 40, 10, and 50 percent of the anterior lobe cells, respectively, but more recent observations by both light and electron microscopy have shown that chromophobes are much less numerous or even nonexistent. ''Basophil'' is a misnomer, since these cells are actually characterized by blue staining of their granules with the aniline blue component of triacid stains such as Mallory's. However, an alternative term, ''mucoid,'' which is based on the fact that basophils are periodic acid-Schiff (PAS) positive, has not gained wide acceptance. The nomenclature of Romeis (1940) takes into account that, with appropriate stains, the classic cell types can be further broken down into distinct entities. Romeis thus distinguished between α and ε acidophils, β and δ basophils, γ cells (which were previously regarded as chromophobes but which appear to be a separate type of basophil), and undifferentiated or degranulated chromophobes. Unfortunately, different authors, using a variety of fixatives and staining procedures, have introduced a number of new nomenclatures since Romeis' treatise was published. This and the extension of his terminology to species other than man have created much confusion. Several authors have made attempts to establish the equivalence of cell types among the many nomenclatures applied to the human pars distalis. Table 27-2 shows the presumed correspondence of cell types in three nomenclatures: the classic terminology, Romeis', and Ezrin's. The author recognizes the following cell types: α, η, β_1, β_2, δ, γ, and possible chromophobic cells. It is to be hoped that these designations will be soon replaced by a functional nomenclature. In fact, it already seems safe to call the α cells STH cells, the β_1 cells ACTH-MSH cells, and δ cells gonadotropic cells (see Table 27-2 and the section Histophysiology of the Adenohypophysis).

Among the acidophils of the human hypophysis, Romeis' α type usually predominates. These cells are located preferentially in posterolateral parts of the lobe; they are smaller than most basophils and rounded. The granulation may vary from sparse to extremely dense. The granules are small and highly refractile. During pregnancy and lactation large, poorly granulated acidophils (pregnancy cells, η cells of Romeis) are numerous. Their relationship to the generally inconspicuous ε cells is not clear.

Table 27-2   Cell types of the human pars distalis

Nomenclature	Stain	Cell type (staining of granules)				
Classic	Mallory's trichrome	Acidophil (red)			Basophil (blue)	
Romeis	Kresazan	α (red)	ε (orange)*	β (purple)		δ (blue)
Ezrin	AT-PAS-orange G	α (orange)	?	β_1 (red)	β_2 (blue)†	$\delta_{1,2}$ (blue)‡
Hormone probably secreted by each cell type		STH	?	MSH ACTH	TSH	Gonadotropins (LH, FSH)

Abbreviations: AT, aldehyde thionin; PAS, periodic acid-Schiff.   Arrows indicate presumed identity.

* The pregnancy cell (Romeis' η cell) also has granules that stain orange with Kresazan.   It is the probable source of prolactin.

† Some believe that the β_2 cells were included among Romeis' δ cells.

‡ The distinction between δ_1 and δ_2 cells is precarious.

§ There seems to be no reason for abandoning the term γ cell.   This cell type may be heterogeneous: Some seem to be derived from β_2 cells, others from δ cells.

The typical basophil is of Romeis' β type.   Such cells are most common in the central, anterior part of the lobe.   They are generally larger than the average α cell, and often angular, especially the β_2 cells.   The number of granules in the cytoplasm of β cells is quite variable, but most of them are less heavily granulated than the α cells; the individual granules, however, appear larger.   The intermediate lobe basophils in the pars nervosa resemble β (more specifically β_1) cells in most of their staining characteristics.   Romeis' δ basophils (which may also be a heterogeneous group; see Table 27-2) are generally smaller than the β cells, round, and often sparsely granulated.   They are more frequent than β cells in lateral parts of the lobe. Romeis' γ cells, when fully grown, are the largest cells of the pars distalis (Fig. 27-5).   They are most numerous near the intermediate lobe and the pars tuberalis.   Their few granules are found predominantly in the Golgi region.   Although colloid droplets may be seen in any cell type of the anterior lobe, they are most frequently encountered in γ cells.

True *chromophobes* are much less common than counts based on Mallory-stained material indicate, if they indeed exist.   Most of the apparently chromophobic cells certainly have a few specific granules.   It is commonly believed that the cells of the pars distalis show cyclic secretory activity, that is, that they first accumulate and then release their specific granules.   "Chromophobes" therefore may be transitionally degranulated cells.   Transformation of a differentiated cell type into another seems unlikely.   Since large shifts in the distribution of granulated cells may occur and mitoses are infrequent in the anterior lobe, the apparent "chromophobes" are the probable reservoir from which more fully granulated cells of different types originate.

ULTRASTRUCTURE OF THE ADENOHYPOPHYSEAL CELLS

The descriptions given are based on the rat hypophysis, for want of adequate information on the human gland.

Acidophils   Two types of acidophils are seen in the rat hypophysis (Fig. 27-6).   One is smaller, on an average, and possesses numerous densely packed secretory granules whose maximum diameter is 350 nm.   It is the most likely source of growth hormone (STH).   The other type of acidophil is

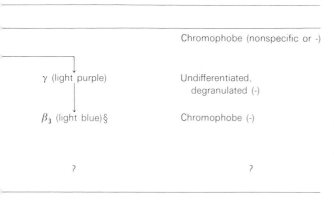

more prominent during pregnancy, lactation, and after estrogen treatment. Cells of this kind have few but large secretory granules, up to 900 nm in diameter, and often show an exceptionally well-developed rough ER whose sacs may be flattened. These cells are the probable producers of prolactin.

Basophils   Two types of basophils are distinguishable with the electron microscope:

1. Angular or stellate cells (Fig. 27-7A) with small granules (maximal diameter about 100 to 200 nm). These are thyrotropic cells.

2. Large, spherical cells with a prominent Golgi apparatus, dark mitochondria, round or confluent ER membrane profiles, and granules whose maximal diameter seldom exceeds 250 nm are gonadotropic, but efforts to separate them into cells producing luteinizing hormone (LH) and follicle-stimulating hormone (FSH) have not been conclusive (Fig 27-7B).

Others   The adrenocorticotropic (ACTH) cells seem to be elongated or stellate cells whose sometimes ovoid granules (usually less than 300 nm in dia-

meter) are lined up along the plasma membrane (Fig. 27-7A).

Cells that are chromophobic (devoid of granules) by electron-microscopic criteria are sparse. Some chromophobic cells with microvilli line small lumina. The cells of the pars intermedia have distinct cell boundaries and a sizable complement of uniformly small granules variable in size.

The rat hypophysis has many pericapillary spaces filled by loose connective tissue, whose macrophages may protrude into the capillary lumen. The fenestrated endothelium of the capillaries and the parenchymal cells rest on separate basement membranes. Extrusion of secretory granules into the pericapillary space can be observed, but they seem to disintegrate there promptly.

HISTOCHEMISTRY OF THE ADENOHYPOPHYSIS

The basophilic cells of the adenohypophysis, including the γ cells, can be best defined as the cells whose secretory granules give a positive PAS reaction after digestion with amylase; that is, they contain glycoproteins. These granules, which usually appear coarse, must correspond to aggregates of those seen under the electron microscope. Recent studies of thin sections from glutaraldehyde-fixed human pituitaries have shown scattered PAS-positive granules in most nonbasophilic cells too. Basophilic cells are (at least in the rat) the source of glycoprotein hormones (thyrotropin, gonadotropins). It is therefore likely that these hormones contribute to the PAS-positive nature of their granules. In man, however, the cells with the most markedly PAS-reactive granules, the β_1 cells, produce the peptide hormones ACTH and β MSH. The colloid droplets seen in hypophyseal cells are intensely PAS-positive and sudanophilic, and they may contain a lipid pigment. Intercellular colloid stains similarly. Basophilia due to rough ER is found in the cytoplasm of anterior lobe cells. It is most pronounced in active acidophils.

HISTOPHYSIOLOGY OF THE ADENOHYPOPHYSIS

Hormones produced by different cell types   Since the adenohypophysis is known to produce a number of hormones and contains several cell types, many

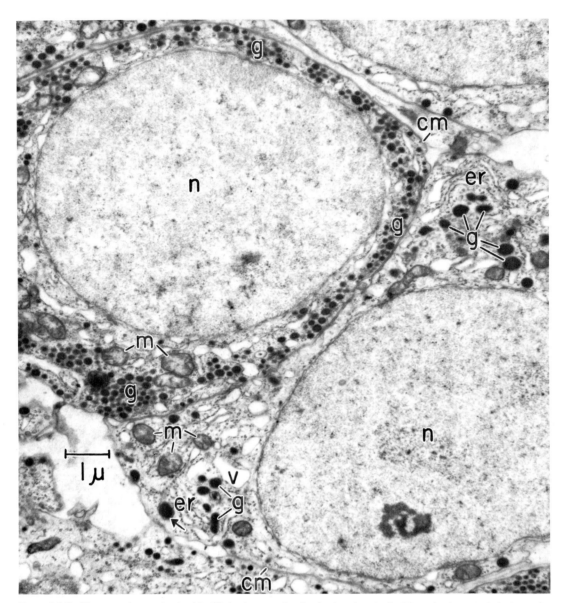

Figure 27-6 Electron micrograph of acidophils in the pars distalis of a female rat. In this and subsequent electron micrographs, the labeled structures are the following: secretory granules (g), endoplasmic reticular vacuoles (v), mitochondria (m), cell membrane (cm), ergastoplasmic sacs (er), and nucleus (n). Arrow points to the membranous envelope of a secretory granule. The cell at the upper left is a somatotropic (STH) cell. Granules abound and do not exceed 350 nm in diameter. The cell at the lower right is a prolactin cell. Note sparse, large granules and prominent endoplasmic reticulum. (Courtesy of E. G. Rennels.)

efforts have been made to identify the cellular source of individual hormones. Procedures used in such endeavors include the following:

1. Attempts to correlate typical histologic changes in various physiologic or pathologic states and under experimental conditions with altered hormone storage or secretion; since target organ hormones act back on the cells that produce the tropic hormones, experimental changes in the levels of the former have been especially useful in eliciting characteristic responses in the latter.

2. Bioassays of different parts of large hypophyses in which cell types are unevenly distributed.

3. Localization of antibodies produced against purified hormones in vivo and labeled with fluorescent dyes or peroxidase, upon incubation with pituitary sections in vitro.

Growth hormone (somatotropin, STH) Somatotropin is a simple protein that enhances body growth after birth. Its absence results in *pituitary dwarfism;* its oversecretion in childhood leads to *gigantism* and during adult life to *acromegaly* (enlargement of hands, feet, mandible, and viscera). Human STH has been totally synthesized. The following evidence leaves little doubt that STH is produced by acidophils—in rats, specifically by the somatotropic cells (see Fig. 27-8, upper left, see color insert), and in man, by the α cells. (1) In gigantism or acromegaly, acidophilic tumors are commonly found. (2) Thyroidectomized rats show degranulation of acidophils (Fig. 27-8C, see color insert) and stunted growth that can be corrected with STH. (3) In a strain of dwarf mice, the hypophysis is severely deficient in acidophils. (4) Antibodies against human STH attach to the acidophils. (5) STH is found predominantly in "acidophilic" regions of the bovine hypophysis. For STH, animal studies and observations in man are in good accord.

Prolactin Prolactin is a simple protein that promotes mammary development and lactation. It also participates in the maintenance of corpora lutea in rodents, whose prolactin has therefore been called *luteotropin* (*LTH*). In the pituitary of a number of species (for example, rabbit, cat), staining with azocarmine and orange G reveals two types of acidophils, carmine cells and orange cells. The former are consistently prominent when prolactin secretion is enhanced (Fig. 27-9, see color insert). They correspond to the acidophils with large granules (Fig. 27-6, lower right) in the rat hypophysis (which, however, do not stain with azocarmine), since these are also active when prolactin production is great—for example, during pregnancy, lactation, and after estrogen administration. It is tempting to suggest that in man the α cells secrete STH and the η cells secrete prolactin, even though in the human being the α cell rather than the η cell stains distinctly with azocarmine. The separate identities of prolactin and STH have not been chemically proved for the human being; however, biologic evidence for the existence of a prolactin distinct from STH in man is increasing. Separate STH and prolactin cells have been identified in monkeys by immunofluorescence.

Thyrotropin (thyroid-stimulating hormone, TSH) This glycoprotein hormone stimulates many functions of the thyroid. Its cell of origin in rodents is an angular basophil which stains with the PAS procedure and aldehyde fuchsin (Fig. 27-8A, see color insert). (See Fig. 27-7A for its submicroscopic features.) In thyroidectomized rats this cell type produces large, hyperactive, vacuolated "thyroidectomy" cells that are agranular (Fig. 27-8C, see color insert), and pituitary TSH stores decline concomitantly. Thyroid hormones cause involution of the aldehyde fuchsin-positive "thyrotrops" and a parallel decrease in pituitary TSH content. In human beings with primary thyroid failure, hypersecretion of TSH is accompanied by the appearance of large, lightly granulated basophils containing colloid droplets. These are said to be derived from β_2 cells.

Gonadotropins: follicle-stimulating hormone (FSH) and luteinizing hormone (LH) or interstitial-cell-stimulating hormone (ICSH). FSH, a glycoprotein, stimulates the growth of ovarian follicles past the primordial stage and activates the spermatogenic epithelium of the testis. LH, also a glycoprotein, is necessary for ovulation and perhaps for the secretion of estrogen by the follicle;

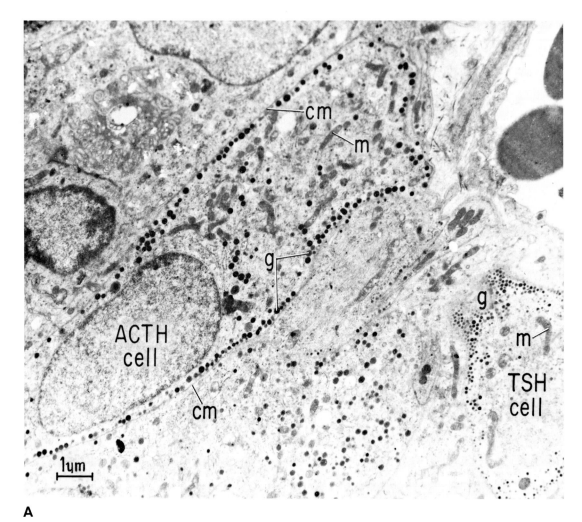

A

Figure 27-7 A. ACTH cell and thyrotropic (TSH) cell in the pars distalis of a male rat. In the former, note the elongated shape and the predominant disposition of the dark, ovoid granules along the cell membrane. In the latter, see the irregular outlines and the small size of the granules. B. Gonadotropic cell in the pars distalis of a male rat. Note the large size, rounded shape, indented nucleus, prominent Golgi apparatus, clustered granules, and many ergastoplasmic vesicles. (Courtesy of Gwen Moriarty.)

it also stimulates the Leydig cells of the testis to secrete androgen. In rats, gonadotropins are produced by basophils that ordinarily do not stain with aldehyde fuchsin (Fig. 27-8A, see color insert), only with the PAS procedure. These cells enlarge and multiply after castration (Fig. 27-8B, see color insert) and eventually form so-called "signet-ring" or castration cells with a single vacuole. The gonadotropin content of the hypophysis rises con-comitantly after gonadectomy. Sex hormones depress pituitary gonadotropin content and cause regression of the aldehyde fuchsin-negative baso-phils ("gonadotrops"). Separate FSH- and LH-producing cells can be unequivocally distinguished in seasonal breeders such as bats, in which the two hormones are secreted at different times. Rennels has convincingly identified the FSH and LH cells of sheep by immunohistologic means.

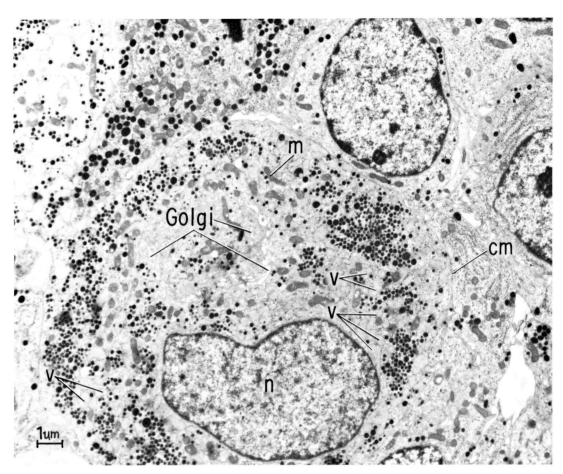

B

Some human δ cells and pars tuberalis cells react with antibodies against chorionic gonadotropin (which is known to overlap immunologically with LH) and are therefore believed to secrete LH. The cells of origin of FSH in man have not yet been identified but may well be the same ones that produce LH.

Adrenocorticotropin (adrenocorticotropic hormone, ACTH)   ACTH is a polypeptide containing 39 amino acids. It has been totally synthesized. ACTH stimulates the adrenal cortex to secrete glucocorticoids such as cortisol. According to Siper-

stein (1970), certain large "chromophobes" of the rat pituitary respond to adrenalectomy with increased protein turnover that can be radioautographically displayed by means of [³H] glycine. These cells are evidently the same as the ACTH cells, of which one is shown in Fig. 27-7A. In man, β_1-cell tumors are often associated with hyperadrenocorticism (Cushing's disease) due to oversecretion of ACTH. Further, antibodies against ACTH attach to human (anterior and posterior lobe) β_1 cells. Finally, Cushing's disease or administration of corticoids leads to a pathognomonic alteration in the β_1 cells; their granules are replaced

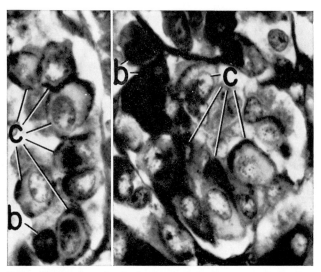

Figure 27-10 Pars distalis from a patient who was treated with large doses of cortisone before his death. Note contrast between fully granulated basophils (b) and basophils showing Crooke's hyaline change (c). The annular distribution of the hyaline material is particularly obvious in the cell near the left lower corner. PAS-hematoxylin-orange G.

in part or totally by PAS-negative, homogeneous material (Crooke's hyaline change, Fig. 27-10). This change is seldom seen in posterior lobe basophils. The functional significance of Crooke's change is obscure. The evidence linking the human β_1 cell with the production of ACTH is quite convincing.

Melanocyte-stimulating hormone (MSH) MSH is a polypeptide whose structure partially overlaps with that of ACTH. It occurs in two forms, α and β MSH, both of which have been synthesized. Only β MSH occurs in significant amounts in the human hypophysis. MSH causes dispersal of melanin in the melanophores of amphibians. Its physiologic role in mammals is not clear, although its injection into human beings causes hyperpigmentation. In species with a distinct pars intermedia, MSH is undoubtedly produced in that part of the hypophysis. In man, MSH is found in both the pars distalis and the pars nervosa when the latter is invaded by basophils. Purves and Herlant believe that MSH in man is secreted by the β_1 cells, with whose number its concentration seems to correlate. They consider these cells to be dispersed pars intermedia cells rather than true

pars distalis components. The implication that β_1 cells secrete both ACTH and MSH now seems quite attractive, since the two hormones are secreted in a parallel fashion in man, and recent studies in animals have located ACTH in the pars intermedia (previously believed to be only the source of MSH), not only the ACTH cells of the pars distalis.

HYPOTHALAMIC REGULATION OF THE ADENOHYPOPHYSIS

Many of the functions of the adenohypophysis depend on its connections with the hypothalamus. Furthermore, some of the negative feedback effects of target gland hormones on the respective tropic hormones are mediated by way of the hypothalamus. Hypophyseal transplants of rats show total or substantial loss of gonadotropic, thyrotropic, and adrenocorticotropic function. The basophils in such grafts are decreased in number and size or are absent. When such transplants are placed back under the median eminence and reestablish normal vascular connections, their structural and functional integrity returns. More or less selective interference with the secretion of various hypophyseal hormones can be achieved by appropriately placed hypothalamic lesions. These functional changes are accompanied by corresponding morphologic alterations of the adenohypophysis. It is likely that circumscribed hypothalamic regions produce specific substances that govern the release (and also the production) of different hypophyseal principles. These factors must reach the adenohypophysis via the portal vessels. The thyrotropin-releasing factor has been chemically identified as pyroglutaminyl-histidyl-prolinamide and synthesized. Prolactin secretion seems to be inhibited rather than stimulated by the hypothalamus. Transplanted pituitaries of rats are eventually transformed so as to consist largely of acidophils of the prolactin-producing type. In such animals corpora lutea are maintained much beyond the normal physiologic limit. Even tissue cultures of pituitary cells secrete prolactin and respond to estrogen, which is also a stimulus to prolactin production in vivo. The intermediate lobe also seems to be restrained by the hypothalamus. Section of the hypophyseal stalk or transplantation of the adenohypophysis in amphibians leads to hyperplasia of the isolated pars intermedia and to blackening of the skin due to enhanced production of MSH.

TUMORS OF THE ADENOHYPOPHYSIS

Tumors of the anterior lobe can be produced by total body irradiation, total or partial removal of target organs, or estrogen treatment. Target gland ablation abolishes the negative feedback which keeps in check the cells producing the respective tropic hormones. These cells then proliferate and may eventually become tumorous. Adenomas of the gonadotropic cells have been found in rats after castration, and tumors of the thyrotropic cells have been found in mice whose thyroid was destroyed with radioactive iodine.

Experimentally produced pituitary tumors may be at first dependent on the stimulus that leads to their formation; later they can become autonomous and transplantable into normal hosts. Functional hypophyseal tumors extensively studied include producers of TSH obtained by thyroidectomizing mice, ACTH-secreting and prolactin + STH-producing neoplasms found in irradiated mice, and prolactin-secreting tumors in rats treated with estrogen. If they grow large enough, most of these tumors become chromophobic by light-microscopic criteria. The absence or paucity of granules merely indicates relatively low levels of stored hormone, compatible with intensive secretory activity. (This is also exemplified by the thyroidectomy cell of the rat, an agranular "thyrotrop" which is hypersecretory but contains little TSH.) Some prolactin + STH-producing tumors are unequivocally acidophilic, and the electron microscope has revealed scattered granules in apparently chromophobic TSH-secreting tumors.

Acidophilic pituitary tumors of man that produce STH and ACTH-producing tumors of the β_1 cells which lead to Cushing's disease have already been mentioned. A few cases of TSH-secreting β_2 cell adenomas have been observed. Most pituitary tumors of man are hormonally inactive and may actually destroy functional portions of the hypophysis by compression. These are usually described as chromophobic tumors, but recent studies have shown that most of them consist of poorly granulated acidophils.

Neurohypophysis

The neurohypophysis releases two hormones into the systemic circulation: *vasopressin* (antidiuretic hormone, ADH) and *oxytocin*. In addition, it is in this part of the pituitary that the "release" and inhibitory hypophysiotropic factors which regulate functions of the adenohypophysis are discharged into the portal vascular system that feeds the pars distalis.

STRUCTURE

The neurohypophysis is best understood as a complex of structures that include the axon terminations of secretory nerve cells of the hypothalamus. The neurosecretory cells are distinct from other neurons in that their axons do not terminate upon other nerve cells or upon other effector cells but store the secretory product and release it into the bloodstream.   Neurosecretory cells which conform to this definition, and which produce secretory material with similar staining characteristics, have been described in many arthropods, as well as in the hypothalamus of vertebrates.   Although their staining characteristics are similar and although similar elementary granules of the order of 100 to 300 nm have been identified in these cells with the electron microscope, a variety of physiologic activities has been linked to the neurosecretory systems of the different species studied.

Developing, as they do, from the floor of the diencephalon behind the optic chiasma, the *infun-*

Figure 27-11   The primate neurohypophysis. Sagittal section of the neurohypophysis of a cynomolgus monkey, in situ in meninges and sella turcica. Protargol silver stain shows rostral and caudal contributions to the hypothalamohypophyseal tract, which sweeps from the infundibulum into the pars nervosa. ot, optic tract; III, third ventricle; me, median eminence; tub, pars tuberalis; i, pars intermedia; pd, pars distalis; pn, pars nervosa; s tr, supraopticohypophyseal tract; t tr, tuberohypophyseal tract; d, diaphragma sellae; ds, dorsum sellae.   × 12. (Bodian.)

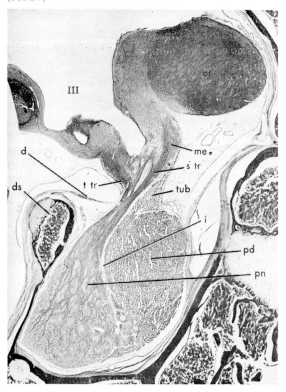

dibulum (median eminence and infundibular stem) and the *pars nervosa* at first contain the continuation of the cavity of the third ventricle (infundibular recess).   This cavity is usually obliterated during development, except for remnants lined by ependymal cells.   Following this obliteration, the hilar or central portion of the pars nervosa is formed by a densely packed bundle of nonmyelinated fibers known as the *hypothalamohypophyseal tract* (Fig. 27-11).   The number of these fibers, estimated by Rasmussen to be at least 50,000, was thought by him "to be out of all proportion to the cellular content of the neural lobe, and to the amount of epithelium in pars tuberalis, pars infundibularis and pars intermedia."

The origins of the nerve fibers of the hypothalamohypophyseal tract have been precisely determined by experiments in animals in which the hypophyseal stalk was sectioned.   The resultant interruption of the nerve fibers in the infundibular stem is followed by chromatolysis and retrograde degeneration of their nerve cell bodies in the supraoptic and paraventricular nuclei of the hypothalamus, and in more scattered nerve cells caudally in the tuber cinereum.   There is evidence from animal experiments that nerve fibers arising from cell bodies in the infundibular and tuberal regions (*tuberohypophyseal tract*) terminate mainly in the median eminence, whereas nerve fibers originating in the supraoptic and paraventricular nuclei (*supraopticohypophyseal tract*) terminate mainly in the pars nervosa.   In man, however, the median eminence is not prominently developed, and it does not have the characteristic neurohypophyseal structure seen in other vertebrates, including lower primates.   The nerve endings of the human tuberohypophyseal tract can presumably be found around the capillary loops in the infundibular stem.

The hypothalamohypophyseal tract branches as it enters the hilum of the pars nervosa, and the branches are dispersed to form the core of the irregular lobules of which the pars nervosa is composed.   An analysis of the structure of the pars nervosa of a primitive mammal, the opossum, has revealed the fundamental plan of the neurohypophyseal lobule (Fig. 27-12).   In the "typical" lobule, the central core of nerve fibers extends to the margin of the lobule as parallel arrays of blindly ending nerve fiber terminals, the *palisade zone*.   The lobule is surrounded by a *septal zone* of loose collagenous tissue containing a rich network of capillary vessels, which in some fashion receive the secretory products contained in the nerve terminals. Among the nerve fibers are dispersed the dominant intrinsic cells of the neurohypophysis, the neuroglia-like *pituicytes,* whose short processes often extend out to the septal zone between the nerve terminals. They have been described in detail by Romeis (1940), who emphasized the occurrence of a variety of pituicytes and a variety of inclusions within them. In most mammals, including man, the lobular pattern is greatly distorted, but careful inspection may reveal "typical" lobules as well as lobules so modified as to appear "inverted," with a central rather than peripheral septal or vascular zone.

In about 5 percent of human hypophyses, aggregates of large, round cells with coarse PAS-positive granules can be seen in the neurohypophysis. The origin and significance of these so-called *choristomas* are not known.

A histologic key to the role of the neurohypophysis was supplied by the finding of Bargmann (1966) that the abundant gelatinous material in the pars nervosa, erroneously described by Herring as a product of the pars intermedia, could be selectively stained and shown to be present not only in the pars nervosa but also in the nerve fibers of the hypothalamohypophyseal system. In some mammals the stainable material is also readily demonstrable in nerve cell bodies in the hypothalamus. By means of certain stains (chrome-alum-hematoxylin, aldehyde fuchsin, or aldehyde thionin after permanganate oxidation), this *neurosecretory substance* (Figs. 27-12 and 27-13) is stained a brilliant blue or purple. Thickenings, outpocketings, and terminals of the axons in the hypothalamohypophyseal tract, the so-called *Herring bodies* (Fig. 27-13), have similar staining characteristics. Conclusive evidence for the relation of the neurosecretory substance to the active principles of the neurohypophysis was obtained by the demonstration that the substance can be depleted by certain osmotic stimuli, such as salt ingestion or water deprivation, which have an antidiuretic effect (Fig. 27-14). Moreover, depletion of the stainable substance is concomitant with depletion of the antidiuretic activity of extracts of the pars nervosa.

FINE STRUCTURE

Electron-microscopic studies have revealed that electron-dense, membrane-bounded granules of the order of 100 to 300 nm, contained within axons and axon terminals in the neurohypophysis, disappear in response to and are restored by the same stimuli which cause depletion and restoration of the neurosecretory substance and of posterior lobe hormones, respectively. Electron-microscopic studies of the secretory process in the neurohypophysis have revealed that neurosecretory granules are found only within the cytoplasm of nerve cells, and especially in the nerve fiber terminals (Fig. 27-15). These granules are reminiscent of membrane-bounded granules of smaller size found in adrenal medulla (catecholamine granules) (Fig. 31-16) and in adrenergic nerve endings. In addition to neurosecretory granules, smaller vesicles (30 nm) have also been observed in the nerve fiber terminals in the pars nervosa. These resemble synaptic vesicles. The specific granules of the posterior pituitary have been isolated in relatively pure form by centrifugal sedimentation in a fraction containing most of the hormone of the gland. Some evidence was obtained that vasopressin and oxytocin are stored in different granules.

In light-microscopic preparations stained with silver, the Herring bodies are revealed as greatly expanded axon portions, containing a more densely stained core. In electron-microscopic preparations (Fig. 27-15), the core appears as a densely osmiophilic mass of tightly packed concentric membranes, or it may contain a number of smaller laminated bodies. The peripheral axoplasm contains numerous neurosecretory granules that are usually more electron-opaque than those seen in the palisade zone terminals. Depletion of granules of Herring bodies by means of osmotic stimulation is more difficult to achieve than is the depletion of those in the palisade zone.

HISTOCHEMISTRY

The localization of the active principles of the neurohypophysis by chemically specific methods rests upon the finding that both ADH and oxytocin (which were synthesized by du Vigneaud) are octapeptides which contain cystine. Histochemical techniques for the disulfide groups of cystine (for example, performic acid–Alcian Blue) have been

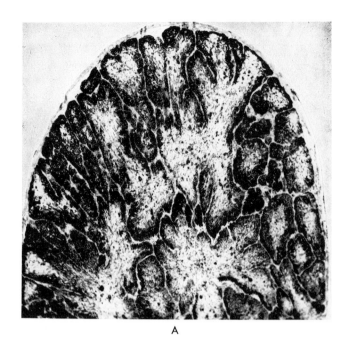

A

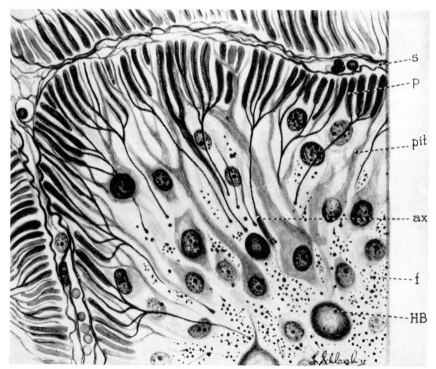

B

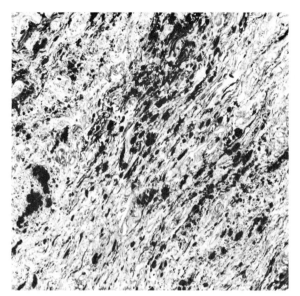

Figure 27-13 Neurosecretion-laden fibers of the human infundibular stem are shown in contact with or near Herring bodies (dark, irregular blobs). Aldehyde thionin after permanganate oxidation. ×160.

successfully applied to the demonstration of neurosecretory substance. No rational basis has been found for the selectivity of chrome-alumhematoxylin and of other staining methods mentioned for the neurosecretory substance. They evidently demonstrate the carrier proteins (neurophysins I, II, and III) to which at least part of the hormones is attached within the axons, and which are secreted into the blood along with the hormones.

HISTOPHYSIOLOGY

Of the two hormones of the neurohypophysis, *vasopressin* was named after its pharmacologic blood-pressure-raising effect; the term *antidiuretic hormone* (ADH) is preferable since it refers to a physiologic function of the hormone: It makes the distal convoluted tubules and collecting ducts of the kidney permeable to water and thereby enables the solute pool in the renal medulla to cause water absorption from these ducts. In the absence of ADH, a large volume (sometimes 20 liters per day or more) of dilute urine is voided (diabetes insipidus). *Oxytocin* (the spelling should be ocytocin) is named after the effect relatively large doses of this hormone have on the parturient uterus: by enhancing contractions to "speed up birth." Whether this is a normal physiologic function of the hormone is questionable. However, oxytocin is known to play a role in the evacuation of the lactating breast, from whose alveoli it squeezes milk by causing contraction of the myoepithelial cells surrounding them.

Although it was originally believed that the hormones of the neurohypophysis are produced by pituicytes, which are stimulated by the fibers of the hypothalamohypophyseal tract that terminate around them, the prevalent view is that of Bargmann, who first suggested that the hormones are manufactured in the perikarya of the supraoptic and paraventricular nuclei and travel with the axoplasmic flow along the axons arising from these, to be discharged at or near the nerve endings in the posterior lobe. Section of the pituitary stalk or removal of the posterior lobe alone does not cause permanent diabetes insipidus: The median eminence in experimental animals subjected to these procedures is readily transformed into a miniature infundibular process. ADH and oxytocin are extractable from the hypothalamus, not only the neurohypophysis, although in small amounts. The classic observations of Fisher, Ingram, and Ranson (1938), who produced diabetes insipidus by placing

Figure 27-12 Opossum neural lobe. A. Low-power view. The lobules are outlined by the dense staining of the palisade zone surrounding the pale hilum of each lobule. Note deeply stained Herring bodies in the hilum of each lobule. Chrome-alumhematoxylin. ×70. B. Schematic representation of the histologic organization of a neural lobe lobule. Nerve fibers of the hypophyseal tract (f), pituicyte cell bodies (pit), and three Herring bodies (HB) are shown in the hilum of the lobule (lower right). Surrounding this, the palisade zone (p) is seen to be formed by rod-like nerve fiber terminals containing the stained neurosecretory substance. Although light micrographs have suggested that the nerve fiber terminals are coated with neurosecretory substance, electron micrographs indicate that the granules which probably represent neurosecretory substance are confined within the plasma membrane of the axon terminals. The central core of the cylindrical axon terminals often contains a cluster of neurofilaments which may represent the axon terminal as seen in silver impregnations at the light-microscopic level. Interspersed among axon terminals are pituicyte fibers which extend to the vascular-collagenous septal layer (s). Axon (ax). (Bodian.)

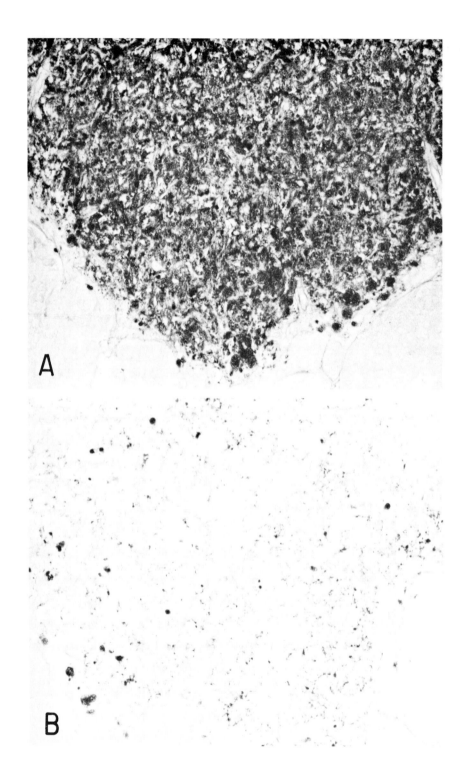

lesions in the hypothalamus of cats, are easily explained: By severing the hypothalamohypophyseal tract before it reaches the neurohypophysis, such lesions prevent the normal flow of hormones to their site of delivery into the blood and even cause retrograde degeneration of the nerve cells in the supraoptic and paraventricular nuclei. There is evidence that ADH is produced primarily in the former and oxytocin in the latter. According to Sachs (1969), the hormones are synthesized as larger molecules (linked to the neurophysins, one of which is relatively specific for ADH and another for oxytocin), and split off while being transported along the axons. Hormone content and the density per area of neurosecretory granules (which also contain neurophysins) correlate well if measured along the hypothalamohypophyseal tract, or during dehydration experiments (Fig. 27-14). Release of ADH and oxytocin (which can occur independently) takes place when the neurosecretory granules rupture at the nerve terminals: The contents enter the perivascular spaces and there quickly lose their electron density. Only in exceptional circumstances, as after stimulation with nicotine, does stainable neurosecretory material appear in the blood vessels. The role of the small synaptic-like vesicles in the nerve endings of the hypothalamohypophyseal tract is not clear: Some believe they are remnants of the membranes of burst neurosecretion granules; others believe that they produce acetylcholine which is involved in hormone discharge. What role, if any, the pituicytes play in the release of neurohypophyseal hormones is obscure.

The stimuli for ADH secretion are an increase in plasma osmolality and a decrease of blood volume in certain pressure-sensitive portions of the vascular system. The perikarya of the supraoptic nucleus themselves may be osmoceptors, since they are in unusually intimate contact with capillaries. The question arises why secretion of neurohypophyseal hormones cannot occur into such hypothalamic capillaries themselves. It may be pertinent that the hypothalamus has and the neuro-hypophysis lacks a blood-brain barrier; for example, the former does not and the latter does stain with vital dyes injected into animals. It is conceivable that the blood-brain barrier permits the passage of the constituent amino acids of the peptide hormones but prevents the entry of these hormones into blood after their synthesis, whereas this is not impeded in the neurohypophysis. ADH discharge also occurs in response to stressful stimuli or upon electrical excitation of the hypothalamus. Oxytocin is released after stimulation of the nipple, as by suckling, or after vaginal distension. These stimuli are conveyed to the hypothalamus along neural pathways.

Bargmann's concept of hypothalamic perikarya as the sole site of synthesis of neurohypophyseal hormones has been challenged. When the infundibular process is depleted of neurosecretory substance after dehydration (Fig. 27-14) and reaccumulates it upon rehydration, this is not necessarily preceded by an increase in this substance (as estimated by light microscopy) in the perikarya of the supraoptic nuclei and the axons coursing through the stalk. However, there is normally so little neurosecretion in the latter locations that such estimates are not reliable, and more sophisticated studies with ^{35}S have not shown its incorporation (presumably into the disulfide-containing hormones) anywhere else than in the cell bodies of the supraoptic and paraventricular neurons.

It is believed that the hypophysiotropic "release" and inhibitory factors, through which the hypothalamus exerts control over the adenohypophysis, are elaborated in the perikarya of scattered tuberal nuclei and then travel to the capillaries of the median eminence and the infundibular stem along the axons of the tuberohypophyseal tract, much as described for the hormones released into the systemic circulation in the infundibular process. However, neither the sites of production of the hypophysiotropic factors nor the histophysiology of their transport and release have been sufficiently well studied to permit positive statements.

Figure 27-14. A. Normal pars nervosa of a rat. It is loaded with neurosecretory substance. B. Pars nervosa of a rat which had received a 2.5 percent sodium chloride solution instead of drinking water for 4 days. Note almost complete disappearance of the neurosecretory substance. Aldehyde fuchsin after permanganate oxidation. ×160.

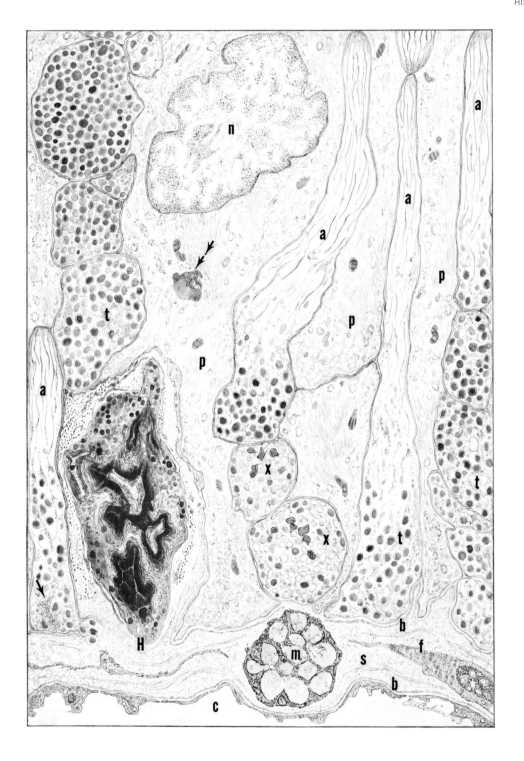

References

GENERAL

DANIEL, P. M.: The Anatomy of the Hypothalamus and Pituitary Gland, in L. Martini and W. F. Ganong, (eds.), "Neuroendocrinology," vol. 1, pp. 15–80, Academic Press, Inc., New York, 1966.

FAWCETT, D. W., J. A. LONG, and A. L. JONES: The Ultrastructure of Endocrine Glands, *Recent Progr. Hormone Res.*, **25**:315–380 (1969).

GANONG, W. F., and L. MARTINI (eds.): "Frontiers in Neuroendocrinology," Oxford University Press, New York, 1969.

MEITES, J. (ed.): "Hypophysiotropic Hormones of the Hypothalamus: Assay and Chemistry," The Williams & Wilkins Company, Baltimore, 1970.

ROMEIS, B.: Hypophyse, in W. von Möllendorff (ed.), "Handbuch der mikroskopischen Anatomie des Menschen," vol. 6, pt. 3, Springer-Verlag OHG, Berlin, 1940.

ADENOHYPOPHYSIS

BAIN, J., and C. EZRIN: Immunofluorescent Localization of the LH Cell of the Human Adenohypophysis, *J. Clin. Endocr.*, **30**:181–184 (1970).

BAKER, B. L.: Studies on Hormone Localization with Emphasis on the Hypophysis, *J. Histochem. Cytochem.*, **18**:1–8 (1970).

BECK, J. S., and A. R. CURRIE: Immunofluorescence Localization of Growth Hormone in the Human Pituitary Gland and of a Related Antigen in the Syncytiotrophoblast, *Vitamins Hormones* (*NY*), **25**:89–121 (1967).

EZRIN, C., and S. MURRAY: The Cells of the Adenohypophysis in Pregnancy, Thyroid Disease and Adrenal Cortical Disorders, in J. Benoit and C. da Lage (eds.), "Cytologie de l'Adénohypophyse," pp. 183–200, Editions du C. N. R. S. (no. 128), 1963.

FRANTZ, A. G., and D. L. KLEINBERG: Prolactin: Evidence That It Is Separate from Growth Hormone in Human Blood, *Science*, **170**:745–747 (1970).

FURTH, J., and K. H. CLIFTON: Experimental Pituitary Tumors, in G. W. Harris and B. T. Donovan (eds.), "The Pituitary Gland," vol. 2, pp. 460–497, University of California Press, Berkeley, 1966.

GOLUBOFF, L. G., and C. EZRIN: Effect of Pregnancy on the Somatotroph and the Prolactin Cell of the Human Hypophysis, *J. Clin. Endocr.*, **29**:1533–1538 (1969).

HALMI, N. S., W. F. MC CORMICK, and D. A. DECKER, JR.: The Natural History of Hyalinization of ACTH-MSH Cells in Man, *Arch. Path.*, **91**:318–326 (1971).

Figure 27-15 Diagram illustrating, at the electron-microscopic level, the principal features of organization of the zone of hormone transfer in the opossum. Capillary lumen (c) lined by endothelium with abundant vesicles indicating active pinocytosis, and numerous "pores"; septal zone (s), composed of collagen space, bounded by basement membranes (b), and separating palisade axon terminals (t) from endothelium. Septal zone contains fibroblasts (f) and mast cells (tip of mast cell shown at m) Isolated depleted palisade terminals (x) occur in the normal animal, unassociated with an increase of synaptic microvesicles. Such vesicles (arrow) typically occupy the tips of palisade terminals near the septal zone. Axons (a) are generally free of neurosecretory granules, which occur almost wholly within the expanded palisade axon terminals. Axons and palisade axon terminals are interspersed with pituicytes and their processes (p), which may extend down to the septal zone. Pituicytes occasionally contain dense inclusions (double arrow). Nucleus of pituicyte (N). Herring bodies (H) are axon terminals apparently formed by development of a central cavity, which becomes surrounded by densely packed membranous lamellae. The cytoplasmic matrix is characteristically electron-dense and contains neurosecretory granules and multivesicular bodies. Herring bodies are found not only in the hilum of pars nervosa but as far distally as the border of the septal zone, where they may be surrounded by membranous processes of the pituicytes. Approximately ×8,000. (Bodian.)

HERBERT, D. C., and T. HAYASHIDA: Prolactin Localization in the Primate Pituitary by Immunofluorescence, *Science,* **169:**378–379 (1970).

HERLANT, M., and J. L. PASTEELS: Histophysiology of Human Anterior Pituitary, *Meth. Achievm. Exp. Path.,* **3:**250–305 (1967).

KUROSUMI, K.: Functional Classification of Cell Types of the Anterior Pituitary Gland Accomplished by Electron Microscopy, *Arch. Histol. Jap.,* **29:**329–362 (1968).

NAKANE, P.: Classifications of Anterior Pituitary Cell Types with Immunoenzyme Histochemistry, *J. Histochem. Cytochem.,* **18:**9–20 (1970).

PHIFER, R. F., and S. S. SPICER: Immunohistologic and Immunopathologic Demonstration of Adrenocorticotrophic Hormone in the Pars Intermedia of the Hypophysis, *Lab. Invest.,* **23:**543–550 (1970).

PHIFER, R. F., S. S. SPICER, and D. N. ORTH: Specific Demonstration of Human Hypophysial Cells Which Produce Adrenocorticotropic Hormone, *J. Clin. Endocr.,* **31:**347–361 (1970).

PURVES, H. D.: Cytology of the Adenohypophysis, in G. W. Harris and B. T. Donovan (eds.), "The Pituitary Gland," vol. 1, pp. 147–232, University of California Press, Berkeley, 1966.

SIPERSTEIN, E. R., and K. J. MILLER: Further Evidence for the Identity of the Cells That Produce Adrenocorticotrophic Hormone, *Endocrinology,* **86:**451–486 (1970).

NEUROHYPOPHYSIS

BARGMANN, W.: Neurosecretion, *Int. Rev. Cytol.,* **19:**183–201 (1966).

BINDLER, E., F. S. LA BELLA, and M. SANWAL: Isolated Nerve Endings (Neurosecretosomes) from the Posterior Pituitary. Partial Separation of Vasopressin and Oxytocin and the Isolation of Microvesicles, *J. Cell Biol.,* **34:**185–205 (1967).

BODIAN, D.: Cytological Aspects of Neurosecretion in Opossum Neurohypophysis, *Bull. Hopkins Hosp.,* **113:**57–93 (1963).

BOUDIER, J. L., J. A. BOUDIER, and D. PICARD: Ultrastructure du lobe postérieur de l'hypophyse du rat et ses modifications au cours de l'excrétion de vasopressine, *Z. Zellforsch.,* **108:**357–379 (1970).

CHRIST, J. F.: Nerve Supply, Blood Supply and Cytology of the Neurohypophysis, in G. W. Harris and B. T. Donovan (eds.), "The Pituitary Gland," vol. 3, pp. 62–130, University of California Press, Berkeley, 1966.

FISHER, C. V., W. R. INGRAM, and S. W. RANSON: Diabetes Insipidus and the Neurohumoral Control of Water Balance: A Contribution to the Structure and Function of the Hypothalamicohypophysial System, J. W. Edwards, Publisher, Incorporated, Ann Arbor, Mich., 1938.

SACHS, H., P. FAWCETT, Y. TAKABATAKE, and R. PORTANOVA: Biosynthesis and Release of Vasopressin and Neurophysin, *Recent Progr. Hormone Res.,* **25:**447–491 (1969).

SCHARRER, B.: Neurohumors and Neurohormones: Definitions and Terminology, *J. Neuro-Visc. Rel., Suppl.,* **9:**1–20 (1969).

SCHARRER, B.: The Neurosecretory Neuron in Neuroendocrine Regulatory Mechanisms, *Amer. Zool.,* **7:**161–169 (1967).

SLOPER, J. C.: The Experimental and Cytopathological Investigation of Neurosecretion in the Hypothalamus and Pituitary, in G. W. Harris and B. T. Donovan (eds.), "The Pituitary Gland," vol. 3, pp. 130–288, University of California Press, Berkeley, 1966.

chapter 28

The pineal gland

WILLARD D. ROTH

Origin

The pineal body (epiphysis cerebri) arises early in the second month of gestation as a dorsal outgrowth of the caudal diencephalon, much as the pituitary pars nervosa (hypophysis cerebri) arises ventrally from the same brain segment. The pineal body develops into a flattened conical structure, which in the adult is 5 to 8 mm in length and 3 to 5 mm in breadth, and remains attached to the brain by a short hollow stalk lined with ependyma (Fig. 28-1). Differentiation and growth of the pineal body continue several years postnatally. In rats, mitosis occurs during the first two postnatal weeks, and the pineal continues to enlarge via cellular hypertrophy until shortly after puberty. The pineal body in man continues to enlarge during childhood.

The mammalian pineal is recognized as a modified remnant of much more extensive and often photoreceptive sensory epiphyseal systems of cold-blooded vertebrates. Because of lack of known function for the human pineal body it has been neglected in modern studies, with recent knowledge of mammalian pineal organs arising from investigations on laboratory animals.

Connective tissue and blood and nerve supply

The pineal body has a thin capsule, formed of pia mater, from which trabeculae of connective tissue extend inwardly to divide the organ into irregular lobules (Fig. 28-2). Many blood vessels traverse these septa and give rise to a rich capillary network. Quay (1962) has shown the pineal blood supply in rats to be relatively nearly as great as that of the adenohypophysis. Wislocki and Leduc (1952) found the pineal body stained after intravitam injection of trypan blue or ingestion of silver nitrate. Therefore, the blood vessels of the pineal organ, as those of the neurohypophysis, act like

Habenular   Pineal   Habenular   Pineal
nucleus   stalk   commissure   body·   Capsule

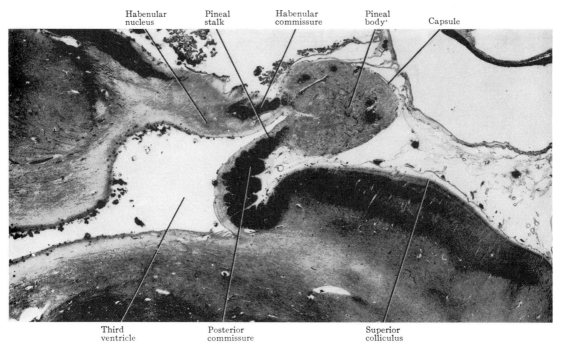

Third   Posterior   Superior
ventricle   commissure   colliculus

Figure 28-1   Sagittal section of the human pineal organ and neighboring structures in the epithalamus, near the midline. Loyes iron-hematoxylin technique for myelin.   ×8.   (Courtesy of P. I. Yakovlev.)

peripheral vessels in their permeability to these substances, and the pineal body must be regarded as lying outside the blood-brain barrier. The endothelium of pineal capillaries is fenestrated much like that in the pituitary and thyroid glands.

Scattered nerve fibers from various regions in the dorsal diencephalon enter the pineal organ, but distinct nerve tracts have not been observed. Ariëns-Kappers (1962) has found most, if not all, nerve fibers in the pineal stalk of rats to be aberrant commissural fibers; it appears unlikely that the gland, at least in that species, receives significant innervation from the brain.

Principal innervation of the organ is via autonomic fibers originating in the superior cervical ganglia and entering the pineal substance through two large tracts, the nervi conarii, coursing through the tentorium cerebelli. Ariëns-Kappers points out that the innervation of the organ is more extensive than could be accounted for by the innervation of the pineal blood vessels. In addition, he has produced light micrographs, and others have produced electron micrographs, suggesting that some autonomic fibers terminate on pineal cells (see Fig. 28-3).

Cells

The cells of the pineal body are neuroectodermal (embryonic ependymal layer) but bear little semblance to nerve cells when fully differentiated. At least two distinct types of cells are recognizable: *parenchymal,* or *chief cells* (pinealocytes, pineocytes, epiphyseal cells) (Fig. 28-4), and stellate

interstitial cells (Fig. 28-5), considered by most microscopists to be astrocytic neuroglial cells.

PARENCHYMAL OR CHIEF CELLS
The parenchymatous cells predominate. Light microscopy reveals them as large, clear cells with

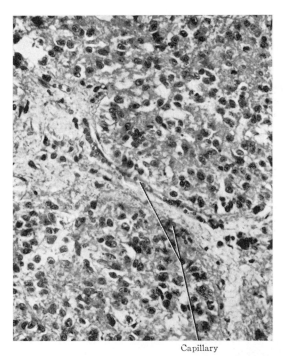

Figure 28-2 Adult human pineal, showing two lobules separated by a trabecula passing diagonally from left to right. Bouin's H&E. ×250.

slender processes having club-shaped endings usually in interstitial trabeculae or perivascular spaces. The nuclei are vesicular, frequently highly indented or lobate, and contain prominent nucleoli. The parenchymal cells display a moderate to strong cytoplasmic basophilia and often contain conspicuous lipid droplets. By electron microscopy (Fig. 28-6) parenchymal cell nuclei are markedly indented and often have deep, slender invaginations of cytoplasm containing cytoplasmic organelles. Very probably these small fingers of cytoplasm account for many of the acidophilic "nuclear secretion droplets" of traditional microscopy. Some intranuclear inclusion bodies are found but appear to be artefacts of fixation. The cytoplasm contains a number of mitochondria, variably developed Golgi complexes, rough and smooth endoplasmic reticulum (ER) in varying amounts, and fairly numerous free ribosomes. Parenchymal cell cytoplasm also contains lipid inclusions, which often have an irregular scalloped form and are frequently seen in association with membranes of the granular reticulum.

Typical lysosomes have also been identified. Wolfe (1965) describes distinctive tight bundles of microtubules which might be centriolar derivatives. Centrioles and rare flagella may also be present. Although various types of membrane-limited inclusions can be found in the cytoplasm of parenchymal cells (Fig. 28-7), none as yet can be

Figure 28-3 A. Large bundles of autonomic nerve fibers coursing in several directions beneath the dorsal surface of rat pineal. ×250. (Romanes.) B. Interfollicular nerve bundle giving rise to individual intrafollicular fibers in rat pineal. Arrow indicates interstitial cell nucleus. ×800. (Bodian.) (Courtesy of J. Ariëns-Kappers, 1960, by permission of *Zeitschrift fur Zellforschung mikroskopische Anatomie.*)

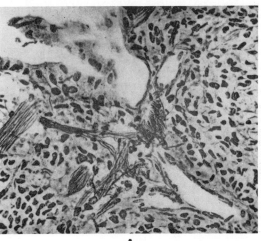

A

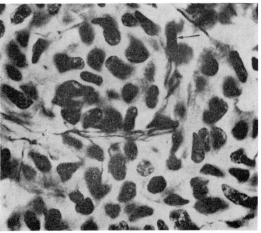

B

Interlobular
septum

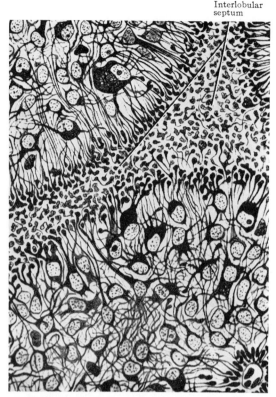

Figure 28-4 Semidiagrammatic representation of adult human pineal body, showing two lobules containing polymorphic parenchymatous cells. Club-shaped prolongations of the parenchymal cells end on blood vessels in the interlobular space. (After Del Rio Hortega.)

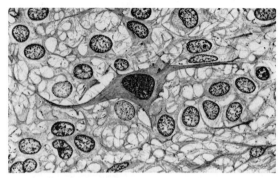

Figure 28-5 Large interstitial cell (astrocyte) in a lobule of adult human pineal. Eosin, methylene blue. (After W. Bargmann, 1943.)

specifically identified as "secretion granules." Indeed, distinction between pinealocyte processes and endings of autonomic nerve fibers is difficult. In any case, it seems clear that pineal parenchymatous cells do not display the prominent evidences of secretion characteristic of other known endocrine cells. A final distinctive feature of the parenchymal cells is the presence of clusters of vesicle-crowned rodlets identical in appearance to the "synaptic ribbons" that occur in many receptor cells. However, they rarely occur in juxtaposition to nerve terminals, and their significance remains in doubt.

INTERSTITIAL OR SUPPORTIVE CELLS

Interstitial cells (Figs. 28-5 and 28-8) of the pineal body are markedly stellate in appearance, with individual extensions often running long distances through the tissue and ending in various relationships to other cellular elements, perivascular spaces, and nerve fibers. These cells have a more dense nucleus and cytoplasm, fewer mitochondria, and more granular reticulum than parenchymal cells. They may possess cilia, basal bodies, and centrioles, and they often contain dense bodies of unknown composition. Interstitial cells are present both in the perivascular spaces and between clusters of parenchymal cells. They constitute approximately 5 percent of the cells in the pineal organ.

Other cells have been described which appear convincingly like neuroglial astrocytes when stained with silver preparations in the light microscope, but glial cells have not been identified with certainty in electron micrographs. In addition, Quay (1962) has described a variety of stellate cells in the rat pineal which are strongly stained by the acid-hematin technique. These have not yet been iden-

Figure 28-6 Electron micrograph of a follicle-like array of parenchymal cells in a rat pineal body. Parenchymal cell nuclei (NP) are markedly indented and contain large, complex nucleoli (NOP). Parenchymal cell cytoplasm (CP) frequently contains irregular lipid inclusions (L). Bulbous apical processes (AP) of parenchymal cells project into the follicular lumen (FL). The much darker nucleus (NI) and cytoplasm (CI) of interstitial cells are seen in the perivascular space (V). ×6,000. (Courtesy of D. Wolfe.)

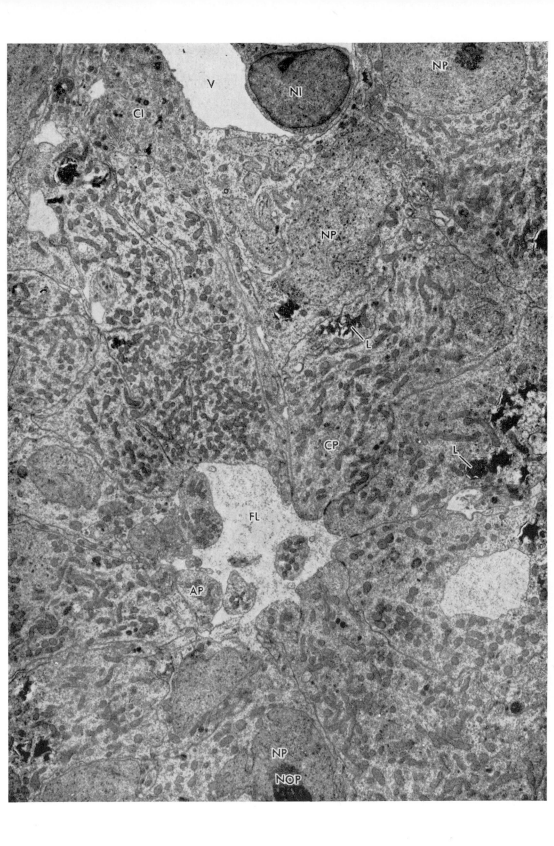

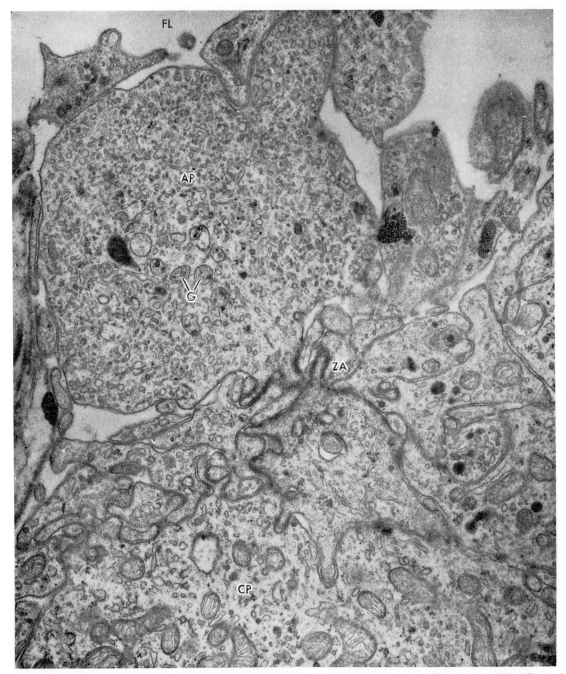

Figure 28-7 Apical process (AP) of parenchymal cell cytoplasm (CP) projecting into the follicular lumen (FL). The bulbous ending contains numerous vesicles and tubular elements as well as some larger coarse granules (G). The process extends between neighboring cells via a thin neck region which is ringed by a zonula adhaerens (ZA). ×30,000. (Courtesy of D. Wolfe.)

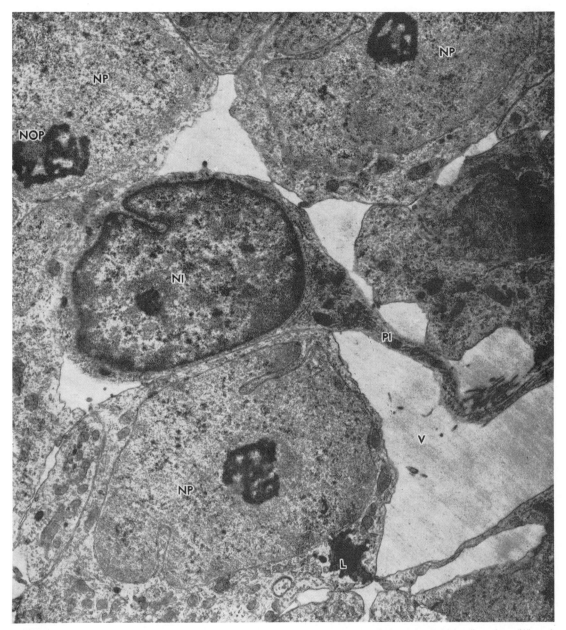

Figure 28-8   Border of the perivascular space (V) with contrasting appearance of dense interstitial cell nucleus (NI) and paler, indented parenchymal cell nuclei (NP).   A narrow process of the interstitial cell (PI) contains much granular endoplasmic reticulum.   L, lipid droplet; NOP, parenchymal cell nucleolus.   ×15,000.   (Courtesy of D. Wolfe.)

tified with the electron microscope. Wolfe (1965) suggests that the interstitial cells of electron microscopy, the astrocytes observed with silver techniques, and the acid-hematin cell of Quay may be identical and that no true neuroglial cells occur in the pineal. It is probable that some species variation exists in the form and number of interstitial or supportive cell elements.

Connective tissue cells, mast cells, Schwann cells, and axons of autonomic nerves are also found in the pineal body, largely along the walls of the vessels. In a number of species, bundles or individual fibers of striated muscle have occasionally been observed in pineal bodies. These are apparently an anomaly of no functional significance.

Concretions

The pineal body in man often contains concretions termed *brain sand* (*acervuli cerebri*, or corpora arenacea) (Fig. 28-9). These concretions are of an as yet unidentified organic matrix mineralized with hydroxyapatite and calcium carbonate apatite. The concretions frequently exhibit concentric layers. They are present in 1 to 2 percent of cases during the first decade of life, about 25 percent in the second, and the proportion increases thereafter to roughly 70 to 80 percent in old age.

Although this chronological incidence has been taken as suggestive of regressive changes commencing at puberty, the significance, if any, is not understood, and they occur only sparingly in most other mammalian species. Even when they are numerous, however, there is much normal parenchymal tissue present; consequently the assumption commonly made that the pineal "calcifies after puberty" is misleading in a histologic sense.

Histochemistry and histophysiology

Although complete understanding of the mammalian pineal body's role in endocrine regulation requires further information, investigations of recent years suffice to establish a physiologic significance that negates former opinions of a mere vestigial structure.

Experimentation with laboratory animals has substantiated earlier theories, based upon cases of precocious puberty shown by boys with parenchymal-cell-destroying tumors, that pineal secretion exercises an antigonadal effect. These investigations have served further to demonstrate that pineal physiology is markedly influenced by daily and, possibly, seasonal photoperiodicity.

Studies with radioisotopes have demonstrated a very high level of phosphorus metabolism and amino acid incorporation, and histochemical methods reveal large amounts of acid phosphatase, succinic dehydrogenase, esterases, and lipases in parenchymal cell cytoplasm. Walls of pineal blood vessels contain substantial quantities of alkaline phos-

phatase and monoamine oxidase. In rats, cytoplasmic basophilia and phosphorus metabolism are reduced by exposure of animals to constant light. Extirpation of the superior cervical ganglia shows that effects of photoperiod are mediated by the autonomic innervation.

Further knowledge of the precise role of the biogenic amines norepinephrine, serotonin, and melatonin is central to a satisfactory elucidation of pineal function. Radioisotope electron micrographs indicate that the norepinephrine is concentrated in the terminals of the autonomic nerve fibers; injection and tissue culture experiments suggest strongly that it serves as the primary neurotransmitter in the system. Fluorescent histochemical methods reveal that the exceptionally large amount of serotonin found in the pineal is contained in two pools, parenchymal cell cytoplasm and nerve endings, although it is not yet clear whether the nerves synthesize the compound or merely absorb it from surrounding parenchymal cells. Finally,

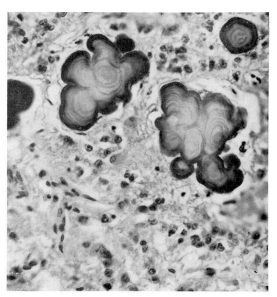

Figure 28-9 Another area of the pineal gland in Fig. 28-1, showing the laminate appearance of the granules of brain sand. ×250.

tory physiology. Melatonin is known to exert a strong blanching of amphibian skin, owing to aggregation of melanin granules in pigment cells, but has no apparent activity on mammalian melanocyte. However, injection of melatonin tends to reduce ovarian weight and alter estrous cycles in rodents. In addition, pineal phospholipid content, serotonin content, and HIOMT activity fluctuate with phases of estrus and during pregnancy. Preliminary findings also suggest an effect of melatonin on pituitary, thyroid, and adrenal function, although further evidence is required to substantiate this.

Consequently, the most widely accepted theory of pineal function at the present time is that the organ functions as a neuroendocrine transducer. It is believed that external stimuli, particularly photic, are relayed to the pineal via the autonomic nervous system. These impulses in turn produce alterations in the synthesis and release of melatonin, and possibly other closely related compounds, which in turn serve to alter the level of endocrine function, particularly by the gonads. It is not yet clear whether the effects of melatonin are primarily on the endocrine target organs directly or are further mediated by specific areas of the central nervous system. Evidence exists to support both hypotheses. Thus it seems clear that the pineal body is a neuroendocrine organ exercising subtle and probably complex regulatory effects on the rhythmic activity of the general endocrine system.

melatonin, an amine synthesized from serotonin and related precursors by the activity of the enzyme hydroxyindole-O-methyl transferase (HIOMT), appears to be the primary secretory product of parenchymal cell cytoplasm. In mammals, HIOMT is found exclusively in the pineal tissue, further substantiating the unique role of this organ in regula-

References

ANDERSON, E.: The Anatomy of Bovine and Ovine Pineals. Light and Electron Microscopic Studies, *J. Ultrastruct. Res.*, **8** (Suppl.):5 (1965).

ARIËNS-KAPPERS, J.: First International Round-table Conference on the Epiphysis Cerebri, *Progr. Brain Res.*, **10**:(1965).

ARIËNS-KAPPERS, J.: The Development, Topographical Relations and Innervation of the Epiphysis Cerebri in the Albino Rat, *Z. Zellforsch.*, **52**:163 (1962).

AXELROD, J., and H. WEISSBACH: Purification and Properties of Hydroxyindole-O-Methyl Transferase, *J. Biol. Chem.*, **236**:211 (1961).

BARGMANN, W.: Die Epiphysis cerebri, in W. von Möllendorff (ed.), "Handbüch mikroskopischen Anatomie des Menschen," vol. 6, Springer-Verlag OHG, Berlin, 1943.

DEL RIO HORTEGA, P.: Pineal Gland, in W. Penfield (ed.), "Cytology and Cellular Pathology of the Nervous System," Paul B. Hoeber, Inc., New York, 1932.

FISKE, V. M., J. POUND, and J. PUTNAM: Effect of Light on the Weight of the Pineal Organ in Hypophysectomized, Gonadectomized, Adrenalectomized or Thiouracil-fed Rats, *Endocrinology,* **71:**130 (1962).

KITAY, J. I., and M. D. ALTSCHULE: "The Pineal Gland," Harvard University Press, Cambridge, Mass., 1954.

LERNER, A. A., and J. D. CASE: Pigment Cell Regulatory Factors, *J. Invest. Derm.,* **32:**221 (1959).

QUAY, W. B.: 24-hour Rhythms in Pineal *S*-hydroxytryptamine and Hydroxy-indole-*O*-Methyl Transferase Activity in the Macaque, *Pro. Soc. Exp. Biol. Med.,* **121:**946 (1966).

QUAY, W. B.: Circadian Rhythm in Rat Serotonin and Its Modifications by Estrous Cycles and Photoperiod, *Gen. Comp. Endocr.,* **3:**473 (1963).

QUAY, W. B.: Experimental and Cytological Studies of Pineal Cells Staining with Acid Hematin in the Rat, *Acta Morph. Neerl. Scand.,* **5:**87 (1962).

REITER, R. J., et al.: Symposium on Comparative Endocrinology of the Pineal, *Amer. Zool.,* **10:**187 (1970).

ROTH, W. D.: Metabolic and Morphologic Studies on the Rat Pineal Organ during Puberty, *Progr. Brain Res.,* **10:**(1965).

ROTH, W. D., R. J. WURTMAN, and M. D. ALTSCHULE: Morphologic Changes in the Pineal Parenchymal Cells of Rats Exposed to Continuous Light or Darkness, *Endocrinology,* **71:**888 (1962).

WARTENBERG, H.: The Mammalian Pineal Organ: Electron Microscopic Studies on the Fine Structure of Pinealocytes, Glial Cells and on the Perivascular Component, *Z. Zellforsch.,* **86:**74 (1968).

WISLOCKI, G. B., and E. H. LEDUC: Vital Staining of the Hematoencephalic Barrier by Silver Nitrate and Trypan Blue, and Cytological Comparisons of the Neurohypophysis, Pineal Body, Area Postrema, Intercolumnar Tubercle and Supraoptic Crest, *J. Comp. Neurol.,* **96:**371 (1952).

WOLFE, D. E.: The Epiphyseal Cell: an Electron Microscopic Study of Intracellular Relationships and Intracellular Morphology in the Pineal Body of the Albino Rat, *Progr. Brain Res.,* **10:**(1965).

WOLSTENHOME, G. E., and J. KNIGHT (eds.): "The Pineal Gland," Ciba Foundation Symposium, Churchill Ltd., London, 1971.

WURTMAN, R. J.: Effect of Light and Visual Stimuli on Endocrine Function, in W. F. Ganong and L. Martini (eds.), "Neuroendocrinology," chap. 18, Academic Press, Inc., New York, 1966.

WURTMAN, R. J., J. AXELROD, and D. E. KELLY: "The Pineal," Academic Press, Inc., New York, 1968.

WURTMAN, R. J., W. D. ROTH, M. D. ALTSCHULE, and J. J. WURTMAN: Interactions of the Pineal and Exposure to Continuous Light on Organ Weights of Female Rats, *Acta Endocr.,* **36:**617 (1961).

ZWEENS, J.: Influence of the Oestrous Cycle and Ovariectomy on the Phospho-lipid Content of the Pineal Gland of the Rat, *Nature (London),* **197:**1114 (1963).

chapter 29

The thyroid gland

NICHOLAS S. HALMI

The most important function of the thyroid is the production of its two iodinated amino acid hormones, L-*thyroxine* (tetraiodo-L-thyronine) and 3, 5, 3'-*triiodo*-L-*thyronine*. (More of the former is secreted but the latter is more potent.) The influences of thyroid hormones on the body can be divided into two main classes: stimulation of metabolism (especially oxidative metabolism in a number of tissues) and maturational effects (for example, promotion of the development of the brain and of ossification centers and acceleration of metamorphosis in amphibian tadpoles). Recently it has been recognized that the thyroid also produces a blood calcium-lowering hormone, *calcitonin* (thyrocalcitonin), which originates from the C cells (light cells, parafollicular cells) (Figs. 29-3 and 29-5).

Origin and gross structure

The thyroid gland owes its name to its position: it lies close to the shield-shaped thyroid cartilage of the larynx. Its parenchyma develops as a median downgrowth of the base of the tongue. The thyroglossal duct, which connects the developing gland with its point of origin, usually becomes obliterated. The foramen cecum marks its junction with the epithelium of the tongue. Remnants of the duct may develop into persisting structures, such as thyroid tissue within the tongue (lingual thyroid), thyroglossal cysts, or the lobus pyramidalis, which is usually a cranial extension of the thyroid isthmus. The thyroid may include such derivatives of the branchial pouches as the parathyroid glands and always contains C cells. The C cells are derivatives of the *ultimobranchial body*, which originates from the fifth branchial pouch. This body also produces a system of tubular structures in the thyroid, which

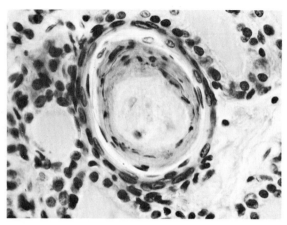

Figure 29-1 Ultimobranchial tubule in a normal rat thyroid. This is the oval cross section of a closed tube lined by stratified squamous epithelium. The lumen contains desquamated cells with pycnotic nuclei, and debris. (Courtesy of C. P. Leblond.)

the follicles, which are variable in shape and size (about 50 to 900 μm in diameter in adult man). Sometimes they resemble branching, blind ducts, around which individual rounded follicles are clustered (without communicating with them). Such units are similar to lobules of an acinar exocrine gland.

The thyroid gland is surrounded by a fibrous capsule. The follicles are separated by stroma, which is typical loose connective tissue. Each follicle is enveloped by a delicate basement membrane consisting of ground substance and reticular fibers.

The exceedingly rich blood supply of the thyroid gland is furnished by the inferior and superior thyroid arteries. The arterioles often have intimal cushions or longitudinal smooth muscle ridges. The extensive capillary network comes in close contact with the basement membranes of the follicles.

An intrinsic plexus of lymphatic vessels arises in the interfollicular spaces and collects into larger vessels beneath the capsule. The regional lymph nodes are cervical or even retrosternal.

Postganglionic sympathetic nerve fibers originating in the middle and superior cervical ganglia enter the thyroid. Parasympathetic fibers also appear to penetrate the gland. These must be partly preganglionic, since the thyroid may contain ganglion cells. All these nerve fibers are likely to be vasomotor, although some are said to end around follicular cells. A secretomotor innervation of the thyroid has not been convincingly demonstrated; transplanted thyroid tissue functions adequately.

are often lined by desquamating stratified squamous epithelium (Fig. 29-1). In the adult human being the thyroid weighs about 15 to 20 gm, on an average, and consists of two lateral lobes connected by an isthmus that lies close to the second and third tracheal rings.

The proliferating mass of entodermal cells that develops into the thyroid parenchyma first forms a network of solid cords or plate-like sheets. These break up into small masses, in each of which a lumen appears. As the lumen enlarges, the cells around it become arranged into a single-layered shell. The lumina and the surrounding cells form

Microscopic structure of the follicle

The fundamental unit of the thyroid is the *follicle,* which consists of a homogeneous, viscous mass, the *colloid,* surrounded by a single layer of epithelial cells. The amount and consistency of the colloid as well as the shape of the cells vary greatly, depending on the functional state of the thyroid. When the thyroid is not stimulated by thyrotropin from the anterior pituitary lobe, the cells are squamous and the abundant colloid dense (Fig. 29-2C). Intense stimulation by thyrotropin, on the other hand, leads to the appearance of tall colum-

nar cells (hypertrophy) which are often in mitosis (hyperplasia), and to liquefaction and partial resorption of the colloid (Fig. 29-2D). The structure of the "normal" follicle is intermediate (Fig. 29-2A).

The human thyroid displays a greater variability in the size and shape of individual follicles than does that of most animals. There are further characteristic species differences: The thyroid of the rat, for example, appears much more "active" than that of the guinea pig if both animals consume the same diet and are exposed to the same ambient

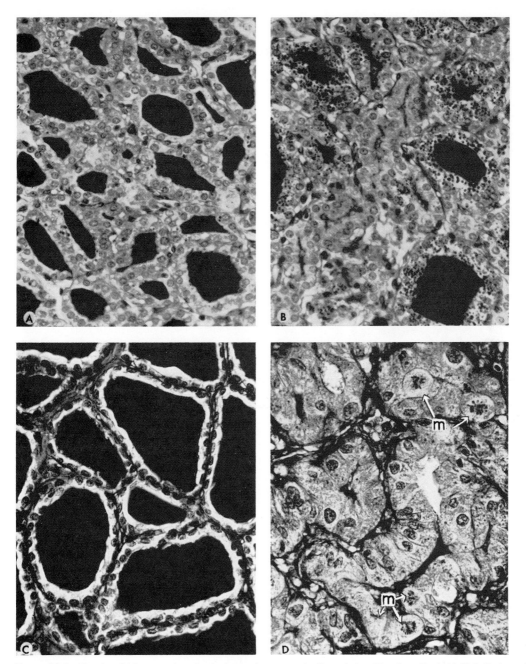

Figure 29-2 Rat thyroid in normal and experimental states. A. Normal thyroid. Note "cuboidal" follicular cells and a few intracellular colloid droplets. B. Thyroid 3 1/2 hr after intravenous injection of 250 mU of thyrotropin. Many follicles contain only traces of colloid. Intracellular colloid droplets are abundant in the follicular cells of follicles which have larger amounts of colloid in their lumina. C. Thyroid several weeks after hypophysectomy. Note distension of lumina by colloid, which shows some shrinkage in the periphery. The follicular cells are flat. D. Thyroid of a rat that was fed an iodine-deficient diet for several weeks and then injected for 10 days with the thiocarbamide propylthiouracil. The collapsed lumina contain little colloid. The follicular cells are tall columnar; several mitoses (m) can be seen. The capillaries are engorged. All sections stained with PAS-hematoxylin. (A and B from S. H. Wollman, J. Cell Biol., **21:**191, 1964.)

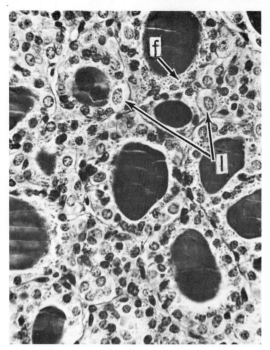

Figure 29-3 Normal rat thyroid. Note differences between follicular cells proper (f), which contain numerous colloid droplets, and the larger C cells (light cells) (l), which do not. PAS-hematoxylin stain. (Courtesy of C. P. Leblond.)

temperature. In the rat thyroid, peripheral follicles are consistently larger than central ones.

The colloid is amphoteric since it stains intensely with eosin and other acid dyes as well as with basic dyes such as methylene blue. Dense colloid is generally more acidophilic; dilute colloid, more basophilic.

There are two kinds of epithelial cells in the thyroid follicles: the follicular cells proper and cells best called C (for calcitonin) cells (Fig. 29-3).

The *follicular cells* border on the lumen and show a definite polarity. The nucleus is near the base of the cell, with the Golgi apparatus lying between it and the lumen. In squamous follicular cells the nucleus is flat; in columnar cells it is spherical and relatively large (Fig. 29-2C and D). Mitochondria are scattered throughout the cell. Colloid droplets are particularly conspicuous after stimulation with thyrotropin (Fig. 29-2B). They were previously believed to be precursors of colloid in the lumen; the best evidence available, however, suggests that they are the result of pinocytosis of luminal colloid by follicular cells. The cytoplasm of follicular cells is basophilic, especially if they are active. Occasionally degenerating cells loaded with large colloid droplets (*colloid cells of Langendorff*) can be seen in the follicular epithelium.

The *C cells* are never in contact with the lumen but lie within the follicular basement membrane, are rather sparse, lack the polarity of follicular cells, do not contain colloid droplets, and may be stimulated by pituitary growth hormone rather than thyrotropin. When appropriately fixed, C cells show many rather small secretory granules of fairly uniform size but variable electron density (Fig. 29-4).

Ultrastructure of the thyroid

The colloid in the lumen is faintly reticular and has moderate electron-scattering properties. Peripheral vacuoles in the colloid often seen under the light microscope are artefacts of shrinkage and do not appear in electron micrographs. The luminal border of the follicular cells shows microvilli (Fig. 29-5) whose height and number increase when the cell becomes more active. Mitochondria are mostly filamentous. The Golgi apparatus is more prominent in active cells than in inactive ones. The endoplasmic reticulum (ER) is also more extensive in stimulated cells, which synthesize large amounts

Figure 29-4 Electron micrograph of the apical portion of a follicular cell stained for acid phosphatase. Note the presence of the enzyme in the darkly stained lysosomes, some of which are closely attached to the much larger colloid droplets (phagosomes) (arrows). The two large droplets with irregular black speckling are phagolysosomes, whose colloid has become intermingled with lysosomal contents, as demonstrated by the irregular staining for acid phosphatase. ×20,000. (From S. H. Wollman, J. Cell Biol., **25**:593, 1965.)

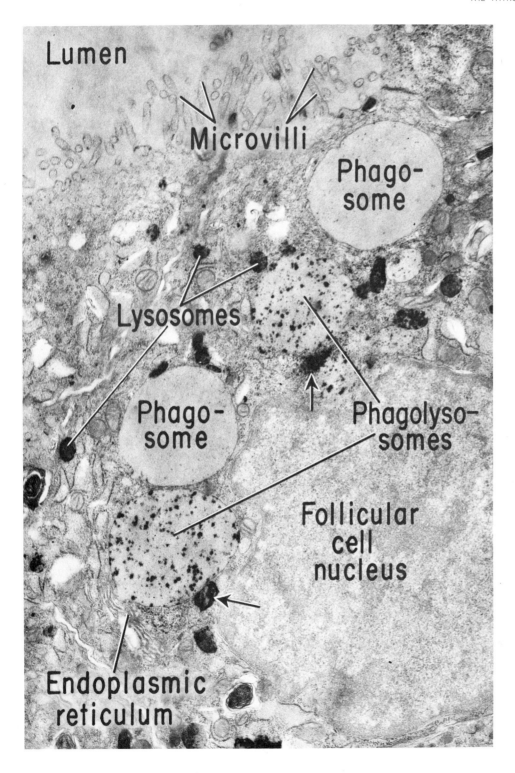

of the protein thyroglobulin. Its sacs may be compressed (Fig. 29-4) or moderately distended (Fig. 29-5). At least three types of rounded bodies occur in the follicular cell, most often above the nucleus: (1) pinocytized colloid droplets (phagosomes), (2) lysosomes (which can be demonstrated by staining for such enzymes as acid phosphatase), and (3) bodies arisen from the fusion of the two previous types (phagolysosomes) (Fig. 29-5).

Small vesicles in the apical part of the cell have been interpreted as representing pinched-off portions of the Golgi apparatus carrying secretion to the lumen.

A structureless basement membrane is clearly evident around the follicles. Next to it collagenous fibrils may be seen. The endothelial cells lining the capillaries frequently show pores in their cytoplasm.

Histochemistry

The luminal colloid is intensely PAS-positive, as are the intracellular colloid droplets (Fig. 29-2B). This reaction, not abolished by previous digestion with amylase, is due largely to the glycoprotein thyroglobulin, which is the main constituent of colloid. Although thyroglobulin contains sialic acid as well as glucosamine, galactose, mannose, and fucose, it does not give the metachromatic reaction with basic thiazine dyes that is characteristic of many acid mucopolysaccharides. Some dense intracellular droplets, unlike colloid in the lumen, exhibit acid phosphatase and esterase reactions; these are evidently lysosomes. Peroxidase activity can also be demonstrated in the thyroid. The role of this enzyme will be described below.

Histophysiology

SYNTHESIS OF THYROID HORMONES
In the follicular cells of the thyroid, the synthesis of hormones proceeds simultaneously in the form of apically and basally directed events. An apically oriented process synthesizes the large (MW 660,000), iodinated glycoprotein thyroglobulin, which is the form in which thyroid hormones are stored in the follicular lumina. A basally directed process starts with the pinocytosis of luminal colloid and terminates with the release of thyroid hormones into the capillaries. Serial radioautographs made at various times after the injection of radioactive forms of ingredients of thyroglobulin, such as ^{131}I or ^{125}I, [^{3}H]-leucine (Fig. 29-6) or [^{3}H]-labeled monosaccharides, have greatly contributed to our understanding of the sequence outlined below.

The basal plasma membrane is the site of active transport of iodide and amino acids into the follicular cell. The synthesis of thyroglobulin precursor proteins and the addition of some of the carbohydrates occur in the rough ER. The carbohydrate component of the molecule is completed and the thyroglobulin precursors are polymerized in the Golgi apparatus. Small vesicles pinched off from this carry the as yet uniodinated glycoprotein to the cell surface. Concurrently, iodide is oxidized to a higher valence state ($I^{+?}$) by a peroxidase: This form of iodine attaches to the tyrosyl groups of thyroglobulin in or near the apical cell membrane. Although some intracellular proteins are also iodinated, radioautography (Fig. 29-7) shows that most of the protein-bound iodine of the thyroid is in the

Figure 29-5   Electron micrograph of a C cell separated from the lumen by two follicular cells. Note the microvilli on the latter, the many unusually electron-opaque lysosomes, the tendency of endoplasmic reticular cisternae to be dilated, and a tight junction between the two cells, near the lumen. The C cell rests on the follicular basement membrane and contains a few dark lysosomes and many secretion granules of varying density, the bounding membrane of some of which is clearly descernible. ×12,000. (Courtesy of S. L. Erlandsen.)

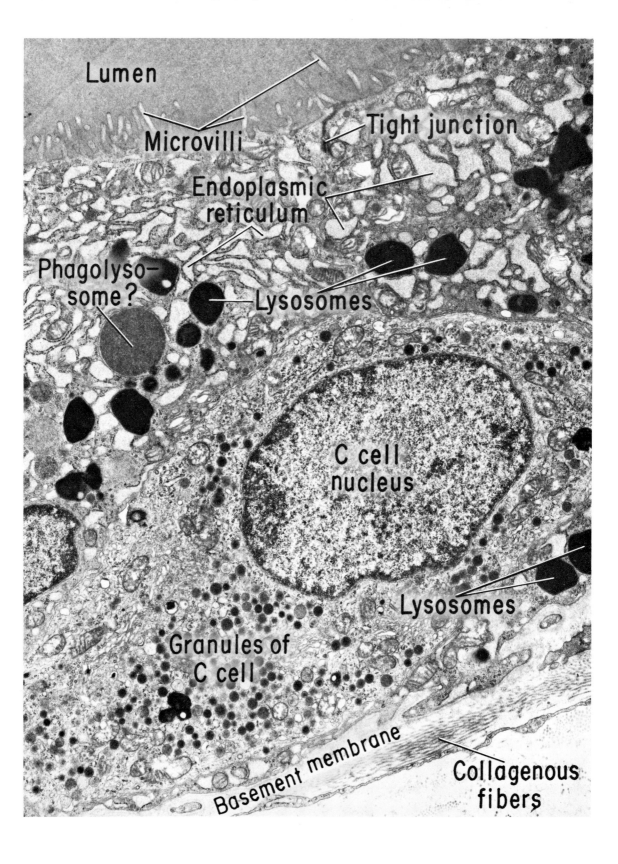

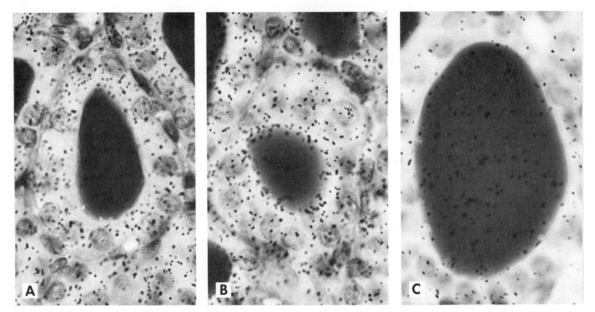

Figure 29-6   Radioautographs of thyroids from rats killed at various time intervals after the injection of [³H]-labeled leucine. The dark grains indicate the locations of proteins (largely thyroglobulin) synthesized from the labeled leucine.   A. At 30 min, the grains overlie the cytoplasm of the follicular cells.   They are located throughout the cell but are scarce at the apical edge in contact with the colloid.   No grains are over the colloid.   B. At 4 hr, the grains predominate in the apical end of the cells.   C. At 36 hr, the grains are distributed uniformly over the colloid.   All three sections are counterstained with PAS-hematoxylin. (Courtesy of N. J. Nadler, K. Harrison, and C. P. Leblond.)

lumina.   Coupling of iodotyrosyl groups within the thyroglobulin molecule produces peptide-linked hormone (iodothyronyl) groups.   Mobilization of hormone thus stored requires that luminal thyroglobulin be pinocytized by the follicular cells, a process which evidently depends on the action of microtubules, since it can be poisoned with colchicine, and on microfilaments, as it can be abolished with cytochalasin B.   Intracellular thyroglobulin in the phagosomes is hydrolyzed to its constituent amino acids as the phagosomes fuse with lysosomes and form phagolysosomes (Fig. 29-4).   The acid pH within the limiting membrane of phagolysosomes makes it possible for thyroglobulin to be digested by acid proteases and peptidases without harm to the rest of the cell.   The iodothyronine hormones thus freed leave the cell at its base.   The iodotyrosine precursors (which account for 70 percent of the iodine in thyroglobulin) are enzymatically deiodinated, and the iodide liberated is reutilized within the thyroid for hormone synthesis.

The origin of calcitonin from the C cells has been documented by immunofluorescent techniques.

REGULATION OF THE THYROID

The most important physiologic regulator of the thyroid, and perhaps the only one that has morphologically demonstrable effects on the gland, is thyrotropin.   The central nervous system, through the hypothalamic thyrotropin release factor (see Chap. 27), stimulates the anterior lobe of the hypophysis to secrete excess thyrotropin in response to lowered levels of thyroid hormone in the blood; elevated levels of circulating thyroid hormone in turn depress thyrotropin secretion, probably by local action on the hypophysis.

The mode and site of action of thyrotropin on the thyroid are not known.   Its first observable effect is a stimulation of colloid pinocytosis; intracellular colloid droplets first appear in apical "streamers" of the follicular cells and later in the cytoplasm itself (Fig. 29-2B); simultaneously the density and amount of colloid in the follicular lumina decrease.   An increase in the blood flow through the gland is another early sequel of thyrotropin action.   While the colloid is resorbed during continued thyrotropic stimulation, the follicular cells hypertrophy and then divide. The morphologic effects of chronic hypersecretion of thyrotropin on the thyroid are spectacular (Fig. 29-2C as against D): It eventually leads to the formation of a big, highly vascular thyroid poor in colloid—a parenchymal (or hyperplastic) goiter. If large amounts of thyrotropin are secreted for many months, benign tumors (adenomas) or even malignant growths (carcinomas) of the thyroid may ensue. In the presence of the hypophysis, any of the following factors that cause sustained lowering of the levels of circu-

Figure 29-7   Radioautograph of the thyroid of a rat which had received ^{125}I-labeled iodide in its drinking water long enough to have its body iodine stores labeled to the same specific redioactivity (that is, the same number of counts per minute per unit mass of iodine). In this condition of so-called radioisotopic equilibrium, the distribution of radioactivity reflects that of nonradioactive iodine faithfully. Note that essentially all the blackening of the emulsion due to the radioactive iodine is over the colloid in the lumina rather than in the follicular epithelium.   ×240.   (From S. H. Wollman, Endocrinology, 81:1074, 1967.)

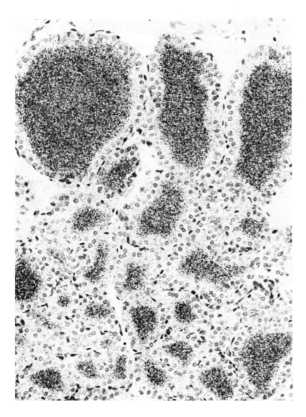

lating thyroid hormones lead to the formation of a parenchymal goiter: (1) iodine-deficient diet; (2) antithyroid agents (goitrogens), such as thiocyanate, which is an inhibitor of thyroidal iodide transport, or thiocarbamides, which interfere with organification of iodine in the thyroid; and (3) perhaps even increased fecal excretion of thyroid hormones due to a high-residue diet. Iodine deficiency prevails in many regions, and goitrogens occur in a number of consumable plants. If the parenchymal goiter becomes large enough to produce normal amounts of hormone despite the underlying impediment to thyroid hormone formation, excessive thyrotropin secretion may subside and the follicles can again accumulate colloid, but their number remains elevated; a colloid goiter is thereby formed. Colloid goiter is often found in people whose diet is deficient in iodine. It has been experimentally produced by feeding iodine to hamsters that had parenchymal goiters owing to iodine deficiency.

Hypothyroidism and hyperthyroidism refer to the level of circulating thyroid hormones, whereas the histologic "activity" of the thyroid reflects the amount of thyrotopin in the blood. If large amounts of exogenous thyroid hormones are given to an experimental animal, the resulting inhibition of thyrotropin production will cause the thyroid to become histologically indistinguishable from that of a hypophysectomized animal. Structural signs of thyroid inactivity can thus be found in the hypothyroid state (after hypophysectomy) or in hyperthyroidism (after injection of thyroid hormones); a morphologically hyperactive thyroid may be found in hypothyroid (that is, goitrogen-treated) or hyperthyroid (thyrotropin-treated) animals.

In the most common form of human hyperthyroidism (Graves' disease), the thyroid shows the histologic criteria of a parenchymal goiter. The blood of such people often contains an IgG immunoglobulin, which is a long-acting thyroid stimulator (LATS) chemically completely unrelated to thyrotropin. The common belief that LATS causes Graves' disease is now being seriously questioned.

The C cells are stimulated to release their granules and the calcitonin contained in them by a rise in plasma Ca^{2+}. Prolonged hypercalcemia can cause C cell hyperplasia. Carcinomas arising from the C cells (medullary carcinomas) contain large amounts of calcitonin and may secrete it in more moderately excessive quantities.

Immunologic reactions of the thyroid

Upon their injection into an animal, thyroglobulin and other thyroidal proteins from the same species or from the animal itself may be treated by the body as if they were foreign proteins (antigens), and antibodies may be produced against them. These antibodies can in turn react with the animal's own thyroid and cause severe inflammation of the gland (thyroiditis), with invasion of the stroma by lympho- cytes and even the appearance of lymphoid nod- ules. Since in a form of human thyroiditis (Hashi- moto's disease) lymphoid infiltration of the thyroid and antithyroid antibodies in blood often occur to- gether, it is possible (but not proved) that this dis- ease is due to an autoimmune reaction against a protein or proteins from the patient's own thyroid gland.

References

ANDROS, G., and S. H. WOLLMAN: Autoradiographic Localization of Radioiodide in the Thyroid Gland of the Mouse, *Amer. J. Physiol.*, **213**:198–208 (1967).

BROWN-GRANT, K.: Regulation of TSH Secretion, in G. W. Harris and B. T. Donovan (eds.), "The Pituitary Gland," vol. 2, pp. 235–269, University of California Press, Berkeley, 1966.

EKHOLM, R.: Thyroid Gland, in S. M. Kurtz (ed.), "Electron Microscopic Anat- omy," pp. 221–237, Academic Press, Inc., New York, 1964.

FOLLIS, R. H., JR.: Experimental Colloid Goiter in the Hamster, *Proc. Soc. Exp. Biol. Med.*, **100**:203–206 (1959).

HEIMANN, P.: Ultrastructure of Human Thyroid: a Study of Normal Thyroid, Untreated and Treated Diffuse Toxic Goiter, *Acta Endocr. (Kobenhavn)*, **53** (Suppl.):110 (1966).

LOEWENSTEIN, J. E., and S. H. WOLLMAN: Distribution of ^{125}I and ^{127}I in the Rat Thyroid Gland during Equilibrium Labeling as Determined by Autoradiog- raphy, *Endocrinology*, **81**:1074–1085 (1967).

NADLER, N. J., S. K. SARKAR, and C. P. LEBLOND: Origin of Intracellular Colloid Droplets in the Rat Thyroid, *Endocrinology*, **71**:120–129 (1962).

NADLER, N. J., B. A. YOUNG, and C. P. LEBLOND: Elaboration of Thyroglobulin in the Thyroid Follicle, *Endocrinology*, **74**:333–354 (1964).

PITT-RIVERS, R., and W. R. TROTTER (eds.): "The Thyroid," Butterworth & Co. (Publishers), Ltd., London, 1964.

SELJELID, R., A. REITH, and K. F. NAKKEN: The Early Phase of Endocytosis in the Rat Thyroid Follicle Cell, *Lab. Invest.*, **23**:595–605 (1970).

TAYLOR, S. (ed.): "Calcitonin: Proceedings of the Symposium on Thyrocalcitonin and the C Cells," Heinemann Educational Books, Ltd., London, 1968.

WETZEL, B. K., S. S. SPICER, and S. H. WOLLMAN: Changes in Fine Structure and Acid Phosphatase Localization in Rat Thyroid Cells Following Thyrotropin Administration, *J. Cell Biol.*, **25**:593–618 (1965).

WHUR, P., A. HERSCOVICS, and C. P. LEBLOND: Radioautographic Visualization of the Incorporation of Galactose-^{3}H and Mannose-^{3}H by Rat Thyroids in vitro in Relation to the Stages of Thyroglobulin Synthesis, *J. Cell Biol.*, **43**: 289–311 (1969).

WOLLMAN, S. H., S. S. SPICER, and M. S. BURSTONE: Localization of Esterase and Acid Phosphatase in Granules and Colloid Droplets in Rat Thyroid Epi- thelium, *J. Cell Biol.*, **21**:191–201 (1964).

chapter 30   The parathyroid gland

ROY O. GREEP

Number, location, and origin

The parathyroid glands in man are paired and are usually four in number, but there may be only two glands or as many as six in an individual. One pair of glands is generally located on the dorsal surface of the lateral lobes of the thyroid gland; the other pair may lie anywhere from just caudal to the lower pole of the thyroid to the anterior or posterior mediastinum. The parathyroids are brownish ovoid bodies, 6 to 7 mm long by 2 to 3 mm thick and weighing, in the adult, about 35 mg each. The variability in number and location of the parathyroid glands and the prevalence of aberrant glands may become matters of critical importance when, as in states of hyperparathyroidism, the location and removal of pathologic parathyroid tissue are necessary. Whereas most mammals, like man, have a superior and inferior pair of glands, the rat and mouse have only the superior pair. In the rabbit the superior (or internal) pair is embedded in the thyroid gland but the inferior (or external) pair lies free in the surrounding tissue.

Microscopic structure

The human parathyroid has a thin external connective tissue capsule from which very fine trabeculae extend into the body of the gland, forming poorly defined irregular lobules, which are further partitioned into sheets or cords by finer septa. In this fibrous stroma are found large blood vessels, nerves, lymphatics, and fat cells. Beginning at puberty, an increasing number of fat cells come to occupy the stroma, until 50 to 80 percent of the gland volume is occupied by fat (Fig. 30-1). The gland cells themselves are enmeshed in reticular fibers which also support a rich network of capil-

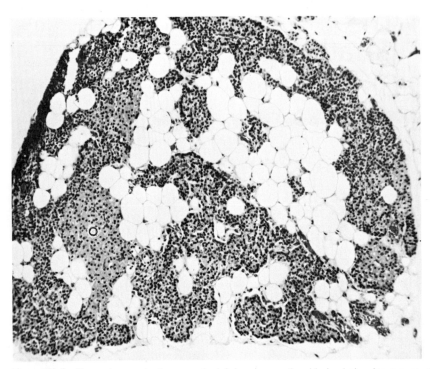

Figure 30-1   Photomicrograph of a normal adult human parathyroid gland showing groups of cords, sheets, and acini of chief cells separated by a stroma containing numerous fat cells.   Oxyphil cell nodules (o) are also seen among the chief cells. H&E.   ×130.   (Courtesy of S. I. Roth.)

laries.   The nerves end mainly on the vascular elements and are not believed to influence the endocrine functions of the parathyroid glands.   At one point on their surface the cells abut on a capillary into which the parathyroid hormone is presumably emptied.   Cell polarity in the normal human parathyroid is not evident.

Two varieties of parenchymal cells are readily identifiable in the adult human parathyroid gland, *chief* cells and *oxyphil* cells (Fig. 30-1).   It will be well to keep in mind, however, that the finding of numerous transitional cells by electron microscopy has raised the possibility that these are not different cells but cytologic modifications of a single type of parenchymal cells.

CHIEF CELLS

The chief cells are considerably more numerous than the oxyphil cells.   By light microscopy they have a round, centrally located nucleus with one or two nucleoli.   The main distinguishing feature is their water-clear and apparently empty cytoplasm, although electron microscopy shows that they contain the usual cytoplasmic organelles such as mitochondria, Golgi apparatus, and endoplasmic reticulum (ER), as well as varying numbers of glycogen granules and lipid droplets (Fig. 30-2).   Cells relatively depleted of glycogen are thought to be in active secretion whereas more abundant glycogen is suggestive of an inactive storage phase.   Several workers have described coated granules or

Figure 30-2   Group of chief cells from a normal human parathyroid gland.   Note the variation in abundance of glycogen and number of mitochondria.   G, glycogen; L, lipid; D, desmosome; M, mitochondria; N, nucleus; RNP, ribonucleoprotein; ER, endoplasmic reticulum.   (Courtesy of R. J. Weymouth and H. R. Seibel.)

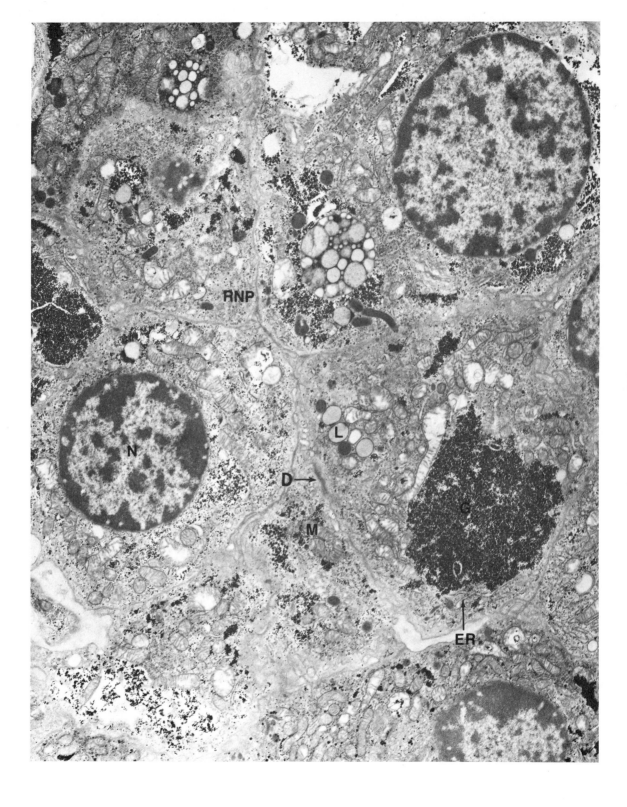

vesicles of varying electron density tentatively thought to represent the secretory product parathyroid hormone (PTH) (Fig. 30-3) probably identical to argyrophilic granules seen earlier by light microscopy.   These coated granules have been observed inside mitochondria and free in the cytoplasm of chief cells, oxyphil cells, and adjacent endothelial cells lining the parathyroid capillaries. Their distribution suggests that they are being secreted into the bloodstream but their relationship to the secretion of parathyroid hormone has not been established.   Localized lamellar arrays of rough ER probably account for the basophilic bodies seen by histologic means.   Lipid vacuoles occur singly or in large, round, membrane-bounded bodies containing lipid vacuoles of various dimensions (Fig. 30-2).   Other lipid bodies, probably representing lipofuscin, the autofluorescent "wear and tear" pigment, are present.

OXYPHIL CELLS

The oxyphil cells are mostly larger than chief cells, their cytoplasm is strongly eosinophilic, and they have relatively small nuclei which may appear pycnotic.   They are usually much fewer in number than chief cells and may occur singly, in nests, or in sizable nodules.   The oxyphil cells do not appear until immediately prior to or at the time of puberty and become somewhat more abundant in old age. Thus far, oxyphils have been found in only two other species, macaque monkeys and cattle; in the latter they likewise are not present in the young.

The most striking feature of the oxyphils is that by histochemical or ultrastructural observations the cytoplasm is seen to be tightly packed with large mitochondria (Fig. 30-3).   Some glycogen granules, bits of ER, and pigment are interspersed between the mitochondria.

TRANSITIONAL CELLS

Cells with intermediate characteristics which appear to be transitional between chief cells and oxyphils are abundant.   Such cells show wide variation in number of mitochondria and content of glycogen granules (Fig. 30-3).   The classification of the parenchymal cells of the human parathyroid gland into chief and oxyphil cells was based on histologic criteria.   Recent electron-microscopic observations tend to favor the concept that there is only one parenchymal cell type, the chief cell.   All others, including the oxyphil, represent modifications of the chief cell.   This concept is supported also by the fact that during the first years of life only chief cells are present.

Desmosomes connect the plasma membranes of both chief and oxyphil cells.   The plasma membranes of adjacent cells are generally smooth although areas of extensive interdigitations do occur.   Intercellular spaces vary in extent and may contain glycogen.

Endocrine function

Parathyroid hormone has been purified and the complete covalent structure determined by Brewer and Ronan.   It contains 84 amino acids and has a molecular weight of 8,500.   The parathyroid hormone serves the vital function of maintaining the calcium content of the blood plasma at an optimal and nearly constant level (10 mg per 100 ml). This is necessary for normal neuromuscular activity.   Following removal of the parathyroids in man and many other mammals, blood calcium falls and neuromuscular irritability increases, eventuating in tetany and often death.   The acute signs, but not all the long-term effects, of hypoparathyroidism are ameliorated by any treatment which will elevate the blood calcium to normal levels.   Injections of calcium salts are immediately effective, and extracts

Figure 30-3   Oxyphil cell in a normal human parathyroid gland shown in comparison with chief cells and a transitional cell. Note the range in density of mitochondria and the presence of glycogen in granules.   OXY, oxyphil cell; C, chief cell; TRA, transitional cell; S, secretory material.   (Courtesy of R. J. Weymouth and M. N. Sheridan.)

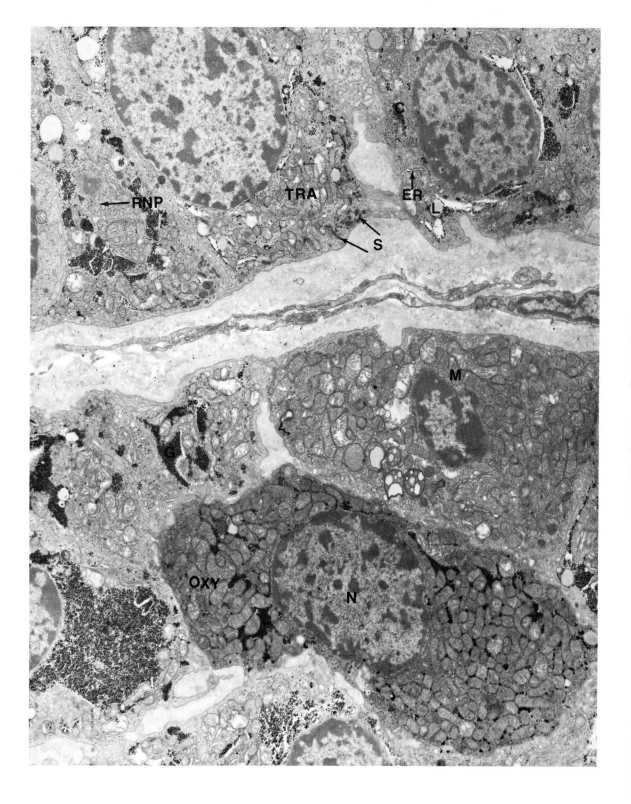

of the parathyroid glands of domestic animals afford relief within a few hours through increased mobilization of calcium from the skeletal depots—an effect brought about by an action of parathyroid hormone on osteocytes and osteoclasts, leading to increased bone resorption.

Parathyroid hormone also has an important regulatory influence on the concentration of blood inorganic phosphate. Excessive secretion of parathyroid hormone leads to a reduction in blood phosphate, and hypoactivity to an increase. These changes are mediated by an effect of the hormone on the kidney. This induced drain of phosphate through the urine is referred to as the *phosphaturic action* of the parathyroid hormone. Work with the purified parathyroid hormone has conclusively demonstrated that the calcemic and the phosphaturic responses are due to a single hormone. It is well established that parathyroid hormone acts directly on the kidney tubules to promote the reabsorption of calcium and inhibit the reabsorption of phosphate from the urine.

The parathyroid hormone, acting systemically, can affect the bones and erupting teeth. Thus, overactivity of the parathyroid glands may lead to osteitis fibrosa cystica, a condition characterized by excessive loss of bone tissue with replacement by fibrous connective tissue. In hypoparathyroidism the calcification of developing bones and teeth may be seriously impaired. Some of the systemic effects are due to the direct action of parathyroid hormone on bone and kidney cells, whereas others stem indirectly from resulting changes in the plasma concentration of calcium and phosphate. A direct effect of the parathyroids on bone was suggested by the production of local erosion under grafts of parathyroid glands onto the surface of bones and conclusively demonstrated by showing that parathyroid hormone stimulates bone resorption in tissue culture.

The functional activity of the parathyroid gland is regulated by the concentration of calcium ions in the blood plasma. Approximately half of the blood calcium is in ionic form and half is bound.

Lowering of the ionic calcium acts as a feedback mechanism, stimulating the parathyroids to secrete more hormone, and if sustained this will result in an enlargement of the glands. Conversely, when the blood ionic calcium is elevated, as by the infusion of calcium salts or excessive intake of vitamin D, the parathyroid glands cease to function and show atrophic changes. Instances of primary hyperparathyroidism in man are due to parathyroid hyperplasia or to an adenoma of one or more of the parathyroid glands. The parathyroids are also stimulated in chronic renal insufficiency where retained phosphate leads to a fall in blood calcium. This is known as secondary hyperparathyroidism.

As noted above, a depression of the blood calcium stimulates the secretion of parathyroid hormone which causes the calcium to rise. The blood calcium is kept from overshooting the optimal level by the only recently discovered second blood-calcium-regulating hormone, calcitonin. In mammals this hormone originates from the thyroid gland and is secreted by the parafollicular or C cells which are derived embryologically from the ultimobranchial body (see Chap. 29). Calcitonin counteracts the action of parathyroid hormone by inhibiting bone resorption and thereby prevents the blood calcium from rising above the optimal level.

The structure of calcitonin has been determined and the hormone synthesized. The molecule consists of a polypeptide of 32 amino acids with a seven-member ring at the N terminus. The sequence of amino acids in calcitonin prepared from different species varies considerably but the function served by the hormone is the same.

In fish, amphibia, reptiles, and birds, the ultimobranchial gland develops separately from the thyroid gland. In these animals, calcitonin is secreted by the ultimobranchial gland and not by the thyroid gland. Although calcitonin has been found in abundance in the ultimobranchial glands of the elasmobranchs, what function, if any, it may serve in these animals having only a cartilaginous skeleton is unknown.

Biologic considerations

The parathyroids appear to have a large reserve functional capacity. Little, if any, compensatory hypertrophy occurs following removal of all but one gland, and parathyroid autografts are successful only when all the glands in situ are excised.

On the phyletic scale, the parathyroid glands are not found in the fishes or gill-bearing amphibia but are constantly present in all other vertebrates. They appear to have originated with the disappearance of the branchial apparatus, that is, at the time the ancestors of our modern amphibia made their appearance on land. (For comparative aspects, see review by Greep, 1963).

References

BAKER, B. L.: A Study of the Parathyroid Glands of the Normal and Hypophysectomized Monkey (*Macaca mulatta*), *Anat. Rec.,* **83:**47 (1942).

BARNICOT, N. A.: The Local Action of the Parathyroid and Other Tissues on Bone in Intracerebral Grafts, *J. Anat.,* **82:**233 (1948).

CHANG, H. Y.: Grafts of Parathyroid and Other Tissues to Bone, *Anat. Rec.,* **111:**23 (1951).

DE ROBERTIS, E.: The Cytology of the Parathyroid Gland of Rats Injected with Parathyroid Extract, *Anat. Rec.,* **78:**473 (1940).

GAILLARD, P. J.: Parathyroid and Bone in Tissue Culture, in R. O. Greep and R. V. Talmage (eds.), ''The Parathyroids,'' Charles C Thomas, Publisher, Springfield, Ill., 1961.

GOLDHABER, P.: Some Chemical Factors Influencing Bone Resorption in Tissue Culture, in R. F. Sognnaes (ed.), ''Mechanisms of Hard Tissue Destruction,'' American Association for the Advancement of Science, Washington, 1963.

GRAFFLIN, A. L.: Cytological Evidence of Secretory Activity in the Mammalian Parathyroid Gland, *Endocrinology,* **26:**857 (1940).

GREEP, R. O.: Parathyroid Glands, in U. S. Von Euler and H. Heller (eds.), ''Comparative Endocrinology,'' vol. 1, Academic Press, Inc., New York, 1963.

GREEP, R. O.: The Chemistry and Physiology of the Parathyroid Hormone, in G. Pincus and K. V. Thimann (eds.), ''The Hormones,'' vol. 1, Academic Press, Inc., New York, 1948.

LANGE, R.: Zur Histologie und Zytologie der Glandula parathyreoidea des Menschen. Licht und Electronenmikroskopische untersuchungen an Epithelkörperadenomen, *Z. Zellforsch.* 53:765 (1961).

LEVER, J. D.: Cytological Appearances in the Normal and Activated Parathyroid of the Rat. A Combined Study by Electron and Light Microscopy with Certain Quantitative Assessments, *J. Endocr.,* **17:**210 (1958).

MARSHALL, R. B., D. K. ROBERTS, and R. A. TURNER: Adenomas of the Human Parathyroid, *Cancer,* **20:**512 (1967).

MECCA, C. E., G. P. MARTIN, and P. GOLDHABER: Alterations of Bone Metabolism in Tissue Culture in Response to Parathyroid Extract, *Proc. Soc. Exp. Biol. Med.,* **113:**538 (1963).

MUNGER, B. L., and S. I. ROTH: The Cytology of the Normal Parathyroid Glands of Man and Virginia Deer. A Light and Electron Microscopic Study with Morphologic Evidence of Secretory Activity, *J. Cell Biol.,* **16:**379 (1963).

POTTS, J. J., JR., G. D. AURBACH, and L. M. SHERWOOD: Parathyroid Hormone: Chemical Properties and Structural Requirements for Biological and Immunological Activity, *Recent Progr. Hormone Res.*, **22:**(1966).

RASMUSSEN, H., and L. C. CRAIG: Isolation and Characterization of Bovine Parathyroid Hormone, *J. Biol. Chem.*, **236:**759 (1961).

ROTH, S. I., and B. L. MUNGER: The Cytology of the Adenomatous, Atrophic, and Hyperplastic Parathyroid Glands of Man. A Light- and Electron-microscopic Study, *Virchow. Arch. Path. Anat.*, **335:**389 (1962).

TALMAGE, R. V., and L. F. BELANGER: ''Parathyroid Hormone and Thyrocalcitonin (*Calcitonin*), Excerpta Medica Foundation, ICS 159, 1968.

TREMBLAY, G., and G. E. CARTIER: Histochemical Study of Oxidative Enzymes in the Human Parathyroid, *Endocrinology*, **60:**658 (1961).

TRIER, J. S.: The Fine Structure of the Parathyroid Gland, *J. Biophys. Biochem. Cytol.*, **4:**13 (1958).

WEYMOUTH, R. J., and H. R. SEIBEL: An Electron Microscopic Study of the Parathyroid Glands in Man: Evidence of Secretory Material, *Acta Endocr. (Kobenhavn)*, **61:**334 (1969).

WEYMOUTH, R. J., and M. N. SHERIDAN: Fine Structure of Human Parathyroid Glands: Normal and Pathological, *Acta Endocr. (Kobenhavn)*, **53:**539 (1966).

chapter 31   The adrenal gland   JOHN A. LONG

The *adrenal glands* constitute one of the major homeostatic organs of the mammalian body. They are composed of two separate endocrine organs which differ in embryologic origin, type of secretion, and function. In mammals, the two organs are arranged as an outer cortex and an inner medulla surrounded by a common capsule (Fig. 31-1, see color insert). In the other vertebrate classes, the two tissues may be completely unassociated or intermingled to a greater or lesser degree. In these cases the homologue of the mammalian medulla is referred to as *chromaffin tissue* whereas the tissue corresponding to the cortex of mammals is called *interrenal tissue*.

The *cortex*, whose secretory rate is controlled by hormones produced in the adenohypophysis and the kidney, produces steroid hormones that affect carbohydrate and protein metabolism, resistance to physiologic stresses, and electrolyte distribution. The *medulla*, which is under nervous control, secretes catecholamines that affect heart rate and smooth muscle function in blood vessels and other viscera, as well as influencing various aspects of carbohydrate and lipid metabolism.

It is convenient to describe the two components of the gland separately; however, it should be kept in mind that there appears to be a phylogenetic trend toward the more intimate structural relationship between the two glandular tissues as seen in mammals. In addition, an interesting functional relationship has been described which will be referred to later.

Gross anatomy

The adrenal glands (called *suprarenal glands* in man because of his upright posture) lie retroperitoneally near the anterior poles of the kidneys and embedded in the perirenal adipose tissue. The right and left glands are of somewhat different shape in man, with the left gland being somewhat broader. The combined weight of the adrenals from adult human beings dying immediately of accidental causes is about 8 gm. It should be borne in mind that both weight and size of the glands may vary considerably with age and physiologic condition of the organism. In gross section, the cortex, which constitutes the largest part of the gland, appears yellow due to the presence of lipids. The medulla, which represents approximately 10 percent of the weight of the adrenal, is reddish or brown.

BLOOD SUPPLY

Three main groups of arteries supply the human adrenal gland: (1) superior suprarenal arteries which arise as branches of the inferior phrenic artery and which are the major blood supply, (2) middle suprarenals arising from the aorta, and (3) inferior suprarenals which arise from the renal artery (Fig. 31-2). The adrenal arteries form a plexus in the capsule from which three types of intraglandular vessels arise. (1) Arteriae capsulae supply the connective tissue capsule of the organ. (2) Arteriae corticis arise from the capsular plexus by repeated branching and then descend into the cortex and break up into the capillary bed supplying the cortical parenchyma. These capillaries anastomose in the inner cortex and empty into the medullary vascular bed via relatively few, small channels. (3) Arteriae medullae penetrate the cortex via connective tissue trabeculae and directly supply the medullary tissue (Fig. 31-3). Thus, the medulla has two blood supplies—one via the cortical capillaries and the other from the direct medullary arteries. Several orders of venules ultimately join to form the large central vein which, in man, has conspicuous bundles of longitudinally oriented smooth muscle in the intraglandular portions of its wall. The adrenal vein exits at the hilum of the gland and on the left side empties into the left renal vein; the right adrenal vein joins the vena cava directly.

LYMPHATICS

The lymphatic drainage is not well known but it appears that the capsule possesses a set of lymphatics which pass out along the adrenal arteries; the central vein has a separate set which follows this vein to the exterior of the gland. No small lymphatic vessels have been detected within the parenchyma of the adrenal.

INNERVATION

The main innervation of the adrenal is composed of preganglionic sympathetic fibers arising from T_8 to T_{11} and passing to the gland via the greater and lesser splanchnic nerves. These fibers penetrate to the medulla and synapse with the chromaffin cells, which are thus homologous with sympathetic ganglion cells. Recent ultrastructural studies have revealed efferent nerve endings (possibly adrenergic) on the endocrine parenchymal cells of the adrenal cortex in several species including man. The role of these nerves in the physiology of the adrenal cortex has not been determined.

Histology of the adrenal cortex

In all mammals, except monotremes, the adrenal cortex can be divided into three concentric zones which were named *zona glomerulosa, zona fasciculata,* and *zona reticularis* by Arnold in 1866 (Fig. 31-4). These structural subdivisions of the cortex have functional implications which will be referred to later. In man, the zona glomerulosa accounts for approximately 15 percent of the total cortical volume, the zona fasciculata about 78 percent, and the zona reticularis about 7 percent. The gland is surrounded by a capsule composed of fibroblasts, collagen, and elastic fibers as well as a few smooth muscle fibers in some species. Connective tissue trabeculae penetrate the cortex, carrying nerves and blood vessels to the medulla. Reticular fibers which are continuous with the fibers

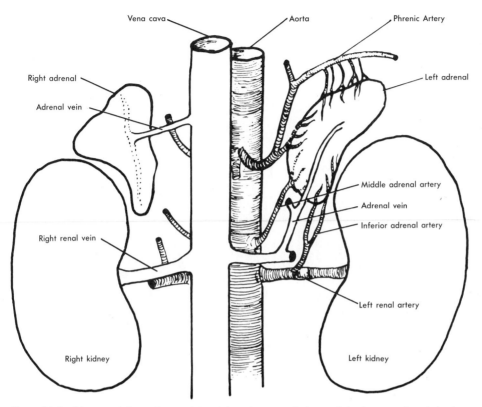

Figure 31-2 Diagram of the major arterial supply and venous drainage of the human adrenal gland.

of the capsule form a meshwork around the parenchymal cells of the cortex and medulla.

Lying immediately beneath the capsule, the cells of the zona glomerulosa are ovoid to columnar in shape and are arranged in spherical masses or arcades. These cells are relatively small (12 to 15 μm in diameter), contain a single spherical nucleus, and possess a small amount of homogeneously staining cytoplasm in which are suspended a few small lipid droplets. In the adrenal of man, the zona glomerulosa may be absent in restricted areas of the cortex; in these regions, cells of the zona fasciculata are found immediately beneath the capsule.

The zona fasciculata is composed of long, radially arranged cords which are generally one or two cells thick and are separated from adjacent cords by capillary vessels which form the blood supply of the cortex. The cells are larger than those of the other zones (approximately 20 μm in diameter) and are packed with numerous large lipid droplets in the

living state. After treatment with the organic solvents necessary for the preparation of routine histologic sections, lipids are extracted, leaving spaces which give the cytoplasm a reticulated appearance and a poor affinity for the usual histologic stains. These cells have sometimes been called *spongiocytes* or *clear cells* because of this artefact of specimen preparation.

The innermost zone of the adrenal cortex, the zona reticularis, is characterized by the breaking down of the regular, parallel alignment of the cords of the zona fasciculata and the formation of an anastomosing network of cellular cords interspersed by capillaries. The component cells are smaller than those of the zona fasciculata and contain relatively few, small lipid inclusions. Hence, the cytoplasm is compact and readily stained. Cells of this zone are notable for large accumulations of lipofuscin pigment which is visible with the light microscope as golden-brown droplets.

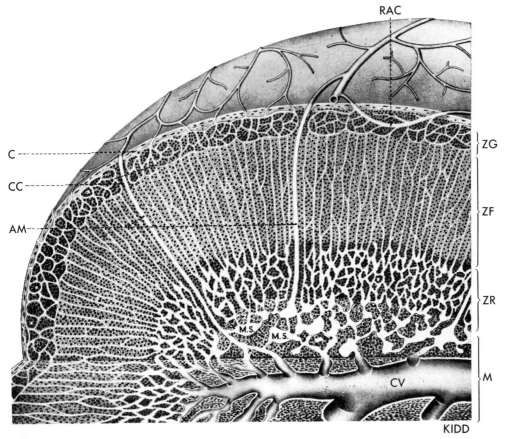

Figure 31-3 Stereogram of a mammalian adrenal gland, showing the medulla (M) with its central vein (CV), and the cortex with its three zones, the zona glomerulosa (ZG), zona fasciculata (ZF), and zona reticularis (ZR) enclosed by the capsule (C). Two arteriae medullae (AM) and an arteria corticis (RAC) are shown. (Reproduced by permission from R. G. Harrison, "A Textbook of Human Embryology," 1st ed., Blackwell Scientific Publications, Ltd., Oxford, 1959.)

Ultrastructure of the adrenal cortex

The ultrastructure of adrenocortical cells is similar in many ways to that of other steroid-secreting cells, including the corpus luteum of the ovary and interstitial cells of the testis. These similarities include the abundance of smooth ER, numerous lipid inclusions, and the frequent occurrence of mitochondria with tubular or vesicular cristae. Despite these general similarities, cells of each of the zones of the adrenal cortex are sufficiently different to warrant separate description.

Each cell of the zona glomerulosa possesses a spherical nucleus with one or two nucleoli bounded by a typical nuclear envelope. The cytoplasm is full of smooth ER membranes (Fig. 31-5) which form a tubular, anastomosing network. A few profiles of rough ER are seen; most of the ribosomes are free in the cytoplasm, and many are arranged in spirals and rosettes. Stacks of smooth membrane-bounded cisternae associated with numerous small vesicles constitute the Golgi complex, usually seen close to the nucleus. A pair of centrioles is present. The mitochondria are usually elongated, and the cristae are broad, flattened extensions of the inner mitochondrial membrane.

Cells of the zona fasciculata differ from those of the zona glomerulosa in several respects. Most prominent is the large number of lipid droplets which may be so numerous as to almost fill the cell (Fig. 31-6). Mitochondria are distinctive in this zone, usually being more rounded than those of the zona glomerulosa. Their cristae are short, tubular extensions of the inner mitochondrial membrane.

Figure 31-4   Cross section of the adrenal gland of a rhesus monkey, showing division of the cortex into three concentric zones. ×100.

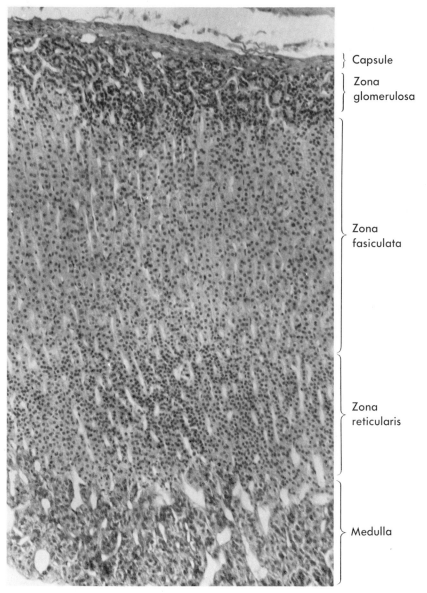

Capsule

Zona glomerulosa

Zona fasiculata

Zona reticularis

Medulla

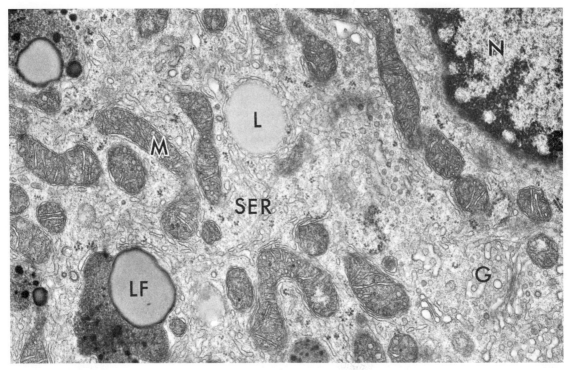

Figure 31-5   Electron micrograph of a cell of the zona glomerulosa of the human adrenal cortex.   N, nucleus; M, mitochondrion; SER, smooth-surfaced endoplasmic reticulum; L, lipid droplet; LF, lipofuscin; G, Golgi complex.   ×22,500.

The rough ER is well developed. It is common to find several cisternae aligned parallel to one another, forming structures which may be seen, in appropriate light-microscopic preparations, as basophilic bodies. The plasma membrane is thrown into short, irregular microvilli over parts of the cell surface whereas in other regions the membranes of adjacent cells are parallel and separated by a space of approximately 200 Å. In restricted regions, the membranes of adjacent cells are much closer and form "gap junctions" which, in other cell types, are thought to be sites of high electrical conductivity between cells.

The ultrastructure of the zona reticularis differs only slightly from that of the zona fasciculata. In the reticularis, mitochondria tend to be more elongate and fewer lipid droplets are present (Fig. 31-7). Large numbers of membrane-bounded inclusions with heterogeneous contents are present. These structures correspond to the lipofuscin pigment granules seen by light microscopy. They

seem to be accumulations of waste materials, some of which are probably oxidized, polymerized products of unsaturated lipids. Acid phosphatase, a typical lysosomal enzyme, has been detected in lipofuscin granules. Their number increases with age.

Certain ultrastructural changes of adrenocortical cells can be observed when the rate of synthesis of adrenocortical steroids is caused to decrease or increase (for example, when the animal is hypophysectomized or is injected with adrenocorticotropic hormone). When adrenocortical cells are stimulated, their cytoplasmic volume enlarges and the quantity of smooth ER increases. The fate of the lipid droplets depends upon the degree of stimulation. With a severe stimulus, the droplets may completely disappear, whereas with a more moderate stimulus, they become smaller than usual but very numerous. These responses reflect the fact that stainable lipid is stored precursor material, not the hormone itself. If the cell secretes hormone at the same rate that it manufactures the precursor, no storage occurs (Fig. 31-8).

When stimulation is withdrawn, as in hypophysectomy, there is an atrophy of the cell and a decrease in the quantity of smooth ER. Lipid droplets at first enlarge and coalesce, reflecting decreased utilization for hormone production. Eventually lipid disappears altogether, as though the cell had utilized this material for its own nutrition.

Close study of adrenocortical cells has not revealed visible evidence for the mechanisms of intracellular transport and release of secretory products, the various steroid hormones. Present evidence indicates that steroid hormones are not stored in large quantity in adrenocortical cells and that they are released continuously as individual molecules and not discontinuously in packets, as is the case in many protein-secreting cells.

Capillary endothelium

The endothelium of the capillary vessels of the cortex is of the fenestrated or visceral type (Fig. 31-9). The cell is quite thin except near the nucleus where thickenings occur to accommodate the nucleus and most of the other cytoplasmic organelles such as Golgi material and mitochondria.

Individual profiles of granular reticulum are sometimes found in the thin cytoplasmic extensions. At intervals, the wall becomes so thin that it appears to be a single layer which does not have the structure of a unit membrane. These regions are termed *fenestrae*. A continuous basal lamina is present

Figure 31-6   Electron micrograph of a cell of the zona fasciculata from the human adrenal cortex.   M. mitochondrion; RER, rough-surfaced endoplasmic reticulum; SER, smooth-surfaced endoplasmic reticulum; L, lipid droplet; LF lipofuscin pigment. ×19,250.

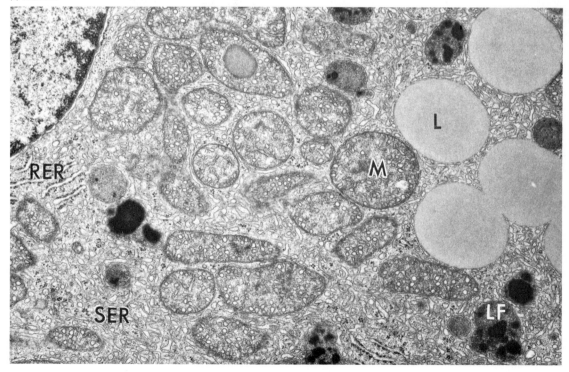

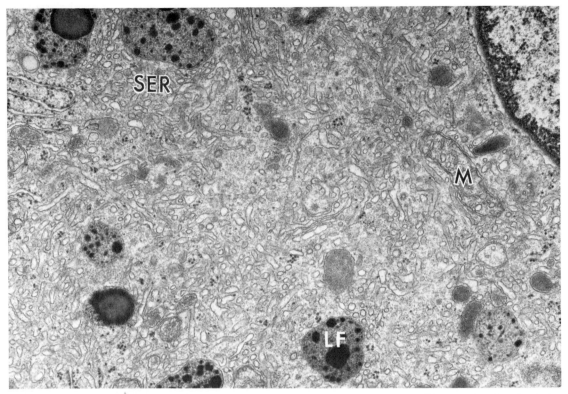

Figure 31-7 Electron micrograph of a cell from the zona reticularis of the human adrenal cortex. SER, smooth-surfaced endoplasmic reticulum; M, mitochondrion; LF, lipofuscin pigment. ✕32,500.

beneath the endothelium. A space which may be occupied by fibroblasts and macrophages is present between the endothelium and the endocrine parenchyma. Individual fibrils with the characteristic 640-Å repeat of collagen are present in the subendothelial space. They correspond to the elements demonstrated by silver impregnation methods and termed *reticular fibers* by light microscopists. A basal lamina is present on the surfaces of parenchymal cells which abut on the subendothelial space.

Histophysiology of the adrenal cortex

A wide variety of steroid hormones are secreted by the adrenal cortex. They are derived from cholesterol which is stored in the lipid inclusions as fatty acyl esters of cholesterol. However, in man, the most important source of substrate for adrenocorticoid biosynthesis is cholesterol taken up from the blood plasma.

Although almost 100 different steroids have been extracted from adrenal glands of man and experimental animals, only a few are normally released from the gland and are hormonally active. In man the most important adrenal steroid is cortisol, an example of a class of hormones called *glucocorticoids* because of their pronounced effects on carbohydrate metabolism. Another member of this class is corticosterone which is secreted in small amounts by the human adrenal gland but which is the principal glucocorticoid secreted by the rat. Aldosterone is the most potent *mineralocorticoid,* so called because of the effects of this class of corticosteroids on electrolyte balance. Other hormones secreted by the adrenal cortex include *estrogens* (for example, estrone and estradiol) and *androgens* (for example, dehydroepiandrosterone sulfate and testosterone).

The morphologic zonation of the adrenal cortex is paralleled by an important *functional zonation.* By this is meant the specialization of cells of a given zone for the synthesis and release of certain classes of steroid hormones. Thus, aldosterone is secreted by cells of the zona glomerulosa, cortisol and estrogens are formed in both the zona fasciculata and zona reticularis, and adrenal androgen synthesis is most active in the zona reticularis although some synthesis can be detected in the zona fasciculata.

Steroid hormones are formed from cholesterol by removal of a six-carbon fragment of the side chain followed by a dehydrogenation at carbon 3 and a series of hydroxylations at specific loci. A simplified scheme showing the biosynthesis of the principal adrenal steroids is given in Fig. 31-10. In addition, the subcellular localization of the enzymes involved is given. Note that a precursor may move from one compartment to another (for example, mitochondria to microsome) several times before the final product is formed. How this is accomplished in a controlled fashion is not understood at present.

Figure 31-8 Some of the cytologic changes in typical lipid-containing adrenocortical cells (A) when their activity is stimulated or inhibited. Left: With stimulation, adrenocortical cells, their nuclei, and the nucleoli enlarge. With acute (B) or prolonged (D) stimulation, there may be a loss of lipid stores; with more moderate but chronic (C) stimulation, the lipid droplets become small and lose detectable cholesterol stores but retain a high titer of unsaturated fatty acids. Right: With removal of stimulus, adrenocortical cells, their nuclei, and their nucleoli shrink (E to G). The lipid droplets apparently coalesce and gradually disappear. Initially there may be an increase in cholesterol concentration. Gradually both the fatty acids and the cholesterol stores decline. Both the severely stimulated and long-term inactive cells lack lipid stores; they are distinguishable only by size. (From Deane, 1962, by permission from Springer-Verlag.)

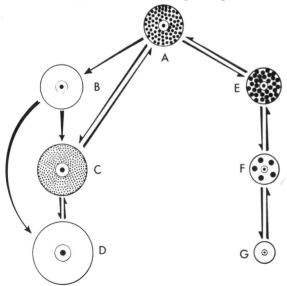

CONTROL OF SECRETION

The adenohypophysis is essential for the maintenance of the structure and function of the adrenal cortex. If the pituitary is removed from an animal, a striking decline in the weight of the adrenal gland ensues and is paralleled by a decline in secretion of most of the adrenal hormones. Upon histologic examination, it is seen that the inner zones of the cortex are atrophied but that the zona glomerulosa is well maintained (Fig. 31-11). The hormone secreted by the adenohypophysis which maintains the adrenal cortex is adrenocorticotropic hormone or ACTH. ACTH is a polypeptide composed of 39 amino acids whose sequence is known for a number of species including man. The main effects of ACTH are to stimulate steroid synthesis and release, to promote growth of the adrenal cortex, to increase blood flow through the adrenal, and to cause ascorbic acid depletion in a few species, most notably the rat.

If ACTH is given to a hypophysectomized animal, it will prevent the decline in weight and secretory activity of the adrenal cortex which would ordinarily ensue. If ACTH is given to an animal with an intact pituitary gland, this hormone will cause a hypertrophy of the inner zones of the adrenal cortex and an elevation of the circulating levels of many of the adrenal corticoids. ACTH will not cause a hyper-

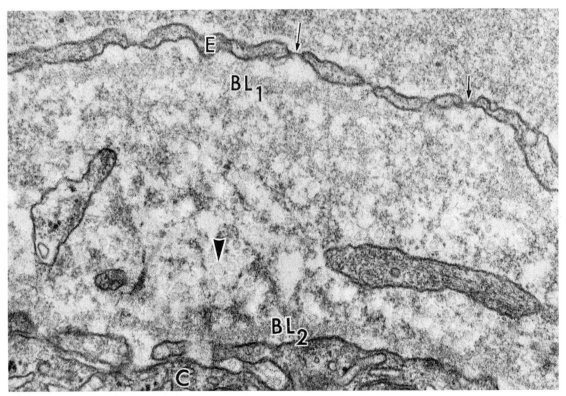

Figure 31-9   Electron micrograph of capillary endothelium in the human adrenal cortex.   Endothelial cell (E) with fenestrae at arrows; basal lamina beneath endothelium labeled BL_1.   Cross sections of reticular fibers are faintly seen at the end of the arrow head.   Basal lamina adjacent to cortical parenchymal cell (C) labeled BL_2. $\times 66,000$.

trophy of the zona glomerulosa nor will it increase the secretory rate of aldosterone except when given in large doses.   It has been concluded that the inner zones of the adrenal cortex, the zona fasciculata and the zona reticularis, are regulated by ACTH and that the zona glomerulosa is controlled by a different mechanism.   This evidence also indicates that aldosterone is formed only by cells of the zona glomerulosa, and careful microchemical investigations have shown that the enzymes necessary for the final steps in aldosterone biosynthesis are found only in these cells.   The zona glomerulosa is also found to hypertrophy if the animal is maintained on a sodium-deficient diet, but if a potent mineralocorticoid such as aldosterone or deoxycorticosterone is given over a long period, the zona glomerulosa will atrophy and the other zones will remain normal.

If experimental animals or human beings are given large quantities of a glucocorticoid such as cortisol over a long period of time, subsequent histologic examination of the adrenal glands will reveal a pronounced atrophy of the zona fasciculata and zona reticularis.   For many years it was thought that the high levels of glucocorticoids directly suppressed the synthesis and release of ACTH by the adenohypophysis which led, in turn, to the observed atrophy.   It is now known that an additional link in the feedback loop is present: the hypothalamus.   Certain neurons in this region of the brain are believed to produce a low-molecular-weight peptide called *corticotropin releasing factor* (CRF).   The rate of secretion of CRF is inversely related to the circulating levels of glucocorticoids to which these neurons are exposed.   The axons of these hypothalamic neurons end on portal blood vessels in the

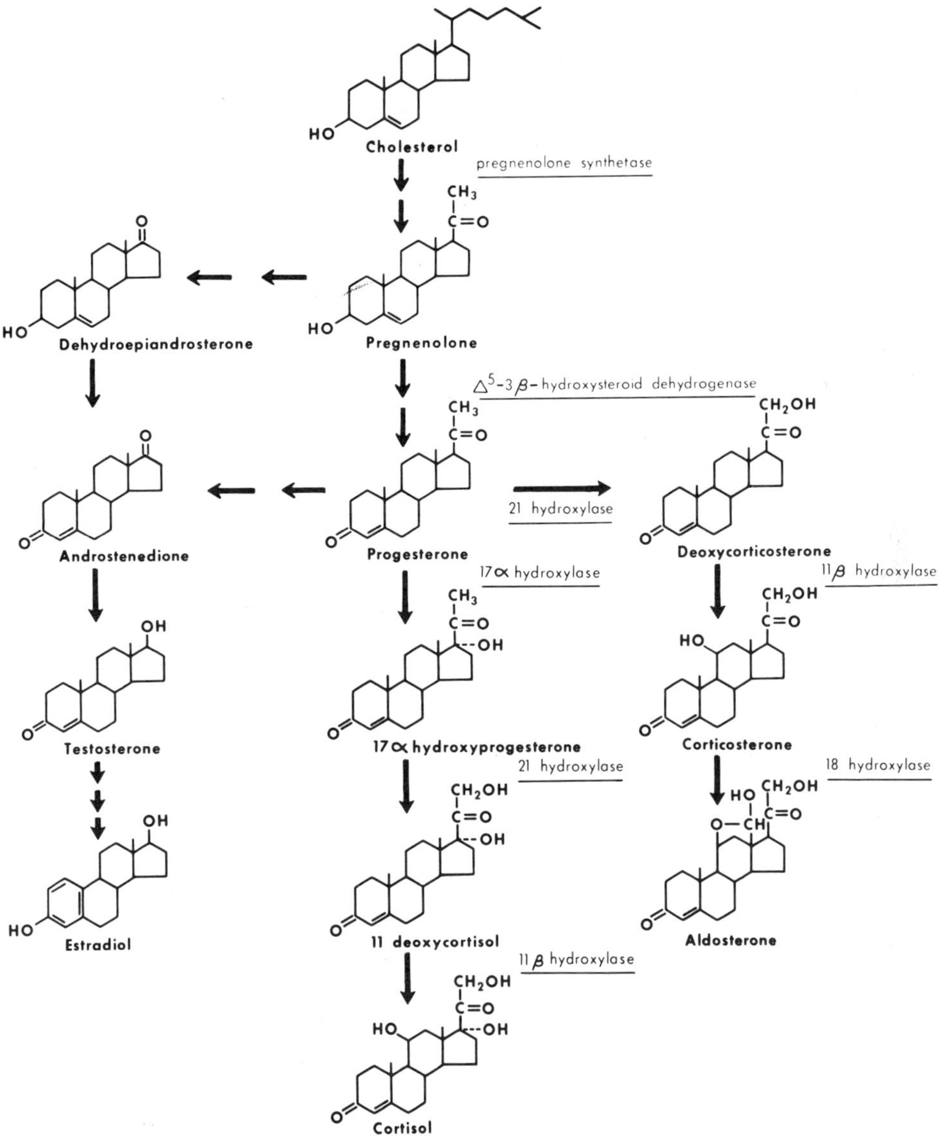

Figure 31-10 Diagram showing the pathways taken in the biosynthesis of the principal corticosteroids. The zonal distribution and subcellular distribution of the most important enzymes are given in the table.

Enzyme	Zonal Localization	Subcellular Localization
Pregnenolone synthetase	All zones	Mitochondria
Δ^5-3β-hydroxy-steroid dehydrogenase	All zones	Microsomes
21 hydroxylase	All zones	Microsomes
11 β hydroxylase	All zones	Mitochondria
17 α hydroxylase	Fasciculata and reticularis	Microsomes
18 hydroxylase	Glomerulosa	Mitochondria

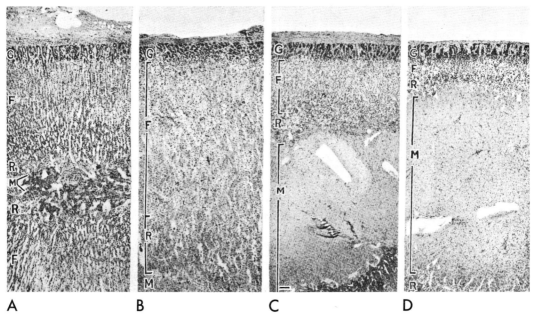

Figure 31-11   Sections of rhesus monkey adrenal glands.   A. Normal adrenal cortex.   B. After treatment with ACTH.   Note the increase in width of zonae fasciculata (F) and reticularis (R).   C. After treatment with cortisone.   The inner zones are reduced in width.   D. Hypophysectomized for 90 days.   Extensive atrophy of inner zones.   Note that the width of the zona glomerulosa (G) is the same in each instance.   M. medulla ×36.   (By permission from Knobil et al. Acta Endocr. (Kobenhavn), **17:**229, 1954.)

Figure 31-12   Diagram illustrating current concepts of the neuroendocrine control of the adrenal cortex.

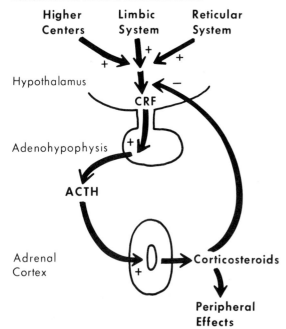

median eminence which transport CRF to the adeno-hypophysis.   Here, CRF stimulates the synthesis and release of ACTH.   Figure 31-12 diagrams this feedback loop.

The peripheral effects of glucocorticoids are numerous and diverse.   Cortisol causes accelerated gluconeogenesis and deposition of glycogen in the liver and, at the same time, suppresses peripheral utilization of glucose (anti-insulin effect) with a consequent hyperglycemia.   This hormone also causes an increased release of fatty acids from adipose tissue.   The increased urinary nitrogen excretion seen after cortisol administration may be due to increased catabolism of protein but is more probably due to a suppression of protein synthesis which, together with normal protein turnover, could account for the increased nitrogen excretion.   An important effect of cortisol already mentioned is its effect on those hypothalamic neurons which produce corticotropin releasing factor.

Aldosterone, the principal secretory product of cells of the zona glomerulosa, is a potent mineralocorticoid first identified in 1953.   Aldosterone promotes the resorption of sodium ions in the distal

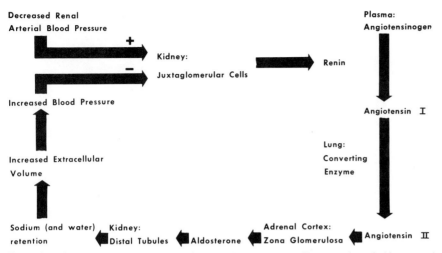

Figure 31-13   Diagram illustrating one of the mechanisms controlling secretion of aldosterone by the zona glomerulosa.

tubule of the nephron, increases potassium excretion by the kidney, and causes a lowering of the sodium concentration in sweat, saliva, and intestinal secretions.

The rate of aldosterone secretion is controlled by several mechanisms, the most important of which is a complex feedback loop involving the kidney (Fig. 31-13). The signal sensed by the juxtaglomerular apparatus is not known with certainty. It may be a decrease in the degree of stretch of the juxtaglomerular cells themselves or it may be a decrease in the sodium load at the macula densa. In either case, this signal causes

a release of renin from the juxtaglomerular cells. Renin is an enzyme which catalyzes the conversion of angiotensinogen, a circulating α_2 globulin, to angiotensin I. Angiotensin I is then converted to angiotensin II, which acts on the zona glomerulosa of the adrenal to stimulate the secretion of aldosterone. Aldosterone acts on the distal tubules of the nephron to promote sodium retention leading to an increase in intravascular fluid volume and consequent increase in blood pressure. This, in turn, stretches the receptor cells of the juxtaglomerular apparatus, thus closing the feedback loop.

Adrenal medulla

The adrenal medulla is composed of an endocrine parenchyma (chromaffin cells) supported by connective tissue elements and profusely supplied with nerves and blood vessels (Fig. 31-14). Ganglion cells are present but are usually difficult to find in routine sections. Chromaffin cells have been defined by Coupland (1965) as cells derived from neurectoderm, innervated by preganglionic sympathetic fibers, and which synthesize and release catecholamines (epinephrine and norepinephrine). These cells show a brown coloration when exposed to an aqueous solution of potassium dichromate. This "chromaffin reaction" is thought to result from

the oxidation and polymerization of catecholamines contained within granules in the cells. Catecholamines also form yellow-green fluorescent compounds after reacting with formaldehyde (Fig. 31-15, see color insert). This technique has been of great value in recent years in mapping the distribution of catecholamines in organs such as the adrenal medulla and the nervous system.

Chromaffin cells are arranged as epithelioid cords in close association with vascular spaces. The cells are round, polyhedral, or, in some species, columnar in shape. In most species, the application of a battery of histochemical methods permits the

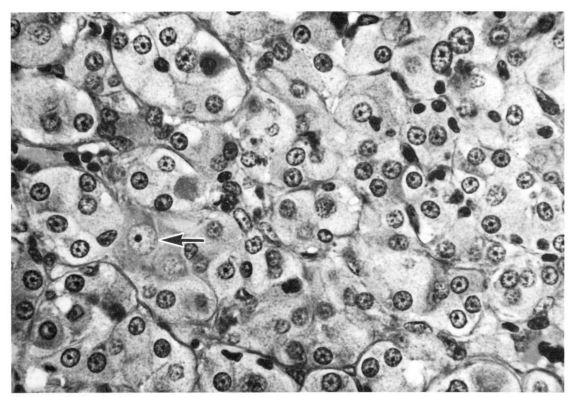

Figure 31-14   Photomicrograph of a section of the human adrenal medulla.   A ganglion cell is indicated by the arrow.   ×600.

identification of two types of cells, one of which contains norepinephrine and the other epinephrine. When viewed in the electron microscope, the most prominent feature of these cells is the abundance of membrane-bounded electron-dense granules, 150 to 350 nm in diameter, which are thought to be the site of storage of catecholamines (Fig. 31-16). These granules also contain high concentrations of ATP, a specific protein called chromogranin, as well as dopamine β-oxidase, the enzyme responsible for converting dopamine to norepinephrine. After special preparative methods, it is possible to demonstrate with the electron microscope that two populations of cells exist. Some of the cells possess granules of very high electron density which are thought to be the sites of storage of norepinephrine, whereas most of the cells possess granules of lesser electron density and correspond to epinephrine-storing cells (Fig. 31-17).

Typical elongate mitochondria and rough ER are present in both cell types. A Golgi apparatus is situated close to the nucleus, and within the cisternae of this organelle a dense material may be seen. It is believed that the chromaffin granules are formed in the Golgi complex in a manner similar to that described for zymogen granules in pancreatic acinar cells. A few microvilli may be present at the cell surface, and a single cilium is probably present on each cell. Maculae adhaerantes are frequently seen at the surface of adjacent parenchymal cells. Each chromaffin cell is innervated by a cholinergic preganglionic sympathetic nerve whose stimulation initiates the release of stored catecholamine from the medullary cell (Fig. 31-18).

Morphologic events accompanying the release of catecholamines are the subject of controversy. Some workers have reported that chromaffin granules retain their integrity and that catecholamine diffuses out of, or is actively transported out of, the granules and the cell. Others have reported that the granule membrane fuses with the plasmalemma and that the entire content of the granule is emptied into the extracellular space and eventually enters the circulation (quantal release). Physiologic evidence is consistent with the quantal release mechanism.

As previously noted, the adrenal medulla receives a dual blood supply, one from the arteriae medullae and the other formed by vessels which are continuous with the capillaries of the cortex. It has been reported that norepinephrine-storing cells are usually more closely associated with vessels arising from arteriae medullae whereas epinephrine-storing cells are supplied with blood which has previously perfused the cortex and which thereby contains a higher concentration of corticosteroids. There is

evidence that phenylethanolamine-*N*-methyl transferase, the enzyme which transfers a methyl group from *S*-adenosyl methionine to norepinephrine, yielding epinephrine, is induced in the presence of glucocorticoids (Fig. 31-19).

In a hypophysectomized animal which does not secrete ACTH and thus does not secrete normal levels of glucocorticoids, the amount of epinephrine which can be isolated from the adrenal medulla declines, with a concomitant slight rise in the concentration of norepinephrine. In rat and rabbit fetuses, the accumulation of epinephrine in the adrenal medulla coincides with the initiation of adrenocortical function. If the fetus is deprived of its hypophysis by decapitation in utero, the rise in epinephrine content is not seen, but the levels of norepinephrine are above normal. Injection of ACTH or cortisol into the decapitated fetuses restores the normal ratio of epinephrine to norepi-

Figure 31-16   Electron micrograph of an epinephrine-storing adrenal medullary cell from the rat. C, chromaffin granules; M, mitochondrion; G, Golgi complex.   ×14,700.

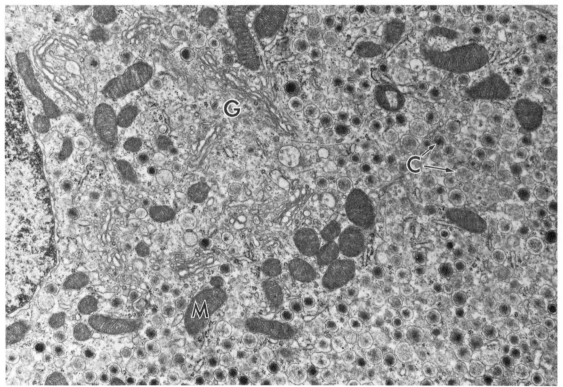

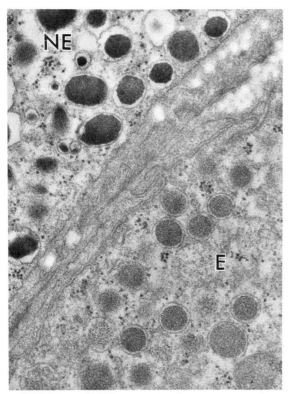

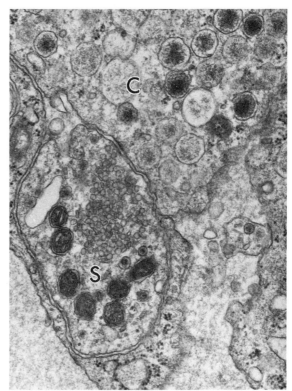

Figure 31-17   Electron micrograph to compare the chromaffin granules in a norepinephrine-storing cell (upper left, NE) and an epinephrine-storing cell (lower right, E) in the cat adrenal medulla. ×33,600.

Figure 31-18   Electron micrograph showing cholinergic preganglionic fiber (S) ending on a chromaffin cell (C) in the rat adrenal medulla. ×34,700.

nephrine.   Comparative histologic and endocrinologic studies lend support to this interesting interaction between cortex and medulla.   In the shark, where interrenal and chromaffin tissues are separate, norepinephrine is the main catecholamine, whereas in mammals, where the cortex (interrenal tissue) surrounds the medulla (chromaffin tissue), the principal catecholamine is epinephrine.

The effects of the hormones of the adrenal medulla are widespread and will be touched upon only briefly here.   Epinephrine causes glycogenolysis in the liver and skeletal muscle, with a consequent rise in blood glucose levels.   Free fatty acids are mobilized from adipose tissue under the influence of catecholamines.   Epinephrine causes an elevation of blood pressure, acceleration of the heart, cutaneous vasoconstriction, dilation of coronary and skeletal muscle vessels, but vasoconstriction in other organs such as the intestinal tract.   Under the influence of catecholamines, the threshold of the reticular activating system of the brain is lowered and the subject becomes more alert.   It can be seen that all these effects have an obvious adaptive value when the organism is confronted with an emergency situation.

Secretion of adrenal medullary hormones is under sympathetic nervous control.   During sleep or narcosis, little or no secretion can be detected but while the organism is carrying on normal activities, low quantities of catecholamines can be detected in the circulation.   When the animal is exposed to pain, cold, anoxia, hypoglycemia, emotional excitement, or other stress, the secretion of catecholamines rises sharply and the homeostatic mechanisms mentioned above are brought into play.

Development

In 4-to 5-week human fetuses mesothelial cells in the region of the dorsal mesentery and near the cranial pole of the mesonephros begin to proliferate and penetrate into the subjacent, highly vascular mesenchyme. Continued growth of these primordia results in bilaterally placed organs which protrude into the coelomic cavity and become encapsulated. The gland becomes differentiated into two regions: an outer zone composed of small, compact cells which form the definitive cortex of the adult and an inner zone of large, eosinophilic cells which is termed the fetal zone (Fig. 31-20). The fetal zone constitutes approximately 80 percent of the cortex at term but it undergoes rapid degeneration after birth whereas the definitive cortex enlarges and eventually becomes differentiated into the familiar three zones of the adult gland.

Chromaffin cells from the neural crest begin to migrate into the adrenal anlagen at 6 to 7 weeks of fetal life and subsequently aggregate in the center of the gland to form the adrenal medulla.

Cells of the fetal cortex have the ultrastructural appearance of other steroid-secreting cells (Fig. 31-21). The smooth ER is elaborately developed, lipid droplets are abundant, and the Golgi complex is prominent. The appearance of the mitochondria in cells of the fetal zone is similar to that of mitochondria on the adult zona fasciculata.

The fetal adrenal is under the control of ACTH secreted by the pituitary of the fetus. Anencephalic monsters possess very small adrenal glands, and the fetal zone is lacking. The physiologic role of the fetal zone of human adrenals in intrauterine life is slowly becoming clearer but progress in this area is hampered by the fact that none of the commonly used experimental animals has a comparable fetal zone.

The human fetal adrenal gland is a steroidogenic organ which is part of a "fetal-placental" unit. The fetal adrenal is incapable of carrying out certain steroidogenic reactions; in particular, the Δ^5-3β-hydroxysteroid dehydrogenase system has a very low activity in the gland. This enzyme is present in high quantity in the placenta. The products of this enzymatic reaction are transferred to the fetus where the adrenal gland carries out a series of

Figure 31-19 Biosynthetic pathway of catecholamines in the adrenal medulla.

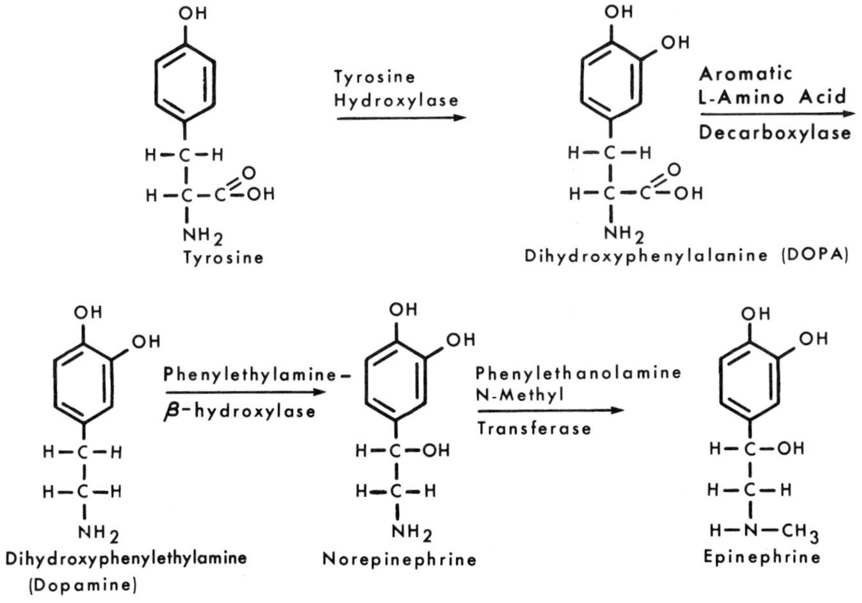

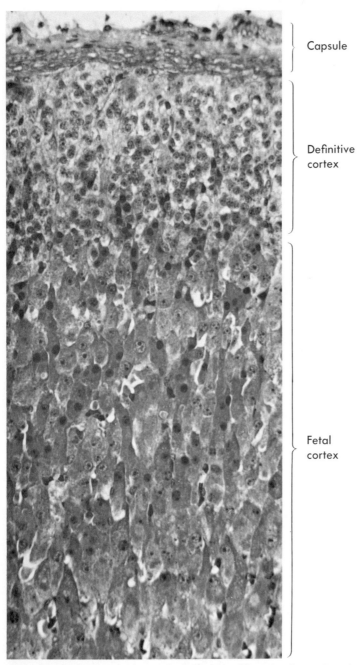

Capsule

Definitive
cortex

Fetal
cortex

Figure 31-20 Section of a human fetal adrenal at 18 weeks of gestation, showing the division into fetal and definitive cortex. ×300.

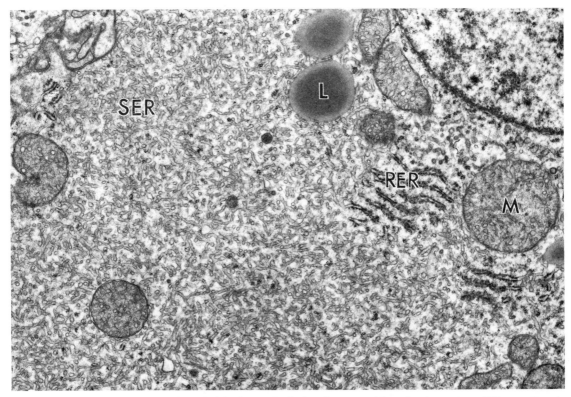

Figure 31-21 Electron micrograph of a cell of the human fetal adrenal cortex at 14 weeks of gestation. SER, smooth-surfaced endoplasmic reticulum; RER, rough-surfaced endoplasmic reticulum; M, mitochondrion; L, lipid inclusion. ×13,000. (Courtesy of Dr. N. S. McNutt and Dr. A. L. Jones.)

hydroxylations which result in the production of cortisol, corticosterone, deoxycorticosterone, and aldosterone. A 17-21 lyase is present which converts C_{21} steroids to C_{19} products, particularly dehydroepiandrosterone (DHA). This enzyme is not found in the placenta. A sulfokinase is present in the adrenal which converts DHA to DHA sulfate, the principal precursor of placental estrogens.

Although much has been learned about the role of the fetal adrenal in steroidogenesis, the full biological significance of this activity during pregnancy remains to be elucidated.

References

COUPLAND, R. E.: "The Natural History of the Chromaffin Cell," Longmans, Green & Co., Ltd., London, 1965.

DEANE, H. W.: The Anatomy, Chemistry, and Physiology of Adrenocortical Tissue, "Handbuch der Experimentellen Pharmakologie," vol. 14, pt. 1, pp. 1–185, Springer-Verlag OHG, Berlin, 1962.

EISENSTEIN, A. B. (ed.): "The Adrenal Cortex," Little, Brown and Company, Boston, 1967.

GRIFFITHS, K., and E. H. D. CAMERON: Steroid Biosynthetic Pathways in the Human Adrenal, *Advances Steroid Biochem. Pharmacol.*, **2:**223–265 (1970).

IDELMAN, S.: Ultrastructure of the Mammalian Adrenal Cortex, *Int. Rev. Cytol.*, **27:**181–281 (1970).

JOHANNISSON, E.: The Foetal Adrenal Cortex in the Human, *Acta Endocr. (Kobenhavn)*, **130** (Suppl.):(1968).

JONES, I. CHESTER: "The Adrenal Cortex," Cambridge University Press, New York, 1957.

LANMAN, J. T.: The Fetal Zone of the Adrenal Gland, *Medicine,* **32:**389–430 (1953).

LONG, J. A., and A. L. JONES: Observations on the Fine Structure of the Adrenal Cortex of Man, *Lab. Invest.,* **17:**355–370 (1967).

POHORECKY, L. A., and R. J. WURTMAN: Adrenocortical Control of Epinephrine Synthesis, *Pharmacol. Rev.,* **23:**1–35 (1971).

SYMINGTON, T.: "Functional Pathology of the Human Adrenal Gland," The Williams & Wilkins Company, Baltimore, 1969.

chapter 32   The eye

DAVID G. COGAN
AND
TOICHIRO KUWABARA

Structure

The human eye is an approximate sphere, 2.5 cm in diameter. It forms an image of the environment on its photoreceptive layer, the retina, and transmits the information from that image to the optic nerve and thence to the brain. Human eyes have a wide range of motility. They can scan the visual field or track a moving object while maintaining precise coordination with one another. The histologic architecture of the eye serves these optical, photoreceptive, and motility requirements.

The eye is often compared to a camera. The rigid box of the camera is analogous to the corneoscleral coat; the black lining of the camera is the uvea of the eye; and the photosensitive film of the camera is the retina of the eye. The mechanism for focusing differs, however, in that the lens of the camera moves back and forth whereas the lens of the eye changes its accommodation by varying its convexity in situ. The diaphragm of the camera is analogous to the iris of the eye; both

control the amount of entering light and the depth of field. With extremes of pupillary size at 2 mm and 7 mm, the *f* stop of the eye varies from 12.0 to 3.5.

PARTS OF EYE AND ADNEXA
The eyes and adnexa lend themselves to the following divisions:

Protective tissues These consist of lids, conjunctiva, and surface of the cornea (Fig. 32-1). To these must be added lacrimal glands in the orbit and adnexal sebaceous glands of the lids.

Tissue giving form and relative rigidity to the eye This is chiefly the corneoscleral coat which, together with the intraocular pressure, maintains the relatively constant size and shape of the eye.

Nutritional and light-excluding tissue This layer lies just internal to the sclera and is called the

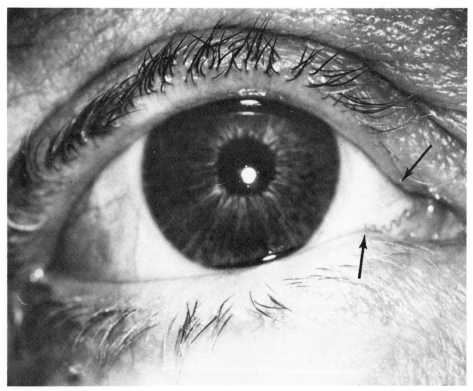

Figure 32-1 Lids and eye. Noteworthy are the conspicuous fold of the upper lid, with the eyelashes coming from the anterior portion of the lid margin; the puncta (arrows) for drainage of tears; the white sclera covered by transparent conjuctiva; the iris with its characteristic radial structure; and the central black pupil. The cornea, being transparent, is not visible but the central light spot reflected from the surface of the cornea indicates its smooth and convex surface.

uvea. Its major anatomic divisions are choroid, ciliary body, and iris.

Photoreceptive and neural tissues These are located in a membrane called the *retina* lining much of the interior of the eye and connected with the brain by way of the optic nerve (Fig. 32-2).

Optical or refractive tissues These consist of the smooth anterior surface of the cornea (where most

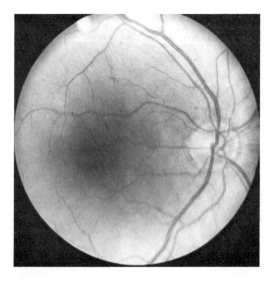

Figure 32-2 Ophthalmoscopic view of the interior of the eye. The nerve head, measuring about 1.5 mm in diameter, is the light, circular structure to the right of center. The blood vessels emerge from the center of this nerve. The smaller and lighter vessels are the arteries; the larger and darker vessels are the veins. The central, relatively dark area corresponds to the macula.

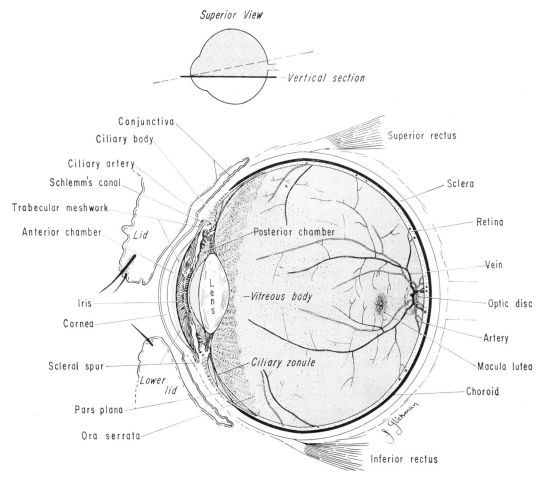

Superior View

Vertical section

Conjunctiva
Ciliary body
Ciliary artery
Schlemm's canal
Trabecular meshwork
Anterior chamber
Lid
Iris
Cornea
Scleral spur
Lower lid
Pars plana
Ora serrata

Superior rectus
Sclera
Retina
Posterior chamber
Vein
Lens
Vitreous body
Optic disc
Ciliary zonule
Artery
Macula lutea
Choroid
Inferior rectus

Figure 32-3 Schematic drawing of lids and eye. The interior of the eye has been exposed by removal of a calotte from the nasal side of the globe, as indicated in the insert.

of the stationary refraction occurs), the lens (where the variable refraction occurs), and clear ocular media, consisting of aqueous humor in front of the lens and vitreous humor behind the lens (Fig. 32-3).

Intraocular fluid Most of the fluid turnover in the eye occurs by way of the aqueous humor. This is secreted by the ciliary body into the posterior chamber, a pyramidal space bounded anteriorly by the iris, posteriorly by the lens and zonular fibers, and laterally by the ciliary body. The aqueous humor drains out of the eye at the periphery of the anterior chamber through the trabecular meshwork and Schlemm's canal.

Ocular motor system There are seven *extraocular muscles* that move each eye with remarkable precision: the levator; the medial and lateral recti in the horizontal orbital plane; the superior and inferior recti in the sagittal plane; and the superior and inferior oblique muscles in a vertical plane extending from the inner angle of the orbit toward the equator of the eye (Fig. 32-4). Except for the levator muscle, which has a smooth muscle component (Müller's muscle) attached to the tarsus, the extraocular muscle fibers are entirely voluntary or skeletal (Fig. 32-51). However, they differ from most skeletal muscle fibers in being finer and more variable in size and in having more nerves and myoneural junctions.

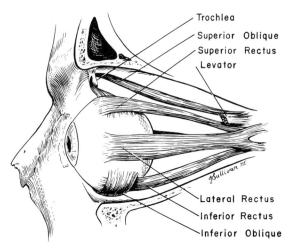

Figure 32-4   Origins and insertions of the ocular muscles. (Reprinted with permission of Charles C Thomas, Publisher.)

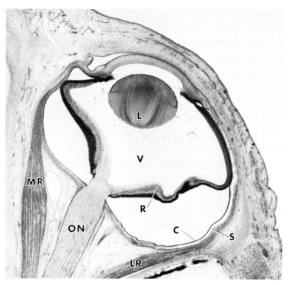

Figure 32-5   Horizontal section of the eye and adjacent structures of a 3-month human embryo.   MR, medial rectus; LR, lateral rectus; ON, optic nerve; S, sclera; C, choroid; R, retina; V, vitreous; L, lens.   The retina is artefactitiously separated, as is frequently the case in histologic preparations.   The lens is surrounded by many small vessels, the tunica vasculosa lentis, which partly disappear and partly become incorporated in the iris during later stages of development.   The choroid and ciliary body are recognizable but the iris does not develop until a later stage.   Compare this section with that of an adult eye (Fig. 32-6).

ORIGIN

The anlagen of the eyes are recognizable early in the embryo as a pair of lateral outpouchings of the diencephalon.   As it approaches the surface ectoderm, each pouch invaginates to form an optic cup.   The inner layer of this cup is destined to form the retina, and the outer layer is destined to form the pigment epithelium of the choroid.

The surface ectoderm overlying the optic cup thickens, invaginates, and eventually becomes the lens.   The embryonic tissue surrounding the optic vesicle and lying in front of the lens then differentiates to form the other structures of the eye.

By the third month of gestation, the eye has already attained its definitive shape and structure (Fig. 32-5); it differs from the eye of a full-term fetus chiefly in having an elaborate vascular system within the vitreous body and about the lens.   This embryonic hyaloid system, as it is called, disappears almost entirely prior to birth.

Lids

The upper and lower lids both protect and lubricate the anterior portions of the eyeballs.   The skin surface is covered by stratified squamous epithelium like that of the rest of the face but the connective tissue stroma is more delicate and contains little fat (Fig. 32-6).   Superficial muscle fibers, constituting the *orbicularis oculi,* are innervated by the VIIth nerve and serve to close the lids.   The superficial dermis also contains lymph vessels, sweat glands, and sebaceous glands.

The deep stroma of the upper and lower lids contains a plaque of compact connective tissue containing large sebaceous glands that open onto the lid margins.   These plaques, called the *tarsal plates,* give a measure of solidity to the lids.   The sebaceous structures within the plates are called *Meibomian glands;* they secrete oily materials that seal the lid margins when the eyes are closed and prevent overflow of tears when the eyes are open. The superior margin of the tarsus of the upper lid also serves for attachment of the *levator palpebrae muscle* that raises the upper lid (Fig. 32-6).

The posterior surfaces of the lids are covered by a mucous membrane, the *palpebral conjunctiva,* that has a stratified epithelium only two to three cells thick and a variable abundance of subepithelial lymphoid tissue. This palpebral conjunctiva has many mucous goblet cells. The transitional zones where the palpebral conjunctiva is reflected onto the eye to become bulbar conjunctiva form cul-de-sacs or *fornices.* The mucus-forming cells are especially abundant in these fornices.

The lid margins mark the transition between skin and mucous membranes. The stratified squamous ectoderm of the former becomes the mucous epithelium of the latter. But the most noteworthy structures of these lid margins are the eyelashes, which emerge from the anterior edge of the lid margin and the 15 to 20 orifices of the Meibomian glands that open into the intermarginal space.

The most medial portions of the upper and lower lid margins contain the orifices and canals that conduct the tears into the lacrimal sac and thence into the nose. These canals, called the *upper* and *lower canaliculi,* are lined by a stratified epithelium somewhat thicker than that of the conjunctiva.

Figure 32-6 Vertical section of lids, globe, and orbit of an adult human being. The upper lid has been somewhat displaced forward but otherwise shows an approximately normal relationship of structures. UL, upper lid; LL, lower lid; C, cornea; AC, anterior chamber; I, iris; L, lens (artefactitiously fragmented); CB, ciliary body; R, retina (artefactitiously separated from choroid); V, vitreous body; ON, optic nerve; Lev, levator muscle; MM, Müller's muscle; SR, superior rectus; CN, ciliary nerve; OF, orbital fat.

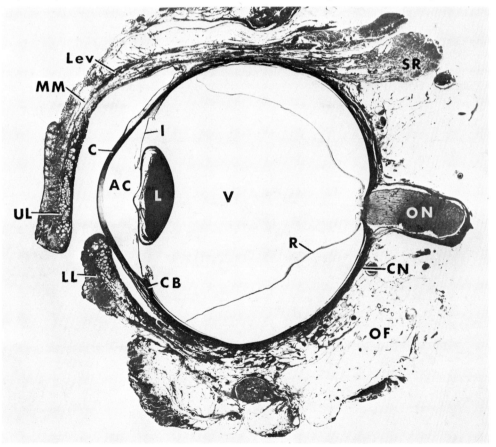

Conjunctiva

Except for the cornea with which it is continuous, the conjunctiva provides the mucous membrane cover for the eye (*bulbar conjunctiva*) and posterior portion of the lids (*palpebral conjunctiva*). The bulbar portion contains goblet cells and has many folds (Fig. 32-7). The goblet cells are most abundant in the nasal portions of the conjunctiva. The connective tissues and blood vessels do not appear unusual histologically, but clinical evidence has shown that they have a great capacity for reversible swelling and congestion.

The epithelium of the bulbar conjunctiva is four to five cells thick, but this increases to as many as ten cells at the junction with the cornea. The epithelium of the conjunctiva is continuous with that of the cornea; the zone of transition is known as the *limbus*.

The nasal or inner angle of the conjunctiva is modified to form the *caruncle* and *semilunar folds*. These are prominent structures consisting of sebaceous glands covered by stratified squamous epithelium.

Cornea

The clear window comprising the most anterior portion of the eye is the *cornea*. In the adult it is about 11 mm in diameter and slightly more than 0.5 mm thick. Having a greater curvature than the sclera, the cornea has the gross appearance of a watch crystal (Fig. 32-3).

When examined with the polarizing microscope, the corneal fibers show a birefringence that differs from that of most collagenous structures in being unusually fine and regular.

It is important, although possibly disappointing, to note that the cornea shows no histologic basis for its transparency. With routine stains the corneal stroma is much like that of the sclera, with no clear-cut demarcation at the limbus corresponding to the sharp optical difference that exists

Figure 32-7 Conjunctiva near caruncle, showing abundant goblet cells. The stroma shows blood vessels and lymph vessels in loose connective tissue. H&E.

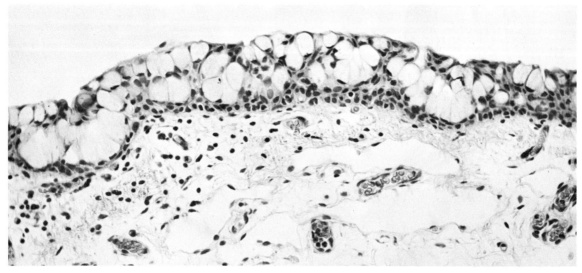

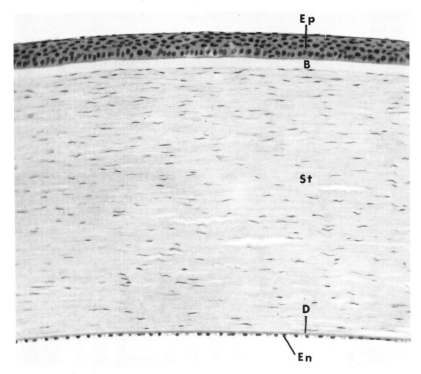

Figure 32-8 Cross section of the cornea.   Ep, epithelium; B, Bowman's membrane; St, stroma; D, Descemet's membrane; En, endothelium.

between cornea and sclera. The basis for transparency is physiologic rather than anatomic; the optical homogeneity is maintained by a continual pumping out of the interstitial fluid across the semipermeable surface membranes so that the cornea is kept in a deturgesced state.

The histologic composition of the cornea is notably uniform (Fig. 32-8). The constituent layers listed in an anterior to posterior direction are *epithelium, Bowman's membrane, stroma, Descemet's membrane,* and *endothelium* (or, as it is called by some authors, "mesenchymal epithelium").

EPITHELIUM
The *epithelium,* accounting for about one-tenth of the total corneal thickness, is five cells deep, with a uniquely smooth anterior surface. The columnar basal layers have a robust basement membrane, as delineated by the PAS reagent, but this has only

a tenuous attachment to the underlying Bowman's membrane. Except for stratification, the epithelial cells show no differentiation toward either mucous cell formation or other specialization. Mitoses are rarely seen in conventional sections but are readily found in flat whole mounts of the cornea.

BOWMAN'S MEMBRANE
Named in honor of a nineteenth-century ophthalmologist and anatomist, *Bowman's membrane* is not a distinct membrane in the usual sense but is compact collagen with the same tinctorial and physical properties as the rest of the corneal stroma (Figs. 32-8 and 32-15). It lies immediately beneath the epithelium throughout the entire extent of the cornea and terminates abruptly at the limbus. Most highly developed in the human eye, Bowman's membrane maintains the optical smoothness of the anterior corneal layers.

STROMA

The *stroma* constitutes the bulk of the cornea and accounts for its characteristic shape and resistance. It consists of laminae of collagen parallel to the surface, with fibroblasts sandwiched between them (Fig. 32-8). Except for occasional wandering cells and inconspicuous nerves in its most anterior layers, the stroma shows no specialized elements. Specifically no blood vessels, lymphatics, or other formed structures are present in the normal cornea. The stroma stains, however, in a characteristically metachromatic fashion with toluidine blue and other thiazine dyes. The metachromatic substances, which have been identified chemically, are chondroitin sulfate and keratosulfate; they probably aid the reversible swelling properties (and transparency) of the cornea. These sulfated polysaccharides are not present in the sclera.

DESCEMET'S MEMBRANE

Descemet's membrane, named for a Parisian ophthalmologist, botanist, and general physician of the eighteenth century, is an acellular hyaline layer about 10 μm thick, situated just posterior to the corneal stroma (Fig. 32-9). It stains lightly with eosin (less than the stroma), lightly although definitely with elastic tissue dyes, but heavily with the PAS reagent (like the lens capsule and certain other hyaline membranes). It does not stain metachromatically. When incised or ruptured, Descemet's

membrane coils inward like a watch spring. At the periphery of the cornea it is frequently thickened by a bundle of circular fibers, forming *Schwalbe's line.*

The anterior border of Descemet's membrane is smooth and firmly attached to the deep corneal stroma. Its posterior surface is also smooth, but wart-like excrescences develop regularly with age toward the periphery of the cornea.

Because of its coiling tendency, Descemet's membrane can take up slack with the reversible swelling of the cornea. Like the elastic lamina of blood vessels, it distributes tension evenly and prevents gross deformation of the tissue.

ENDOTHELIUM

The *endothelium* covering the posterior surface of the cornea is a single layer of cells which are thin and inconspicuous in conventional cross sections (Fig. 32-9) but which appear as a regular mosaic of hexagonal cells in flat preparations. Despite its thinness, the endothelium is an essential structure for the maintenance of normal deturgescence and transparency of the cornea. Mitoses are rarely seen, although the endothelium has the capacity for vigorous proliferation in pathologic states.

At the periphery of the cornea, approximately 1 mm central to the termination of Descemet's membrane, the normally thin endothelium becomes even more tenuous and then extends over the pores of the trabecular meshwork.

Figure 32-9   Posterior portion of the cornea treated with the PAS reagent which stains Descemet's membrane an intense red. St, stroma; D, Descemet's membrane; En, endothelium.

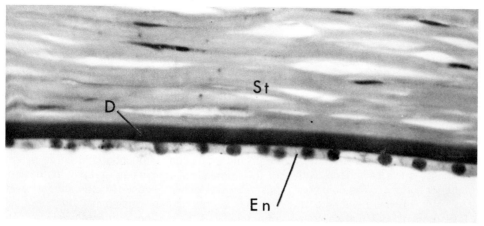

Corneal fine structure

By electron microscopy the epithelium is seen to consist of closely packed cells having a fine fibrillary cytoplasm with relatively few mitochondria and little endoplasmic reticulum (Figs. 32-10 to 32-12). The cell boundaries show interlacing undulations and an abundance of desmosomes. Bowman's membrane and corneal stroma consist of a felt-like network of collagen fibrils and an amorphous interfibrillar substance. In Bowman's membrane the fibrils are somewhat finer and not regularly arranged into laminae, as they are in the stroma (Fig. 32-15). The stromal cells are similar to fibroblasts elsewhere in the body but are packed between dense bundles of collagen fibrils (Fig. 32-13 and 32-14).

Descemet's membrane, which appears structureless by light microscopy, also shows little structure by electron microscopy (Fig. 32-16). It is made up chiefly of ground substance similar to basement membrane. Toward the periphery of the cornea, however, there are fibers with a periodicity of 1000 Å. These are thought to be a unique form of collagen. There are also many fine clefts in the peripheral cornea, permitting processes of endothelial cells to insinuate into the cornea.

In electron micrographs the endothelium is seen to consist of overlapping cells (Fig. 32-10) without the interdigitations or abundant desmosomes such as are present in the epithelium. Also in contrast to the epithelium, the endothelial cells are rich in mitochondria, vesicles, and granules but lack the finely filamentous cytoplasm metabolically; this endothelium appears to be the more active tissue.

Limbus

An imaginary line connecting the peripheral terminations of Bowman's and Descemet's membranes is the boundary of the cornea with the sclera (Fig. 32-17). The region of this line is called the *limbus;* it corresponds to the abrupt optical change from the transparent cornea to the opaque sclera. Aside from the terminations of Bowman's and Descemet's membranes, it contains the sites of transition of conjunctival epithelium into corneal epithelium, the peripheral boundary of metachromatic staining of the corneal stroma, and the important trabecular meshwork in the angle of the anterior chamber.

TRABECULAR MESHWORK AND SCHLEMM'S CANAL

Just peripheral to the end of Descemet's membrane is the *trabecula,* or *trabecular meshwork,* that marks the site for drainage of aqueous humor (Fig. 32-17). The trabecular strands which are continuous with Descemet's membrane and endothelium enclose spaces, called the *spaces of Fontana,* that communicate with the anterior chamber. The central or axial border of the trabecula coincides with Schwalbe's line and the peripheral border coincides with a prominent ridge, the *scleral spur,* from which the ciliary muscle arises.

Anterior and lateral to the trabecular meshwork are one or more endothelium-lined channels coursing circumferentially about the cornea. These are collectively called *Schlemm's canal* (Fig. 32-18, see color insert). They collect the aqueous humor which has filtered through the spaces of Fontana and which then passes out of the eye and into the episcleral vessels. It is obstruction of drainage in these structures at the angle of the anterior chamber that causes a pathologic rise in the intraocular pressure and the eye disease *glaucoma.*

Electron microscopy shows the trabecular meshwork to consist of central cores of collagenous fibers ensheathed by homogeneous ground substance, and a lining of endothelial cells. The central cores become less conspicuous toward Schlemm's canal and may disappear altogether, leaving a meshwork of endothelial cells. The spaces within the trabecula communicate with each other by pores 0.5 to 1.5 μm in diameter, with decreasing apertures toward Schlemm's canal. It is a moot question whether or not these spaces open directly into Schlemm's canal.

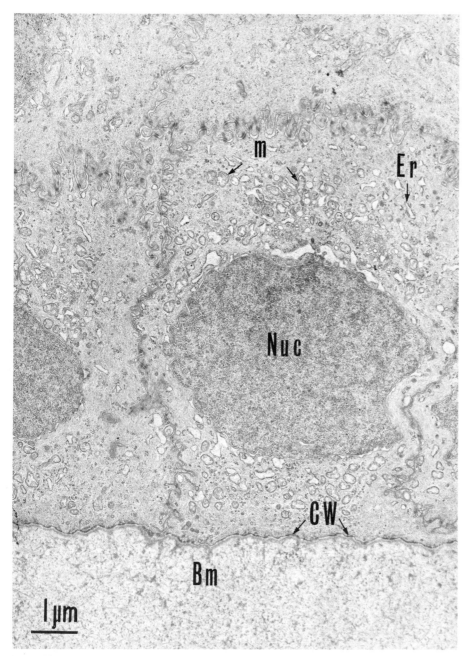

Figure 32-10 Electron micrograph at the junction of basal epithelial cells and Bowman's membrane. Bm, Bowman's membrane; CW, cell wall; Er, endoplasmic reticulum; m, mitochondria; Nuc, nucleus.

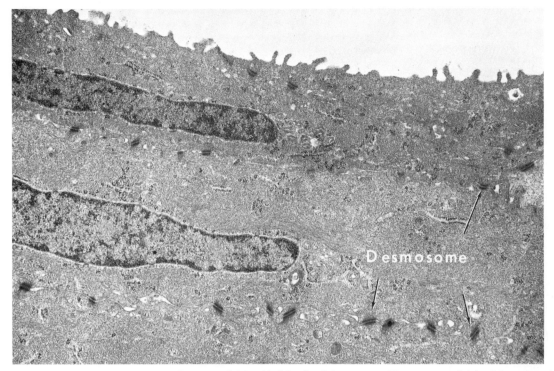

Figure 32-11   Electron micrograph of the superficial epithelial cells of the cornea.   The most superficial cell is nucleated.   The cells appear to be attached loosely at the sites of desmosomes.   The surface cells have fine ridges.

Figure 32-12   Higher magnification of a corneal epithelial cell.   The cytoplasm contains rich keratofibrils and glycogen particles. Mitochondria are sparse.   Cell membranes are joined by conspicuous desmosomes.

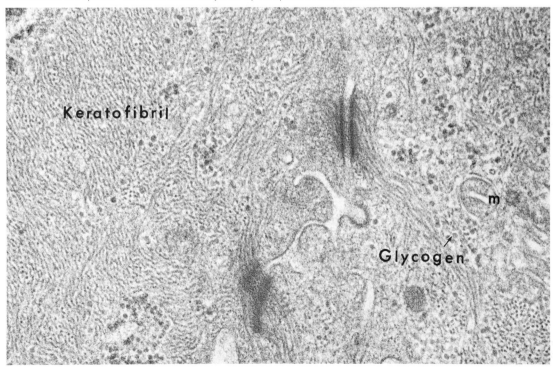

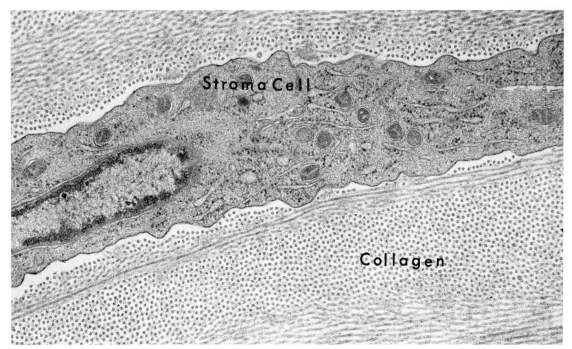

Figure 32-13 Electron micrograph of a portion of a stromal cell between collagenous laminae. The cell contains rich mitochondria and rough endoplasmic reticulum.

Anterior and posterior chambers

The *anterior chamber* is the area bounded by the cornea anteriorly and by the iris and lens posteriorly (Fig. 32-18, see color insert). It has a depth of approximately 3-mm at its center, a volume of 0.2 ml, and a fluid turnover rate of 2 mm^3 per min. The *aqueous humor*, which fills the anterior chamber, is a water-clear fluid containing most of the soluble constituents of the blood with an extremely small concentration of proteins (0.02 percent, in contrast to 7 percent in the blood).

The *posterior chamber* is the pyramidal area bounded by the iris anteriorly, the lens and zonules posteriorly, and the ciliary body laterally. The aqueous humor which fills the posterior chamber is secreted by the ciliary epithelium and circulates through the pupil into the anterior chamber. The pupillary margin of the iris rests on the lens and thereby provides a ball valve which allows fluid to pass from posterior chamber to anterior chamber but not in the reverse direction.

Sclera

The *sclera* is that portion of the outer tunic of the eye extending posteriorly to constitute about four-fifths of the eye's capsule (Fig. 32-3). With an average thickness of 0.5 mm, it varies from a maximal thickness at the posterior pole to a minimal thickness beneath the extraocular muscles. Like

the corneal stroma with which it is continuous, the sclera consists chiefly of compact fibrous tissue. In contrast to the cornea, however, the collagenous laminae are less regularly arranged (seen especially well with crossed polaroids); there is more elastic tissue; blood vessels are present (especially at the

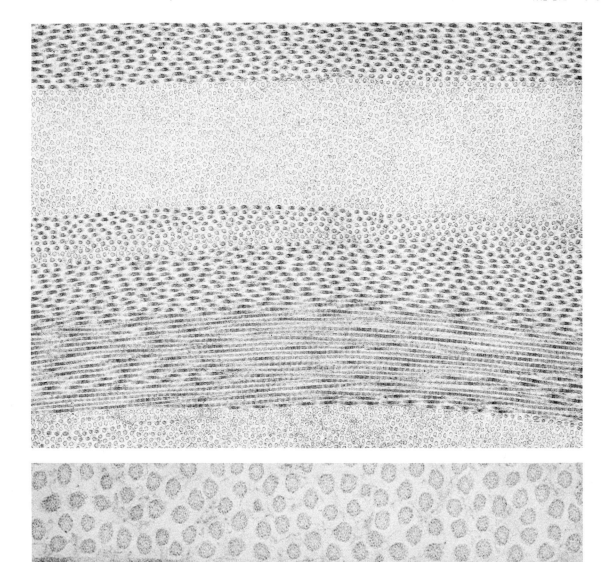

Figure 32-14 Lamellar arrangement of the corneal collagen fibers. Fibers are uniform in size (about 300 Å in diameter) and regularly spaced. Fibers are arranged parallel to the surface of the cornea.

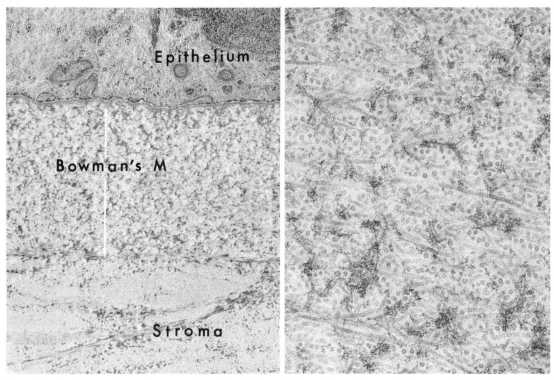

Figure 32-15 Bowman's membrane consists of fine fibrils and short collagen fibers. Higher magnification on the right shows their randomly intermingled arrangement.

Figure 32-16 Electron micrograph of the posterior portion of the cornea of a newborn monkey.

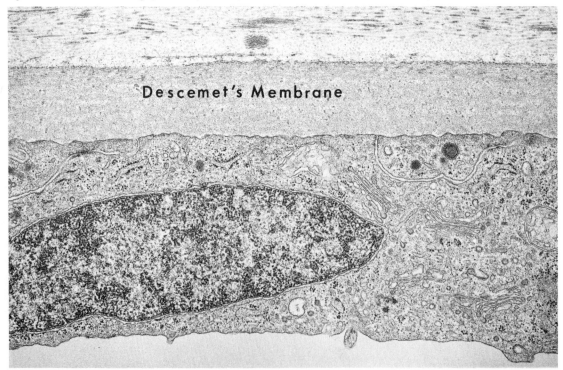

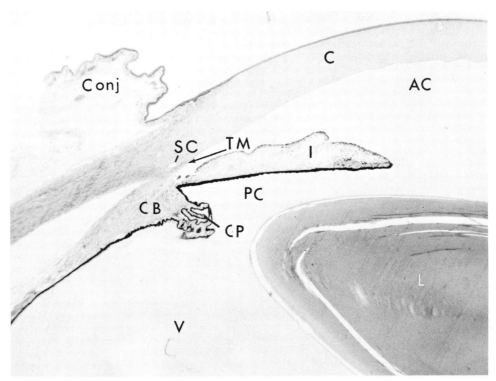

Figure 32-17 Portion of the anterior segment of the eye. C, cornea; Conj, conjunctiva; SC, Schlemm's canal; TM, trabecular meshwork; AC, anterior chamber; PC, posterior chamber; I, iris; CP, ciliary process; CB, ciliary body (artefactitiously separated from sclera); L, lens; V, vitreous.

limbus); the acidic mucopolysaccharides are absent; and there is no tendency to imbibe water.

The sclera shows several regional modifications. Abutting the limbus, the sclera contains a fairly rich plexus of blood vessels in anastomotic connection with Schlemm's canal and with the anterior ciliary vessels. The four rectus muscles insert in the superficial layers of the sclera at 5 to 8 mm from the limbus and the two oblique muscles insert farther posteriorly. But the most noteworthy modification is at the site of exit of the optic nerve. Here the sclera is reduced to a fenestrated membrane, the *lamina cribrosa,* through which the nerves pass like filaments through a sieve (Fig. 32-18, see color insert). This "hole" has a diameter of little more than 1 mm and is situated about 3 mm nasal to the posterior pole of the eye. It represents a weak spot in the sclera's resistance, and its fibers become bowed outward with abnormal elevations of the intraocular pressure (glaucoma).

Together with the corneal stroma, the sclera maintains the size and form of the eye. That this is of the utmost optical importance is evident from the observation that increasing the axial length of the eye by only 1 mm would cause a person to be severely incapacitated by nearsightedness (*myopia*) whereas a decrease of the length by only 1 mm from the norm would cause him to have a refractive deviation (*hyperopia*) of the same magnitude in the opposite direction.

Uvea

The *uvea* is the pigmented and predominantly vascular coat of the eye. It is divided into the *iris,* the *ciliary body,* and the *choroid.*

IRIS

The *iris,* the most anterior portion of the uvea, extends from the angle of the anterior chamber to the pupillary margin (Fig. 32-17). It thus has the form of a disc with a hole in its center (Fig. 32-1). Because of its reaction to light, it is properly considered the *diaphragm* of the eye.

The iris consists of a *spongy stroma* facing the anterior chamber, constituting the bulk of the iris, and a *pigment epithelial layer* facing the posterior chamber and resting on the lens at the pupillary margin. In addition, the iris contains a substantial *sphincter muscle* near its pupillary margin and a tenuous *dilator muscle* lying just anterior to the pigment epithelium.

The iris stroma is a loose and spongy connective tissue with tissue spaces that are continuous with the anterior chamber (Fig. 32-19). Aside from the fibroblasts, the stroma contains pigmented cells of two distinctive shapes. First there are the *melano-*

Figure 32-19 Contrasting irises of lightly pigmented (blonde) and heavily pigmented (Negro) eyes. The former has a delicately spongy stroma whereas the latter has a relatively compact stroma in which the pigment is concentrated anteriorly. The abundant blood vessels with their characteristically thick walls are especially well seen in the pigmented iris. The sphincter muscle forms a delicate lamina of smooth muscle fibers near the pupillary edge (to the left of center). Both irises contain a heavily pigmented epithelium lining their posterior surfaces.

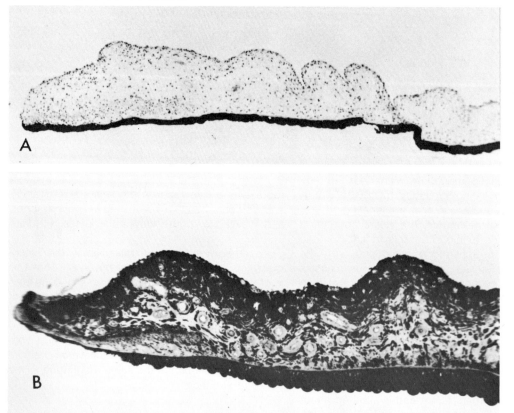

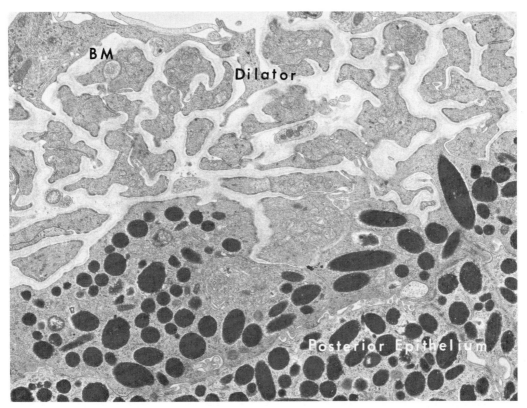

Figure 32-20   Dilator muscle is developed within the basal infolds of the anterior epithelial cell.   Apical portion of the dilator muscle cell is heavily pigmented.

phores, with elongated processes and light-brown pigment granules; they are most heavily concentrated along the anterior border layers of the iris. Then there are the round and more heavily pigmented *clump cells,* which are more numerous toward the sphincter regions of the iris. The relative number of pigment cells varies with the individual's complexion. In dark-skinned persons with brown eyes the pigment cells are abundant; in light-skinned persons with blue eyes the stromal pigment may be absent altogether.

The blood vessels of the iris are noteworthy for having a thick, although not compact, adventitial layer about them. This forms a fibrous acellular "wall" that is unique for vessels of the iris.

The *sphincter muscle* comprises a compact bundle of smooth muscle fibers arranged circularly near the pupillary margin (Fig. 32-19). It receives in-nervation for contraction from the parasympathetic ganglion in the orbit by way of the long ciliary nerves within the eye. The *dilator muscle* is formed within the basal portion of the anterior epithelial cell (Fig. 32-20). Although the muscle fibers are surrounded by basement membranes, they are so indistinct that they can scarcely be identified by light microscopy. These dilator muscle fibers are arranged radial to the pupil, run the full length of the iris, and receive their innervation for positive contraction from the sympathetic nervous system.

The dilator and sphincter muscles function reciprocally and provide an excellent example of the opposite action of the two components of the autonomic nervous system.

The *pigment epithelium* on the posterior surface of the iris is a double layer of cells which are attached to each other apically. The posterior surface is covered with the basement membrane. Cells of both layers are heavily pigmented, whether the eye is that of a light- or dark-skinned person. The details of the cells are normally masked by the pigment, but bleaching of the cells permits recognition of two layers of cuboidal cells, of which the anterior layer cells have dilator fibers in their basal portions. At the pupillary margin, the cells extend centrally more than does the stroma; hence the pupillary border of the iris normally has a collarette of pigment epithelial cells.

CILIARY BODY

The *ciliary body* is the intermediate portion of the uvea extending from the root of the iris anteriorly to the beginning of the retina at the ora serrata posteriorly (Fig. 32-17).

In cross section the ciliary body has a roughly triangular shape, occupied chiefly with smooth muscular mass, the *ciliary muscle,* which controls the focal power of the lens. The muscle is subdivided into a circular band situated at the inner anterior angle of the triangle and a radial-meridional portion that extends from the scleral insertion just behind the trabecular meshwork to the posterior and inner portions of the ciliary body (Fig. 32-21). The circular fibers, called *Müller's muscle,* relax the tension on the lens and cause the lens to accommodate for near vision; they are innervated by the parasympathetic system through the ciliary ganglion. The radial and meridional fibers (sometimes called *Brücke's muscle*) have no clearly proved function; some evidence suggests that they are innervated by the sympathetic system and cause the lens to focus for distant vision.

The inner lining of the ciliary body comprises two layers of cuboidal cells (Fig. 32-22) of neuroectodermal origin derived in the embryo from the optic

Figure 32-21   Electron micrograph of the ciliary muscle. Smooth muscle cells are divided by thick basement membranes. Cells have rich mitochondria and smooth endoplasmic reticulum. Marginal patches are apparent (arrow). N, nerve fibers.

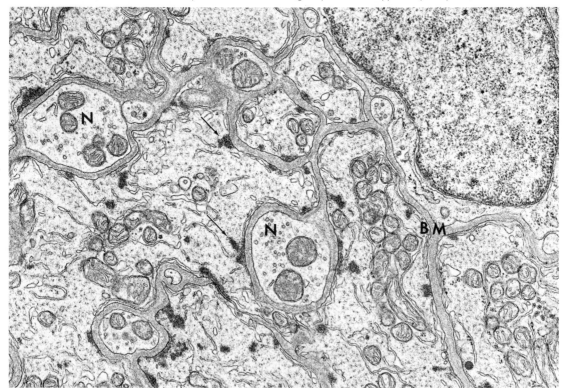

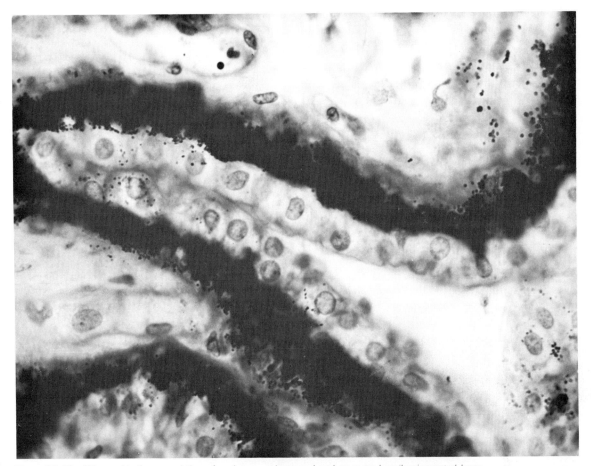

Figure 32-22   Ciliary epithelium consisting of an inner unpigmented and an outer heavily pigmented layer.

vesicle.   The inner layer with basement membrane abutting the vitreous is nonpigmented whereas the outer layer with basement membrane abutting the stroma is, for the most part, pigmented.

The anterior portion of the ciliary body is arranged in approximately 70 sagittally oriented folds or processes (*pars plicata*).   In the opened eye these form regular ridges radiating posteriorly (Fig. 32-23).   These folds or processes contain a highly vascular stroma and are believed to be the main sites for the formation of the aqueous humor (Fig. 32-18, see color insert).

The posterior portion of the ciliary body is flat; accordingly it is called *pars plana*.   If the whole eye is cut coronally at its equator, the pars plana may be seen to join abruptly with the retina in a characteristically scalloped manner; this anatomic landmark is called the *ora serrata*.

The anterior portion of the ciliary body contains a circular artery that provides the main blood supply to the iris and ciliary body.   It is in turn connected with the anterior ciliary arteries and the long posterior ciliary arteries.

Electron microscopy of the ciliary body shows the double layer of ciliary epithelium containing basement membrane on both sides, with zonular fibers inserting on the innermost membrane.   The basement membrane lining the inner surface of the epithelium often contains an amorphous substance in its interstices.   The basement membrane lining the outer surface is thick and dissected by processes of the basal epithelial cells. Characteristic of the inner ciliary epithelium is the elaborate interdigitation of the walls of adjacent cells and the extensive infolding of the surface facing the posterior chamber (Fig. 32-24A and B). Pigment granules are especially abundant in the outer pigment epithelium (Fig. 32-24A).

CHOROID

The *choroid* is that portion of the uvea extending from the region of the ora serrata posteriorward (Fig. 32-3). It lies immediately beneath the sclera and comprises a heavily vascularized and variably pigmented layer of choroid proper, a hyaline membrane called *Bruch's membrane,* and a pigment epithelial layer.

The choroid proper contains relatively large vessels, mostly veins, in its outer portions and a single layer of small sinuses called the *choriocapillaris* just beneath Bruch's membrane in its inner portions

(Fig. 32-25). The veins drain out of the choroid by the four vortex vessels, one in each posterior quadrant, and, to a lesser extent, by way of the ciliary body into the anterior ciliary vessels. The arterial supply to the choroid comes in part from the short ciliary arteries entering about the optic nerve and in part from anterior ciliary arteries entering the eye from the extraocular muscles. In addition, the choroid contains two long ciliary arteries and two long ciliary nerves passing to the ciliary body in the horizontal meridian.

The *stroma* of the chroid contains pigment cells, the *melanophores,* that vary in abundance according to the complexion of the individual. These cells are also the sites of the common melanotic tumors of the eye. Less common in the choroid are mast cells, seen best with metachromatic stains, and, rarely, isolated ganglion cells.

Bruch's membrane is a hyaline lamina that interdigitates with the choriocapillaris on its posterior surface and constitutes the basement membrane of

Figure 32-23   View of the lens and ciliary body from the back of the eye. The most central, white disc corresponds to the pupil; the lozenge-shaped structure is the lens; the radiating ridges comprise the processes of the ciliary body (pars plicata). Peripheral to the white ridges is the flat portion of the ciliary body (pars plana) ending most peripherally in the ora serrata.

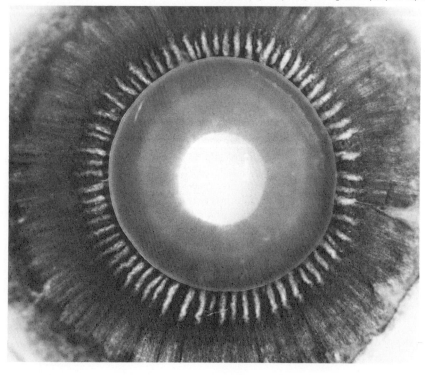

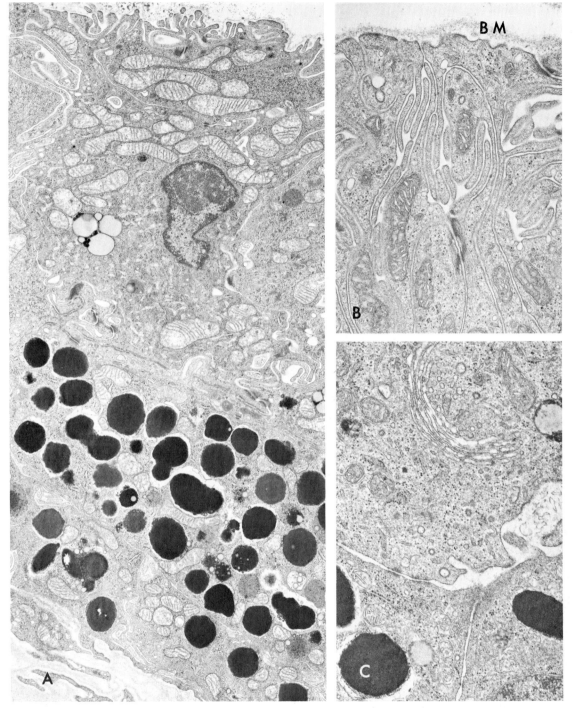

Figure 32-24 Electron micrograph of the epithelium of the ciliary body. Two-cell-layer epithelium has basement membranes on both surfaces. A. Outer layer cells contain abundant melanin pigment. Inner layer is rich in mitochondria. Base of the inner layer cell forms the posterior chamber surface. B. Inner layer adjacent to posterior chamber, showing abundant infolding of the cell wall. C. Intercellular space is formed between the apical ends of the two cell layers.

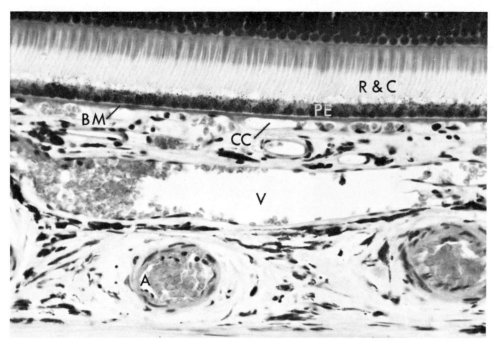

Figure 32-25   Choroid and outermost layers of retina. R & C, rod and cone layer; PE, pigment epithelium; BM, Bruch's membrane; CC, choriocapillaris; V, vein; A, artery.

the pigment epithelium on its anterior surface. The portion adjacent to the choriocapillaris contains elastic tissue.

The *pigment epithelium* is a single layer of cuboidal cells situated just internal to Bruch's membrane. The cells contain a heavy concentration of melanin granules in the apical portion.

The inner surface of the pigment epithelium has a multitude of processes that extend forward to interdigitate with the rods and cones. Between these rods and cones is a mucoid cement substance that stains with alizarin blue. Thus the rods and cones are not anatomically bound to the outer coats of the eye, and most histologic sections show artefactitious separation of the retina from the choroid (Fig. 32-6). Separation of the retina is also a common clinical entity. The retina is, however, attached anatomically to the choroid at the nerve head and at the ora serrata.

Electron microscopy of the pigment epithelium shows the pigment to consist of round or oval granules several times larger than the granules of melanocytes and concentrated along the inner aspects of the epithelium (Fig. 32-26). Also contained occasionally within the epithelial cells are myelin bodies (with a laminated structure similar to that seen in photoreceptors), secretory granules, and numerous mitochondria.

Zonules

The *zonules* are hairlike filaments that connect the ciliary body with the lens. They insert, on the one hand, into the inner surface of the ciliary body and, on the other hand, into the lens capsule just in front of and just behind the lens equator. They can be seen during life to be the suspensory filaments by which the lens is held in place and through which tension is varied on the lens by contraction of the ciliary muscle. The zonules stain poorly with acid dyes but well with the PAS reagent (Fig. 32-27).

The zonules form the posterior boundary of the posterior chamber and the anterior demarcation of the vitreous space.

By electron microscopy the zonules are dense aggregates of the filaments similar to those constituting the vitreous structure.

Lens

The *lens* is a transparent structure situated behind the iris and in front of the vitreous; it is held in place by the zonular fibers (Fig. 32-28). In the adult human eye it measures approximately 10 mm in diameter and 5 mm in thickness. The anterior surface of the lens has an approximately spherical convexity, whereas the posterior surface has a paraboloid convexity.

Changes in refraction of the lens occur by the interplay between its inherent tendency to become more spherical and the tension on the zonules which flatten it.

Figure 32-26 Electron micrograph of the junction between choroid and retina. In the lower left corner is a vessel of the choriocapillaris adjacent to Bruch's membrane. The endothelium of the choriocapillaris is fenestrated (arrows). Occupying the center portion of the photograph is the pigment epithelium. The photoreceptor outer segments are interdigitating with microvilli of the pigment epithelium.

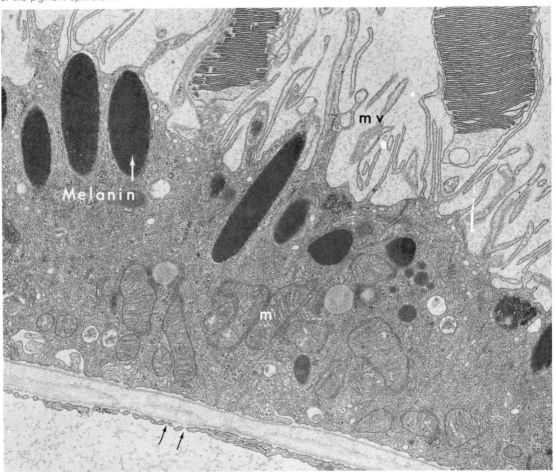

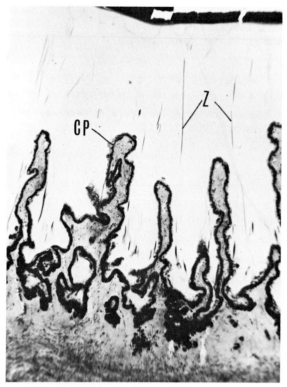

Figure 32-27   Meridional section showing zonules (Z) and ciliary processes (CP).

The outer surface of the lens is bounded by a hyaline capsule that has the same physical and tinctorial properties as Descemet's membrane (Fig. 32-29). The anterior portion of the capsule averages approximately 10 μm in thickness (disregarding minor regional variations) whereas the posterior portion is less than half this.

Beneath the anterior capsule is a layer of cuboidal epithelial cells (Fig. 32-29) that are remarkable for their uniformity and mode of differentiation. At the equator these cells elongate and insinuate beneath the lens epithelial layer anteriorly and beneath the posterior capsule posteriorly (Fig. 32-30). These differentiated cells are called *lens fibers*. The lens grows throughout life by continual addition of these fibers superficially. (As in the growth of a tree trunk, the youngest fibers are just beneath the capsule.) The nuclei of these fiber-like cells undergo progressive pycnosis as they are displaced inward, forming the *lens bow* which radiates from the equator toward the center of the lens. Mitoses are practically never seen in conventional sections of the lens but a few mitoses may be found in the equatorial regions in flat preparations of the epithelium.

The *lens substance* consists of concentrically arranged cells, the lens fibers, that have undergone varying degrees of condensation. The individual

Figure 32-28   Anterior segment of the eye, showing the position of the lens behind the iris. The lens is held in place by delicate zonules (not visible in the photograph) connected with the ciliary body. Because of its dense proteinaceous substance, the adult lens usually shows artefactitious clefts such as are evident in this section.

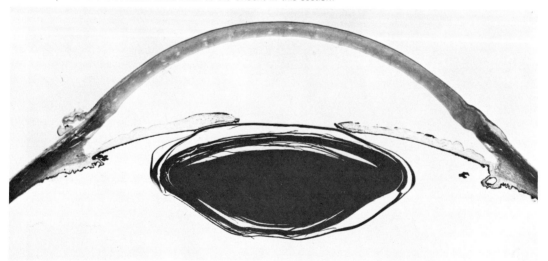

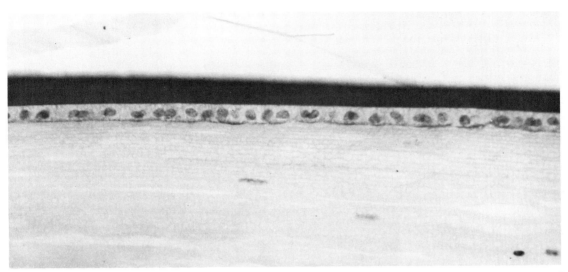

Figure 32-39 Anterior portion of the lens stained with the PAS reagent. The capsule stains a deep red. The subadjacent epithelium forms a monocellular layer of cuboidal cells. Beneath this epithelium are the lens fibers with a few nuclei.

fiber structure is most evident in the superficial layers of the lens substance, called the *cortex;* toward the center or *nucleus* of the lens, the fibers become progressively more homogeneous and less readily distinguishable as fibers. The adult lens

Figure 32-30 Equator of the lens of a child. The lens epithelial cells are differentiating into recognizable lens fibers. The nuclei are found at considerable depth in the cortex of the young lens.

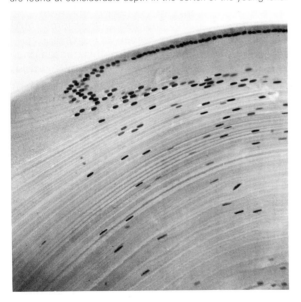

substance represents one of the most dense concentrations of protein in any tissue of the body. It stains strongly with eosin and other acid dyes. Because of its density, the adult lens substance is poorly infiltrated by ordinary embedding media; hence it is rare, except with embryonic or fetal specimens, to obtain sections of the lens without disturbing artefacts (Fig. 32-28).

Electron microscopy of the lens shows marked regional variations. The monocellular epithelium forms thick basement membrane (capsule), and its apical end attaches to the lens fibers inwardly. The cells have conspicuous interdigitations, especially toward the equator. The cortical lens fibers are closely packed without appreciable interspaces. The cells have an abundance of interdigitations (Fig. 32-31). Except for occasional microorganelles in the cells at the bow zone, the lens cells contain only a uniform sprinkling of granules. Toward the center of the lens, the cytoplasm becomes extremely homogeneous and dense (Fig. 32-32). Cortical cells contain microtubules. The paucity of mitochondria accords with the relative insignificance of respiratory metabolism in the lens substance.

One of the intriguing features of the lens is its isolation not only from a blood supply but from interchange of cells with the rest of the body. The lens epithelium is derived from surface ectoderm

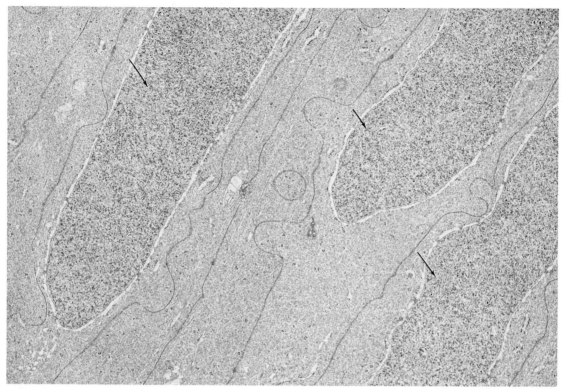

Figure 32-31   Electron micrograph of the bow zone of the lens.   Lens cells have nuclei in this area (arrow).   Cell membranes are markedly interdigitated.   Microtubules are seen frequently.   Other microorganelles are sparse.

and is enclosed in a permanent capsule early in gestation. This capsule is impermeable to cells and permits no ingress of macrophages nor egress of the lens' own cells; the lens carries on its metabolism throughout life in a sort of tissue culture. Moreover, it permits an isolation of antigenic pro-

teins that are foreign to the rest of the body.

Another intriguing feature is the remarkable transparency of the lens despite its densely protein-aceous nature. With age some of this transparency is lost; opacification of the lens sufficient to disturb vision is called *cataract*.

Vitreous

The large space between the lens, retina, and pars plana of the ciliary body contains a viscid transparent fluid called the *vitreous* (Fig. 32-6). This space is lined by basement membranes of the adjacent tissues. It is made up of minute amounts of collagen and hydrophilic polysaccharides (especially hyaluronic acid) that stain faintly with the PAS reagent. It is most dense anteriorly in the region

of the ciliary body and behind the lens. The vitreous shows considerable shrinkage with most fixatives, however, so that one does not ordinarily find the normal distribution of vitreous in microscopic preparations.

A few wandering cells may be present, and metachromatic dyes frequently reveal cells affixed to the outermost portions of the vitreous or between the vitreous and the retina. It has been suggested that these cells are concerned with the formation and regeneration of the vitreous.

Electron microscopy of the vitreous is complicated by artefacts because of high water content (99.9 percent). However, such specimens as do survive the process of fixation, drying, and staining show thin fibrils that have a periodicity of 120 Å and an interfibrillary substance. Some of this interfibrillary substance disappears after treatment by hyaluronidase and is therefore presumed to be hyaluronic acid; the rest must be residual protein. The anterior border of the vitreous comprises an especially dense packing of the filaments, thereby constituting the layer which in other types of microscopy is known as the *hyaloid membrane*. The fibrils in the posterior vitreous merge with the internal limiting membrane of the retina without forming any special condensation.

Figure 32-32 A. Cross section of lens fibers or cells in the superficial cortex. The cytoplasm consists of fine granular substance. Except for scanty ribosomes, no microorganelles are seen. Cell membranes interdigitate. B. Cross section of the center of the lens. Cell membranes are attenuated. The cytoplasm is extremely compact and homogeneous.

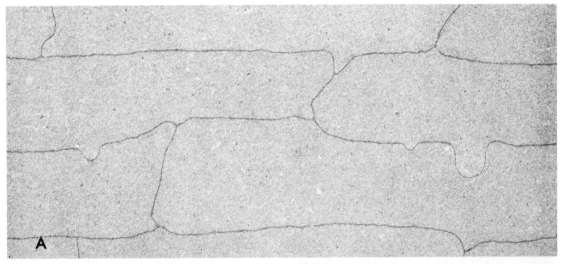

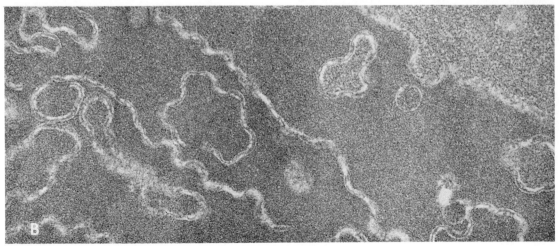

Retina

Perhaps the most remarkable tissue of the eye, if not of the body, is the *retina*. In this membrane, which is no more than 0.5 mm thick, a light stimulus is received, converted into a neural impulse, integrated to some extent locally, and transmitted to the optic nerve for relay to the brain. All this is accomplished with an extraordinary degree of adaptability to varying light intensities, discrimination of images, and color perception.

PHOTORECEPTORS
The photoreceptors are the *rods* and *cones* situated on the outer surface of the retina (Figs. 32-33 and

Figure 32-33 Cross section of the retina. ILM, internal limiting membrane; NFL, nerve fiber layer; GCL, ganglion cell layer; IPL, inner plexiform layer; INL, inner nuclear layer; SL, synaptic layer; OPL, outer plexiform layer; ONL, outer nuclear layer; OLM, outer limiting membrane; R & C, rods and cones.

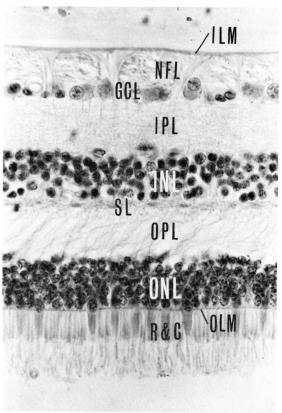

32-34). These rods and cones consist of an *outer segment* that stains with the PAS reagent and with Baker's stain (for phospholipids) and an *inner segment* that stains well with eosin and other acid dyes. The outer segment contains the photoreceptive substance (*rhodopsin*, or visual purple, in the rods and *iodopsin* in the cones) and is responsible for the absorption of light that triggers off the visual stimulus. The inner segment of each photoreceptor contains a concentration of mitochondria in a body called the *ellipsoid*.

By electron microscopy the outer segments have a series of *laminated plates* concerned with photoreception (Figs. 32-35 to 32-38). The ellipsoids, with the packed mitochondria, are connected to the outer segment by a few cilia situated on one side. It is not clear whether these cilia are supportive or conductive. The laminated plates form at the base of the rod outer segments and move centrifugally to be cast off at their outermost tips. They are then phagocytized by the pigment epithelium. In each monkey rod, there are approximately 1,300 plates, each with a life expectancy of about 10 days (Young, 1967).

As their name implies, the rods have long, thin bodies whereas the cones have a broad base. The rods have more photoabsorptive pigment which, along with their cumulative neural connections, gives them greater sensitivity for low levels of illumination, that is, night vision. The cones, having less photosensitive pigment and less summation in the retina, permit greater resolution of images and therefore better visual acuity in daylight. The cones are also responsible for color perception.

OUTER NUCLEAR LAYER
The cell bodies and nuclei of the rods and cones constitute the *outer nuclear layer*. The cone nuclei are placed in the outermost portion of this layer. These rod and cone cell bodies are separated from each other by ramifications, the radial glia of the retina called *Müller's cells*. Just anterior to these nuclei, the sites of contact of Müller's cells and the bases of the rods and cones form a series of terminal bars that have long been known as the *external limiting membrane* of the retina (Figs. 32-39 and 32-40). Processes of the Müller's cells extend

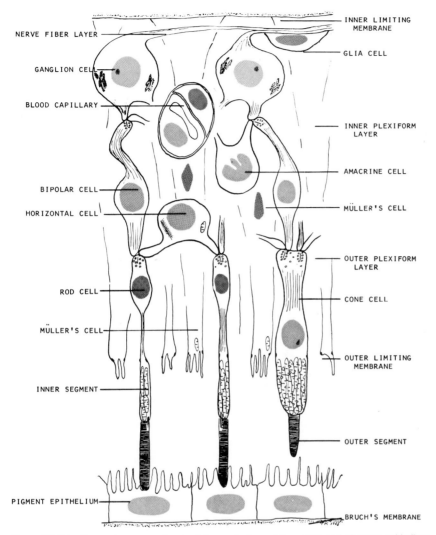

NERVE FIBER LAYER

GANGLION CELL

BLOOD CAPILLARY

BIPOLAR CELL

HORIZONTAL CELL

ROD CELL

MÜLLER'S CELL

INNER SEGMENT

PIGMENT EPITHELIUM

INNER LIMITING MEMBRANE

GLIA CELL

INNER PLEXIFORM LAYER

AMACRINE CELL

MÜLLER'S CELL

OUTER PLEXIFORM LAYER

CONE CELL

OUTER LIMITING MEMBRANE

OUTER SEGMENT

BRUCH'S MEMBRANE

Figure 32-34 The major neuronal and glial organization of the retina and pigment epithelium.

outward, separating the ellipsoids of the individual rods and cones.

The rod and cone cells are often called the *neuroepithelial portion* of the retina. They are analogous to the sensory receptors of the skin or to the first neurons in the efferent arc of other sensory systems. The bipolar cells are analogous to the cells in the dorsal ganglia; the ganglion cells of the retina are analogous to the relay in the spinal cord and brain stem. The optic nerves, the counterparts of the lemnisci in the brain stem, conduct their impulses to the lateral geniculate bodies and thalami. The same number of neuronal relays are thus operative in the retina as in other sensory pathways.

Anterior to the outer nuclear layer is the outer plexiform layer providing synaptic connections (Figs. 32-41 and 32-42) between the axons of the rod and cone cells and the dendrites of the next order of cells.

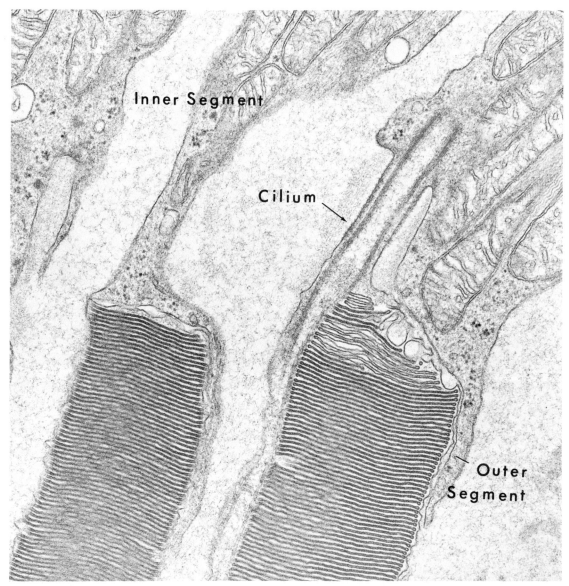

Figure 32-35 Electron micrograph through the junctions of the outer and inner segments of the rods. The upper portion of the photograph comprises the inner segments, or ellipsoids, containing dense concentrations of mitochondria, whereas the lower portion comprises the outer segments, or photoreceptive end organs, containing laminated plates. The two portions are connected by modified cilia.

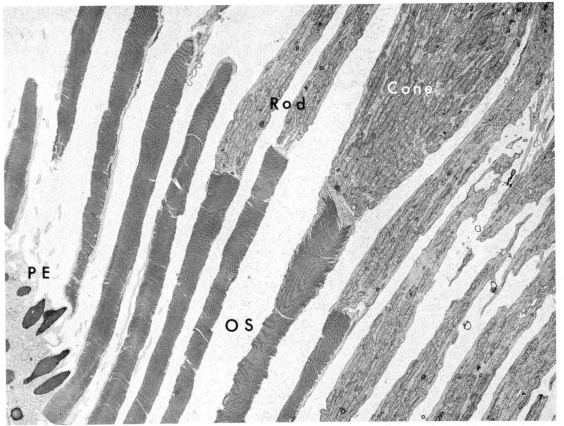

Figure 32-36 Photoreceptor elements of the retina. Inner segments of rods and cones contain packs of mitochondria. Outer segments (OS) consist of lamellar membranes. Pigment epithelium (PE) touches lightly at the tips of the outer segments.

Figure 32-37 Higher magnification of the rod outer segment. Saccular discs are separated from each other.

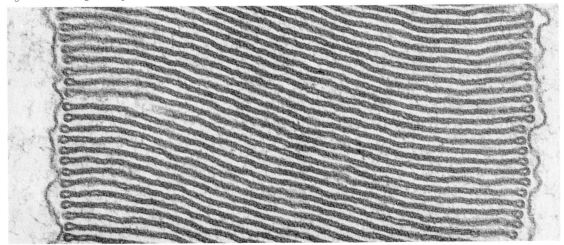

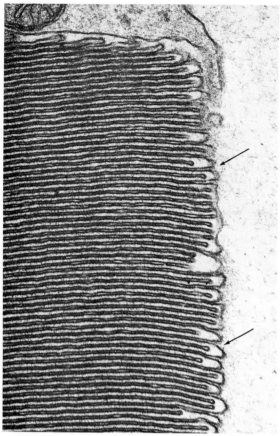

Figure 32-38 Cone outer segment. Many membranes of the saccular discs constitute the outer wall of the photoreceptor. Inner side of the disc may communicate with the outside of the cell (arrow).

BIPOLAR LAYER

The middle lamina of cells is called the *bipolar cell layer* because it is chiefly made of bipolar neurons that relay impulses from the rod and cone cells to the next layer of cells inward. It also contains the nuclei of Müller's cells, horizontal cells, large monopolar amacrine cells, and a few ganglion cells. This layer effects some integration of the rods and cones and, in the case of the rods, a summation of impulses.

Although Müller's cells form an inconspicuous fraction of the bipolar cell layer when stained routinely, special histochemical studies have shown them to play an important metabolic role in addition to their supportive and insulative functions. They and their fibers are the chief reservoirs for glycogen and for many of the oxidative enzymes concerned with energy metabolism.

Anterior to this bipolar cell layer is the *inner plexiform layer* for the synapses of the bipolar layer and the next order of cells. This plexiform layer also contains a few glial cells and some blood vessels.

GANGLION LAYER

The *ganglion cell layer* is the most anterior lamina of cells (Fig. 32-43, see color insert). It consists of cells that are distinctive in having a relative abundance of cytoplasm containing rough ER organized in masses called *Nissl bodies* (Fig. 32-44). Its dendrites connect with the bipolar cells in the outer plexiform layer and its axons form the nerve fiber layer and optic nerve. The ganglion cell layer may be eight to ten cells thick at the posterior pole of the eye (about the macula) but it becomes reduced anteriorly to single scattered cells.

NERVE FIBER LAYER

The *nerve fiber layer* comprises axons of the ganglion cells that leave the eye by way of the optic nerve. It is, of course, thickest as it approaches the optic nerve. Along with the nerve fibers, this layer also contains blood vessels, miscellaneous glia, and a plexus of *Müller's fibers* that departmentalize the nerve fibers and fan out toward the innermost surface of the retina.

INTERNAL LIMITING MEMBRANE

The inner boundary of the retina is the *internal limiting membrane,* a basement membrane that stains nonspecifically with acid dyes but stands out conspicuously with the PAS reagent. Flat preparations of the internal limiting membrane show a gyrate design impressed on it by the arborization of Müller's fibers.

MACULA

The overall architecture of the retina is modified particularly in two areas. One of these is at the posterior pole of the eye where it forms the *macula,* or *fovea.* This is an area about 1.5 mm in diameter at the posterior pole and constitutes the zone of greatest visual acuity (Fig. 32-45). It is the zone

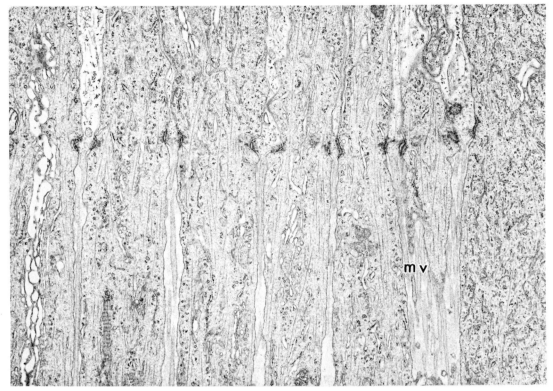

Figure 32-39 External limiting membrane is a chain of apical junctions of Müller's cells. Microvilli of Müller's cells (mv) extend beyond the limiting membrane.

Figure 32-40 Horizontal section at the level of the external limiting membrane. Apical ends of Müller's cells form a sieve-like structure through which photoreceptor cells extend. Junctions are formed between Müller's cells and photoreceptor cells.

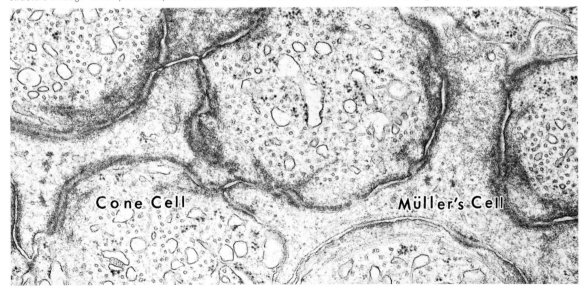

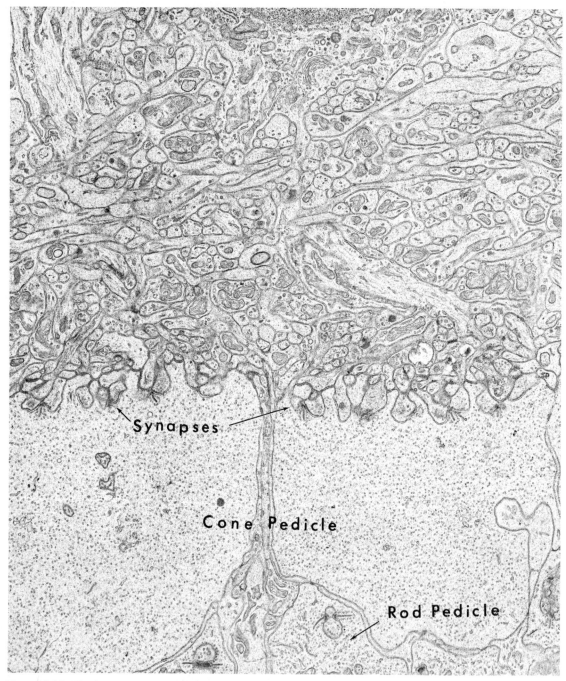

Figure 32-41   Electron micrograph of a section of the retina through the outer plexiform layer.   Pedicles of cones and rods contain abundant vesicles.   Synaptic junctions are seen in the terminal ends of the pedicles.   The upper portion of the photograph is occupied by processes of bipolar and horizontal cells.

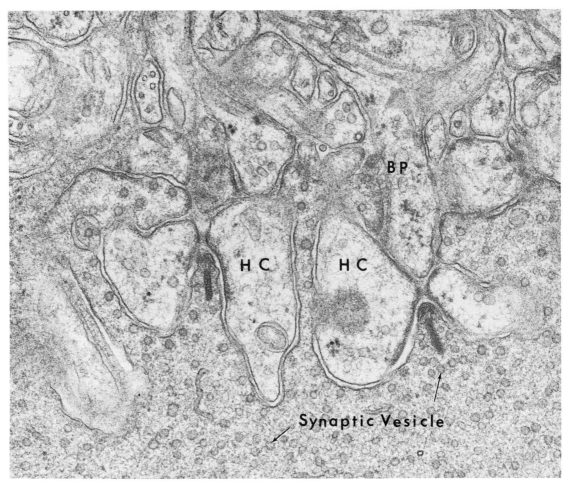

Figure 32-42 Higher magnification of cone synapsis. The synapsis consists of the axonal end of the cone cell in which synaptic vesicles and synaptic bars are seen. Large horizontal cell processes (HC) and the dendritic end of the bipolar cell (BP) invaginate the cone pedicle.

of optimal image formation.   (The name *macula lutea* refers to the yellow carotenoid pigment in the retina of this region which can be seen in the gross specimen but which is not visible by ordinary histologic examination.)   At the macula the photoreceptors are modified into long, thin elements called *cones*.   Morphologically they resemble rods more closely than cones.   The overlying retinal layers are greatly reduced at the center of the macula so that the inner surface of the retina forms a pit-like depression called the *foveola*.   The nerve fibers from the regions of the retina lateral to the

macula arch about it; the ganglion cells, inner plexiform layer, and bipolar cells are displaced away from it; and the inner plexiform layer has a radiating pattern that has been called *Henle's fiber layer*. However, the most distinctive feature of the macula is the increased number of ganglion cells about the foveola.

The thinning of the retina at the macula serves the interests of visual acuity by reducing to a minimum the overlying tissue through which light must pass before reaching the photoreceptors.

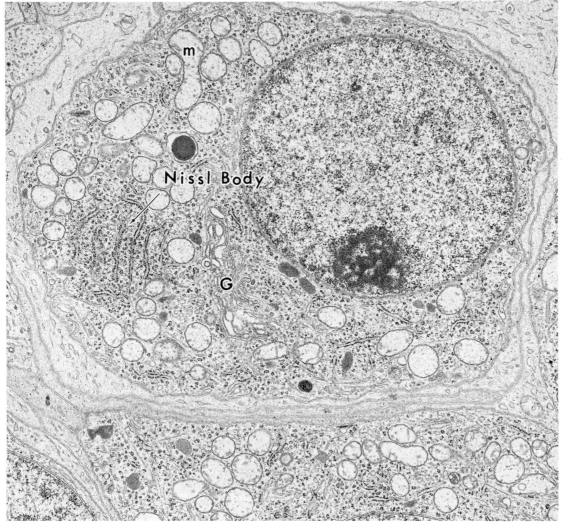

Figure 32-44   Ganglion cell in the macula area.   The cell contains marked Nissl bodies.   The nucleus is located at one edge of the cell and contains a prominent nucleolus.

Figure 32-45   Cross section through macula.   In the human eye the macula comprises a central fossa in which all the layers, except that of the rods and cones, are displaced to the side.   R, retina; Ch, choroid; S, sclera.

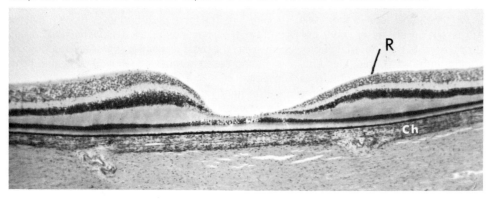

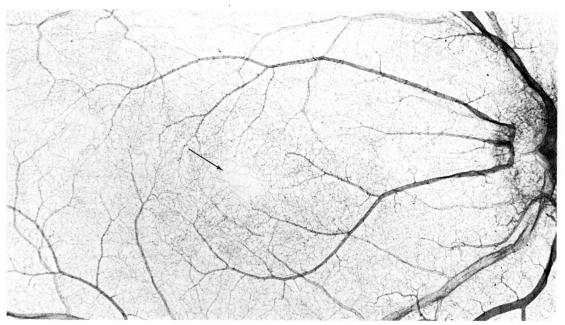

Figure 32-46   Flat preparation of the retinal vessels.   Fine capillaries form a uniform meshwork.   Arrow indicates the avascular zone of the fovea.

Figure 32-47   Capillary wall is made of two types of cells, regularly distributed.   Endothelial nuclei are ellipsoidal in shape. Mural cells (arrow) have dark round nuclei.

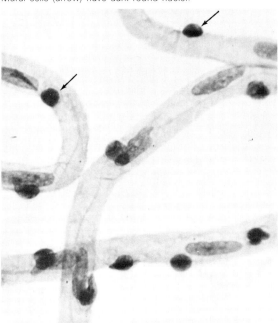

NERVE HEAD

The second modification of retinal architecture occurs at the *nerve head,* or *papilla.*   This is an area about 1 mm in diameter where the nerve fibers leave the eye to form the optic nerve (Fig. 32-48). The retina is absent in this region, and the visual field shows a corresponding "blind spot."   The center of the nerve head is situated about 3 mm nasal to the center of the macula.   Only those cross sections of the eye cut near the horizontal meridian will show both macula and optic nerve.   Cross sections through the center of the nerve head show a central depression, the *physiologic cup,* through which the central vessels pass.

RETINAL VESSELS

The retinal arteries and veins traverse the nerve head but show immediate branching once they are within the eye.   The larger vessels course horizontally in the nerve fiber and ganglion cell layers but develop elaborate branching and *capillary plexuses* in all the inner layers of the retina (Fig. 32-46).

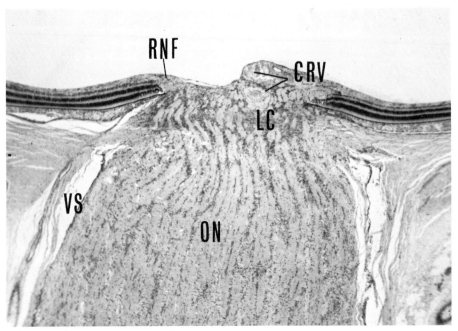

Figure 32-48 Cross section through the nerve head. ON, myelinated optic nerve; VS, vaginal space; LC, lamina cribrosa; CRV, central retinal vessels; RNF, retinal nerve fibers which are nonmyelinated.

Figure 32-49 Cross section of the optic nerve just behind the eye. In the orbital structures surrounding the optic nerve are the ciliary arteries and nerves. DM, dura mater; Ar, arachnoid; P, pia; NF, nerve fibers; CV, central vessels.

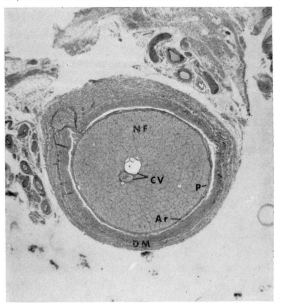

The retinal-vascular tree may be studied as whole mounts either through injection of some opaque material or by digestion of the rest of the retina with trypsin. The latter permits subsequent staining of the vessels by ordinary dyes. The capillaries are then seen to contain an unusually thick basement membrane and two types of cells, one the endothelium lining the capillary lumina and the other enclosed within the basement membrane, whence the name *mural cell* (Fig. 32-47). Cells of the latter type are believed to control flow through the capillaries.

The outer plexiform layer and outer nuclear layers of the retina are vessel-free zones that can derive sufficient nutrition from the choroid to survive when the retinal arteries are obstructed. The fovea is also a capillary-free zone that presumably derives its nutrition from the choriocapillaris.

Optic nerve

The *optic nerve* begins at the lamina cribrosa where on leaving the eye the nerve fibers first acquire myelin. Up to this point myelin is absent. With the acquisition of myelin, the optic nerve becomes a tract comparable to white matter of the brain. It is surrounded by *meningeal sheaths:* a robust dura (continuous with the sclera), a delicate arachnoid, and a thin pia (Fig. 32-49). The subdural and subarachnoid spaces, called collectively the *vaginal spaces* of the optic nerve, are continuous with those of the intracranial spaces.

The optic nerve contains approximately a million fibers. Having no sheath of Schwann, these fibers are unlike peripheral nerves but are analogous to those of the brain.

Ocular adnexa and orbit

Surrounding the eye is a sheath of connective tissue called *Tenon's capsule.* Although this is often looked upon as a socket within which the eye rotates, it has no synovial membrane and no other resemblance to joint structures.

The *lacrimal gland* is an acinous structure (Fig. 32-50) similar to salivary glands, situated in the upper outer portion of the oribt and opening onto the conjunctiva by 10 to 20 separate ducts. Histologically it consists of serous glandular cells, surrounded by myoepithelial elements, and ducts containing mucus-forming cells.

The *nasolacrimal sac* is situated in the bony fossa at the side of the nose. It consists of stratified squamous epithelium, about 10 cells thick, connected with canaliculi from the upper and lower lids and with a nasolacrimal duct that opens into the middle meatus of the nose. The canaliculi, sac, and duct constitute the effluent channels for tears.

The *extraocular muscles* are seven in number; the levator, the four recti (medial, superior, lateral, and inferior) (Fig. 32-51), and the two obliques (superior and inferior).

Fat is abundant in the orbit but since it is similar to adipose tissue elsewhere, it requires no special comment. Rarely, sections of the orbit will reveal the *ciliary ganglion* embedded in fat, medial and inferior to the optic nerve.

Regular changes with age

Certain changes occur with age so regularly that they may be considered normal. These will be mentioned briefly.

1. Sudanophilia of the circumferential portions of Descemet's membrane and, to a lesser extent, of the circumferential stroma of the cornea and of Bowman's membrane. This causes an opacity of the cornea that is known clinically as *arcus senilis.*

2. Hyalinization of the stroma in the ciliary processes and between the ciliary muscle and epithelium.

3. Condensation of lens fibers with loss of malleability of the lens substance. This results in a progressive decrease of accommodative power (*presbyopia*), becoming so marked in middle age that supplementary glasses are needed for near focusing.

4. Occlusion of the capillaries in the peripheral retina with cyst formation in the most anterior portions of the retina.

5. Sudanophilia and basophilia of Bruch's membrane in the posterior portions of the eye.

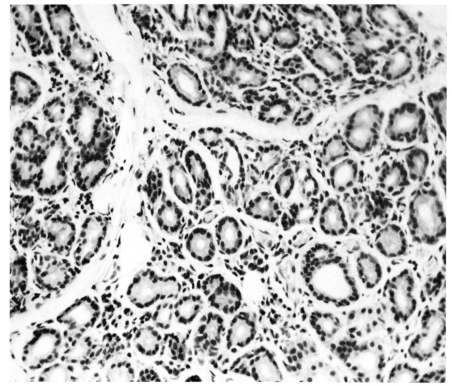

Figure 32-50 Lacrimal gland.

Figure 32-51 Rectus muscle showing fine muscle fibers (MF), abundant nerves (N), and considerable connective tissue.

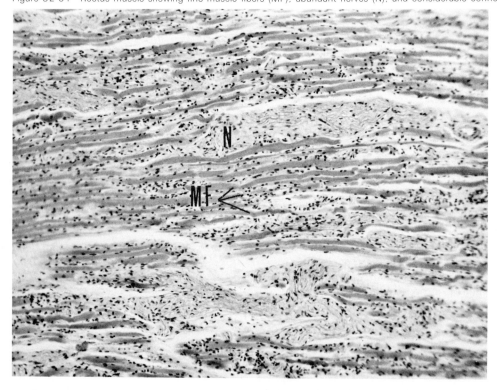

References

DUKE-ELDER, S., and K. C. WYBAR: in S. Duke-Elder (ed.), "The Anatomy of the Visual System. System of Ophthalmology," vol. 2, The C. V. Mosby Company, St. Louis, Mo., 1961.

EISLER, P.: Die Anatomie des menschen Auges, in F. Schieck and A. Brückner (eds.), "Kurzes Handbuch der Ophthalmologie," vol. 1, Berlin, Springer-Verlag OHG, 1930.

FINE, B. S., and M. YANOFF: "Ocular Histology," Harper & Row, New York, 1972.

HOGAN, M. J., J. A. ALVARADO, and J. E. WEDDELL: "Histology of the Human Eye," W. B. Saunders Co., Philadelphia, 1971.

MANN, I.: "The Development of the Human Eye," 2d ed., Grune & Stratton, Inc., New York, 1950.

POLYAK, S.: "The Retina," The University of Chicago Press, Chicago, 1941.

SALZMANN, M.: "The Anatomy and Histology of the Human Eyeball in the Normal State," trans. E. V. L. Brown, The University of Chicago Press, Chicago, 1912.

SMELSER, G. K. (ed.): "The Structure of the Eye," Academic Press, Inc., New York, 1961.

WALLS, G. L.: "The Vertebrate Eye and Its Adaptive Radiation," Cranbrook Institute of Science, Bloomfield Hills, Mich., 1942.

WOLFF, E.: "The Anatomy of the Eye and Orbit," 5th ed., McGraw-Hill Book Company, New York, 1961.

YOUNG, R. W.: The Renewal of Photoreceptor Cell Outer Segments, *J. Cell Biol.,* **33:**61 (1967).

chapter 33   The ear

ÅKE FLOCK

General structure

The ear is composed of three parts, which are illustrated schematically in Fig. 33-1:

1. The external ear, which includes the auricle, or pinna, projecting from the head and the external auditory meatus leading from the surface to the ear drum

2. The middle ear, including the tympanic cavity, the drum, and the chain of three bones extend-ing from the drum to the medial wall of the tympanic cavity, which communicates with the nasopharynx by means of the auditory (eustachian) tube

3. The internal ear, which consists of the membranous labyrinth containing the organs of hearing and equilibrium, the bone surrounding these sense organs, and the acoustic nerve

External ear

AURICLE
The *auricle* consists of an irregular flap of elastic cartilage. On the lateral surface, the skin adheres tightly to the perichondrium which contains abundant elastic fibers, whereas on the posterior surface a subcutaneous layer is present. Sebaceous glands are often quite large and are associated with small hairs.

EXTERNAL AUDITORY MEATUS
The *external meatus* is lined with skin continuous with the cutaneous layer of the tympanic mem-

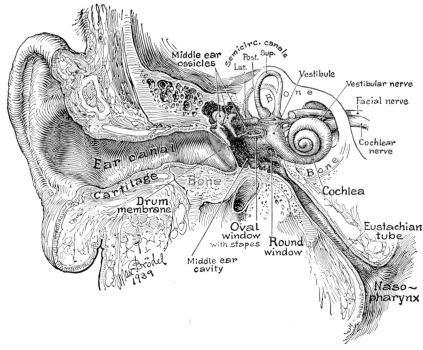

Figure 33-1   Schematic drawing of the human ear, illustrating the anatomic relations of the various parts of the ear and the surrounding and connecting structures.   (Courtesy of Brödel, three unpublished drawings of the anatomy of the human ear. W. B. Saunders Company, Philadelphia.)

brane.   In the deep or osseous portion, the skin is very thin and without hairs or glands except along its upper wall.   There, and in the outer or cartilaginous part, ceruminous glands that secrete a wax (cerumen) are abundant.   They are branched, tubuloalveolar glands which in many respects resemble large sweat glands.   Their ducts are lined with stratified epithelium, and their coils consist of a single layer of secreting cells, generally cuboid,

surrounded by smooth muscle fibers and a well-defined basement membrane.   They differ from sweat glands in that their coils have a very large lumen, especially in the adult, and their gland cells, often with a distinct cuticular border, contain many pigment granules and lipid droplets.   Their narrow ducts end on the surface of the skin or they open together with sebaceous glands into the neck of hair follicles.

Middle ear

TYMPANIC CAVITY

The air-filled *tympanic cavity,* or *tympanum,* is lined with a mucous membrane closely connected with the surrounding periosteum.   It consists of a thin layer of connective tissue covered generally with simple cuboidal epithelium.   In places the epithelial cells may be flat or tall, with nuclei in two rows.

Cilia are sometimes widely distributed and are usually found on the floor of the cavity.   In the anterior part of the tympanic cavity, small alveolar mucous glands occur very sparingly.   Capillaries form wide-meshed networks in the connective tissue, and lymphatic vessels are found in the periosteum.

TYMPANIC MEMBRANE

The tympanic cavity is separated from the external auditory canal by the *tympanic membrane* or *ear drum* which consists of the following strata: the outermost cutaneum, the radiatum, the circulare, and the innermost mucosum. The stratum cutaneum is a thin skin without papillae in its corium, except along the handle or manubrium of the malleus. There it is a thicker layer, containing the vessels and nerves which descend along the manubrium and spread from it radially. In addition to the venous plexus which accompanies the artery there, a plexus of veins at the periphery of the membrane receives tributaries from both the stratum cutaneum and the less vascular stratum mucosum. The radiate and circular strata consist of compact bundles of fibrous and elastic tissue which are so arranged as to suggest tendon. The fibers of the radial layer blend with the perichondrium of the hyaline cartilage covering the manubrium. Peripherally the fiber layers form a fibrocartilaginous ring which connects with the surrounding bone. The stratum mucosum is a thin layer of connective tissue covered with a simple, nonciliated, flat epithelium continuous with the lin-

ing of the tympanic cavity. Peripherally, in children, its cells may be taller and ciliated. As a whole, the tympanic membrane is divided into tense and flaccid portions. The latter is a relatively small upper part in which the fibrous layers are deficient. The tensor tympani muscle is attached by a tendon to the center of the tympanic membrane.

AUDITORY OSSICLES

The tympanic membrane is connected to the inner ear through a chain of three small bones, the *malleus, incus,* and *stapes* (Fig. 33-1). They articulate against each other by regular joints and are supported in the middle ear cavity by connective tissue strands. The *manubrium* of the malleus attaches to the tympanic membrane; the footplate of the stapes is held by an annular fibrous ligament in the *fenestra vestibuli,* or oval window, which opens into the inner ear. The *stapedius muscle* attaches to the head of the stapes (Fig. 33-2).

AUDITORY TUBE

The *auditory,* or *eustachian tube* (Fig. 33-1) includes an osseous part toward the tympanum and a cartiliginous part toward the pharynx. Its mucosa

Figure 33-2 Cat stapes with stapedius muscle. The stapes in the oval window. The stapedius muscle is attached to the head of the stapes. Note the sesamoid bone between the head of the stapes and the incus. The facial nerve cut in cross section. TC, tympanic cavity; FN, facial nerve; SB, sesamoid bone; I, incus; HS, head, stapes; FS, footplate, stapes; CS, crura stapes; V, vestibule; SM, stapedius muscle. ×15. (Courtesy of Lurie.)

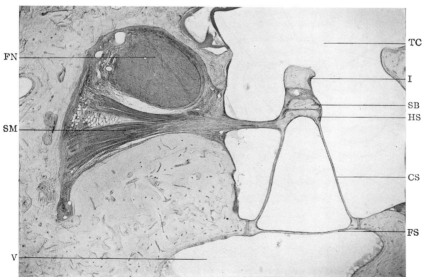

consists of fibrillar connective tissue, with a ciliated columnar epithelium which becomes stratified as it approaches the pharynx. The stroke of the cilia is toward the pharyngeal orifice. In the osseous portion, the mucosa is without glands and very thin; it adheres closely to the surrounding bone. Along its floor there are pockets containing air, the cellulae pneumaticae. In the cartilaginous part the mucosa is thicker; near the pharynx it contains many mixed glands. Lymphocytes are abundant in the surrounding connective tissue, forming nodules near the end of the tube which blend with the pharyngeal tonsil. The cartilage, which only partly surrounds the auditory tube, is hyaline near its junction with the bone of the osseous portion. Here and there are coarse nonelastic fibers. Toward the pharynx the matrix contains thick nets of elastic tissue, so the cartilage there is elastic.

Inner ear

BONY AND MEMBRANOUS LABYRINTH

The inner ear is located in the pars petrosus of the temporal bone. The bone is pierced by a system of tortuous canals and cavities, the *bony labyrinth,* which is shaped to lodge the *membranous labyrinth.* The bony labyrinth is filled with a fluid, *perilymph* and communicates with the cerebrospinal space by a narrow canal, the *vestibular aqueduct.*

The membranous labyrinth (Fig. 33-3) has two subdivisions. The *vestibular labyrinth* contains the organs of equilibrium: the *semicircular canals,* the *utricle,* and *saccule.* The *cochlea* contains the organ of hearing: the *organ of Corti.* The membranous labyrinth is filled with a fluid called *endolymph.*

VESTIBULAR LABYRINTH

The *utricle* is an elliptical sac which lies in the upper posterior part of the bony vestibule, a cavity on the

Figure 33-3   Schematic drawing of the membranous labyrinth.   Within each sensory area the orientation of the sensory cells is indicated.   (Modified from Ebner.   Reproduced with permission of W. Engelmann.)

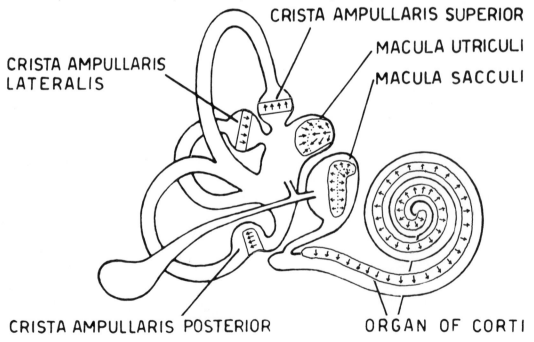

CRISTA AMPULLARIS SUPERIOR

MACULA UTRICULI

MACULA SACCULI

CRISTA AMPULLARIS LATERALIS

CRISTA AMPULLARIS POSTERIOR

ORGAN OF CORTI

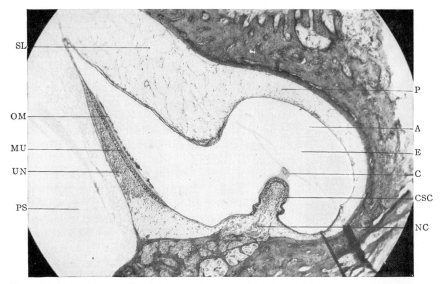

Figure 33-4 Macula utriculi and the ampulla of a semicircular canal. Supporting ligaments run from the membranous semicircular canal and utricle to the bony walls of the cavity. The utricle is suspended in the vestibule. PS, perilymphatic space; SL, supporting ligaments; MU, macula utriculi; UN, utricular nerve; OM, otolithic membrane; A, ampulla; CSC, crista, semicircular canal; C, cupula; NC, nerve to crista; E, endolymph; P, perilymph. Guinea pig. ×40. (Courtesy of Lurie.)

bony labyrinth. The spherical saccule lies anterior and medial to the utricle and is connected to it by the utriculosaccular duct. From the utriculosaccular duct arises the endolymphatic duct. The three membranous semicircular canals communicate with the utricle. These three canals lie at right angles in the three dimensions of space. Each one has an ampullated end. The ampullae of the anterior (vertical) and lateral (horizontal) canals lie close to each other and open into the superior end of the utricle, whereas the ampulla of the posterior (vertical) canal opens into its inferior end. The common end of the two vertical canals, the *crus commune,* enters the midportion of the utricle, as does also the nonampullated end of the horizontal canal.

The connective tissue layer of the utricle, saccule, and membranous canals consists of a finely fibrillated intercellular substance and spindle-shaped or stellate fibroblastic cells (Fig. 33-4). From its outer surface trabeculae run through the perilymphatic spaces to the inner periosteum of the osseous vestibule and the bony semicircular canals. These support the semicircular canals, utricle, and saccule. The spaces and periosteum

are lined with a layer of flattened connective tissue cells, which is a mesothelium.

The neuroepithelial areas of the utricle and saccule are called *maculae.* The macula of the utricle, which is about 2 by 2 mm, lies in the superior anterior part of the utricle, approximately in the plane of the base of the skull and also in the plane of the horizontal semicircular canal. The macula of the saccule, which is about 2 by 3 mm, lies in a sagittal plane of the head, and so the two maculae are perpendicular to each other.

Semicircular canals Each semicircular canal is provided with a sense organ responding to angular acceleration in the plane of the canal. This is the *crista ampullaris* (Figs. 33-5 and 33-6), a ridge of connective tissue which projects into the ampulla of the canal and is covered by a neuroepithelium consisting of sensory *hair cells* and supporting cells (Fig. 33-7). At both ends, where the crista joins the wall of the ampulla, is a region of tall cylindrical cells called *planum semilunatum.* Each hair cell has a bundle of sensory hairs which project from the luminal surface (Fig. 33-8) and are attached to a gelatinous structure, the *cupula,* which rides

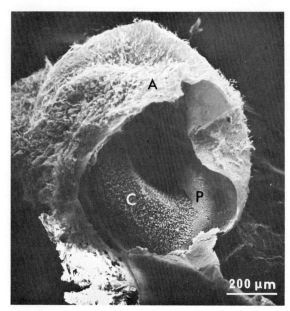

Figure 33-5 Ampulla of the semicircular canal cut open to expose the sensory epithelium of the crista. The cupula has been removed during dissection. A, ampulla; C, crista; P, planum semilunatum. Scanning microscopy. (Courtesy of Wersäll, Björkroth, Flock, and Lundquist. Reproduced with permission of Springer-Verlag.)

on top of the crista and reaches to the roof of the ampulla. The cupula acts as a swinging door to the motion of endolymph and excites the sensory cells by displacing the sensory hairs.

Two types of hair cells are distinguished in vestibular sensory epithelia (Fig. 33-7). *Type I cells* have a constricted neck and a round cell body, most of which is enclosed in a chalice-like afferent nerve terminal. The nerve chalice, in turn, is contacted by endings of efferent nerve fibers which contain abundant vesicles and probably have an inhibitory function. *Type II cells* are cylindrical cells innervated at their base by terminals of afferent and efferent fibers. At the afferent synapse of both types of cells are regions of ultrastructural specialization with a presynaptic dense bar surrounded by vesicles similar to those seen where neurochemical synapatic transmission occurs.

Each sensory hair bundle is composed of 40 to 80 *stereocilia* which progressively increase in length toward one pole of the cell (Fig. 33-7). These

sensory hairs are modified microvilli with a core of fibrils, 30 Å in diameter, which continue as a rootlet into a *cuticular plate* in the apical cytoplasm. The cuticular plate is absent near the longest stereocilia, where a single *kinocilium* that has the "9 + 2" pattern of microtubules seen elsewhere is situated, although motility is not expected in this cilium. Each hair cell can thus be given a direction in which the kinocilium is facing. This is functionally important since the sensory nerve fiber connected to that cell increases its firing rate when the sensory hairs are bent in the direction of the kinocilium, whereas opposite displacement causes a decrease in firing frequency. In each crista all hair cells face the same direction: in the horizontal crista toward the utricle and in the two vertical cristae away from the utricle (Fig. 33-3).

The supporting cells have basal nuclei, an apical cytoplasm containing secretory granules, and a luminal surface provided with microvilli. Their secretory product forms the matrix of the cupula.

Utricle and saccule The sensory epithelium of the macula utriculi and macula sacculi has the same structure as that of the crista (Figs. 33-7, 33-9, and 33-10). The surfaces of the maculae are covered with a layer of gelatinous substance, the *otolithic membrane*, into which the sensory hair bundles penetrate. In the free surface of the otolithic membrane lie many crystals of calcium carbonate, called *otoconia* (Fig. 33-11). Because the otoconia are denser than endolymph, gravitational forces can cause a shear motion of the otolith membrane relative to the sensory epithelium and thus excite or inhibit the sensory cells. Linear acceleration and changes of the position of the head are adequate stimuli. As appears in Fig. 33-3, the pattern of orientation of hair cells is quite complicated in the two maculae. For each direction of motion there is a region of hair cells which will be excited. At the same time other cells will be inhibited; it is likely that the sensory neurons from different regions project specifically via brain stem nuclei to appropriate muscles which control posture.

COCHLEA
The bony cochlea provides a rigid protective covering for the membranous cochlea (ductus cochlearis)

with its delicate sense organ for hearing. The canal of the bony cochlea makes $2\frac{1}{2}$ turns around its axis, which is a pillar of spongy bone called the *modiolus* (Figs. 33-1 and 33-12). The base of the modiolus (the largest turn) forms the anterior wall of the internal acoustic meatus. The cochlear nerve and blood vessels enter the cochlea through the base of the modiolus. The bony canal is partially divided by a projection of bone from the modiolus, called the *lamina spiralis ossea*. In radial section of the cochlea through the modiolus, this projection looks like the thread of a screw. The lamina spiralis ossea has two lips separated by a sulcus, an upper vestibular lip, or *limbus spiralis,* and a lower tympanic lip (Figs. 33–13 and 33–14).

Attached to the osseous lamina and the outer wall of the canal lies the membranous cochlea which separates the bony cochlear canal into two partitions, the *scala vestibuli,* which opens into the vestibule, and the *scala tympani,* which ends basally

Figure 33-6   Sensory epithelium of the crista ampullaris contains hair cells with apical sensory hairs coupled to the cupula.   (Courtesy of Wersäll.)

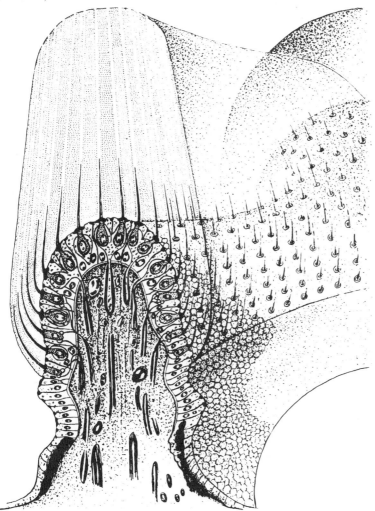

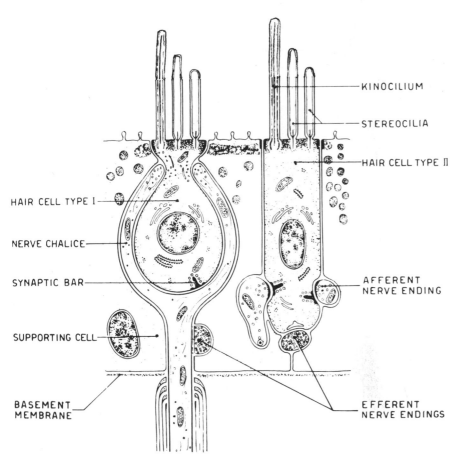

KINOCILIUM

STEREOCILIA

HAIR CELL TYPE Ⅱ

HAIR CELL TYPE I

NERVE CHALICE

SYNAPTIC BAR

SUPPORTING CELL

AFFERENT
NERVE ENDING

BASEMENT
MEMBRANE

EFFERENT
NERVE ENDINGS

Figure 33-7   Schematic drawing of vestibular sensory cells.   (Modified from Wersäll.   Reproduced with permission of Pergamon Press.)

at the *round window.*   The round window faces the middle ear cavity.   The lumen of the membranous cochlea is referred to as the *scala media.*   It is delimited toward the scala vestibuli by the *Reissner's membrane* and toward the scala tympani by the *basilar membrane.*   The membranous cochlea filled with endolymph ends as a blind sac (lagena or cecum cupulare) at the apex of the cochlea. Just beyond this point the scala vestibuli and scala tympani, which had been separated by the membranous cochlea, join; this is called the *helicotrema.*   The aquaeductus cochleae stems from the scala tympani at the base of the cochlea near the round window and passes to the subarachnoid space near the jugular fossa.

The membranous cochlea, which is triangular in shape when seen in cross section, is attached inwardly to the lamina spiralis ossea and outwardly by the *spiral ligament* to the outer wall of the bony canal.   The base of the membranous cochlea is made of the tympanic lip of the lamina spiralis ossea and the basilar membrane, which connects the tympanic lip with the spiral ligament.   At the attachment of the basilar membrane to the spiral ligament there is a small sulcus called the *external sulcus.*   The vestibular lip of the lamina spiralis ossea has attached to it Reissner's membrane and the *tectorial membrane.*   The space between the limbus and the tympanic lip is called the *internal sulcus.*

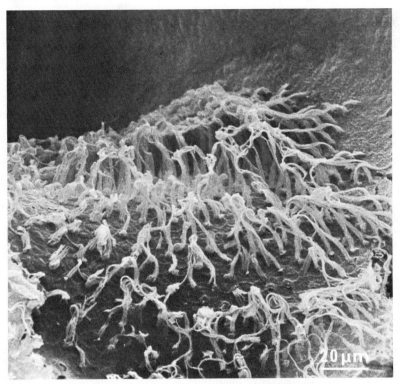

Figure 33-8 Scanning picture of the crista toward the planum semilunatum shows sensory hair bundles projecting from the neuroepithelium. The cupula has been removed. (Courtesy of Wersäll, Flock, and Lundquist. Reproduced with permission of Killisch-Horn Verlag.)

Figure 33-9 Sensory epithelia of the macula utriculi and sacculi have identical structure. (Courtesy of Iurato. Reproduced with permission of Pergamon Press.)

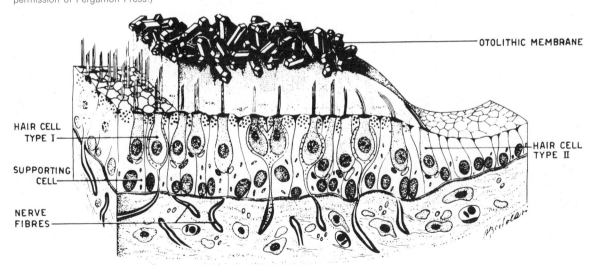

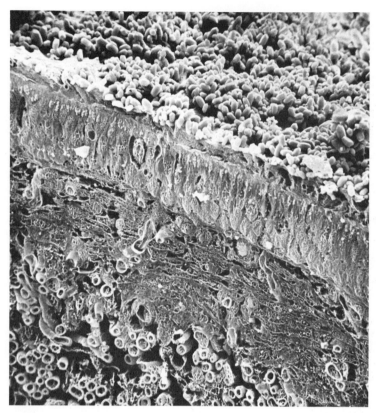

Figure 33-10 Freeze fracture through the macula utriculi shows the otolith membrane overlying the sensory epithelium below which myelinated nerve fibers are seen in cross section. Human. (Courtesy of Lundquist, Flock, and Wersäll.)

Figure 33-11 Otoconia from the human utricle.

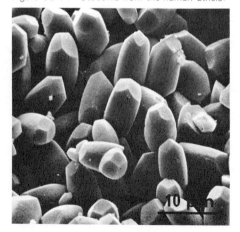

The basilar membrane is sometimes considered to have two parts, the zona arcuata (inner zone) and the zona pectoralis (outer zone). Its middle layer is formed by fibers which run through both zones. The basilar membrane varies in width from the basal coil at the round window to the apex. It is smallest at the round window, 0.16 mm, and widest at the helicotrema, 0.52 mm. The length of the basilar membrane in man is about 31 mm. On its scala tympani aspect, mesothelial cells and connective tissue line the basilar membrane. There is a small artery running under it, the *vas spirale*. On the upper surface of the basilar membrane in the scala media rests the organ of Corti. Reissner's membrane is attached to the inner superior surface of the vestibular lip of the lamina spiralis ossea and goes to the outer wall of the bony cochlea at the

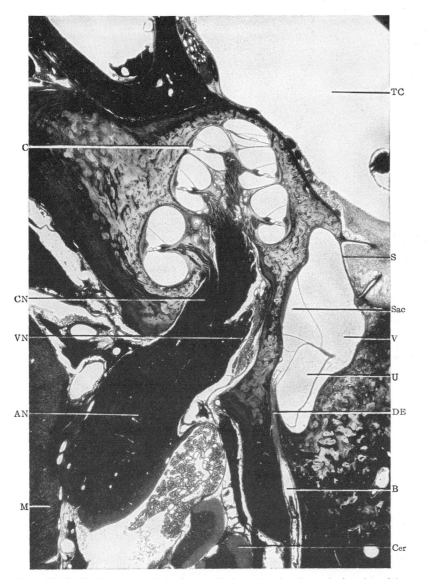

Figure 33-12 Cochlea and vestibule of a cat. Horizontal section shows the footplate of the stapes in the oval window, the vestibule showing the relationship of saccule and utricle to the oval window, and the large perilymphatic space around the footplate of the stapes. The ductus endolymphaticus can be followed in the aquaeductus vestibuli. The bulb of the ductus lymphaticus can be seen. The cochlea is cut to show three turns. The cochlear nerve and vesitubular nerve can be seen in their course from the spiral and Scarpa's ganglion into the medulla. TC, tympanic cavity; S, stapes; V, vestibule; Sac, saccule; U, utricle; DE, ductus endolymphaticus; B, bulb (sarcus) of ductus endolymphaticus; C, cochlea; CN, cochlear nerve and spiral ganglia; VN, vestibular nerve, Scarpa's ganglion; AN, auditory nerve; Cer, cerebellum. ×12. (Courtesy of Lurie.)

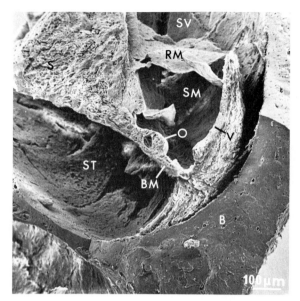

Figure 33-13 Freeze fracture through the cochlear portion shows the scala vestibuli (SV), scala media (SM), scale tympani (ST) separated by Reissner's membrane (RM), and the basilar membrane (BM). O, organ of Corti; S, spiral ganglion; B, bone; V, stria vascularis.

upper end of the spiral ligament. It is two cell layers in thickness and is lined with epithelium on its surface facing the scale media and with mesothelium on its surface facing the scala vestibuli.

The third wall of the scala media is called the *stria vascularis*. It runs from the attachment of Reissner's membrane to the external sulcus. It has a low pseudostratified epithelium in intimate contact with the capillaries. The stria vascularis is believed to secrete the endolymph that fills the membranous cochlea. It runs the whole length of the scala media.

Organ of corti On the basilar membrane lies the organ of Corti, which is built up by hair cells and supporting cells arranged in a complicated manner (Figs. 33-15 to 33-22). It runs from the round window to the helicotrema of the cochlea. There are no blood vessels in the organ of Corti. A portion of it rests on the tympanic lip of the lamina spiralis ossea, but most of it lies on the basilar membrane. Between these parts is a free triangular space called the *tunnel*, which is delimited by two rows of supporting cells, the *inner pillar cells*

Figure 33-14   Organ of Corti of a mouse. First turn of the cochlea, showing the relationship of scala vestibuli, scala media, and scala tympani. Reissner's membrane; the stria vascularis; the organ of Corti; techtorial-membrane; inner hair cell; pillar cells; outer hair cells; basilar membrane; the spiral ligaments; and the spiral ganglia. SV, scala vestibuli; RM, Reissner's membrane; STV, stria vascularis; SPL, spiral ligament; LSO, lamina spiralis ossea; VL, vestibular lip; TL, tympanic lip; TM, tectorial membrane, ISC, inner sulcus cells; IHC, inner hair cell; EHC, external hair cells; BM, basilar membrane; ST, scala tympani; SpG, spiral ganglia ×120   (Courtesy of Lurie.)

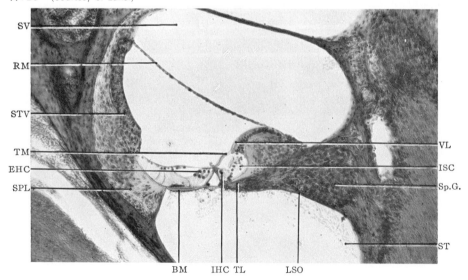

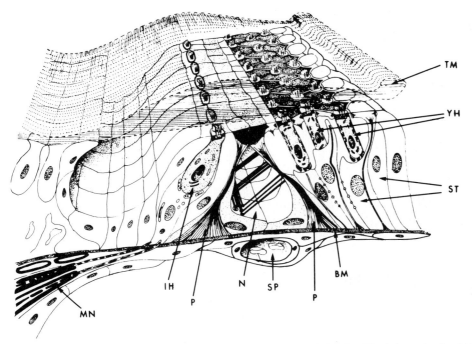

Figure 33-15   Organ of Corti.   TM, tectorial membrane; YH, outer hair cells; ST, phalangeal cells; BM, basilar membrane; P, outer and inner pillars; SP, spiral vessel; N, tunnel of Corti; IH, inner hair cell; MN, myelinated nerve fibers.   (Courtesy of Wersäll, Flock, and Lundquist.   Reproduced by permission of Cold Spring Harbor Laboratories.)

resting on or near the tip of the tympanic lip and the *outer pillar cells* on the basilar membrane.   The pillar cells have a broad base in which the nucleus lies.   The body of the pillar cell contains rigid tonofibrils.   The top of the pillar cells is enlarged and covered on its free surface with a cuticular plate. The head of the internal pillar cell is concave so that the rounded head of the external pillar cell can fit into it, like a ball-and-socket joint.   There are about 6,000 inner pillar cells and about 4,000 external pillar cells, so that three inner cells articulate with two external cells.

The sensory cells are in two groups: the *inner hair cells,* a single row of about 3,500 cells close to the inner pillar cells, and the *outer hair cells,* about 20,000 cells in three to four rows external to the outer pillar.   The outer hair cells are cylindrical with a rounded lower end (Fig. 33-17).   They are slanted relative to the surface of the organ of Corti.   From the apical end of each outer hair cell a bundle of about 100 stereocilia (Figs. 33-18 and

33-19) project from a cuticular plate in a W pattern (Fig. 33-20), with the row of tallest hairs facing away from the modiolus toward the stria vascularis.   The cuticular plate is near the stria vascularis.   Here is a centriole which sits with its axis perpendicular to the cell membrane and with its upper end close to the membrane (Figs. 33-17 and 33-20).   Consequently, the hair cells in the organ of Corti are morphologically polarized like the vestibular hair cells and with similar functional implications.   At their base the outer hair cells are innervated by a few afferent nerve endings and several large efferent nerve endings containing abundant vesicles.

The inner hair cells have a roundish cell body (Fig. 33-17), their sensory hairs are lined up in straight rows (Fig. 33-18), and their centriole also faces the stria vascularis.   They are innervated by several afferent and a few efferent terminals.   The inner hair cells are totally enclosed by supporting cells called *inner phalangeal cells* and the outer hair

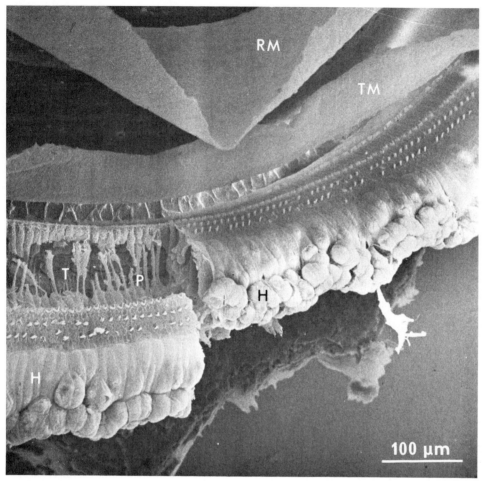

Figure 33-16 Scanning micrograph of the organ of Corti. RM, Reissner's membrane; TM, tectorial membrane; H, Hensen cells; P, outer pillar cells; T, tunnel of Corti.

cells are held by supporting *outer phalangeal cells*. These cells extend as a slender curved process toward the surface of the organ of Corti (Figs. 33-21 and 33-22). At the surface they form a rhomboid plate which interlocks with its neighbors to form the *reticular membrane* that holds the apical ends of the hair cells. Outwardly the phalangeal cells are succeeded by tall *Hensen's cells*. Hensen's cells then pass into a layer of cuboidal *cells of Claudius,* which terminate in the external sulcus just under the spiral prominence.

Lying above the organ of Corti is a gelatinous *tectorial membrane* whose lower surface rests on the tips of the tallest row of stereocilia in each hair bundle (Figs. 33-15 and 33-22). It is attached to the limbus spiralis which contains the *interdental cells* that secrete the substance of the membrane.

NERVE SUPPLY

The VIIIth cranial (auditory) nerve supplies the sensory areas of the membranous labyrinth. It divides into a superior posterior part, the *vestibular nerve,* and an inferior anterior part, the *cochlear nerve.*

The vestibular nerve has a superior portion which

supplies the macula of the utricle and the cristae of the anterior vertical and the horizontal canals, and an inferior portion which supplies the macula of the saccule and the cristae of the posterior semicircular canals. The ganglion of the vestibular nerve, called the *vestibular ganglion,* or *Scarpa's ganglion,* lies in the internal auditory canal. There is also a small branch from the inferior portion of the vestibular nerve that joins the cochlear nerve and is called the *nerve of Oort.* Scarpa's ganglion cells are bipolar. The axons of the ganglion cells enter the medulla and end in the vestibular nuclei of the medulla in the region of the fourth ventricle. The vestibular nuclei have connections with the

cerebellum and the third, fourth, and sixth eye nuclei, through the posterior longitudinal bundle. They then send nerves down the spinal cord through the vestibular spinal tracts.

The cochlear nerve enters the cochlea through the modiolus, and its ganglion (the *spiral ganglion*) lies in the lamina spiralis ossea. The sensory neurons are bipolar. The nerve fibers go to the hair cell through canals in the lamina spiralis ossea and enter the organ of Corti through small openings called the *foramina nervosa.* When the nerve fibers leave the foramina nervosa, they lose their myelin sheaths.

The pattern of innervation is very complex and

Figure 33-17   Inner (A) and outer (B) hair cells. C, centriole; IP, inner pillar cell; Eff.NE, efferent nerve ending; Aff.NE, afferent nerve ending; H, sensory hairs; M, mitochondria; Nu, nucleus. (Courtesy of Wersäll, Flock, and Lundquist. Reproduced by permission of Cold Spring Harbor Laboratories.)

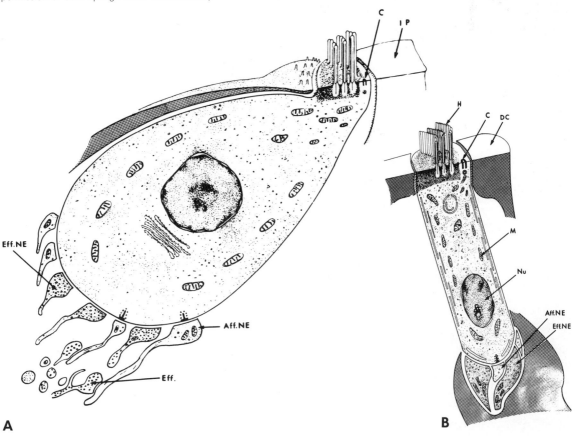

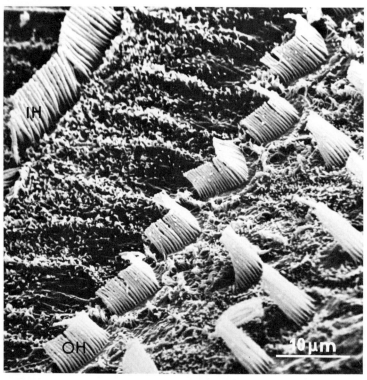

Figure 33-18   Sensory hair bundles of inner (IH) and outer (OH) hair cells project from the surface of the organ of Corti.   Supporting cells of the reticular lamina have microvilli.

Figure 33-19   Sensory hair bundle of an outer hair cell seen from the modiolus side.   Human.   (Courtesy of Lundquist, Flock, and Wersäll.   Reprinted with permission from Urban & Schwarzenberg, Vienna.)

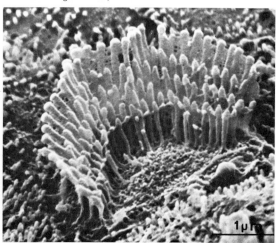

is not yet fully understood.   It seems that several afferent neurons innervate each inner hair cell, to which they take a direct course (Fig. 33-23). Other fibers cross the tunnel of Corti, turn toward the base of the cochlea, and run as outer spiral fibers to innervate several outer hair cells.

The cochlear nerve enters the medulla and terminates in the cochlear nuclei.   From the cochlear nuclei there are connections with other nuclei; the main portion of the cochlear nuclei fibers goes to the medial geniculate of the thalamus and then radiates to the auditory centers of the brain, which lie in the temporal lobe.

The organ of Corti also receives an efferent innervation, as does the vestibular apparatus (Fig. 33-24).   These fibers, the olivocochlear bundle, have their cell bodies in the superior olivary nucleus.   Fibers from the contralateral side cross the midline of the medulla at the bottom of the fourth ventricle.   The efferent fibers leave the medulla with

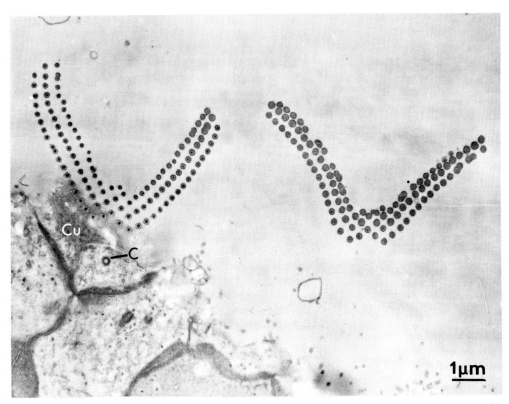

Figure 33-20 Section through the sensory hairs of one outer hair cell and through part of the cuticular plate (Cu) and the centriole (C) of its neighbor. (Courtesy of Flock, Kimura, Lundquist, and Wersäll. Reproduced by permission of American Institute of Physics, New York.)

the vestibular nerve and then pass over to the cochlear nerve in Oort's anastomosis. Within the cochlea they travel along a spiral course in the spiral ganglion. Efferent fibers pass the tunnel of Corti to innervate several outer hair cells. Inner hair cells are not as well supplied with efferents.

Sympathetic fibers innervate the blood vessels of the inner ear and also form a plexus of fibers independent of blood vessels. These free fibers have terminals in the vestibular ganglion and in the peripheral vestibular nerve branches. Terminals are seen also in the spiral ganglion and are conspicuous at the point of demyelinization of cochlear nerve fibers in the foramina nervosa of the lamina spiralis ossea. The sympathetic fibers originate in the superior cervical ganglion and reach the inner ear via arteries and via the plexus tympanicus. Their function is as yet unknown.

Figure 33-21 Phalangeal cells have slender twisted processes which reach the surface of the organ of Corti where their heads form the reticular lamina. (Courtesy of Wersäll, Flock, and Lunquist. Reproduced with permission from Killisch-Horn Verlag.)

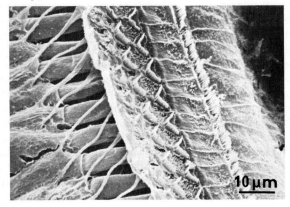

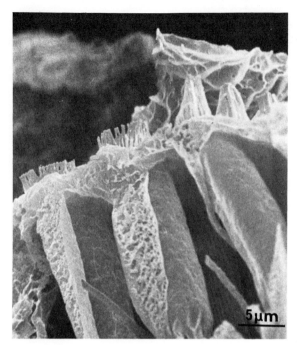

5μm

Figure 33-22 Tectorial membrane is in contact with the sensory hair bundles. The phalangeal processes are seen. (Courtesy of Wersäll, Flock, and Lundquist. Reproduced with permission from Killisch-Horn Verlag.)

ENDOLYMPHATIC SAC

Utriculus and sacculus are joined by a short duct, the *ductus utriculo saccularis* (Fig. 33-3), from which springs the *ductus endolymphaticus* which terminates as the endolymphatic sac under the dura. The epithelium outlining the endolymphatic sac is specialized for absorption. The sac often contains cellular debris, and active phagocytosis has been demonstrated.

VESSELS OF THE LABYRINTH

The internal auditory artery is a branch of the basilar artery. It arises along with branches which are distributed to the underside of the cerebellum and the neighboring cerebral nerves, and it passes through the internal acoustic meatus to the ear. It divides into vestibular and cochlear branches. The *vestibular artery* supplies the vestibular nerve and the upper lateral portion of the sacculus, utriculus, and semicircular ducts. The *cochlear artery* sends a vestibulocochlear branch to the lower and

medial portion of the sacculus, utriculus, and ducts. This branch also supplies the first third of the first turn of the cochlear. The capillaries formed by the vestibular branches are generally wide-meshed, but near the maculae and cristae the meshes are narrower. The terminal portion of the cochlear artery enters the modiolus and forms three or four spirally ascending branches which divide into about 30 radial branches distributed to three sets of capillaries—to the spiral ganglion, to the lamina spiralis, and to the outer walls of the scalae and the stria vascularis of the cochlear duct.

The veins of the labyrinth form three groups:

1. The *vena aquaeductus vestibuli* receives blood from the semicircular ducts and a part of the utriculus. It passes toward the brain in a bony canal along with the ductus endolymphaticus and empties into the superior petrosal sinus.

2. The *vena aquaeductus cochleae* receives blood from parts of the utriculus, sacculus, and cochlea. It passes through a bony canal to the internal jugular vein. It arises from small vessels, including the vas prominens and the vas spirale. Branches derived from these veins pass toward the modiolus. There are no vessels in Reissner's membrane of the adult, and the vessels in the wall of the scala tympani are arranged so that only veins occur in the part toward the membranous spiral lamina. Thus the latter is not affected by arterial pulsation. Within the modiolus the veins unite in an inferior spiral vein, which receives blood from the basal and a part of a second turn of the cochlea, and a superior spiral vein, which proceeds from the apical portion. These two spiral veins unite with vestibular branches to form the vena aquaeductus cochleae.

3. The *internal auditory vein* arises within the modiolus from the veins of the spiral lamina. These anastomose with the spiral veins. It receives branches also from the acoustic nerve and from the bones and empties into the *vena spiralis anterior*.

Lymphatic spaces within the internal ear are represented by the perilymph spaces, which communicate through the aquaeductus cochleae with the arachnoid space. The connecting structure, or *ductus perilymphaticus*, is described as a lymphatic vessel.

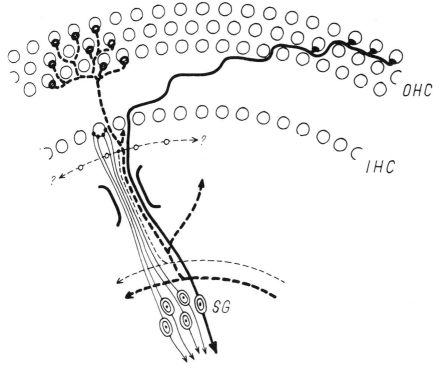

Figure 33-23 Innervation pattern of the organ of Corti in the cat. Interrupted lines are afferent fibers; full lines are efferent fibers. OHC, outer hair cells; IHC, inner hair cells; SG, spiral ganglion. (Courtesy of Spoendin. Reproduced with permission from Karger.)

Figure 33-24 Efferent nerve supply to the inner ear. (Modified by Iurato from Rossi and Cortesina. Reproduced with permission from Pergamon Press.)

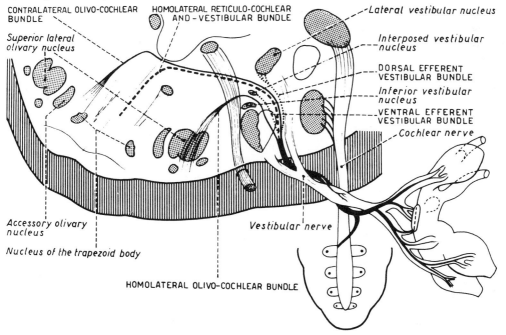

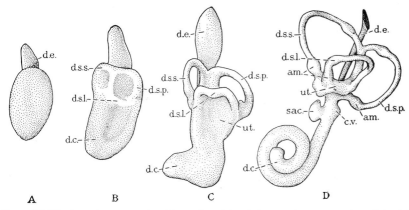

Figure 33-25   Lateral or external surfaces of models of the membranous portion of the left internal ear from human embryos. Different enlargements.   A. From an embryo of 6.9 mm. B. 10.2 mm. C. 13.5 mm. D. 22 mm. am, ampulla; cv, cecum vestibulare of dc, cochlear duct; de, endolymphatic duct; dsl, dsp, and dss, horizontal, posterior vertical, and anterior vertical semicircular ducts, sac, sacculus; ut, utriculus.   (His, Jr.)

Embryologic development

The sense organs are derivatives of the ectoderm. The internal ear first appears as a bilateral local thickening of ectoderm opposite that part of the medullary tube which is destined to become the pons. The thickened areas invaginate, as shown in Fig. 33-25, and the pockets thus formed separate from the ectoderm and develop into auditory vesicles (*otocysts*). The point where they become detached from the epidermis is marked by an elevation on the medial side of the vesicle, which elongates and produces the endolymphatic duct.

In two places the medial and lateral walls of the auditory vesicle approach one another and fuse, and the epithelial plates thus formed become thin and are absorbed, leaving two loops, each attached at both ends to the parent vesicle. These are the vertical semicircular canals. Similarly, a third canal forms soon afterward. The lower portion of the otocyst elongates and coils to make $2\frac{1}{2}$ revolutions, forming the ductus cochlearis. A constriction separates the sacculus from the utricle and the cochlea. The surrounding mesenchyme becomes cartilage and then bone.

The middle ear develops from the first pharyngeal pouch and the external ear from the first branchial cleft. At an early stage the ectoderm of the branchial cleft and the entoderm of the pharyngeal pouch meet and fuse to form the tympanic membrane.

References

BAST, T. H., and B. J. ANSON: "The Temporal Bone and the Ear," Charles C Thomas, Publisher, Springfield, 1949.

BÉKÉSY, G. VON: "Experiments in Hearing," McGraw-Hill Book Company, New York, 1960.

DE BURLET, H. M.: Vergleichende Anatomie des stato-akustischen Organs, in Bolk et al. (eds.), "Handbüch der Vergleichenden Anatomie der Wirbelthiere," vol. 2, p. 1293, Urban & Schwarzenberg, Vienna, 1934.

DAVIS, H.: A Model for Transducer Action in the Cochlea, *Cold Spring Harbor Symp. Quant. Biol.*, **30**:181 (1965).

ENGSTRÖM, H., H. ADES, and A. ANDERSON: "Structural Pattern of the Organ of Corti," Almqvist and Wiksell, Stockholm, 1966.

FLOCK, Å.: Sensory Transduction in Hair Cells, in W. R. Loewenstein (ed.), "Handbook of Sensory Physiology," vol. 1, "Principles of Receptor Physiology," p. 396, Springer-Verlag OHG, Berlin, 1971.

FLOCK, Å., KIMURA, R., P.-G. LUNDQUIST, and J. WERSÄLL: Morphological Basis of Directional Sensitivity of the Outer Hair Cells in the Organ of Corti, *J. Acoust. Soc. Amer.*, **34**:1351 (1962).

HELD, H.: Die Cochlea der Säuger und der Vögel, Entwicklung und ihr Bau, "Handbüch der normale und pathologische Physiologie," vol. 11, p. 467, Julius Springer, Berlin, 1926.

IURATO, S. (ed.): "Submicroscopic Structure of the Inner Ear," Pergamon Press, New York, 1967.

KIMURA, R. S., H. F. SCHUKNECHT, and I. SUNDO: Fine Morphology of the Sensory Cells in the Organ of Corti in Man, *Acta Otolaryng. (Stockholm)*, **58**:390 (1965).

KOLMER, W.: Gehörorgan, in W. von Möllendorff and W. Bargmann (eds.), "Handbüch der mikroskopischen Anatomie des Menschen," vol. 3, p. 250, Springer-Verlag OHG, Berlin, 1927.

LINDEMAN, H.: Studies on the Morphology of the Sensory Regions of the Vestibular Apparatus, *Advances Anat. Embryol. Cell Biol.*, **42**:1 (1969).

LORENTE DE NÓ, R.: Anatomy of the Eighth Nerve, *Laryngoscope*, **43**:3 (1933).

LUNDQUIST, P-G.: The Endolymphatic Duct and Sac in the Guinea Pig, *Acta Otolaryng. (Stockholm)*, **201** (Suppl.): 1 (1965).

LUNDQUIST, P-G., Å. FLOCK, and J. WERSÄLL: Rasten-Elektronen-mikroskopie des Menschlichen Labyrinths. Österreich, Monatsschr. HNO, **105**:285 (1971).

POLYAK, S., G. MCHUGH, and D. K. JUDD, JR.: "The Human Ear in Anatomical Transparencies," T. H. McKenna, Inc., New York, 1946.

RAMÓN Y CAJAL, S.: Histologie du systéme nerveux de l'homme et des vertébrés, 2 vols., A. Maloine, Paris, 1909–1911.

RASMUSSEN, G., and W. F. WINDLE (eds.): "Neural Mechanisms of the Auditory and Vestibular Systems," Charles C Thomas, Publisher, Springfield, Ill., 1961.

SPOENDLIN, H.: The Organization of the Cochlear Receptor, in "Advances in Oto-Rhino-Laryngology," vol. 13, S. Karger, Basel, Switzerland, 1966.

TAKASAKA, T., and C. SMITH: The Structure and Innervation of the Pigeons Basilar Papilla, *J. Ultrastruct. Res.*, **35**:20 (1971).

WERNER, U. F.: "Das Gehörorgan der Wirbeltiere und des Menschen," Thieme Verlag, Leipzig, Georg 1960.

WERSÄLL, J.: Studies on the Structure and Innervation of the Sensory Epithelium of the Cristae Ampullares in the Guinea Pig, *Acta Otolaryng. (Stockholm)*, **126** (Suppl.): (1956).

WERSÄLL, J., Å. FLOCK, and P-G. LUNDQUIST: The Vestibular Sensory Areas and the Organ of Corti. A Scanning Electron Microscopic Study, *Z. Hörgeräte Akustik*, **9**:56 (1970).

WERSÄLL, J., Å. FLOCK, and P-G. LUNDQUIST: Structural Basis for Directional Sensitivity in Cochlear and Vestibular Sensory Receptors, *Cold Spring Harbor Symp. Quant. Biol.*, **30**:133 (1965).

Index

Page references in **boldface** indicate figures.